PEDIATRIC NEUROSURGERY

THIRD EDITION

PEDIATRIC NEUROSURGERY

Surgery of the Developing Nervous System

Editor-in-Chief

WILLIAM R. CHEEK, M.D.

Chief, Section of Pediatric Neurosurgery
Professor of Clinical Neurosurgery
Baylor College of Medicine
Houston, Texas

Section Editors

ARTHUR E. MARLIN, M.D.

Chief, Section of Pediatric Neurosurgery
Santa Rosa Children's Hospital
Clinical Professor of Pediatrics
University of Texas Health Science Center
San Antonio, Texas

DAVID G. McLONE, M.D., Ph.D.

Head, Division of Pediatric Neurosurgery
Children's Memorial Medical Center
Professor of Surgery (Neurosurgery)
Northwestern University Medical School
Chicago, Illinois

DONALD H. REIGEL, M.D.

Director, Pediatric Neurosurgery
Allegheny General Hospital
Professor of Surgery (Neurosurgery)
Medical College of Pennsylvania
Pittsburgh, Pennsylvania

MARION L. WALKER, M.D.

Chief, Division of Pediatric Neurosurgery
Primary Children's Medical Center
Professor of Neurosurgery
University of Utah School of Medicine
Salt Lake City, Utah

AMERICAN SOCIETY OF PEDIATRIC NEUROSURGEONS
SECTION OF PEDIATRIC NEUROSURGERY OF THE
AMERICAN ASSOCIATION OF NEUROLOGICAL SURGEONS

W.B. SAUNDERS COMPANY

A Division of Harcourt Brace & Company

PHILADELPHIA, LONDON, TORONTO, MONTREAL, SYDNEY, TOKYO

W.B. SAUNDERS COMPANY

A Division of
Harcourt Brace & Company

The Curtis Center
Independence Square West
Philadelphia, Pennsylvania 19106

Library of Congress Cataloging-in-Publication Data

Pediatric neurosurgery: surgery of the developing nervous system/editor-in-chief, William R. Cheek;
section editors, Arthur E. Marlin. . . . [et al.].—3rd ed.

p. cm.

"Section of Pediatric Neurosurgery of the American Association of Neurological Surgeons [and the]
American Society of Pediatric Neurosurgery."

Includes bibliographical references and index.

0–7216–3767–1

1. Nervous system—Surgery.   2. Children—Surgery.   I. Cheek, William R.   II. American
  Association of Neurological Surgeons. Section of Pediatric Neurosurgery.   III. American Society for
  Pediatric Neurosurgery.   [DNLM: 1. Nervous System Diseases—in infancy & childhood.
  2. Nervous System Diseases—surgery.   3. Neurosurgery—methods.   WL 368 P372 1994]

RD593.P383 1994   617.4′8′0083—dc20

DNLM/DLC   93–38501

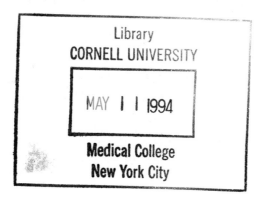
PEDIATRIC NEUROSURGERY
Surgery of the Developing Nervous System   ISBN 0–7216–3767–1

Printed in the United States of America.

Last digit is the print number: 9   8   7   6   5   4   3   2   1

CONTRIBUTORS

RICK ABBOTT, M.D.
Assistant Professor of Neurosurgery, New York University Medical Center, New York, New York.
Brainstem Tumors: Surgical Indications

KEITH E. ARONYK, M.D.
Associate Clinical Professor, University of Alberta; Attending Neurosurgeon, University of Alberta Hospital, Edmonton, Alberta, Canada.
Post-Traumatic Hematomas

JAMES E. BAUMGARTNER, M.D.
Assistant Professor, Department of Neurosurgery, University of Texas Health Science Center, Houston, Texas.
Pineal Region Tumors

DEREK A. BRUCE, M.D, M.B., Ch.B.
Clinical Associate Professor, University of Texas Southwestern Medical School; Attending Neurosurgeon, Children's Medical Center of Dallas, Dallas, Texas.
Techniques of Skull Base Surgery

CAROLYN MARIE CAREY, M.D.
Assistant Professor of Neurosurgery, University of Utah School of Medicine; Pediatric Neurosurgeon, Primary Children's Medical Center, Salt Lake City, Utah.
Hydrocephalus: Etiology, Pathologic Effects, Diagnosis, and Natural History; Stereotactic Neurosurgery; Ventriculoscopy

WILLIAM M. CHADDUCK, M.D.
Professor of Neurosurgery, George Washington University School of Medicine; Chairman, Departent of Neurosurgery, Children's National Medical Center, Washington, D.C.
Craniosynostosis

PAUL H. CHAPMAN, M.D.
Associate Professor of Surgery, Harvard Medical School; Associate Visiting Neurosurgeon, Massachusetts General Hospital, Boston, Massachusetts.
Radiosurgery

WILLIAM R. CHEEK, M.D.
Chief, Section of Pediatric Neurosurgery, Professor of Clinical Neurosurgery, Baylor College of Medicine, Houston, Texas.
Suppurative Central Nervous System Infections

RICHARD A. COULON, Jr., M.D.
Associate Professor of Neurosurgery, Louisiana State University Medical School; Head of Pediatric Neurosurgery, Ochsner Clinic and Alton Ochsner Medical Foundation, New Orleans, Louisiana.
Extramedullary Spinal Tumors

ROBERT CREIGHTON, M.D., F.R.C.P.C.
Associate Professor of Medicine, University of Toronto; Senior Anaesthetist, Hospital for Sick Children, Toronto, Ontario, Canada.
Pediatric Neuroanesthesia

MARK S. DIAS, M.D.
Assistant Professor of Neurosurgery, State University of New York at Buffalo; Chief, Department of Pediatric Neurosurgery, Children's Hospital of Buffalo, Buffalo, New York.
Normal and Abnormal Early Development of the Nervous System; Normal and Abnormal Development of the Spine

DAVID J. DONAHUE, M.D.
Clinical Instructor, Department of Neurosurgery, University of Tennessee, Memphis, Tennessee.
Intraventricular Tumors

ANN-CHRISTINE DUHAIME, M.D.
Assistant Professor, Neurosurgery, University of Pennsylvania School of Medicine; Associate Neurosurgeon, Children's Hospital of Philadelphia, Philadelphia, Pennsylvania.
Phakomatoses: Surgical Considerations

CHARLES C. DUNCAN, M.D.
Associate Professor of Surgery/Neurosurgery and Pediatrics, Yale University School of Medicine; Chief of Pediatric Neurosurgery, Yale University and Yale–New Haven Hospital, New Haven, Connecticut.
Posthemorrhagic Hydrocephalus in the Premature Infant

MICHAEL S. B. EDWARDS, M.D.
Professor of Neurological Surgery and Pediatrics, School of Medicine, University of California, San Francisco, California.
Pineal Region Tumors

HOWARD M. EISENBERG, M.D.
Professor, University of Maryland; Chairman, Division of Neurosurgery, Maryland Institute of Emergency Medical Services, Baltimore, Maryland.
Late Complications of Head Injury

FRED J. EPSTEIN, M.D.
Professor, New York University Medical School; Director, Pediatric Neurosurgery, New York University Medical Center, New York, New York.
Brainstem Tumors: Surgical Indications; Intramedullary Tumors of the Spinal Cord

SARAH J. GASKILL, M.D.
Resident in Neurosurgery, Duke University Medical Center, Durham, North Carolina.
Cerebrospinal Fluid Shunts: Complications and Results

JAMES T. GOODRICH, M.D., Ph.D.
Associate Professor of Neurological Surgery, Pediatrics, and Plastic and Reconstructive Surgery, Albert Einstein College of Medicine; Director, Division of Pediatric Neurosurgery, Montefiore Medical Center, Bronx, New York
Management of Scalp Injuries

HAROLD J. HOFFMAN, M.D., B.Sc.(Med.), F.R.C.S.(C.), F.A.C.S.
Professor of Surgery, Division of Neurosurgery, University of Toronto; Chief of Neurosurgery, The Hospital for Sick Children, Toronto, Ontario, Canada.
Craniofacial Surgery; Craniopharyngiomas

ROBIN P. HUMPHREYS, M.D., F.R.C.S.(C.), F.A.C.S.

Professor, Department of Surgery, Faculty of Medicine, University of Toronto; Associate Surgeon-in-Chief and Senior Neurosurgeon, Hospital for Sick Children, Toronto, Ontario, Canada.

Encephalocele and Dermal Sinuses; Vascular Malformations of the Brain

DENNIS L. JOHNSON, M.D.

Associate Professor of Neurosurgery, Penn State University; Milton S. Hershey Medical Center, Hershey, Pennsylvania.

Optic Nerve Gliomas and Other Tumors Involving the Optic Nerve and Chiasm

BRUCE A. KAUFMAN, M.D.

Assistant Professor of Neurological Surgery, Department of Neurology and Neurological Surgery, Washington University School of Medicine; Attending Neurosurgeon, St. Louis Children's Hospital, St. Louis, Missouri.

Tumors of the Skull and Metastatic Brain Tumors

JOHN R. W. KESTLE, M.D., B.Sc., M.Sc., F.R.C.S.(C.)

Assistant Professor, Department of Surgery, Division of Neurosurgery, University of British Columbia; Pediatric Neurosurgeon, British Columbia Children's Hospital, Vancouver, British Columbia, Canada.

Craniofacial Surgery; Craniopharyngiomas

ALI KRISHT, M.D.

Chief Resident, Emory University Hospitals, Department of Neurosurgery, Atlanta, Georgia.

Cerebellar Astrocytomas

JOHN P. LAURENT, M.D., F.A.C.S., F.A.A.P.

Associate Professor of Neurosurgery, Baylor College of Medicine; Chief of Neurosurgery Service, Texas Children's Hospital, Houston, Texas.

Peripheral Nerve Injuries

HARVEY S. LEVIN, Ph.D.

Professor of Neurological Surgery, University of Maryland; Director of Neuropsychology Service, University Center, Baltimore, Maryland.

Late Complications of Head Injury

N. SCOTT LITOFSKY, M.D.

Assistant Professor of Surgery, Department of Neurosurgery, University of Massachusetts Medical Center, Worcester, Massachusetts.

Skull Fractures

THOMAS G. LUERSSEN, M.D.

Associate Professor of Neurosurgery, Indiana University School of Medicine; Director, Pediatric Neurosurgery, James Whitcomb Riley Hospital for Children, Indianapolis, Indiana.

Acute Traumatic Cerebral Injuries; Late Complications of Head Injury

TIMOTHY B. MAPSTONE, M.D.

Associate Professor of Neurosurgery, Division of Pediatric Neurosurgery, The University of Alabama at Birmingham, Birmingham, Alabama.

Congenital CSF Anomalies of the Posterior Fossa

ARTHUR E. MARLIN, M.D.

Clinical Professor of Pediatrics, University of Texas Health Science Center; Chief, Section of Pediatric Neurosurgery, Santa Rosa Children's Hospital, San Antonio, Texas.

Cerebrospinal Fluid Shunts: Complications and Results

MICHEL E. MAWAD, M.D.

Clinical Associate Professor of Radiology, Neurosurgery and Ophthalmology, Baylor College of Medicine; Director of Neuroradiology, The Methodist Hospital, Houston, Texas.
Interventional Neuroradiology

J. GORDON McCOMB, M.D.

Professor of Neurosurgery, University of Southern California School of Medicine; Head, Division of Neurosurgery, Children's Hospital of Los Angeles, Los Angeles, California.
Arachnoid Cysts; Cerebrospinal Fluid and the Blood-Brain Interface

DAVID C. McCULLOUGH, M.D.*

Optic Nerve Gliomas and Other Tumors Involving the Optic Nerve and Chiasm

ROBERT L. McLAURIN, M.D., J.D.

Professor Emeritus, Neurosurgery, University of Cincinnati; Attending Staff, Children's Hospital Medical Center, Cincinnati, Ohio.
Ethical and Legal Considerations in Developmental Anomalies of the Nervous System

M. ELIZABETH McLEOD, M.D., F.R.C.P.C.

Assistant Professor of Medicine, University of Toronto; Staff Anaesthetist, The Hospital for Sick Children, Toronto, Ontario, Canada
Pediatric Neuroanesthesia

DAVID G. McLONE, M.D., Ph.D.

Professor of Surgery (Neurosurgery), Northwestern University Medical School; Head, Division of Pediatric Neurosurgery, Children's Memorial Medical Center, Chicago, Illinois.
Normal and Abnormal Early Development of the Nervous System; Normal and Abnormal Development of the Spine; Tethered Spinal Cord

ARNOLD H. MENEZES, M.D., F.A.C.S., F.A.A.P.

Professor and Vice-Chairman, Division of Neurosurgery, University of Iowa College of Medicine; Professor of Neurosurgery and Vice-Chairman, University of Iowa Hospital and Clinics, Iowa City, Iowa.
Abnormalities of the Craniocervical Junction; Spinal Cord Injury

LAURA R. MENT, M.D.

Professor of Pediatrics and Neurology, Yale University School of Medicine, New Haven, Connecticut.
Posthemorrhagic Hydrocephalus in the Premature Infant

WILLIAM J. MORRIS, M.D.

Chief, Neurosurgery, Madigan Army Medical Center, Tacoma, Washington.
Intracranial Hypertension: Mechanisms and Management

IAN R. MUNRO, M.A., M.B., B.Chir., F.R.C.S.(C).

Director, Humana Advanced Surgical Institutes, Dallas, Texas.
Techniques of Skull Base Surgery

MARK S. O'BRIEN, M.D.

Chief, Neurosurgery Section, Egleston Children's Hospital at Emory, Atlanta, Georgia.
Cerebellar Astrocytomas

---

*Deceased

CHRISTOPHER S. OGILVY, M.D.
Assistant Professor of Surgery, Harvard Medical School; Assistant Visiting Neurosurgeon, Massachusetts General Hospital, Boston, Massachusetts.
Radiosurgery

RICHARD K. OSENBACH, M.D.
Resident in Neurosurgery, University of Iowa Hospitals and Clinics, Iowa City, Iowa; Neurosurgery Service, Walter Reed Army Medical Center, Washington, D.C.
Spinal Cord Injury

ROGER J. PACKER, M.D.
Professor of Neurology and Pediatrics, George Washington University; Chairman, Department of Neurology, Children's National Medical Center, Washington, D.C.
Medulloblastomas; Postsurgery Management of Brain Tumors

TAE SUNG PARK, M.D.
Professor of Neurological Surgery and Pediatrics, Department of Neurology and Neurological Surgery, Washington University School of Medicine; Neurosurgeon-in-Chief, St. Louis Children's Hospital, St. Louis, Missouri.
Tumors of the Skull and Metastatic Brain Tumors

WARWICK J. PEACOCK, M.D., B.Sc., M.B., Ch.B., F.R.C.S.
Professor and Director of Pediatric Neurosurgery, University of California Los Angeles School of Medicine, Los Angeles, California.
Surgical Treatment of Epilepsy

JOSEPH PETRONIO, M.D.
Assistant Professor of Neurosurgery and Pediatrics, Emory University School of Medicine, Atlanta, Georgia.
Stereotactic Neurosurgery; Ventriculoscopy

COREY RAFFEL, M.D., Ph.D.
Associate Professor of Neurosurgery, University of Southern California, School of Medicine; Staff Neurosurgeon, Children's Hospital Los Angeles, Los Angeles, California.
Arachnoid Cysts; Skull Fractures

JOHN RAGHEB, M.D., M.A.
Clinical Instructor of Pediatric Neurosurgery, University of Maryland Medical System, Baltimore, Maryland.
Brainstem Tumors: Surgical Indications; Intramedullary Tumors of the Spinal Cord

DONALD H. REIGEL, M.D.
Professor of Surgery (Neurosurgery), Medical College of Pennsylvania; Director, Pediatric Neurosurgery, Allegheny General Hospital, Pittsburgh, Pennsylvania.
Spina Bifida; Tethered Spinal Cord

HAROLD L. REKATE, M.D.
Clinical Professor of Neurosurgery, University of Arizona School of Medicine, Tucson, Arizona; Chief, Pediatric Neurosurgery, Barrow Neurological Institute, Phoenix, Arizona.
Treatment of Hydrocephalus

KENNETH L. RENKENS, Jr., M.D.
Clinical Instructor in Neurosurgery, Indiana University School of Medicine, Indianapolis, Indiana.
Ischemic Strokes and Moyamoya Syndrome

STEVEN N. ROPER, M.D.
Assistant Professor, Department of Neurological Surgery, University of Florida, Gainesville, Florida.
Surgical Treatment of Epilepsy

LUCY BALIAN RORKE, M.D.
Clinical Professor of Pathology and Neurology, University of Pennsylvania School of Medicine; Neuropathologist, The Children's Hospital of Philadelphia, Philadelphia, Pennsylvania.
Introductory Survey of Brain Tumors

DEBORAH ROTENSTEIN, M.D.
Assistant Professor of Pediatrics, Medical College of Pennsylvania; Director, Pediatric Endocrinology and Diabetes, Allegheny General Hospital, Pittsburgh, Pennsylvania.
Spina Bifida

TIMOTHY C. RYKEN, M.D.
Resident in Neurological Surgery, Division of Neurosurgery, University of Iowa Hospitals and Clinics, Iowa City, Iowa.
Abnormalities of the Craniocervical Junction

ROBERT A. SANFORD, M.D.
Associate Professor, University of Tennessee Medical School; Neurosurgery Consult, St. Jude Children's Research Hospital; Le Bonheur Children's Medical Center, Memphis, Tennessee.
Intraventricular Tumors

LUIS SCHUT, M.D.
Professor, Neurosurgery and Pediatrics, University of Pennsylvania School of Medicine; Chief, Neurosurgical Services, Children's Hospital of Philadelphia, Philadelphia, Pennsylvania.
Phakomatoses: Surgical Considerations

R. MICHAEL SCOTT, M.D.
Professor of Surgery, Harvard Medical School; Director, Pediatric Neurosurgery, The Children's Hospital of Boston, Boston, Massachusetts.
Ischemic Strokes and Moyamoya Syndrome

KENNETH SHAPIRO, M.D.
Clinical Associate Professor, University of Texas, Southwest Medical School, Attending Neurosurgeon, Children's Medical Center, Dallas, Texas.
Intracranial Hypertension: Mechanisms and Management; Techniques of Skull Base Surgery

BRUCE B. STORRS, M.D.
Associate Professor of Neurosurgery and Pediatrics, Medical University of South Carolina; Chief, Pediatric Neurosurgery, Medical University of South Carolina Children's Hospital, Charleston, South Carolina.
Spasticity

LESLIE N. SUTTON, M.D.
Associate Professor of Neurosurgery and Pediatrics, University of Pennsylvania School of Medicine; Associate Neurosurgeon, Children's Hospital of Philadelphia, Philadelphia, Pennsylvania.
Medulloblastomas; Phakomatoses: Surgical Considerations

CHARLES TEO, M.D.
Assistant Professor, Division of Pediatric Neurosurgery, Arkansas Children's Hospital, Little Rock, Arkansas.
Intracranial Hypertension: Mechanisms and Management

TADANORI TOMITA, M.D.

Associate Professor of Surgery (Neurosurgery), Northwestern University Medical School, Chicago, Illinois.

Miscellaneous Posterior Fossa Tumors

MICAM W. TULLOUS, M.D.

Assistant Professor, Section of Pediatric Neurosurgery, University of Texas Health Sciences Center; Attending, Santa Rosa Children's Medical Center, San Antonio, Texas.

Hydrocephalus: Etiology, Pathologic Effects, Diagnosis, and Natural History

JOAN VENES, M.D.

Professor of Surgery (Neurosurgery), University of Michigan, Ann Arbor, Michigan.

Intracranial Hemorrhage Due to Nonstructural Causes

MARION L. WALKER, M.D.

Professor of Neurosurgery and Pediatrics, University of Utah School of Medicine; Chief, Division of Pediatric Neurosurgery, Primary Children's Medical Center, Salt Lake City, Utah.

Hydrocephalus: Etiology, Pathologic Effects, Diagnosis, and Natural History; Stereotactic Neurosurgery; Ventriculoscopy

JEFFREY H. WISOFF, M.D.

Assistant Professor, Division of Pediatric Neurosurgery, New York University Medical Center, New York, New York.

Tumors of the Cerebral Hemispheres

BERISLAV V. ZLOKOVIC, M.D., Ph.D.

Professor of Neurosurgery, Physiology and Biophysics, University of Southern California School of Medicine; Director, Laboratories for Neurosurgery Research, University of Southern California School of Medicine, Los Angeles, California.

Cerebrospinal Fluid and the Blood-Brain Interface

To Kenneth Shulman, M.D.

Kenneth Shulman was born on September 6, 1928. He was first introduced to medicine while working in the family drugstore where his father was a pharmacist.

Ken Shulman graduated from Clark University, with Honors, in 1952, and from Washington University School of Medicine, with Honors, in 1954. He received his neurosurgical training at the Neurological Institute in New York City, under the guidance of J. Lawrence Pool, M.D. Dr. Shulman first became seriously interested in the evolving subspecialty of pediatric neurosurgery toward the end of his residency training, and he spent 3 months with Dr. Donald Matson at the Children's Hospital in Boston, Massachusetts. In 1961 Dr. Shulman became the director of the pediatric neurosurgical service at New York University Medical Center, where he spent 3 years. From 1964 to 1967 he was the Director of Pediatric Neurosurgery at the Children's Hospital of Philadelphia. He returned to New York in 1967 at the Albert Einstein College of Medicine where he ultimately became Professor and Chairman of the Department of Neurological Surgery.

One of Dr. Shulman's accomplishments was his early research, which reflected his complete commitment to pediatric neurosurgery. He also was a leader in the organization and establishment of the Pediatric Section of the American Association of Neurological Surgeons, of which he was President pro-tem from 1971 to 1972 and Chairman from 1975 to 1976. More recently, he supervised a large laboratory complex within his department that was investigating intracranial pressure, brain tissue pressure, and brain edema and its biomechanics.

Dr. Shulman had a brilliant mind as well. He was capable of expressing his thoughts succinctly and thereby imparting knowledge to all who either worked with him or attended his many lectures. His gift for poetic and philosophical thought brought an additional dimension to his scientific contributions. Most of all, he was a sensitive and compassionate human being who was admired, respected, and regarded with affection by everyone who had the opportunity to know him.

With Dr. Shulman's death we have lost a teacher, colleague, and friend; yet we are all the better for having been associated with him. It is in the spirit of friendship and respect that we acknowledge the masterful and talented contributions he made to pediatric neurosurgery and to the publication of this volume.

FRED EPSTEIN, M.D.

To Donald Darrow Matson, M.D.

Although Donald Darrow Matson was not the founder of pediatric neurosurgery, he was its undisputed champion for nearly two decades until his premature death in 1969. It is with the deepest admiration and respect that this volume is dedicated to his memory by those who have attempted to expand the frontiers that he originally explored.

Donald Matson was born in 1913 at Fort Hamilton, New York. His college education was obtained through a scholarship at Cornell University, and his medical education continued at Harvard. Except for a three-year distinguished period of service in the armed forces and a year as chief neurosurgical resident at Duke University, he remained at Harvard for the rest of his career.

The major part of his neurosurgical training was obtained at Peter Bent Brigham and Children's Hospitals, where he developed an interest in pediatrics under the guidance of Dr. Franc Ingraham. Dr. Matson was invited to join Dr. Ingraham after completing his medical training. This alliance resulted in an impressive productivity of laboratory investigation and clinical progress relating to pediatric neurosurgery. One of the by-products of their work was a textbook published in 1954, *Neurosurgery of Infancy and Childhood*. Following Dr. Ingraham's retirement, Dr. Matson became the first Ingraham Professor of Neurosurgery at Harvard, a chair he held until his death.

In addition to his dedication to pediatric neurosurgery, he was equally committed to teaching and the improvement of neurosurgical training. He was a superb teacher himself, not didactic, but rather he set forth a method of approaching, investigating, and resolving clinical problems. Although his knowledge was not overwhelming, his ability to reach the correct diagnostic and therapeutic answers was uncanny. Dr. Matson's interest in neurosurgical training was not confined to his own program; throughout his term on the American Board of Neurological Surgery he attempted to exert an impact on all programs to improve standards of training and medical care.

Dr. Matson's experience in pediatric neurosurgery was eloquently recorded in his volume, *Neurosurgery of Infancy and Childhood* (2nd ed.), published in 1969, the year of his death. This textbook has remained the most complete and influential work in the field. The authors of this book, therefore, humbly dedicate this effort to the principle of excellence in pediatric neurosurgery which Donald Matson so clearly defined.

ROBERT L. McLAURIN, M.D.

PREFACE

Because of continued developments in the field of pediatric neurosurgery and the increasing numbers of neurosurgeons devoting their careers to the subspecialty, it was decided that *Pediatric Neurosurgery* should be updated. This Third Edition was done under the auspices of the Pediatric Section of the American Association of Neurological Surgeons in conjunction with the American Society of Pediatric Neurosurgeons. There are many changes in the current volume with the first two chapters extensively dealing with normal and abnormal development of the nervous system and spine. Hydrocephalus is thoroughly covered in the second section by a number of highly respected authors in this field. The sections on trauma and tumors have been increased and updated with current knowledge. The vascular disease section includes information on interventional neuroradiology, as well as the current thinking on the treatment of ischemic problems, hemorrhage, and vascular malformations in children. The final section on the application of newer technologies contains information relative to those advances that have occurred in recent years in the treatment of spasticity and epilepsy, as well as radiosurgery, skull base surgery, ventriculoscopy and stereotaxis. The editors have picked authors for each of the chapters in the book who have expertise and knowledge for the particular subject at hand. The section editors have done an outstanding job in assimilating the material and working with the individual authors. I wish to thank the section editors for the tremendous amount of work they have done, as well as all of the individual authors for their contributions to this volume. All of us believe that this has become an important publication of interest to anyone in the field of neurosurgery, neurology, or pediatrics.

WILLIAM R. CHEEK, M.D.

CONTENTS

PART VII

APPLICATION OF NEWER TECHNOLOGIES

PART

I

DEVELOPMENTAL ABNORMALITIES

NORMAL AND ABNORMAL EARLY DEVELOPMENT OF THE NERVOUS SYSTEM

DAVID G. McLONE, M.D., Ph.D, and MARK S. DIAS, M.D.

Disorders of neural development comprise a significant proportion of pediatric neurosurgical disorders, and the treatment of these malformations is the sine qua non of the pediatric neurosurgeon. It is important for those who treat these children to be thoroughly familiar with both the normal development of the nervous system and the ways in which neural development might go awry. With this in mind, we have attempted to present a more detailed description of early neural development and its associated malformations than has usually been provided. Although this has been an ambitious undertaking, we feel that it is only through an intimate understanding of normal and abnormal neuroembryology that we as pediatric neurosurgeons can identify the many malformations with which we are confronted and appropriately treat those children so afflicted.

Most of what we know of the mechanisms of normal human neural development is derived from the study of nonhuman embryos including those of amphibian, avian, and other mammalian species. These studies have elucidated many of the details concerning the mechanisms of early neural development in these animals, and although many interspecies differences exist, they provide considerable insight into the mechanisms underlying early *human* neural development. Several recent reviews provide more detailed information on selected topics than can be covered here.[1-6]

In addition to the information provided through the study of animal development, a considerable volume of descriptive information has been derived through the study of early human embryos such as those of the Carnegie collection. The development of these embryos has been chronicled by O'Rahilly and Müller in *Developmental Stages in Human Embryos,* Carnegie Institution of Washington, Publication Number 637, available

through the Government Printing Office in Washington, D.C. The interested reader is referred to this work for more detailed information. The ages of these embryos have been estimated by comparing their morphologic features with those of nonhuman primate embryos of known age. The date of fertilization is assumed to coincide with the date of ovulation; therefore, all developmental events are measured in terms of *postovulatory days* (POD).

In order to standardize the study of human development, a variety of embryonic staging systems have been employed. The most recent and the most comprehensive is that of O'Rahilly (Table 1–1), which postdates the developmental stages of Mall,[7] the horizons of Streeter,[8] and other staging systems (discussed in O'Rahilly, 1973[9]). It provides a timetable for each of the important events in early neural morphogenesis and is the staging system that will be used throughout this chapter. According to this staging system, the embryonic period begins at conception with stage 1, encompasses approximately the first 56 to 57 days of human development, and ends at stage 23 with the appearance of bone marrow within the humerus.[10] Beyond this time, the developing human enters the fetal period.

NORMAL EARLY HUMAN NEURAL DEVELOPMENT

During the first four days after fertilization (POD 1 to 4, stages 1 to 3), the human embryo undergoes about five cell divisions to form a mass of approximately 32 cells (the blastocyst), which surrounds a central cavity (the blastocystic cavity). The blastocyst contains an eccentrically located inner cell mass, the embryonic cell proper, and a thinner surrounding ring of cells, the

TABLE 1–1. DEVELOPMENTAL STAGES IN HUMAN EMBRYOS*

CARNEGIE STAGE	PAIRS OF SOMITES	SIZE (MM)	AGE (DAYS)†	FEATURES
1		0.1–0.15	1	Fertilization.
2		0.1–0.2	1½–3	From 2 to about 16 cells.
3		0.1–0.2	4	Free blastocyst.
4		0.1–0.2	5–6	Attaching blastocyst.
5		0.1–0.2	7–12	Implanted although previllous.
5a		0.1	7–8	Solid trophoblast.
5b		0.1	9	Trophoblastic lacunae.
5c		0.15–0.2	11–12	Lacunar vascular circle.
6		0.2	13	Chorionic villi: primitive streak may appear.
6a				Chorionic villi.
6b				Primitive streak.
7		0.4	16	Notochordal process.
8		1.0–1.5	18	Primitive pit; notochordal and neurenteric canals; neural folds may appear.
9	1–3	1.5–2.5	20	Somites first appear.
10	4–12	2–3.5	22	Neural folds begin to fuse; 2 pharyngeal bars; optic sulcus.
11	13–20	2.5–4.5	24	Rostral neuropore closes; optic vesicle.
12	21–29	3–5	26	Caudal neuropore closes; 3–4 pharyngeal bars; upper limb buds appearing.
13	30–?	4–6	28	Four limb buds; lens disc; otic vesicle.
14		5–7	32	Lens pit and optic cup; endolymphatic appendage distinct.
15		7–9	33	Lens vesicle; nasal pit; antitragus beginning; hand plate; trunk relatively wider; future cerebral hemispheres distinct.
16		8–11	37	Nasal pit faces ventrally; retinal pigment visible in intact embryo; auricular hillocks beginning; foot plate.
17		11–14	41	Head relatively larger; trunk straighter; nasofrontal groove distinct; auricular hillocks distinct; finger rays.
18		13–17	44	Body more cuboidal; elbow region and toe rays appearing; eyelid folds may begin; tip of nose distinct; nipples appear; ossification may begin.
19		16–18	47½	Trunk elongating and straightening.
20		18–22	50½	Upper limbs longer and bent at elbows.
21		22–24	52	Fingers longer; hands approach each other, feet likewise.
22		23–28	54	Eyelids and external ear more developed.
23		27–31	56½	Head more rounded; limbs longer and more developed.

*From O'Rahily R, Miller F: Development Stages in Human Embryos. Washington D.C., Carnegie Institution of Washington, Publication 637, 1987.
†Olivier and Pineau (1962) for stages 11–23; miscellaneous sources for stages 1–10.

trophoblast (Fig. 1–1). By stage 3 (POD 4), the inner cell mass develops two distinct layers: cells on the dorsal surface, adjacent to the trophoblast, form the *epiblast* while cells on the ventral surface, adjacent to the blastocystic cavity, form the *hypoblast*.[11]

By stage 5 (POD 7 to 12), two additional cavities develop (Fig. 1–1): the *amnionic cavity* appears between the epiblast and the overlying trophoblast cells, and the *umbilical vesicle* (or *yolk sac*) appears below the hypoblast.[11] The epiblast is therefore adjacent to the amnionic cavity, and the hypoblast is adjacent to the umbilical vesicle. By stage 6 (POD 13), the hypoblast thickens cranially; this portion of the hypoblast is the prochordal plate and is the first morphologic feature of craniocaudal orientation. The prochordal plate eventually will give rise to the cephalic mesenchyme and to portions of the foregut;[11] maldevelopment of the prochordal plate may be responsible for the malformations associated with holoprosencephaly and agenesis of the corpus callosum.[12]

The primitive streak first develops at the caudal end of the blastocyst at stage 6 (POD 13) and elongates cranially over the next three days (Fig. 1–2). It reaches its full length by stage 7 (POD 16), at which time it occupies the midline in the caudal half of the human embryo; beyond this time, the primitive streak begins to regress—that is, it becomes shorter and moves back toward the caudal pole of the embryo.[11] The primitive streak is contiguous cranially with the *primitive knot*, or *Hensen's node;* in the middle of Hensen's node is a small indentation, the *primitive pit*. Along the length of the primitive streak is located a midline trough, the *primitive groove*, which is contiguous cranially with the primitive pit. Hensen's node is regarded as the cranial extension of the primitive streak, and the primitive pit as the cranial extension of the primitive groove.

During both primitive streak elongation and regression, cells of the epiblast migrate toward the primitive streak and invaginate through the primitive groove (Fig. 1–2). In the chick embryo studied by electron microscopy, this ingression of epiblast cells is accompanied by a loss of the basement membrane in the region of the primitive groove; epiblast cells lose their attachments with one another and ingress through this gap in the basement membrane.[13–17] The first cells to ingress are the prospective endodermal cells, which intercalate with the hypoblast and displace the hypoblast cells laterally. The prospective endoderm cells will form the

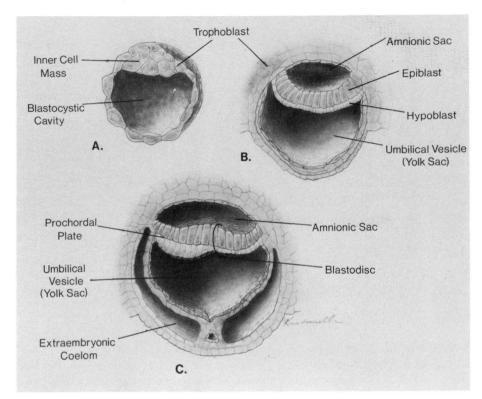

FIGURE 1–1. Development of the blastocyst; midsagittal illustrations. *A,* Continued proliferation of cells produces a sphere containing a blastocystic cavity surrounded by an eccentrically located inner cell mass and a surrounding ring of trophoblast cells. *B,* The inner cell mass develops further into a two-layered structure, the blastodisc, containing the epiblast adjacent to the amnionic cavity and the hypoblast adjacent to the yolk sac. *C,* With further development, the blastodisc thickens cranially to form the prochordal plate.

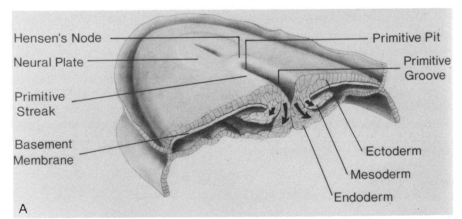

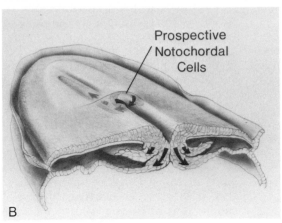

FIGURE 1–2. Normal human gastrulation. *A,* Prospective endodermal and mesodermal cells of the epiblast migrate toward the primitive streak and ingress *(arrows)* through the primitive groove to become the definitive endoderm and mesoderm. *B,* Prospective notochordal cells in the cranial margin of Hensen's node will ingress through the primitive pit during primitive streak regression to become the notochordal process. (From Dias MS, Walker ML: The embryogenesis of complex dysraphic malformations: a disorder of gastrulation? J Pediatr Neurosurg 18:229, 1992.)

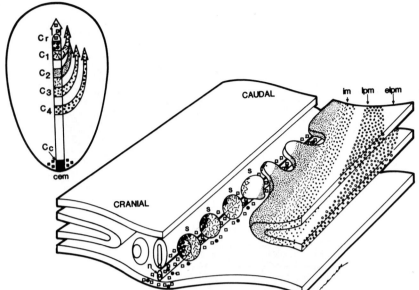

FIGURE 1–3. Composition of the primitive streak (PS) and Hensen's node in avian embryos; Cr, C1, C2, C3, C4, and Cc represent sites of grafting used for fate mapping studies (n = notochord, s = somite, im = intermediate mesoderm, lpm = lateral plate (somatic) mesoderm, elpm = extraembryonic lateral plate mesoderm, cem = caudal extraembryonic mesoderm). Hensen's node contributes to notochord and endoderm. The most cranial regions of the primitive streak (just posterior to Hensen's node) contribute to the somitic mesoderm, whereas consecutively more caudal regions of the streak contribute to sequentially more lateral (intermediate and lateral plate) mesoderm. The most caudal regions of the streak contribute to extraembryonic mesoderm. (From Schoenwolf GC, Garcia-Martinez V, Dias MS: Mesoderm movement and fate during avian gastrulation and neurulation. Dev Dynamics 193:235, 1992.)

definitive endoderm, while the displaced hypoblast cells ultimately will form extraembryonic tissues.[18–22] A short time later, prospective mesodermal cells ingress between the epiblast and the newly formed endoderm to become the mesoderm.[20, 21] The remaining epiblast cells migrate medially to replace the cells that have ingressed through the primitive groove; these remaining epiblast cells will form the ectoderm (both neuroectoderm and surface ectoderm). Embryonic endoderm, mesoderm, and ectoderm are thus all derived from the epiblast. This process, referred to as *gastrulation,** transforms the embryo from a two-layered structure containing an epiblast and a hypoblast into a three-layered structure containing ectoderm, mesoderm, and endoderm.[23]

The composition of the primitive streak varies along its craniocaudal length (Fig. 1–3). In the avian embryo, the caudal half of the primitive streak contains ingressing cells that are destined to form *extraembryonic* mesoderm, whereas the cranial half contains cells that are destined to form *embryonic* mesoderm and endoderm.[23] Prospective endoderm is contained in Hensen's node and the cranial-most portions of the progressing primitive streak, whereas prospective mesoderm is located more caudally, in the midportion of the primitive streak. The prospective *segmental plate* (or *somitic*) *mesoderm* (i.e., that mesoderm which will form the somites) is located more cranially in the primitive streak than is the prospective *lateral plate mesoderm* (i.e., that which will form the somatic mesoderm).[20, 21, 23]

---

*Strictly speaking, gastrulation, as defined in amphibian embryos, refers to the formation of the archenteron, which does not occur in avian or mammalian embryos. Instead, the term *germ layer formation* is more correct when describing the formation of the ectoderm, mesoderm, and endoderm in mammalian embryos. However, the term gastrulation is so widely understood that it will be retained throughout the text.

The composition of the primitive streak and Hensen's node also varies with time. In the chick, the primitive streak initially contains only prospective endodermal cells, which ingress through the streak from its earliest appearance until full primitive streak elongation (definitive primitive streak stage). Prospective mesodermal cells ingress later, beginning at intermediate and late stages of primitive streak elongation and continuing throughout streak regression.

Hensen's node in the chick initially contains only prospective endodermal cells, but as the streak elongates, these cells ingress and are gradually replaced by prospective mesodermal cells. By the time the streak is fully elongated, mesodermal cells predominate[20, 23] and consist chiefly of prospective notochord cells, which ingress through the cranial end of Hensen's node during full primitive streak elongation and subsequent regression, and are laid down in the midline as the *notochordal process* (Fig. 1–2B).

LOCALIZATION OF PROSPECTIVE NEUROECTODERM

Recent fate-mapping studies[24] have localized the prospective neuroectoderm to an area of the epiblast which surrounds and flanks Hensen's node and the cranial half of the primitive streak (Fig. 1–4A). Earlier mapping studies suggested that the prospective neuroectoderm is organized in a craniocaudal sequence, so that prospective forebrain cells are located more cranially than prospective midbrain cells.[25] However, more recent studies suggest a different organization. Instead of contributing to a single neuraxial level, each region of the neuroepithelium contributes to multiple neuraxial levels. For example, marking the most cranial regions of the prospective neuroectoderm results in a strip of label which extends through all craniocaudal subdivisions of the neuraxis from forebrain to spinal

FIGURE 1–4. Location of prospective neuroepithelium. *A,* Dorsal view of an avian embryo during gastrulation. Striped region illustrates localization by earlier mapping studies, which used carbon particles; hatched area illustrates additional caudal areas demonstrated by more recent mapping studies using horseradish peroxidase (HRP) injections and chimeric transplantation. (From Dias MS, Walker ML: The embryogenesis of complex dysraphic malformations: a disorder of gastrulation? J Pediatr Neurosurg 18:229, 1992.) *B,* Mediolateral organization of the developing neural tube. Median hingepoint (MHP) cells arise from an area just cranial to Hensen's node and extend caudally the length of the neuraxis in the midline. MHP cells are flanked bilaterally by paired lateral (L) cell regions, which arise from areas adjacent to Hensen's node and extend caudally between the MHP cells and surface ectoderm (SE). MHP cells will form the floor of the future neural tube, whereas L cells will contribute to the lateral walls. Horizontal lines indicate the primitive streak (FB = forebrain). (From Alvarez IS, Schoenwolf GC: Patterns of neuroepithelial cell rearrangement during avian neurulation are determined prior to notochordal inductive interactions. Dev Biol 143:78, 1991.)

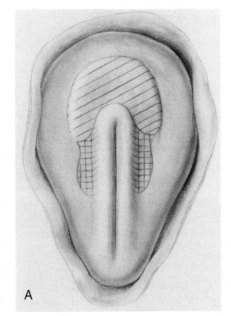
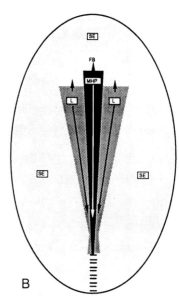

cord; marking more caudal levels results in similar strips, which, although beginning at more caudal levels, extend caudally through all subsequent levels of the neuraxis (Fig. 1–4*B*). These more recent studies suggest a mediolateral, rather than a craniocaudal, organization to the developing neural tube.[24]

REGRESSION OF THE PRIMITIVE STREAK AND FORMATION OF THE NOTOCHORD

In the human, the formation of the notochordal process from cells in Hensen's node begins at stage 7 (POD 16); concomitantly, the primitive streak begins to regress (Fig. 1–5).[11] To what extent does the notochordal process extend cranially from Hensen's node, and to what extent does it elongate caudally by addition of cells to its caudal end from the regressing Hensen's node? In the chick, the notochordal process grows largely by the latter mechanism.[25] Much less is known about mammalian notochord formation; however, the available evidence suggests that the situation is much more complex than in the chick (C. Lawson, personal communication). The mechanism of notochord elongation in man is unknown.

The notochordal process at stage 7 consists of a median cord of cells, located between the ectoderm and endoderm cranial to Hensen's node;[26] in cross section, the cells of the notochordal process are radially arranged about a central lumen called the *notochordal canal* (Fig. 1–6*A*).[11] This central canal is continuous dorsally with the amnionic cavity through the primitive pit.[27] The notochordal canal is present in human[11] and nonhuman primate[28] embryos but has not been de-

FIGURE 1–5. Formation of the notochord in avian embryos. The notochord is formed through the addition of cells to its caudal end as the primitive streak regresses; true cranial growth of the notochord is minimal. (Adapted from Spratt NT: Regression and shortening of the primitive streak in the explanted chick blastoderm. J Exp Zool 104:69, 1947.)

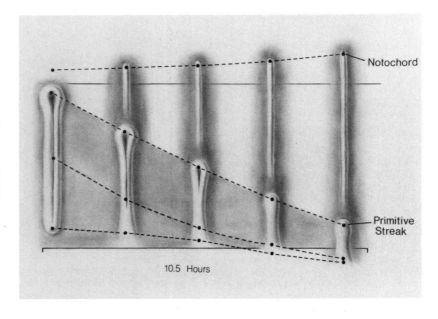

scribed in amphibian, avian, or nonprimate mammalian embryos. Its function is not known.

The notochordal process continues to elongate during stage 8 (POD 17 to 19) and reaches its full length at stage 9 (POD 19 to 21).[11, 29] It initially is rod-shaped and separate from both the overlying neuroectoderm and the underlying endoderm; however, during stage 8 (POD 17 to 19) it fuses, or *intercalates,* with the endoderm to form the *notochordal plate* (Fig. 1–6B). Intercalation begins in the middle third and subsequently extends both cranially and caudally to involve the entire notochordal process.[29] The notochordal plate is incorporated into the roof of the yolk sac, and the notochordal canal becomes continuous with the yolk sac. The most caudal portion of the notochordal canal is continuous both with the amnion through the primitive pit and with the yolk sac as a result of intercalation; this

communication is called the *neurenteric canal.*[11] The neurenteric canal first appears during stage 8 (POD 17 to 19) and continues during stages 9 and 10 (POD 19 to 23).[11, 29–31]

During stage 10 (POD 21 to 23) the notochordal plate begins to fold dorsoventrally, and by stage 11 (POD 23 to 25) it has completely separated once again from the underlying endoderm;[11, 31, 32] this process is termed *excalation* (Fig. 1–6C). Accordingly, the neurenteric canal is obliterated, and the amnionic and yolk sacs are once again separate. Excalation proceeds from caudal to rostral; the pharynx is the last area of endoderm to dissociate from the notochordal plate.[32] After excalation, a solid rod of notochordal cells forms the true *notochord.*[32] Like the notochordal canal, intercalation and excalation of the notochordal process have been described only in human[11, 29–31] and nonhuman primate[28] embryos.

Although most of the notochordal cells are derived from Hensen's node, the caudal-most notochordal cells arise from the *caudal eminence* or *end bud* at the caudal end of the embryo;[32, 33] the process of secondary notochord formation accompanies *secondary neurulation* and will be described subsequently.

FORMATION OF THE NEURAL TUBE

In the human embryo, the neuroectoderm is first discernible at stage 7 (POD 16) as a pseudostratified columnar epithelium composed of three or four rows of nuclei; it is taller than the surrounding cutaneous ectoderm.[9] By stage 8 (POD 17 to 19), a shallow midline fold, the *neural groove,* is present and represents the beginning of neurulation.[29] The neural groove is intimately adherent to the underlying notochord throughout its length, being separated from the latter by only a basement membrane. This close association continues until after neural tube closure, whereupon the notochord separates from the neural tube.[33]

By stage 9 (POD 19 to 21), the neural groove has deepened considerably, and neural folds are developing laterally.[30] Although the neural tube at this stage is not yet closed, 80 per cent of embryos exhibit clear craniocaudal subdivisions including prosencephalon (forebrain), mesencephalon (midbrain), rhombencephalon (hindbrain), and spinal cord. The rhombencephalon can be further subdivided at this stage into four *rhombomeres (Rh).* Rhombomere A lies between the mesencephalon cranially and the otic plates caudally, RhB lies opposite the otic plates, RhC lies between the otic plates cranially and the first somite caudally, and RhD lies opposite and caudal to the first somite.[30] The brain occupies 70 to 85 per cent of the total length of the neuraxis at stage 9, while the spinal cord occupies only 15 to 30 per cent; the spinal cord merges caudally with the regressing Hensen's node. From one to three pairs of somites are present in stage 9 embryos.[30]

The neural folds continue to elevate and converge toward the midline during stages 9 and 10. The initial apposition of the neural folds to form a closed neural tube occurs during stage 10 (POD 21 to 23). The timing

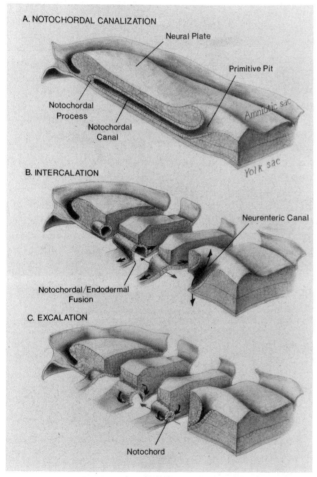

FIGURE 1–6. Notochordal canalization, intercalation, and excalation. *A,* The notochordal process contains a central lumen (the notochordal canal), which is continuous with the amnionic cavity through the primitive pit. *B,* During intercalation, the canalized notochordal process fuses with the underlying endoderm; the communication of the amnion with the yolk sac forms the *primitive neurenteric canal. C,* During excalation, the notochord rolls up and separates from the endoderm to become the definitive notochord; the primitive neurenteric canal becomes obliterated. (From Dias MS, Walker ML: The embryogenesis of complex dysraphic malformations: a disorder of gastrulation? J Pediatr Neurosurg 18:229, 1992.)

and manner of neural tube closure are species-specific. In the chick, the midbrain is the first region of the neural tube to close, whereas in the mouse, rat, and hamster, the point of initial closure is at the junction between the rhombencephalon and cranial spinal cord.[31] In the human, the point of initial closure is most commonly at the level of the caudal rhombencephalon or cranial spinal cord, and usually occurs when five pairs of somites are present; closure involves apposition and fusion of first the cutaneous ectoderm, then the neuroectoderm.[11, 31] Closure of the remaining neural tube continues throughout stages 10 to 12, and extends over 4 to 6 days. Neural tube closure often occurs simultaneously at several places along the neural tube, rather than as a sequential "zippering up" of the neural tube cranial and caudal to the point of initial closure.[31] In the past, the intervening open areas have been mistaken for areas of dysraphism, but they too eventually close.[11] Neural tube closure keeps pace with the cranial to caudal development of the somites, so that the cranial end of the caudal neuropore lies adjacent or just caudal to the last-formed somite.[34]

Closure of the cranial neuropore occurs during stage 11 (POD 23 to 25) and is bidirectional;[32] closure advances cranially from the rhombencephalon and meets a second wave of closure, which begins at the future optic chiasm and advances caudally. The site of final closure is the commissural plate located immediately anterior to the prospective lamina terminalis, at the site of the future anterior commissure.[11, 35]

The caudal neuropore closes during stage 12 (POD 25 to 27) in a craniocaudal direction.[33] At the time the caudal neuropore closes, approximately 25 somites have formed; the caudal neuropore at this stage is located caudal to the last visible somite. Therefore, the site of closure has been estimated by measuring the space between the last visible somite and the caudal

neuropore and calculating the number of somites that would subsequently form in this space. Using this method, the site of closure has been estimated to be opposite somites 30/31,[33] which corresponds to both a spinal ganglion and a vertebral level of S2.[36] It therefore appears that, in the human, the majority of the nervous system (as far caudal as the second sacral spinal cord segment) forms by primary neurulation, and the filum terminale and perhaps the lower sacral spinal cord form by secondary neurulation. Accordingly, one can deduce that *all central nervous system malformations that arise cranial to S2, whether open or closed, involve regions of the neural tube that are formed from primary neurulation.*

OCCLUSION OF THE SPINAL NEUROCELE

During neural tube closure in amphibians,[37] birds,[38–40] mice,[41] rats,[42] and humans,[43] the lateral walls of the neural tube in the region of the spinal cord become apposed and obliterate the lumen of the spinal neurocele (Fig. 1–7). In the human, this *spinal occlusion* begins concomitant with the closure of the anterior neuropore at stage 11 (POD 23 to 25), continues throughout the period of caudal neuropore closure at stage 12 (POD 25 to 27), and ends at stage 14 (POD 32). Occlusion of the neurocele begins cranial to the first pair of somites, extends as far caudal as the ninth somite, and involves approximately 60 per cent of the neuraxis.[43] Occlusion always occurs in regions of the neural tube that are adjacent to somites, suggesting an important function for somites in initiating occlusion.[40, 44, 45]

Concurrent with spinal occlusion, the neural tube cranial to the point of occlusion begins to undergo rapid expansion due to (1) growth of the neural tube and (2) expansion of the ventricular system.[46, 47] This has led several authors to suggest that spinal occlusion may

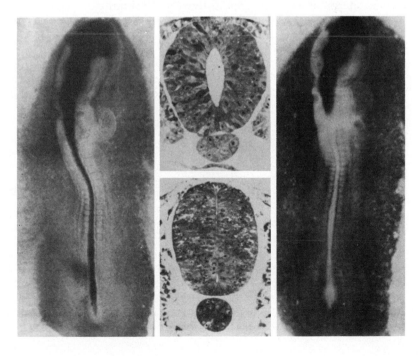

FIGURE 1–7. Spinal occlusion in avian embryos. *Left,* Chick embryo before occlusion of the neurocele; dye injected into the ventricular system cranially shows communication throughout the central canal of the entire neural tube. *Upper middle,* A photomicrograph of the spinal neurocele at this stage shows a patent central canal. *Right,* A chick embryo during the period of neurocele occlusion shows, at the level of the hindbrain, a complete block to more caudal flow of dye. *Lower middle,* A photomicrograph of the spinal neurocele at this stage shows complete obliteration of the central canal. (Modified from Desmond M: *In* Gilbert, SF: *Developmental Biology,* 2nd ed. Sunderland, MA, Sinauer Associates Inc., 1988, p. 163.)

play an important role in the initial expansion of the brain and ventricular system.[38–41, 43–45, 48] Cranial neuropore closure and spinal occlusion isolate the cranial ventricular system from the external environment and establish a closed, fluid-filled space. Once established, the isolated ventricular system is subjected to an intraluminal pressure,[49, 50] which provides a driving force for brain enlargement. When the intra- and extraluminal pressures are equalized by cannulating the cranial neural tube lumen with a hollow glass rod during the period of rapid brain enlargement, brain expansion is significantly reduced; the resultant neural tube is collapsed and folded, and its walls contain fewer cells.[38, 51, 52] As we shall see, a failure to maintain this driving pressure in patients with open neural tube defects also appears to be responsible for the myriad cranial and mesenchymal abnormalities seen in the Chiari malformation.

FORMATION OF THE NEURAL CREST

The neural crest in human embryos first develops at stage 9 (POD 19 to 21) with the appearance of the mesencephalic and rhombencephalic (principally facial) neural crest cells.[30] The formation of mesencephalic and facial neural crest cells reaches a peak at stage 10 (POD 21 to 23). The remaining neural crest cells begin to develop at stage 11; the order of appearance is facial, mesencephalic, trigeminal, vagal, occipital, and glossopharyngeal neural crest.[31] Formation of cranial neural crest continues during stage 12 (POD 25 to 27) and ends during stage 13 (POD 28).[33, 53] The trunk neural crest first appears during stage 11 (POD 23 to 25) and continues until at least stage 14 (POD 32).[54]

Neural crest cells in human,[8, 32] mouse,[55] and rat[56] embryos are thought to arise from the neural tube at the junction between the neural folds and adjacent surface ectoderm; at least in humans, however, a simultaneous origin for some neural crest cells from the adjacent surface ectoderm cannot be excluded.[31] The initial formation of the cranial neural crest in the human begins during neural fold elevation (at stage 9) *before* the neural folds fuse, and continues from the closed neural tube *after* the neural folds fuse.[31, 32] More caudal neural crest cells arise exclusively from the neural tube following neural tube closure.[11, 33] A similar sequence has been described in the rat.[56]

Neural crest cells undergo terminal differentiation into a bewildering variety of cell types. In the human, cranial neural crest cells contribute to the cephalic mesenchyme associated with the pharyngeal arches, to the primary meninx giving rise to both the pia and arachnoid,[57] to the cranial Schwann cells and melanocytes, and to the cranial ganglia.[32, 33, 53] Both the optic and mesencephalic neural crest contribute to the optic primordium and form the optic nerve sheath.[58] The mesencephalic neural crest may also contribute to the trigeminal ganglion,[33] along with a contribution from the rhombencephalic (Rh2) neural crest.[33] Neural crest from Rh4 contributes to the faciovestibulocochlear ganglion, that from Rh6 to the glossopharyngeal ganglion, and that from Rh7 to the vagal ganglion. No neural crest cells develop from either Rh3 or Rh5.[11]

The trunk neural crest cells contribute to melanocytes of the body wall and limbs, to the Schwann cells investing the peripheral nerves, to the primary meninx of the spinal cord, and to dorsal root and autonomic ganglion cells of the spinal nerves. In addition, these cells give rise to the adrenal medulla.[1] In both avian and mammalian (and presumably human) embryos, trunk neural crest cells choose either a dorsal or a ventral migratory pathway shortly after they leave the neural tube. Neural crest cells that follow the dorsal, or "subepidermal migratory" pathway will form the melanocytes of the skin, while those that follow the ventral migratory pathway will form the remaining neural crest derivatives.[59] The neural crest cells in the "ventral migratory pathway" advance between the neural tube and adjacent somites. These cells traverse the somite, where they are restricted to the rostral half of the sclerotomal portion. At this point, some of the ventral neural crest cells remain near the neural tube and become dorsal root ganglion cells, while others advance farther ventrally to become sympathetic ganglion and adrenal cells.[60] Further details regarding the control of migration and terminal differentiation of neural crest cells can be found in several recent reviews.[3, 59, 61]

SECONDARY NEURULATION

Following the closure of the caudal neuropore at stage 12 (POD 25 to 27), the entire nervous system is skin covered and further neural development takes place by *secondary neurulation*.[33] The primitive streak has regressed concomitant with neural tube formation and by stage 9 forms a mass of pluripotent cells referred to as the *caudal eminence*[30] or *end bud*.[62] By stage 12, the caudal eminence extends from the site of the former neurenteric canal to the cloacal membrane; it will give rise to all tissues of the caudal embryo including the *neural cord* (the caudal continuation of the neural tube) and caudal neural crest cells, the caudal notochord and somites (including somite 32 and all more caudal somites), caudal mesenchyme, and hindgut.[33] The caudal eminence contains two types of tissue: a more compact, dorsally located tissue, which will contribute to the neural cord, notochord and somites; and a less compact, ventrally located tissue, which will contribute to the hindgut.[33]

Studies of secondary neurulation in chick[62] and mouse[63] embryos have revealed several important interspecies differences. In the chick embryo (Fig. 1–8A), secondary neurulation results in the formation of a *medullary cord* (the equivalent of the neural cord in the human) from the end bud. The medullary cord is composed of two cell types: an outer layer of tightly packed cells surrounds an inner cluster of more loosely arranged cells. Cavitation begins cranially between the outer and inner cell groups and forms multiple lumina between the two cell groups. The outer cells become

Secondary Neurulation

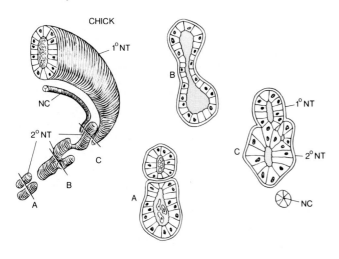

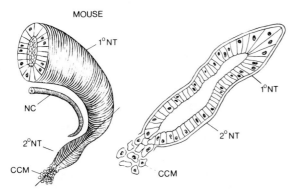

FIGURE 1–8. Secondary neurulation. Upper illustration depicts secondary neurulation in avian embryos. *A*, The medullary cord consists of multiple lumina, each surrounded by an outer layer of tightly packed, radially oriented cells and containing an inner group of more loosely packed cells. *B*, Adjacent cords coalesce to form larger aggregates; simultaneously, the inner cells are lost. Eventually a single structure is formed, having a single lumen which is *not* yet in direct communication with the lumen formed by primary neurulation. *C*, Later, the neural tube formed by secondary neurulation (2° NT) fuses with that formed from primary neurulation (1° NT); at this point, the lumina of the two neural tubes communicate directly (NC = notochord). Lower illustration depicts secondary neurulation in mouse embryos. A medullary rosette is composed of cells radially arranged about an empty central lumen. The lumen is always in communication with the central canal formed by primary neurulation. Growth of the secondary neural tube occurs by additional cavitation of the secondary lumen and by recruiting additional cells from the caudal cell mass (CCM).

radially arranged about each lumen, are joined together at both apex and base by gap junctions, and are surrounded by a basal lamina, while the inner cells lie within the lumina. Eventually, the inner cells are lost, perhaps by incorporation with the outer cell group, by cell death, or by migration away from the medullary cord; the outer cells then surround multiple empty lumina. These smaller lumina coalesce to form larger cavities; eventually a single lumen is formed and is surrounded by the outer cell group. This *secondary* neural tube lies adjacent to the primary neural tube in an

overlap zone, with the primary neural tube located dorsally and the secondary neural tube located ventrally; these two tubes fuse to form a single structure. In summary, secondary neurulation in the chick involves five major processes: (1) formation of a medullary cord from the tail bud, (2) segregation of the inner and outer cell groups, (3) cavitation to form multiple lumina between the inner and outer cell groups, (4) coalescence of the lumina to form a single lumen, and (5) fusion of the secondary and primary neural tubes.[64]

Secondary neurulation in the mouse (Fig. 1–8B) begins with the formation of a *medullary rosette,* a cluster of cells radially arranged about a central lumen formed by cavitation. The cells of the medullary rosette are thought to be the homologue of the outer cell group in the chick embryo; the inner cell group seen in the chick does not appear to be present in the mouse. A basal lamina surrounds the basal surfaces of the rosette cells, and intercellular gap junctions develop between the cells of the rosette, as they do between the outer cells in the chick. Caudal growth of the secondary neural tube occurs by additional cavitation of the medullary rosette and recruitment of additional cells from the end bud. In summary, secondary neurulation in the mouse involves only two steps: (1) formation of the medullary rosette, which is continuous with the primary neural tube, and (2) cavitation of the rosette to form a central lumen, which similarly communicates with the central canal of the primary neural tube.[63]

In review, then, secondary neurulation in the mouse and chick differ in several respects. First, the secondary neural tube in the mouse is always directly continuous with the primary neural tube and develops caudally from the posterior neuropore; in contrast, the secondary neural tube in the chick develops independently and only later fuses with the primary neural tube. Second, the lumen of the secondary neural tube in the mouse is single and is always continuous with that of the primary neural tube; in contrast, multiple lumina are initially formed in the chick and only later communicate with one another and with the lumen of the primary neural tube. Finally, there is no overlap zone in the mouse, as there is in the chick.

There is some debate about whether secondary neurulation in the human more closely resembles that of the chick or mouse. According to Müller and O'Rahilly, human secondary neurulation more closely resembles that of the mouse; in their study, the neural cord was continuous with the primary neural tube, a single lumen was present and was continuous with the central canal of the primary neural tube, and no overlap zone was present.[33] In contrast, Lemire and associates[65] and Bolli[66] propose that human secondary neurulation more closely resembles that of the chick. These authors describe multiple independent secondary tubes having separate lumina and no discernible connection either with one another or with the primary neural tube. Lemire suggests that these independent tubes later coalesce to form a single secondary neural tube, which then fuses with the primary neural tube, as occurs in the chick.[65]

ASCENT OF THE CONUS MEDULLARIS

Beginning at about stage 18 to 20 (POD 43 to 48), and continuing into later fetal development and postnatal life, the caudal neural tube undergoes several morphogenetic changes collectively referred to as the "ascent of the conus medullaris" (Fig. 1–9).[67, 68] The neural tube caudal to the 32nd vertebra regresses beyond stage 18 to become more slender and fibrous;[67] this tissue ultimately becomes the filum terminale, within which is located an ependyma-lined central canal, the *ventriculus terminalis*.[69] The ventriculus terminalis is present in embryos beyond stage 20, reaches its maximum diameter at two years of age, and frequently persists into adulthood; it usually occupies the cranial end of the filum, as well as the caudal end of the conus medullaris, and has no communication with the subarachnoid space.[70] The transition between caudal spinal cord and filum terminale is abrupt, usually occupying only one spinal segment.

The ascent of the conus medullaris has been chronicled by Streeter[68] and by Barson.[71] The ascent has been thought to occur by two mechanisms: (1) differential growth of the spinal cord and adjacent vertebral column, and (2) "retrogressive differentiation." The degree to which differential growth of the vertebrae and spinal cord contributes to ascent can be estimated by measuring the distance between the exit site of the nerve root from the spinal cord on the one hand and the site of the dorsal root ganglion (which marks the spinal segment) on the other; any additional length discrepancy is attributed to retrogressive differentiation.[68] Before stage 22 (POD 54), ascent involves primarily retrogressive differentiation; thereafter, ascent takes place largely by differential growth.[67, 68]

Retrogressive differentiation is a little-understood

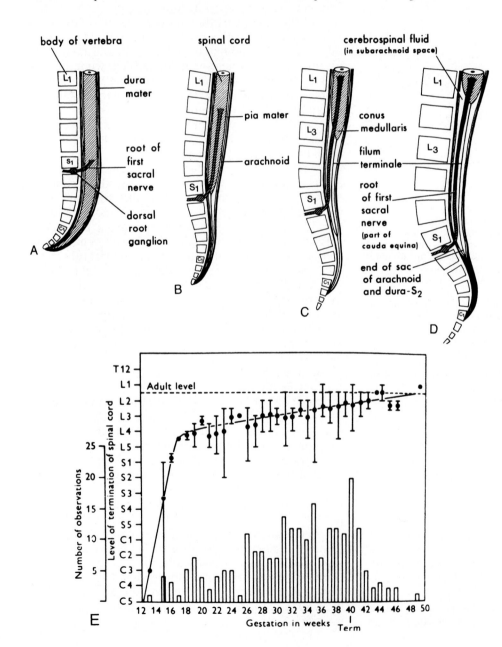

FIGURE 1–9. Ascent of the conus medullaris. Progressive ascent of the conus medullaris during embryogenesis and the immediate postnatal period: *A*, 8 weeks' gestation; *B*, 24 weeks' gestation; *C*, newborn; *D*, adulthood. (From Moore KL: The Developing Human, 5th ed. Philadelphia, WB Saunders Co, 1993, Fig. 10–10, p 394.) *E*, Vertebral level of termination of the conus medullaris during fetal and early postnatal life. (From Barson AJ: The vertebral level of termination of the spinal cord during normal and abnormal development. J Anat 106:489, 1970.)

process in which the postcoccygeal neural tube loses much of its diameter, fails to develop a distinct mantle zone, exhibits only a thin, rudimentary marginal zone, and "generally appears less well developed" than it did at earlier embryonic stages.[68] Little is known about the processes that underlie this fascinating event.

The period of time during which the conus medullaris ascends has been studied by Barson[71] and is reproduced in Figure 1–9B. Most of the ascent occurs prenatally, between 8 and 25 weeks of gestation; at birth, the conus medullaris lies approximately opposite the L2–L3 disc space, and by 1 year of age has reached its "adult" level opposite or cranial to the L1–L2 disc space in the majority of humans. A more caudally located conus, at or below the L2–L3 disc space, suggests that the spinal cord is abnormally tethered.

MECHANISMS OF PRIMARY NEURULATION

Primary neurulation is not the simple all-or-none process depicted in standard textbooks, in which a flat sheet of cells rolls up into a tube. Rather, neurulation is a complex morphogenetic process composed of several interdependent events, all of which overlap temporally to some degree. These include (1) shaping of the neuroepithelium to form a neural plate; (2) bending of the neural plate, first in the midline neural groove and later along the lateral edges of the neural tube, which results in elevation and apposition of the neural folds in the midline; and (3) fusion of the neural folds to close the neural tube.[6] The mechanisms of normal neurulation will be reviewed here; the interested reader is referred to an excellent recent monograph by Schoenwolf and Smith[6] for a more comprehensive treatise.

Shaping of the Neural Plate

The developing neural plate undergoes changes in its shape during which it (1) thickens apicodorsally, (2) narrows transversely, and (3) lengthens craniocaudally. These changes convert the neural plate from a relatively flat, discoid shape to a narrower and more elongated structure. Three cellular mechanisms account for this neural plate shaping: (1) changes in neuroepithelial cell height, (2) oriented cell divisions, and (3) cell rearrangements.

The first morphologic feature of the induced neuroepithelium involves a cell shape change from a simple cuboidal to a pseudostratified columnar epithelium. It has long been recognized that this neuroepithelial cell elongation is the result of a reorganization of intracellular longitudinally (or paraxially) oriented microtubules. These microtubules are abundant in neuroepithelial cells of many species including amphibians,[72–75] birds,[64, 76–81] and mammals.[63, 82–84] Moreover, agents that depolymerize microtubules (such as colchicine, nocodazole, or cold treatment) invariably result in a loss of neuroepithelial cell height when applied to embryonic neuroepithelium.[73, 77, 85–88]

Although microtubules are important, they are prob-

ably not the only forces that play a role in neuroepithelial cell elongation. In chick embryos, microtubule depolymerization with colchicine, nocodazole, or cold results in only a 25 per cent loss of neuroepithelial cell height.[81] Other mechanisms that may be important in neuroepithelial cell elongation include differential cell-cell adhesion[89, 90] and "cortical tractoring."[91]

In addition to the apicodorsal thickening discussed above, neural plate shaping involves two other morphologic changes: transverse narrowing and craniocaudal elongation.[6] As we have seen, changes in neuroepithelial cell height account for some of the apicodorsal thickening of the neural plate. However, these changes can account for only 15 per cent of the transverse narrowing and none of the craniocaudal elongation that occur during neural plate shaping.[92] Two other cellular events also contribute substantially to these morphologic changes: cell division (at least in avian and mammalian embryos) and cell rearrangement (intercalation). Computer modeling studies (Fig. 1–10) suggest that these three processes (cell elongation, cell division,

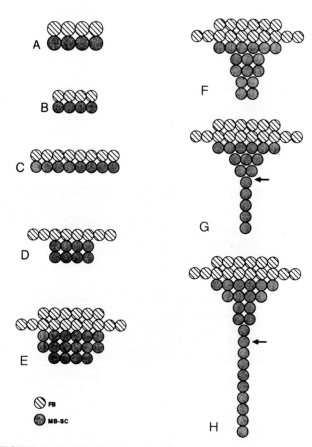

FIGURE 1–10. Contributions of cell shape changes, oriented cell division, and intercalation to the shaping of the neuroepithelium. Computer simulation shows one possible mechanism by which neural plate shaping might be brought about by a 30 per cent increase in neuroepithelial cell height (and a corresponding approximate 15 per cent decrease in cell diameter, leaving cell volume constant), two to three rounds of oriented cell divisions, and two rounds of cell rearrangement (FB = forebrain; MB–SC = midbrain–spinal cord). (From Schoenwolf GC, Alvarez IS: Roles of neuroepithelial cell rearrangement and division in shaping of the avian neural plate. Development 106:427, 1989.)

and cell rearrangement) can account for most of the changes in the shape of the avian neural plate.[92]

Bending of the Neural Plate

Most embryology texts equate neurulation with neural plate bending, during which the flat neural plate is converted to a neural tube. The morphogenetic events and underlying mechanisms of neural plate bending have been extensively studied in avian embryos, in which bending can be subdivided into several discrete steps (Fig. 1–11): (1) cells located in the midline of the neural plate and overlying the notochord change from spindle to wedge shape and are associated with the formation of a *median hingepoint*, or neural groove (Fig. 1–11A); (2) the neural folds elevate on either side of the median hingepoint to form a characteristic V shape; (3) additional cell shape changes develop in discrete, bilaterally paired regions of the dorsolateral neural tube and are associated with the formation of the *dorsolateral hingepoints* (DLHP), around which the neural folds converge toward the midline (Fig. 1–11B); and (4) the converging neural folds meet in preparation for neural fold fusion (Fig. 1–11C).[6] Similar morphologic changes have been observed in mammalian embryos[93] but have not been as well characterized as in the chick.

The driving forces behind each of these processes are complex and have been the focus of considerable scientific investigation. Traditional theories have held to three fundamental concepts: (1) ". . . all forces for neurulation are intrinsic to the neuroepithelium," (2) ". . . neurulation is driven by changes in the shape of neuroepithelial cells," and (3) ". . . [the] forces for cell shape changes are generated by the cytoskeleton of neuroepithelial cells."[6] However, each of these concepts has been challenged by more recent experimental evidence. More recent theories emphasize the importance of forces both intrinsic and extrinsic to the nervous system in neural plate bending; these forces are summarized in Figure 1–12.

Roux first proposed in 1885 that neurulation was a process intrinsic to the neuroepithelium; he demonstrated that the neural plate could roll up into a tube when cultured in isolation.[94] However, as Schoenwolf has pointed out, the neural tubes in these experiments (1) roll up sooner than expected, (2) do not undergo the characteristic shaping movements described above, and (3) often roll up *backward*—that is, with the apical side of the neuroepithelium on the *outside* of the neural tube.[6] This investigator has argued that the bending movements of isolated neuroepithelium are nonspecific and do not represent neurulation.[6]

More recent experimental evidence suggests that forces extrinsic to the neuroepithelium may play an important role in promoting neural tube bending.[95] Extrinsic forces that might contribute to neural plate bending include compression of the neural folds by the medial convergence of the surface ectoderm,[6, 95] elevation of the neural folds by the accumulation of underlying mesodermal cells or expansion of the underlying extracellular matrix,[96–105] and passive (so-called "Eulerian") buckling of the neural tube by the elongation of the notochord and/or "notoplate" (floorplate) of the

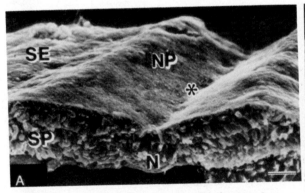

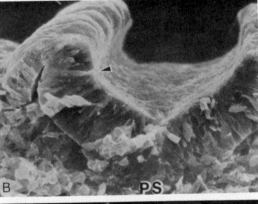

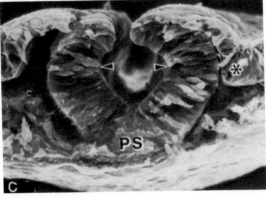

FIGURE 1–11. Bending of chick neuroepithelium. *A,* Scanning electron micrograph (SEM) of the neural plate of a stage 8 chick embryo. Median hingepoint (MHP) cells overlying the notochord (N) become wedge shaped and form the neural groove. Asterisk denotes the developing neural folds. (SE = superficial ectoderm, SP = somatopleure, NP = neural plate.) *B,* SEM of neural folds of a stage 10 chick embryo. Dorsolateral hingepoint (DLHP) cells undergo wedging to form bilateral dorsolateral furrows *(arrowhead).* Neural fold elevation is well under way (PS = primitive streak). *C,* SEM of the neural tube of a stage 11 chick embryo. Dorsolateral furrows *(arrowheads)* are well developed; neural fold elevation is nearly complete, and the neural folds are nearly apposed in the midline in preparation for fusion. Asterisk denotes surface ectoderm (PS = primitive streak). (From Schoenwolf GC: On the morphogenesis of the early rudiments of the developing central nervous system. Scanning Electron Microsc 1982; Pt 1:289.)

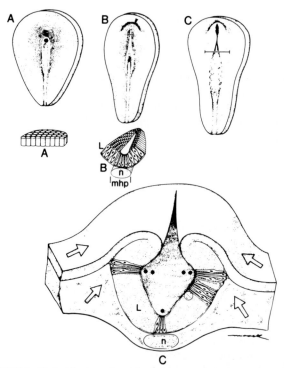

FIGURE 1–12. Intrinsic and extrinsic forces contributing to neural tube closure in the chick. *A and B,* Neural plate shaping. Prospective neuroepithelium is indicated by heavy stippling, surface ectoderm by lighter stippling, and head fold by the arrowhead. MHP cells *(shaded area)* arise from the area immediately cranial to Hensen's node (*), extend the length of the midline, and are flanked bilaterally by L (lateral) cells (*B,* cross-sectional view). Initial stages of neural plate bending involve the formation of a median hingepoint, during which MHP cells increase in height, lengthen their cell cycle times, and become wedge shaped; this results in the formation of a median furrow. *C,* Later stages of neural plate bending involve continued MHP wedging and formation of bilaterally paired DLHPs (**). Neural fold elevation occurs around the MHP (*), and convergence occurs around the DLHPs (**). Available evidence suggests that the forces for neural plate bending are generated both intrinsic (cell wedging in the MHP and DLHP regions) and extrinsic to the neuroepithelium. Extrinsic forces *(open arrows)* are provided by surrounding non-neuroepithelial tissues including the surface ectoderm, underlying mesodermal cells, and mesenchymal stroma. (From Schoenwolf GC, Smith JL: Mechanisms of neurulation: traditional viewpoint and recent advances. Development 109:243, 1990.)

neural tube.[4, 5, 106, 107] The importance of these extrinsic forces in neural tube formation has been debated by Gordon[4] and by Schoenwolf and Smith;[6] the interested reader is referred to these reviews for additional information.

The second tenet of traditional dogma, that neural plate bending is driven by changes in neuroepithelial cell shape, was first proposed by His in 1894, who suggested that if cells in a flat sheet were to become wedge-shaped, either through apical constriction or basal expansion, the sheet would fold into a tubular structure.[108] Wedging of neuroepithelial cells during neural plate bending has been documented in amphibian,[109, 110] avian,[111] and mammalian[112] embryos. However, cell wedging does not occur in all neuroepithelial cells; in the chick, only 10 per cent of cells become wedge-

shaped during neural plate bending.[111] These cells are largely restricted to the median hingepoint (MHP) and dorsolateral hingepoint (DLHP) regions of the neural tube.[111]

The relationship between neural plate bending and cell shape changes in the hingepoint regions has been carefully studied in avian embryos.[111] Chick neuroepithelial cells are of four types, depending upon their shape: (1) spindle cells have a bulbous waist and a tapering apex and base, (2) wedge-shaped cells have a bulbous base and a tapering apex, (3) inverted wedge-shaped cells have a bulbous apex and a tapering base, and (4) globular cells have a spherical shape. These cell shapes are associated with the location of the nucleus, which resides in the widest portion of the cell body; in the case of the globular cells, the nucleus is more centrally located and is in the mitotic (M) phase of the cell cycle. Schoenwolf and Franks studied the distribution of these four cell types throughout the avian neural plate during bending. Before neural plate bending begins, the distribution of the four cell types is random. However, concurrently with formation of the neural groove, most MHP cells change from spindle to wedge shape. A similar shape change occurs slightly later in the DLHP cells as the neural folds converge toward the midline. Most cells in the intervening regions of the neural tube remain spindle shaped. The cell shape changes in the hingepoint regions result in focal areas of neural plate bending at these points.[111]

Although MHP wedging may assist in neural plate bending, experimental evidence suggests that it is neither necessary nor sufficient for neurulation to occur.[6] First, neural plate bending can occur in the absence of MHP wedging; when prospective notochordal cells are destroyed by X-irradiation[113, 114] or prevented from forming by excising Hensen's node,[115] MHP cells do not undergo wedging, yet neural plate bending occurs in many cases. Second, when the neural plate is separated from more lateral tissues, MHP cells still undergo wedging on schedule, but neural fold elevation and convergence fail to occur.[95] It has been suggested that, rather than *driving* neural plate bending, MHP wedging may *direct* bending toward a specific site.[6] In this respect, the MHP region may provide a "crease" upon which neural plate bending may occur.

According to Schoenwolf, the DLHP may play a more important role in neural plate bending, at least in the chick.[6] In one study, wedging of DLHP cells did not occur in approximately one third of chick embryos treated with cytochalasin D (an agent that disrupts microfilaments). The neural folds in these embryos failed to converge about the DLHP, and these embryos consequently were dysraphic.[116] A failure of neural fold convergence about the DLHP region is also a common feature of many animal models of dysraphism (G. Schoenwolf, personal communication).

The third tenet of traditional dogma proposes that cell wedging is the result of changes in cytoskeletal components within the neuroepithelial cells. One example of this mechanism has already been described—neural plate thickening is brought about in part by elongation of paraxially oriented microtubules. Similarly, neural plate bending is thought to be due to cell wedging brought about by the contraction of *circumferentially oriented apical microfilaments.*

A large body of observational and experimental evidence suggests an important role for apical microfilaments in neural plate bending. Apical microfilaments are present in neuroepithelial cells of amphibians,[72, 117, 118] birds,[77, 118, 119] and mammals,[42, 83, 120] and are better seen during neural plate bending, suggesting a "sliding filament" action.[117] Actin and myosin are both localized to the apices of neuroepithelial cells,[121, 122] and the apical microfilaments bind heavy meromyosin,[119] a component of the actin-myosin complex. When embryos are treated with cytochalasins or vinblastine, agents known to disrupt microfilaments, neurulation often fails to occur.[73, 74, 77, 88, 123–134] Finally, calcium, a mediator of microfilament contraction, has been localized to coated vesicles in the apices of neuroepithelial cells,[135] and is released during neurulation;[136] papaverine, which inhibits calcium release, impairs neural plate bending, while the ionophore A23187, which enhances calcium release, promotes it.[137, 138]

However, agents used to disrupt microfilament action may adversely affect many other cellular processes;[133, 139–141] moreover, they may interfere with many non-neuroepithelial cells, which also contain microfilaments. In one study in which embryos were treated with cytochalasin D, neuroepithelial apical microfilaments were not demonstrable, yet two thirds of treated embryos underwent normal neurulation.[116] It is therefore unclear whether the effect of these agents on neurulation is due to a specific disruption of microfilament-mediated, neuroepithelial cell apical constriction.

An alternative (or perhaps complementary) mechanism whereby cells could become wedge-shaped is the expansion of the cell base.[6, 73, 142, 143] Burnside proposed that translocation of cytoplasm or subcellular organelles toward the base of the neuroepithelial cell could expand the base and result in cell wedging;[73] there is no evidence to support or refute this theory. More recent evidence in the chick suggests that changes in neuroepithelial cell shape are closely correlated with the position of the cell nucleus.[142] The nuclear position varies with the cell cycle (due to interkinetic nuclear migration); nuclei of cells in both the DNA-synthetic (S) and non—DNA-synthetic (non-S) phases of the cell cycle are located near the cell base, while those in the M (mitotic) phase are located more centrally.[144–146] During cell wedging, the nucleus is translocated toward the cell base; this translocation is associated with a prolongation of both the S and non-S phases of the cell cycle.[142] Moreover, this change in cell cycle appears to be induced, at least in the MHP, by the notochord. When an accessory notochord is transplanted beneath a more lateral region of the neuroepithelium, a second hingepoint develops over the accessory notochord;[115, 147] this second hingepoint exhibits a lower cell cycle time than the corresponding contralateral region.[147] The stimulus for DLHP formation is unknown. Although these findings are important, it is not known whether such changes in neuroepithelial cell cycle times are the *cause* or the *result* of changes in cell shape.

However intriguing, neither apical microfilament contraction nor changes in cell cycle time have been *proven* to drive changes in neuroepithelial cell shape. Other cellular mechanisms of potential importance in neuroepithelial cell wedging include the "cortical tractoring" of adjacent neuroepithelial cells as proposed by Jacobson and colleagues,[91] and interactions between adjacent neural fold and surface ectodermal cells at the point of divergence of the neural fold from cutaneous ectoderm as proposed by Martins-Green and colleagues.[93]

Neural Fold Fusion

Apposition and fusion of the converging neural folds is probably the least understood event in neurulation. The behavior of opposing neuroepithelial cells may involve molecule-molecule, molecule-cell, or cell-cell interactions.[148] At least three cellular mechanisms may contribute, alone or in combination, to neural fold fusion: (1) interactions of cell surface glycoproteins such as glycosaminoglycans (GAGs) and/or cell adhesion molecules (CAMs), (2) interdigitation of cell surface filopodia or "blebs," and (3) formation of intercellular junctions. All three of these processes may be involved at different times during neural fold fusion. Cell surface recognition may be the initial event that brings the neural folds into apposition. Interdigitating cell processes may aid further in establishing connections between opposing cell surfaces. Finally, intercellular junctions may serve to establish more permanent connections between adjacent neuroepithelial cells.[149]

Several lines of evidence suggest an important role for cell surface glycoproteins in neural fold fusion. A carbohydrate-rich "surface coat material," which stains readily with ruthinium red and lanthanum (which bind to polyvalent anions), and with HRP-labeled concanavalin A (which binds to terminal glycosyl and mannosyl residues), has been demonstrated on the neural folds of amphibian,[150] chick,[151] and mouse[152] embryos. This "surface coat material" is largely composed of *glycosaminoglycans* (GAGs)—complex glycoproteins that contain multiple carbohydrate residues. Both the temporal and spatial distribution of cell surface glycoproteins change during neurulation. The labeling of cell surface glycoproteins is scant in early neural groove stages, progressively increases as the neural folds elevate and converge, reaches a maximum just before neural fold fusion, and declines thereafter.[149] Labeling initially is present along the floor and walls of the neural plate, but moves dorsally during neural fold elevation and becomes restricted to the prospective fusion areas of the neural folds.[149] The character of GAGs on the neuroepithelial cell surface also changes during neurulation. Hyaluronic acid (HA) is the predominant GAG before neural fold fusion is complete, whereas chondroitin sulfate (CS) predominates following neural fold fusion.[149]

Several experimental observations suggest that these

cell surface glycoproteins participate in neural fold fusion. Exposing mouse embryos to phospholipase C, which removes surface-coat glycoproteins;[153] or treating rat embryos with heparatinase, which degrades heparan sulfate, or β-D-xyloside, which interferes with chondroitin synthesis;[100, 105] or exposing chick embryos to concanavalin A (Con A), which binds to carbohydrate residues and interferes with GAG function[154] all result in neural tube defects. Finally, GAG expression is defective in the splotch mouse (Sp/Sp) mutant; both HA and CS are present in approximately equal amounts in the open neural tube of affected animals, whereas HA predominates in the normal open neural tube and CS predominates in the normal closed neural tube.[149]

More recently, a 30-kilodalton (Kd) GAG has been discovered on mouse neuroepithelium during neural tube closure, and has been implicated in neural fold fusion. This glycoprotein binds with several exogenously administered carbohydrate binding lectins; the pattern of lectin binding suggests that this molecule is a complex N-linked glycoprotein containing an N-acetyllactosamine oligosaccharide chain structure.[155] Following the maternal administration of vitamin A, mouse embryos having open neural tube defects exhibit decreased binding of the 30-Kd glycoprotein to carbohydrate-binding lectins compared with littermates having closed neural tubes.[156] A similar decrease in lectin binding of the 30-Kd glycoprotein occurs in the delayed splotch mouse mutant (Spd/Spd); binding in the dysraphic regions of the neural tube is decreased compared with closed regions of the neural tube of Spd/Spd mutants or with neural tubes of control mice.[155]

The second cellular mechanism that may contribute to neural fold fusion is the interaction of cell membrane processes. Variably described as filopodia, "ruffles," and "blebs," these processes have been described on the luminal surfaces of neuroepithelial cells in amphibian,[157] chick,[158–160] and mammalian[161, 162] embryos. Like cell surface glycoproteins, these processes become more prominent throughout neurulation, reach a peak at about the time of neural fold fusion, and decline thereafter; they are most conspicuous on the luminal surfaces of the converging neural folds.[157, 162] The temporal appearance and spatial distribution of these filopodia suggest a role in neural fold fusion, either by aligning the converging neural folds or by drawing the apposed surfaces together.[157, 158]

Eventually, intercellular connections are established between neuroepithelial cells of the apposed neural folds.[163–165] Neither the nature of these junctions (tight or gap) nor their function (cell adhesion, intercellular communication) are known with certainty. Much more work is needed to elucidate the roles of these intercellular junctions, as well as the importance of cell surface glycoproteins and filopodia, in promoting and maintaining neural fold fusion.

The forces underlying secondary neurulation are even less well understood than those underlying primary neurulation. In the chick, the outer cells of the medullary cord elongate during secondary neurulation to become columnar cells; these shape changes rely at least in part upon microtubules, as do those that occur during primary neurulation.[81] The forces that drive cavitation to form secondary lumina are not understood; however, at least in the chick, cavitation appears not to rely upon hydrostatic pressure from the lumen of the primary neural tube, since these secondary lumina form without a direct connection with the lumen of the primary neural tube.[64] Moreover, when closure of the caudal neuropore is prevented in the chick, the hydrostatic pressure from the primary neural tube lumen is negated, yet secondary neurulation occurs normally.[166]

ABNORMAL EARLY NEURAL DEVELOPMENT

A large number of human neural malformations have been ascribed to disorders of early neural embryogenesis (Table 1–2). Many theories have been proposed to explain the origin of these various anomalies; it is important to recognize that all of these theories are speculative, as none of them have been validated experimentally. We have grouped the malformations according to the proposed embryopathic mechanism(s). We begin with a discussion of the open neural tube defects (myelomeningoceles and anencephaly) and follow with a discussion of the occult dysraphic malformations.

FAILURE OF NEURAL TUBE CLOSURE—NEURAL TUBE DEFECTS (NTD)

At present, two major theories have been proposed to explain the open neural tube defects of myelomeningocele and anencephaly. The "nonclosure theory," elaborated in 1886 by von Recklinghausen,[167] proposes that neural tube defects are the result of a primary failure of the neural tube to close. The "overdistention theory," introduced in 1769 by Morgagni[168] and more recently popularized by Gardner,[169–172] proposes that neural tube defects are the result of overdistention and

TABLE 1–2. HUMAN DYSRAPHIC CENTRAL NERVOUS SYSTEM MALFORMATIONS

Open Dysraphic Malformations (Spina bifida aperta)
  Anencephaly
  Myelomeningoceles
  Hemimyelomeningoceles
  Cervical myelomeningoceles
  Combined (anterior and posterior) spina bifida
Closed Dysraphic Malformations (Spina bifida clausus)
  Lipomyelomeningoceles
  Dermal sinus tract, dermoid/epidermoid tumors
  Myelocystoceles
  Split cord malformations
  Neurenteric cysts
  Thickened filum terminale
  Caudal agenesis syndrome
  "Complex dysraphic malformations"
  Encephaloceles

rupture of a previously closed neural tube, perhaps due to hydrodynamic forces driven by production of a proteinaceous "neural tube fluid."

Since its introduction, the "nonclosure theory" has gained almost universal acceptance, whereas the "overdistention theory" has been virtually discarded. The "nonclosure theory" is consistent with observations of early human embryos in which neural tube defects have been described during or shortly after neural tube closure, and with most animal models of dysraphism, which display a primary defect in neural tube closure. However, overdistention cannot be excluded as a cause of some neural tube defects.[173]

The nature of the disorder that results in a failure of neural tube closure is a matter of speculation. As we have seen, neural tube closure is dependent, at least in part, on a variety of embryonic processes; a disruption in any of these processes will, in certain instances, result in a failure of neurulation. However, while experimental manipulations (reviewed by Schoenwolf[6]) and dysraphic animal models (reviewed by Campbell[2]) have suggested a number of possible mechanisms whereby neural tube defects might arise, the cause of *human* malformations remains elusive. Neural tube defects are most likely etiologically heterogeneous[2] and represent the end result of a variety of embryonic disorders.

The nature and severity of the resultant malformations are determined by both the location and the length of the un-neurulated segment. A failure of cranial neurulation results in anencephaly, whereas failure of more caudal neurulation produces a myelomeningocele. The term *myelomeningocele* has referred to an open caudal neural tube in association with a fluid-filled sac, whereas *myeloschisis* has been defined as a completely open caudal neural tube having no evidence of a central canal[174] or investing meninges.[175] However, we find this classification to be confusing and imprecise. In both cases, a portion of the neural tube has failed to close, the neural folds remain attached to the adjacent cutaneous ectoderm, and some portion of the neural plate (the placode) is therefore exposed on the dorsal surface of the embryo (Fig. 1–13). Because the exposed placode remains attached to the cutaneous ectoderm, cerebrospinal fluid (CSF) can form only in the subarachnoid space beneath the placode. We feel that the extent to which the CSF displaces the placode dorsally determines the type of resultant malformation. In the case of the myelomeningocele, the accumulation of CSF displaces the neural placode to the top of a fluid-filled sac (Fig. 1–13A). In the case of myeloschisis, CSF does not accumulate beneath the placode (perhaps because it is vented instead through the central canal or through a tear in the attenuated surrounding tissues); the placode in this instance lies flat on the dorsal surface (Fig. 1–13B). These two malformations therefore reflect differences, not in their origin, but only in subsequent development. We therefore suggest that the term myeloschisis be discarded and all such lesions be referred to as myelomeningoceles.

Whereas myelomeningoceles are most frequently the result of a failure of neural tube closure, meningoceles

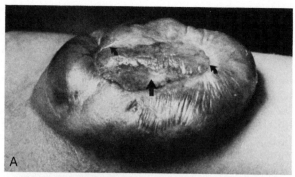

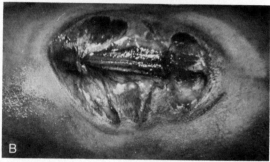

FIGURE 1–13. Human neural tube defects. *A*, Lumbosacral myelomeningocele in a newborn infant. The placode *(straight arrow)* has been pushed dorsally by the underlying cerebrospinal fluid (CSF) and sits atop a small CSF-containing sac; the placode is attached circumferentially *(curved arrows)* to the adjacent surface ectoderm. *B*, Thoracolumbar "myeloschisis" in an infant. The open placode, much larger in this infant, is not displaced by underlying CSF, which has been vented either through the central canal or through small tears in the adjacent tissues, and lies flush with, but still attached to, the adjacent surface ectoderm. (From McLone DG, Dias MS: Complications of myelomeningocele closure. Pediatr Neurosurg 17:267, 1991–92.)

are thought to be the products of a *postneurulation* disorder. In these malformations, both neurulation and dysjunction of the cutaneous ectoderm have occurred normally; the neural tube therefore is normally formed beneath the cutaneous lesion. However, the subsequent development of the overlying mesenchymal tissues and cutaneous ectoderm is aberrant and results in a cutaneous and mesenchymal defect which contains only CSF. The embryogenesis of meningoceles is unclear.

Anomalies Resulting from Incomplete Dysjunction—Dermal Sinus, Dermoid and Epidermoid Tumors

Dermal sinuses incorporate a tract of cutaneous ectoderm from the dorsal midline skin, which extends for a variable distance into the underlying mesenchymal tissues and, in many instances, penetrates the dura to end within the thecal sac adjacent to, or contiguous with, the neural tube. Approximately 60 per cent of dermal sinuses incorporate or end in a dermoid or epidermoid tumor; conversely, approximately 30 per cent of dermoid and epidermoid tumors occur in association with dermal sinus tracts.[176, 177] Cutaneous anomalies are frequently present and include skin dimples, hairy patches, and cutaneous nevi or hemangiomas.

The most widely accepted theory regarding the embryogenesis of dermal sinus tracts and related anomalies proposes that they arise through a faulty separation of neuroectoderm from the overlying cutaneous ectoderm at the time of dysjunction.[178] As a result, a tongue of cutaneous ectoderm becomes sequestered between the dorsal ectodermal surface and the neural tube. Differentiation of this tract may produce a number of cutaneous ectodermal abnormalities including epithelium-lined sinuses (dermal sinus tracts), epidermoid tumors (containing only ectodermal tissue as pseudostratified squamous epithelium), or dermoid tumors (containing both ectodermal tissue and associated mesodermal structures such as sebaceous glands and hair follicles) located anywhere between the skin and neural tube.

Dermal sinuses may involve any level of the neuraxis; a predilection for the lumbosacral region at the site of the caudal neuropore, and for the frontonasal region at the site of the anterior neuropore, underscores the complex nature underlying closure of these two areas of the neural tube. Lumbosacral dermal sinuses arise in the dorsal midline skin cranial to the intergluteal cleft (Fig. 1–14A) and traverse the underlying mesenchyme to a variable degree (Fig. 15A). Some end blindly within the soft tissues superficial to the underlying laminae. Most penetrate the vertebral canal (usually between the laminae of two adjacent vertebrae, or between bifid laminae) and enter the dura immediately beneath, or just caudal to, the cutaneous lesion (Fig. 1–15B); from this point, they extend cephalad to a variable degree, ending as high as the conus medullaris. Associated dermoid or epidermoid tumors, composed of desquamated keratinized debris and, variably, other mesodermal tissues, may accompany the dermal sinus tract and may be found anywhere along its length (Fig. 1–15B).

It is important to distinguish between the sacral der-

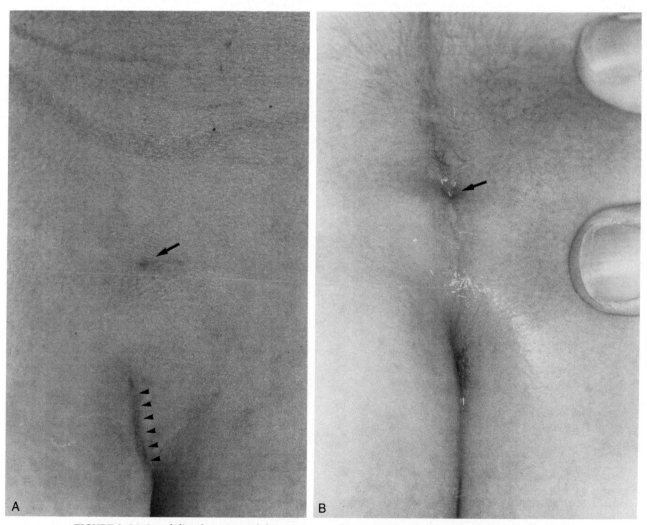

FIGURE 1–14. Sacral dimples. *A,* Sacral dermal sinus tract in a newborn infant. The tract *(arrow)* is located well above the gluteal crease. The upper end of the gluteal crease is abnormally deflected toward the left *(arrowheads).* *B,* An innocent coccygeal dimple in a newborn infant. The gluteal folds have been pulled apart to reveal this small dimple within the folds of the gluteal cleft, overlying the coccyx. Note that the gluteal cleft is normally positioned in the midline.

mal sinus and the innocent coccygeal dimple. Dermal sinuses usually are larger, more complex cutaneous anomalies having uneven margins and associated skin dimples, hemangiomas, or tufts of hair; the intergluteal cleft is often abnormal as well. Most importantly, dermal sinuses almost always lie cranial to the intergluteal cleft (Fig. 1–14A). In contrast, coccygeal dimples usually are simple blind sinuses, have no associated cutaneous abnormalities, and are located more caudally within the intergluteal cleft (Fig. 1–14B). Dermal sinuses are pathologic anomalies that often cause spinal cord tethering and require surgical treatment. In contrast, coccygeal dimples are thought to be vestiges of the primitive pit and cells of the surrounding caudal cell mass and are of no clinical consequence.

Cranial dermal sinuses most commonly involve either the frontobasal skull or the occipital squama, locations that are also frequent sites for encephaloceles.[179, 180] However, it is important to emphasize that although many authors have suggested that cranial dermal sinus anomalies (dermal sinuses, dermoid/epidermoid tumors, and "nasal gliomas"—small sequestered neuroglial masses located along nasal dermal sinus tracts) and encephaloceles share a common em-

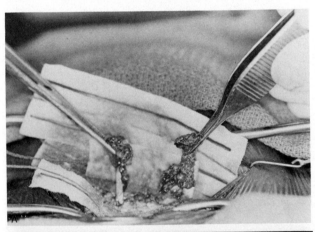

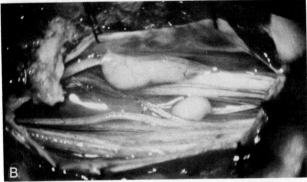

FIGURE 1–15. Lumbosacral dermal sinus tracts. *A,* Two separate dermal sinus tracts in a child with two sacral dimples; each extended down to the underlying dural sac. *B,* Associated dermoid tumors located within the dural sac, adjacent to the cauda equina, in another patient with a sacral dimple and a dermal sinus tract. (From McLone DG, Naidich TP: The tethered spinal cord. *In* McLaurin RL, Schut L, Venes JL, Epstein F [eds]: Pediatric Neurosurgery. 2nd ed. Philadelphia, WB Saunders Co, 1989.)

bryonic origin, several lines of evidence suggest otherwise: (1) encephaloceles usually contain differentiated neural (basifrontal or occipital cortex, cerebellum, and brainstem) and mesenchymal (choroid plexus, pia-arachnoid) tissues,[180, 181] whereas heterotopic "nasal gliomas" along frontobasal dermal sinus tracts are composed of only disorganized neuroglial tissue;[182] (2) the neural tissue within encephaloceles most commonly takes origin from the frontobasal or occipital cortex; in many instances, elements of *both* frontal and occipital lobes are present and suggest a disorder that occurred *after* the division of the telencephalon; in contrast, the intracranial origin of frontobasal dermal sinus tracts is from the region of the lamina terminalis and commissural plate,[183] the site of the anterior neuropore; (3) frontobasal encephaloceles are common among Asian populations,[180] whereas frontobasal dermal sinuses, dermoids, and nasal gliomas are not. As discussed below, encephaloceles are now thought by most to be the result of a *postneurulation* disorder of the cephalic mesenchyme[179, 184, 185] and, we feel, are therefore pathogenetically distinct from frontonasal dermal sinuses and related malformations.

The embryogenesis and surgical anatomy of frontonasal dermal sinuses are predicted by the normal development of the anterior cranial base (Fig. 1–16). The prosencephalic primordium, olfactory epithelium, adenohypophysis, and facial cutaneous ectoderm all share a common embryonic origin (at least in avian embryos) from the region of the anterior neuropore.[186, 187] The frontal bones later develop from bilaterally paired mesenchymal anlagen and are separated by the metopic suture. Simultaneously, nasal bones develop along the nasal spine and are separated from the frontal bones by a fibrous capsule, the *fonticulus nasofrontalis.* The nasal spine is separated from the deeper nasal cartilaginous capsule by the *prenasal space.* During normal embryogenesis, a tongue of dura extends ventrally from the inferior aspect of the anterior cranial fossa and is interposed anteriorly between the frontal and nasal bones at the fonticulus nasofrontalis and inferiorly between the prenasal cartilage and the nasal bones within the prenasal space. During normal development, this dural reflection becomes surrounded by ossifying bone and regresses; remnants of the tract persist as the *foramen cecum* along the floor of the anterior cranial fossa, between the insertion of the falx cerebri anteriorly and the crista galli posteriorly.[188]

The nasal dermal sinus tract arises from the anterior neuropore at the commissural plate and connects the cranial neural tube with the midline nasal skin. Subsequent development, around the tract, of the craniofacial structures described above gives rise to the characteristic course of the nasal dermal sinus (Fig. 1–16D), which passes along the floor of the anterior fossa through the prospective foramen cecum and extends either through the fonticulus nasofrontalis to present at the glabella (Fig. 1–17A) or, to a variable degree, within the prenasal space to present anywhere along the bridge of the nose (Fig. 1–17B). The tract may end extracranially, having no intracranial component, or it

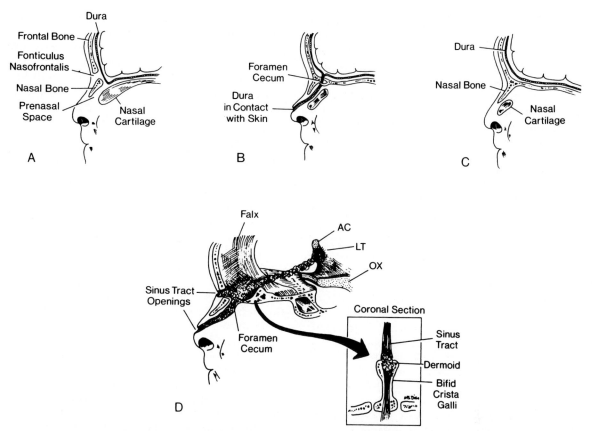

FIGURE 1–16. Normal frontonasal development (*A–C*) and the embryology of frontonasal dermal sinus tracts (*D*). *A,* During normal embryogenesis, the fonticulus nasofrontalis forms between the frontal and nasal bones; the prenasal space forms between the nasal bone and nasal cartilage. *B,* A tongue of dura extends through the foramen cecum toward the midline nasal skin. *C,* Later, this tongue of dura is obliterated and the anterior cranial base is formed; the foramen cecum remains as a vestige of this embryonic tract. *D,* Abnormal dysjunction during closure of the anterior neuropore leaves a tract of cutaneous ectoderm between the commissural plate and the midline nasal skin. Formation of the anterior frontobasal structures results in a tract whose cutaneous opening may be located at the fonticulus naso-frontalis or anywhere along the dorsum of the nose, and which extends through the foramen cecum, between the two halves of a bifid crista galli, and along the anterior cranial base; in rare instances, the tract extends all the way to the commissural plate. (Adapted from Sessions RB: Nasal dermal sinuses: new concepts and explanations. Laryngoscope 92[Suppl 29]:1, 1982.)

FIGURE 1–17. Nasal dermal sinus tracts. *A,* Dermal sinus tract in an infant, opening onto the nasion at the site of the fonticulus naso-frontalis. *B,* Dermal sinus tract extending to the nasal tip.

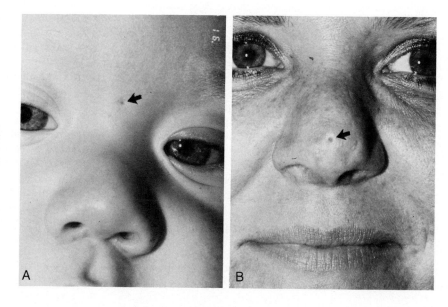

may extend intracranially to a variable degree in close association with the foramen cecum, anterior cranial base, and/or the anterior commissure and lamina terminalis (Fig. 1–16D). Associated dermoid tumors may occur anywhere along the dermal sinus tract and involve extra- or intracranial sites.[183, 188–192] Finally, sequestered neuroepithelium within the prenasal space may develop independently into a mass of neuroglial tissue, the nasal cerebral heterotopia or "nasal glioma."[182, 193, 194]

Dermal sinuses occasionally occupy the posterior parietal region. These lesions arise in the region of the quadrigeminal cistern in close proximity to the posterior and habenular commissures, pass posterior to the splenium of the corpus callosum, and extend dorsally between the cerebral hemispheres within the leaves of the falx cerebri to end in the parietal midline, occasionally fenestrating the superior sagittal sinus. Between the parietal region and the fonticulus nasofrontalis, midline dermal sinuses with intracranial extension have not been described. This distribution is predicted by the embryology of the anterior neuropore, the locus of the prospective commissural plate. We postulate that dermal sinuses arising from the region of the commissural plate (the cranial neuropore) may have one of two fates. If the disorder involves the cranial rim of the anterior neuropore, the tract remains anteriorly placed and in close relationship to the floor of the anterior cranial fossa. If, on the other hand, the disorder involves the caudal lip of the anterior neuropore (that is, at the caudal margin of the future commissural plate), it will be swept posteriorly by the explosive growth of the telencephalic vesicles and the associated posterior growth of the corpus callosum, and will arise at the opposite end of the commissural plate, posterior to the splenium and adjacent to the posterior and habenular commissures.

Finally, dermal sinuses also are relatively common in the occipital region,[195, 196] where they typically arise from either the roof of the fourth ventricle, the cerebellar vermis, or the subdural space posterior to the cerebellum; penetrate the dura below the tentorium; and end in the occipital skin. These occipital lesions do *not* involve the anterior neuropore, as has been suggested, but rather involve the *rhombencephalic* neural tube. Why dermal sinuses have a predilection for this region of the neuraxis is unclear. The rhombencephalon in humans is among the first regions of the neural tube to undergo neural fold fusion and may therefore be particularly vulnerable to disorders of neurulation; in addition, the presence of the pontine flexure may lend additional stress to the neural tube at this site. Finally, the frequent occurence of dermal sinuses may simply reflect the relatively large size of this region of the neural tube at the time of neurulation.

ANOMALIES RESULTING FROM PREMATURE DYSJUNCTION—SPINAL LIPOMAS

Spinal lipomas are perhaps the most frequent occult dysraphic malformations and most frequently involve the lumbosacral spinal cord, conus medullaris, and filum terminale. Some lipomas lie exclusively within the thecal sac in association with the conus medullaris but without an associated dural defect (Fig. 1–18B). More frequently, these lesions occupy both intradural and extradural sites (Fig. 1–18C);[197–200] in these, a subcutaneous mass (Fig. 1–18A) is contiguous, between bifid laminae and a dural defect, with the thecal space and the caudal spinal cord.

The spinal cord in the region of the lipoma is dorsally dysraphic; the lipoma arises from within this area of dysraphism, occupying the central canal of the terminal cord and occasionally extending cephalad within the central canal to a variable degree. Ventrolateral to the lipoma are located the displaced neural folds, from which the dorsal nerve roots emerge (Fig. 1–18C). This last point is critical to understanding the surgical anatomy of these lesions.

The commonly held belief is that lipomas also arise through a disorder of dysjunction.[201, 202] In contrast to the dermal sinus tract, in which the cutaneous ectoderm *incompletely* separates from the neural tube, lipomas are thought to arise when the cutaneous ectoderm *prematurely* separates from the neuroepithelium prior to neural fold fusion (Fig. 1–19). Under these circumstances, the surrounding mesenchyme ingresses between the neural tube and overlying cutaneous ectoderm and gains access to the ependymal surface of the developing neural tube. Whereas mesenchyme adjacent to the outer (basal) surface of the neural tube is normally induced to form dura, the fate of the anomalous mesenchyme within the central canal may instead be redirected to form fat.[201]

While some lipomas may be the result of disordered primary neurulation, others, particularly terminal lipomas involving the filum terminale and myelocystoceles containing lipomatous elements, represent disorders of secondary neurulation.[174, 201] As such, these malformations are most likely to take origin from an abnormality of the caudal cell mass. In support of this concept, the character of terminal lipomas differs from that of more cranially located malformations. Whereas the more cranial lipomas discussed above usually contain only fat cells, terminal lipomas, as belies their origin from the caudal cell mass, more frequently contain striated muscle and other disparate tissue types.[201] The nature of the underlying disorder of secondary neurulation that results in terminal lipomas is unknown at present.

ANOMALIES RESULTING FROM DISORDERS OF GASTRULATION—COMBINED SPINA BIFIDA, SPLIT CORD MALFORMATIONS, NEURENTERIC CYSTS

A number of seemingly unrelated disorders, including combined (anterior and posterior) spina bifida, split cord malformations, neurenteric cysts and certain other intestinal anomalies, and a number of other *complex dysraphic malformations* exhibiting disorders of all three primary germ layers, are all thought to have a common embryogenesis, variously described as the "split noto-

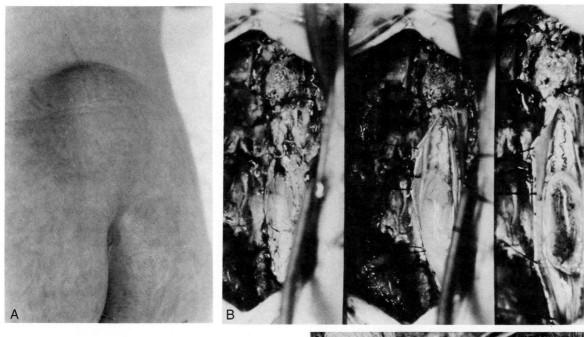

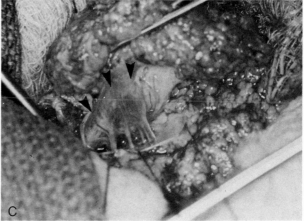

FIGURE 1–18. Spinal lipomas. *A,* Photograph of the back and buttocks of an infant with an obvious spinal lipoma. *B,* Operative photograph of a completely intradural lipoma: *left,* the lipoma can be seen through the thinned but intact dura; *center,* the dura has been opened and the lipoma arises from the dorsal cord; *right,* the lipoma has been removed. (From McLone DG, Naidich TP: The tethered spinal cord. *In* McLaurin RL, Schut L, Venes JL, Epstein F [eds]: Pediatric Neurosurgery, 2nd ed. Philadelphia, WB Saunders Co, 1989.) *C,* Operative photograph of a lipoma with both intra- and extradural components. The lipoma arises from the dorsal surface of the spinal cord, between the neural folds and (therefore) medial to the dorsal root entry zones *(arrowheads).*

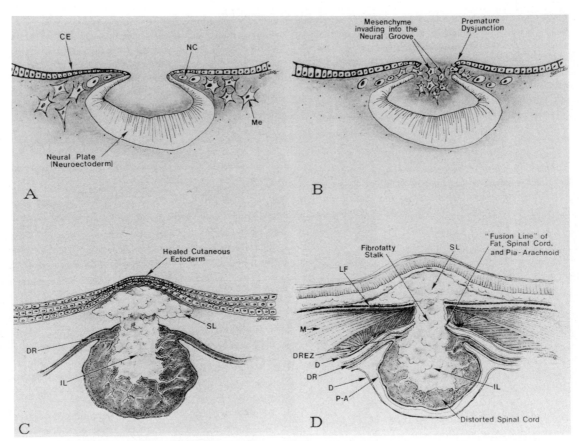

FIGURE 1–19. Embryogenesis of spinal lipomas. *A,* Neural plate during latter stages of neurulation. *B,* Premature dysjunction allows adjacent mesenchyme (Me) to ingress into the central canal of the neural tube. *C,* The ingressing mesenchymal cells are induced to form fibrofatty tissue, whereas extramedullary mesenchymal cells are induced to form pia-arachnoid (P-A). The cutaneous ectoderm is intact overlying the malformation. *D,* Dorsal roots (DR) and dorsal root ganglia arise from neural crest cells (derived from the neural folds) and are located immediately lateral to the fibrofatty mass. The pia-arachnoid (P-A) surrounds the neural tube except where the fatty mass fuses with the adjacent neural folds (the "fusion line"). CE = cutaneous ectoderm; NC = neural crest; SL = subcutaneous lipoma; IL = intramedullary lipoma; DREZ = dorsal root entry zone; D = dura; M = paraspinous muscles. (From Pang D: Tethered cord syndrome. *In* Neurosurgery: State of the Art Reviews. Philadelphia, Hanley & Belfus, 1986, vol 1, pp 45–79.

chord syndrome,"[203] the "endodermal-ectodermal adhesion syndrome";[204] or the "accessory neurenteric canal syndrome."[205] The common element in many of these anomalies is a split cord malformation that involves some portion of the neuraxis.

Split cord malformations (SCM) may occur either in association with open neural tube defects or, more commonly, as occult malformations developing either in isolation or in conjunction with other associated anomalies. Early classification schemes have done little to foster our understanding of the embryogenesis of these lesions. Hertwig first used the term "diastematomyelia" (from the Greek "diastema" meaning cleft and "melos" meaning medulla) to describe malformations in which the spinal cord is "split" into two "hemicords," each containing only a *single* set of dorsal and ventral nerve roots. In contrast, Herren and Edwards introduced the term "diplomyelia" to describe a complete *duplication* of the spinal cord with each side containing *two* sets of ventral and dorsal nerve roots.[206–208]

The confusion has been further compounded by dividing these malformations according to the composition of their dural coverings or by the presence or absence of tethering midline structures. Each of the "hemicords" in diastematomyelia lies within its own dural sheath (Fig. 1–20A), whereas both of the duplicated spinal cords in diplomyelia are thought to be contained within a common, single dural sheath (Fig. 1–21A). Midline bony, cartilaginous, or fibrous spurs are present between the two "hemicords" in diastematomyelia (Fig. 1–20A), whereas no such midline structures are thought to be present in diplomyelia. Thus, the widespread belief is that diastematomyelia involves a splitting of the spinal cord into two half-cords lying within two separate dural sheaths and separated by an osseous or fibrocartilaginous tethering spur; in contrast, diplomyelia is thought to involve a true spinal cord duplication within a common dural tube, with no interposed mesenchymal tissue.[206, 207]

However, several observations suggest a common

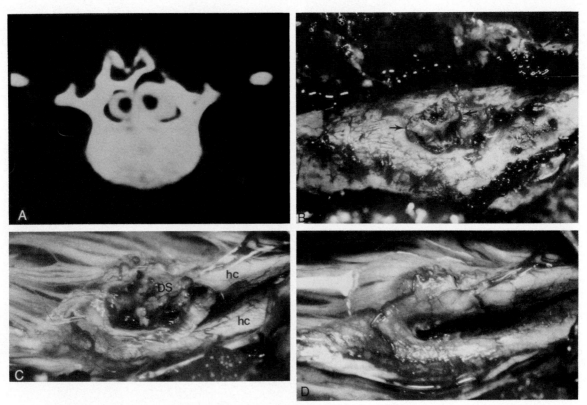

FIGURE 1–20. Diastematomyelia (type I split cord malformation). *A,* Axial view of a metrizamide CT myelogram shows two "hemicords" separated by a thick, midline bony spur. Each "hemicord" is contained within its own separate dural sheath. *B,* Operative photograph of a patient with a type I split cord malformation, before opening the dura. The bony spur *(arrows)* transfixes the two "hemicords" between the two dural sheaths. *C,* Same patient, after opening the dura. After the bony spur has been removed, the surrounding dural sleeve (DS) is tightly wedged between the two "hemicords" at the site of caudal reunion. *D,* After resection of the median dural sleeve, the two "hemicords" lie freely without tethering. (*B, C,* and *D* from Pang D: Split cord malformation. Part II: Clinical syndrome. Neurosurgery 31:481, 1992.)

embryonic origin for these two malformations. James and Lassman's original description of diastematomyelia includes 11 cases of "single dural tube" malformations; midline fibrous "bands," analogous to the bony spurs of the double dural tube malformations, were described in at least eight of these malformations.[209] These "bands" have also been reported by Pang and colleagues (Fig. 1–21B). The bands originate in the cleft between the two "hemicords" and traverse the subarachnoid space to end more caudally on the dura; they are composed of tough, fibrous connective tissue, prominent blood vessels, and dystrophic median nerve roots that originate from one or both of the "hemicords."[210]

Just as the single dural tube malformations of diastematomyelia may have midline fibrous bands, so too can diplomyelia have double dural sheaths and osseous or fibrocartilaginous spurs. Herren and Edwards described several cases of "diplomyelia" with such midline spurs, and both double and single dural tube malformations were described with approximately equal frequency.[207]

Finally, dystrophic median nerve roots projecting from one or both "hemicords" have been described in both diastematomyelia and diplomyelia (Fig. 1–21C);[207, 209–212] these dystrophic roots originate from one

or both "hemicords" and insert onto the midline osseous spurs or fibrous "bands." Both dorsal and ventral roots, as well as ganglion cells, have been described (Fig. 1–21B and C).[210, 212] The presence of both lateral and median sets of nerve roots arising from each "hemicord" strongly suggests the presence of at least a partial spinal cord duplication in both malformations.* Moreover, close examination of illustrations of the "hemicords" from published examples of both diastematomyelia and diplomyelia demonstrate neither absolute splitting nor complete duplication of the cord in any instance. Rather, the "hemicords" are *incomplete duplications*, with relatively well preserved lateral halves and dystrophic medial halves (Fig. 1–22).[206, 207, 212–214]

These observations suggest that diastematomyelia and diplomyelia represent different ends of a spectrum

---

*Alternatively, it could be argued that median dorsal nerve roots arise through aberrant migration of neural crest cells from the lateral half of a split cord; similarly, ventral roots could arise through redirection of motoneuron axons from the ventral horn of the lateral half of a split cord. This issue could be resolved with postmortem examinations of diastematomyelia spinal cords using lipophilic fluorescent markers such as DiI, which insert into the cell membrane and are therefore capable of labeling axons even after death.

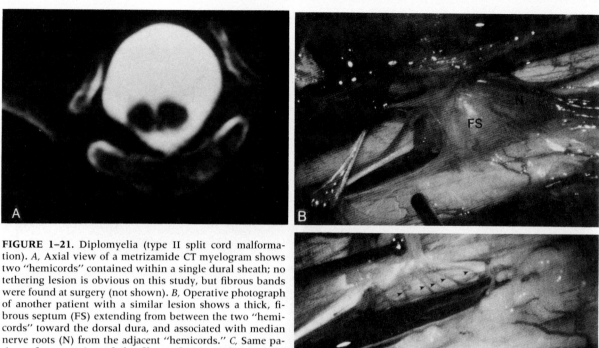

FIGURE 1–21. Diplomyelia (type II split cord malformation). *A,* Axial view of a metrizamide CT myelogram shows two "hemicords" contained within a single dural sheath; no tethering lesion is obvious on this study, but fibrous bands were found at surgery (not shown). *B,* Operative photograph of another patient with a similar lesion shows a thick, fibrous septum (FS) extending from between the two "hemicords" toward the dorsal dura, and associated with median nerve roots (N) from the adjacent "hemicords." *C,* Same patient after resection of the fibrous band; median ventral nerve rootlets *(arrowheads)* travel dorsally from the ventral surface of the left "hemicord" and coalesce (at the ball dissector) to join the median septum. (*B* and *C,* from Pang D, Dias MS, Ahab-Barmada M: Split cord malformation. Part I: A unified theory of embryogenesis for double cord malformations. Neurosurgery 31:451, 1992.)

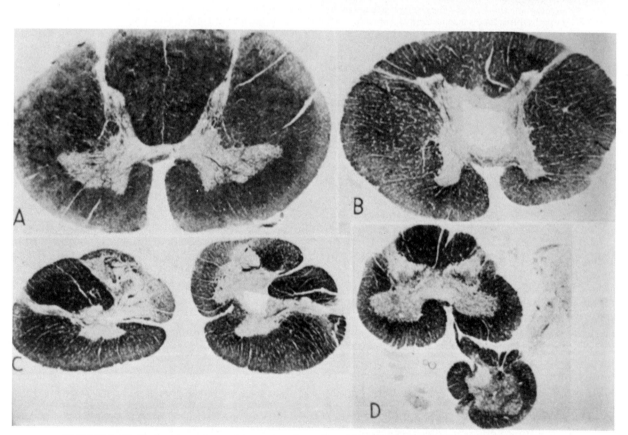

FIGURE 1–22. Postmortem photomicrographs of a split cord malformation. The two "hemicords" in *C* represent incomplete duplications, with each "hemicord" containing a relatively well-preserved lateral half and a dystrophic medial half. (From Herren RY, Edwards JE: Diplomyelia (duplication of the spinal cord). Arch Pathol 30:1203, 1940.)

of SCMs having a common embryonic mechanism (Fig. 1–23). SCMs are seen in association with a variety of anomalies, including combined (anterior and posterior) spina bifida (Fig. 1–24); hemimyelomeningoceles; myelomeningoceles (occurring in up to one third of cases at autopsy); cervical myelomeningoceles; neurenteric cysts; some examples of the Klippel-Feil anomaly, iniencephaly, and caudal agenesis; and certain intestinal duplications and diverticula. All of these *complex dysraphic malformations* have in common stereotypical anomalies involving tissues derived from all three primary germ layers and are thought to share a common embryonic origin.[172, 215] Four theories have attempted to explain the underlying embryopathy:

Theory 1. Beardmore and Wigglesworth proposed that prior to or during notochordal outgrowth, an adhesion could develop between the epiblast and hypoblast.[216] This "endodermal-ectodermal adhesion" would provide a barrier to subsequent notochordal elongation and result in a splitting of the notochord around the adhesion; independent development of paired neuroepithelial anlagen would then form two "hemicords." Associated remnants of the adhesion could give rise to endodermal remnants located anywhere between the gut and cutaneous ectoderm. This mechanism could work only if the notochord extends cranially from Hensen's node; if, on the other hand, the notochord grows by addition of cells to its caudal end during Hensen's node regression, an adhesion of this type would not provide a barrier to notochordal outgrowth. Prop and associates have consequently modified this theory by postulating an adhesion within the primitive streak caudal to Hensen's node, around which the notochord might be split during node regression.[204]

Theory 2. Bremer studied patients with combined spina bifida (or the "split notochord syndrome"),[205] which is characterized by an open neural tube defect and widespread underlying vertebral anomalies. The involved vertebrae are split midsagittally to form two

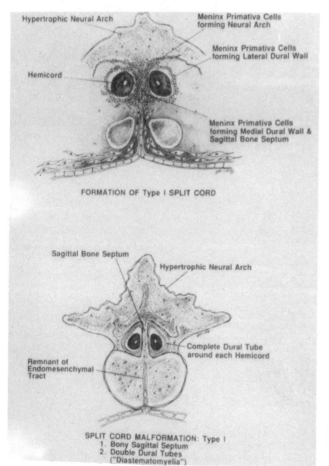

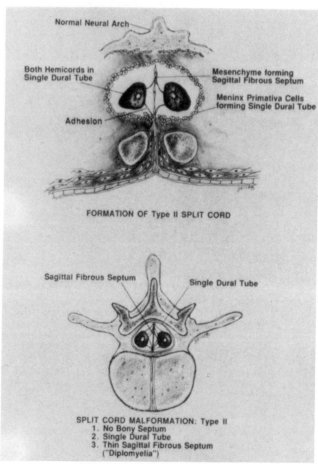

FIGURE 1–23. Embryogenesis of split cord malformations. *Left,* A type I malformation (diastematomyelia) in which the midline mesenchymal tract forms a median bony spur between the two "hemicords"; the surrounding meninx primitiva is induced to form two separate dural sheaths, each of which surrounds one of the two "hemicords". *Right,* A type II malformation (diplomyelia) in which the mesenchymal tract is thinner and more delicate, forming only a fibrous midline septum, which bisects and is frequently adherent to the medial aspect of the two "hemicords." The meninx primitiva is induced to form a single dural sheath, within which are contained both "hemicords." (From Pang D, Dias MS, Ahab-Barmada M: Split cord malformation. Part I: A unified theory of embryogenesis for double cord malformations. Neurosurgery 31:451, 1992.)

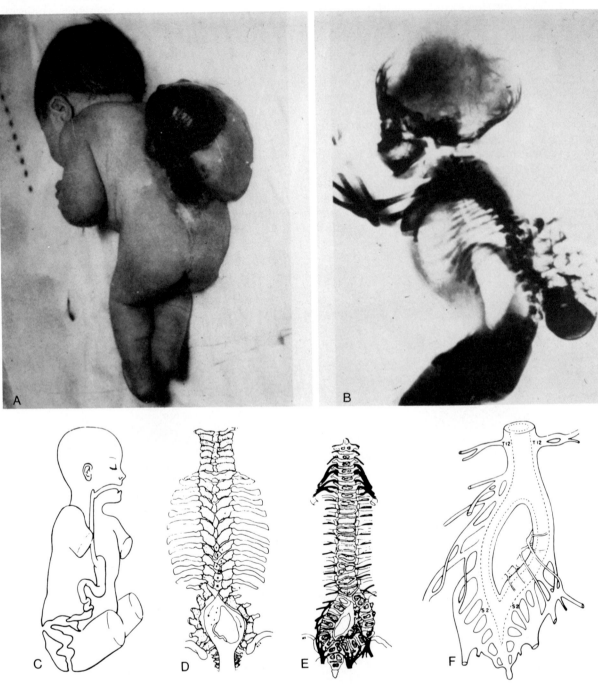

FIGURE 1–24. Combined (anterior and posterior) spina bifida (the "split notochord syndrome"). *A,* Infant with a large mass arising from the thoracolumbar spine. *B,* Radiograph of same infant shows bowel loops within the sac. (From Dénes J, Honti J, Léb J: Dorsal herniation of the gut: a rare manifestation of the split notochord syndrome. J Pediatr Surg 2:359, 1967.) *C,* Schematic of a similar malformation in another child shows communication between bowel and the dorsal surface. *D, E,* and *F,* Diagrams show widely split bony vertebral (*D, E*) and spinal cord (*F*) elements around a central cleft, through which the loops of bowel were extruded. (From Saunders RL: Combined anterior and posterior spina bifida in a living neonatal human female. Anat Rec 87:255, 1943.)

laterally displaced "hemivertebral" columns, which surround a central cleft (Fig. 1–24). This cleft connects the dorsum with the peritoneal cavity; through the cleft passes a variable amount of endodermal tissue (ranging from a neurenteric cyst to entire loops of bowel). The intra-abdominal intestine also may contain variable duplications or diverticula. In virtually every instance an associated SCM is present, with the two "hemicords" surrounding the central cleft. Associated visceral malformations are exceedingly common.[216, 217]

Bremer noted the similarities between the central cleft in combined spina bifida and the neurenteric canal of normal embryos. However, the two entities differ in that the dorsal opening of the neurenteric canal is the primitive pit that ultimately comes to occupy a coccygeal level, whereas combined spina bifida (and other variants of SCMs) arise at more cranial levels of the neuraxis. Bremer proposed that such malformations arise through the formation of an "accessory neurenteric canal" caused by a dorsal herniation of endoderm that splits the notochord and neuroepithelium. However, the impetus for such a dorsal herniation is unknown.

Theory 3. McLetchie[218] and Saunders[219] suggested that duplication of the notochord is the initial abnormality and is followed by a secondary endodermal-ectodermal interaction between the duplicated notochords. Dodds suggested that during normal embryogenesis, bilaterally paired prospective notochordal cell anlagen are integrated into a single midline structure during primitive streak regression.[220] Feller and Sternberg proposed that abnormal rests of undifferentiated cells in Hensen's node might interfere with proper midline integration and result in paired notochords;[221] subsequent differentiation of these cell rests could give rise to a variety of midline anomalies comprising tissues derived from any of the three primary germ cell layers.

Theory 4. Dias and Walker have recently proposed that these complex dysraphic malformations arise during a time when prospective anlagen from all three germ layers are in intimate association—that is, while they are being laid down during *gastrulation*.[215] The events of this model are contrasted with those of normal development in Figure 1–25. During normal development, paired notochordal anlagen are integrated to form a single notochordal process; in contrast, during the formation of complex dysraphic malformations, these notochordal precursors remain separate and develop independently over a variable portion of their length. Similarly, during normal development, bilaterally paired prospective neuroepithelial cells flanking both sides of the primitive streak are integrated to form a single midline neural plate; in contrast, during the formation of complex dysraphic malformations, these cells remain separate and develop independently to produce two "hemicords." Laterally displaced somitic tissue would form an abnormally widened spinal canal with numerous associated vertebral segmentation anomalies including sagittally clefted ("butterfly") vertebrae, fused vertebrae (either single, or multiple as is seen in the Klippel-Feil syndrome), hemivertebrae, absent vertebrae (either single, or multiple as is seen in the caudal agenesis syndrome), or finally, if displaced widely enough, incompletely duplicated vertebrae (as is seen in combined spina bifida). The intervening space between the paired "hemicords" is composed of pluripotent primitive streak cells and could give rise to a variety of tissue types from any of the three primary germ layers, including enteric structures (neurenteric cysts; loops of bowel), mesenchymal tissues (the bony or fibrous midline structures, blood vessels, muscle and fat encountered in SCMs; anomalous vertebrae; immature renal tissues) and ectodermal tissues (dermoid and epidermoid tumors), as well as pathologic tissues such as teratomas and Wilms' tumors.[222–224]

Similar malformations have been reproduced in chick embryos by splitting Hensen's node midsagittally

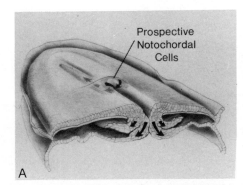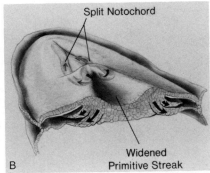

FIGURE 1–25. Proposed embryogenesis of split cord malformations and other "complex dysraphic malformations." *A*, Normal human gastrulation. Prospective notochordal cells located along the anterior margin of Hensen's node ingress through the primitive pit to become the notochordal process. The neuroectoderm flanking the node and primitive streak is integrated to form a single neural tube. *B*, Abnormal gastrulation results in a failure of midline axial integration. The primitive streak is abnormally wide; prospective notochordal cells therefore begin ingressing more laterally than normal. As a result, two notochordal processes are formed. The caudal neuroepithelium flanking the primitive streak also fails to become integrated to form a single neuroepithelial sheet, and instead forms two "hemineural plates." (From Dias MS, Walker ML: The embryogenesis of complex dysraphic malformations: a disorder of gastrulation? J Pediatr Neurosurg 18:229, 1992.)

into two "heminodes" during gastrulation.[215] Double neural tube malformations of variable extent are produced by these maneuvers and are associated with widespread open neural tube defects and multiple somitic abnormalities. Splitting the node during midgastrulation (when the primitive streak is at full extension) produces more cranial malformations, whereas manipulations performed slightly later, during primitive streak regression, result in more caudal malformations. Although preliminary, these data support the theory that complex dysraphic malformations are the result of disordered gastrulation.

Anomalies Resulting from Disorders of Secondary Neurulation—Thickened Filum Terminale, Myelocystocele

Abnormalities of secondary neurulation are thought to produce only skin-covered malformations, since secondary neurulation occurs after closure of the caudal neuropore and separation of cutaneous from neuroectoderm. Since the sacral spinal cord segments (below S2) and filum terminale are the only parts of the nervous system to develop from the caudal cell mass,[36] disorders of secondary neurulation produce malformations that involve only these caudal-most structures.

Common malformations include shortened filum terminale and terminal myelocystocele. The embryology of the shortened filum terminale is entirely unknown, but may represent either an abnormal formation of the secondary neural tube from the caudal cell mass or an abnormality of retrogressive differentiation. The filum terminale is abnormally thickened and frequently is infiltrated with adipose tissue; in the extreme, this lesion merges with the terminal lipoma described above.

Terminal myelocystoceles (Fig. 1–26) are rare occult dysraphic lesions in which the central canal of the caudal spinal cord expands to become a CSF-containing, glial- or ependyma-lined terminal cyst (or myelocystocele).[225, 226] The dilated terminal cord is surrounded, in turn, by a dilated and ectatic dural sleeve. This produces a "double sac" in which the contents of the inner sac communicate with the central canal of the more cranial spinal cord, while the contents of the outer sac communicate with the more cranial subarachnoid space (Fig. 1–26B and C).[225] Ordinarily, there is no free communication between the inner and outer sacs.[225] An associated lipoma is almost universal. Malformations of other caudal organ systems (all derived from the caudal cell mass) are frequent[225–227] and include cloacal exstrophy, imperforate anus, ambiguous genitalia, and multiple caudal vertebral malformations including segmentation anomalies and caudal agenesis.

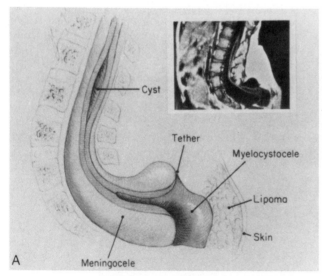

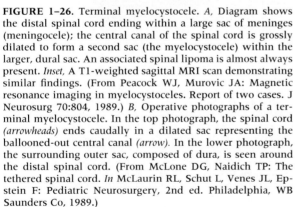

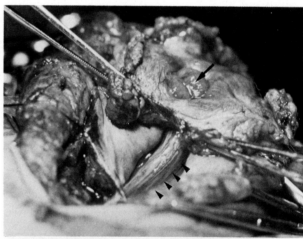

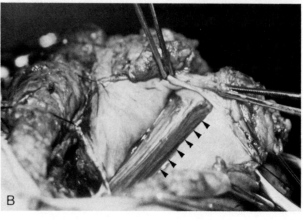

FIGURE 1–26. Terminal myelocystocele. _A,_ Diagram shows the distal spinal cord ending within a large sac of meninges (meningocele); the central canal of the spinal cord is grossly dilated to form a second sac (the myelocystocele) within the larger, dural sac. An associated spinal lipoma is almost always present. _Inset,_ A T1-weighted sagittal MRI scan demonstrating similar findings. (From Peacock WJ, Murovic JA: Magnetic resonance imaging in myelocystoceles. Report of two cases. J Neurosurg 70:804, 1989.) _B,_ Operative photographs of a terminal myelocystocele. In the top photograph, the spinal cord _(arrowheads)_ ends caudally in a dilated sac representing the ballooned-out central canal _(arrow)._ In the lower photograph, the surrounding outer sac, composed of dura, is seen around the distal spinal cord. (From McLone DG, Naidich TP: The tethered spinal cord. _In_ McLaurin RL, Schut L, Venes JL, Epstein F: Pediatric Neurosurgery, 2nd ed. Philadelphia, WB Saunders Co, 1989.)

Myelocystoceles are one component of the OEIS complex (omphalocele, exstrophy, imperforate anus, and spinal malformations).[227]

Terminal myelocystoceles are thought to arise during the period of secondary neurulation from the caudal cell mass.[225, 226, 228] The juxtaposition of cells in the caudal cell mass that give rise to multiple organ rudiments probably accounts for the frequent association of myelocystocele with other hindgut and cloacal anomalies.[225] One proposal is that CSF, unable to exit from the central canal, is vented into the terminal portion of the central canal during canalization of the secondary neural tube.[225] This, of course, assumes that the central canals of the primary and secondary neural tubes are in continuity during canalization, as occurs in the mouse[33] (alternatively, CSF could distend the terminal neural tube secondarily following integration of the caudal cell mass with the cranial neural tube). Progressive accumulation of CSF would then distend the central canal. Continued growth of the terminal cyst distends the surrounding arachnoid to produce the enveloping outer sac. The cyst ultimately disrupts the overlying mesenchyme (but not the cutaneous ectoderm) and results in a dorsal bony dysraphism and mesenchymal abnormality with intact overlying skin.[225] The nature of the underlying CSF disturbance is uncertain. It is important to note that hydrocephalus is extremely uncommon in patients with terminal myelocystoceles, suggesting that the disturbance in CSF dynamics is local rather than global.

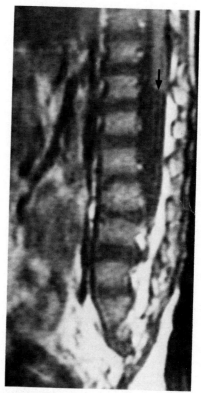

FIGURE 1–27. Caudal agenesis sequence. The distal sacral and coccygeal vertebral segments are absent; the distal spinal cord ends abruptly *(arrow)* in the midportion of the conus medullaris; the distal aspect of the conus as well as the filum terminale are absent.

ANOMALIES RESULTING FROM FAILURE OF CAUDAL NEURAXIAL DEVELOPMENT—CAUDAL AGENESIS

The term caudal agenesis was suggested by Passarge and Lenz in 1966[229] to describe a group of caudal malformations characterized by partial or complete absence of a variable number of lumbar and/or sacral vertebrae, together with corresponding regions of the caudal neural tube. The vertebral anomalies are striking; in addition to agenesis, other complex vertebral anomalies are sometimes present cranial to the absent regions and include hemivertebrae, wedge-shaped vertebrae, fused vertebrae, sacralization of lumbar vertebrae, posterior spina bifida, midline bony spurs, and abnormal rib articulations.[230–237] In some cases, bizarre, complex vertebral anomalies are present. The spinal canal is sometimes widened; in the extreme, combined spina bifida occurs.[172, 238–240]

The distal spinal cord is absent (Fig. 1–27), with the terminal spinal cord ending in a dysplastic glial nodule.[231, 241, 242] Motor deficits usually correspond to the level of the agenesis. In contrast, sensory sparing is characteristic* and suggests a relative preservation of neural crest cells; alternatively, migration of neural crest cells from more cranial spinal segments may occupy the territory rendered vacant by the agenesis. Associated myelomeningoceles are present in up to 50 per cent of cases;[235, 237, 244] conversely, sacral agenesis is re-

ported in up to 24 per cent of patients with myelomeningoceles.[247] SCMs (both single and double dural tube malformations) have been reported in several patients.[235, 240, 248–250]

Associated limb anomalies are common and include flattened buttocks, gluteal atrophy, and equinovarus deformities. The legs are wasted distally, imparting an "inverted champagne bottle" appearance.[234] Histologic examination of involved muscles demonstrates a virtual absence of myocytes with relative preservation of connective tissues[231, 236, 241, 242] and suggests either denervation atrophy[234, 246] or a failure of somitic development to contribute myoblasts to prospective muscle masses.

Associated visceral malformations are present in 35 per cent of patients with caudal agenesis[232] and most commonly include intestinal (tracheoesophageal fistulas, Meckel's diverticulum, cloacal exstrophy, omphalocele, intestinal malrotations) and urogenital (renal agenesis, horseshoe kidney, ureteral and bladder duplications, anomalies of external genitalia) malformations.*

The etiology of caudal agenesis is not completely known, although most authors agree that the malformation arises during early embryogenesis, probably prior to the tenth week.[234] The association of caudal agenesis with myelomeningoceles suggests a disorder that arises prior to or during caudal neural tube closure.

---

*References 232, 233, 235–237, 240, 243–246.

*References 235, 236, 239, 242, 246, 251, 252

The frequent occurrence of caudal agenesis in offspring of diabetic mothers is well described.[229, 241, 243, 253] "Rumpless" chickens exhibiting similar malformations have been produced by exposing embryos to insulin or other sulfur-containing compounds during early embryogenesis.[254-256] Similar malformations have been produced in mice by exposing embryos to hyperglycemic medium or to β-hydroxybutyrate, a ketone body that is elevated during periods of ketoacidosis.[257] The optimum time for producing such anomalies is during late gastrulation, when caudal neuraxial structures are first being formed. Sadler and colleagues have invoked an interference with the structure and/or function of glycoproteins known to be involved in early embryonic development.[257]

Duhamel has proposed a common etiology for a wide spectrum of malformations involving the caudal urogenital and gastrointestinal systems, including imperforate anus at the one extreme and sirenomelia (characterized by caudal spinal agenesis, multiple visceral anomalies, and associated fusion of both hindlimbs into a single appendage—the so-called "mermaid" syndrome) at the other; caudal agenesis is thought to represent an intermediate form of these disorders.[258] Sirenomelia has been produced in chickens by destroying the caudal axial mesoderm,[259] which has led to the suggestion that a disorder of an axial mesodermal "developmental field," which is responsible for orchestrating the migration and determination of prospective caudal mesodermal cells during gastrulation, might be responsible for caudal agenesis. According to this theory, malformations arise when epiblast cells migrating through the primitive streak ". . . fail to make, at the proper time, the proper transition whereby they come to acquire mesodermal characteristics."[260] Such a caudal "organizer" has been implicated by others in the pathogenesis of caudal agenesis[232, 235, 261] and may act

through cell-cell interactions mediated by cell surface "morphogenesis proteins."[260, 262]

The association of caudal agenesis with the broader group of malformations collectively referred to above as "complex dysraphic malformations" suggests that caudal agenesis may perhaps represent another expression of a disorder of midline axial integration during gastrulation.[215] In this case, regression of the primitive streak and caudal cell mass cease altogether; midline neuraxial structures (neural tube and notochord) are therefore deficient, and somitic development, which is dependent upon proper notochordal development, is also severely impaired.

ANOMALIES RESULTING FROM DISORDERS OF POSTNEURULATION DEVELOPMENT—ENCEPHALOCELES

The embryology of encephaloceles has recently been reviewed by Chapman and colleagues.[179] Encephaloceles were initially thought by von Recklinghausen to arise from a failure of closure of the cranial neuropore.[263] However, unlike anencephaly (in which the involved neural tissue is completely disorganized), these malformations contain well developed neural (uni- or bilateral basifrontal or occipital cortex, cerebellum, or brainstem) and mesenchymal (choroid plexus, pia-arachnoid) tissues[180, 181] that have undergone considerable histogenesis and therefore could not be the products of failed neural tube closure. Rather, encephaloceles are thought to arise from a *postneurulation* disorder in which fully neurulated, and often relatively normally formed, neural tissue herniates through a defect in the anterior basal (in the case of anterior encephaloceles) or occipital (as in the case of occipital encephaloceles) mesenchyme (Fig. 1–28). Marin-Padilla has suggested that a mesodermal insufficiency may

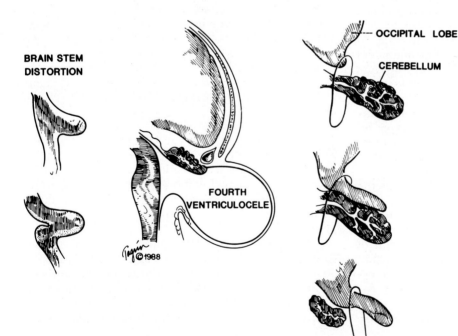

BRAIN STEM DISTORTION

OCCIPITAL LOBE

CEREBELLUM

FOURTH VENTRICULOCELE

©1988

FIGURE 1–28. Occipital encephaloceles. Diagrammatic representation of various anatomic configurations. Note that in every case the tissue that is within the encephalocele sac has undergone significant histogenesis to form either brainstem or cerebellar and/or cerebral tissues; in several cases, *both* cerebellum and occipital lobe are present in the encephalocele sac, implying that the malformation arose at least after the differentiation of the three primary cerebral vesicles. (From Chapman PH, Swearingen B, Caviness VS: Subtorcular occipital encephaloceles. Anatomical considerations relative to operative management. J Neurosurg 71:375, 1989.)

result in growth impairment of the chondrocranium and a delay in closure of the membranous neurocranium.[97, 98] The subsequent explosive growth of the telencephalon may eventually surpass the accommodative capacity of the neurocranium, and neural tissues may then herniate through the mesenchyme to end extracranially. Microcephaly is a common concomitant of encephaloceles; however, it is uncertain whether this is a primary or secondary event. Alternatively, all that may be necessary is a focal area of mesenchymal insufficiency or weakness to allow the rapidly growing telencephalon to herniate; occipital encephaloceles may be produced in chickens simply by incising the occipital mesenchyme overlying the cranial neural tube after neurulation is complete (McLone, unpublished observations). Chapman has suggested that associated hydrocephalus may contribute to the genesis of encephaloceles.[179] However, encephaloceles may occur in the absence of hydrocephalus; moreover, associated hydrocephalus may be merely a consequence rather than the cause of the encephalocele.

TABLE 1–3. CHIARI-ASSOCIATED CENTRAL NERVOUS SYSTEM MALFORMATIONS

Disorders of the Skull
"Lückenschädel" of the skull
Small posterior fossa
Low-lying tentorium cerebelli with large incisura
Scalloping of the petrous bone
Shortening of the clivus
Enlargement of the foramen magnum
Disorders of the Cerebral Hemispheres
Polymicrogyria
Cortical heterotopias
Dysgenesis of the corpus callosum
Large massa intermedia
Disorders of the Posterior Fossa
Descent of the cerebellar vermis through foramen magnum
Caudal displacement of pons and medulla
Rostral displacement of superior cerebellum through the tentorium
"Kinking" of the brainstem
Loss of pontine flexure
Aqueductal stenosis or forking
"Beaking" of the tectum

SECONDARILY "ACQUIRED" CENTRAL NERVOUS SYSTEM ANOMALIES RESULTING FROM MYELODYSPLASIA—CHIARI II MALFORMATION

The Chiari II malformation is a complex disorder that, to a variable extent, encompasses anomalies of virtually the entire neuraxis (Fig. 1–29). Most prominent among these are caudal displacement of the cere-

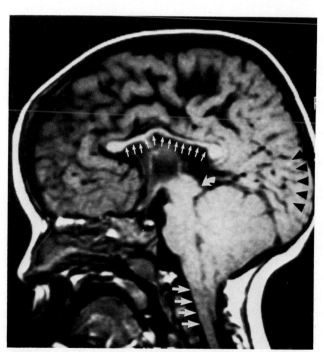

FIGURE 1–29. Chiari II malformation in a child with a myelomeningocele. The cerebellar vermis, fourth ventricle, and caudal brainstem have all descended into the cervical canal *(white arrows).* Additionally, the midbrain tectum is beaked *(curved white arrow),* the corpus callosum is thin and misshapen *(small white arrows),* and several areas of cortical dysplasia *(black arrowheads)* are present.

bellar vermis and tonsils into the cervical canal; elongation, kinking, and caudal displacement of the lower brainstem below the foramen magnum; and upward displacement of the superior cerebellum through a dysplastic, low-lying tentorial incisura. A small posterior fossa and lückenschädel of the skull, as well as many associated telencephalic and diencephalic anomalies (Table 1–3), suggest a pancerebral disorder involving much of the cranial neuraxis and chondrocranium.[264]

Theories regarding the embryology of Chiari malformations can generally be grouped into four types.[264] The first group, regarded as the dysgenesis/developmental arrest theories, presumes the Chiari malformation to be the result of a primary dysgenesis of the neuraxis[265] or a failure of the pontine flexure to form.[266, 267] Neither of these theories can account for the frequent associated cerebral malformations.

The second group, referred to as the hydrocephalus/hydrodynamic theories, relies upon the presence of "fetal hydrocephalus," which, because of a presumed imbalance (either static or dynamic) between supra- and infratentorial compartments, displaces the posterior fossa contents caudally. However, these theories ignore the small cranial volumes and absence of hydrocephalus in all early human fetuses with dysraphism and Chiari malformations.[268] Moreover, they fail to explain the small size of the posterior fossa, *upward* herniation of the superior cerebellar vermis, and associated cerebral anomalies.

The third group, referred to as the traction theories, suggests that traction on the caudal spinal cord by a myelomeningocele may pull the hindbrain caudally.[269, 270] However, experimental evidence suggests that the forces generated by spinal cord traction are dissipated within four spinal segments.[271] Moreover, these theories do not explain the upwardly herniated superior cerebellar vermis, the medullary kink and vermian peg, or associated cerebral anomalies.

The fourth group, referred to as the small posterior fossa/overgrowth theories, suggests that the Chiari malformation is caused by a primary disorder of paraxial mesoderm that results in a small posterior fossa that cannot adequately accommodate the burgeoning cerebellum and brainstem.[272] Padget and colleagues suggested that leakage of cerebrospinal fluid from an open neural placode might result in an acquired microcephaly with a small posterior fossa; this leads to premature fusion of the cerebellar primordia and, with subsequent growth of the posterior fossa contents, produces a Chiari malformation.[273, 274]

Although each of these theories explains certain elements of the Chiari malformation, none of them fully explains all of the observed features. McLone and Knepper have recently proposed a unifying theory of embryogenesis for Chiari malformations which incorporates elements of each of the preceding theories.[264, 268] According to this model, an open neural placode allows CSF to escape from the central canal of the caudal neural tube. In addition, spinal occlusion (which, in normal animals and in humans, precedes and appears to be responsible for rapid brain enlargement) is incomplete in animal models of dysraphism and allows further leakage of CSF from the ventricles through the central canal. Finally, CSF continues to leak from the still open placode after spinal occlusion ends at stage 14 (POD 32). This persistent venting of CSF interferes with proper ventricular enlargement and eventually results in multiple central nervous system anomalies. For example, incomplete dilatation of the telencephalic ventricles provides less support for the telencephalic hemispheres and results in disorganized migration of neurons from the ventricular zone, producing cortical heterotopias, gyral anomalies, and callosal dysgenesis. Inadequate distention of the third ventricle results in extended contact between the two thalami and an enlarged massa intermedia. Finally, inadequate enlargement of the rhombencephalic ventricle may similarly influence brainstem development and produce abnormalities of cranial nerve nuclei and their afferent and efferent connections.[264]

Most importantly, impaired ventricular enlargement has effects on the development of the chondrocranium; this is most evident in the development of the posterior fossa. The growth and development of the chondrocranium are normally dependent upon cues provided by the expansion of the underlying neural mass (the developing brain and ventricular system) during early embryogenesis.[50, 51] Incomplete distention of the rhombencephalic ventricle leaves the posterior fossa chondrocranium without an adequate inductive force; the posterior fossa is therefore smaller than normal, and the tentorium is low-set and deficient.[264, 268] This small posterior fossa is incapable of later accommodating the explosive growth of the rhombencephalon; as a result, the posterior fossa contents are displaced both cephalad through the tentorial incisura and caudad through the foramen magnum. Impaction of neural tissues at these levels impairs CSF flow through the foramina of Luschka and Magendie, as well as through the sub-arachnoid space at the foramen magnum and tentorial incisura, and results in hydrocephalus.

SUMMARY

We have tried to give a detailed and comprehensive description of normal early human neural development and to discuss the scientific basis for the many theories that speak to the mechanisms underlying these processes. It is our contention that a thorough understanding of normal anatomy and embryology provides a solid background for the accurate diagnosis and rational treatment of children with dysraphic malformations. Within this context, we have discussed the current state of knowledge regarding the mechanisms underlying these malformations. As we have seen, a variety of theories have been offered to explain the origin of these malformations; some have advanced our understanding of dysraphism, while others have fallen short of the mark. It is important for the reader to understand that while each of these theories is plausible, none has been rigorously tested experimentally. It is our fervent hope that the next generation of pediatric neurosurgeons, armed with a knowledge of normal embryonic mechanisms, will begin to provide some answers to the many unanswered questions that remain.

REFERENCES

1. Bronner-Fraser M: The neural crest: what can it tell us about cell migration and determination? Curr Top Dev Biol 15:1, 1980.
2. Campbell LR, Dayton DH, Sohal GS: Neural tube defects: a review of human and animal studies on the etiology of neural tube defects. Teratology 34:171, 1986.
3. Erickson CA: Morphogenesis of the neural crest. In Browder LW (ed): Developmental Biology, Vol. 2. New York, Plenum Publishing Corp., 1986, pp 481–543.
4. Gordon R: A review of the theories of vertebrate neurulation and their relationship to the mechanics of neural tube birth defects. J Embryol Exp Morphol 89(Suppl):229, 1985.
5. Jacobson AG: Morphogenesis of the neural plate and tube. In Connelly TG, Brinkeley LL, Carlson BM (eds): Morphogenesis and Pattern Formation. New York, Raven Press, 1981, pp 233–263.
6. Schoenwolf GC, Smith JL: Mechanisms of neurulation: traditional viewpoint and recent advances. Development 109:243, 1990.
7. Mall FP: On stages in the development of human embryos from 2 to 25 mm. long. Anat Anz 46:78, 1914.
8. Streeter GL: Developmental horizons in human embryos. Description of age group XI, 13 to 20 somites, and age group XII, 21 to 29 somites. Contrib Embryol 30:211, 1942.
9. O'Rahilly R: Developmental stages in human embryos, including a survey of the Carnegie collection. Part A: embryos of the first three weeks (stages 1 to 9). Washington, D.C., Carnegie Institution of Washington, Publ 631, 1973.
10. Streeter GW: Developmental horizons in human embryos (fourth issue). A review of the histogenesis of cartilage and bone. Contrib Embryol 34:165, 1949.
11. O'Rahilly R, Müller F: Developmental Stages in Human Embryos. Washington, D.C., Carnegie Institution of Washington, 1987.
12. Jellinger K, Gross H, Kaltenbäch E, Griswold W: Holoprosen-

cephaly and agenesis of the corpus callosum: frequency of associated malformations. Acta Neuropathol 55:1, 1981.

13. Duband JL, Thiery JP: Appearance and distribution of fibronectin during chick embryo gastrulation and neurulation. Dev Biol 94:337, 1982.

14. Mitrani E: Primitive streak-forming cells of the chick invaginate through a basement membrane. Wilhelm Roux Arch 191:320, 1982.

15. Sanders EJ: Labelling of basement membrane constituents in the living chick embryo during gastrulation. J Embryol Exp Morphol 79:113, 1984.

16. Sanders EJ: Ultrastructural immunocytochemical localization of fibronectin in the early chick embryo. J Embryol Exp Morphol 71:155, 1982.

17. Sanders EJ, Prasad S: Epithelial and basement membrane responses to chick embryo primitive streak grafts. Cell Differ 18:233, 1986.

18. Fontaine J, Le Douarin NM: Analysis of endoderm formation in the avian blastoderm by the use of quail-chick chimaeras. The problem of the neurectodermal origin of the cells of the APUD system. J Embryol Exp Morphol 41:209, 1977.

19. Modak SP: Experimental analysis of the origin of the embryonic endoblast in birds. Rev Suisse Zool 73:877, 1966.

20. Nicolet G: Analyse autoradiographique de la localisation des différentes ébauches présomptives dans la ligne primitive de l'embryon de poulet. J Embryol Exp Morphol 23:79, 1970.

21. Rosenquist GC: A radioautographic study of labeled grafts in the chick blastoderm. Development from primitive streak stages to stage 12. Contrib Embryol 38:73, 1966.

22. Vakaet L: Some new data concerning the formation of the definitive endoblast in the chick embryo. J Embryol Exp Morphol 10:38, 1962.

23. Nicolet G: Avian gastrulation. Adv Morphol 9:231, 1971.

24. Schoenwolf GC, Sheard P: Fate mapping the avian epiblast with focal injections of a flourescent-histochemical marker: ectodermal derivatives. J Exp Zool 255:323, 1990.

25. Spratt NT: Regression and shortening of the primitive streak in the explanted chick blastoderm. J Exp Zool 104:69, 1947.

26. Hill JP, Florian J: A young human embryo (embryo Dobbin) with head-process and prochordal plate. Philos Trans R Soc Lond (Biol) 219:443, 1931.

27. Shaw W: Observations on two specimens of early human ova. Br Med J 1:411, 1932.

28. Hendrickx AG: Description of stages IX, X, and XI. In Hendrickx AG (ed): Embryology of the Baboon. Chicago, The University of Chicago Press, 1971, pp 69–85.

29. O'Rahilly R, Müller F: The first appearance of the human nervous system at stage 8. Anat Embryol 163:1, 1981.

30. Müller F, O'Rahilly R: The first appearance of the major subdivisions of the human brain at stage 9. Anat Embryol 168:419, 1983.

31. Müller F, O'Rahilly R: The first appearance of the neural tube and optic primordium in the human embryo at stage 10. Anat Embryol 172:157, 1985.

32. Müller F, O'Rahilly R: The development of the human brain and the closure of the rostral neuropore at stage 11. Anat Embryol 175:205, 1986.

33. Müller F, O'Rahilly R: The development of the human brain, the closure of the caudal neuropore, and the beginning of secondary neurulation at stage 12. Anat Embryol 176:413, 1987.

34. Bartelmez GW, Evans HM: Development of the human embryo during the period of somite formation, including embryos with 2 to 16 pairs of somites. Contrib Embryol 17:1, 1926.

35. Müller F, O'Rahilly R: Cerebral dysraphia (future anencephaly) in a human twin embryo at stage 13. Teratology 30:167, 1984.

36. Müller F, O'Rahilly R: Somitic-vertebral correlation and vertebral levels in the human embryo. Am J Anat 177:3, 1986.

37. Löfberg J, Ahlfors K, Fallstrom C: Neural crest cell migration in relation to extracellular matrix organization in the embryonic axolotl trunk. Dev Biol 75:148, 1980.

38. Desmond ME, Jacobson AG: Embryonic brain enlargement requires cerebrospinal fluid pressure. Dev Biol 57:188, 1977.

39. Desmond ME, Schoenwolf GC: Timing and positioning of occlusion of the spinal neurocele in the chick embryo. J Comp Neurol 235:479, 1985.

40. Schoenwolf GC, Desmond ME: Descriptive studies of occlusion and reopening of the spinal canal of the early chick embryo. Anat Rec 209:251, 1984.

41. Kaufman MH: Occlusion of the neural lumen in early mouse embryos analysed by light and electron microscopy. J Embryol Exp Morphol 78:211, 1983.

42. Freeman BG: Surface modifications of neural epithelial cells during formation of the neural tube in the rat embryo. J Embryol Exp Morphol 28:437, 1972.

43. Desmond ME: Description of the occlusion of the spinal cord lumen in early human embryos. Anat Rec 204:89–93, 1982.

44. Desmond ME, Schoenwolf GC: Evaluation of the roles of intrinsic and extrinsic factors in occlusion of the spinal neurocele during rapid brain enlargement in the chick embryo. J Embryol Exp Morphol 97:25, 1986.

45. Schoenwolf GC, Desmond ME: Timing and positioning of reopening of the occluded spinal neurocele in the chick embryo. J Comp Neurol 246:459, 1986.

46. Desmond ME, O'Rahilly R: The growth of the human brain during the embryonic period proper. 1. Linear axes. Anat Embryol 162:137, 1981.

47. Schoenwolf GC, Desmond ME: Neural tube occlusion precedes rapid brain enlargement. J Exp Zool 30:405, 1984.

48. Pacheco MA, Marks RW, Schoenwolf GC, Desmond ME: Quantification of the initial phases of rapid brain enlargement in the chick embryo. Am J Anat 175:403, 1986.

49. Jelínek R, Pexieder T: The pressure of encephalic fluid in chick embryos between the 2nd and 6th day of incubation. Physiol Bohemoslov 17:297, 1968.

50. Jelínek R, Pexieder T: Pressure of the CSF and the morphogenesis of the CNS. I. Chick embryo. Folia Morphol 18:102, 1970.

51. Coulombre AJ, Coulombre JL: The role of mechanical factors in brain morphogenesis. Anat Rec 130:289, 1958.

52. Pexieder T, Jelínek R: Pressure of the CSF and the morphogenesis of the CNS. II. Pressure necessary for normal development of brain vesicles. Folia Morphol 18:181, 1970.

53. Müller F, O'Rahilly R: The development of the human brain from a closed neural tube at stage 13. Anat Embryol 177:203, 1988.

54. Müller F, O'Rahilly R: The first appearance of the future cerebral hemispheres in the human embryo at stage 14. Anat Embryol 177:495, 1988.

55. Nichols DH: Formation and distribution of neural crest mesenchyme to the first pharyngeal arch region of the mouse embryo. Am J Anat 176:221, 1986.

56. Tan SS, Morris-Kay G: The development and distribution of the cranial neural crest in the rat embryo. Cell Tissue Res 240:403, 1985.

57. O'Rahilly R, Müller F: The meninges in human development. J Neuropathol Exp Neurol 45:588, 1986.

58. Bartelmez GW, Bount MP: The formation of neural crest from the primary optic vescicle in man. Contrib Embryol 233:57, 1954.

59. Perris R, Bronner-Fraser M: Recent advances in defining the role of the extracellular matrix in neural crest development. Comments Dev Neurobiol 1:61, 1989.

60. Bronner-Fraser M: Analysis of the early stages of trunk neural crest migration in avian embryos using monoclonal antibody HNK-1. Dev Biol 115:44, 1986.

61. Anderson DJ: The neural crest cell lineage problem: Neuropoiesis? Neuron 3:1, 1989.

62. Schoenwolf GC: Histological and ultrastructural observations of tail bud formation in the chick embryo. Anat Rec 193:131, 1979.

63. Schoenwolf GC: Histological and ultrastructural studies of secondary neurulation in mouse embryos. Am J Anat 169:361, 1984.

64. Schoenwolf GC, DeLongo J: Ultrastructure of secondary neurulation in the chick embryo. Am J Anat 158:43, 1980.

65. Lemire RJ: Secondary caudal neural tube formation. In Lemire RJ, Loeser JD, Leech RW, Ellsworth CA Jr. (ed): Normal and Abnormal Development of the Human Nervous System. Hagerstown, Md, Harper and Row, 1975, pp 71–83.

66. Bolli P: Sekundäre Lumenbildungen im Neuralrohr und Rückenmark menschlicher Embryonen. Acta Anat 64:48, 1966.

67. Kunimoto K: The development and reduction of the tail and of the caudal end of the spinal cord. Contrib Embryol 8:161, 1918.
68. Streeter GL: Factors involved in the formation of the filum terminale. Am J Anat 25:1, 1919.
69. Krause W: Der Ventriculus terminalis des Rückenmarks. Arch fur mikr Anat 11:216, 1875.
70. Kernohan JW: The ventriculus terminalis: its growth and development. J Comp Neurol 38:107, 1925.
71. Barson AJ: The vertebral level of termination of the spinal cord during normal and abnormal development. J Anat 106:489, 1970.
72. Baker PC, Schroeder TE: Cytoplasmic filaments and morphogenetic movement in the amphibian neural tube. Dev Biol 15:432, 1967.
73. Burnside B: Microtubules and microfilaments in amphibian neurulation. Am Zool 13:989, 1973.
74. Karfunkel P: The role of microtubules and microfilaments in neurulation in *Xenopus*. Dev Biol 25:30, 1971.
75. Schroeder TE: Mechanisms of morphogenesis: the embryonic neural tube. Int J Neurosci 2:183, 1971.
76. Handel MA, Roth LE: Cell shape and morphology of the neural tube: implications for microtubule function. Dev Biol 25:78, 1971.
77. Karfunkel P: The activity of microtubules and microfilaments in neurulation in the chick. J Exp Zool 181:289, 1972.
78. Lyser KM: Early differentiation of motor neuroblasts in chick embryo as studied by electron microscopy. II. Microtubules and neurofilaments. Dev Biol 17:117, 1968.
79. Messier P-E: Effects of β-mercaptoethanol on the fine structure of the neural plate cells of the chick embryo. J Embryol Exp Morphol 21:309, 1969.
80. Nagale RG, Lee H: Ultrastructural changes in cells associated with interkinetic nuclear migration in the developing chick neuroepithelium. J Exp Zool 210:89, 1979.
81. Schoenwolf GC, Powers ML: Shaping of the chick neuroepithelium during primary and secondary neurulation: role of cell elongation. Anat Rec 218:182, 1987.
82. Herman L, Kauffman SL: The fine structure of the embryonic mouse neural tube with special reference to cytoplasmic microtubules. Dev Biol 13:145, 1966.
83. Wilson DB, Finta LA: Early development of the brain and spinal cord in dysraphic mice: a transmission electron microscopic study. J Comp Neurol 190:363, 1980.
84. Wilson DB, Finta LA: Fine structure of the lumbosacral neural folds in the mouse embryo. J Embryol Exp Morphol 55:279, 1980.
85. Ferm VH: Colchicine teratogenesis in hamster embryos. Proc Soc Exp Biol Med 112:775, 1963.
86. Karfunkel P: The role of microtubules and microfilaments in neurulation in *Xenopus*. Dev Biol 25:30, 1971.
87. Löfberg J, Jacobson C-O: Effects of vinblastine sulphate, colchicine, and guanosine phosphate on cell morphogenesis during amphibian neurulation. Zoon 2:85, 1974.
88. O'Shea S: The cytoskeleton in neurulation: Role of cations. *In* Harrison RJ (ed): Progress in Anatomy. London, Cambridge University Press, 1981, pp 35–60.
89. Gustafson T, Wolpert L: Cellular mechanisms in the morphogenesis of the sea urchin larva. Change in shape of cell sheets. Exp Cell Res 27:260, 1962.
90. Gustafson T, Wolpert L: Cellular movement and contact in sea urchin morphogenesis. Biol Rev 42:442, 1967.
91. Jacobson AG, Oster GF, Odell GM, Cheng LY: Neurulation and the cortical tractor model for epithelial folding. J Embryol Exp Morphol 96:19, 1986.
92. Schoenwolf GC, Alvarez IS: Roles of neuroepithelial cell rearrangement and division in shaping of the avian neural plate. Development 106:427, 1989.
93. Martins-Green M: Origin of the dorsal surface of the neural tube by progressive delamination of epidermal ectoderm and neuroepithelium: implications for neurulation and neural tube defects. Development 103:687, 1988.
94. Roux W: Beiträge zur entwicklungsmechanik des embryo. Zeitschrift fuer Biologie 21:411, 1885.
95. Schoenwolf GC: Microsurgical analysis of avian neurulation: separation of medial and lateral tissues. J Comp Neurol 276:498, 1988.
96. Anderson CB, Meier S: Effect of hyaluronidase treatment on the distribution of cranial neural crest cells in the chick embryo. J Exp Zool 221:329, 1982.
97. Marin-Padilla M: Mesodermal alterations induced by hypervitaminosis A. J Embryol Exp Morphol 15:261, 1966.
98. Marin-Padilla M, Ferm VH: Somite necrosis and developmental malformations induced by vitamin A in the golden hamster. J Embryol Exp Morphol 13:1, 1965.
99. Morris-Kay G, Tuckett F: Immunohistochemical localisation of chondroitin sulfate proteoglycans and the effects of chondroitinase ABC in 9- to 11-day old rat embryos. Development 106:787, 1989.
100. Morris-Kay GM, Crutch B: Culture of rat embryos with β-D-xyloside: evidence of a role for proteoglycans in neurulation. J Anat 134:491, 1982.
101. Morris-Kay GM, Tuckett F, Solursh M: The effects of Streptomyces hyaluronidase on tissue organization and cell cycle time in rat embryos. J Embryol Exp Morphol 98:59, 1986.
102. Morriss GM, Solursh M: Regional differences in mesenchymal cell morphology and glycosaminoglycans in early neural-fold stage rat embryos. J Embryol Exp Morphol 46:37, 1978.
103. Schoenwolf GC, Fisher M: Analysis of the effects of *Streptomyces* hyaluronidase on formation of the neural tube. J Embryol Exp Morphol 73:1, 1983.
104. Smits-van Prooije A, Poelman R, Dubbeldam J, et al.: The formation of the neural tube in rat embryos, cultured in vitro, studied with teratogens. Acta Histochem 32:41, 1986.
105. Tuckett F, Morris-Kay GM: Heparitinase treatment of rat embryos during cranial neurulation. Anat Embryol 180:393, 1985.
106. Jacobson AG: Some forces that shape the nervous system. Zoon 6:13, 1978.
107. Jacobson AG, Gordon R: Changes in the shape of the developing nervous system analyzed experimentally, mathematically, and by computer simulation. J Exp Zool 197:191, 1976.
108. His W: Über mechanische Grundvorgänge thierischer Formbildung. Arch Anat Physiol u wiss Med: Anat Abthl 1:1, 1894.
109. Brun RB, Garson JA: Neurulation in the Mexican salamander (*Ambystoma mexicanum*): a drug study and cell shape analysis of the epidermis and the neural plate. J Embryol Exp Morphol 74:275, 1983.
110. Schroeder TE: Neurulation in *Xenopus laevis*. An analysis and model based upon light and electron microscopy. J Embryol Exp Morphol 23:427, 1970.
111. Schoenwolf GC, Franks MV: Quantitative analyses of changes in cell shapes during bending of the avian neural plate. Dev Biol 105:257, 1984.
112. Moore P, Stanisstreet M, Evans GE: Morphometric analyses of changes in cell shape in the neuroepithelium of mammalian embryos. J Anat 155:87, 1987.
113. Malacinski GM, Youn BW: Neural plate morphogenesis and axial stretching in "notochord-defective" *Xenopus laevis* embryos. Dev Biol 88:352, 1981.
114. Youn BW, Malacinski GM: Axial structure development in ultraviolet-irradiated (notochord-defective) amphibian embryos. Dev Biol 83:339, 1981.
115. Smith JL, Schoenwolf GC: Notochordal induction of cell wedging in the chick neural plate and its role in neural tube formation. J Exp Zool 250:49, 1989.
116. Schoenwolf GC, Folsom D, Moe A: A reexamination of the role of microfilaments in neurulation in the chick embryo. Anat Rec 220:87, 1988.
117. Burnside B: Microtubules and microfilaments in newt neurulation. Dev Biol 26:416, 1971.
118. Schroeder TE: Cell constriction: contractile role of microfilaments in division and development. Am Zool 13:949, 1973.
119. Nagale RG, Lee H: Studies on the mechanism of neurulation in the chick: microfilament-mediated changes in cell shape during uplifting of neural folds. J Exp Zool 213:391, 1980.
120. Morris GM, New DAT: Effect of oxygen concentration on morphogenesis of cranial neural folds and neural crest in cultured rat embryos. J Embryol Exp Morphol 54:17, 1979.
121. Lee H, Kosciuk MC, Nagale RG, Roisen FJ: Studies on the mech-

anisms of neurulation in the chick: possible involvement of myosin in elevation of neural folds. J Exp Zool 225:449, 1983.

122. Nagale RG, Lee H: Motility-related proteins in developing neuroepithelial cells in the chick. Am Zool 18:608, 1978.

123. Austin WL, Wind M, Brown KS: Differences in the toxicity and teratogenicity of cytochalasin D and E in various mouse strains. Teratology 25:11, 1982.

124. Greenaway JC, Shepard TH, Kuc J: Comparison of cytochalasins (A,B,D, and E) in chick explant teratogenicity and tissue culture systems. Proc Soc Exp Biol Med 155:239, 1977.

125. Lee H, Kalmus GW: Effects of cytochalasin B on the morphogenesis of explanted early chick embryos. Growth 40:153, 1976.

126. Lee H, Nagale RG: Neural tube defects caused by local anesthetics in early chick embryos. Teratology 31:119, 1985.

127. Linville GP, Shephard TH: Neural tube closure defects caused by cytochalasin B. Nature New Biol 236:246, 1972.

128. Messier P-E, Auclair C: Effects of cytochalasin B on interkinetic nuclear migration in the chick embryo. Dev Biol 36:218, 1974.

129. Morris-Kay G, Tuckett F: The role of microfilaments in cranial neurulation in rat embryos: Effects of short-term exposure to cytochalasin D. J Embryol Exp Morphol 88:333, 1985.

130. Morris-Kay GM: Growth and development of pattern in the cranial neural epithelium of rat embryos during neurulation. J Embryol Exp Morphol 65 (Suppl):225, 1981.

131. Shepard TH, Greenaway JC: Teratogenicity of cytochalasin D in the mouse. Teratology 16:131, 1977.

132. Tuckett F, Moriss-Kay GM: The kinetic behavior of the cranial neural epithelium during neurulation in the rat. J Embryol Exp Morphol 85:111, 1985.

133. Webster W, Langman J: The effect of cytochalasin B on the neuroepithelial cells of the mouse embryo. Am J Anat 152:209, 1978.

134. Wiley MJ: The effects of cytochalasins on the ultrastructure of neurulating hamster embryos in vivo. Teratology 22:59, 1980.

135. Nagale RG, Pietrolungo JF, Lee H: Studies on the mechanisms of neurulation in the chick: the intracellular distribution of Ca^{++}. Experientia 37:304, 1981.

136. Moran DJ: A scanning electron microscopic and flame spectrometry study on the role of Ca^{2+} in amphibian neurulation using papaverine inhibition and ionophore induction of morphogenetic movement. J Exp Zool 198:409, 1976.

137. Lee H, Nagale R, Karasanyi N: Inhibition of neural tube closure by ionophore A23187 in chick embryos. Experientia 34:518, 1977.

138. Moran D, Rice RW: Action of papaverine and ionophore A23187 on neurulation. Nature 261:497, 1976.

139. Carter SB: The cytochalasins as research tools in cytology. Endeavour 31:77, 1972.

140. Carter SB: Effects of cytochalasin on mammalian cells. Nature 213:261, 1967.

141. Wessels NK, Spooner BS, Ash JF, Bradley MO, Luduena MA, Taylor EL, Wrenn JT, Yamada KM: Microfilaments in cellular and developmental processes. Science 171:135, 1971.

142. Smith JL, Schoenwolf GC: Cell cycle and neuroepithelial cell shape during bending of the chick neural plate. Anat Rec 218:196, 1987.

143. Smith JL, Schoenwolf GC: Role of cell-cycle in regulating neuroepithelial cell shape during bending of the chick neural plate. Cell Tissue Res 252:491, 1988.

144. Langman J, Guerrant RL, Freeman BG: Behavior of neuroepithelial cells during closure of the neural tube. J Comp Neurol 127:399, 1966.

145. Martin A, Langman J: The development of the spinal cord examined by autoradiography. J Embryol Exp Morphol 14:25, 1965.

146. Sauer FC: The cellular structure of the neural tube. J Comp Neurol 63:13, 1935.

147. van Straaten HWM, Hekking JWM, Wiertz-Hoessels EJLM, Thors F, Drukker J: Effect of the notochord on the differentiation of a floor plate area in the neural tube of the chick embryo. Anat Embryol 177:317, 1988.

148. Edelman GM: Surface modulation in cell recognition and cell growth. Science 192:218, 1976.

149. McLone DG, Knepper PA: Role of complex carbohydrates and neurulation. Pediatr Neurosci 12:2, 1985.

150. Moran D, Rice RW: An ultrastructural examination of the role of cell membrane surface coat material during neurulation. J Cell Biol 64:172, 1975.

151. Lee H, Sheffield JB, Nagele RG, Kalmus W: The role of extracellular material in chick neurulation I. Effects of concanavalin A. J Exp Morphol 198:261, 1976.

152. Sadler TW: Distribution of surface coat material on fusing neural folds of mouse embryos during neurulation. Anat Rec 191:345, 1978.

153. O'Shea KS, Kaufman MH: Phospholipase C-induced neural tube defects in the mouse embryo. Experientia 36:1217, 1980.

154. Lee H, Nagale RG, Kalmus GW: Further studies on neural tube defects caused by concanavalin A in early chick embryos. Experientia 32:1050, 1978.

155. Higbee RG, Fiacco JL, Vanden Hoek T, Goossens W, McLone DG, Knepper PA: Oligosaccharides and abnormal neurulation in the delayed splotch mutant. Neurosci Abstr 14:829, 1988.

156. Ersahin Y, Higbee RG, Vanden Hoek T, McLone DG, Knepper PA: Vitamin A-induced suppression/enhancement of protein glycosylation and neurulation. Pediatr Neurosci 13:293, 1987.

157. Mak LL: Ultrastructural studies of amphibian neural fold fusion. Dev Biol 65:435, 1978.

158. Bancroft M, Bellairs R: Differentiation of the neural plate and neural tube in the young chick embryo. Anat Embryol 147:309, 1975.

159. Gouda JG: Closure of the neural tube in relation to the developing somites in the chick embryo (Gallus gallus domesticus). J Anat 118:360, 1974.

160. Revel JP: Scanning electron microscope studies of cell surface morphology and labelling, in situ and in vitro. IITRI, SEM, 1974, pp 542–548.

161. Waterman RE: SEM observations of surface alterations associated with neural tube closure in the mouse and hamster. Anat Rec 183:95, 1975.

162. Waterman RE: Topographical changes along the neural fold associated with neurulation in the hamster and mouse. Am J Anat 146:151, 1976.

163. Geelen JAG, Langman J: Ultrastructural observations on closure of the neural tube in the mouse. Anat Embryol 156:73, 1979.

164. Santander RG, Cuadrado GM: Ultrastructure of the neural canal closure in the chicken embryo. Acta Anat 95:368, 1976.

165. Schoenwolf GC: Observations on closure of the neuropores in the chick embryo. Am J Anat 155:445, 1979.

166. Costanzo R, Watterson RL, Schoenwolf GC: Evidence that secondary neurulation occurs autonomously in the chick embryo. J Exp Zool 219:233, 1982.

167. von Recklinghausen E: Untersuchungen über die Spina bifida. Arch Pathol Anat 105:243, 1886.

168. Morgagni JB: The Seats and Causes of Disease Investigated by Anatomy. London, A. Millar and T. Cadell, 1769.

169. Gardner WJ: Diastematomyelia and the Klippel-Feil syndrome. Relationship to hydrocephalus, syringomyelia, meningocele, meningomyelocele, and iniencephalus. Cleve Clin Q 31:19, 1964.

170. Gardner WJ: Embryologic origin of spinal malformations. Acta Radiol (Diagn) 5:1013, 1966.

171. Gardner WJ: Hypothesis: overdistention of the neural tube may cause anomalies of non-neural organs. Teratology 22:229, 1980.

172. Gardner WJ: The Dysraphic States from Syringomyelia to Anencephaly. Amsterdam, Excerpta Medica, 1973.

173. Caldarelli M, McLone DG, Collins JA, Suwa J, Knepper PA: Vitamin A induced neural tube defects in a mouse. Concepts Pediatr Neurosurg 6:161, 1985.

174. French BN: Abnormal development of the central nervous system. In McLaurin RL, Venes JL, Schut L, Epstein F (eds): Pediatric Neurosurgery: Surgery of the Developing Nervous System. 2nd ed. Philadelphia, W.B. Saunders Co., 1989, pp 9–34.

175. Humphreys RP: Spinal dysraphism. In Wilkins RH, Rengachary SS (eds): Neurosurgery. New York, McGraw-Hill Book Company, 1985, vol 3, pp 2041–2052.

176. Boldrey EB, Elvidge AR: Dermoid cysts of the vertebral canal. Ann Surg 110:273, 1939.

177. Guidetti B, Gagliardi FM: Epidermoid and dermoid cysts: clinical evaluation and late surgical results. J Neurosurg 47:12, 1977.

178. Walker AE, Bucy PC: Congenital dermal sinuses; a source of

spinal meningeal infection and subdural abscesses. Brain 57:401, 1934.

179. Chapman PH, Swearingen B, Caviness VS: Subtorcular occipital encephaloceles. Anatomical considerations relevant to operative management. J Neurosurg 71:375, 1989.

180. Suwanwela C, Suwanwela N: A morphological classification of sincipital encephalomeningoceles. J Neurosurg 36:201, 1972.

181. Blackwood W, Corsellis JAN: Greenfield's Neuropathology. Chicago, Year Book Medical Publishers, 1976, pp 377–380.

182. Yeoh GPS, Bale PMB, de Silva M: Nasal cerebral heterotopia: the so-called nasal glioma or sequestered encephalocele and its variants. Pediatr Pathol 9:531, 1989.

183. Wardinsky TD, Pagon RA, Kropp RJ, Hayden PW, Clarren SK: Nasal dermoid sinus cysts: association with intracranial extension and multiple malformations. Cleft Palate-Craniofacial J 28:87, 1991.

184. Marin-Padilla M: Notochordal-basichondrocranium relationships: abnormalities in experimental axial skeletal (dysraphic) disorders. J Embryol Exp Morphol 53:15, 1979.

185. Marin-Padilla M: Study of the skull in human cranioschisis. Acta Anat 62:1, 1965.

186. Couly G, Le Douarin NM: The fate map of the cephalic neural primordium at the presomitic to the 3-somite stage in the avian embryo. Development 103(Suppl):101, 1988.

187. Couly G, Le Douarin NM: Mapping of the early neural primordium in quail-chick chimeras. II. The prosencephalic neural plate and neural folds: implications for the genesis of cephalic human congenital malformations. Dev Biol 120:198, 1987.

188. Sessions RB: Nasal dermal sinuses: new concepts and explanations. Laryngoscope 92(Suppl 29):1, 1982.

189. Barkovich AJ, Vandermarck P, Edwards MSB, Cogen PH: Congenital nasal masses: CT and MR imaging features in 16 cases. Am J Neuroradiol 12:105, 1991.

190. McQuown SA, Smith JD, Gallo AE: Intracranial extension of nasal dermoids. Neurosurgery 12:531, 1983.

191. Okuda Y, Shizuo O: Nasal dermal sinus and dermoid cyst with intrafalcial extension. Case report and review of literature. Child's Nerv Syst 3:40, 1987.

192. Pensler JM, Bauer BS, Naidich TP: Craniofacial dermoids. Plast Reconstr Surg 82:953, 1988.

193. Gorenstein A, Kern EB, Facer GW, Laws ER: Nasal gliomas. Arch Otolaryngol 106:536, 1980.

194. Hirsh LF, Stool SE, Langfitt TW, Schut L: Nasal glioma. J Neurosurg 46:85, 1977.

195. Cheek WR, Laurent JP: Dermal sinus tracts. Concepts Pediatr Neurosurg 6:63, 1985.

196. Schijman E, Monges J, Cragnaz R: Congenital dermal sinuses, dermoid and epidermoid cysts of the posterior fossa. Child's Nerv Syst 2:83, 1986.

197. Ehni G, Love JG: Intraspinal lipomas: report of cases, review of the literature, and clinical and pathologic study. Arch Neurol Psychiatry 53:1, 1945.

198. Lassman LP, James CCM: Lumbosacral lipomas: critical survey of 26 cases submitted to laminectomy. J Neurol Neurosurg Psychiatry 30:174, 1967.

199. McLone DG, Mutluer S, Naidich TP: Lipomeningoceles of the conus medullaris. In Raimondi AJ (ed): Concepts in Pediatric Neurosurgery. Basel, S. Karger, 1982, vol 3, pp 170–177.

200. Walsh JW, Markesbery WR: Histological features of congenital lipomas of the lower spinal canal. J Neurosurg 52:564, 1980.

201. McLone DG, Naidich TP: Spinal dysraphism: Experimental and clinical. In Holtzman RN, Stein BM (eds): The Tethered Spinal Cord. New York, Thieme-Stratton, 1985, pp 14–28.

202. Naidich TP, McLone DG, Mutluer S: A new understanding of dorsal dysraphism with lipoma (lipomyeloschisis): radiologic evaluation and surgical correction. Am J Roentgenol 140:1065, 1983.

203. Bentley JFR, Smith JR: Developmental posterior enteric remnants and spinal malformations. The split notochord syndrome. Am J Dis Child 35:76, 1960.

204. Prop N, Frensdorf EL, van de Stadt FR: A postvertebral entodermal cyst associated with axial deformities: a case showing the "entodermal-ectodermal adhesion syndrome." Pediatrics 39:555, 1967.

205. Bremer JL: Dorsal intestinal fistula; accessory neurenteric canal; diastematomyelia. Arch Pathol 54:132, 1952.

206. Cohen J, Sledge CB: Diastematomyelia. An embryological interpretation with report of a case. Am J Dis Child 100:127, 1960.

207. Herren RY, Edwards JE: Diplomyelia (duplication of the spinal cord). Arch Pathol 30:1203, 1940.

208. Naidich TP, Harwood-Nash DC: Diastematomyelia: hemicord and meningeal sheaths; single and double arachnoid and dural tubes. Am J Neuroradiol 4:633, 1983.

209. James CCM, Lassman JP: Diastematomyelia. A critical survey of 24 cases submitted to laminectomy. Arch Dis Child 39:125, 1964.

210. Pang D, Dias MS, Ahab-Barmada M: Split cord malformation. Part I: A unified theory of embryogenesis for double cord malformations. Neurosurgery 31:451, 1992.

211. Pang D: Tethered cord syndrome. In Neurosurgery: State of the Art Reviews. Philadelphia, Hanley & Belfus, 1986, vol 1, pp 45–79.

212. Ross GW, Swanson SA, Perentes E, Urich H: Ectopic midline spinal ganglion in diastematomyelia: a study of its connections. J Neurol Neurosurg Psychiatry 51:1231, 1988.

213. Lichtenstein BW: "Spinal dysraphism." Spina bifida and myelodysplasia. Arch Neurol 44:792, 1940.

214. Rokos J: Pathogenesis of diastematomyelia and spina bifida. J Pathol 117:155, 1975.

215. Dias MS, Walker ML: The embryogenesis of complex dysraphic malformations: a disorder of gastrulation? J Pediatr Neurosurg 18:229, 1992.

216. Beardmore HE, Wigglesworth FW: Vertebral anomalies and alimentary duplications. Pediatr Clin North Am 5:457, 1958.

217. Burrows FGO, Sutcliffe J: The split notochord syndrome. Br J Radiol 41:844, 1968.

218. McLetchie NGB, Purves JK, Saunders RL: The genesis of gastric and certain intestinal diverticula and enterogenous cysts. Surg Gynecol Obstet 99:135, 1954.

219. Saunders RL: Combined anterior and posterior spina bifida in a living neonatal human female. Anat Rec 87:255, 1943.

220. Dodds GS: Anterior and posterior rhachischisis. Am J Pathol 17:861, 1941.

221. Feller A, Sternberg H: Zur Kenntnis der Fehlbildungen der Wirbelsäule. I. Die Wirbelkörperspalte und ihre formale Genese. Virchow Arch Path Anat 272:613, 1929.

222. Cameron AH: Malformations of the neuro-spinal axis, urogenital tract and foregut in spina bifida attributable to disturbances of the blastopore. J Pathol Bact 73:213, 1957.

223. Fernbach SK, Naidich TP, McLone DG, Leestma JE: Computed tomography of primary intrathecal Wilms tumor with diastematomyelia. J Comput Assist Tomogr 8:523, 1984.

224. Ugarte N, Gonzalez-Crussi F, Sotelo-Avila C: Diastematomyelia associated with teratoma. J Neurosurg 53:720, 1980.

225. McLone DG, Naidich TP: Terminal myelocystocele. Neurosurgery 16:36, 1985.

226. Peacock WJ, Murovic JA: Magnetic resonance imaging in myelocystoceles. Report of two cases. J Neurosurg 70:804, 1989.

227. Carey JC, Greenbaum B, Hall BD: The OEIS complex (omphalocele, extrophy, imperforate anus, spinal defects). Birth Defects 14(6B):253, 1978.

228. Lemire RJ, Beckwith JB: Pathogenesis of congenital tumors and malformations of the sacrococcygeal region. Teratology 25:201, 1982.

229. Passarge E, Lenz W: Syndrome of caudal regression in infants of diabetic mothers: observations of further cases. Pediatrics 37:672, 1966.

230. Alexander E, Nashold BS: Agenesis of the sacrococcygeal region. J Neurosurg 13:507, 1956.

231. Frantz CH, Aitken GT: Complete absence of the lumbar spine and sacrum. J Bone Joint Surg 49-A:1531, 1967.

232. Freedman B: Congenital absence of the sacrum and coccyx. Report of a case and review of the literature. Br J Surg 37:299, 1950.

233. Hamsa WR: Congenital absence of the sacrum. Arch Surg 30:657, 1935.

234. Pang D, Hoffman HJ: Sacral agenesis with progressive neurological deficit. Neurosurgery 7:118, 1980.

235. Renshaw TS: Sacral agenesis. A classification and review of twenty-three cases. J Bone Joint Surg 60-A:373, 1978.
236. Sarnat HB, Case ME, Graviss R: Sacral agenesis. Neurologic and neuropathologic features. Neurology 26:1124, 1976.
237. Smith ED: Congenital sacral defects. In Stephens FD (ed): Congenital Malformations of the Rectum, Anus, and Genito-Urinary Tracts. Edinburgh & London, E. & S. Livingstone, 1963, pp 82–105.
238. Rosselet P: A rare case of rachischisis with multiple malformations. Am J Roentgenol 73:235, 1955.
239. Stewart SF: Absence of sacrum with report of a case, and a review of the literature. Arch Surg 9:647, 1924.
240. Williams DI, Nixon HH: Agenesis of the sacrum. Surg Gynecol Obstet 105:84, 1957.
241. Price DL, Dooling EC, Richardson EP: Caudal dysplasia (caudal regression syndrome). Arch Neurol 23:212, 1970.
242. Rusnak SL, Driscoll SG: Congenital spinal anomalies in infants of diabetic mothers. Pediatrics 35:989, 1965.
243. Banta JV, Nichols O: Sacral agenesis. J Bone Joint Surg 51-A:693, 1969.
244. Blumel J, Butler MC, Evans EB, Eggers GWN: Congenital anomaly of the sacrococcygeal spine. Arch Surg 85:982, 1962.
245. Blumel J, Evans EB, Eggers GWN: Partial and complete agenesis or malformation of the sacrum with associated anomalies. J Bone Joint Surg 41-A:497, 1959.
246. Ignelzi RJ, Lehman AW: Lumbosacral agenesis: management and embryological implications. J Neurol Neurosurg Psychiatry 37:1273, 1974.
247. Naik DR, Lendon RG, Barson AJ: A radiological study of vertebral and rib malformations in children with myelomeningocele. Clin Radiol 29:427, 1978.
248. Lausecker H: Beitrag zu den mißbildungen des Kreuzbeines. Virchows Arch Pathol Anat 322:119, 1952.
249. Lichtor A: Sacral agenesis. Report of a case. Arch Surg 54:430, 1947.
250. Sinclair JG, Duren N, Rude JC: Congenital lumbosacral defect. Arch Surg 43:473, 1941.
251. Girard PM: Congenital absence of the sacrum. J Bone Joint Surg 17:1062, 1935.
252. Källén B, Winberg J: Caudal mesoderm pattern of anomalies: from renal agenesis to sirenomelia. Teratology 9:99, 1974.
253. Mills JL: Malformations in infants of diabetic mothers. Teratology 25:385, 1982.
254. Duraiswami PK: Comparison of congenital defects induced in developing chickens by certain teratogenic agents with those caused by insulin. J Bone Joint Surg 37:277, 1955.
255. Landauer W: Rumplessness of chicken embryos produced by the injection of insulin and other chemicals. J Exp Zool 98:65, 1945.
256. Zwilling E: The effects of some hormones on development. Ann NY Acad Sci 55:196, 1952.
257. Horton WEJ, Sadler TW: Effects of maternal diabetes on early embryogenesis: alterations in morphogenesis produced by the ketone body, β-hydroxybutyrate. Diabetes 32:610, 1983.
258. Duhamel B: From the mermaid to anal imperforation: the syndrome of caudal regression. Arch Dis Child 36:152, 1961.
259. Wolff E: La Science des Monstres. Paris, Gallimard, 1948.
260. Gardner RJM, Nelson MM: An association of caudal malformations arising from a defect in the "axial mesoderm" developmental field. Am J Med Genet 2(Suppl):37, 1986.
261. Storm-Mathisen A: Myelodysplasia with absence of sacrum. Acta Psychiatr Neurol Scand 29:145, 1954.
262. Bennett D: The T-locus of the mouse. Cell 6:441, 1975.
263. von Recklinghausen G: Untersuchungen über die Spina bifida. Part 2 (Über die Art un die Entstenhung der Spina bifida, ihre Bezichung zur Ruckenmarks und Darmspalte). Virchows Arch 105:296, 1886.
264. McLone DG, Knepper PA: The cause of Chiari II malformation: a unified theory. Pediatr Neurosurg 15:1, 1989.
265. Cleland J: Contribution to the study of spina bifida, encephalocele, and anencephalus. J Anat Physiol 17:257, 1883.
266. Daniel PM, Strich SJ: Some observations on the congenital deformity of the central nervous system known as the Arnold-Chiari malformation. J Neuropathol Exp Neurol 17:255, 1958.
267. Peach B: The Arnold-Chiari malformation. Morphogenesis. Arch Neurol 12:527, 1965.
268. McLone DG, Nakahara S, Knepper PA: Chiari II malformation: pathogenesis and dynamics. Concepts Pediatr Neurosurg 11:1, 1991.
269. Lichtenstein BW: Distant neuroanatomic complications of spina bifida (spinal dysraphism): hydrocephalus, Arnold-Chiari deformity, stenosis of the aqueduct of Sylvius, etc., pathogenesis and pathology. Arch Neurol Psychiatry 47:195, 1942.
270. Penfield W, Coburn DF: Arnold-Chiari malformation and its operative treatment. Arch Neurol Psychiatry 40:328, 1938.
271. Goldstein F, Kepes JJ: The role of traction in the development of the Arnold-Chiari malformation. An experimental study. J Neuropathol Exp Neurol 25:654, 1966.
272. Marin-Padilla M, Marin-Padilla TM: Morphogenesis of experimentally induced Arnold-Chiari malformation. J Neurol Sci 50:29, 1981.
273. Padget DH: Development of so-called dysraphism: with embryologic evidence of clinical Arnold-Chiari and Dandy-Walker malformations. Johns Hopkins Med J 130:127, 1972.
274. Padget DH, Lindenberg R: Inverse cerebellum morphogenetically related to Dandy-Walker and Arnold-Chiari syndromes: bizarre malformed brain with occipital encephalocele. Johns Hopkins Med J 131:228, 1972.

Chapter 2

NORMAL AND ABNORMAL DEVELOPMENT OF THE SPINE

DAVID G. McLONE, M.D., Ph.D., and MARK S. DIAS, M.D.

The development of the vertebral column begins during gastrulation, within a few days of conception, and continues throughout fetal and postnatal life. To properly understand this process, it is important to know how segmentation occurs in the developing organism.

Segmental organization in higher organisms is necessary during development to allow the independent development of structurally and functionally different body regions. The process of segmentation has been scrutinized at many levels—from gross anatomic dissection at one extreme to an examination of underlying genetic and molecular events at the other. The discovery of particular *homeobox* genes that direct segmental development provides proof of direct genomic control of segmentation; evidence is mounting that the development of single segments of the organism may be under direct control of specific regions of the genome.[1]

NORMAL DEVELOPMENT OF THE SPINE

GASTRULATION AND FORMATION OF THE SOMITES

Humans (along with fishes, reptiles, amphibians, birds, and other mammals) are members of the subphylum *Vertebrata,* which is a division of the phylum *Chordata* and is characterized by the presence of a segmented bony or cartilaginous spinal column. In mammalian embryos, prospective mesodermal cells that will form the vertebral column are located in the epiblast; during gastrulation these cells ingress through Hensen's node and the cranial half of the primitive streak, and spread bilaterally to form the definitive mesodermal layer between the overlying ectoderm and underlying endoderm. As discussed in Chapter 1, prospective mesodermal cells in Hensen's node will form the notochordal process, whereas prospective mesodermal cells of the primitive streak will form the remaining

mesoderm. Mesodermal cells begin ingressing through the primitive streak during mid- to late gastrulation (during Hensen's node regression) and do so in an orderly fashion. Prospective notochordal cells within Hensen's node are the first mesodermal cells to ingress and pass cranially in the midline between the ectoderm and endoderm. Cells located within the primitive streak ingress in a craniocaudal sequence; cells that will form more medial mesodermal structures (e.g., prospective somitic mesoderm) ingress first and are more cranially located within the primitive streak, whereas cells that will form more lateral mesodermal structures (e.g., prospective limb mesoderm) ingress later and are more caudally located.[2]

The definitive mesoderm subsequently becomes organized, from medial to lateral, into paraxial (lying immediately lateral to the notochord) or somitic mesoderm, intermediate mesoderm, and lateral plate mesoderm. The paraxial mesoderm contributes to the formation of the somites, the intermediate mesoderm contributes to the formation of the genitourinary system, and the lateral plate mesoderm contributes to the musculoskeletal components of the limbs.

The somitic mesoderm subsequently becomes segmented to form discrete blocks of tissue, the somites.[3, 4] The somites are bilaterally paired structures that lie on either side of the midline notochord and contribute to the formation of the axial skeleton (vertebrae and ribs), as well as the muscles of the trunk and the dermis of the body wall. The fate of the cells that will form the vertebrae is already specified to a considerable extent at the time of somitic segmentation; however, as Bellairs and colleagues[5] have suggested, these cells must be supplemented by other cells from the primitive streak to fulfill their ultimate fate. The notochord involutes during later development; remnants of the notochord persist as the nucleus pulposus of the mature spine.[6]

The formation of the neural tube both precedes and continues during somitic segmentation. The neural tube provides the principal stimulus for somitic segmentation.[7] Prospective somitic cells within the paraxial mesoderm are located immediately subjacent to the neural plate during early neurulation, extending as far laterally as the lateral edges of the neural plate. As neurulation proceeds, these cells occupy a position immediately lateral to the developing neural tube (Fig. 2–1). Condensation of these paraxial mesodermal cells and cleavage of the cells into discrete masses produce the somites (Fig. 2–2). In chick embryos somitic cells surround a central lumen to form a complete rosette, whereas in mammalian embryos the lumen is incomplete inferomedially. Somitic cells are joined both apically and basally by junctional processes;[8] the apical regions contain actin microfilaments similar to those found in neuroepithelial cells.[9]

The somite is divided into a dorsal dermomyotome and a ventral sclerotome.[10, 11] The dermomyotomal portion gives rise to dermal elements and to the myocytes of the dorsal muscles. The cells of the sclerotomal portion surround the notochord and form the primordia of the developing axial skeleton (vertebrae and ribs).

The number of somites that develop appears to be species-specific and is relatively constant.[12] If somitic mesoderm is removed prior to somitic segmentation, regulation occurs so that the number of somites that form is unchanged, but the size of the somites is somewhat reduced. During later development, even the size

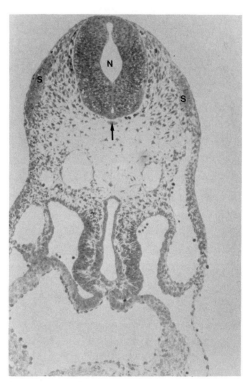

FIGURE 2–2. A transverse section light micrograph of a mouse embryo at 11 days of gestation demonstrates the closed neural tube (N) and bilateral somites (S). The notochord (arrow) lies immediately ventral to the neural tube.

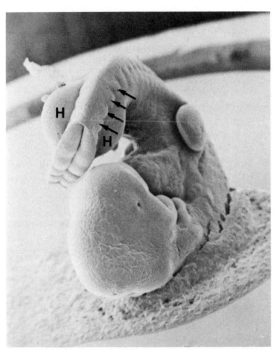

FIGURE 2–1. A scanning electron micrograph of a mouse embryo at 11 days of gestation shows the protrusions caused by the somites lateral to the closed neural tube (arrows) and beneath the un-neurulated portion of the neural tube. Note that the process of neurulation continues beyond the level of the hindlimb bud (H).

of the somites is reconstituted so that the fetus will appear to be normal.[13, 14]

The subsequent development of the somites into the vertebral elements can be divided into three overlapping phases.[15] The initial or *membranous* phase begins at 5 weeks of gestation, the second or *chondrification* phase begins at 6 weeks, and the final or *osseous* phase begins at about 9 weeks of gestation.

MEMBRANOUS PHASE

During the membranous phase, sclerotomal cells move toward and surround the notochord (Fig. 2–3). The cells of the sclerotome are divided into a loosely packed rostral cell mass and a more dense caudal cell mass. The junction between the rostral and caudal portions of the sclerotome forms a cleft, called the fissure of von Ebner. Each vertebra has been thought to receive contributions from two adjacent somites in a process called *resegmentation* (Fig. 2–4).[16] Experiments in which chick vertebrae were excised and replaced with corresponding quail vertebrae (the fate of the transplanted quail tissue can be followed using a nucleolar marker) suggest that during resegmentation the centrum of each vertebral body is formed from the caudal region of the more rostral sclerotome and the rostral region of the more caudal sclerotome.[17] However, the concept of resegmentation has been ques-

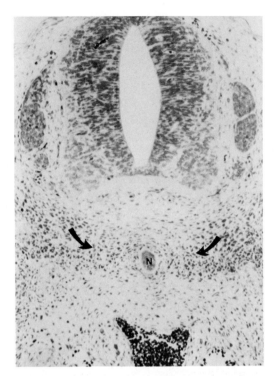

FIGURE 2–3. A light micrograph of a mouse embryo at 11 days of gestation shows the notochord (N) has moved ventrally, away from the neural tube, and mesenchymal cells *(arrows)* are streaming from the adjacent somites to surround the notochord.

tioned by others,[18] and equally plausible mechanisms have been proposed.[15] The fate of the rostral and caudal portions of the sclerotome also differs in that only the caudal sclerotome participates in the formation of the neural arches and costal processes. The cells within the cleft of von Ebner proliferate and contribute to the intervening intervertebral disc.

The contributions of each of the somites to vertebrate development is unclear. Following unilateral removal of as many as 90 per cent of the somites in the chick, the vertebrae are fully or nearly reconstituted from the remaining somitic mesoderm so that normal or only minimally malformed vertebrae (i.e., those missing only a single process) result; hemivertebrae and other complex vertebral malformations of the type usually encountered in clinical practice are rare.[14] Even following bilateral removal of somites at a single level, chick embryos are capable of establishing a normal pattern of vertebrae. This extraordinary ability for embryonic regulation may well explain the infrequent occurrence of vertebral anomalies in clinical practice.

CHONDRIFICATION PHASE

Chondrification centers appear during the sixth week of embryogenesis. Initially, three paired centers of chondrification form (Fig. 2–5). The first pair surrounds the notochord and fuses ventral to the neural tube to form the centrum of the vertebral body. The second pair forms dorsolaterally and fuses dorsal to the neural tube to become the posterior neural arch and spinous process. The final pair develops between the ventral and dorsal pairs and forms the transverse process. Chondrification begins at the cervicothoracic junction and extends both cranially and caudally thereafter. The centrum is the first portion of the vertebra to chondrify; the dorsal neural arch chondrifies later. Chondrification is initiated in response to substances secreted by both the notochord and the ventral portion of the developing neural tube through a process known as "inductive tissue interaction."[19]

The anterior and posterior longitudinal ligaments form during the chondrification phase and are derived from the mesenchyme surrounding the cartilaginous vertebrae. The intervertebral disc develops from densely aggregated somitic mesoderm and receives contributions from both rostral and caudal halves of adjacent sclerotomes. The vertebral cartilages are initially contiguous with the cartilage of the intervertebral discs so that the vertebral column exists as a continuous cartilaginous column. Later, as the vertebrae ossify, the discs become distinct from the adjacent vertebrae; the intervertebral cartilage differentiates to form the fibrocartilaginous component of the intervertebral disc.[6] A ring of perinotochordal tissue forms the annulus fibrosus. Notochordal remnants contribute to the nucleus pulposus and mucoid streak within the vertebral centra.

OSSIFICATION PHASE

Ossification of the vertebral column begins in the second gestational month and continues into postnatal life (Fig. 2–6). Ossification is initiated within four *primary ossification centers,* two in the vertebral centrum and one in each side of the dorsal neural arch. The vertebral body becomes ossified from both dorsal and ventral ossification centers, which fuse during the 20th to 24th gestational week to form a single ossification center. Cartilaginous zones develop rostral and caudal to the vertebral ossification centers and will form the cartilaginous end plates adjacent to the intervertebral discs. At the periphery of the cartilaginous end plates, a C-shaped ring of cartilaginous material, the *ring apophysis,* develops in intimate association with the lateral borders of the vertebral bodies and with the annulus of the intervening discs at the centrum—disc interface and firmly attaches the intervertebral disc to the vertebral bodies. The ring apophysis is similar to the epiphysis of the long bones and eventually fuses with the peripheral portions of the vertebrae during mid-adolescence. However, during childhood the apophyseal ring may become fractured and dislocate posteriorly into the spinal canal; symptoms and signs of neural impingement simulate those of a herniated intervertebral disc.

Ossification of the paired dorsal neural arches proceeds medially within the laminae and ventrally within

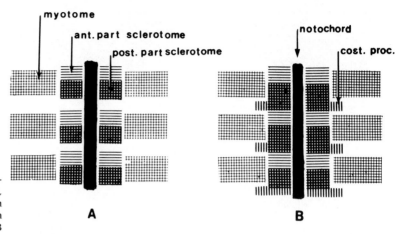

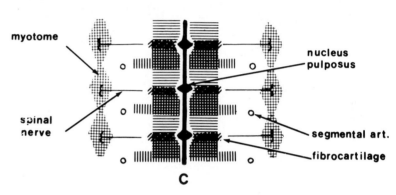

FIGURE 2–4. Schematic illustration showing developmental changes in the sclerotome and notochord. *A,* Embryonic. *B,* Resegmentation. *C,* Mature. (From Parke WW: Development of the spine. *In* Rothman RH, Simeone FA [eds]: The Spine. Philadelphia, WB Saunders Co, 1975, Vol 1, pp 1–17.)

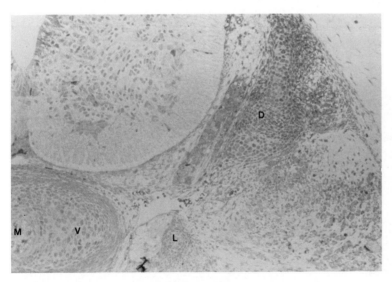

FIGURE 2–5. A mammalian embryo during the chondrification phase shows the three paired centers of chondrification—ventral (V), dorsal (D), and intermediate or lateral (L)—surrounding the mucoid streak (M). (From McLone DG: Development of the spine and spinal cord. *In* Cockard A, Hayward R, Hoff J: Neurosurgery. The Scientific Basis of Clinical Practice, Vol. 1, 2nd ed. London, Blackwell Scientific, 1992, pp 84–91.)

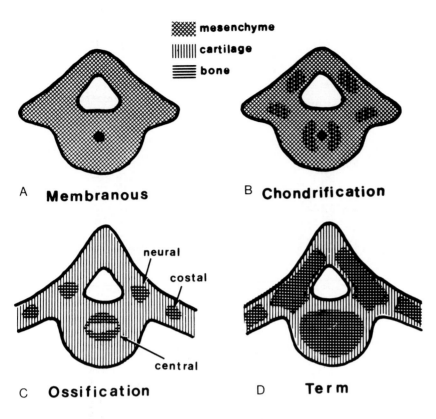

A **Membranous**   B **Chondrification**

C **Ossification**   D **Term**

FIGURE 2–6. Schematic illustration of the sequential development of vertebral components: (a) membranous, (b) chondrification, (c) ossification, (d) term. (From Parke WW: Development of the spine. *In* Rothman RH, Simeone FA [eds]: The Spine. Philadelphia, WB Saunders Co, 1975, Vol 1, pp 1–17.)

the pedicles; the junction of the dorsal and ventral ossification centers marks the neurocentral synchondrosis[20] (Fig. 2–7). This *neurocentral joint* lies within the developing vertebral body; therefore the terms centrum and vertebral body are not equivalent, since the vertebral body contains elements derived from both the centrum and dorsal ossification centers (Fig. 2–8).

Ossification of the vertebral bodies begins in the lower thoracic and upper lumbar spine and proceeds both cranially and caudally from this point. Ossification of the dorsal neural arch begins cranially in the cervical spine and proceeds caudally; however, the final union of the laminae begins in the lumbar spine and proceeds cranially.[21, 22]

Secondary ossification centers appear later during child-

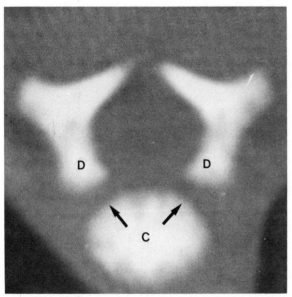

FIGURE 2–7. Computed tomography (CT) scan through the vertebra of a term human infant shows the single ossification center in the centrum (C) and the paired dorsal ossification centers (D). Arrows indicate the cartilaginous neurocentral synchondrosis.

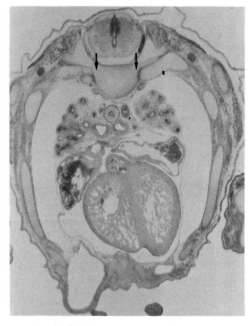

FIGURE 2–8. Light micrograph of a human embryo at 35 days of gestation shows the contribution of the dorsal ossification center to the vertebral body *(arrows)*.

hood and are located in the transverse processes, spinous processes, and ring apophyses. These secondary centers fuse with the primary centers by 15 or 16 years of age.

An understanding of vertebral development allows some insight into how vertebral malformations might arise. For example, hemivertebrae may result from unilateral maldevelopment of a cartilaginous center and, secondarily, a vertebral centrum. In contrast, anterior or posterior anomalies of the vertebral bodies might arise from defects in ventral or dorsal vertebral body ossification centers (Fig. 2–9).

Dorsal laminar fusion usually occurs by 1 to 3 years of age. However, a localized failure of laminar fusion may occur at one or more segments as spina bifida occulta and is seen in as many as 10 per cent of adults.[23] Spina bifida occulta occurs with decreasing frequency at the following vertebral levels: L5, S1, C1, C7, T1, and lower thoracic levels.

DEVELOPMENT OF THE CRANIOVERTEBRAL JUNCTION

While the general developmental plan previously discussed holds true for the majority of the spine, the two ends of the spine (the craniovertebral junction and the sacrum) undergo significant modifications. The development of the craniovertebral junction is particularly complex and embryologically unstable; malformations are therefore more frequent in this location. The development of this region is covered in greater detail in a subsequent chapter; its development will be only briefly summarized here.

The craniovertebral junction (encompassing the basicranium, axis, and atlas) develops from the last four occipital somites and the C1 sclerotome.[24] The basicranium is formed from the first four somites and forms the clivus, occipital condyles, and occipital squama. The C1 vertebral ring develops from the caudal portion of the first cervical sclerotome and the rostral portion of the second cervical sclerotome. This vertebra does not contain a centrum, but rather forms the C1 vertebral ring. The "body" of C1 is actually incorporated into the atlas as the odontoid process. The odontoid also receives a contribution from the fourth occipital sclerotome at its tip. The remainder of the atlas (the body and posterior neural arch) is derived from the second cervical sclerotome.

The atlas ossifies from two ossification centers, one in each of the lateral masses. The axis ossifies from five separate ossification centers: one that gives rise to the tip of the dens (derived from the fourth occipital sclerotome), two that form the dens proper (derived from the first cervical sclerotome), and one each for the body and posterior neural arch (both derived from the second cervical sclerotome). The dens is formed from bilaterally paired ossification centers that are present by 10 to 24 weeks of gestation and that ultimately fuse to give a single structure (Figs. 2–10 and 2–11). Fusion of the dens with the axis body begins at about 4 years of

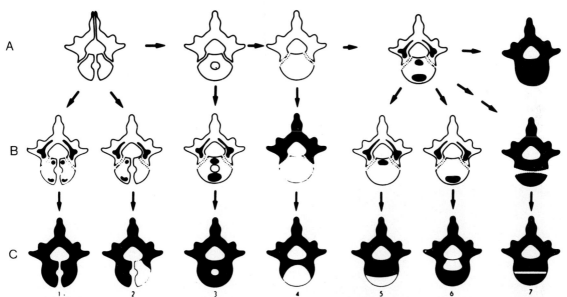

FIGURE 2–9. Normal vertebral development and possible developmental malformations. Cartilaginous development is shown in white, ossification in black: (A) normal sequence; (B) intermediate stage of abnormal development; (C) final stage of abnormality. 1, Sagittal cleft of body (butterfly vertebrae) results from nonfusion of the bilaterally paired cartilaginous centers. 2, Hemivertebrae result from nonfusion of the cartilaginous centers and subsequent nondevelopment of the ossification centers on one side. 3, Notochordal remnants. 4, Absent vertebral body results from nondevelopment of ossification centers. 5, Hypoplastic vertebral body from nondevelopment of the anterior ossification center. 6, Hypoplastic vertebral body from nondevelopment of the posterior ossification center. 7, Failure of fusion of the anterior and posterior ossification centers. (From Harwood-Nash DC, Fitz CR: Neuroradiology of Infants and Children. St. Louis, CV Mosby, 1976.)

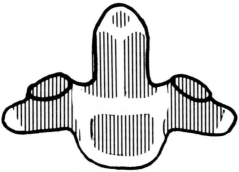

FIGURE 2–10. The ossification centers of the axis. The paired lateral centers and central ossification center are the same as for the remaining vertebrae; however, the odontoid shows two bilaterally paired primary centers and a single secondary apical center. (From Parke WW: Development of the spine. *In* Rothman RH, Simeone FA (eds): The Spine. Philadelphia, WB Saunders Co, 1975, Vol 1, pp 1–17.)

age and is completed by about 8 years; fusion of the tip of the dens with the dens proper does not occur until about 12 years.

A number of anomalies may arise through abnormal development of this complex region. The atlas may fail to separate completely from the basiocciput and remain fused with the clivus, a condition known as assimilation of the atlas. The anterior or posterior atlas ossification centers may fail to develop or to fuse properly and result in bifid or deficient C1 laminae or anterior arch. Failure of the odontoid to properly fuse with the axis body results in an *os odontoideum;* failure of the odontoid tip to fuse with the odontoid proper results in an *ossiculum terminale* (or *os avis*). Failure of the odontoid to properly form from the second cervical sclerotome results in odontoid agenesis or hypoplasia. These malformations are discussed in greater detail in a subsequent chapter.

DEVELOPMENT OF THE SACRUM AND COCCYX

The sacrum and coccygeal vertebrae are the last to develop at 31 days of gestation. In addition to the nor-

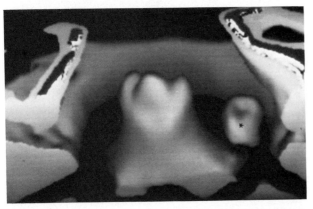

FIGURE 2–11. Three-dimensional CT reconstruction of the atlas and axis in a child demonstrates the three components of the odontoid. Note also the presence of an accessory ossification center *(asterisk).*

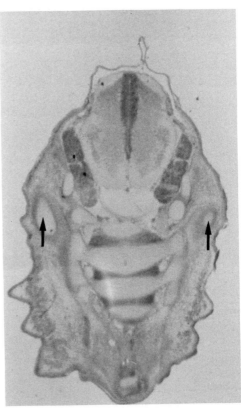

FIGURE 2–12. Photomicrograph of the caudal vertebral segments of a 35-day-old human embryo shows the segmental development of the sacrum with the two additional lateral centers *(arrows).*

mal developmental sequence previously described, the first three sacral elements contain an extra pair of ossification centers (Fig. 2–12). Fusion of the sacral vertebrae begins during early puberty and is complete by the middle part of the third decade.

The coccyx is formed from rudimentary segments; ossification of the first segment begins between 1 and 4 years of age. The remaining coccygeal segments ossify in rostrocaudal order from the fifth through the 20th years. The coccyx is usually segmented, although fusion occasionally occurs.

POSTNATAL DEVELOPMENT OF THE SPINE

The developmental changes of the spine during childhood are readily evaluated with standard radiographs or with computed tomography (CT). Magnetic resonance imaging (MRI) techniques offer a new noninvasive means to study the developing spine. During the first two postnatal years the spine demonstrates changes related to ossification of the cartilaginous end plates, conversion of red marrow to yellow marrow, responses to weight-bearing stresses, and changes in the water content of the disc. During the first 6 months, the spine is relatively straight due in part to the lack of weight-bearing forces. Red marrow occupies the vertebral body and is hypointense on T1- and T2-weighted images. The cartilaginous end plates are hyperintense on T1-, and hypointense on T2-weighted images (Fig. 2–13*A* and *B*; Fig. 2–14*A* and *B*).

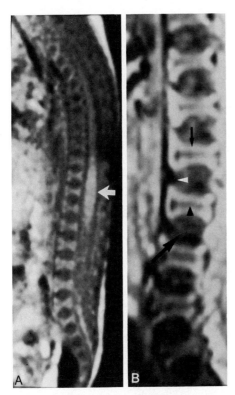

FIGURE 2–13. Magnetic resonance imaging of the spine (T1-weighted, sagittal) in a newborn. *A,* Relatively straight spine with slightly bulbous conus medullaris *(arrow).* *B,* Coned-down view of the lower thoracic-lumbosacral spine demonstrates hypointensity of the red bone marrow *(large arrow)* with intersegmental vessels *(white arrowhead),* hyperintensity of the cartilaginous end plates *(small black arrow),* and hypointensity of the intervertebral discs *(black arrowhead).* (From Byrd SE, Wilczynski MA: Imaging modalities for the pediatric spine. Curr Opin Radiol Dec 3(6):906–918, 1991.)

By six months, the end plates have largely ossified and have become hypointense on both T1- and T2-weighted images. Between 6 and 12 months, the red marrow is replaced by yellow marrow; this gives a mixed signal, which is slightly hyperintense on T1- and hypointense on T2-weighted images. The intervertebral disc at this age is isointense on T1- and hypointense on T2-weighted images (Fig. 2–15*A* and *B;* Fig. 2–16).

The spine during gestation has a C-shaped profile. Postnatally, this curve begins to straighten and a lordotic curve develops in the lumbar region. The final configuration of spinal curvature develops during early childhood.

As the child begins to sit and then to stand, the normal spinal curvatures begin to appear. From 6 months to 2 years of age, the vertebral bodies undergo a normal but unusual change in imaging characteristics. The rostral half of each vertebral body becomes hyperintense on T1-weighted images, whereas the lower half becomes hypointense. This difference is not appreciated on T2-weighted images. By two years of age, these changes have disappeared, and the child has a more characteristic composition and a curvature reminiscent of the adult spine. The ossified cortex of the vertebrae at this age are hypointense on all sequences. The inter-

vertebral disc, annulus fibrosus, and nucleus pulposus can all usually be differentiated by 5 years of age (Fig. 2–17*A* through *C*).

CONGENITAL ANOMALIES OF THE SPINE

As we previously discussed, congenital anomalies of the spine are relatively rare and are perhaps related to the enormous capacity of the embryo to regulate and overcome developmental insults. The cause of many of these vertebral anomalies is obscure; however, extrapolating from what we know of normal spinal development allows some insight into the timing and pathogenesis of these insults.

Vertebral malformations may conveniently be divided into those that arise through a disorder of formation and those that represent a disorder of segmentation. In many instances, disorders of both formation and segmentation will coexist.

Defects of vertebral formation may be partial or complete and may be unilateral or bilateral. Examples of unilateral partial failures of formation include wedge or trapezoid vertebrae, whereas unilateral complete failure would result in hemivertebrae (Fig. 2–18). Complete failure of vertebral development would result in caudal (lumbar and/or sacral) agenesis (Fig. 2–19).

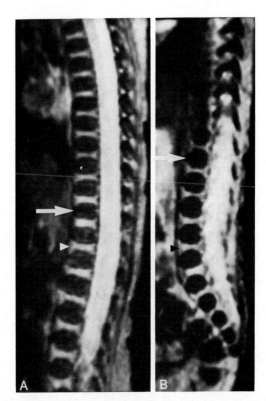

FIGURE 2–14. *A,* T2-weighted sagittal magnetic resonance imaging of lower thoracic-lumbosacral spine in a newborn. *B,* T2-weighted gradient echo image shows hypointensity of the red bone marrow *(large arrow),* hypointensity of the cartilaginous end plates *(small arrow),* and hyperintensity of the intervertebral discs *(arrowhead).* (From Byrd SE, Wilczynski MA: Imaging modalities for the pediatric spine. Curr Opin Radiol Dec 3(6):906–918, 1991.)

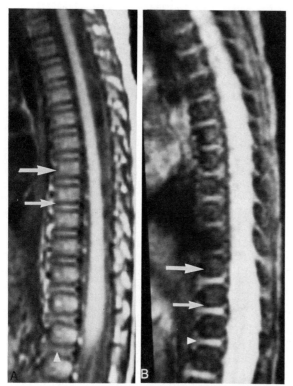

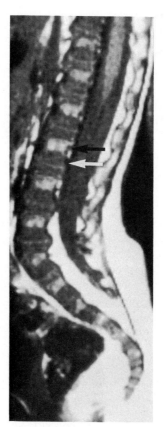

FIGURE 2–15. Magnetic resonance images of thoracic upper lumbar spine (sagittal view) in a 7-month-old infant. *A,* T1-weighted image shows slight hyperintensity of the bone marrow *(large arrow),* hypointensity of the ossifying end plates *(small arrow),* and isointensity of the intervertebral discs *(arrowhead). B,* T2-weighted image shows hypointensity of the bone marrow *(large arrow),* hypointensity of the cortical end plates *(small arrow),* and hyperintensity of the intervertebral discs *(arrowhead).* (From Byrd SE, Wilczynski MA: Imaging modalities for the pediatric spine. Curr Opin Radiol Dec 3(6):906–918, 1991.)

FIGURE 2–16. Magnetic resonance image of lower thoracic and lumbosacral spine (sagittal view) in a 7-month-old infant. T1-weighted image shows a striated appearance to the vertebral bodies with the upper half demonstrating hyperintensity *(black arrow)* and the lower half demonstrating hypointensity *(white arrow).* (From Byrd SE, Wilczynski MA: Imaging modalities for the pediatric spine. Curr Opin Radiol Dec 3(6):906–918, 1991.)

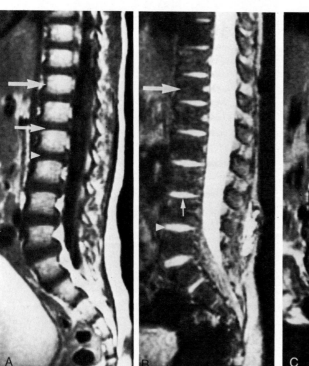

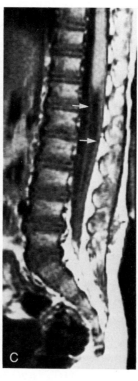

FIGURE 2–17. Magnetic resonance images of the lower thoracic-lumbosacral spine (sagittal view) in a 2-year-old child. *A,* T1-weighted image shows slight hyperintensity of bone marrow *(large arrow),* hypointensity of the cortical end plate *(small arrow),* and hypointensity of the discs *(arrowhead). B,* T2-weighted image shows hypointensity of bone marrow *(large arrow)* and cortical end plates *(small arrow)* and hyperintensity of the discs *(arrowhead). C,* Magnetic resonance image (T1-weighted, sagittal view) of the lower thoracic and lumbosacral spine in a normal child demonstrates the cauda equina as two main bundles *(arrows).* (From Byrd SE, Wilczynski MA: Imaging modalities for the pediatric spine. Curr Opin Radiol Dec 3(6):906–918, 1991.)

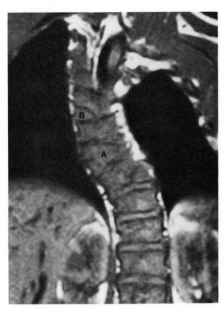

FIGURE 2–18. Magnetic resonance image of the spine in a child shows multiple segmentation anomalies. Both wedge (A) and hemivertebrae (B) are present.

Defects in segmentation result in failure of separation of the vertebrae and various degrees of vertebral fusion. Examples of defective segmentation include block vertebrae and unsegmented bars (Fig. 2–20). The disorder may be limited to two adjacent vertebrae or may extend over several vertebral segments. Anterior, poste-

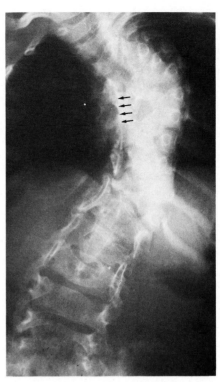

FIGURE 2–20. Radiograph of the midthoracic spine of a child shows an unsegmented bar *(arrows)* and the severe scoliosis due to the restricted growth on the side of the bar.

rior, or combined fusions may exist in isolation or combination. The Klippel-Feil syndrome represents a severe form of multifocal segmentation anomaly in which multiple adjacent vertebrae are fused in various combinations. Lateral segmentation anomalies are thought to arise during membranous and cartilaginous phases of vertebral development, whereas vertebral body segmentation anomalies are thought to arise through disordered ossification.

The outcome from vertebral anomalies is variable. Hemivertebrae or wedge-shaped vertebrae may contribute to asymmetric growth of the spine and result in scoliosis; unilateral segmentation anomalies such as unsegmented bars have a similar fate and carry the worst prognosis for progressive spinal deformity. Bilateral segmentation anomalies such as block vertebrae result in the least spinal deformity, but limit growth at that segment. Symmetric anterior segmentation anomalies generally produce kyphosis, whereas posterior anomalies produce lordosis.

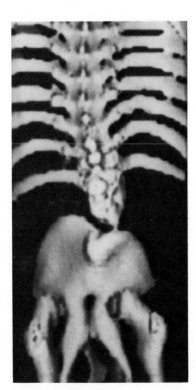

FIGURE 2–19. A reformatted image of a spine CT in a child with caudal agenesis. Note the absence of most of the lumbar vertebrae and all of the sacral spine.

REFERENCES

1. Keynes RJ, Stern CD: Mechanisms of vertebrate segmentation. Development 103:413, 1988.
2. Schoenwolf GC, Garcia-Martinez V, Dias MS: Mesoderm movement and fate during avian gastrulation and neurulation. Dev Dynamics 193:235, 1992.
3. Tam PPL, Meier S: The establishment of a somitomeric pattern in the mesoderm of the gastrulating mouse embryo. Am J Anat 164:209, 1982.

4. Lipton BH, Jacobson AG: Analysis of normal somite development. Dev Biol 38:73, 1974.
5. Bellairs R, Veine M: Experimental analysis of control mechanisms in somite segmentation in avian embryos. II. Reduction of material in the gastrula stages of the chick. J Embryol Exp Morphol 79:183, 1984.
6. Peacock A: Observations on the pre-natal development of the intervertebral disc in man. J Anat 85:260, 1951.
7. Fraser RC: Somite genesis in the chick. III. The role of induction. J Exp Zool 45:151, 1960.
8. Revel JP, Yip P, Chang LL: Cell junctions in the early chick embryo—a freeze etch study. Dev Biol 35:302, 1973.
9. Ostrovsky D, Sanger JW, Lash JW: Light microscope observations on actin distribution during morphogenetic movements in the chick embryo. J Embryol Exp Morphol 78:23, 1983.
10. Christ B, Jacob HJ, Jacob M: On the formation of the myotomes in avian embryos. An experimental and scanning electron microscope study. Experientia 34:514, 1978.
11. Christ B, Jacob M, Jacob HJ, Brand B, Wachtler F: Myogenesis: a problem of cell distribution and cell interactions. *In* Bellairs R, Ede DA, Lash JW (eds): Somites in Developing Embryos. New York, Plenum Press, pp 261–275, 1986.
12. Flint OP, Ede DA, Wilby OK, Proctor J: Control of somite number in normal and amputated mutant mouse embryos: an experimental and a theoretical analysis. J Embryol Exp Morphol 45:189, 1978.
13. Tam PPL: The control of somitogenesis in mouse embryos. J Embryol Exp Morphol 65(Suppl):103, 1981.
14. Bagnall KM, Sanders EJ, Higgins SJ, Leam H: The effects of somite removal on vertebral formation in the chick. Anat Embryol 178:183, 1988.
15. O'Rahilly R, Meyer DB: The timing and sequence of events in the development of the human vertebral column during the embryonic period proper. Anat Embryol 157:167, 1979.
16. Remack R: Untersuchungen über die Entwicklung der Wirbelthiere. Berlin, Reimer, 1855.
17. Bagnall KM, Higgins SJ, Sanders EJ: The contribution made by a single somite to the vertebral column: experimental evidence in support of resegmentation using the chick-quail chimaera model. Development 103:69, 1988.
18. Verbout AJ: A critical review of the ''Neugliederung'' concept in relation to the development of the vertebral column. Acta Biotheor (Leiden) 25:219, 1976.
19. Hall BK: Developmental and Cellular Skeletal Biology. New York, Academic Press, 1978.
20. Sherk HH, Park WW: Developmental anatomy. *In* Bailley RW (ed): The Cervical Spine. Philadelphia, J.B. Lippincott Co., 1983.
21. Noback CR, Robertson GG: Sequences of appearance of ossification centers in the human skeleton during the first five prenatal months. Am J Anat 89:1, 1951.
22. O'Rahilly R, Meyer DB: Roentgenographic investigation of the human skeleton during early fetal life. Am J Roentgenol 76:455, 1979.
23. Schmorl G, Junghanns H: The Human Spine in Health and Disease, 2nd ed. New York, Grune and Stratton, 1971.
24. Jenkins FA: The evolution and development of the dens of the mammalian axis. Anat Rec 164:173, 1969.

Chapter 3

SPINA BIFIDA

DONALD H. REIGEL, M.D., and DEBORAH ROTENSTEIN, M.D.

Spina bifida is the most common central nervous system birth defect encountered by the pediatric neurosurgeon. Although archaeologic observations reveal the presence of spina bifida for 3000 years, the person who first used the term "spina bifida" remains unknown.[1] Traditionally, spina bifida was defined by characteristic developmental abnormalities of the vertebrae and spinal cord. More recently, associated profound changes in the cerebrum, brainstem and peripheral nerves and continuing complications from these abnormalities have been appreciated. The expression of spina bifida encompasses the entire central nervous system, ranging in severity from merely an absent spinous process with normal intraspinal structures to the other extreme of myelomeningocele, Chiari malformation, hydrocephalus, and cortical cytoarchitectural changes. The multisystem abnormalities associated with spina bifida contribute to its widely accepted identity as the most complex developmental defect compatible with long life.

The ongoing debate over the ethics and technique of primary closure has gradually moved on to the recognition of a variety of delayed neurologic and systemic complications of spina bifida. Awareness of one of these complications, tethered spinal cord, has led to improved microsurgical neural tube reconvolution and anatomic closure. Marked advances in neuroimaging techniques have provided a more precise definition of the pathologic anatomy of the spinal cord, Chiari malformation, and the cerebral cortex and its commissures. Ultrasonography has provided us with the opportunity to recognize spina bifida during intrauterine life and to follow the development of these spinal, cerebellar, and ventricular abnormalities. Our increased understanding of the continuum of multidisciplinary care required from the prenatal period through maturity has improved and enhanced the prognosis for a rewarding and meaningful life for each newborn with spina bifida.

TERMINOLOGY

Spina Bifida Occulta. This term refers to anatomic abnormalities of the vertebrae identified on spine x-ray films. The spinous process of one or more vertebrae is absent, along with minor amounts of the vertebral arch (failure of fusion of the posterior arch). This change may be found in 20 to 30 per cent of the general population and is most frequently seen on incidental x-ray films at the L5 and S1 level. Usually, the central nervous system, cauda equina and peripheral nervous system are not involved.

The overlying skin and the neurologic examination are normal. However, when spine x-ray films demonstrating these changes are obtained because of the presence of a skin abnormality, such as dimples, sinus tracts, hypertrichosis, or capillary hemangiomas, the suspicion of an occult intraspinal lesion increases. These abnormalities, including epidermoid and dermoid tumors, lipomas, diastematomyelia, dural bands and tethered spinal cord, are grouped under the terms *occult spinal dysraphism, occult spinal lesions* and *meningocele manqué*.[2, 3]

The high frequency of spina bifida occulta has led many to question the significance of its relationship to back pain, enuresis and scoliosis.[4-6] In recent studies of patients treated in emergency rooms (which excluded those with spine abnormalities, back pain, and enuresis), a 22 per cent incidence of spina bifida occulta was discovered, and the incidence progressively declined with increasing age.[7] The high incidence, with or without associated problems, has not permitted conclusions about the clinical significance of uncomplicated spina bifida occulta. Indeed, many have placed little emphasis upon this isolated finding and have suggested that the diagnosis be omitted from the x-ray report. Perhaps of more overriding concern is the question whether spina bifida occulta is related to the overall spectrum of expressions of spina bifida and therefore deserves special consideration in genetic counseling.[8, 9] Data pertinent to this point are incomplete, and at this time, the increased association of spina bifida occulta with occult intraspinal lesions is the most important consideration.

Spinal Dysraphism. This is a generic term describing pathologic conditions that occur because of improper development (fusion) of the posterior neuropore. These conditions express themselves as abnormalities of ectodermal, mesodermal, and neuroectodermal tissues of the fetus[10] (Chapter 1). The term is frequently used to encompass all conditions associated with spina bifida.

Meningocele. Meningocele designates a skin- or membrane-covered cystic midline mass usually found in the lumbodorsal area, although it has also been found in the cervicothoracic area. Meningocele has also been identified with the Dandy-Walker syndrome.[11, 12] It is most commonly found at the time of birth, and patients with meningocele comprise about 10 per cent of all patients with spina bifida.[13] The dorsal half of one or more vertebrae is absent, and the contents of the bulge are limited to cerebrospinal fluid, meninges, and skin. However, tissue discarded at the time of operative treatment frequently shows histologic evidence of ganglion cells, aberrant peripheral nerve, and occasionally tissue suggestive of spinal cord. As with spina bifida occulta, a high index of suspicion must be maintained regarding associated occult intraspinal lesions, either at the site of the meningocele or at a removed location.[14] Generally, the remainder of the central nervous system is not involved, and the prognosis for development is excellent. Hydrocephalus is associated with meningocele, but much less frequently than the 80 to 90 per cent incidence expected with myelomeningocele.

Myelomeningocele. Including spina bifida cystica and spina bifida aperta, this form of spina bifida is associated with severe neurologic change and is identified at birth by a posterior midline mass covered by a membrane that may or may not incorporate nervous tissue and leak cerebrospinal fluid. Vertebral anomalies include (1) absence of the spinous process and lamina, (2) reduction in the anterior-posterior size of the vertebral body, (3) increased interpedicular distance, (4) decreased height of the pedicle, and (5) large laterally extending transverse processes. Often, adjacent transverse processes fuse and surround the exiting peripheral nerve. The midline mass is most frequently located in the thoracolumbar area and contains cerebrospinal fluid, meninges, cauda equina and abnormal spinal cord (neural plaque) (Fig. 3–1). Several abnormalities of the cerebrum and cerebellum have been described, in addition to the Chiari malformation, which is present in all patients with myelomeningocele. Depending upon the series reported, at least 75 per cent of patients develop hydrocephalus. Clinical examination reveals sensory and motor changes distal to the anatomic level of the lesion that produce varying degrees of anesthesia, weakness of the lower extremities, and urine and fecal incontinence. Orthopedic deformity and other system anomalies are also commonly present.

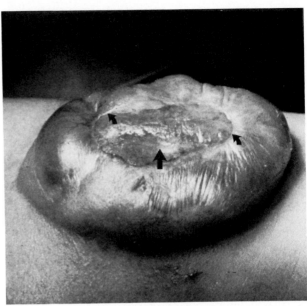

FIGURE 3–1. Thoracolumbar myelomeningocele showing the neuroplaque *(straight arrow)* and the white line that defines the junctional zone of the arachnoid, dura, and skin *(curved arrows).*

Spina bifida cystica refers to either meningocele or myelomeningocele,[15] whereas *spina bifida aperta* (open) implies that the lesion communicates with the environment.

Neural Plaque. Neural plaque indicates the dorsal neural tissue contained within a myelomeningocele, consisting of spinal cord (usually abnormal conus medullaris). A midline groove may be visualized; this is the anterior half of the neural groove that is, embryologically, the central canal of the spinal cord. Often, cerebrospinal fluid exits from the proximal portion of this groove—the distal intact central canal (Fig. 3–2).

Myelocystocele. Myelocystocele occurs at the terminal end of the neural axis and is identified at birth by a midline skin-covered mass in the intragluteal fold. This lesion is thought to evolve secondary to embryonic hydromyelia, which produces a distal trumpeting, or ballooning, of the cord and spinal fluid through a posterior vertebral defect (spina bifida).[16] Therefore, the sacral mass contains dilated spinal cord, spinal fluid, lipoma, fibrous bands, and meninges. The spinal cord is tethered by the terminal expansion of the spinal cord and, in the absence of release, commits the child to progressive neurologic deficit. The embryology is discussed in Chapter 1. Frequently, myelocystocele is associated with exstrophy of the bladder. Imaging studies such as ultrasonography are often required to differentiate myelocystocele from sacrococcygeal teratoma.

Lipomeningocele, Lipomyelomeningocele, Lipomyeloschisis,[17] and Lipomyelolipoma.[18] These refer to the lipomatous content of the spina bifida lesion. The lipoma may be extradural, intradural, or both. Lipoma invades the dorsal spinal cord or conus medullaris, with associated envelopment of the cauda equina (Fig. 3–3). Naidich and co-workers have described the embryologic, radiographic, and surgical anatomy of

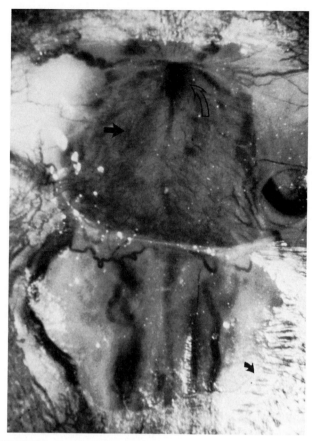

FIGURE 3–2. External appearance at lumbar myelomeningocele. The open arrow points to the central canal, the solid straight arrow identifies neuroplaque, and the curved black arrow indicates junctional zone.

these lesions, and this information aids immensely in surgical considerations.[17]

Anterior Meningocele. This term most commonly refers to a pelvic mass or, rarely, a thoracic mass that communicates with the spinal subarachnoid space through a small opening in the anterior vertebral column. The content of the mass is primarily cerebrospinal fluid; however, a variety of tumors such as teratomas, lipomas, neurofibromas and dermoids have been associated with anterior meningocele. This lesion is also the result of abnormal development of the distal neural tube (Chapter 1).

Rachischisis. Rachischisis describes a condition of the fetus in which the brain and spinal cord are dorsally exposed to the environment. This lesion results from complete lack of closure of the neural groove and occurs at approximately 15 to 23 days of gestation.[19] This rare anomaly is incompatible with survival.

Chiari II Malformation. This term denotes a congenital anomaly of the hindbrain that is almost always associated with myelomeningocele. The medulla oblongata and pons are posteriorly bowed and elongated, frequently extending into the rostral cervical spinal canal, along with the cerebellar vermis. Abnormalities of the posterior skull, dura, medulla oblongata, pons, midbrain, cerebellum, cerebral hemispheres, cisterns, and ventricles have been described[20–22] (Table 3–1).

INCIDENCE AND EPIDEMIOLOGY

Spina bifida occulta is relatively common in our society, with incidence rates reported to be as high as 30 per cent.[7] During the past 50 years, incidence figures for open spina bifida (myelocele and myelomeningocele) have been reported to be declining in many areas of the world. Prior to the early 1980s, the incidence was thought to be as high as 1 to 2 per 1000 live births in the United States and from 4 to 5 per 1000 live births in regions of Ireland.[23, 24] Current figures indicate a drop in the United States from 5.9 per 10,000 births in 1984 to 3.2 per 10,000 births in 1992.[25] The declining incidence may be the result of many factors and could include improved maternal nutrition and availability of prenatal screening and diagnosis, selective pregnancy termination, undetermined environmental changes, and vitamin supplementation. Geographic variations continue to exist, but at a lower incidence. Thus, the incidence decreases from east to west in the United States, and from north to south in the British Isles.[26, 27] Incidence remains higher in females than in males.[28, 29]

FIGURE 3–3. Lipomyelomeningocele. The open arrow points to spinal cord anterior to large lipoma contiguous with conus.

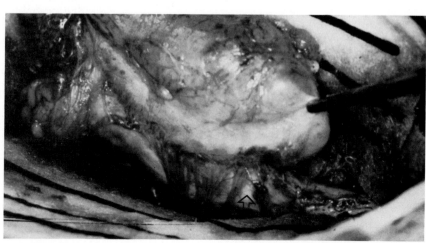

TABLE 3–1. ANOMALIES ASSOCIATED WITH THE ARNOLD-CHIARI–SPINA BIFIDA COMPLEX

Cerebellum	Caudal displacement of vermis and fourth ventricle; cerebellum smaller than normal
Brainstem	Caudal displacement of pons, medulla, and cervicomedullary junction with kink; displaced basilar and vertebral arteries; stretching of lower cranial nerves
Cervical and lower spinal cord	Compression of upper segments; hydrosyringomyelia
Midbrain	Tectal "beak"; aqueduct stenosis and forking
Cerebral hemispheres and third ventricle	Polymicrogyria; cortical heterotopia; enlarged massa intermedia; Meynert's commissure; hydrocephalus
Meninges	Hypoplasia of falx cerebri; low-set tentorium with enlarged incisura; low position of torcula and lateral sinuses; thick, adhesive leptomeninges at foramen magnum
Skull and cervical spine	Craniolacunia; enlarged foramen magnum; small posterior fossa; scalloped petrous bone; enlarged upper cervical spinal canal

The rates of incidence are also much lower in blacks and Asians than in whites.[26] The incidence of spina bifida does seem to increase with poverty and poor nutrition. However, these observations have not led to meaningful etiologic information, and reported clusters, at this time, have been explained by chance.[30] Studies of variations with season, maternal age, and parity do not seem to provide meaningful clues regarding etiology.[31–33] The fact that open spina bifida has been reported to be 13 times more common in spontaneously aborted fetuses than in full-term infants leads one to question what the true risk of neural tube defects may be with conception for any given parent.[34]

GENETICS

There is a familial tendency, or predisposition, to the occurrence of spina bifida.[35] The occurrence statistics do not fit mendelian transmission, although neural tube defects attributable to single genes have been described.[7, 36] Multifactorial inheritance[27] is strongly supported by environmental factors, familial tendency, declining risk with increasing distance of relatives, and the fact that when one or more siblings are affected there is a marked increase in risk for subsequent siblings to be affected. In North America, the risk of having a child with spina bifida is about 0.05 per cent. If there is one sibling with spina bifida, the risk of a sub-

sequent child having spina bifida increases to about 5 per cent, and if there are two, the risk increases to approximately 12 to 15 per cent.[37] Studies of monozygotic and dizygotic twins, consanguinity studies and environmental studies have produced little further information to elucidate genetic inheritance.[27, 38]

The known tendency of neural tube defects to recur in families suggests several possible genetic mechanisms, including a recessive gene, a dominant gene with reduced penetrance, a recessive X-linked gene, cytoplasmic inheritance, and polygenic inheritance. On the basis of pedigree analysis, Jorde and colleagues proposed that spina bifida occulta may be related to an autosomal dominant trait with a 75 per cent penetrance.[39] However, further analysis will be required to test this thesis. The fact that neural tube defects have been observed in chromosomal abnormality syndromes has added to the suspicion that there is a genetic form of spina bifida.[40]

Regardless of the genetic forms of inheritance, genetic counseling should be offered to all parents and close relatives of children with spina bifida. A detailed listing of facilities offering these services may be obtained from the National Foundation of the March of Dimes.[41]

ETIOLOGY

Interest in identifying etiologic factors of spina bifida has been driven by the goal of prevention. The incidence variation with season, geography, ethnic classification, social group, parity, and maternal age has fueled the search for an environmental factor. This search was exemplified by the theory of Renwick that a teratogenic substance existed in blighted potatoes that caused anencephaly and spina bifida.[27, 42] Subsequent trials of potato avoidance and evaluation of exposure patterns failed to produce convincing evidence to support the potato blight teratogen.[43, 44] Since that time, numerous teratogens have been suggested, including valporic acid, phenytoin, trimethadione, haloperidol, alcohol, viral infections, local anesthetics, triamcinolone, infectious diseases, hydroxyurea, hypervitaminosis, dextromethorphan, and maternal fever.[45–55] Despite the abundance of teratogens suggested for spina bifida, conclusive supporting data for a causal factor continue to be missing. Further review of teratogens affecting neural tube development is available from the literature search conducted by the Environmental Teratology Information Center, done at the request of the Teratology Society.[56]

Numerous nutritional deficiency states, including that of folic acid and zinc, have been suggested as etiologic factors for spina bifida. Early reports that folic acid supplementation, given prior to conception and continued afterward, is associated with a statistically significant reduction in neural tube defects when compared with unsupplemented groups have now been confirmed.[57–61] Folic acid, 0.4 mg per day, given before conception and through early pregnancy, appears to substantially reduce, perhaps as much as 72 per cent, occurrence of spina bifida in high-risk and first pregnancies.[62–67] These important results have led people to suggest that folic acid prevents spina bifida, thus inferring that folate deficiency causes spina bifida. However, there have been no studies indicating folate deficiency of mothers of children with spina bifida.[68–71] Furthermore, affected pregnancies have been reported, despite the use of folate supplementation. Therefore, the mechanism appears to be protective rather than preventive because of deficiency. The evidence at this point has permitted the Center for Disease Control and the U.S. Public Health Service to recommend that all women of childbearing age consume the equivalent of 0.4 mg of folic acid per day in order to reduce the risk of having a child with a neural tube defect.[72] Perhaps the greater value from the studies of folic acid will be that they provided an important clue in the search for the cause and pathogenesis of spina bifida.

EMBRYOLOGY

The detailed discussion of the embryology of neural tube defects is contained in Chapter 1.

PATHOLOGY

Although the pathologic abnormalities observed at the site of the neural plaque may be the most obvious, additional changes are frequently found throughout the entire central and peripheral nervous systems.[73] Furthermore, there may be congenital defects in the genitourinary and cardiovascular systems. The variations and combinations are numerous, and awareness of this potential contributes to comprehensive understanding and treatment from the health care team and parents.

Brain

Lobar agenesis, polymicrogyria, holoprosencephaly, and cerebellar dysplasia and necrosis are commonly observed.[74] In addition, defects of cellular migration such as heterotopias, schizencephaly, and gyral anomalies have been described.[75] Agenesis of the corpus callosum, cysts of the septum pellucidum, midline lipoma, and arachnoid cysts have also been observed.[76] Hydrocephalus and associated anomalies of the aqueduct and cerebrospinal fluid pathways occur at a very high frequency (up to 90 per cent).

Spinal Cord

The most common site of spinal cord lesions is the distal thoracic, lumbar, or sacral area. Over 85 per cent of meningoceles and myelomeningoceles are found at these levels. Approximately 10 per cent are detected in the thoracic area, and an additional 5 per cent are found in the cervical area.[11, 15, 77] Occasionally, more than one lesion is observed, and as many as three have been reported.[14]

In about one third of patients, the neural plaque has an appearance like that of an open book, with the midline neural groove and caudal central canal visible at the rostral aspect of the lesion (see Fig. 3–2). The anterior columns of the spinal cord are frequently intact, whereas there are varying degrees of destruction of the dorsal columns and the internuncial pathways.[78] Since the neural plaque represents a splaying out of the neural tube, the dorsal roots exit from what appears to be the lateral anterior half of the spinal cord, and the ventral roots exit from the medial anterior neural plaque. In addition, the angle of exit of the nerve roots is more tangential than that of the rostral nerve roots. In approximately one third of the patients, the spinal cord rostral to the lesion shows diplomyelic changes, and about 40 per cent of patients have hydromyelia or syringomyelia.[78] These studies do not reveal the incidence of hydrocephalus, and therefore it is possible that a high frequency of uncontrolled hydrocephalus could artificially inflate the figures for occurrence of hydromyelia.

The arachnoid forming the cystic wall of the lesion is adherent to the neural plaque, dura, and skin. Intradural and extradural lipoma, dermoid, epidermoid, squamous cell carcinoma, histiocytoma, enterogenous cyst, and teratoma have been observed with myelomeningocele.[79–81]

Neuronal counts in the lumbrosacral spinal cords of children with myelomeningoceles have demonstrated reductions related to the degree of cord damage or of deformity present. Rostral spinal cord segments contain normal numbers of neurons.[82] Studies of the peripheral nervous systems of newborn children with myelomeningoceles have demonstrated reductions in the size of peripheral nerves. However, preservation of some or all the fibers of nerves distal to the plaque has been demonstrated.[83]

In patients with spina bifida, there is a high incidence of congenital malformations of other systems. A study of 434 patients with spina bifida demonstrated an average of 2.2 associated defects per patient.[84] Skeletal anomalies are the most frequent, with clubfeet and hip dislocation being the most common. Table 3–2 lists generally associated anomalies.

NEUROPHYSIOLOGY

In the past, it was commonly thought that the motor lesion of myelomeningocele was at the level of the anterior horn cell. However, clinical observations have revealed upper motor neuron lesions in patients with functioning isolated distal segments.[76] Stark and Drummond have demonstrated that neural plaque simula-

TABLE 3–2. SYSTEMIC ANOMALIES ASSOCIATED WITH SPINA BIFIDA

SKELETAL	GASTROINTESTINAL	PULMONARY	CRANIOFACIAL	CARDIOVASCULAR	GENITOURINARY
Clubfeet	Inguinal hernia	Tracheoesophageal fistula	Synostosis	Ventriculoseptal defect (VSD)	Hydronephrosis
Hip dislocation	Meckel's diverticulum	Situs inversus	Cleft palate	Atrial-septal defect (ASD)	Hydroureter
Rib anomalies	Malrotation		Strabismus	Patent ductus	Horseshoe kidney
Kyphoscoliosis	Omphalocele		Low-set ears	Coarctation	Undescended testes
Pectus excavatum	Imperforate anus		Hypertelorism		Hydrocele
Syndactyly					Malrotation, exstrophy

tion results in involuntary contraction of 80 to 100 per cent of the paralyzed muscles of the lower extremities.[85] The magnitude of contraction was similar to that observed following peripheral nerve stimulation of normal infants. Absence of fibrillation potentials further led Stark and Drummond to conclude that paralysis associated with myelomeningocele was secondary to an upper motor neuron lesion. They postulated that the lesion was either within the plaque itself or just rostral to the plaque.[85] The etiology of the upper motor neuron lesion remains undetermined. Possible explanations include abnormal development and change occurring in the neural plaque before, during, and after birth.

Somatosensory evoked potential studies of newborn children with myelomeningoceles have demonstrated intact sensory pathways to and from the neural plaque. In two of seven patients studied, afferent integrity through the plaque was observed.[86] Therefore, interference with afferent conduction appears to be located at the level of the neural plaque.

The observation of functioning motor and sensory systems within the neural plaque provides further support for meticulous protection and preservation of the neural plaque vascular supply during early surgical care of the patient with myelomeningocele. Furthermore, these findings, coupled with Lendon's observation of normal neuronal populations in the rostral spinal cord,[82] have provided the background data to justify cauda equina reconstruction, as described by Epstein and co-workers, in which proximal intercostal nerves are anastomosed to nerve roots distal to the lesion.[87] Early electromyographic observations have indicated reinnervation of muscle groups within the lower extremities. This exciting technique offers the possibility of bypassing the afferent and efferent interruption that occurs at the level of the plaque but requires further investigation and long-term study.[82, 87]

PRENATAL DIAGNOSIS

Open neural tube defects permit fetal protein (alpha-fetoprotein) to enter amniotic fluid and the maternal bloodstream. Elevations of alpha-fetoprotein peak at about 15 to 18 weeks following the last menstrual period.[88] Separate collaborative studies in the United States and the United Kingdom have shown maternal serum alpha-fetoprotein assays to be an effective way of screening for identification of the fetus with an open neural tube defect.[88–90] This method has an accuracy of 60 to 70 per cent. If alpha-fetoprotein levels are elevated on two separate occasions, sonographic results are negative, and corrections for weight, race, gestational age, multiple gestations, placental bleeding and other anomalies (omphalocele, gastroschisis) are not explanatory, amniocentesis is recommended. Analysis of alpha-fetoprotein and acetylcholinesterase of amniotic fluid have a protection rate of 97 per cent or greater, and a false-positive rate of 0.4 per cent for women with elevated maternal serum alpha-fetoprotein levels.[91, 92] Ultrasonography techniques are so highly developed that some experienced sonographers are reporting nearly 100 per cent detection rates.[93] It has been suggested that for women without a family history of neural tube defects and moderate elevations of alpha-fetoprotein with normal sonograms, amniocentesis may not be required.[93] Despite the presence of excellency of sonography, the occasional small, closed lesion may still go undetected, whether it be spina bifida or encephalocele.[94, 95] Genetic counseling may help to identify couples at high risk for a fetus with open neural tube defects (e.g., those with affected second or third degree relatives). Thus, prenatal screening programs lead to early intrauterine diagnosis, providing parents the opportunity to effectively prepare for the birth of a child with spinal bifida or to decide to terminate the pregnancy. For those electing to complete the pregnancy with a fetus with spina bifida, the route of delivery will become important. Current studies indicating prelabor cesarean section have not been prospective and have not considered variables in surgical treatment.[96, 97] Others having many of the same flaws have suggested that prelabor elective cesarean section carries no demonstrable advantage.[98, 99] Most pediatric neurosurgeons now recommend vaginal delivery in the absence of craniomegaly from hydrocephalus and a large, protruding spinal lesion. The decision to deliver via cesarean section should be based on obstetric indications such as breech presentation. Greater availability of nondirective genetic counseling and the widespread use of screening techniques can only benefit society. Neurosurgeons should be prepared to inform parents and relatives of children with spina bifida and the rapidly growing population of young adults with spina bifida of genetic counseling, screening, and diagnostic centers.

HISTORY OF TREATMENT

It is not known who first used the term spina bifida. It is known that neural tube defects of the sacrum have been identified in skeletons from the fifth millennium B.C.[1] The first description of a child with spina bifida was made by Peter Van Forest in 1587,[1, 100] and Tulp provided the first accurate anatomic illustrations of spina bifida in 1641.[1, 101, 102] In 1761, Morgagni related the clinical changes to the spinal cord lesion, and it was Lebedeff who, in 1881, first suggested failure of the neural tube to close.[1, 103, 104] In 1886, Von Recklinghausen classified the anatomic types of spina bifida and discussed treatment that included surgery.[105]

Although operative treatment for spina bifida may have occurred as early as 1610, when Forestus ligated a sac,[106] significant attempts to treat the lesion surgically did not occur until the twentieth century. Since the report of Fraser that of 131 patients operated upon, 63 per cent were discharged between 1898 and 1923, and 23 per cent were still alive in 1929,[107] there has been a steady succession of reports indicating continuously improving results with operative treatment. With the advent of aseptic surgical technique and antibiotics, an increasing number of surgeons began to consider operative closure of spina bifida. Care in selecting candidates for surgery was exercised, and often, extensive paralysis and hydrocephalus were contraindications to surgery. Operative delay was recommended in order to permit epithelialization of the lesion.[108, 109] While these measures led to a marked reduction in operative mortality, infection and hydrocephalus were still the leading causes of death in children with spina bifida.

With the introduction of antibiotics, cerebrospinal fluid shunts, modern pediatric anesthesia, and improved neonatal care came new hope and enthusiasm for children with spina bifida as exemplified by Matson, Nulsen, and Spitz, and by Sharrad and co-workers.[15, 110, 111] These improvements in care resulted in an unprecedented number of survivors with spina bifida. However, many early survivors had significant physical and mental disabilities. Care and support systems were not prepared for the continuum of associated problems such as a chronic urinary tract infection, reduced intellect, intractable shunt infections, unrelenting scoliosis, and psychosocial maladjustment. This led to a second wave of pessimism and the advancement of the concept of selecting ideal children for treatment while permitting (if not actively supporting) others who might not be expected to achieve an acceptable quality of life to die without treatment.[112] The criteria for withholding treatment included extensive paralysis, severe hydrocephalus, kyphosis, and associated major anomalies. Proponents of these criteria reported that death uniformly followed selection. Contrary to the original reports, numerous investigators found that significant numbers of these children denied treatment survived. These discussions catapulted the care of children with spina bifida into the center of an international medical ethics debate.[113] Frequently, the rhetoric was based on disproportionately small experiences and scientific

analysis. Since 1959, however, several studies of treatment results of unselected newborns have been completed. McLone analyzed these studies[114–117] and found that if selected patient populations are compared on the basis of continence, renal function, ambulation, mortality, and IQ, the results are distinctly better for current unselected series than for the highly selected series reported by Lorber.[118] Quite simply, the results of treatment and comprehensive continuing care are of such high quality that they have led most treatment centers to provide aggressive multidisciplinary care from infancy to adulthood. The outlook and potential for rewarding, meaningful existence now extends to all patients with spina bifida and puts the selection discussion to rest because it cannot be supported on the basis of clinical experience or ethical principles.

Thus, it is clear that the potential for a high quality of life has been documented and should give comfort to neurosurgeons, who have seen the operative mortality of primary closure go down to zero per cent and the survival rate for the first 2 years of life exceed 95 per cent. Nonetheless, despite these favorable survival statistics, two studies report that 35 per cent of 69 and 24 per cent of 58 children died within 6 months when treatment was withheld.[119, 120] The justification for no treatment in these reports was not the quality of life of the infant but the opportunity of making a decision and the quality of life for the parents. It is the experience of most large centers that families can cope, that financial support is available, and that increasing comprehensive programs for educational and psychosocial enrichment offer excellent opportunities for the child with spina bifida and the family.[121] We can now assure Father McCormick that infants with spina bifida will survive in relative comfort and will be able to experience our caring and love.[122]

CLINICAL ASSESSMENT

PRENATAL ASSESSMENT

Meningocele and myelomeningocele are usually evident at birth. With advances in prenatal diagnosis, such as alpha-fetoprotein analysis, amniocentesis, and ultrasound imaging, increased numbers of fetuses with spina bifida are being identified during intrauterine life. This has led parents to consult with a neurosurgeon during pregnancy. Often, these sessions include social workers, obstetricians, and neonatologists in order to fully prepare the parents and to plan for timely delivery, often by cesarean section. Most pediatricians and neurosurgeons now agree that prompt closure of the open lesion is associated with decreased mortality and morbidity rates. When prenatal diagnosis has been made and the parents have been prepared and informed, the baby should be taken to the operating room as soon as possible after delivery. Ultrasonography of the brain and general pediatric evaluation are completed promptly, preferably in the delivery room.

POSTNATAL ASSESSMENT

Initial Examination. If birth occurs at another hospital, infants are usually transferred as soon as possible. If the receiving hospital has the facilities, it is preferable to transfer the mother as well. This system of child-maternal transfer leads to complete participation of the parents in health care and to early acceptance and bonding to the mother. Routine intensive neonatal care is started immediately, and oral intake is withheld. Normothermia is rigorously maintained by continuous temperature monitoring. Lesions are covered with sterile, saline-moistened dressings, and the patient is kept in the prone or lateral decubitus position in order to protect exposed neural tissue. The initial evaluation includes prompt assessment of the infant's general pediatric condition and the degree of neurologic deficit or the functional level.

With the aid of the neonatalogist or the pediatrician, the possibility of associated cardiopulmonary, genitourinary, and gastrointestinal conditions that would interfere with early operation is ruled out. Occasionally, delivery is complicated by unexpected abnormal fetal presentation or hydrocephalus. Thus, initial observation should include a search for trauma. After general neurologic examination, the size and location of the lesion is noted. The rostral level of spinal cord involvement provides a general estimate of the level of the spinal cord lesion. The sensory-motor examination of a child with myelomeningocele is complicated by the presence of numerous normal and abnormal reflexes and possibly an element of spinal cord shock.[76, 85, 114] An understanding of this phenomenon is mandatory to prevent the parents and medical staff from developing an overly optimistic or pessimistic opinion about the motor potential of the child. Such understanding is also important for the surgeon, since the disappearance of reflex activity following the operation may be misinterpreted as a significant loss of function, or conversely, the appearance of motion that was previously absent may be falsely credited to operative treatment. Light pressure stimulation, motion, and sound may elicit abnormal reflex activities in the lower extremities that may have no bearing on future appearance of volitional motor function.

The sensory examination requires that the child be relaxed and quiet or even sleeping. The cutaneous dermatomes are stimulated sharply from distal to proximal until one identifies the dermatome that produces facial or upper extremity response characteristic of pain perception. Some have advocated that dermatomal somatosensory evoked potentials be used to evaluate and follow sensory function in children with myelomeningocele, and have suggested that these potentials may help to identify more precisely the future sensory level.[123]

The motor examination is also done with the child at rest and begins with sharp or painful stimulation of the torso or upper extremities, with observation for voluntary motion below the level of the lesion. Hip flexion and knee extension require the innervation of L1–L3, and adduction requires the innervation of L2–L4. Hip abduction, hip extension, and knee flexion require the presence of L5–S2. Plantar flexion and intrinsic muscle action of the feet require the preservation of the sacral roots.[124] Orthopedic deformities may also provide clues to the motor level. Patients with levels above T12, for example, often have flaccid hips and feet, whereas patients with lesions below L1–L2 have flail feet. Sharrad has described the limb and spinal deformities associated with neurologic deficit in detail.[124–127] Additional aid in identifying the sensory level may come in the future with the application of somatosensory evoked potentials.

Bladder Dysfunction. Over 90 per cent of patients with myelomeningocele have a form of neurogenic bladder. It is extremely difficult to predict the type of bladder dysfunction at the time of neonatal examination. Because of the presence of abnormal reflexes, anal wink and tone cannot be used as a reliable indication of perineal sensation. One must rely on observation to determine the presence of spontaneous voiding and the nature of the urinary stream. It is easy to perform Credé's maneuver on children with lower motor neuron defect (approximately 30 per cent), and they often remain dry. However, in patients with sphincter or bladder spasticity, Credé's maneuver may be extremely difficult to perform and cause ureteral reflux and subsequent infection. Reliable determination of bladder function may not be possible for months after closure. It is important that the high incidence of neurogenic bladder be recognized and that appropriate steps be taken to ensure that the bladder is intermittently and completely emptied. Usually, bowel incontinence is associated with bladder incontinence, and generally, lower motor neuron lesions produce anal relaxation and prolapse. As the child develops, bladder and bowel training programs offer the possibility of achieving socially acceptable continence.

DISCUSSIONS WITH PARENTS

Once the initial evaluation of the infant is completed, early repair of all lesions is recommended unless there are overriding pediatric complications or death is imminent (less than 1 per cent). Clearly, the parents always make the final decision concerning surgery, but it is the neurosurgeon's responsibility to provide current factual data on the natural untreated course and the prognosis with aggressive prompt management. Whether the diagnosis is made during the prenatal period or at the time of birth, the majority of couples will experience immense emotional turmoil and sadness. Their primary worries are related to prognosis for intellectual development, ambulation, and survival. The parents should be given the current data that 90 per cent or more of newborn children with myelomeningocele will survive, 80 per cent or more will have normal intelligence, and 85 per cent will walk with or without some form of assistance.[117] Extreme caution should be exercised regarding motor function in the lower extremities, and one should repeatedly emphasize that surgery will not restore function but will preserve existing function. The neurosurgeon will find it necessary to teach the parents about hydrocephalus, which develops in 80 to 90 per cent of infants with spina bifida, and to explain the meaning of neurogenic bowel and bladder. Today, it can be expected that 80 per cent of patients will become socially continent with the use of drugs and clean intermittent catheterization.[117] At the present time it is difficult to predict the patients who will have complete independence.

One must be continually cognizant of the fact that these are devastated parents with dashed dreams and that the responsibility of a "caring" surgeon is to provide the facts and to repeatedly teach the parents about the problem, the proposed treatment, and the support systems. Especially in the case of first-born children so affected, parents experience self-doubt and fears of inadequacy, along with profound guilt. It is helpful to assure the parents that these feelings are not unique to the parents of children with spina bifida, but that all parents feel guilt when their children are ill or injured. They also experience a natural universal doubt about parental competency. Assuring the parents that they can cope and introducing them to the team concept of continuing care and compassion of the entire multidisciplinary health care team will be of help. Finally, the parents are seeking guidance and help, and the neurosurgeon who has negative personal opinions about meaningful life for children with spina bifida will convey hesitancy, tentativeness, and doubt, which will only impair quality care and further unsettle the parents. The care team should assure the parents that it has confidence in them and in the prospects for a rewarding existence for their child. This requires a continuing commitment, through all phases of life, to the well-being of the child and the family. Given this approach, most parents request aggressive management and care.

Most people now believe that closure is not a surgical emergency and that a limited period of time should be used to inform and counsel parents.[128] Simultaneously, the pertinent members of the multidisciplinary team—nurses, social workers, orthopedists, urologists, and therapists—begin to participate in the care of the child and the family.

If the lesion is open and draining cerebrospinal fluid and surgery cannot be performed within 24 hours, or if the lesion is closed and surgery cannot be performed in 48 hours, surgery should be delayed until three negative, consecutive 24-hour cultures are obtained from the surface of the lesion. The lesion can usually be sterilized with good local care. If signs of sepsis or ventriculitis develop, treatment should consist of external ventricular drainage and systemic and intrathecal antibiotics until sterilization of the cerebrospinal fluid and lesion is achieved.[129]

OPERATIVE TECHNIQUE

The purposes of surgery are to preserve intellectual, motor, and sensory function by restoring the spinal cord to its normal cerebrospinal fluid environment and to prevent central nervous system infection. Meningitis and ventriculitis produce intellectual and developmental delay.[130] An additional purpose is to restore the normal contour of the back, which contributes to ease of care and future bracing.

The operative technique for primary closure of myelomeningocele has been described by many; modern methods include the use of the microscope, laser, and kyphectomy.[131–133] The general guidelines for closure include protection and preservation of exposed neural tissue, reconvolution of the spinal cord within the spinal canal, and a five-layer closure. Potentially neurotoxic scrubs and topical antibiotics are avoided. The five-layer closure begins with the reconvolution of the spinal cord by closing the pia-arachnoid and continues with sequential closure of the dura, iliocostal fascia, subcutaneous tissue, and skin. The operating microscope, microinstruments, and laser are used for reconvolution of the spinal cord while all forms of traction are avoided. Magnification leads to preservation of the vascular supply of the neural plaque, and the use of bipolar cautery is mandatory to avoid unnecessary neural trauma.

The child is placed in the prone position on bilateral, firm chest rolls so that the abdomen is suspended freely and femoral pulsation is maintained. The initial incision follows the circumferential white line formed by the junction of the arachnoid and the skin (Figs. 3–4A and B and 3–5). This leads to isolation of the neural plaque and the immediately rostral spinal cord. At this point, one may observe arachnoidal adhesions to the ventral, lateral intradural surface, and these are lysed by sharp dissection.

Following identification of the neural plaque and arachnoid investment, the dura is isolated. To identify the dura, the skin defect is extended rostrally in the midline in order to observe the inferior aspect of the most caudal intact lamina and, immediately beneath it, the intact dorsal dura (Fig. 3–6). With the normal rostral dura thus identified, the dura is then isolated by dissecting laterally and inferiorward in the epidural space to the caudal margin of the defect (Fig. 3–4C and D). The caudal defect is extended in the midline in order to identify the termination of the defect and the inferior dorsal dural surface.

With the use of the operating microscope and carbon dioxide laser, dural remnants, fat, and excess arachnoid are now sharply dissected free from the circumference of the neural plaque. Inclusion of these tissues in the intradural repair may lead to subsequent intraspinal lipoma and epidermoid tumor.[134, 135] Magnification is required at this point because it is the area of the alar plate or dorsal root entry zones. The medial aspect of the plaque represents the basilar plate, or area of the anterior horn cells. The lateral arachnoidal edges are now approximated in the midline with 7-0 suture or with CO_2 laser welding, thus reconstituting the neural plaque to a tubular structure resembling the remainder of the spinal cord (Figs. 3–4E and 3–7A). The interior of this tube is the continuation of the central spinal canal.

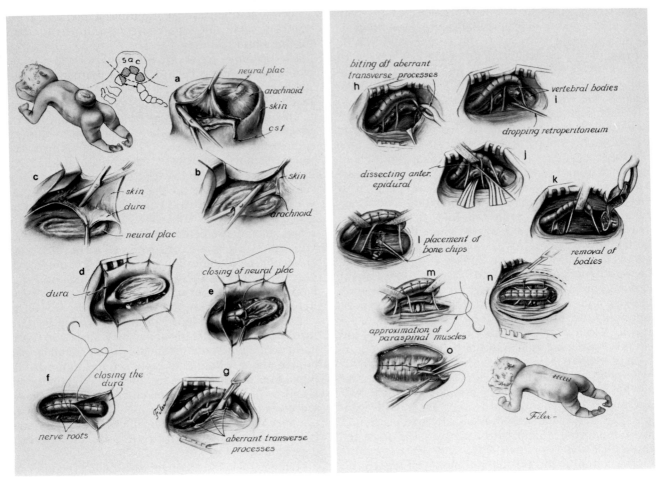

FIGURE 3–4. Diagrammatic illustration of technique for closure of myelomeningocele. (With permission from Reigel DH: Kyphectomy and myelomeningocele repair. *In* Ransohoff J [ed]: Modern Technics in Surgery. Neurosurgery, Vol. 13. Mt. Kisco, NY, Futura Publishing Co., 1979, pp 1–9.)

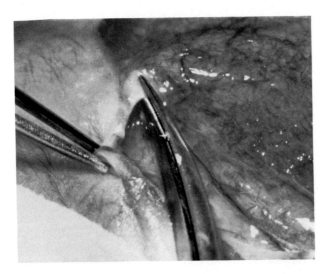

FIGURE 3–5. Operative photograph demonstrating the line of incision along the junctional zone.

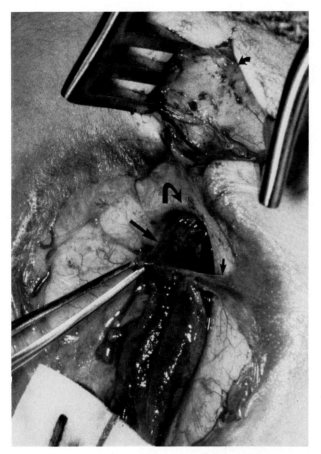

FIGURE 3–6. Intraoperative photograph demonstrating the rostral skin incision *(curved arrow)*, the last normal lamina *(reversed arrow)*, the intact dorsal dural sac overlying spinal cord *(large straight arrow)*, and the point of dural dissection *(small straight arrow)*.

patulous and water-tight. Constriction at any point could contribute to ischemia of the neural plaque, subsequent tethering, or both. Some have advocated plastic and other forms of dural substitute in order to maintain a patulous intradural space. Unfortunately, many of these also carry the risk of arachnoiditis and secondary tethering.

The lumbosacral fascia is identified at its attachment to the posterior iliac crest and sacrum. The fascia is bilaterally incised and dissected free from the posterior iliac crest and the underlying sacrospinalis muscle (Fig. 3–4N). The sacral attachment of the fascia is not disturbed. Attenuated fascia may be protected by including some of the superficial fibers of the sacrospinalis muscle. The lateral edges of the fascial flaps are then folded medially and sutured in the midline over the dorsal dural surface (Fig. 3–4O). Again, attention must be given to avoiding constriction of the dural sac.

The subcutaneous tissue is closed in the midline, and the skin margins are then sharply incised to form a vertical midline incision. With closure of the skin, the five-layer closure is completed.

Recently, there has been increasing interest in a variety of myocutaneous reconstructive procedures designed to obtain full-thickness skin covering for larger myelomeningocele defects.[136–143] These procedures, while obtaining excellent skin coverage, have the potential to interfere significantly with muscle function of the upper torso and shoulders, which is vital for daily activities and ambulation. Furthermore, such procedures extend the operation and increase the risk for significant blood loss. In a recent series of 358 consecutive patients with myelomeningocele, we were able to obtain primary skin coverage in all patients without the use of flaps.[144] There were no dehiscences, and the average blood loss was 29 cc.

Approximately 15 per cent of patients with myelomeningocele have thoracolumbar kyphosis (Figs. 3–4A and 3–8). The width of the vertebral bodies is increased, and they may actually protrude posterior to the dermal surface of the back. With growth and devel-

The dura is then approximated in the midline with sutures, thus restoring the continuity of the dural sac to a tubular structure surrounding the reconstituted spinal cord (Figs. 3–4F and 3–7B).

Every effort should be made to make the dural sac

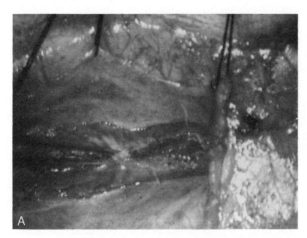 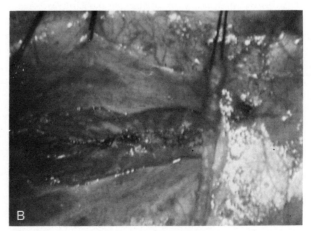

FIGURE 3–7. *A,* Neuroplaque reconvoluted. Laser weld beginning at caudal extent. *B,* Neuroplaque. Laser welded into cylindrical form (cauda equina to the left).

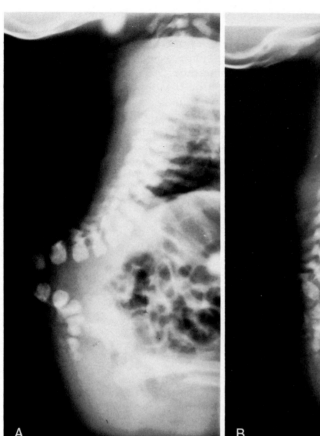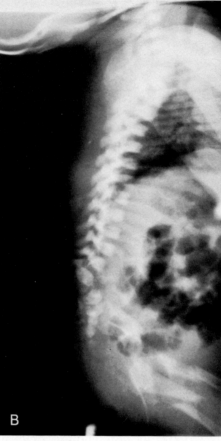

FIGURE 3–8. *A*, X-ray film of lumbar kyphosis, prekyphectomy, at birth. *B*, Postoperative x-ray film following kyphectomy and primary closure.

opment, the natural course of this defect is progressive angulation and deformity. The presence of kyphosis complicates early repair in that it is difficult to obtain adequate subcutaneous tissue and skin coverage over the defect, which causes skin necrosis and, in turn, postoperative infections and ventriculitis. However, even in the presence of adequate skin coverage, the progression of the underlying kyphosis leads to the recurring complication of skin ulceration and vertebral angulation. Bracing becomes difficult, ambulatory capacity declines, and ultimately life expectancy is reduced because of associated progressive cardiopulmonary complications.

Primary spinal osteotomy for kyphosis associated with myelomeningocele was proposed by Sharrad in 1968.[145] He was able partially to correct the deformity and obtain good skin coverage. The author has found that kyphectomy can be done safely at birth, during the time of primary operation, and that it enables one to obtain good skin coverage and vertebral alignment, leading to reduced hospitalization time and early ambulation (Fig. 3–4*H* through *M*).[133, 146, 147]

POSTOPERATIVE MANAGEMENT

Following surgery, the infant is returned to the Isolette, with no restriction on positioning. Every effort should be made to have the mother hold the baby within the first postoperative day. As soon as bowel sounds are present, routine feeding is started. Prophylactic antibiotics are not used.

The wound is observed closely for signs of infection and wound breakdown. If an early, meticulous, five-layer closure is achieved, it is unlikely that superficial infection or necrosis will be followed by meningitis and attendant ventriculitis. However, cellulitis and wound breakdown will delay insertion of a cerebrospinal fluid shunt for hydrocephalus. If wound infection develops, the patient should be treated with appropriate local drainage, surgical scrubs, and high-dose systemic antibiotics selected on the basis of cultures and sensitivity studies. If ventriculitis develops in the presence of hydrocephalus, prompt clearing of the infection and control of the hydrocephalus can be achieved by means of external ventricular drainage and the addition of intrathecal antibiotics.[129] Meticulous closure, as described, is associated with significant reduction in the incidence of postoperative cerebrospinal fluid leak or fistula. When fistulas do occur, most will close spontaneously. In the rare event that a fistula does not spontaneously close, secondary closure is performed immediately. External ventricular drainage of hydrocephalus has been proposed to control leaks, but it predisposes to secondary infection, with meningitis and ventriculitis. Insertion of a shunt is ill-advised in the presence of cerebrospinal fluid leaks, since the incidence of infection may be increased because of failure to recognize early infection at the site of the leak.

Although the etiology of hydrocephalus associated with myelomeningocele has been ascribed to aqueductal stenosis, many surgeons have noted exacerbation of hydrocephalus following repair of myelomeningocele. Perhaps as few as 15 per cent of patients with myelomeningocele are born with signs of hydrocephalus, but 80 per cent or more will develop them in early infancy.[117, 148] One explanation is that the hydrocephalus may be aggravated by a shift in the brainstem after repair, which produces changes in the aqueduct or the Chiari malformation, leading to further alterations in the cerebrospinal fluid flow pathways. Aqueductal stenosis may be a secondary phenomenon of hydrocephalus rather than the primary cause.[148, 149] It is doubtful that the sac serves as a site of absorption and that its removal aggravates the hydrocephalus.

For patients with signs of hydrocephalus at birth, ultrasonographic brain scans should be obtained before transfer to the operating room. With the verification of significant hydrocephalus, a ventriculoperitoneal shunt is inserted prior to closure of the myelomeningocele. The morbidity (i.e., infection) with pre-repair insertion of a shunt has not exceeded that with delayed insertion, and the average length of hospitalization in the absence of complication has been reduced to approximately 5 days.

The onset of hydrocephalus after closure may be indicated by intermittent short periods of apnea, decreased spontaneous activity, and poor feeding patterns. The onset of hydrocephalus can usually be verified by serial examinations, transcephalic impedance, and ultrasonography.[150, 151] Marked hydrocephalus may be present with only minimal cranial enlargement. Only in rare cases should these children be discharged without a computerized tomographic (CT) scan.[148] As soon as clinical suspicion is high that progressive hydrocephalus is present, a CT or MRI scan should be performed. If clinical examinations indicate the absence of wound infection, and there are no signs and symptoms of meningitis or ventriculitis, insertion of a ventriculoperitoneal shunt is recommended because of its described advantages over ventriculoatrial shunts.[152, 153] We do not predispose a child to porencephaly by ventricular taps preoperatively for cerebrospinal fluid culture. In the rare event that cultures and analysis of cerebrospinal fluid obtained at the time of the shunt insertion indicate ventriculitis, externalize the shunt and treat with systemic and intrathecal antibiotics. McLaurin has demonstrated successful treatment with only high-dose intravenous and intrathecal antibiotics.[154]

POSTOPERATIVE RESULTS AND TREATMENT

The operative mortality rate is approaching zero, and 95 per cent or greater survival rates for the first 2 years of life have been reported.[115, 117, 144, 151] In a recent review of the primary closure of 358 consecutive myelomeningoceles, the average blood loss was 29 cc, and postoperative ileus (3 per cent), wound effusion (2.7 per cent), and pneumonia (6.3 per cent) were infrequent complications. Wound infection occurred in 12 per cent, but there were no dehiscences.[144] In this recent series, the incidence of cerebrospinal fluid leak was rarely associated with infection. It closed spontaneously and was thought to be increased because of special efforts to obtain a patulous dural closure in order to prevent tethered spinal cord. A total of 18 per cent of patients developed ventriculitis, and all were promptly and successfully treated with external drainage and intrathecal and systemic antibiotics.[129] Prophylactic antibiotics have had no significant effect on the frequency of ventriculitis. The risk of postoperative ventriculitis is increased for patients with delayed primary operations and remote sources of infection such as the urinary tract. The most common cause of early demise is pulmonary infection, often related to the Chiari malformation and ventriculitis.[117, 155]

Although the prognosis for intellectual development is difficult to determine for any given infant, it now appears that, in the absence of ventriculitis and intracerebral hemorrhage, children with myelomeningocele, with or without hydrocephalus, will have IQ test results within normal range.[117, 130, 156, 157] However, of those with myelomeningocele and a history of cerebrospinal fluid shunt infections, only 31 per cent will have IQ test results within the norm. There is no correlation between degree of hydrocephalus and the presence of lacunar skull deformity.[158, 159] Despite these encouraging observations, discussion of prognosis for intellectual development must be tempered by other emerging findings that children with myelomeningocele have significant disturbance in hand function, perhaps related to neurologic change, incoordination, delayed hand dominance, and delayed use of the hands for balance during crucial development phases. Furthermore, significant problems with visual perception and eye-hand coordination have been documented in this group of patients.[157, 160] All these findings may partially account for the frequently reported verbal-performance discrepancies in IQ testing. Additionally, memory deficits have now been documented for children with myelomeningocele.[157, 160] Therefore, an early awareness of these possible impairments may lead to improved family counseling and educational opportunity for the child.

For parents of the newborn child with myelomeningocele, concerns about ambulation are superseded only by those about intelligence. Improved recognition and treatment of tethered spinal cord, with reduction in the incidence of scoliosis and maintenance of motor function; orthopedic care of extremity deformity; and appropriate orthosis when required means that more than 80 per cent will be ambulatory.[116, 117, 144, 161]

The management of urinary incontinence has been markedly improved with the advent of pharmacologic treatment of neurogenic bladder and the introduction of nonsterile intermittent catheterization. Continence (staying dry for 3 to 4 hours) rates of 85 per cent are now possible.[162–168] For the small percentage of patients who remain incontinent, the artificial sphincter holds promise.[169] Intelligent and comprehensive management of urinary incontinence contributes significantly to the development of social relationships.

Frequently, parents inquire about the patient's sexual development and activity. The sacral (S2–S4) innervation is required for erection and ejaculation. An individual's ability in these areas is highly variable, and with certain lesions, reflex erection and ejaculation are possible.[170] Shurtleff and Sousa have indicated that 18 per cent of patients of a group of 60, aged 16 to 24, were sexually active.[171] Counseling has been urged for all of these patients.

It is clear that one of the major handicaps imposed upon children with myelomeningocele is that of psychosocial problems originating within themselves, their families, and society. These forms of stress can be reduced by bringing the child into the educational mainstream, personal and family counseling, improved understanding of the patient's potential, and increased public awareness of spina bifida.

MENINGOCELE

In addition to the routine assessment described with myelomeningocele, other recommended methods include preoperative ultrasonography,[172] metrizamide myelography with CT, and magnetic resonance imaging (MRI) to identify dermoid tumor, diastematomyelia, lipoma, or tethered spinal cord. After complete evaluation, surgery is recommended to prevent infection and to restore continuity of the back. Delaying surgery until the child is older predisposes the patient to irreversible neurologic deficit and psychologic trauma. Therefore, surgery at the time of diagnosis, which is usually at birth, is encouraged. Then, the child can begin a healthy normal development process with the parents and family.

The operative technique follows the guidelines described for myelomeningocele. The neck of the dural sac is often significantly smaller than the sac and may be surprisingly narrow. Occasionally, nerve roots of the filum terminale may be involved within the sac. Nerve roots should be replaced and the filum terminale sectioned. The spinal cord is normal. Excessive dura is excised, and the remainder is closed in the midline. The fascia and skin closures are similar to those for myelomeningocele. The postoperative management requires all the same precautions and observations as with the child with myelomeningocele. However, the incidence of hydrocephalus is markedly reduced, and the prognosis for normal development is very good.

ANTERIOR SACRAL MENINGOCELE

This form of meningocele extends anteriorly into the presacral retroperitoneal space and usually communicates with the sacral subarachnoid space through a narrow anterior sacral defect. The natural course of this meningocele is one of progressive enlargement of the intrapelvic sac, secondary to hydrostatic pressure of cerebrospinal fluid. The sacral canal also may be enlarged secondary to lipoma, dermoid tumor, teratoma, or intrasacral meningocele. The lesion is probably more common in females than in males and is often associated with other pelvic organ anomalies such as bicornate uterus, vaginal septation, rectovaginal fistula, duplication of the kidneys, changes in the ureter, and imperforate anus.

These patients may appear with chronic constipation, obstetric complications, or pelvic masses.[173–175] Incontinence, recurrent urinary tract infection, headache, dysmenorrhea, dyspareunia, and radicular pain may also alert one to this diagnosis. The mass may be palpable by abdominal, rectal, or pelvic examination. The differential diagnosis includes most pelvic tumors. Plain x-ray films of the sacrum show the posterior aspect of the pelvis to be intact and the classic "scimitar" (sickle-shaped) sacrum.[176] Intravenous pyelography and ultrasonography may identify changes in the kidneys, ureter, and bladder. The diagnosis is established by metrizamide myelography. Ultrasonography, computerized tomography, and MRI verify the diagnosis.[177]

Generally, sacral laminectomy has been primarily recommended because it permits visualization of the intraspinal contents and direct anterior suture closure of the opening into the sacral canal. With aspiration of the meningocele and obliteration of the dural communication, the pelvic mass disappears. Occasionally, dural graft may be required to close the meningocele.[173] Rarely, because of intrameningocele neural structures, a delayed anterior abdominal operation may be required to obliterate the meningocele.[178] Barring complications such as infection, the results of surgical treatment should be gratifying.

ANTEROLATERAL MENINGOCELE

These meningoceles appear at the thoracic and lumbar levels, protrude through enlarged intervertebral foramina and are often associated with vertebral scalloping and scoliotic deformity. This form of meningocele is often associated with neurofibromatosis, Marfan's syndrome, or both.[179, 180] Myelography, CT scanning, and MRI permit establishment of the diagnosis and exclusion of neoplasm. Operative treatment in collaboration with the orthopedist is designed to obliterate the meningocele and ensure spinal stability.

DELAYED COMPLICATIONS

Even with improved care and prognosis, it has become evident that spina bifida is a dynamic birth defect of the entire central nervous system and that optimal development of the child requires serial examinations of all systems for delayed complications. These complications include esotropia, auditory deficits, swallowing disorders, apnea, cranial nerve dysfunction, seizure, cervical medullary compression, kyphoscoliosis, hydromyelia, intraspinal tumor, tethered spinal cord, urinary tract change, nutrition and growth disturbances, psychosocial adjustment problems, and skin breakdown. Early recognition of the potential onset of these complications often leads to their prevention or the interruption of their progression. Aggressive identification and treatment of these problems enhances development and performance.

HINDBRAIN DYSFUNCTION AND CHIARI II MALFORMATION

The major cause of death during the first two decades of life of children with myelomeningocele appears to be related to the brainstem.[117, 181] During early infancy, these problems frequently include intermittent apnea, cyanosis, bradycardia, swallowing disorders and aspiration, nystagmus, vocal cord paralysis, torticollis, opisthotonos, hypotonia, and spasticity. Older children frequently demonstrate increasing scoliosis, spasticity, and recurrent vomiting. Thus, with age, the symptoms of primary brainstem dysfunction appear to become less important and changes related to the cervical spinal cord become more prominent. However, symptoms of hindbrain abnormality may occur at any time in the life of a person with myelomeningocele. They may be aggravated by hydrocephalus and shunt failure, or they may spontaneously appear.

The main pathologic features of the Chiari malformation affect the cerebellum, brainstem, and spinal cord. The cerebellum is small and caudally displaced along with the pons and medulla into the cervical spinal cord.[182, 183] There are numerous anomalies of the remaining spinal cord, cerebrum, and ventricular system.[21, 22] As many as 75 per cent of patients have structural changes of the brainstem, which include hypoplasia of the cranial nerve nuclei and aplasia of the olives, pontine nuclei, and tegmentum.[73] Neuronal migration anomalies such as heterotopias and heterotaxias are common.[73, 184]

The evaluation of this problem is directly related to the principal complaints and neurologic findings. In addition to specialized imaging studies with MRI, which should include the entire central nervous system, otolaryngologic and ophthalmologic evaluation of lower cranial nerve function, brainstem evoked potentials, swallowing studies, and laryngoscopy may be of help. The standard study for evaluation of the posterior fossa and cervical medullary junction is MRI (Fig. 3–9).[185, 186] It not only reveals the hindbrain anomalies, but provides opportunity to evaluate the ventricular system and spinal cord for associated rostral and caudal anomalies. With the array of possible pathologic changes in all areas of the central nervous system, it is not surprising that a wide variety of treatments have been advocated for the symptoms and neurologic changes thought to be secondary to the Chiari malformation.

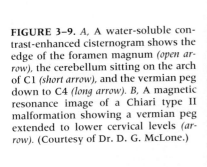

FIGURE 3–9. *A,* A water-soluble contrast-enhanced cisternogram shows the edge of the foramen magnum *(open arrow),* the cerebellum sitting on the arch of C1 *(short arrow),* and the vermian peg down to C4 *(long arrow). B,* A magnetic resonance image of a Chiari type II malformation showing a vermian peg extended to lower cervical levels *(arrow).* (Courtesy of Dr. D. G. McLone.)

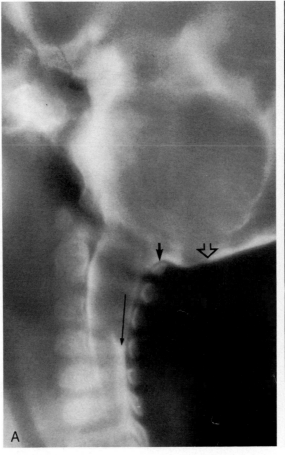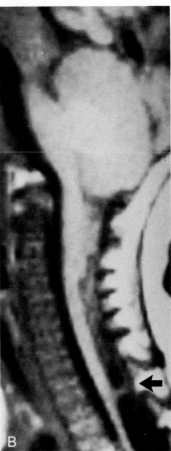

Irrespective of the pathologic anatomy of Chiari malformation, the surgical treatment of hydrocephalus takes precedence over other surgical procedures such as posterior fossa craniotomy and spinal cord operations. Hall has demonstrated that for hydromyelia, which communicates with the ventricular system, the treatment with ventricular shunt is effective for treating scoliosis, cranial nerve findings, and spasticity.[187–189] Preceded by Gardner's work suggesting the hydrodynamic mechanism for hydromyelia, many have suggested caudal laminectomy and plugging of the obex.[190–192] Resection of atrophic cerebellar tissue, myelotomy, and insertion of a foramen of Munro subarachnoid stent has also been proposed.[193, 194] The results of operative treatment of hindbrain-origin abnormalities have been mixed and of controversial non-uniform benefit. Clearly, improvement has been reported, but most studies are limited in their capacity to relate the patient's subsequent postoperative course directly to intervention. It appears that every effort should be made to connect clinical abnormalities with demonstrable abnormalities revealed by modern neuro-imaging studies. The operative treatment should then be designed to alter the abnormality in the hope of reversing the pathologic process. Therefore, cerebrospinal fluid shunts should be used in the presence of uncontrolled hydrocephalus. Decompression should be considered in the presence of impaction or compression of structures, which may account for the clinical abnormalities such as quadriparesis, spasticity, and hydromyelia—which are unresponsive to treatment of hydrocephalus. The surgeon should be cautious in suggesting posterior fossa operation for abnormalities primarily of cranial nerve origin. The rare patient who becomes apneic secondary to Chiari malformation and mechanical factors may respond to decompressive operations. During infancy, many patients demonstrate progressive improvement associated with maturation. In the absence of prospective control studies, the controversy and dilemma of choosing the appropriate surgical treatment for this often desperate population is destined to continue.

TETHERED SPINAL CORD

This subject is fully discussed in Chapter 4.

HYDROMYELIA (SYRINGOHYDROMYELIA)

Hydromyelia refers to a centrally originating cavitation of the spinal cord which is lined by ependyma (Fig. 3–10). It has been compared to hydrocephalus and described as "hydrocephalus of the spinal cord." Syringo-

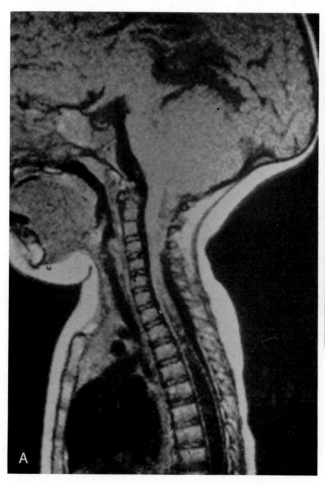

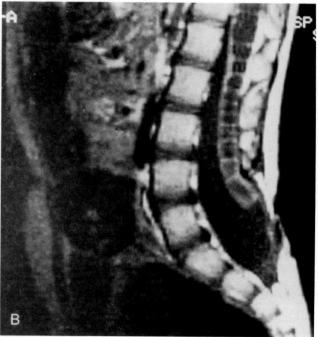

FIGURE 3–10. Magnetic resonance images show severe hydromyelia. In A, it is associated with the Chiari type II malformation. B shows the common haustral pattern in the hydromyelia cavity and a distal spinal cord that appears tethered. (Courtesy of Dr. D. G. McLone.)

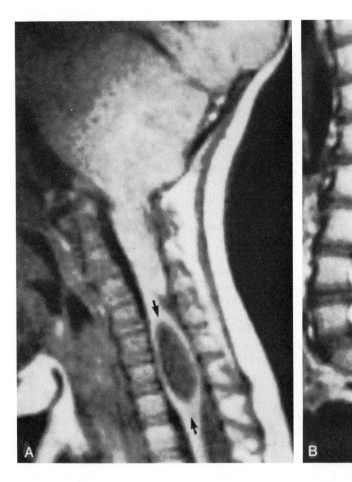

FIGURE 3–11. Magnetic resonance images of two children with segmental hydromyelia (syringomyelia?) *(arrows).* *A* also shows a Chiari type II malformation. In *B,* the terminal spinal cord appears tethered into the myelomeningingocele repair. (Courtesy of Dr. D. G. McLone.)

myelia defines an eccentric cavitation of the spinal cord not lined by ependyma. Both conditions may involve the entire spinal cord, but syringomyelia tends to be more focal (Fig. 3–11). For patients with myelomeningocele, hydromyelia is often thought to originate when spinal fluid passes through the iter of the central canal at the level of the obex. Therefore, it is frequently associated with inadequately treated hydrocephalus or cerebral spinal fluid shunt malfunction. It may be that syringomyelia develops from an outpouching through the ependyma of the central canal. These descriptive conditions are associated with numerous primary problems such as Chiari malformation, posterior fossa cyst, platybasia, spinal cord tumors, inflammatory diseases, disc disease, and trauma. This variability of causes and the observation that many cavitations do not communicate with the fourth ventricle suggest that the pathogenesis is not solely related to cerebrospinal fluid flowing from the fourth ventricle to act as a dilating force of the central canal as described by Gardner.[190, 195] In addition to the Gardner hydrodynamic theory, others have suggested pressure dissociations with cerebrospinal fluid being sucked into the central canal, or cerebrospinal fluid flowing into the central canal through the Virchow-Robinson spaces.[196, 197] Probably the most attractive current theory is that cerebrospinal fluid flows in a caudal to rostral direction and that the unifying factor in development of cavitation of the cord,

perhaps with the exception of trauma, is a compression or interference with the central canal flow of cerebrospinal fluid with subsequent intramedullary accumulation.[198]

The most common symptoms and findings of spinal cord cavitary lesions include muscle weakness, spasticity, pain, sensory changes, incontinence, scoliosis, and kyphosis.

Recently, treatment recommendations have become more defined as a result of improved imaging of these lesions with MRI. The treatment paradigms have been recommended on the basis of etiology and on the presence or absence of communication with the fourth ventricle.[198, 199] For patients with myelomeningocele and hydromyelia, the first line of therapy is adequate control of ventricular enlargement, and in the absence of ventricular enlargement and persistent hydromyelia, hydromyelic shunts, usually plural, are recommended.[198–200] With these two procedures, the vast majority of patients with Chiari II and hydromyelia will be effectively treated and reversal of deficit and disappearance of the cavity fully expected. For the occasional patient who fails these procedures, cervical medullary decompression is recommended to release the obstruction to caudal-rostral flow of cerebrospinal fluid. It is possible that dynamic video MRI studies will confirm this observation in the future.

MRI has demonstrated and confirmed the high incidence of small syrinxes of the spinal cord long described by pathologists. These lesions are usually asymptomatic and do not change with time.

As with the clinical picture of hindbrain malformations, one operation is not suitable for all patients, and operative treatment recommendations should be designed on the basis of the pathology demonstrated by MRI.

SPASTICITY

Spasticity in the upper and lower extremities may be a complicating factor for up to 40 per cent of patients with myelomeningocele and sensorimotor levels above L5.[201, 202] Spasticity may significantly interfere with sitting balance and ambulation. Spasticity usually appears and becomes a problem during the first decade of life.[202] It is associated with a high incidence of foot deformity, hip dislocation, and contracture. Hip flexion contractures may play a role in the etiology of subsequent scoliosis and lordosis. Evaluation for the cause of spasticity such as tethered spinal cord, hindbrain abnormalities, hydromyelia, and hydrocephalus should be prompt and operative treatment pursued in order to prevent increasing disability. Despite a search for these causes there is a significant percentage of patients who will show continuing evidence of spasticity and its associated morbidity. These patients should be considered for dorsal root rhizotomy.[203, 204]

OPHTHALMOLOGIC COMPLICATIONS

Ophthalmologic complications occur in 70 to 80 per cent of children with spina bifida during the first decade of life. These abnormalities include papilledema, defects in visual acuity, amblyopia, optic atrophy, nystagmus, strabismus, movement disorders, and cortical blindness.[205, 206] Frequent ophthalmologic evaluation will identify these problems, often beginning within the first years of life. These changes often indicate the onset of cerebral spinal fluid shunt malfunction. They may also be associated with hindbrain abnormalities. Prompt neurosurgical treatment is associated with reversal of abnormality and preservation of visual acuity.

SEIZURE

Seizure has been reported in as many as 30 per cent of patients with myelomeningocele.[207] The manifestations of seizure may be associated with respiratory change, bradycardia, and change in level of consciousness, all of which must be distinguished from changes associated with shunt malfunction and hindbrain malformations. Hack et al. reported that 9 per cent of patients admitted with increased ventricular pressures had seizures as one of the initial symptoms.[208] They concluded, as many have observed, that seizure may be temporally related to shunt malfunction. Therefore, the occurrence of unexplained seizure or recurrence of seizure should precipitate not only the usual neurologic evaluation, but also a critical evaluation of shunt function.

URINARY INCONTINENCE

Ninety per cent or more of patients with myelomeningocele have neurogenic bladder. Vigorous urologic evaluation and treatment are required. Prior to the 1970s, urinary diversion was the accepted form of management. However, since that time the widespread use of clean intermittent catheterization has virtually eliminated diversion. Comprehensive urodynamic evaluation, pharmacologic therapy of bladder tone, new surgical procedures to alter bladder size, electrical stimulation, biofeedback, undiversion, and prostheses have enabled over 80 per cent of patients to achieve social continence.[117, 209–217]

BOWEL INCONTINENCE

The vast majority of patients with myelomeningocele have rectal incontinence, which has the potential to produce social isolation and rejection. The key goals in management include predictability of bowel evacuation to limit soilage and accidents. This is usually achieved with a regular enema program.[218] Dietary guides to increase fiber in order to alter and increase fecal consistency are also of benefit. A regular enema program and dietary controls constitute an effective method for attaining fecal continence in virtually all cases.

GROWTH AND DEVELOPMENT

Within the past decades, the approach and management of children with abnormal closure of the posterior neural tube have varied between nonintervention and aggressive early treatment.[219] As a result, the investigation of the endocrine aspects of open neural tube defects (ONTD) has been limited.

There are reasons to suspect altered endocrine function in these patients. Anterior midline lesions such as septo-optic dysplasia, cleft palate, and transphenoidal encephalocele have been associated with growth hormone deficiency.[219] Patients with altered intracranial pressure may have altered growth hormone neuroregulatory systems. Shunt catheters necessary to control hydrocephalus may impinge on the third ventricle, possibly causing injury to several hypothalamic nuclei. The Chiari deformity, which is associated with abnormalities of the midbrain and ventricles, is frequently observed in these patients.

With these concepts in mind, one can consider the severe short stature of this population, early pubertal progression, and body composition as well as adult stature from an endocrine perspective.

Children with myelomeningocele are extremely short.[220, 221] It has been assumed that underdevelopment of the lower limbs or spinal deformities explain small size.[222] The presence of a tethered spinal cord contributes to scoliosis and may explain some of the apparent short stature. In addition, these children are extremely difficult to measure in a standing position owing to the frequent necessity of braces and appliances.

Because of such difficulty, alternate approaches to measurement using arm span or arm length have been attempted.[223] However, current comparison normative data are lacking. Measurement of recumbent length on a horizontal stadiometer in comparison to the normative lengths of the Fels Research Institute data, which represent a modern cohort of children, is a difficult but more accurate method for following growth.[224] Both right and left lengths can be obtained for those with leg length discrepancies.

For the early part of childhood, length for males and females with ONTD overlap with normals and then diverge at about age 4 years.[225] After ages 10–12 years, the mean length for both males and females are well below the 5th percentile. Stratification of stature by function level of lesion has been observed.[226] Those with occipital and sacral lesions are tallest, followed by those with L3–L5 lesions, and finally by those with thoracic level lesions to L3.[221]

Evaluation of growth hormone secretion and response to treatment of seven prepubertal children with ONTD was reported in 1989.[227] Alterations in the frequency and amplitude of growth hormone secretion were observed in the three males and four females from the Fels Research Institute who had a mean length of 104.9 cm, which is an average of 28 cm less than the expected length adjusted for age and sex. The mean nocturnal growth hormone value was 1.88 ± 1.37 mg/ml with a mean of one peak greater than 7 ng/ml in 12 hours of nocturnal sampling, which is less than expected. As a group, these patients produce a variable amount of growth hormone.[222]

RESPONSE TO GROWTH HORMONE TREATMENT

The mean growth rate of these children prior to treatment was $1.7 \pm .17$ cm/year, which increases to 7.9 ± 3.5 cm.year on growth hormone treatment for 6 months ($p < .05$).[228] Children normally grow at a rate of 5 to 6 cm/year, depending on age. Somatomedin-C (also known as IGFI) is the second messenger after growth hormone, and it also increased significantly in these patients during treatment ($p < .03$). For many years it has been assumed that those children could not be growth-delayed on a hormonal basis, as some investigators noted long upper extremities.[229] Presumably a hormonal etiology would affect all extremities. The arm lengths of the seven treated patients, as indicated by the lengths of the radius and ulna on radiographs, was significantly less than expected for each patient ($p < .03$). In addition, bone maturation of these children

was altered with a mean bone age delay of 3 ± 1.3 years.[220]

The length of the upper extremity (using the lengths of the radius and ulna from radiographs) does not appear to grow in excess of recumbent length during treatment with growth hormone.[230] Thirteen poorly growing children with spina bifida who produced a variable amount of growth hormone were treated and followed for three 8-month intervals. They responded with an acceleration in growth; however, no differences in the observed and expected rated of growth for the radius, ulna, and recumbent length were seen. Their bone age did not advance excessively while on treatment, appearing in fact to decrease in rate from interval I (16.2 month/yr) to interval II (7.5 months/yr), which raises the question of the interrelationships between growth hormone treatment and the tempo of puberty.

Longer-term treatment of 18 children with ONTD treated for a mean of 27.1 ± 15.8 months has demonstrated an increase in growth rate from 3.1 ± 1.2 cm/yr to 8.2 ± 2.7 cm/yr, with significant improvement in the standard deviation score for stature from -2.9 ± 1.3 to -1.6 ± 1.5 through 36 months.[231] Seven of these 18 children were prepubertal for the duration of treatment with .3 mg/kg per week of growth hormone. While receiving treatment, five of the 18 children required surgical correction of tethered spinal cord, which presented as growth arrest. None of this cohort of patients had progression of their scoliosis. However, 12 of 18 children had a total of 35 symptomatic urinary tract infections. Multiple factors influence the response of children to RHGH in this complex patient group, and a multidisciplinary approach is essential.

Thyroid function of this group is normal, with a prevalence of subclinical hypothyroidism of approximately 2.5 per cent, which is similar to the normal population. However, puberty occurs early in children with neural tube defects. Greene et al. observed significant advancement of bone age after age 10 for males and females with concomitant early pubertal progression.[232] The precocious puberty is central in origin and is responsive to treatment with analogues of LHRH on an anecdotal basis.

A major and frequent handicap for children with myelomeningocele is obesity, the etiology of which is unknown.[233] Weight for age may not be a useful measure of obesity since it does not compensate for the significant short stature. Body mass index (BMI weight/meters²) is altered in patients with ONTD. There is clearly an increase in adipose tissue after age 4, which suggests a developmental or matrilinear influence.[234] It is possible that in addition to reduced activity and a mismatch between food intake and energy expenditure, the altered tempo of puberty may influence obesity.

Adults with spina bifida are also exceedingly small. Little information exists on adult stature and anthropomorphic measurements. The recumbent length of 23 adult females and 24 adult males of mean age 23.7 ± 5.4 years was reported and compared to the 50th percentile recumbent length values for 18-year-old males and females by the Fels Research Institute. The recumbent length for females was 141.3 ± 12.9 cm, with an expected length of 167 cm, and for males, 151.6 ± 14.7 cm, with an expected length of 182 cm.[235] Sitting height correlated best with recumbent length in comparison to arm span or arm length. The correlation coefficient (r) or sitting height to recumbent length was .87, significant at p <.001. The recumbent length of these adults was significantly less than the midparental height. Recumbent length correlated with weight, level of lesion, arm span, and arm length. Arm length was also significantly less than the 50th percentile values for males and females, using the t-test for independent samples. Therefore, adults with open neural tube defects are significantly short and the etiology is not solely a function of orthopedic abnormalities, as sitting height and arm length are also subsequently decreased.

Further study will be necessary to determine whether therapeutic intervention with respect to growth and pubertal progression will increase final stature with minimal complications. Through various endocrine interventions, puberty of closer-to-normal duration, decrease in adiposity, and taller adult stature may aid this group on an emotional and functional level as they strive toward self-sufficiency.

HYDROCEPHALUS

Hydrocephalus is either present or will develop in 80 to 90 per cent of patients with myelomeningocele.[144] The primary indications for shunt insertion are symptoms and findings related to increasing ventricular and cranial size. These findings are verified by ultrasound and CT or MRI. Some of the symptoms and findings commonly include an enlarging head, full fontanelle, vomiting, stridor, reflux, poor head control, spasticity, and ocular motor changes. The treatment of hydrocephalus is discussed in Chapter 13. Except in the presence of extreme ventriculomegaly, intellectual development for this population of patients does not correlate with degree of hydrocephalus.[236]

LATEX ALLERGY

There is increasing evidence that repeated exposure to latex contained in products such as gloves, catheter, balloons, and products used during surgical procedures has predisposed people with spina bifida to an increased incidence of sensitization (18 to 20 per cent). Anaphylaxis during surgical procedures, characterized by bronchospasm, hypotension, anoxia, and macular papillary rash, has been reported.[237–242] Therefore, preoperative preparations probably should include prick tests or a Rast test.[243]

ORTHOPEDICS

The objectives of orthopedic treatment of patients with spina bifida are to prevent deformity and provide methods (orthoses or surgery) to achieve maximal mobility and ambulation. Deformity of the lower extremities, alterations in hip function, and spinal curvature all interfere with these goals. Orthopedic changes should always precipitate neurologic evaluation. It is now clear that tethered spinal cord, hydromyelia, Chiari malformation, and hydrocephalus play a dynamic role in orthopedic deformity, and frequently neurosurgical treatment is required prior to orthopedic reconstruction or spinal fusion.

Children with myelomeningocele have a high risk of lower extremity flexure and epiphyseal injury (12 per cent).[244] The incidence declines during adulthood. Prevention is aided by ambulation and care in activities.

To achieve ambulation within their communities, many people with spina bifida require a variety of orthotic assistive devices including braces, canes, and walkers. With age and increase in body weight, many increasingly rely on wheelchairs for mobility. Ability to achieve ambulation is related to intellectual performance, and a high percentage with retardation require wheelchairs. Similarly, higher lesions (thoracic) increasingly cause people to become wheelchair-dependent. However, for the remainder, 50 to 75 per cent will be community ambulators.[117, 144]

LIFE SKILLS

Intellectual Performance. Research to date has emphasized intellectual quotient of patients with myelomeningocele with and without shunts.[115, 130, 157, 245, 246] These studies have consistently shown that patients with myelomeningocele and absence of hydrocephalus have IQ scores comparable to those of their peers without myelomeningocele. Furthermore, those with hydrocephalus and myelomeningocele who have not had episodes of infection or hemorrhage have IQs equal to those of children with myelomeningocele without hydrocephalus.[130] Studies by McLone have demonstrated that 75 per cent have an IQ within normal range which will remain stable through grade school; two thirds of these children are in mainstream education programs.[117] Many of these existing studies are somewhat flawed by the heterogeneity of the study groups such as variability of testing method, failure to consider pathologic changes in the brain that are unrelated to hydrocephalus, upper extremity discoordination, seizure, and anti-epileptic medications. IQ testing has also demonstrated that performance IQ scores are consistently lower than verbal IQ scores.[157, 247]

Education. With increasing numbers of children with spina bifida surviving and participating in mainstream education, a wide array of complex learning disabilities have been uncovered. Many of these require committed remedial efforts in order to permit the child to experience full educational opportunity.[157, 160] These include discrepancies in verbal and nonverbal cognitive skills, reduction in memory, conceptual and problem-solving deficits, deficient linguistic performance, short attention span, and difficulty in grasping abstract concepts. There is also a high frequency of uncoordinated hand function and abnormalities of visual-motor coordination.[248] In order to enhance education of these children, comprehensive quality neuropsychological testing is required to identify these abnormalities, plan treatment, and design individual education plans. In summary, despite reasonable intelligence, these abnormalities threaten the heart of education: reading, writing, and arithmetic.

Family. Spina bifida and its chronic disabilities predispose family members to ongoing stress, which begins with the birth of the child. Instead of joy at birth, the process begins with grief and guilt, which is reinforced by repeated hospitalizations. Therefore, extensive uncontrolled medical problems lead the family to social, economic, and psychological strain. Intensification of family relationships, isolation, and additional burden posed by the chronically disabled child may threaten the marriage. With increased awareness of these family stressors, programs of advocacy and support with family counseling will enable many to reach family structures of reward and joy.

Social Life. Many children with spina bifida have weak social skills and competence. They are often not chosen as friends and playmates and acquire limited social acceptance after early childhood. Indeed, many find themselves isolated and rejected. This social deprivation is complex and not confined to the disability of spina bifida. The origins are complex and extend to all strata of our society. The psychological sequelae are significant.[155, 249–251] The behaviors of the child with these experiences reflect lack of self esteem and assertiveness. Academic and vocational performance is threatened. Depression follows. Clinicians must be prepared to recommend psychiatric counseling.

Independence and Vocation. Over 80 per cent of young adults with spina bifida continue to live within dependent or semi-dependent settings.[250, 251] Although the majority are now completing secondary school and perhaps one third are receiving additional education, less than 10 per cent of our patients are economically independent. The vast majority of adults have had modest dating experience and most are not married. A surprising group have had experience with chemical abuse, and as many as 80 per cent of young adults in our transition program have required intensive psychiatric therapy. These developments, while discouraging, do not present events mandated by the disability but rather signify an indictment of our society's negative interaction with the disabled. The Disabilities Act and societal awareness combined with advances in medical care promise to make the future brighter for people with spina bifida.

CONCLUSION

The prognosis of newborn infants with myelomeningocele is better at this time that at any time in history. New operative methods of closure of the neural plaque and early kyphectomy preserve existing neural function and reduce the incidence of wound breakdown and infection. The development of new shunting systems and diagnostic tools such as ultrasonography, computerized tomography, and MRI have made possible critical determination of shunt function, leading to earlier revision and thus preventing irreversible pathologic and functional change of the brain. Multimodality neuropsychological testing has confirmed normal intellectual performance in many of these children. Intermittent, clean catheterization and pharmacologic treatment of the neurogenic bladder have drastically reduced the incidence of unrelenting urinary tract infection and renal failure. Early recognition and treatment of tethered spinal cord have reduced the incidence of delayed neurologic deterioration and scoliosis. Advances in the selection and the technique of orthopedic procedures with improved orthotics have enabled most children with myelomeningocele to achieve ambulation. The quality of the patient's life and prognosis appear to be related directly to comprehensive health care. Advances in community understanding and interaction have allowed children with spina bifida to attain social acceptance, educational and vocational opportunities, and rewarding lives.

REFERENCES

1. Gool JB, Gool JD: A Short History of Spina Bifida. Netherlands, Society for Research into Hydrocephalus and Spina Bifida, 1986.
2. Till K: Occult spinal dysraphism. The value of prophylactic surgical treatment. Recent Progress in Neurological Surgery. Amsterdam, Excerpta Medica ICS, No. 320, 1973, pp 61–66.
3. Lassman LP, James CCM: Meningocele manqué. Child's Brain 3:1, 1977.
4. Eckstein HB: Neuropathic bladder. In Williams DI (ed): Urology in Childhood. Berlin, Springer Verlag, 1974, p 250.
5. Gillespie HW: The significance of congenital lumbosacral anomalies. Br J Radiol 22:270, 1949.
6. Wynne-Davies R: Congential vertebral anomalies. Etiology and relationship to spina bifida cystica. J Med Genet 12:280, 1975.
7. Boone D, Pansons D, Lochman SM, et al: Spina bifida occulta: Lesion or anomaly? Clin Radiol 36:159, 1985.
8. Fineman RM, Jorde LB, Martin RA, et al.: Spinal dysraphia as an autosomal dominant defect in four families. Am J Med Genet 12:457, 1982.
9. Rudd LN: Genetics. In Hoffman HJ, Epstein F (eds): Disorders of the Developing Nervous System: Diagnosis and Treatment. Boston, Blackwell Scientific Publications, 1986, p 47.
10. Lichtenstein BW: Spina dysraphism (spina bifida and myelodysplasia). Arch Neurol Psychiatry 99:792, 1940.
11. Steinbok P, Cochrane DD: The nature of congenital posterior cervical or cervicothoracic midline cutaneous mass lesions. J Neurosurg 75:206, 1991.
12. Bindal AK, Storrs BB, McLone DG: Occipital meningoceles in patients with the Dandy-Walker syndrome. Neurosurgery 6:844, 1990.
13. Laurence KM, Tew BJ: The natural history of spina bifida cystica: Detailed analysis of 407 cases. Arch Dis Child 39:41, 1964.
14. Tryfonas G: Three spina bifida defects in one child. J Pediatr Surg 8:75, 1973.
15. Matson DD: Neurosurgery of Infancy and Childhood. 2nd ed. Springfield, IL, Charles C Thomas, 1969.
16. McLone DG, Naidich TP: Terminal myelocystocele. Neurosurgery 16:36, 1985.
17. Naidich TP, McLone DG, Mutluer S: A new understanding of dorsal dysraphism with lipoma (lipomyeloschisis): Radiologic evaluation and surgical correction. Am J Radiol 140:1065, 1983.

18. Chapman PH, Beyerl B: The tethered spinal cord, with particular reference to spinal lipoma and diastematomyelia. *In* Hoffman HJ, Epstein F (eds): Disorders of the Developing Nervous System: Diagnosis and Treatment. Boston, Blackwell Scientific Publishers, 1986, p 119.

19. Lemire RJ: Causes of neural tube defects. *In* McLaurin RL (ed): Spina Bifida: A Multidisciplinary Approach. New York, Praeger Publishers, 1986, pp 2–7.

20. Naidich TP, Publowski RM, Naidich JB: Computed tomographic signs of Chiari II malformation. II. Midbrain and cerebellum. Radiology 134:391, 1980.

21. Naidich TP, Publowski RM, Naidich JB: Computed tomographic signs of Chiari II malformation. III. Ventricles and cisterns. Radiology 134:657, 1980.

22. Naidich TP, Publowski RM, Naidich JB, et al.: Computed tomographic signs of the Chiari II malformation. Part I: Skull and dural partitions. Radiology 134:65, 1980.

23. Elwood JH: Major central nervous system malformations notified in Northern Ireland, 1964–1968. Dev Med Child Neurol 14:731, 1972.

24. Laurence KM: A declining incidence of neural tube defects in the U.K. Z Kinderchir 44:51, 1989.

25. CDC: Spina bifida incidence at birth—United States. MMWR 41:497, 1992.

26. Elwood JM, Elwood JH: Epidemiology of Anencephalus and Spina Bifida. New York, Oxford University Press, 1980.

27. Thompson MW, Rudd NL: The genetics of spinal dysraphism. *In* Morley TP (ed): Current Controversies in Neurosurgery. Philadelphia, W. B. Saunders, 1976, pp 126–146.

28. Greene WB, Terry RC, DeMasi RA, et al.: Effect of race and gender on neurological level in myelomeningocele. Dev Med Child Neurol 33:110, 1991.

29. Sever LE, Saunders M, Monsen R: An epidemiologic study of neural tube defects in Los Angeles County. I. Prevalence at birth based on multiple sources of case ascertainment. Teratology 25:315, 1982.

30. Shurtleff DB, Lemire RJ, Warkany J: Embryology, etiology and epidemiology. *In* Shurtleff DB (ed): Myelodysplasias and Exstrophies: Significance, Prevention, and Treatment. New York, Grune & Stratton, pp 39–64, 1986.

31. Carter CO, Evans KA: Spina bifida and anencephalus in greater London. J Med Genet 10:209, 1973.

32. Leck I: The geographical distribution of neural tube defects and oval clefts. Br Med J 40:309, 1984.

33. Till K: Paediatric Neurosurg. London, Blackwell, 1975.

34. Osaka K, Tanimiwa T, Hivayama A, et al.: Myelomeningocele before birth. J Neurosurg 49:711, 1978.

35. Toriello HV, Higgins JV: Occurence of neural tube defects among first-, second-, and third-degree relatives of probands: Results of a United States study. Am J Med Genet 15:601, 1983.

36. Toriello HV, Warran ST, Lindstrom JA: Brief communication: Possible X-linked anencephaly and spina bifida—report of a kindred. Am J Med Genet 6:119, 1980.

37. Fraser F: Genetic counseling in some common paediatric diseases. Am J Hum Genet 26:636, 1974.

38. Laurence KM, Carter CO, David PA: Major central nervous system malformations in South Wales II: Pregnancy factors, seasonal variation, and social class effects. Br J Prev Soc Med 22:212, 1968.

39. Jorde LB, Fineman RM, Martin RA: Epidemiology and genetics of neural tube defects: An application of the Utah Genealogical Data Base. Am J Phys Anthropol 62:23, 1983.

40. Rodríguez JI, García M, Morales C, et al.: Trisomy 13 syndrome and neural tube defects. Am J Med Genet 36:513, 1990.

41. Birth Defects. Genetic Services International Directory, 8th ed. The National Foundation-March of Dimes, 1986.

42. Renwick JH: Hypothesis: Anencephaly and spina bifida are usually preventable by avoidance of a specific but unidentified substance present in certain potato tubers. Br J Prev Soc Med 26:67, 1972.

43. Clarke CA, McKendrick OM, Sheppard PM: Spina bifida and potatoes. Br Med J 3:251, 1973.

44. Nevin NC, Merrett JD: Potato avoidance during pregnancy in women with a previous infant with either anencephaly or spina bifida. Br J Prev Soc Med 29:111, 1975.

45. Janerich DT: Influenza and neural-tube defects. Lancet ii:551, 1971.

46. Layde PM, Edmonds LD, Erickson JD: Maternal fever and neural tube defect. Teratology 21:105, 1980.

47. Leck I, Hay S, Witte JJ, et al.: Malformations recorded on birth certificates following A2 influenza epidemics. Public Health Rep 84:971, 1969.

48. Leck I: Maternal hyperthermia and anencephaly. Lancet i:671, 1978.

49. Lee H, Nagele RG: Neural tube defects caused by local anesthetics in early chick embryos. Teratology 31:119, 1985.

50. Michejda M, Hodgen GD: Induction of neural-tube defects in nonhuman primates in prevention of physical and mental congenital defects, Part B: Epidemiology, early detection and therapy and environmental factors. Prog Clin Biol Res 163:243, 1985.

51. Miller P, Smith DW, Shepard TH: Maternal hyperthermia as a possible cause of anencephaly. Lancet i:519, 1978.

52. Milunsky A, Ulcickas M, Rothman KJ, et al.: Maternal heat exposure and neural tube defects. JAMA 7:882, 1992.

53. Paulson RB, Sucheston ME, Hayes TG, et al.: Teratogenic effects of valporate in the CD-1 mouse fetus. Arch Neurol 42:980, 1985.

54. Seller MJ: The cause of neural tube defects: Some experiments and a hypothesis. J Med Genet 20:164, 1983.

55. Strassburg MA, Saunder G, Wang S: A correctional study of neural tube defects and infectious diseases. Public Health (London) 97:275, 1983.

56. ETIC Search Subject, Neural Tube Environmental Teratology Information Center (F Jordan), PO Box 12233, NIEHS, Maildrop 18-01 Research Triangle Park, North Carolina, 27709.

57. Laurence KM: In prevention of neural tube defects by improvement in maternal diet and preconceptional folic acid. Supplementation in prevention of physical and mental congenital defects. Part B: Epidemiology, early detection and therapy and environmental factors. Prog Clin Biol Res 163:383, 1985.

58. Nevin NC: The role of periconceptional vitamin supplementation in the prevention of neural tube defects. Part B: Epidemiology, early detection and therapy and environmental factors. Prog Clin Biol Res 163:389, 1985.

59. Scharah CJ, Wild S, Hartley R, et al.: The effect of periconceptional supplementation on blood vitamin concentrations in women of recurrence risk for neural tube defect. Br J Nutr 49:203, 1983.

60. Hibbard ED, Smithells RW: Folic acid metabolism and human embryology. Lancet i:1254, 1965.

61. Smithells RW, Sheppard S, Schorah CJ: Possible prevention of neural-tube defects by periconceptional vitamin supplementation. Lancet i:647, 1980.

62. MRC Vitamin Study Research Group. Prevention of neural tube defects: Results of the Medical Research Council Vitamin Study. Lancet 338:131, 1991.

63. Smithells RW, Nevin NC, Seller MJ, et al.: Further experience of vitamin supplementation for the prevention of neural tube defect recurrences. Lancet i:1027, 1983.

64. Mulinare J, Cordero JF, Erickson JD, Berry RJ: Periconceptional use of multivitamins and the occurrence of neural tube defects. JAMA 260:3141, 1988.

65. Milunsky A, Jick H, Jick SS, et al.: Multivitamin/folic acid supplementation in early pregnancy reduces the prevalence of neural tube defects. JAMA 262:2847, 1989.

66. Czeizel AE, Dudás I: Prevention of the first occurrence of neural-tube defects by periconceptional vitamin supplementation. N Engl J Med 26:1832, 1992.

67. Werler M, Shapiro S, Mitchell AA: Periconceptional folic acid exposure and risk of occurrent neural tube defects. JAMA 10:1257, 1993.

68. Economides DL, Ferguson J, Mackenzie IZ, et al.: Folate and vitamin B_{12} concentrations in maternal and fetal blood, and amniotic fluid in second trimester pregnancies complicated by neural tube defects. Br J Obstet Gynaecol 99:23, 1992.

69. Gardiki-Kouidou P, Seller SM: Amniotic fluid folate, vitamin B_{12} and transcobalamins in neural tube defects. Clin Genet 33:441, 1988.

70. Hall MH: Folic acid deficiency and congenital malformations. J Obstet Gynaecol Br Commonw 79:159, 1972.

71. Yates JRW, Ferguson-Smith MA, Shenkin A, et al.: Is disordered folate metabolism the basis for the genetic predisposition to neural tube defects? Clin Genet 31:279, 1987.

72. CDC. Recommendations for the use of folic acid to reduce the number of cases of spina bifida and other neural tube defects. MMWR 41:1, 1992. No. RR-14.

73. Gilbert JN, Jones KL, Rorke LB, et al.: Central nervous system anomalies associated with myelomeningocele, hydrocephalus and the Arnold-Chiari malformation: Reappraisal of theories regarding the pathogenesis of posterior neural tube closure defects. Neurosurgery 18:559, 1986.

74. Variend S, Emery JL: The pathology of the central lobes of the cerebellum in children with myelomeningocele. Dev Med Child Neurol 16:99, 1974.

75. Yakolev PI, Wadsworth RC: Schizencephalies. J Neuropathol Exp Neurol 5:116, 1946.

76. Stark GD, Baker GCW: The neurological involvement of the lower limbs in myelomeningocele. Dev Med Child Neurol 9:732, 1967.

77. MacKenzie NG, Emery JL: Deformities of the cervical cord in children with neurospinal dysraphism. Dev Med Child Neurol 13:58, 1971.

78. Emery JL, Lendon RG: Clinical implications of cord lesions in neurospinal dysraphism. Dev Med Child Neurol 14:45, 1972.

79. Chadduck WM, Uthman EO: Squamous cell carcinoma and meningomyelocele. Neurosurgery 14:601, 1984.

80. Helle TL, Hanbury JW, Becker DH: Meningeal malignant fibrous histiocytoma arising from a thoracolumbar myelomeningocele. J Neurosurg 58:593, 1983.

81. Mickle JP, McLennan JE: Malignant teratoma arising within a meningomyelocele. J Neurosurg 43:761, 1975.

82. Lendon RG: Neuron population in the lumbosacral cord of myelomeningocele children. Dev Med Child Neurol 20:82, 1969.

83. Ralis J, Ralis HM: Morphology of peripheral nerves in children with spina bifida. Dev Med Child Neurol 109:101, 1972.

84. Brown SF: Congential malformations associated with myelomeningocele. J Iowa Med Soc 65:101, 1975.

85. Stark GD, Drummond M: The spinal cord lesion in myelomeningocele. Dev Med Child Neurol 13:1, 1971.

86. Reigel DH, Dallmann DE, Scarff TB, et al.: Intraoperative evoked potential studies of newborn infants with myelomeningocele. Dev Med Child Neurol 18:42, 1977.

87. Epstein F, Spielholz N, Battista A, et al.: Delayed cauda equina reconstruction in myelomeningocele. Neurosurgery 6:540, 1980.

88. Globus MS, Loughman WD, Epstein CJ, et al.: Prenatal genetic diagnosis in 3000 amniocenteses. N Engl J Med 300:157, 1979.

89. Milunsky A, Alpert E, Neff RK, et al.: Prenatal diagnosis of neural tube defects. IV. Maternal serum alpha-fetoprotein screening. Obstet Gynecol 55:60, 1980.

90. Wald NJ, Cuckle H, Brock JH, et al.: Maternal serum alpha-fetoprotein measurement in antenatal screening for anencephaly and spina bifida in early pregnancy. (Report of United Kingdom collaborative study on alpha-fetoprotein in relation to neural tube defects.) Lancet i:1323, 1977.

91. Wald NJ, Cuckle H, Nanchahal K: Amniotic fluid acetylcholinesterase measurement in the prenatal diagnosis of open neural tube defects: Second report of the Collaborative Acetylcholinesterase Study. Prenat Diagn 9:813, 1989.

92. Brock DJH, Barron L, Von Heyningen V: Prenatal diagnosis of neural tube defects with monoclonal antibody specific for acetylcholine esterase. Lancet i:8419, 1985.

93. Nadel AS, Green JK, Holmes LB, et al.: Absence of need for amniocentesis in patients with elevated levels of maternal serum alpha-fetoprotein and normal ultrasonographic examinations. N Engl J Med 9:557, 1990.

94. Wald NJ, Cuckle HS, Haddow JE: Letters to the Editor. N Engl J Med 11:769, 1991.

95. Brock DJH, Sutcliffe RG: Alpha-fetoprotein in the antenatal diagnosis of anencephaly and spina bifida. Lancet ii:197, 1972.

96. Luthy DA, Wardinsky T, Shurtleff DB, et al.: Cesarean section before the onset of labor and subsequent motor function in infants with myelomeningocele diagnosed antenatally. N Engl J Med 10:662, 1991.

97. Robertson P: Operative and assisted delivery. Curr Opinion Obstet Gynecol 3:769, 1991.

98. Cochrane D, Aronyk K, Sawatzky B, et al.: The effects of labor and delivery on spinal cord function and ambulation in patients with myelomeningocele. Child's Nerv Sys 7:312, 1991.

99. Sakala EP, Andree I: Optimal route of delivery for myelomeningocele. Obstet Gynecol Surv 4:209, 1990.

100. Forestus P: De capitis et cerebre morbis ac symptomatis. Observationum Medicinalium, libri III. Leiden, Ex Off Plantiniana Raphelemgii, 1587.

101. Tulpius N: Cum aetieis figuris. Observationum Medicinalium, libri III. Amsterdam, Apud Ludovican Elzevirium, 1641.

102. Tulpius N: Observationum Medicinalium, libri III, Cap. XXIX, XXX. Amsterdam, Apud Ludovican Elzevirium, 1641, p. 229.

103. Lebedeff A: Uber che Enstehurg der Anencephalie und Spina Bifida dei Vogelin und Menschen. Virchows Arch Pathol Anat Physiol 86:263, 1881.

104. Morgagni J-B: De sedubis et causis morborum per anatomen indigatis, libri V. Venice, Ex Typographia Remondiona, 1761.

105. Von Recklinghausen F: Untersuchungen ubev che Spina Bifida. Arch Pathol Anat 105:243, 1886.

106. Forestus P: Observation chir., libri V, lib III, obs VII, 1610.

107. Fraser J: Spina bifida. Edinburgh Med J 36:284, 1929.

108. Ingram FD, Swan H: Spina bifida and cranium bifidum: I: A survey of five hundred forty-six cases. N Engl J Med 228:559, 1943.

109. Moore JE: Spina bifida with a report of 385 cases treated by excision. Surg Gynecol Obstet 1:137, 1905.

110. Nulsen FE, Spitz EB: Treatment of hydrocephalus by direct heart shunt from ventricle to jugular vein. Surg Forum 2:399, 1951.

111. Sharrad WJW, Zachary RB, Lorber J, et al.: A controlled trial of immediate and delayed closure of spina bifida cystica. Arch Dis Child 38:18, 1963.

112. Lorber J: Results of treatment of myelomeningocele: An analysis of 524 unselected cases with special references to possible selection for treatment. Dev Med Child Neurol 13:279, 1971.

113. Black PM: Selective treatment of infants with myelomeningocele. Neurosurgery 5:334, 1979.

114. McLone DG: Treatment of myelomeningocele and arguments against selection. Clin Neurosurg 33:359, 1986.

115. McLone DG, Dias L, Kaplan WE, et al.: Concepts in the management of spina bifida. In Humphreys RP (ed): Concepts in Pediatric Neurosurgery. 5th ed. Basel, S. Karger, 1985, pp 97–106.

116. McLone DG: Results of treatment of children born with a myelomeningocele. Clin Neurosurg 30:407, 1983.

117. McLone DG: Continuing concepts in the management of spina bifida. Pediatr Neurosurg 18:254, 1992.

118. Lorber J, Salfield S: Results of selective treatment of spina bifida cystica. Arch Dis Child 56:822, 1981.

119. Charney EB, Miller SC, Sutton LN, et al.: Management of the newborn with myelomeningocele: Time for a decision-making process. Pediatrics 75:58, 1985.

120. Gross HR, Cox A, Tatyrek R, et al.: Early management and decision making for the treatment of myelomeningocele. Pediatrics 72:450, 1983.

121. Freeman JM: Early management and decision making for treatment of myelomeningocele: A critique. Pediatrics 73:564, 1984.

122. McCormick RA: To save or let die. JAMA 229:172, 1974.

123. Scarff TB, Toleikis JR, Bunch WH, et al.: Dermatomal somatosensory evoked potentials in children with myelomeningocele. Z Kinderchir 28:384, 1979.

124. Sharrad WJW: The mechanism of paralytic deformity in spina bifida. Dev Med Child Neurol 4:310, 1962.

125. Sharrad WJW: The segmental innervation of the lower limb muscles in man. Ann R Coll Surg Engl 35:106, 1964.

126. Sharrad WJW: Neuromotor evaluation of the newborn. In American Academy of Orthopaedic Surgeons: Symposium on Myelomeningocele. St. Louis, C. V. Mosby, 1972, pp 26–40.

127. Sharrad WJW: Assessment of the myelomeningocele child. In McLaurin RL (ed): Myelomeningocele. New York, Grune & Stratton, 1977, pp 389–410.

128. Venes JL: Letter to the Editor. Pediatrics 74:948, 1984.

129. Scarff TB, Nelson P, Reigel DH: External drainage for ventricular infection following cerebrospinal fluid shunts. Child's Brain 5:129, 1979.

130. McLone DG, Czyzewski D, Raimondi AJ, et al.: Central nervous system infections as a limiting factor in the intelligence of children born with myelomeningocele. Pediatrics 70:338, 1982.

131. Amacher L: The microsurgical anatomy of lumbar rachischisis. Adv Ophthalmol 37:197, 1978.

132. McLone DG: Technique for closure of myelomeningocele. Child's Brain 6:65, 1980.

133. Reigel DH: Kyphectomy and myelomeningocele repair. Modern techniques in surgery. Neurosurgery 13:1, 1979.

134. Reigel DH: Tethered spinal cord. In Humphreys RP (ed): Concepts in Pediatric Neurosurgery. Vol. 4. Basel, S. Karger, 1983, pp 142–164.

135. Storrs BB: Are dermoid and epidermoid tumors preventable complications of myelomeningocele repair? Accepted for publication in Pediatr Neurosurg, 1994.

136. Bannister CM: A method of repair of myelomeningoceles. Br J Surg 59:445, 1972.

137. Blaiklock CR, Demetriou EL, Rayner CRW: The use of a latissimus dorsi myocutaneous flap in the repair of spinal defects in spina bifida. Br J Plast Surg 34:358, 1981.

138. Cruz NI, Ariyan S, Duncan CC, et al.: Repair of lumbosacral myelomeningoceles with double Z-rhomboid flaps. J Neurosurg 59:714, 1983.

139. Lehrman A, Owen MP: Surgical repair of large meningomyeloceles. Ann Plast Surg 12:501, 1984.

140. McDevitt NB, Gillespie RP, Woolsey RE, et al.: Closure of thoracic and lumbar dysraphic defects using bilateral latissimus dorsi myocutaneous flap transfer with extended gluteal fasciocutaneous flaps. Child's Brain 9:394, 1982.

141. Mustarde JC: Meningomyelocele: The problem of skin cover. Br J Surg 53:36, 1966.

142. Zook EG, Dzenitis AJ, Bennett JE: Repair of large myelomeningoceles. Arch Surg 98:41, 1969.

143. Zide BM: How to reduce the morbidity of wound closure following: 1. Extensive & complicated laminectomy, 2. Tethered cord surgery. Pediatr Neurosurg 18:157, 1992.

144. Reigel DH, McLone DG: Myelomeningocele: Operative treatment and results. In Marlin AE (ed): Concepts in Pediatric Neurosurg. Vol. 8. Basel, S, Karger, 1987.

145. Sharrad WJW: Spinal osteotomy for congenital kyphosis in myelomeningocele. J Bone Joint Surg 50:466, 1968.

146. Reigel DH: Indications for and techniques of kyphectomy. In McLaurin RL (ed): Spina Bifida: A Multidisciplinary Approach. New York, Praeger Publishers, 1986, pp 140–145.

147. Reigel DH, McLone DG: Spina bifida. In Mustarde JC, Jackson IT (eds): Plastic Surgery in Infancy and Childhood, 3rd ed. London, Churchill Livingstone, 1988.

148. McMillan JJ, Williams B: Aqueduct stenosis: Case review and discussion. J Neurol Neurosurg Psychiatry 40:521, 1977.

149. Williams B: Is aqueduct stenosis the result of hydrocephalus? Brain 96:399, 1973.

150. Reigel DH, Dallmann DE, Scarff TB, et al.: Transcephalic impedance measurement during infancy. Dev Med Child Neurol 19:295, 1977.

151. Sauerbrei EE, Harrison PB, Ling E, et al.: Neonatal intra-cranial pathology demonstrated by high-frequency linear array ultrasound. JCU 9:33, 1981.

152. Robertson JS, Maraqa MI, Jennett V: Ventriculoperitoneal shunting for hydrocephalus. Br Med J 2:289, 1973.

153. Stark GD, Drummond MB, Poneprasert S, et al.: Primary ventriculoperitoneal shunts in treatment of hydrocephalus associated with myelomeningocele. Arch Dis Child 29:112, 1974.

154. McLaurin RL: Treatment of infected ventricular shunts. Child's Brain 1:306, 1975.

155. Holinger PC, Holinger LD, Reichert TJ, et al.: Respiratory obstruction and apnea in infants with bilateral abductor vocal cord paralysis, meningomyelocele, hydrocephalus, and Arnold-Chiari malformation. Pediatrics 92:368, 1978.

156. Raimondi AJ, Soare P: Intellectual development in shunted hydrocephalic children. Am J Dis Child 127:664, 1974.

157. Shaffer J, Wolfe L, Friedrich W, et al.: Developmental expectations: Intelligence and fine motor skills. In Shurtleff DB (ed): Myelodysplasias and Exstrophies: Significance, Prevention, and Treatment. New York, Grune & Stratton, 1986, pp 359–372.

158. Cull C, Wyke MA: Memory function of children with spina bifida and shunted hydrocephalus. Dev Med Child Neurol 26:177, 1984.

159. Lonton AD: The relationship between intellectual skills and the computerized axial tomograms of children with spina bifida and hydrocephalus. Z Kinderchir 28:368, 1977.

160. Rowley-Kelly FL, Reigel DH: Teaching the Student with Spina Bifida. Baltimore, P. L. Brooks, 1993.

161. Reigel DH, Tchernoukha K, Bazmi B, et al.: Change in spinal curvature following release of tethered spinal cord associated with spinal bifida. Pediatr Neurosurg 20:5, 1994.

162. Action Committee on Myelodysplasia, Section of Urology: Current approaches to evaluation and management of children with myelomeningocele. Pediatrics 63:663, 1979.

163. Awad SA, Downie J, Kiruluta H: Pharmacologic treatment of disorders of bladder and urethra: A review. Can J Surg 22:515, 1979.

164. Hannigan KF: Teaching intermittent self-catheterization to young children with myelodysplasia. Dev Med Child Neurol 21:365, 1979.

165. Kaplan WE: Clear intermittent catheterization. In McLaurin RL (ed): Spina Bifida: A Multidisciplinary Approach. New York, Praeger Publishers, 1986; pp 274–276.

166. Lapides J, Diokno AC, Lowe BS, et al.: Follow-up of unsterile intermittent self-catheterization. J Urol 111:184, 1974.

167. Scott FB, Bradley WE, Timm GW: Treatment of urinary incontinence by an implantable prosthetic sphincter. Urology 1:252, 1973.

168. Whitehead WE, Parker LH, Masek BJ, et al.: Biofeedback treatment of fecal incontinence in myelomeningocele. Dev Med Child Neurol (in press).

169. Burch DM: The artificial sphincter to correct sphincter incontinence in the myelodysplastic child. In McLaurin RL (ed): Spina Bifida—A Multidisciplinary Approach. New York, Praeger Publishers, 1986, pp 277–280.

170. Wabrek AJ: Myelodysplasia and interpersonal and sexual aspects. In McLaurin RL (ed): Spina Bifida: A Multidisciplinary Approach. New York, Praeger Publishers, 1986, pp 332–340.

171. Shurtleff DB, Sousa JC: The adolescent with myelodysplasia: Development, achievement, sex and deterioration. In McLaurin RL (ed): Myelomeningocele. New York, Grune & Stratton, 1977, pp 809–835.

172. Naidich TP, McLone DG, Shkolnik A, et al.: Sonographic evaluation of caudal spine anomalies in children. AJNR 4:661, 1983.

173. Anderson TM, Burke BL: Anterior sacral meningocele. A presentation of three cases. JAMA 237:30, 1977.

174. Oren M, Lorber B, Lee SH, et al.: Anterior sacral meningocele: Report of five cases and review of the literature. Dis Colon Rectum 20:492, 1977.

175. Vogel EH: Anterior sacral meningocele as a gynecologic problem: Report of a case. Obstet Gynecol 36:766, 1970.

176. Silvis RS, Riddle LR, Clark GG: Anterior sacral meningocele. Am Surg 22:554, 1956.

177. Chamaa MT, Berney J: Anterior-sacral meningocele; value of magnetic resonance imaging and abdominal sonography. Acta Neurochir (Wien) 109:154, 1991.

178. Amacher AL, Drake CG, McLachlin AD: Anterior sacral myelocele. Surg Gynecol Obstet 126:986, 1968.

179. O'Neill P, Whetmore WJ, Booth AE: Spinal meningoceles in association with neurofibromatosis. Neurosurgery 13:82, 1983.

180. Stroud RD, Eisenburg HM: Anterior sacral myelocele in association with Marfan's syndrome. Radiology 99:653, 1971.

181. Tomita T, McLone DG: Acute respiratory arrest: A complication of malfunction of the shunt in children with myelomeningocele and Arnold-Chiari malformation: A report of three cases. Am J Dis Child 137:142, 1983.

182. Peach B: Arnold-Chiari malformation: Anatomic features of 20 cases. Arch Neurol 12:113, 1965.

183. Peach B: Arnold-Chiari malformation: Morphogenesis. Arch Neurol 12:527, 1965.

184. Rorke LB, Fogelson MH, Riggs HE: Cerebellar heterotopia in infancy. Dev Med Child Neurol 10:664, 1968.

185. Naidich TP, Maravilla K, McLone DG: The Chiari II malforma-

tion. *In* McLaurin RL (ed): Proceedings of the Second Symposium on Spina Bifida. New York, Praeger Publishing, 1986, pp 164–173.

186. Naidich TP, McLone DG, Fulling KH: The Chiari II malformation. Part IV: The hindbrain deformity. Neuroradiology 25:179, 1983.

187. Hall PV, Campbell RL, Kalsbek JE: Meningomyelocele and progressive hydromyelia. Progressive paresis in myelodysplasia. J Neurosurg 43:457, 1975.

188. Hall PV, Lindseth RE, Campbell RL, et al.: Myelodysplasia and developmental scoliosis. A manifestation of syringomyelia. Spine 1:48, 1956.

189. Hoffman HJ, Neill J, Crone KR, et al.: Hydrosyringomyelia and its management in childhood. Neurosurgery 21:347, 1987.

190. Gardner WJ: Hydrodynamic mechanisms of syringomyelia: Its relationship to myelomeningocele. J Neurol Neurosurg Psychiatry 28:247, 1965.

191. Hoffman HJ, Hendrick EB, Humphreys RP: Manifestations and management of Arnold-Chiari malformations in patients with myelomeningocele. Child's Brain 1:255, 1975.

192. Park TS, Hoffman HJ, Hendrick EB, et al.: Experience with surgical decompression of the Arnold-Chiari malformation in young infants with myelomeningocele. Neurosurgery 13:147, 1983.

193. Williams B: A critical appraisal of posterior fossa surgery for communicating syringomyelia. Brain 101:223, 1978.

194. Venes JL, Black KL, Latack JT: Preoperative evaluation and surgical management of the Arnold-Chiari II malformation. J Neurosurg 64:363, 1986.

195. Gardner WJ, Goodall RJ: The surgical treatment of Arnold-Chiari malformation in adults. An explanation of its mechanism and importance of encephalography in diagnosis. J Neurosurg 7:199, 1950.

196. Ball MJ, Dayan AD: Pathogenesis of syringomyelia. Lancet ii:799, 1972.

197. Williams B: Progress in syringomyelia. Neurol Res 8:139, 1986.

198. Milhorat TH, Johnson WD, Miller JI, et al.: Surgical treatment of syringomyelia based on magnetic resonance imaging criteria. Neurosurgery 31:231, 1992.

199. Wisoff JH, Epstein F: Management of hydromyelia. Neurosurgery 25:562, 1989.

200. Park TS, Cail WS, Broaddus WC, et al.: Lumboperitoneal shunt combined with myelotomy for treatment of syringohydromyelia. J Neurosurg 70:721, 1989.

201. Venes JL: Spasticity in a myelodysplasia clinic population—report on a work in progress. Conc Pediatr Neurosurg 8:57, 1988.

202. Mazur JM, Stillwell A, Menelaus M: The significance of spasticity in the upper and lower limbs in myelomeningocele. J Bone Joint Surg 68B:213, 1986.

203. McLaughlin TP, Banta MD, Gahm NH, et al.: Intraspinal rhizotomy and distal cordectomy in patients with myelomeningocele. J Bone Joint Surg 68A:88, 1986.

204. Park TS, Cail WS, Maggio WM, et al.: Progressive spasticity and scoliosis in children with myelomeningocele. J Neurosurg 62:367, 1985.

205. Biglan AW: Ophthalmologic complications of meningomyelocele: A longitudinal study. Trans Am Ophthalmol Soc 88:389, 1990.

206. Gaston H: Ophthalmologic complications of spina bifida and hydrocephalus. Eye 5:279, 1991.

207. Shurtleff DB, Dunne K: Adolescents with meningomyelocele. *In* Shurtleff DB (ed): Myelodysplasias and Exstrophies: Significance, Prevention, and Treatment. New York, Grune & Stratton, 1986, pp 39–64.

208. Hack CH, Enrile BG, Donat JF, et al.: Seizures in relation to shunt dysfunction in children with myelomeningocele. J Pediatr 116:57, 1990.

209. Kaplan WE, Richards TW, Richards I: Intravesical transurethral bladder stimulation to increase bladder capacity. J Urol 142:600, 1989.

210. Kaplan GW: Myelomeningocele and related disorders. J Continuing Ed Urol 17:15, 1978.

211. Gonzalez R, Koleilat N, Austin C, et al.: The artificial sphincter AS 800 in congenital urinary incontinence. J Urol 142:512, 1989.

212. Gonzalez R, Nguyen DH, Koleilat N, et al.: Compatibility of enterocystoplasty and the artificial urinary sphincter. J Urol 142:502, 1989.

213. Mulcahy JJ, James HE, McRoberts JW: Oxybutynin chloride combined with intermittent clean catheterization in the treatment of myelomeningocele patients. J Urol 118:95, 1977.

214. Spindel MR, Bauer SB, Dyro FM, et al.: The changing neurologic lesion in myelodysplasia. JAMA 258:1630, 1987.

215. Pike JG, Berardinucci G, Hamburger B, et al.: The surgical management of urinary incontinence in myelodysplastic children. J Pediatr Surg 26:466, 1991.

216. Rudy DC, Woodside JR: The incontinent myelodysplastic patient. Urol Clin North Am 18:295, 1991.

217. Lindehall B, Claesson I, Hjälmås K, et al.: Effect of clean intermittent catheterization on radiological appearance of the upper urinary tract in children with myelomeningocele. Br J Urol 67:415, 1991.

218. Blair GK, Djonlic K, Fraser GC, et al.: The bowel management tube: An effective means for controlling fecal incontinence. J Pediatr Surg 27:1269, 1992.

219. Leonard CO, Freeman JM: Spina bifida: A new disease. Pediatrics 68:136, 1981.

220. Rimoin DL: Genetic disorders of the pituitary gland. *In* Emery AEH, Rimoin DL (eds): Principles and Practice of Medical Genetics. New York, Churchill Livingston, 1983, pp 1134–1151.

221. Hayes-Allen MC: Obesity and short stature in children with myelomeningocele. Dev Med Child Neurol 14(Suppl 27):59, 1972.

222. Rosenblum MF, Finegold DN, Charney EB: Assessment of stature of children with myelomeningocele and usefulness of arm-span measurement. Dev Med Child Neurol 25:338, 1983.

223. Belt-Niedbala BJ, Ekvall S, Cook C, et al.: Linear growth measurement: A comparison of single arm-lengths and arm span. Dev Med Child Neurol 28:319, 1986.

224. Hamill PVV: NCHS growth curve for children, birth to 18 years: United States. Hyattsville, MD: National Center for Health Services. DHEW publication No. 78-1650. Vital and Health Statistics 1977, Series 11, No. 165, pp 20–23.

225. Rotenstein D, Cottington E, Henry J, et al.: Growth curves of children with open neural tube defect. Clin Res 40:760A, 1992.

226. Roberts D, Shepherd RW, Shepherd K: Anthropometry and obesity in myelomeningocele. J Paediatr Child Health 27:83, 1991.

227. Rotenstein D, Flom LL, Reigel DH: Growth hormone treatment accelerates growth of short children with neural tube defects. J Pediatr 115:417, 1989.

228. Rotenstein D, Reigel DH, Flom LL: Growth hormone treatment accelerates growth of short children with neural tube defects. Ann Rev Hydrocephalus 8:152, 1990.

229. Rotenstein D: Anthropometry and obesity in myelomeningocele. J Paediatr Child Health 3:270, 1992.

230. Rotenstein D, Flom L, Reigel DH, et al.: Growth hormone treatment of children with spina bifida does not accelerate growth of the upper extremity in excess of recumbent length. 73rd Annual Meeting of the Endocrine Society, June 1991, Abstract 1314, p. 359.

231. Rotenstein D, Reigel DH, Flom LL, et al.: Growth hormone treatment of children with open neural tube defects: Treatment beyond the first 6 months. 74th Annual Meeting of the Endocrine Society, June 1992; 705:228. Program and abstracts.

232. Greene SA, Frank M, Zachmann M, Prader M: Growth and sexual development in children with myelomeningocele. Eur J Paediatr 144:146, 1985.

233. Shepherd K, Roberts D, Golding S, et al.: Body composition in myelomeningocele. Am J Clin Nutr 53:1, 1991.

234. Rotenstein D, Flom LL, Reigel DH, Cottington E: Obesity and Body Mass Index (BMI) of children with open neural tube defects. 71st Annual Meeting of the Endocrine Society, June 1989, Abstract 1191, p. 3200.

235. Rotenstein D, Adams M, Reigel DH: Adult stature and anthropomorphic measurements of patients with neural tube defects. 72nd Annual Meeting of the Endocrine Society, June 1990, Abstract 1107, p. 301.

236. Storrs BB, McLone DG: Ventricular size and intelligence in my-

elodysplastic children. *In* Marlin AE (ed): Concepts in Pediatric Neurosurg. Vol. 8. Basel, S. Karger, 1988, pp 51–56.

237. CDC. Anaphylactic reactions during general anesthesia among pediatric patients—United States, January 1990–January 1991. MMWR Vol. 40, No. 26, p. 437, 1991.

238. Meerpol E, Kelleher R, Bell S, et al.: Allergic reactions to rubber in patients with myelodysplasia. Letter to the Editor. N Engl J Med 323:1072, 1990.

239. Merguerian PA, Klein RB, Graven MA, et al.: Intraoperative anaphylactic reaction due to latex hypersensitivity. Urology 4:301, 1991.

240. Moneret-Vautrin DA, Laxenaire MC, Bavoux F: Allergic shock to latex and ethylene oxide during surgery for spina bifida. Anesthesiology 73:556, 1990.

241. Moneret-Vautrin DA, Mata E, Gueant JL, et al.: High risk of anaphylactic shock during surgery for spina bifida. Letters to the Editor. Lancet 335:865, 1990.

242. Slater JE: Rubber anaphylaxis. N Engl J Med 315:1126, 1989.

243. Slater JE: Routine testing for latex allergy in patients with spina bifida is not recommended. Letters to the Editor. Anesthesiology 74:391, 1991.

244. Parsch K: Origin and treatment of fractures in spina bifida. Eur J Pediatr Surg 1:298, 1991.

245. Soare PL, Raimondi AJ: Intellectual and perceptual motor characteristics of treated myelomeningocele children. Am J Dis Child 131:199, 1977.

246. Hunt GM, Holmes AE: Some factors relating to intelligence in treated hydrocephalic children. Am J Dis Child 127:664, 1974.

247. Fletcher JM, Francis DJ, Thompson NM, et al.: Verbal and nonverbal skill discrepancies in hydrocephalic children. J Clin Exp Neuropsychol 14:593, 1992.

248. Rogosky-Grassi MA: Working with perceptual-motor skills. *In* Rowley-Kelly FL, Reigel DH (eds): Teaching the Student With Spina Bifida. Baltimore, P. L. Brooks, 1993.

249. Pless IB, Power C, Peckham CS: Long-term psychosocial sequelae of chronic physical disorders of childhood. Pediatrics 91:1131, 1993.

250. Shaffer J, Friedrich W: Young adult psychosocial development. *In* Shurtleff DB (ed): Myelodysplasias and Exstrophies: Significance, Prevention, and Treatment. New York, Grune & Stratton, 1986, pp 359–372.

251. Kokkonen J, Saukkonen AL, Timonen E, et al.: Social outcome of handicapped children as adults. Dev Med Child Neurol 33:1095, 1991.

Chapter 4

TETHERED SPINAL CORD

DONALD H. REIGEL, M.D., and DAVID G. McLONE, M.D., Ph.D.

The term tethered spinal cord describes a condition in which the spinal cord is fastened to an immovable structure, such as a lipoma, vertebra, dura, or skin. The spinal cord is fixed between two points: first at the tethering element and second at the base of the brain or dentate ligaments. Thus, vertebral structures that move as a result of growth, daily activity, and pathologic skeletal change (scoliosis) stretch the spinal cord, producing abnormal tension. The result is that the intervening segment of spinal cord is stretched beyond its tolerance, and vascular, neuronal, and axonal changes ensue. Furthermore, these neurologic changes alter function of the structures served by the involved area of spinal cord. Thus, a characteristic clinical syndrome evolves that frequently consists of muscle weakness, change in bowel and bladder control, pain, sensory deficit, and skeletal deformity. A heterogeneous group of congenital lesions have been recognized as causes for this group of symptoms and physical findings. They may be classified as in Tables 4–1 and 4–2. Thus, the clinical syndrome of tethered cord is tied together by a similar pathophysiology, embryologic origin, morbid anatomy, and clinical picture. The pathologic anatomy can be recognized because of the unique physical appearance and diagnostic findings. These lesions have often been described as occult, primarily because the physical findings were considered to be hidden and of little consequence despite the ability of the abnormality to insidiously produce profound disability for children and adults. Deficit associated with this family of problems was often accepted and described as fixed or static. Furthermore, operative treatment was thought to only increase disability and disappointingly fail to alter the fate of these patients. These opinions have evolved and persisted for the past 100 years despite literature supporting a contrary opinion.

In 1891, Mr. Jones published a report entitled "Spina Bifida Occulta: No Paralytic Symptoms Until Seventeen Years of Age; Spine Trephined to Relieve Pressure on the Cauda Equina; Recovery."[1] A patient with the neonatal history of spina bifida had been ignored from childhood and "rediscovered" when the patient developed intense pain and paresis. The skin was "puckered and covered with short hairs." At the time of operation in 1890, a "dense adventitious fibrous band" crossed the "spinal canal compressing the cauda equina." The lower border of the band was continuous with "cicatricial tissue which represented the old spina bifida." This band was transected and removed. Six months following surgery, the patient was free of pain and able to micturate and walk without difficulty.

In 1918, Brickner referred to Elsberg's description of stretching of nerve roots as the "disproportion in length between the bony and medullary columns developed with the growth of the individual."[2] Brickner went on to recommend operation for infants and children with spina bifida occulta, congenital lipoma, or hypertrichosis even in the absence of symptoms "in the hope of obviating the development of symptoms during adolescence." During the last 40 years there has been a

TABLE 4–1. DESCRIPTIVE CLASSIFICATION

Primary causes
Dermal sinus tract
Diastematomyelia
Dural bands (meningocele manqué)
Intraspinal lipoma
Intraspinal tumors (dermoid, epidermoid, ependymoma, teratoma, astrocytoma)
Meningocele
Myelomeningocele
Neurenteric cyst
Terminale myelocystocele
Tight filum terminale

Secondary causes
Arachnoiditis
Dermoid
Retethered spinal cord syndrome
Suture granuloma
Trauma

TABLE 4–2.   EMBRYOLOGIC CLASSIFICATION

Deranged primary neurulation
    Dermal sinus
    Diastematomyelia
    Lipomyelomeningocele
    Myelomeningocele
    Secondary neurulation

Deranged retrogressive differentiation
    Terminal myelocystocele
    Tight filum terminale

Caudal regression syndrome
    Atresias
    Agenesis of lumbosacral spine
    Enteric fistula
    Exstrophies
    Sirenomelia

Persistent notochord canal
    Diverticuli
    Enteric cords
    Anterior spina bifida
    Neurenteric cysts
    Diastematomyelia

long succession of published reports indicating that the following points should be emphasized in the treatment of lesions associated with tethered spinal cord:

1. The natural course of congenital spinal lesions that cause tethered spinal cord is associated with progressive neurologic deterioration and disability.

2. Early recognition, evaluation, and diagnosis are possible and of extreme importance.

3. Early operative treatment prevents deterioration and may result in neurologic recovery.

4. Operation in the absence of symptoms and findings may preserve normal neurologic, orthopedic, and urologic status.[3–24]

EMBRYOLOGY

During the first 3 weeks of fetal development, the spinal cord evolves from ectodermal cells above the notochord. The notochord induces formation of the neural plate and guides formation of the vertebral column. Through a process of elevation and rolling upon itself, the neural tube develops and thereafter a series of events leads to the formation of the spinal cord (neurulation and canalization) (Chapter 1). The superficial ectoderm separates from and covers the neural tube and then forms the skin. Mesoderm migrates between the skin and neural tube to form the tissues surrounding the spinal column. Derangement during neurulation produces the group of congenital anomalies outlined in Table 4–2.

Early in intrauterine development the fetal spinal cord extends caudally to the tail fold of the embryo. The distal spinal cord and notochord form from the caudal cell mass. This cell mass undergoes canalization to form the initial conus medullaris and filum terminale. The process of involution has been termed "ret-

rogressive differentiation." A better term is *secondary neurulation*. At its completion the spinal cord is located at the coccygeal level. Thereafter, the spinal column elongates more rapidly than the spinal cord. Therefore, at birth the conus rests at L2–L3 and, within the first 2 months of infancy, comes to rest at its adult location of L1–L2.[25] Thus, the spinal cord does not ascend, but the ascending location of the conus is a result of disproportionate longitudinal growth between the vertebrae and the spinal column. Abnormalities during the period which affect secondary neurulation lead to the anomalies described in Table 4–2. Combinations of abnormalities affecting the caudal cell mass and secondary neurulation result in the syndrome of embryonic deformation and caudal suppression (see Table 4–2). For further detailed discussion of the embryology of the spine and spinal cord, see Chapter 1.

PATHOPHYSIOLOGY

The morbid anatomy of these congenital lesions sets the stage for the forces that produce the pathophysiologic changes which cause the clinical symptoms and deficits. In all of these conditions, the spinal cord is fixed at a point distal to the brain so that the demands for tolerance of motion or traction in the adjacent areas exceed the tolerance of the cord. It must be emphasized that in the normal newborn the conus rests at L1–L3 and little further change in its rostral caudal location occurs with growth. Therefore, tethered cord is not failure of the spinal cord to ascend.

The evidence that metabolic, vascular, and mechanical factors play a role in deteriorating function arise from intraoperative and laboratory observations. During surgery, the rostral to caudal decrease in diameter, pallor, and absence of pulsation of the spinal cord, which extends tightly across the posterior thecal sac, suggest traction (Fig. 4–1). Retraction of the distal

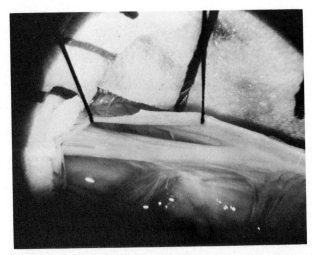

FIGURE 4–1. Tethered spinal cord. Note decreasing diameter, pallor, and linear dorsal blood vessels. The nerve roots depart the spinal cord at a right angle.

spinal cord to a more rostral level following release also suggests abnormal stretch. The increase of the angle of the axilla of nerve roots, often exceeding 90 degrees, further suggests a rostrocaudal tension. Barry et al. have shown an increase of intraspinal cord segment length immediately rostral to the points of tethering, which would also indicate that stretch is a factor in the pathology.[26] The dorsal vasculature of the spinal cord is frequently linear and of reduced diameter (Fig. 4–2). The dorsal nerve roots are stretched, and the small radicular vessels appear narrow and elongated.[20] The spinal cord appearance and vascular pattern suggesting traction are observed to increase when, during the surgery, the pelvis is flexed and to decrease when the pelvis is extended. The elongation of the vertebral column and spinal curvature have the potential to further increase tension on the spinal cord and peripheral nerves near the point of fixation. Weakness of muscles of the pelvis, which is often associated with myelomeningocele, may increase the magnitude of neural stretch caused by pelvic motion. Thereafter, daily activity associated with pelvic motion increases the frequency of intermittent stretch and its detrimental effect. The symptoms and signs of tethered spinal cord can be traced to the lumbosacral spinal cord and cauda equina. Experimental and clinical studies have indicated that this area is most susceptible to stretch and elongation, which may initiate metabolic, vascular, and conduction changes.[27] Further experimental studies have shown the lumbosacral cord to be maximally sensitive to stretch and that angulation of the axilla of the nerve roots disappears within five segments.[28–30] Yamada et al. used reflection spectrophotometry to evaluate mitochondria of the spinal cord in *in vivo* determination of redox changes of cytochrome A1, A3 in animals and humans at the time of surgery for tethered spinal cord.[31] Their findings indicated decreased mitochondrial metabolism associated with tethering. They suggested a decrease in production of adenosine triphosphate (ADP), which altered neural function. These observations, coupled with a simultaneous finding of decreased intraneuron potentials characteristic of hypoxia, suggest a primary mechanism of decrease in blood supply precipitated by mechanical factors.[32] Clinical and experimental studies have shown decreases in somatosensory evoked potentials which are similar to those observed in ischemia.[20, 32]

Intraoperative observations of the peripheral nerve support the possibility that in addition to spinal cord changes, peripheral nerve or axon abnormalities may also contribute to neurologic changes of the tethered spinal cord syndrome. Peripheral nerves and their vessels are demonstrably altered and stretched in their course. Following release, the radicular arteries increase in diameter and become undulating as the angle between the peripheral nerve and the cord decreases (Fig. 4–3).[20] With the use of laser doppler flowmetry, spinal cord blood flow has been evaluated in humans before and after tethered cord release.[33, 34] Following release of the cord there is a threefold increase in blood flow within an area of 2 to 3 cm rostral to the tether. Additionally, spinal cord ischemia has been shown to alter axonal transport of cholinergic enzymes, and this mechanism may further contribute to neurologic change observed with tethering.[35] Thus, the origin of change seems to be both axonal and neuronal, both being adversely affected by traction, ischemia, and mechanical distortion. For some patients with associated mass lesions such as lipomas, dermoids, neurenteric cysts, and arachnoidal pouches, compression may also produce adverse alteration in neuronal and axonal function.[36] Fujita and Yamamoto have shown in animal studies with nerve root, segmental spinal, and conductive spinal evoked potentials that both the spinal cord and the nerve roots are injured.[32] The morbid anatomy of tether, whether primary or secondary, sets the stage for clinical change of tethered cord, and the appearance and rate of change are directly related to the mechanical forces such as growth, physical activity, and compression, which precede the ischemia and metabolic

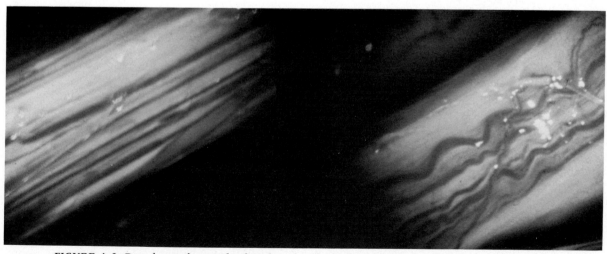

FIGURE 4–2. Dorsal vasculature of tethered cord. *Left,* Pre-release. *Right,* Post-release. Note change in contour and size of vessels.

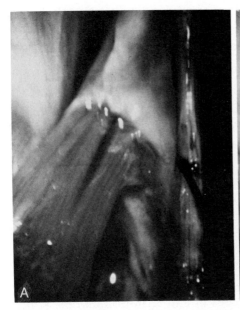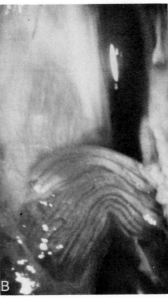

FIGURE 4–3. *A,* Peripheral nerve pre-release of spinal cord. *B,* Post-release. Note change in tension and vasculature of the root.

change. Finally, it is possible that some of the small caudal spinal cord syrinxes observed on the MRI of newborns with myelomeningoceles may be secondary to intrauterine tether and ischemia.

CLINICAL MANIFESTATIONS

Since, for the majority of patients with tethering lesions, the lumbosacral spinal cord is the focus of traction or tensile forces, it is not surprising that the clinical changes occur in function subserved by this area of the spinal cord and its associated nerve roots. Therefore, the most common alterations occur in motor strength of the lower extremities, bowel and bladder control, attitude of the lower extremities, and spinal curvature, which begins with change in the muscles with attachments between the vertebral column, pelvis, and lower extremities. The appearance and progression of these changes are highly variable and are dependent upon age, growth, physical activity, type of lesion producing the tether, and preexisting fixed deficit. Recognition may be facilitated by obvious signs, such as the onset of neurogenic bladder; conversely, identification may be masked by preexisting fixed deficit, slow change, and acceptance of subtle complaints. Furthermore, minor cutaneous changes, small dimples, and subcutaneous masses may be overlooked in a child with normal findings on neurologic examination. Cutaneous markers such as midline dimples, dermal sinuses, nevi, capillary hemangiomas, cutaneous lipomas, small tufts of hair, gluteal asymmetry, or indentation should immediately produce suspicion of potential for hidden lesions. These minor skin markers should be sought in all children with recurrent meningitis of unknown etiology and recurrent unexplained urinary tract infections. Back and leg pain, and the emergence of minor changes in bladder control such as enuresis, stress incontinence, and delayed toilet training, should not be taken casually by the observer. Lower extremity fatigue requiring rest periods during play, refusal of long walks, and a stumbling, unsteady running gait should prompt a careful neurologic examination and a search for cutaneous markers. Postural changes and varus, valgus, and cavus deformities of the foot are important signs of tether. Lower extremity rotation, hip dislocation, and knee flexion with lordotic wide-based gait, although obvious, should not escape combined neurologic and orthopedic evaluation. Finally, no patient with scoliosis, lordosis, or kyphosis should escape scrutiny for lesions that cause tethering of the conus and cauda equina. Recently the literature has emphasized that this constellation of problems is not confined to childhood and adolescence.[37–40]

Although there are many similarities in clinical appearance of the tethered cord syndrome between childhood and adulthood, some distinctive features appear during adulthood. The history frequently includes precipitating activity such as trauma, lithotomy position, leg raising, and sitting, all of which presumably stretch the conus and cauda equina.[37–40] Clinical changes begin suddenly and generally include pain, sensory and motor change, and deterioration of bladder function.

TETHERING LESIONS

DERMAL SINUS

Examination of the skin of the back frequently provides important clues to the presence of tethering lesions of all types. Dermal sinus tracts should be suspected when a dimple or a pinpoint hole is discovered at the caudal lumbar or presacral area. About 70 per cent are located in these areas, with an occasional one located in the thoracic cavity and the remainder located in the cervical and occipital areas. Dermal sinus tracts are most frequently located above S2 level and can be distinguished from pilonidal sinus tracts, which tend to be closer to the anus. Usually the fibrous band associated with pilondial sinus tracts extends to the coccyx. Occasionally there may be more than one dermal sinus, and they may be found slightly off the midline. Small tufts of hair are frequently found within the opening, and cutaneous capillary hemangiomas may surround the area of the dimple or skin opening. Larger capillary hemangiomas have been reported to be associated with tethering caused by tight filum terminale and intraspinal lipomas.[41] A high percentage (60 per cent) of dermal sinus tracts may point to the presence of intraspinal dermoids and epidermoids.[42–45] The skin lesions are continuous with an ectodermal tract which extends through the midline subcutaneous tissue and into the spinal canal though a bifid vertebra. Often the ectodermal sleeve becomes continuous with a dural stem, which enters the intradural compartment. These usually extend from a caudal skin location to a rostral intraspinal level (Fig. 4–4). Occasionally they may end external to the dura. However, most frequently they enter the dura, becoming continuous with dural bands, fibrous nodules, lipoma, dermoids, or epidermoids,

which attach to components of the cauda equina and/or conus. These lesions participate in tethering and the potential for occult progressive neurologic change. Dermal sinuses may also function as a conduit for bacterial infection of the central nervous system, causing meningitis, arachnoiditis, and intraspinal abscess (Fig. 4–4). During infancy, recurring fever and/or meningitis of unknown origin should lead to a search for previously unrecognized skin markers that identify dural sinuses.[46–49] Leaking dermoids and epidermoid cysts may produce a similar clinical picture of meningitis, not of bacterial origin but of chemical etiology.

Although rare, neurologic deficits such as changes in gait, control of rectum and bladder, and orthopedic deformity of the lower extremities may be associated with solo dermal sinuses, especially during later childhood.

Dermal sinus tracts can be readily identified with MRI. The intradural course may be hard to follow, and associated lesions such as extramedullary dermoid and epidermoid may be difficult to identify because of their variable spinal intensity. Iso intensity has been the limiting factor. However, intramedullary dermoid and epidermoids associated with dermal sinus tracts form a contrast with the spinal cord and therefore can be identified. CT with contrast may be helpful in the identifi-

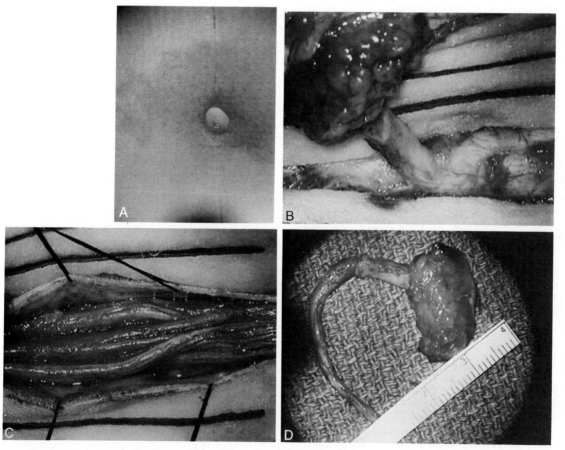

FIGURE 4–4. *A,* Dermal sinus with central ostium, cerebrospinal fluid leak, and surrounding hemangioma. *B,* Subcutaneous tissue surrounding sinus and dural stalk which extends to dura surrounding cauda equina. *C,* Inflamed cauda equina secondary to bacterial meningitis. *D,* Skin lesion and dural stalk after removal.

cation of extramedullary lesions. Invariably the conus is abnormally caudal (below L2) and the filum may be a thickened and tethering structure.[50]

DIASTEMATOMYELIA

Diastematomyelia was described in 1837 by Olliver, who defined it as a sagittal division or split of the spinal cord over one or more segments.[51] A fissure separates the two halves of the spinal cord and frequently contains a bony spicule or fibrocartilaginous septum (Fig. 4–5). These structures arise from the dorsal surface of the vertebral body and posteriorly become continuous with the lamina. The two hemichords are narrow and usually reunite distally to form a single cord structure below the cleft. Frequently, the two hemicords are asymmetric in diameter and each is associated with its own set of dorsal and ventral roots, which may not be equal in number. The cleft spinal cord may be housed in a single arachnoid and dural sleeve (50 per cent), and similarly each hemicord may reside in its own distinct arachnoid-dural sleeve. In the former bony spurs are absent, whereas in the latter bony structures or fibrocartilaginous septa are invariably present between the two dural sleeves. The bony spur is usually located at the caudal end of the cleft; thus, with this lesion, tethering of the cord arises at several levels—the fibrous medial portions of the separate dural sleeves, the cartilaginous or osseous septum at the rostral point where the spinal cord reunites, and the filum terminale. These structures may produce traction leading to ischemia and mechanical distortion of the cord and nerve roots.

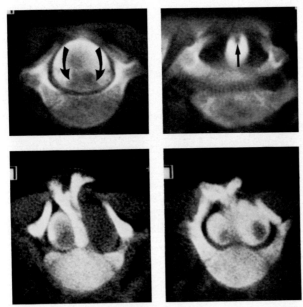

FIGURE 4–5. A water-soluble contrast-enhanced CT myelogram shows the bony spur dividing the canal and attached to the abnormal lamina. Each hemicord has its own canal. Note that distally the hemicords unite (curved arrows) and end in thickened filum terminale (arrow). Dorsally between the curved arrows is a Wilms's tumor, a rare additional lesion in congenital anomalies of the spine.

TABLE 4–3. CUTANEOUS CHANGES

Hypertrichosis
Nevus
Dimples
Sinus tract
Capillary hemangioma
Lipoma
Pilonidal cyst
Meningocele

Diplomyelia occurs very rarely and is defined as duplication of the spinal cord. There are two spinal cords, and they are usually associated with duplication of the spine. Second lesions such as dermal sinus tracts, lipoma, and meningocele have been described.[16, 52–54] Occasionally diastematomyelia may be associated with myelomeningocele and should be considered as a cause for delayed neurologic deterioration. The embryology of this lesion is described in Chapter 1.

Diastematomyelia is two to three times more common in females than in males and is heralded by cutaneous changes such as nevi and characteristic areas of silky hypertrichosis ("fawn's tail") in up to 80 per cent of patients (Table 4–3).[10, 16, 52, 53] The absence of skin change does not exclude the diagnosis of diastematomyelia.[53, 54] Often the clinical history and physical findings are slowly progressive and complaints often include back and leg pain, weakness, incontinence, and foot deformity. The physical findings have been divided into orthopedic and neurologic[10, 55] (Tables 4–4 and 4–5). Abnormal spine curvature and hydromyelia may occur in as many as 90 per cent of patients with diastematomyelia.[56–58] In contrast to neurogenic scoliosis associated with myelomeningocele, scoliosis of diastematomyelia is mechanical or congenital in origin. The neurologic findings are frequently dominant in one lower extremity, but mixed findings of reflex and sensory change frequently occur. Occasionally neurogenic changes in bowel and bladder control may be the only indication of the diagnosis.

Plain spine x-rays are invariably abnormal, and the most pathognomonic finding, depending on age is the calcified midline spur that may be identifiable in as many as 60 per cent of patients.[59, 60] The most commonly observed spine changes are shown in Table 4–6. The combination of vertical intralaminar fusion and adjacent spina bifida is highly suggestive of diastematomyelia.[60] Although 70 per cent of diastematomyelia is located in the lower lumbar area, the malformation has

TABLE 4–4. ORTHOPEDIC CHANGES

Congenital elevation of scapula
Scoliosis
Kyphosis
Lordosis
Hip dislocation
Leg length asymmetry
Foot size asymmetry
Valgus, varus, and cavus foot deformity

TABLE 4–5. NEUROLOGIC CHANGES

Leg muscle weakness and atrophy
Gait disturbance
Deep tendon reflex change
Sensory deficit
Neurogenic bowel and bladder

been described in all areas of the spine including the cervical and skull base.[61, 62] Ultrasonography during early infancy as a screening device may help to identify a split cord, septum, or hydromyelia.[63] Furthermore, prenatal ultrasonography has been reported to identify diastematomyelia.[64, 65] MRI is the method of choice for definition of the anatomic features of diastematomyelia. With axial or coronal sections the hemicords, the septum, the spur, hydromyelia, and the filum can be identified. Association lesions such as lipoma may also be defined. Sagittal images may falsely suggest a normal cord when only one hemicord is visualized. With severe scoliosis, multiple coronal images may be required to define the pathologic anatomy. The increasingly evident progressive deterioration, the poor potential for restoration of neurologic function, the skeletal deformity, and the inability to predict onset of deterioration have lead many to recommend surgical treatment for all patients with diastematomyelia.[10, 16, 52, 53, 55, 66] Therefore, the primary goal of surgery is prevention of further adverse change. Additional goals include relief of pain, treatment of associated lesions, and possibly stabilization of skeletal changes such as extremity deformity and scoliosis. Finally, there is increasing evidence that surgical treatment is of little benefit in restoring neurologic bowel and bladder function. Therefore, prophylactic surgical treatment is of greater importance.

SPINAL LIPOMAS

Spinal lipomas are tumors comprised primarily of fat and a variety of other tissues (connective, cartilage, bone, neural). They may be partially encapsulated and connect with the dura, filum terminale, or spinal cord (Fig. 4–6). Therefore, they have been classified in three groups: (1) intradural lipomas, (2) lipomyelomeningoceles (dorsal cleft of the spinal cord containing lipoma), and (3) fibrolipoma of the filum terminale. The embryologic development of these lesions is described in Chapter 1.

Intradural Lipomas. Intradural lipomas (intact dura) make up approximately 4 per cent of spinal lipomas; they are surrounded by pia within the dural sac and are located in a juxtamedullary position in relation to the cervical and thoracic spinal cord (Fig. 4–6).[67, 68] The spinal canal is modestly altered with segmental anomalies and bifida deformity. The canal may be widened at the level of the tumor. The dura is thin but intact and displaced laterally by the mass effect of the cord and the tumor. The lipoma involves the dorsal surface of the cord and causes the cord to rotate upon

itself, thus giving the appearance that the tumor is lateral to the spinal cord. Occasionally the lipoma may be anterior to the spinal cord, which usually is anteriorly compressed and displaced. Occasionally a small syrinx will be associated with these lesions.

Lipomyelomeningocele. The most common forms of spinal lipoma (84 per cent) are associated with definite defects in the dura, through which the lipoma may extend from the spinal cord to the subcutaneous tissue (Fig. 4–7).[8, 69–74] In patients so affected, the subcutaneous component of the lipoma typically forms a large skin-covered, lumbosacral mass that lies cephalad to the intergluteal crease. The subjacent spinal canal usually shows a wide spina bifida. Sacral anomalies and segmentation anomalies are present in nearly 50 per cent of patients.[75]

The spinal cord, which is low and usually tethered by the lipoma, is cleft dorsally (partial dorsal myeloschisis) and closely resembles the neural plate of a myelomeningocele. The dura that normally forms a complete tube around the spinal cord is deficient in the dorsal midline, deep to the lipoma.[74, 76] The medial edges of the dural defect are not just free margins of a tube. Rather, the dura appears to attach to the edges of the neural plate, just dorsal to the entry zones of the dorsal roots. Thus the raw, cleft surface of the neural plate lies medial to and outside the dural sac (i.e., it is extradural). The arrangement of pia-arachnoid and of nerve roots in such lipomas is identical with that seen in myeloceles and myelomeningoceles. The lipoma inserts into the exposed dorsal "extradural" face of the neural plate and extends from there to the subcutaneous space (Fig. 4–7). Since the dorsal extradural surface of the neural plate is directly continuous with the central canal of the normal cord above, lipoma may also extend in continuity from the plate into the central canal of the cord. Although the portion of lipoma within the central canal is certainly intramedullary, it is also extradural in the sense that it is not surrounded on all sides by dura. Rather, it is directly continuous with the extradural portion of the lipoma. This intramedullary component may increase in size as the child gains weight and may function as an expanding intramedullary tumor,[65, 70] in which case a dorsal myelotomy and partial resection of the lipoma may be re-

TABLE 4–6. PLAIN SPINE X-RAY CHANGES

Midline density, calcified spur
Spina bifida
Hemivertebrae
Scalloping
Vertebral body fusion
Narrow intervertebral space
Small vertebra
Hemilamina and lamina hypertrophy
Fused lamina
Increased interpedicular distance
Prominent, split, or absent spinous process
Scoliosis
Kyphosis
Lordosis

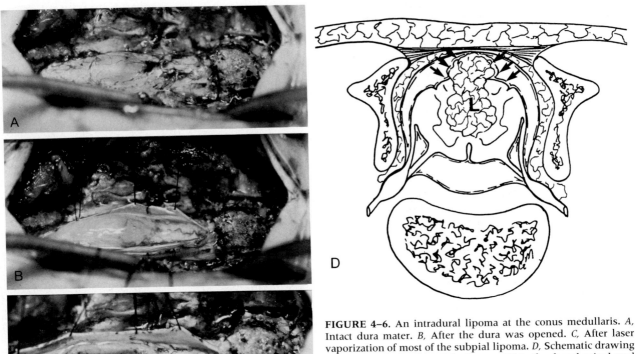

FIGURE 4–6. An intradural lipoma at the conus medullaris. *A,* Intact dura mater. *B,* After the dura was opened. *C,* After laser vaporization of most of the subpial lipoma. *D,* Schematic drawing shows the relationship of the lipoma (L) to the dorsal spinal cord and the pial covering *(arrows).*

quired to preserve function in the surrounding neural tissue.

The junction of the lipoma and the spinal cord may be entirely within the spinal canal, may lie entirely outside the spinal canal, or may bridge the spina bifida to lie both inside and outside the spinal canal. When the spinal cord remains completely within the spinal canal, the lipoma extends into the canal before entering into the cleft in the cord. In these cases, the anatomic

arrangement of the neural tissue is similar to that of the myelocele, except that the raw dorsal surface of the neural plate is covered by fat, and the entire complex lies within the bifid spinal canal underneath the intact surface of skin. These lesions may be designated lipomyelocele.

When the cord herniates out of the canal, so that the junction of fat and cord is at least partially outside the canal, the anatomic arrangement of the neural tissue is

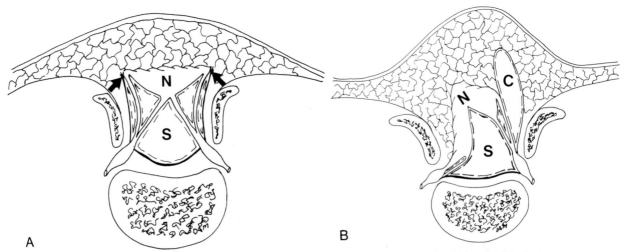

FIGURE 4–7. Schematic drawings of a lipomyelomeningocele, showing the neural placode (N), the junction of the dorsal root entry zone, neural tissue, and the lipoma *(A, arrows). A* shows the subarachnoid space (S) in a more normal position. *B* shows the subarachnoid space (S) and a meningocele (C) herniating into the lipoma.

similar to that of the myelomeningocele, except that the dorsal surface of the neural tissue is covered by fat and the entire complex is buried deep to intact skin. These lesions may be designated lipomyelomeningocele. In these cases, gross expansion of the subarachnoid space pushes the cord and the liponeural junction out of the canal into the sac (Fig. 4–8). The dura remains attached to the edges of the neural plate, so that the lipoma itself remains extradural.

Typically, the neural plate rotates as it herniates out of the canal, causing the dorsal surface to face posterolateral or lateral rather than directly posterior. The lipoma then lies dorsolateral or lateral to the neural tissue, while the sac bulges to the contralateral side. The left and right pairs of nerve roots become markedly different in length. The roots arising from the superficial side of the rotated spinal cord are long. The roots arising from the deep side of the rotated spinal cord are far shorter. These deep roots may be so short that they act to tether the spinal cord inferiorly.[19]

Lipomas of Filum. Lipomas of the filum terminale are observed incidentally in 4 to 6 per cent of normal adults and may be considered a normal variation if they are not associated with spinal cord tethering and neurologic change.[77] Persistence of caudal cells that differentiate toward fat may produce lipoma of the filum. Filar lipomas may involve the intradural, extradural, or both portions of the filum (Fig. 4–9). Extradural lipomas of the filum are more diffuse and may merge with the extradural fat, making identification difficult with MRI. Filar lipomas may be associated with lipomas of the distal half of the conus medullaris—the portion of the conus medullaris that is also formed by cannulization and retrogressive differentiation. In some instances, accessory fila are present and may also contain lipomatous tissue. It has been suggested that fat in the filum occurs in 90 per cent of patients with the clinical findings of tethered spinal cord and in 19 per cent of

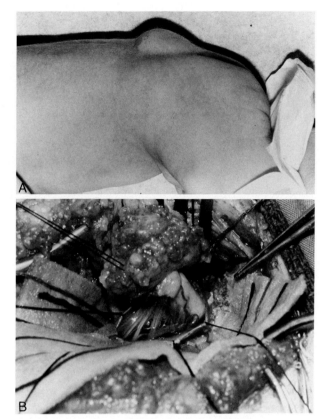

FIGURE 4–8. *A,* Lipomyelomeningocele. *B,* Lipoma and spinal cord extending out of canal.

asymptomatic adults.[78] This fat within the filum is not necessarily a cause of tethering, but it may certainly point to tethering and indeed, if it does involve the distal conus, may lead to neurologic deterioration.

Spinal lipomas seem to equally affect females and males and are often associated with a skin lesion. Most

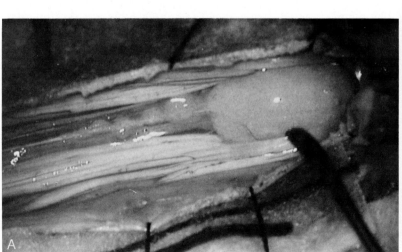

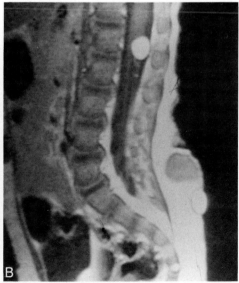

FIGURE 4–9. *A,* Conus lipoma with daughter lipomas of filum. *B,* MRI.

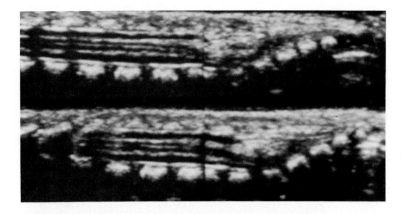

FIGURE 4–10. An ultrasound scan of an infant shows the low-lying spinal cord with its central echo fusing and passing under the echoic mass of the lipoma and the dermoid tumor.

commonly there is a cutaneous fatty mass located in the midline of the lumbar spinal area, and it is often associated with cutaneous markers of occult spina bifida such as dimples, tags, nevi, hypertrichosis, ostia, and hemangiomas.[19, 21, 76, 79] Cutaneous lipomas are rarely associated with intradural lipomas and fibrolipomas of the filum. Conversely, the absence of subcutaneous lipomas in the presence of spinal lipoma has been reported to be as high as 30 per cent.[76] The child with a spinal lipoma may have no neurologic deficit or a variety of changes including alterations in reflexes, gait change, motor weakness, wasting, bowel and bladder incontinence, pain, and sensory loss. Orthopedic deformity is common and may include varus, valgus, cavus deformities of the foot, asymmetry of the lower extremities, dislocation of the hip, and scoliosis. Trophic ulceration of the skin may be part of the foot deformity. The neuro-orthopedic abnormalities increase in frequency and magnitude with age.[19, 67] Chiari malformation and hydrocephalus are extremely rare.

Intradural lipomas and lipomyelomeningoceles constitute 20 to 50 per cent of all cases of occult spinal dysraphism. In these patients, computed tomography reveals a large lucent subcutaneous mass of fat, posterior spina bifida, insertion of the lucent lipoma into the dorsal surface of the cleft spinal cord, and any associated meningocele. The liponeural junction may be relatively smooth or stellate. A variable thick band of increased density is often observed at the liponeural junction and appears to represent fibrous tissue at the interspace between the neural tissue and fat. MRI demonstrates the same anatomic features. The fat has high signal intensity on T1-weighted images and stands out distinctly from low-signal CSF and intermediate-signal neural tissue. In T2-weighted images the signal intensity of fat decreases while that of CSF increases, so that the CSF may become as bright or brighter than the fat. Currently CT and MRI both display spinal lipoma satisfactorily.[80–82] MRI displays the sagittal plane more clearly than CT, whereas CT displays the axial plane more clearly than MRI.

Ultrasonography has been extremely useful in determining the structure of many of these congenital spinal lesions in infants. Because the immature bone allows ultrasound to penetrate and give excellent structural detail, tethering and the extent of the lesion can be determined (Fig. 4–10).

The current prevailing opinion is that spinal lipomas produce progressive neuro-orthopedic and neurologic deterioration at all ages.[6, 19, 21, 67, 76, 79, 83, 84] Furthermore, the course of adverse change is unpredictable in terms of onset, rate, and magnitude. There is little information to suggest reversal of fixed deficit following operative treatment, and the benefit of operative treatment is measured in terms of interrupting progression of deterioration. Therefore, early and prophylactic operative treatment is recommended.

TIGHT FILUM TERMINALE

The tight filum terminale syndrome refers to patients with the characteristic clinical findings associated with tethered spinal cord in which the filum is short and thickened (greater than 2 mm) and tethers the conus medullaris in an abnormally caudal position.[9, 12, 24, 85] The tip of the conus is below L2 in 86 per cent of patients, and fibrolipomas may be present in as many as 90 per cent.[78, 86] In 10 to 15 per cent of patients, the conus is attached to the distal thecal sac. The most common clinical findings include weakness (76 per cent), pain (42 per cent), bladder dysfunction (35 per cent), sensory loss (21 per cent), and kyphoscoliosis (25 per cent).[50] Over half the patients have the neurocutaneous signs of occult spinal lesions, as described with other forms of tethering. Plain spine x-rays invariably demonstrate a midline arch defect at one or more level in the lumbosacral area. Indeed, normal spine x-rays may exclude this diagnosis.[11] Both CT and MRI identify

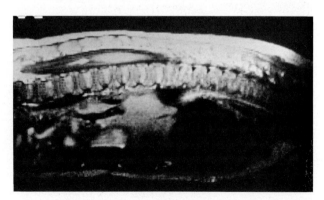

FIGURE 4–11. MRI. Tight filum containing lipoma.

the low conus and the thick filum while excluding other causes of tethering. Lipomas within the filum appear as lucent or high-signal areas that are easily identified (Fig. 4–11). Axial images should always be part of MRI evaluation for an abnormal filum since sagittal constructions may miss these changes. With this group of patients, complaints and findings often are distinct and point to the diagnosis. Therefore, the decision to treat with laminectomy and release of the filum is less controversial than for other areas of occult spina bifida.

SYNDROME OF EMBRYONIC DEFORMATION AND CAUDAL SUPPRESSION (SACRAL AGENESIS; CAUDAL REGRESSION)

Children with the syndrome of caudal suppression (regression) exhibit anomalies of the hind end of the trunk, including partial agenesis of the thoracolumbosacral spine, imperforate anus, malformed genitalia, bilateral renal dysplasia or aplasia, pulmonary hypoplasia, and (in the most severe deformities) extreme external rotation and fusion of the lower extremities (sirenomelia).[87] There is a definite but incomplete association with diabetes mellitus: 1 per cent of offspring of diabetic mothers have a form of this syndrome; 16 per cent of patients with this syndrome have diabetic mothers (rarely diabetic fathers).[88, 89]

Isolated agenesis of the coccyx is an incidental finding in some patients. In patients with more extensive agenesis of the distal spine, the lowest vertebra present is T11 or T12 in one third of the patients, L1 to L4 in 40 per cent of the patients, and L5 or below in 27 per cent of the patients.[90] The distal agenesis may be bilaterally symmetric or unilateral. Unilateral agenesis leads to marked pelvic tilt and scoliosis.

Recently, studies have suggested that in malformations with the majority of the sacrum absent (below S1), the spinal cord ends in a "club" shaped blunt fasion at T11–T12, whereas low sacral malformations are correlated with low-lying conus, which is frequently tethered.[91] Segmentation anomalies have been reported in 22 per cent of these patients and in 33 per cent of patients with spina bifida.[92] Associated lesions such as myelomeningocele, lipomas, dermoids, meningoceles, fibrous bands, and bony stenosis have been identified and carry the potential to cause delayed neurologic deficit. Surprisingly, patients with high malformations seem to remain neurologically stable,[91] in which case urologic and surgical treatment frequently take precedence over neurosurgical evaluation and treatment. Thereafter, MRI will identify the spinal abnormalities associated with this complex malformation.[91, 93] Since this constellation of tethering lesions may be expected to produce progressive neurologic change, operative treatment is often required in order to preserve function.[91, 94]

NEURENTERIC CYSTS

Neurenteric cysts appear within the spinal canal, most commonly in the cervical and thoracic areas (Fig.

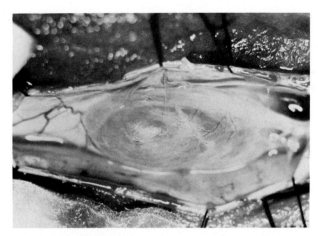

FIGURE 4–12. Neurenteric cyst of thoracic cord. *(Courtesy of Dr. John Woodford.)*

4–12).[95] However, they have been reported in the lumbar area.[96] They are lined by enteric tissues, which may include intestine, stomach, and pancreas. Defects in the vertebral bodies are common, and the cyst may also be simultaneously located in the thorax or abdomen with and without communication between the spinal cyst and the extraspinal cyst. Thus, they may (1) communicate around a hemivertebra or through a butterfly vertebra with the extraspinal component of cyst in the mesentery or mediastinum, (2) attach by a fibrous stalk to the vertebra, mesentery, or gut, or (3) do both. They have been reported to communicate with intestine.[97] Neurenteric cysts are usually discovered during the first decade of life. Complaints of pain, weakness, and bowel and bladder incontinence may call attention to the lesion. During infancy, fever and meningitis of unknown origin may be caused by these cysts. Furthermore, cardiorespiratory change may be caused by the intrathoracic mass or cervical cord compression. Conus compression seems to be more common in older patients.[98]

The vertebral column usually exhibits a wide spinal canal with a widened interpedicular distance.[99] Spina bifida and segmentation anomalies of the bodies are common, but not invariable. In older patients the vertebrae may be normal, except for pressure erosion. The cyst usually lies ventral or ventrolateral to the spinal cord and may be deeply invaginated into the cord. CT and MRI display the cyst, the displaced spinal cord, bone abnormalities, and associated mediastinal or mesenteric lesions. Complete removal is the treatment of choice, and residual cyst has the potential to produce chemical inflammation of the meninges.

ANTERIOR MENINGOCELE

Anterior meningocele refers to a pelvic mass that communicates with the spinal subarachnoid space through a small opening in the anterior sacrum. The content of the mass is usually limited to cerebrospinal fluid. In rare instances, this mass has been observed in the thoracic area.

Although not a direct cause of tethering of the spinal

cord, this lesion occasionally is associated with spinal lipomas, dermoid tumors, and thickened filum terminale. Familial cases have been reported.

Nearly all the children in our experience have been girls with a history of chronic constipation. Many of these children have been under observation for years and have had multiple gastrointestinal studies. Review of previous x-rays usually reveals the characteristic scimitar sacrum. Myelography, CT, or MRI shows the extent of this meningocele and associated lesions.[100]

MYELOMENINGOCELE (RETETHERING OF THE SPINAL CORD)

Tethered spinal cord that occurs following repair of myelomeningocele is the form of tethering which most classically displays the pathophysiology and clinical findings of the syndrome. With this condition the spinal cord and, frequently, the cauda equina are densely scarred to the tissues used in the primary closure (dura, fascia, or skin) by thick arachnoiditis and fibrous adhesions. The spinal cord is invariably located in a caudal position, frequently as low as S1; in perhaps 40 per cent of the patients there is a second lesion, such as inclusion lipomas and epidermoids, hydromyelia, dural bands, and diastematomyelia. The spinal cord frequently appears stretched like a "bow string" and extends along the shortest pathway across the dorsal dural sac, which is usually patulous. The termination of the cord may be indistinguishable from the dorsal tissues, and the conus may not be identifiable as a distinct structure. The nerve roots are often reversed in angulation and, indeed, travel from caudal to rostral with axillary angles exceeding 90 degrees in contrast to the normal 20 degrees (see Fig. 4–3).[101] Surgical observation reveals a pale narrow distal spinal cord with linear stretched dorsal vasculature (see Figs. 4–1 and 4–2). Similarly, the spinal cord roots are stretched and pale with the radicular arteries also appearing attenuated (Fig. 4–13). The most common symptoms associated with this form of tethering are progressive weakness and gait change, orthopedic deformity, scoliosis, and pain. Since most of these patients have neurogenic bladders, subjective complaints of change in control are infrequent. However, serial urodynamic studies may reveal changes that coincide with more obvious forms of neurologic deterioration and further suggest retethering of the spinal cord of patients with myelomeningocele.[102] A small percentage, 6 to 10 per cent, demonstrate a bent knee or flexed posture as an indication of tethering. Progressive scoliosis and perhaps lordosis also indicate onset of tethering.[103, 104] Serial somatosensory evoked potentials may provide a method for early recognition of tethering.[20] MRI, the study of choice, demonstrates tethering and the associated lesions. Surgical correlation has been excellent. The magnitude of arachnoiditis and density of adhesions are frequently underestimated on the basis of MRI evaluation.[18, 63, 105, 106] The radiologic (MRI) imaging of tethering probably occurs relatively quickly (perhaps in months) following primary repair of myelomeningocele. The constellation of adverse clinical change does not occur immediately, nor does it occur in all patients. As many as 25 per cent or more do not develop signs of retether in up to 20 years of follow-up.[103] Growth and daily activity produce stretch and associated mass lesions, which in turn produce compression, causing unrelenting neurologic and orthopedic changes that later become evident. Although many had hoped that combining the surgical return of the neural tube to a cylindrical structure with a pia anastomosis and patulous dural closure would prevent tethering, the effect appears to have been modest at best.[107] Operative release of tethered spinal cord has been shown to interrupt and reverse neuro-orthopedic changes in many children.

DIAGNOSTIC EVALUATION

If the presence of a tethering lesion is suspected, further diagnostic evaluation is indicated to identify the

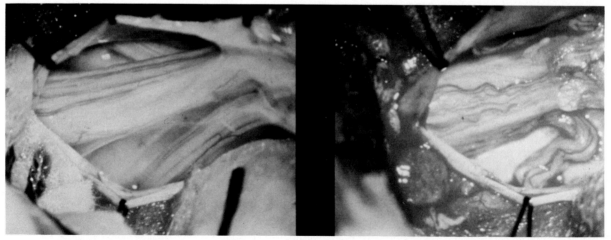

FIGURE 4–13. Spinal cord with characteristic changes pre-release *(left)* and post-release *(right)* of tethered spinal cord.

specific anatomy. Occasionally serial evaluation uncovers subtle changes of potential significance. Currently indications for operative treatment require clinical change to be coupled with characteristic findings on imaging studies. For instance, almost all patients with a history of myelomeningocele repair have the appearance of tethering on MRI, but may not have clinical change to suggest alteration in spinal cord function. Operations to treat tethering lesions associated with myelomeningocele have not been recommended on the sole basis of identification as it has been with lipomas, sinus tracts, dural bands, and diastematomyelia—all of which inevitably lead to neurologic change.

SPINE X-RAYS

Routine spine x-rays of patients suspected of having occult lesions almost invariably show one or more vertebral anomalies.[38] These include hemivertebrae, fused verebrae, and wedge-shaped vertebrae; scalloped vertebral margins; absent spinous processes; alterations in intrapedicular distance (widened spinal canal); erosion of the pedicles; absent lamina; midline spurs; and incomplete development of the sacrum. Early change in curvature, such as scoliosis or lordosis, is often detected.[17] The presence of any of these changes is an indication for additional imaging studies such as ultrasonography, CT, or MRI.

ULTRASONOGRAPHY

Sonography has proved effective in screening for spinal cord location and tethering, meningocele, sacral coccygeal teratoma, diastematomyelia, and lipoma.[63, 108, 109] Ultrasonography has also been used to search for absence of spinal cord motion as an indication of pathologic tethering.[110] Although the concept is attractive, the prognostic value of cord motion determination has not been demonstrated.

MAGNETIC RESONANCE IMAGING (MRI)

MRI is known to be effective for evaluating the level and location of the conus. The thickness of the filum terminale can also be readily determined,[111] the normal thickness being 2 mm or less.[86] Intramedullary lipoma, lipomyelomeningocele, and lipoma of the filum may be easily identified.[78, 80, 112, 113] Dermal sinus tracts have been detected with MRI as they traverse the skin, subcutaneous tissue, and lamina. They have been difficult to follow within the dural sac.[42] Tumors characteristically associated with dermal sinus tracts—such as lipomas, dermoids, and epidermoids—can be quickly recognized. Dermoids and epidermoids usually appear isodense within cerebrospinal fluid. MRI is effective in defining the characteristic features of diastematomyelia, such as bony spur, lamina abnormalities, and cleft of the spinal cord. In the absence of the bony spur, fibrous

bands may traverse the cleft, producing tethering, but this has been difficult to demonstrate. With MRI, it can be determined whether the dural sheath is divided into two distinct structures.[113] MRI has replaced myelography for the evaluation of tethering following primary repair of myelomeningocele. The low-lying spinal cord can be traced to its point of attachment whether it be the dura, subcutaneous tissue, or other lesions associated with the repair. Associated lesions such as lipomas, dermoids, epidermoids, cysts, and diastematomyelia may also be defined in relation to the myelomeningocele. Meningoceles are usually demonstrated with MRI, and except for small nerve fibers, the presence of major neural structures can be excluded from the interior of the sac.

Meningocele manqué refers to dorsal fibrotic or neural bands associated with dysraphic lesions.[114] They are frequently encountered at the time of operation for more obvious lesions. Kaffenberger has recently shown that they can be identified by MRI and CT with metrizamide.[115] Finally, cavitations of the spinal cord, which are often associated with tethered spinal cord, can also be clearly visualized. Hydromyelia, a longitudinal cavitation lined by ependyma, may extend to the tethered conus, and its presence requires consideration of a cerebrospinal fluid shunt insertion or revision prior to tethered cord release. Focal enlargement of the conus lined by ependyma has been called ventricularis terminalis and may be recognized by MRI.[116, 117] Focal cavitations at other sites in the spinal cord not lined by ependyma frequently appear on MRI obtained as part of tethered cord evaluation. Serial MRI has demonstrated that most of these syrinxes are static and of little consequence. MRI is effective in the evaluation of sacral agenesis particularly when tethered cord and associated lesions such as lipoma and meningocele are suspected. The presence of rostrally terminating subarachnoid space may also be identified with sacral agenesis.[91, 113] MRI has added a new dimension to the evaluation of the split notochord syndrome or neurenteric cyst in that the intraspinal mass, paravertebral mass, and intra-abdominal mass may be fully appreciated.[97, 118] Likewise MRI has been helpful in searching for the occasional patient with tethered cord and caudal deformation syndrome. These patients may have meningocele, myelomeningocele, lipoma of the filum, lipomyelomeningocele, diastematomyelia, and dural bands. With MRI, Barkovich found tethered cord in 2 of 13 patients with caudal regression syndrome, and Pang has demonstrated an even higher incidence of associated lesions in patients with this malformation.[91, 93]

In summary, MRI for the study of conditions which produce spinal cord and cauda equina tethering is excellent for identifying the configuration and location of the conus medullaris and, with the occasional exception of defining intra- versus extradural fat, clearly defines lipoma within the cord, filum terminale, and the relationship of lipoma to the conus medullaris. Hydromyelia and syringomyelia cavities are prominent. The size of the filum can be determined, but axial view may be required. Tumors within the cauda equina may be well defined. Small lesions and abnormalities of the filum may be difficult to appreciate during infancy because of motion artifact related to respiration. Spinal curvature of older patients may require close correlation of multiple sagittal and axial views to detect some lesions and precisely locate the conus. Bone detail usually is not a problem, but if it is of importance, axial CT will augment MRI. Surgical observations have consistently revealed dense arachnoiditis and fibrolipomatous scar that exceeds estimates based on preoperative MRI. Enmeshment of roots of the cauda equina within the scar tissue is frequently invisible on MRI. Dermoid and epidermoid tumor may also be hidden when they rest within the neural plaque repair or masses of scar tissue. All in all, MRI is still the definitive study.[18]

SOMATOSENSORY EVOKED POTENTIALS

Serial somatosensory evoked potentials obtained with peroneal nerve stimulation may reveal decreasing amplitude and increasing latency of response. Asymmetry may reflect static neurologic change, but serial changes in asymmetry may also suggest deterioration secondary to tether. Reversal of these abnormal changes have been observed following surgical release.[20]

URODYNAMICS

Alterations in bladder function associated with tethered spinal cord may be insidious or overt. Unfortunately, untethering rarely reverses fixed deficit. Therefore, early diagnosis and treatment assume greater importance. Cystometrograms and pelvic electromyography may detect early neuro-urological change. Abnormal pressure volume curves, detrusor dysfunction, and sphincter dyssynergia may be an early signal of tethered cord.[102, 119] Pre- and postoperative urodynamics have demonstrated the urologic benefit of tethered cord release.[102, 119, 120]

SURGICAL TREATMENT AND OUTCOME

GENERAL PRINCIPLES

The decision to recommend operation for treatment for tethered spinal cord must be preceded by a careful evaluation of the clinical history, findings on neurologic examination, and focused imaging studies. The decision requires that all of the findings be correlated with high confidence. The contemplated operation can then be planned with a clear understanding of the pathologic anatomy. The indications for surgery are based upon an understanding that the specific lesion and tethered spinal cord are producing symptomatology and neurologic change which is unacceptable and that operation has the potential to produce relief of

symptoms and neurologic improvement. The decision to operate requires acceptance that tethered spinal cord is destined to produce neurologic, orthopedic, and urologic disability, and that surgical treatment will interrupt this progression. In a significant group of these patients, we can anticipate reversal of neurologic, orthopedic, and urologic deterioration.

Prior to surgery, all patients should have a neurologic and urologic evaluation. Preoperative muscle testing, electromyography, evoked potentials, and cystometrography document the preoperative status of the patient and provide a base from which to evaluate postoperative results. Since some of these patients have hydrocephalus, particularly those with myelomeningocele, preoperative verification of shunt function is mandatory.

Preparation for operation should follow the guidelines of good pediatric surgical practice. An understanding of nutrition and the unique physiology of the infant, such as small blood volume, is required. Collaborative preoperative communication among the pediatrician, the pediatric intensivist, and the anesthesiologist improves preoperative evaluation and intraoperative and postoperative care.

Adherence to a variety of pediatric neurosurgical principles will improve operative results. Special efforts to ensure that the abdomen is free of pressure in the prone position will reduce the loss of valuable blood. This may be difficult in the presence of spinal curvature and hip contracture, and a variety of materials should be available to ensure position support without risking cutaneous pressure necrosis. A midline incision is planned which begins at least two normal vertebral levels rostral to the lesion and extends caudally to the sacrum or at least two levels beyond the primary location of the tether. The incision should not be carried through cutaneous manifestations of the lesion, such as sinuses or fat, until the normal anatomy rostral or caudal to the lesion has been defined. In planning the midline incision, special attention to scoliosis should be given, and the incision should follow the palpable midline of the scoliotic spine. The golden principle of pediatric neurosurgical treatment of congenital defects is to identify the normal anatomy and work from normal to abnormal while always using the normal as a reference point. This can be from rostral to caudal or vice versa. Therefore, when dissecting dura from surrounding tissues, one should always work from normal dura to abnormal, and frequently this means working from the lateral gutters of the spinal canal toward the midline. Since the rostral spinal canal is usually in the midline, the dural incision should begin rostrally and lateral to the midline (the lateral posterior quadrant).

The operating microscope, high-speed drill, carbon dioxide laser, and ultrasonic dissector are all valuable adjuncts and reduce blood loss, risk of tissue trauma, and operative time. The laser is used for dissection and excision with a 0.2-mm spot size and power from 0.5 to 10 watts, depending on area of use. Pulsed delivery enables increased power density and improved hemostasis, whereas a broader beam is used for vaporization of fatty tissues. The dura can be opened with the laser without disrupting the arachnoid, and often one is able to seal the arachnoid to the pia in an effort to reduce rostral CSF contamination with blood and tissue products. Laminotomy and replacement of lamina have limited application and should be carefully considered in the presence of multiple arch defects. If the dura is carefully dissected from surrounding tissue it can always be primarily closed. However, when subsequent dural closure will produce a small dural sac and compromise neural tissues or enhance retether, artificial dura should be used to expand the volume of the thecal sac. Usually a midline iliocostalis muscle and fascial closure is possible, and the subcutaneous tissue and skin are closed in the midline. It should be noted that some have proposed intraoperative urodynamic studies, rectal monitoring (EMG and pressure), and intraoperative somatosensory evoked potentials as methods of preserving functioning neurologic tissue.[40, 121–124] Patients are kept supine for approximately one hour following surgery, and thereafter they are allowed to be in any position. Narcotic analgesia is provided routinely for all age groups for 36 to 48 hours. The average hospital stay is 2 to 3 days.

DERMAL SINUS

The sinus tract should be traced through the midline of the iliocostalis and preserved during the laminectomy since it then can be traced to the dural entrance. Often a dural band or small aberrant root will extend to the conus. These should be transected and removed. Associated lesions such as dermoids and lipomas should be removed with magnification and the laser (Fig. 4–14). If the filum is tethered and contains lipoma, it should be transected with the laser and a section removed. The dura can always be closed in the midline. Arachnoidal adhesions caused by previous infection should not deter one from the dissection. There is little or no morbidity with the operation, and long-term neurologic stability of the patient can be fully expected.

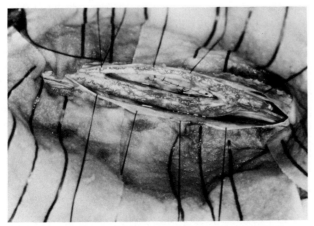

FIGURE 4–14. Diastematomyelia with anterior dural closure.

DIASTEMATOMYELIA

The primary purpose of surgery for this condition is the prevention of inevitable neurologic and orthopedic deterioration.[10, 16, 52, 53] Occasionally, reversal of preexisting neurologic and urologic deficit will follow the operation. Pain will be invariably relieved. Furthermore, the removal of associated lesions such as tumors will also prevent potential adverse change. In the event that scoliosis is the primary complaint and fusion is required, operation for diastematomyelia should precede fusion.[125] Laminectomy should be planned to include 1 or 2 laminae rostral and caudal to the cleft and the cord. It is extremely important to remember the abnormal posterior arch anatomy of this lesion, particularly the fact that the septum (bony or cartilaginous) usually joins with the abnormal laminar arch and the interpedicular distance is always widened at the cleft levels. Therefore, laminectomy should proceed from the normal lamina to the abnormal lamina and should *not* begin at the medial portion of the abnormal lamina. As one works from the lateral to medial, the dorsum of the septum may be safely removed by rongeur dissection, assuming that pulling and stretching of intraspinal adhesions and structures are avoided. One should anticipate that vigorous arterial and venous bleeding may originate from the dorsal septum, and this should be carefully controlled prior to further dissection. Frequently there are bands of adhesions between the septum and medial surfaces of the dural sleeves, and these should be transected and associated bleeding meticulously controlled. With microscopic magnification and the high-speed drill, the spur can be safely removed. Microinstrumentation and laser can be used to remove the nonosseous septum.

The dura is opened to the full extent of both dural sleeves and the incision is extended rostral to normal cord and caudally in sufficient length to release the tethered reunited cord and conus from the filum, which is invariably a factor. Associated arachnoidal and dural bands are released from their attachments to the cord. Similarly, lesions such as dermoids, lipomas, and sinuses are also removed. Extraneous medial dura is excised, and the remaining dura is closed anteriorly in the midline (Fig. 4–15). If the anterior dura cannot be closed without risk of trauma to the cord, closure should not be attempted. The dorsal dura is closed in the midline. The outlook for patients treated prophylactically is distinctly superior to the outlook for those treated expectantly, and operative treatment should be advocated following diagnosis.[10, 15, 16, 19, 52, 53, 126, 127]

LIPOMYELOMENINGOCELE AND LIPOMYELOCELE

Large series now document that spinal cord lipomas can be untethered successfully and that the intramedullary portion of the lipoma can be resected successfully, with nearly zero morbidity and no mortality.[6, 8, 19, 21, 67, 76, 79, 83, 84] Further, the series prove that such operations lead to recovery of neurologic and urologic func-

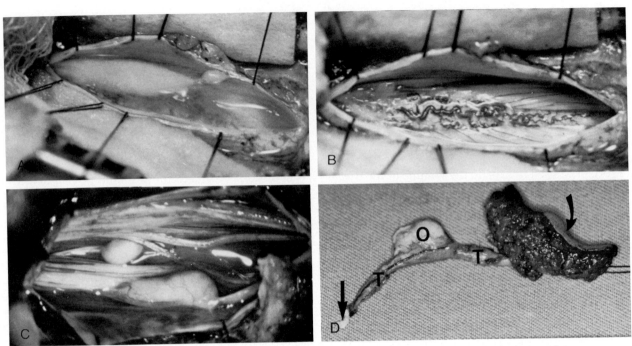

FIGURE 4–15. Operative photographs show a dermoid attached to the spinal cord *(A)*, the same area after laser resection *(B)*, and a patient with multiple dermoids *(C)*. A specimen *(D)* shows skin dimple *(curved arrow)*, tract (T), dermoid (O), and point of attachment to the conus medullaris *(arrow)*.

tion in a significant number of patients with preexisting deficits.[127] In our study, for example, 40 per cent of those with motor deficits and 12 per cent of those with incontinence recovered normal function after effective operation.

Surgery is carried out with the child prone. A scalpel is used to incise the skin, and a scalpel or laser is used for the dura mater. All other dissection and all resection of lipoma are performed with a laser, with the beam focusing for cutting and for vaporization. No attempt is made to resect the lipoma in toto. Rather, lipoma is vaporized progressively until an interface between lipoma and neural tissue can be identified. Certainly this operation can be done without the laser, but the laser has real advantages in removing the lipoma (see Fig. 4–6). When possible, the neural tube is re-formed and the arachnoid and dural tubes are closed around the spinal cord. Artificial dura mater is used, if necessary, to ensure a capacious subarachnoid space and that ample dura surrounds the spinal cord. Then, the wound is closed in layers. Patients are maintained in a supine position for 12 to 24 hours to reduce the incidence and the degree of the common, transient accumulations of cerebrospinal fluid in the subcutaneous pocket left by the lipoma resection.

In all patients, untethering of the spinal cord is the goal. In a few patients, the lipoma is resected, and the spinal cord is freed from lipoma. However, congenitally short nerve roots on one side may still anchor the spinal cord to the root sleeves. Such unilaterally short roots are encountered in three circumstances: (1) in patients with unilateral, partial sacral agenesis (on the side of agenesis), (2) in patients with conjoint neural

foramina, and (3) in patients in whom the lipoma has rotated the cord 90 degrees, so that the left and right dorsal roots lie anterior and posterior to each other in a (nearly) sagittal plane, rather than side by side in a coronal plane. In such patients, roots that are displaced and rotated anteriorly are invariably short, whereas those that come to lie posterior to the rotated spinal cord are unusually long. These circumstances can be anticipated in most patients by careful evaluation of plain roentgenograms, computed tomograms, and MRI.

TIGHT FILUM, SACRAL AGENESIS, AND NEURENTERIC CYST

The strength of indications for operative treatment of these lesions is similar to other tethering lesions and rest with recovery of function and relief of symptoms.[85] Certainly prevention of further adverse change is also a major benefit of surgery. Improved prognosis is also obtained by removal of associated lesions. The laminectomy should be adequate to obtain rostral and caudal exposure of the intradural lesion. The tight filum can usually be distinguished from spinal roots by its color and its obvious dorsal vein. Complete removal of neurenteric cysts is required in order to prevent residual tissue secretion and subsequent inflammation. The extraspinal portion may require an additional procedure for removal.

RETETHERING OF THE SPINAL CORD

The prevention of progressive deterioration in gait, muscle strength, urinary control, orthopedic deformity, and scoliosis are the primary indications for release of the retethered spinal cord.[4, 5, 11, 12, 15, 17, 20, 22, 31, 37, 40, 104, 111, 128] Improvement in gait, strength, and occasionally bladder function can be anticipated. Tethered spinal cord release markedly reduces the incidence and magnitude of scoliosis, lordosis, and kyphosis associated with myelomeningocele.[103, 104] As with other operations, the vertical midline incision is extended above and below the area of previous repair. The skin incision is kept superficial over the site of previous repair until the dura can be identified. Rostral normal dura is identified beneath the most caudal normal lamina, and dissection of the repaired dural sac is carried caudally in a circumferential fashion, working from lateral normal dura to its medial point of adhesion to the fascia and/ or skin. Often the spinal cord extends posteriorly and superficially, resting adjacent to the subcuticular tissues. Failure to consider this abnormality could lead to spinal cord injury with the primary incision. Under the operating microscope, the dura is opened vertically within a posterior lateral quadrant most distal from the spinal cord and its adhesive attachment. By means of laser and magnification, the spinal cord, peripheral nerves, and associated vessels are dissected free from the point of attachment to the dura. Lipoma is completely removed with laser dissection. Similarly, dermoids and epidermoids can be completely removed intact from intra- or extramedullary locations. If possible, the spinal cord is reconvoluted with pia to pia laser welding. If the dural sac appears small, expansion is accomplished with interpositioning of an artificial dural graft. The dura, fascia, subcutaneous tissue, and skin are then sequentially closed. Twenty-year follow-up has now demonstrated that neurologic stability follows aggressive release of tethered spinal cord.[103] An additional threat to stability may occur with recurrent retether, which should be promptly treated. Improvement in muscle strength may be anticipated in 50 per cent or more, and 15 per cent will have improvement in bladder function. The incidence of scoliosis greater than 30 degrees is 20 per cent of all patients with sensory motor levels below L1.[103, 104] Virtually all patients are relieved of pain syndromes.

SUMMARY

The experience of comparing patients who are not treated surgically and deteriorate over time to patients who have gratifying recovery following surgery compels us to consider offering surgery to the asymptomatic child with tethered spinal cord syndrome. Early intervention is effective prophylaxis against later, often irreparable damage. Long-term studies have now demonstrated that neurologic stability and maximal function may be anticipated when tethered spinal cord is aggressively and expectantly treated. The time of onset and rate of progressive neurologic deficit cannot be predicted. The common experience of pediatric neurosurgeons confirms that the decline in function may be either insidious or precipitous. It is no longer tenable to advocate delayed anticipatory observation. Early prophylactic operation is now the standard of care even in asymptomatic infants. Continuing follow-up has shown normal development in infants with tethering lesions who have been promptly treated with surgery.

Release of the spinal cord from tethering lesions is the aim of the surgical procedure. Occasionally a surgeon will be required to stop short of this goal in order to avoid causing further neurologic deficit. This occurrence should be extremely rare. In conclusion, when deterioration occurs in any child or adult who previously underwent surgery to untether the spinal cord, one must conclude that the spinal cord has become retethered. These patients should be reevaluated, and if the cause of deterioration appears to be retethering, operative treatment should be promptly recommended. To accept neurologic, orthopedic, and urologic deterioration is to accept preventable deficit. Therefore, aggressive operative treatment of tethering lesions is always recommended.

REFERENCES

1. Jones: "Spina bifida occulta: No paralytic symptoms until seventeen years of age; spine trephined to relieve pressure on the cauda equina; recovery." Reports on the medical and surgical practice in the hospitals and asylums of Great Britain, Ireland, and the Colonies. Br Med J 1:173, 1891.
2. Brickner WM: Spina bifida occulta. Am J Med Sci 155:474, 1918.
3. Anderson F: Occult spinal dysraphism: A series of 73 cases. Pediatrics 55:826, 1975.
4. Bakker-Niezen S, Walder H, Merx J: The tethered spinal cord syndrome. Z Kinderchir 39H:100, 1984.
5. Balasubramaniam C, Laurent J, McCluggage C, et al.: Tethered cord syndrome after repair of myelomeningocele. Child's Nerv Sys 6:208, 1990.
6. Bruce D, Schut L: Spinal lipomas in infancy and childhood. Child's Brain 5:192, 1979.
7. Burrows F: Some aspects of occult spinal dysraphism: A study of 90 cases. Br J Radiol 41:496, 1968.
8. Ehni G, Love JG: Intraspinal lipomas: Report of cases, review of the literature, and clinical and pathologic study. Arch Neurol Psychiatry 53:1, 1945.
9. Garceau GJ: The filum terminale syndrome (the cord-tration syndrome). J Bone Joint Surg (Am) 35A:711, 1953.
10. Guthkelch AN: Diastematomyelia with median septum. Brain 97:729, 1974.
11. Hendrick EB, Hoffman HJ, Humphreys RP: The tethered spinal cord. Clin Neurosurg 30:457, 1983.
12. Hoffman H, Hendrick E, Humphreys R: The tethered spinal cord: Its protean manifestations, diagnosis and surgical correction. Child's Brain 2:145, 1976.
13. James M, Lassman L: Spinal dysraphism: The diagnosis and treatment of progressive lesions in spina bifida occulta. J Bone Joint Surg 44:828, 1962.
14. Lagae L, Verpoorten P, Casaer P, et al.: Conservative versus neurosurgical treatment of tethered cord patients. Z Kinderchir 45(Suppl 1):16, 1990.
15. Lapras C, Patet J, Huppert J, et al. The tethered cord syndrome (Experience of 58 cases). J Pediatr Neurosci 1:39, 1985.
16. Matson DD, Woods RP, Campbell JB, Ingraham FD: Diastematomyelia (congenital clefts of the spinal cord). Pediatrics 6:98, 1950.
17. Merx J, Niezen-Bakker S, Thijssen H, Walder H: The tethered spinal cord syndrome: A correlation of radiological features and preoperative findings in 30 patients. Neuroradiology 31:63, 1989.

18. Moufarrij N, Palmer J, Hahn H, Weinstein M: Correlation between magnetic resonance imaging and surgical findings in the tethered spinal cord. Neurosurgery 25:341, 1989.
19. Pierre-Kahn A, Lacombe J, Pichon J, et al.: Intraspinal lipomas with spina bifida. J Neurosurg 65:756, 1986.
20. Reigel DH: Tethered spinal cord. In Concepts in Pediatric Neurosurgery. Vol. 4. Basel, S. Karger, 1983, pp 142–164.
21. Schut L, Bruce D, Sutton L: The management of the child with a lipomyelomeningocele. Clin Neurosurg 30:464, 1983.
22. Tamaki N, Shirataki K, Kojima N, et al.: Tethered cord syndrome of delayed onset following repair of myelomeningocele. J Neurosurg 69:393, 1988.
23. Till K: Occult spinal dysraphism: The value of prophylactic surgical treatment. In Recent Progress in Neurological Surgery. Amsterdam, Excerpta Medica, 1974, pp 60–66.
24. Yashon D, Beatty A: Tethering of the conus medullaris within the sacrum. J Neurol Neurosurg Psychiatry 29:244, 1966.
25. Barson A: The vertebral level of termination of the spinal cord during normal and abnormal development. J Anat 106:489, 1970.
26. Barry A: A quantitative study of the prenatal changes in angulation of the spinal nerves. Anat Rec 126:97, 1956.
27. Breig A: Overstretching of and circumscribed pathological tension in the spinal cord: A basic cause of symptoms in cord disorders. J Biomechanics 3:7, 1970.
28. Sarwar M, Crelin E, Kier E, et al.: Experimental cord stretchability and the tethered cord syndrome. Am J Neuroradiol 4:641, 1983.
29. Sarwar M, Virapongse C, Bhimani S: Primary tethered cord syndrome: A new hypothesis of its origin. Am J Neuroradiol 5:235, 1984.
30. Tani S, Yamada S, Knighton R: Extensibility of the lumbar and sacral cord. J Neurosurg 66:116, 1987.
31. Yamada S, Zinke D, Sanders D: Pathophysiology of "tethered cord syndrome." J Neurosurg 54:494, 1981.
32. Fujita Y, Yamamoto H: An experimental study on spinal cord traction effect. Spine 14:698, 1989.
33. Reigel DH, Kortyna R, Quigley MR: Cerebral blood flow following release of the tethered spinal cord. Joint section on Disorders of the Spine and Peripheral Nerves. AANS/CNS 7:104, 1991.
34. Schneider S, Rosenthal A, Greenberg B, Danto J: A preliminary report on the use of laser-doppler flometry during tethered spinal cord release. Neurosurgery 32:214, 1993.
35. Malatova Z, Chavko M, Marsala J: Effect of spinal cord ischemia on axonal transport of cholinergic enzymes in rabbit sciatic nerve. Brain Res 481:31, 1989.
36. Gelfan S, Tarlov I: Physiology of spinal cord, nerve root and peripheral nerve compression. J Neurophysiol 18:170, 1955.
37. Baldwin H, Rekate H, Sonntag V: Diagnosis, surgical management, and outcome of the adult tethered cord syndrome. BNI Quarterly 7:16, 1991.
38. Kaplan J, Quencer R: The occult tethered conus syndrome in an adult. Radiology 137:387, 1980.
39. Oi S, Yamada H, Matsumoto S: Tethered cord syndrome versus low-paced conus medullaris in an over-distended spinal cord following initial repair of myelodysplasia. Child's Nerv Sys 6:264, 1990.
40. Pang D, Wilberger J: Tethered cord syndrome in adults. J Neurosurg 57:32, 1982.
41. Albright A, Gartner J, Wiener E: Lumbar cutaneous hemangiomas as indicators of tethered spinal cords. Pediatrics 83:977, 1989.
42. Barkovich A, Edwards M, Cogen P: MR evaluation of spinal dermal sinus tracts in children. Am J Neuroradiol 12:123, 1991.
43. Naidich TP, McLone DG, Harwood-Nash DC: Spinal dysraphism. In Newton TH, Potts DG (eds): Computed Tomography of the Spine and Spinal Cord. San Anselmo, CA, Clavadel Press, 1983.
44. Guidetti B, Gagliandi FM: Epidermoid and dermoid cysts: Clinical evaluation and late surgical results. J Neurosurg 47:12, 1977.
45. Wright RL: Congenital dermal sinuses. Prog Neurolog Surg 4:175, 1971.
46. Cardell BS, Laurence B: Congenital dermal sinus associated with meningitis: Report of a fatal case. Br Med J 2:1558, 1951.
47. El-Gindi S, Fairburn B: Intramedullary spinal abscess as acomplication of a congenital dermal sinus: Case report. J Neurosurg 30:494, 1969.
48. Matson DD, Jerva MJ: Recurrent meningitis associated with congenital lumbo-sacral dermal sinus tract. J Neurosurg 25:288, 1966.
49. Mount LA: Congenital dermal sinuses as a cause of meningitis, intraspinal abscess and intracranial abscess. JAMA 139:1263, 1949.
50. Naidich T, McLone D: Congenital pathology of the spine and spinal cord. In Taveras JM, Ferrucci JT (eds): Radiology: Diagnosis, Imaging, Intervention. Vol. 3. Philadelphia, JB Lippincott, 1988.
51. Olliver CP: Traite des Maladies de la Moelle Epiniere. 3rd ed. Vol. 1. Paris, Mequignon-Marvis, 1837.
52. Till K: Occult spinal dysraphism: The value of prophylactic surgical treatment. In Recent Progress in Neurological Surgery. Amsterdam, Excerpta Medica, 1974, pp 60–66.
53. Humphreys RP, Hendrick EB, Hoffman HJ: Diastematomyelia. Clin Neurosurg 30:436, 1983.
54. Sedzimir CB, Roberts JR, Occleshaw JV: Massive diastematomyelia without cutaneous dysraphism. Arch Dis Child 48:400, 1973.
55. James CCM, Lassman LP: Spinal Dysraphism: Spina Bifida Occulta. London, Butterworth, 1972, pp 61–76.
56. Keim HA, Greene AF: Diastematomyelia and scoliosis. J Bone Joint Surg (Am) 55A:1425, 1973.
57. Schlesinger AE, Naidich TP, Quencer RM: Concurrent hydromyelia and diastematomyelia. AJNR 7:473, 1986.
58. Winter RB, Haven JJ, Moe JH, Lagaard SM: Diastematomyelia and congenital spine deformities. J Bone Surg 56:1:27, 1974.
59. Agnoli AL, Schonmayr R, Popovic M, et al: The value of neuroradiological investigations in intraspinal malformations of the lumbosacral spine in childhood. Neuroradiology 16:91, 1978.
60. Hilal SK, Marton D, Pollack E: Diastematomyelia in children. Radiology 112:609, 1974.
61. Herman TE, Siegel MJ: Cervical and basicranial diastematomyelia. Am J Radiol 154:806, 1990.
62. Rawanduzy A, Murali R: Cervical spine diastematomyelia in adulthood. Neurosurgery 28:459, 1991.
63. Raghavendra B, Epstein F, Pinto R, et al.: The tethered spinal cord: Diagnosis by high-resolution real-time ultrasound. Radiology 149:123, 1983.
64. Caspi B, Gorbacz S, Appelman Z, Elchalal U: Antenatal diagnosis of diastematomyelia. J Clin Ultrasound 18:721, 1990.
65. Pachi A, Maggi E, Giancott A, et al.: Prenatal sonographic diagnosis of diastematomyelia in a diabetic woman. Prenatal Diag 12:535, 1990.
66. James CCM, Lassman LP: Diastematomyelia with median septumin spina bifida occulta: Indications for surgery. Z Kinderchir 22:460, 1977.
67. McLone D, Naidich T: Laser resection of fifty spinal lipomas. Neurosurgery 18:611, 1986.
68. Ammerman BJ, Henry JM, De Girolami U, et al.: Intradural lipomas of the spinal cord: Clinicopathological correlation. J Neurosurg 44:331, 1976.
69. Lassman LP, James CCM: Lumbosacral lipomas: Critical survey of 26 cases submitted to laminectomy. J Neurol Neurosurg Psychiatry 30:174, 1967.
70. Bassett RC: The neurologic deficit associated with lipomas of the cauda equina. Ann Surg 131:108, 1950.
71. Rogers HM, Long DM, Chou SN, et al.: Lipomas of the spinal cord and cauda equina. J Neurosurg 34:349, 1971.
72. Villarejo FJ, Blazquez MG, Gutierrez-Diaz JA: Intraspinal lipomas in children. Child's Brain 2:361, 1976.
73. Walsh J, Markesbery W: Histological features of congenital lipomas of the lower spinal canal. J Neurosurg 52:564, 1980.
74. McLone DG, Mutluer S, Naidich TP: Lipomeningoceles of the conus medullaris. In Raimondi AJ (ed): Concepts of Pediatric Neurosurgery. Vol. 3. Basel, S. Karger, 1982.
75. McAlister WH, Siegel JJ, Shackelford GD: A congenital iliac anomaly often associated with sacral lipoma and ipsilateral lower extremity weakness. Skeletal Radiol 3:161, 1978.
76. Chapman P, Beyerl B: The tethered spinal cord, with particular

reference to spinal lipoma and diastematomyelia. *In* Hoffman HJ, Epstein F (eds): Disorders of the Developing Nervous System: Diagnosis and Treatment. Boston, Blackwell Scientific, 1986, pp 109–131.

77. Emery JL, Lendon RG: The local cord lesion in neuro-spinal dysraphism (meningomyelocele). J Pathol 110:83, 1973.

78. McLendon R, Oakes W, Heinz E, et al.: Adipose tissue in the filum terminale: A computed tomographic finding that may indicate tethering of the spinal cord. Neurosurgery 22:873, 1988.

79. Hoffman H, Taecholarn C, Hendrick E, Humphreys R: Management of lipomyelomeningoceles. J Neurosurg 62:1, 1985.

80. Naidich T, McLone D, Mutluer S: A new understanding of dorsal dysraphism with lipoma (lipomyeloschisis): Radiologic evaluation and surgical correction. Am J Neuroradiol 4:103, 1983.

81. Naidich TP, McLone DG, Mutluer S, et al.: Presurgical evaluation of lipomyelomeningoceles. Presented at the 19th Annual Meeting of the American Society of Neuroradiology. Chicago, April 1981. Am J Neuroradiol 3:93, 1982.

82. Resjo IM, Harwood-Nash DC, Fitz CR, et al.: Computed tomographic metrizamide myelography in spinal dysraphism in infants and children. J Comput Assist Tomogr 2:549, 1978.

83. Kanev PM, Lemire RJ, Loeser JD, Berger MS: Management and long-term follow-up review of children with lipomyelomeningocele, 1952–1987. J Neurosurg 73:48, 1990.

84. Stolke D, Zumkeller M, Seifer V: Intraspinal lipomas in infancy and childhood causing a tethered cord syndrome. Neurosurg Rev 11:59, 1988.

85. Jones P, Love J: Tight filum terminale. AMA Arch Surg 73:556, 1956.

86. Fitz C, Harwood-Nash D: The tethered conus. Am J Roentgenol 125:515, 1975.

87. Price DL, Dooling EC, Richardson EP Jr.: Caudal dysplasia (caudal regression syndrome). Arch Neurol 23:212, 1970.

88. Passarge E: Congenital malformations and maternal diabetes. Lancet i:324, 1965.

89. Passarge E, Lenz W: Syndrome of caudal regression in infants of diabetic mothers: Observations of further cases. Pediatrics 37:672, 1966.

90. McKusick VA: Mendelian Inheritance in Man. 2nd ed. Baltimore, Johns Hopkins Press, 1988.

91. Pang D: Sacral agenesis and caudal spinal cord malformation. Neurosurgery 5:755, 1993.

92. Smith ED: Congenital sacral defects. *In* Stephens FP (ed): Congenital Malformations of the Rectum, Anus, and Genitourinary Tracts. Edinburgh, E&S Livingstone, 1963, p 82.

93. Barkovich A, Raghavan N, Chuang S, Peck W: The wedge-shaped cord terminus: A radiographic sign of caudal regression. Am J Neuroradiol 10:1223, 1989.

94. Warf B, Scott R, Barnes P, Hendren W: Tethered spinal cord inpatients with anorectal and urogenital malformations. Pediatr Neurosurg 19:25, 1993.

95. Ebisu T, Odake G, Fujimoto M, et al.: Neurenteric cysts with meningomyelocele or meningocele. Child's Nerv Sys 6:465, 1990.

96. LeDoux MS, Faye-Petersen O, Aronin PA, et al.: Lumbosacral neurenteric cyst in an infant. J Neurosurg 78:821, 1993.

97. Fernandes E, Custer M, Burton E, et al.: Neurenteric cyst: Surgery and diagnostic imaging. J Pediatr Surg 1:108, 1991.

98. Holmes GL, Traders S, Ignatiadis P: Intraspinal enterogenous cysts: A case report and review of pediatric cases in the literature. Am J Dis Child 132:906, 1978.

99. Neuhauser EBD, Harris GBC, Berrett A: Roetgenographic features of neurenteric cysts. Am J Roentgenol 79:235, 1958.

100. Chamaa MT, Berney J: Anterior-sacral maningocele; value of magnetic resonance imaging and abdominal sonography. Acta Neurochir (Wien) 109:154, 1991.

101. Heinz ER, Rosenbaum AE, Scarff TB, et al.: Tethered spinal cord following meningomyelocele repair. Radiology 131:153, 1979.

102. Kaplan W, McLone D, Richard I: The urological manifestations of the tethered spinal cord. J Urol 140:1285, 1988.

103. Reigel DH, Tchernoukha K, Bazmi B et al.: Change in spinal curvature following release of the tethered spinal cord. Pediatr Neurosurg 20(I), 1994.

104. McLone D, Herman J, Gabrieli A, Dias L: Tethered cord as a cause of scoliosis in children with a myelomeningocele. Pediatr Neurosurg 16:8, 1990–1991.

105. Just M, Ermert J, Higer HP: Magnetic resonance imaging of postrepair myelomeningocele: Findings in 31 children and adolescents. Neurosurg Rev 10:47, 1987.

106. Hall WA, Albright AL, Brunberg JA: Diagnosis of tethered cords by magnetic resonance imaging. Surg Neurol 30:60, 1988.

107. McLone DH: Technique for closure of myelomeningoceles. Child's Brain 6:65, 1980.

108. Braun I, Raghavendra B, Kricheff: Spinal cord imaging using real-time high-resolution ultrasound. Radiology 147:459, 1983.

109. Naidich T, Fernbach S, McLone D, Shkolnik A: Sonography of the caudal spine and back: Congenital anomalies in children. Am J Radiol 142:1229, 1984.

110. DiPietro MA, Venes JL: Real-time sonography of the pediatric spinal cord: Horizons and limits. Concepts Pediatr Neurosurg 8:120, 1988.

111. Raghavan N, Barkovich A, Edwards M, Norman D: MR imaging in the tethered spinal cord syndrome. Am J Radiol 152:843, 1989.

112. Brophy J, Sutton L, Zimmerman R, et al.: Magnetic resonance imaging of lipomyelomeningocele and tethered cord. Neurosurgery 25:336, 1989.

113. Brunberg J, Latchaw R, Kanal E, et al.: Magnetic resonance imaging of spinal dysraphism. Radiol Clin North Am 2:181, 1988.

114. Lassman LP, James CCM: Meningocele manqué. Child's Brain 3:1, 1977.

115. Kaffenberger D, Heinz E, Oakes J, Boyko O: Meningocele manqué: Radiologic findings with clinical correlation. Am J Neuroradiol 12:1083, 1992.

116. Kernohan JW: The ventriculus terminalis: Its growth and development. J Comp Neurol 38:107, 1924.

117. Sigal R, Denys A, Halimi P, et al.: Ventriculus terminalis of the conus medullaris: MR imaging in four patients with congenital dilatation. Am J Neuroradiol 12:733, 1991.

118. Gilchrist B, Harrison M, Campbell J: Neurenteric cyst: Current management. J Pediatr Surg 25:1231, 1990.

119. Khoury A, Hendrick E, McLorie G, et al.: Occult spinal dysraphism: Clinical and urodynamic outcome after division of the filum terminale. J Urol 144:426, 1990.

120. Kondo H, Kato K, Kanai S, et al.: Bladder dysfunction secondary to tethered cord syndrome in adults: Is it curable? J Urol 135:313, 1986.

121. Delatis V, Vodusek DB, Abbott R et al.: Intraoperative monitoring of the dorsal sacral roots: Minimizing the risk of iatrogenic micturition disorders. Neurosurgery 30:72, 1992.

122. Nuwer MR: Electrophysiologic evaluation and monitoring of spinal cord and root function. Neurosurg Clin North Am 3:533, 1990.

123. Sathi S, Madsen J, Bauer S, Scott RM: The effect of surgical repair on the neuro-urologic function in infants with lipomeningocele. Pediatr Neurosurg 19:256, 1993.

124. Shinomiya K, Fuchioka M, Matsuoka T, et al.: Intraoperative monitoring for tethered spinal cord syndrome. Spine 16:1290, 1991.

125. Frerebeau Ph, Dimeglio A, Grass M, Harbi H: Diastematomyelia: Report of 21 cases surgically treated by a neurosurgical and orthopedic team. Child's Brain 10:328, 1983.

126. Begeer J, Wiertsema P, Breukers M, et al.: Tethered cord syndrome: Clinical signs and results of operation in 42 patients with spina bifida aperta and occulta. Z Kinderchir 44:5, 1989.

127. Linder M, Rosenstein J, Sklar F: Functional improvement after spinal surgery for the dysraphic malformations. Neurosurg 11:622, 1982.

128. Venes J, Stevens EA: Surgical pathology in tethered cord secondary to myelomeningocele repair. Concepts Pediatr Neurosurg 4:165, 1983.

Chapter 5

ENCEPHALOCELE AND DERMAL SINUSES

ROBIN P. HUMPHREYS, M.D.

ENCEPHALOCELE

Encephalocele, a neural tube defect that occurs less commonly than those in the spinal axis, is nevertheless one potentially associated with substantial neurologic harm. It invokes great anxiety in the parents, an unpredictable course in the child, and great prognostic frustration for the surgeon. How striking it is that half the distance of the cranium should make such a difference in the artistic repair and prognostic implications of encephalocele. Hence, the lesions known as sincipital, which lie along the skull base, may be difficult to diagnose but can be beautifully managed with delicate anterior fossa surgery, and usually they carry an excellent prognosis. None of this is necessarily true for the encephalocele that is located in the posterior half of the skull.

The various developmental defects involving scalp, bone, brain, and its coverings have been defined.[1] With regard to the "cephalocele," this chapter will consider those forms known as "cranial meningocele," "meningoencephalocele," and "atretic cephalocele."

INCIDENCE

The world-wide incidence of encephalocele is at least 1 per 5,000 live births.[2] Among the many populations of the World Health Organization study, this incidence was markedly consistent. Even Belfast, notorious for its high incidence of central nervous system (CNS) malformations, reported only six encephaloceles among 28,091 births.[2] The incidence may be even less frequent in North America.

Sex incidence seems to vary with location of the defect. About three fourths of children with occipital encephaloceles are females, whereas males predominate when the malformation is anteriorly located.[3]

CLASSIFICATION OF ENCEPHALOCELES

Encephalocele classification has become more elaborate.[1, 4–8] Davis and Alexander, in 1959, neatly grouped the encephaloceles that occur along the skull base as well as in the upper and anterior portions of the forehead into the *basal* and *sincipital* types, respectively.[4] Subsequently, Suwanwela subclassified the frontoethmoidal encephaloceles.[8] But even now, the workable simplicity of Matson's clinical classification of all the lesions has much to recommend it[6] (Table 5–1).

Basal Encephaloceles. This type of encephalocele exists in the base of the skull and is named according to its site of presentation. The *sphenopharyngeal* lesion presents through the sphenoid bone into the epipharynx and may be recognized as a pulsating mass, sometimes visible transorally through an associated cleft palate. The *intranasal* mass passes through the cribriform plate into the nasal cavity and presents as a mass be-

TABLE 5–1. CLASSIFICATION OF ENCEPHALOCELE

Basal
    Sphenopharyngeal
    Intranasal
    Spheno-orbital
    Sphenomaxillary
Sincipital
    Nasofrontal
    Frontoethmoidal
    Naso-orbital
Convexity
    Frontal
    Parietal (or sagittal)
    Occipital
    Cervico-occipital
Atretic
    Alopecic (parietal)
    Nodular (occipital)

tween the middle turbinate bone and the nasal septum. This lesion or its forme fruste is being encountered more frequently during major craniofacial surgery performed for correction of hypertelorism. Two uncommon lesions are the *spheno-orbital* encephalocele, which passes through the superior orbital fissure into the orbital cavity, and the *sphenomaxillary* encephalocele, which penetrates the inferior orbital fissure and enters the pterygopalatine fossa from the medial side of the ramus of the mandible.

Sincipital Encephaloceles. The sincipital lesions are located in the anterior and upper part of the forehead. The *nasofrontal* lesion is found directly in the midline between the frontal and nasal bones at the glabella, whereas the *frontoethmoidal* mass presents between the frontal, nasal, and ethmoid bones—being obvious at the side of the nose. In either circumstance, the superficial mass is of a variable size, often skin-covered, and must be distinguished from a dermoid cyst. Hypertelorism is often present. The *naso-orbital* variety passes between frontal, lacrimal, and ethmoid bones to enter the anteromedial portion of the orbital cavity.

Convexity Encephalocele. These represent the most common group and are found in the frontal, parietal, or occipital bones of the skull convexity, usually in its midline. These encephaloceles may be located rostral to or at the level of the anterior fontanelle, between it and the posterior fontanelle (hence "sagittal" encephalocele), or, most frequently in the Western Hemisphere, caudal to the latter—"occipital encephalocele." While there has been an attempt to subclassify the latter into "superior," "inferior," and even those crossing the "cervico-occipital" region, such division becomes unworkable during the clinical evaluation of the infant with a large sac and small head[1, 9] (Fig. 5–1). These subdivisions are proposed in an attempt to identify the tissues most likely to be contained within the sac; the "superior" lesion probably contains supratentorial structures; the "inferior," cerebellum and perhaps a portion of brainstem; and the "cervico-occipital," any combination of fourth ventricle, adjacent stem, and cervical cord tissues.

Atretic Encephalocele. The atretic lesion has a much more innocent appearance. Its "alopecic" form occurs in the parietal midline, has dorsal cyst malformations, and is *not* associated with normal development.[10] The "nodular" type is found in the occipital midline and is unassociated with other cerebral anomalies; the child usually develops normally.

DEVELOPMENTAL PATHOLOGY

Malformations that closely approximate the occipital encephalocele found in humans can be induced in animals by the administration of three different teratogens—sodium arsenate, clofibrate, and vitamin A. In the laboratory setting it is critical that these substances be introduced into the pregnant dam when the hamster embryos are at the primitive streak stage of development.[11]

There is little doubt that encephalocele is related to a disorder in the closure of the primitive neural tube, a phenomenon that is well under way if not complete by the sixth week. However, by this time there is only a minute cerebral hemisphere and cerebellum within the forming cranium. Hence, if there were a failure of closure of the neural tube at this early stage as proposed by von Recklinghausen, one might expect the cerebral hernia to contain tissues of the tectum, but not of the cerebral hemispheres.[12] However, as encephaloceles (notably those in the occipital region) do contain cerebral cortex (and often much of cerebellum), one must consider altered timing for this developmental abnormality which occurs at a later stage of fetal maturation.[4] That is, there appears not to be a local failure of fusion of the neural tube but rather a failure of development of the overlying mesenchymal tissue with a local cerebral "blow-out" occurring—at the earliest—at 8 to 12 weeks of gestation. With regard to occipital encephaloceles, the experimental administration of one of the identified teratogens results in a decrease in the rate and degree of growth of the basal bones of the skull, in particular the basioccipital component of the sphenoid bone (clivus).[11]

The lesions that lie in the anterior half of the skull over its convexity probably do not arise as a result of a "blow-out," but rather from small cell rests left in the closing neural groove. These lesions in skin communicate through the skull with the pia-arachnoid and dura and often do not have a direct communication with the cerebral tissue. The frequent association of anomalies of the face, optic system, and brain concomitant with the trans-sphenoidal encephalocele are assumed to be formed together in the same stage in the embryonic period, and to arise from neighboring areas in the ventral surface of the cephalic end of the neural tube around the anterior neuropore.[13]

Dilatation of the cerebral ventricles from the usual obstructing, dysplastic causes generally is not an early feature with encephalocele. Paradoxically, hydrocephalus, which tends to become clinically obvious after birth and in many instances after the operation on the encephalocele, can appear in a skull that otherwise is regarded as microcephalic.

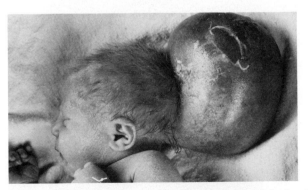

FIGURE 5–1. The encephalocele sac exceeds the size of the head. Its origin through the occipital region is uncertain, thus making classification unsure. Its contents also are unknown. In this instance the sac was filled almost exclusively with CSF.

PATHOLOGY OF THE OCCIPITAL ENCEPHALOCELE

The bony defect of the occipital encephalocele may be localized to the occipital squame or extend into the foramen magnum and involve the posterior arch of the atlas.[14] The skull base can be deformed with small anterior and middle cranial fossae and a large or small posterior fossa.[11, 14] The falx and tentorium are often abnormal in layout.

The masses vary considerably in size, from that of an acorn to a lesion substantially larger than the skull itself. The sac may be sessile or pedunculated and completely or only partially covered with normal skin. If a covering parchment membrane is present, it varies in thickness and may weep blood or burst and gush cerebrospinal fluid (CSF). The brain tissue present in the encephalocele sac contains an asymmetric herniation of the cerebral hemispheres. As much as one half of a hemisphere may be so displaced. Although the cerebral cortex may be histologically indistinguishable from normal regions of brain, hemorrhage and ischemic necrosis are usually present.[4] Defects in the commissural system and accompanying hydrocephalus are sufficiently common. The latter may be due to the presence of a ventricle within the hernia sac, aqueduct distortion, or obliteration of the usual posterior fossa CSF pathways.

The hernia sac or "cyst" in severe cases contains parts of cerebellum, brainstem, occipital lobes, vascular structures, or only cerebrospinal fluid and glial remnants.[11] Simpson found that 37 per cent of occipital encephaloceles contained cerebral tissue but no cerebellum, 21 per cent had cerebral and cerebellar tissue, 5 per cent had cerebellum only, and 37 per cent had nodules of glia or other dysplastic neural tissue.[7] Any of the solid structures may show (in addition to elongation and distortion) various degrees of disorganization.

CLINICAL EVALUATION

Children with basal or sincipital encephaloceles may be diagnosed only on a delayed basis, at a later stage in life when they are being evaluated for a nasal or glabellar mass, nasal congestion or snoring, hypertelorism, or craniofacial abnormality. The child's development up to the time of assessment may be entirely normal and the neurologic examination unremarkable. Specific to the latter, deficiencies in olfaction must be ascertained preoperatively. The mass itself is clinically described and the children then meticulously examined with sophisticated neuro-imaging studies.

By contrast, the presence of an occipital encephalocele can be detected by certain prenatal tests.[7, 15] While it is moot whether alpha-fetoprotein levels are increased in amniotic fluid from a fetus with an encephalocele, the prenatal ultrasound examination can outline the sac, its location, the associated ventricular dilatation, and other constructional abnormalities in brain formation.[7, 15] At birth, the encephalocele is immediately apparent unless it is small and of the atretic type. Spuriously, the infant who functions at a brainstem capacity sucks, feeds, cries, and sleeps as a normal neonate. The subsequent neurologic features of psychomotor delay, ocular palsies, and limb and trunk spasticity are not obvious at this early stage.

A number of determinations that are made on the size and contents of the sac as well as the skull size and shape and the presence of hydrocephalus all have prognostic implications (Fig. 5–2). For example, a large sac filled only with spinal fluid does not imply a dismal prognosis, but the infant who shows a small head with forehead sloping posteriorly has a poor prognosis.

RADIOLOGY

The modern neuro-imaging features of encephaloceles have been published recently.[1] Standard skull radiography may delineate the limits of the bony skull defect that is associated with the encephalocele, be it in the base or over the vault. Bony windows of computed tomography or three-dimensional (3-D) reconstructs in the sagittal, coronal, and axial planes are often a useful adjunct to examine the frontoethmoidal and basal encephaloceles.

The CT scan will also show the amount of cerebral tissue within the sac, the extent of the CSF spaces, and perhaps the nature of the blood channels about the sac itself. If one is concerned about the latter, arteriography should be performed. For example, the tissue from the frontal lobe and nasal encephaloceles may contain peripheral branches of the fronto-polar arteries, whereas the larger occipital lesions can be associated with a bizarre array of major tributaries from anterior, middle, and occasionally posterior cerebral supply. Frequently the superior sagittal sinus, which remains intracranial, is split by the sac attachments.

Magnetic resonance imaging (MRI) outlines the herniated cerebral tissues, and especially their relationship with each other. The herniated tissue can be traced back to the intracranial compartment and its union

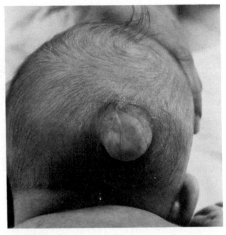

FIGURE 5–2. The small encephalocele is of the "superior occipital" type and contained almost no solid tissue. The child is normal.

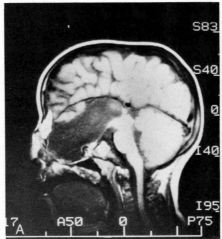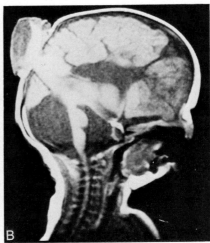

FIGURE 5–3. *A,* This child with orbital hypertelorism has a large sphenopharyngeal encephalocele. The MRI midsagittal T1 image shows a large CSF space communicating from basal cisterns to the nasopharynx. *B,* The MRI study of this infant's "superior occipital" encephalocele shows cerebrum extending externally from above the tentorium. Generous subtentorial CSF spaces also exist.

with anatomic structures therein. In addition, other constructional defects such as callosal agenesis, Dandy-Walker malformation, dorsal cysts, and porencephaly may be noted (Fig. 5–3*A* and *B*).

DECISIONS

When presenting the treatment program for the child with an encephalocele, the surgeon will have little difficulty advocating operative care for the patient with a basal or sincipital lesion. The smaller masses at these sites may be excised for cosmetic reasons or to minimize the threat of retrograde infection. The larger anterior encephaloceles may be repaired at the time of a more major craniofacial reconstruction. In either event, these cases are managed on an elective basis and in anticipation of an excellent prognosis.

On the other hand, one might presume that infants with occipital encephaloceles would present the same ethical dilemma as the child with myelodysplasia. Such is not the case. The child with an encephalocele does not usually have a severe, fixed neurologic deficit obvious at birth or early and obvious hydrocephalus, either of which might allow the clinician to accurately predict the child's future. Encephalocele prognosis is much more difficult to determine. Furthermore, it seems that these children are not as susceptible to contaminating meningitis as are infants with neural tube defects of the spine, even though the encephalocele sac may bleed, rupture, discharge CSF, and then reseal. One cannot expect therefore that nature will aid with the ultimate decision. In short, virtually all children with occipital encephalocele will require operative obliteration of the lesion. The practical reasons for this decision are as follows:

1. The sac is not only grossly disfiguring (potentially producing considerable parental anxiety), but its unwieldy character interferes with infant positioning, feeding, and nursing care.

2. With the passage of time, the sac tends to expand in size, usually as a consequence of CSF accumulating within it. Even the skin that was originally normal and covered the sac can, in time, become considerably thinned until the sac bursts. Hemorrhage or the release of CSF is at any time a messy occurrence.

3. Some infants with smaller dura-covered lesions may show extreme sensitivity to simulation of the dome of their sac. The infant's irritability usually can only be relieved by reconstituting normal tissue barriers and covering the defect with normal skin.

4. Progressive hydrocephalus will in time become more of a threat to the intracranial nervous tissue, possibly harming its further development.

Hence, most infants with occipital encephaloceles are subjected to early operative repair of this lesion and to early or interval treatment of the hydrocephalus if present.

OPERATIVE TREATMENT

When operating upon the infant with an encephalocele, the surgeon not only must consider factors related to the encephalocele and its position, but also must observe the principles relevant to surgery performed on the newborn. Thus the operative positioning must permit the placement of monitoring lines and control of body temperature. The immediate hazard of operation upon midline skull defects, especially for the more posteriorly positioned lesions, is blood loss because of the encephalocele's relationship to the superior sagittal sinus, torcula, and/or an enlarged occipital sinus. However, unless the surgeon is unnecessarily rough or becomes lost, the major venous channels need not be encountered.

For anterior lesions, the child is placed supine with the head and neck extended, and intubation is performed via the oral route. In all likelihood, a neurosurgeon and plastic surgeon will have consulted on the case together and will have decided whether operation is to be performed simultaneously or at an interval.[7] If a single procedure is scheduled, the neurosurgeon must *first* explore the anterior cranial fossa and midline structures from both the extradural and the *intradural* approaches. The dural defects, CSF pools, and anterior falcine abnormalities must be identified on all sides. For lesions in the region of the foramen cecum or cribriform plate, the stalk or herniated tissue can usually be isolated from the walls of the dural tunnel through which they leave the skull. The stalk must be transected intradurally and a fascial patch placed to occlude the dural trough. Thereafter, the associated surgeon can dissect the lesion downward into the nose.

The identification and fascial repair of sphenopharyngeal encephaloceles or meningoceles is also performed intradurally. The extent of the defect can be alarming and fraught with postoperative problems pertaining to continued CSF leakage. It is often difficult to obtain a watertight closure, and despite meticulous attention the patient may experience CSF rhinorrhea postoperatively. The patient's condition during these difficult postoperative days may be further complicated by previously unrecognized hypopituitarism.

By contrast, the repair of the newborn's occipital encephalocele is relatively standard. The mass is usually sizable and pendulous, and its location renders positioning of the patient difficult for operative exposure. Surgery is usually performed with the infant placed prone on a small padded bolster, with the head positioned in the traditional headrest. After the encephalocele sac is manipulated to allow proper preparation of the skin, the surgeon can incise the sac at almost any site except its margin with the surrounding scalp (Fig. 5–4). That is, the skin incision should be made on the stalk or over the dome of the sac, preferably on its lateral extremes, to be certain that there will be enough skin present at the conclusion of the procedure to approximate the scalp edges. The first incision will enter the intradural space directly, releasing a gush of CSF and allowing the sac to collapse. Once the surgeon can visualize the inside of the sac, he can determine the amount of dura required for closure over the encephalocele remnant (if this is his choice) and then circumscribe the entire encephalocele with either scalpel or dissecting scissors.

At this stage, a fundamental decision must be made whether the herniated cerebral tissue should be saved. Guthkelch feels that ". . . cerebral tissue should, if possible, be dealt with conservatively" by detaching it from its arachnoid adhesions and replacing it within the cranial cavity.[16] Others argue that to amputate herniated brain tissue might jeopardize intracranial blood supply if errant vessels within the sac then re-enter the skull to supply vital regions of brain.[17] Simpson has endeavored to minimize the ablation of herniated tissue and has tried duraplasty and expansion of the cranial cavity. Unfortunately, ". . . the results have been very disappointing."[7] However, as this extracranial tissue is usually severely gliotic and ischemic and in very few areas shows viable neurons, and as it is frequently difficult to replace cerebral tissue within the cranial cavity through what usually amounts to a small skull defect located directly over the sagittal sinus, it is usual practice to excise all of the herniated tissue flush with

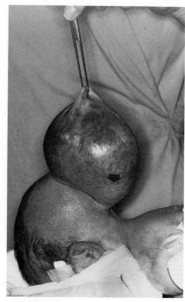

FIGURE 5–4. The encephalocele sac must be held aloft during skin preparation and draping. There is an abundant and full-thickness skin cuff at its base through which the incision is made *(arrow)*.

the surrounding skull (Fig. 5–5). A small dural flap is then sewn across the remaining stalk covering the site of bony defect. The marginal skin edges can then be trimmed appropriately and the scalp closed most easily, as a rule, in the transverse plane.

Should hydrocephalus arise, a bypass CSF shunt will be required. The hydrocephalus can be determined early with the technical ease of ultrasound or CT and a shunt inserted at the same operation as encephalocele excision if necessary. This usually has a dramatic effect on diminishing CSF volume and pressure within the encephalocele sac.

It may be necessary many years later for the surgeon to repair a persisting midline skull defect with a re-

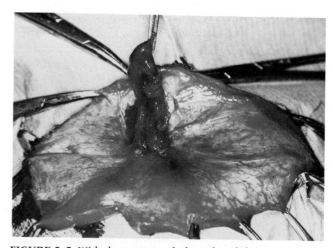

FIGURE 5–5. With the sac opened, the only solid tissue proves to be a small projection of glial and venous tissue. This was amputated and the glistening surrounding dura closed over the small skull defect. (Same patient as in Figure 5–1.)

placement cranioplasty. This should be kept in mind at the time of the initial surgery so that bony edges and dural closure are easily defined later on.

RESULTS OF TREATMENT

Historically, there have been three major determinants of a child's survival and development following early treatment of occipital encephalocele. In the past few years these have been subject to critical analysis.[3, 18, 19]

The original unfavorable influence on postencephalocele recovery was *hydrocephalus*. Even though the encephalocele surgery had proceeded smoothly, the subsequent development of hydrocephalus was the major cause of death prior to introduction of sophisticated shunt devices. With the expectation that 60 to 70 per cent of infants with occipital encephalocele will develop hydrocephalus, diversionary shunts are required.[3, 18] Death is averted by their early placement, and while hydrocephalus is a serious associated malady, its presence now has little bearing on the child's quality of survival.[3, 19]

Microcephaly is present in at least 20 per cent of children with occipital encephalocele and is an unfavorable feature.[3, 18] When the child's head circumference remains below the tenth percentile, one can expect cognitive delay.[3]

The single most important prognostic factor is the *presence or absence of brain tissue in the sac.* This statement begs the differentiation between occipital encephaloceles and meningoceles. Obviously, children born with cranium bifidum and a leptomeningeal sac filled with spinal fluid should be expected to have a better quality of survival (60 per cent normal in Lorber's study and about 80 per cent in Guthkelch) than those whose sacs harbor cerebral substance (only 10 per cent are completely normal in Lorber's series and approximately 25 per cent in the series of Guthkelch and Simpson).[3, 7, 16]

SUMMARY

One thus concludes about encephaloceles that the basal lesions are often insidious in presentation and difficult to repair, and the sincipital masses are somewhat obvious, amenable to precise anterior fossa corrective surgery, and characterized by an excellent prognosis (containing as they do portions of relatively ''silent'' frontal lobe), whereas the vertex lesions (particularly those in the occipital area) are obvious at birth and easy to repair but carry a questionable prognosis.

DERMAL SINUSES

The dermal sinus tract represents an abnormal communication between the dermis and the intracranial structures. Although it is conceivable that the tract may

halt its migration in any tissue plane superficial to the intradural compartment, the surgeon must accept that the lesion can proceed to the underlying arachnoid and brain, with the potential hazards that this process creates.

Sinus tracts that enter the anterior portion of the skull are often occult and infrequently are a source of infection.[20] Instead, they present as a cosmetic blemish. The intradural extension of the sinus is interesting but usually not dramatic as it terminates on midline anterior fossa dura or within the leaves of the falx.[21] By contrast, the posterior fossa dermal sinus is capable of inciting purulent meningitis or empyema, or it may declare itself as a mass within the posterior fossa (the midline dermoid cyst). The investigations and treatments for these lesions of the skull have to be individualized according to their location.

PATHOLOGY

If an epithelial defect occurs during separation of the neuroectoderm from the surface ectoderm between the third and fifth week of fetal life, such a defect may extend to any depth through the layers of the skin down to neural tissue.[6] Chronologically this phenomenon is most likely to occur between the third and fifth weeks of intrauterine life; defects in the posterior fossa are likely to be produced by a failure of the anterior neuropore to close toward the end of the fourth gestational week. The midline placement is determined by the interrelationship of mesodermal and neuroectodermal structures during their migration and ultimate midline closure.[5] In reality, the sinus tract can run through tissues from the bony nasal bridge to the sacrum, although it is uncommon to find one between the glabella and inion.

The sinus may be constructed as a single, fine tubular structure lined by hair-bearing epithelium, or it may be forked with side passages that end blindly. Any degree of local inflammatory response is an added feature, and the sinus may terminate as an expansion into either an epidermoid or dermoid cyst, which contains its characteristic contents. If infection has occurred, the arachnoid barrier and the cyst margin are enveloped in a reactive inflammatory scar.

CLINICAL FEATURES

The features typical of a dermal sinus of the skull range from the innocuous-appearing cutaneous cosmetic blemish to those that herald an intracranial infectious process or tumor.

Cosmetic Blemish. Usually a midline phenomenon, the tiny dermal pit may be situated at the nasion, or just off the midline near the inner canthus of one eye, or posteriorly in the midline scalp just above the hairline. The dermal sinus at the nasion is characterized by a tiny dimple from which a fine black hair frequently issues, and the lesion may be reported to become intermittently and superficially infected. A white pultaceous discharge is occasionally noted. The sinus located in the posterior scalp may not be discovered until the imaging studies have suggested its presence and the hair is shaved. Again the dermal pit is noted, and it is often surrounded by a hemangioma flare. On rare occasions the sinus may be located laterally in the region of the pterion and in turn be associated with intradural extensions to the temporal lobe.

Hypertelorism. In some instances the investigation or correction of an older child's orbital hypertelorism demonstrates that as a part of the midline abnormality there is an intrafalcine dermoid cyst, or a fine dermal stalk is found extending through the foramen cecum.[21] The unanticipated appearance of the intradural dermal sinus at operation need not deter the completion of the craniofacial procedure.

Meningismus. The cranial sinus tract, like those of the spine, is capable of inciting either a purulent or an aseptic meningitic reaction. Bacterial infection most commonly occurs from *Staphylococcus aureus*.[22] If the intradural cyst leaks, an aseptic reaction may be encountered, but it will be difficult, based on clinical characteristics, to distinguish it from bacterial infection.

Posterior Fossa Mass. The intradural dermoid cyst may produce symptoms typical for a posterior fossa tumor. Modern neuro-imaging usually suggests the preoperative diagnosis; indeed, a routine Towne skull radiograph frequently demonstrates the bony defect through which the sinus stalk passes. Failing that, the diagnosis becomes apparent after the subocciput is shaved and the characteristic sinus opening is noted.

RADIOGRAPHY

It is unlikely that the anterior sinus tract will be detected by plain skull radiography, but those in the sub-occiput will be detailed as noted above. Axial views of the CT scan may show the sinus penetrating various tissue layers as well as the dermoid or epidermoid cyst associated with it. The latter are hypodense lesions owing to the cholesterol and keratin of their epithelial cells, and they have well-defined hyperdense margins with a slight postcontrast peripheral enhancement.[22] MRI may not be as specific with regard to bone penetration by the stalk. The cyst on this study may appear lobulated and have slightly inhomogeneous signal and indistinct margins.[23]

TREATMENT

The principle that governs treatment of any dermal sinus of the cranium or spine dictates that the lesion be excised before it becomes infected. To take on this task after infection has occurred creates a difficult situation for the patient and surgeon, and the operative result is usually less than optimum.[6]

The nasal dermal sinus can be excised as a staged procedure with a plastic surgeon. If there is little radiologic evidence that the sinus penetrates the midline skull base, the plastic surgeon can excise the sinus portion in skin and intranasal structures. If it happens that the stalk extends through bone, the intranasal stump is marked with a tiny hemostatic clip, and the neurosurgeon, after an interval, can proceed with a routine midline anterior fossa exploration. The intradural compartment and olfactory structures are examined first; the lesion, if it has reached that far, usually lies within a 2-cm radius of the foramen cecum. Afterward, the extradural space is searched.

If details of the anterior dermal sinus and/or cyst are noted on the preoperative imaging of a child with orbital hypertelorism, the neurosurgeon at the craniofacial procedure must first disengage the intra- and extra-

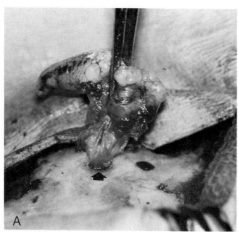
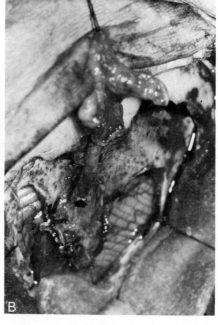

FIGURE 5–6. *A,* Posterior fossa dermoid cyst. The forceps grasp the excised ellipse of skin, and the stalk is traced to its entry through the skull defect *(arrow)*. *B,* The stalk is pursued to its entry through dura *(arrow),* which is partially opened.

dural components of the lesion before the craniofacial surgeon places the para-cribriform bony cuts and manipulates the nasal and orbital structures.

The dermal lesion of the posterior cranial fossa must be approached with all the preparations for a formal intradural exploration and "tumor" removal. Wide suboccipital scalp preparation and bony exposure are required. The cutaneous stalk is excised circumferentially and the integrity of the stalk preserved so that it can be traced as it passes through bone. A generous suboccipital craniectomy is necessary, and the bone removal proceeds centripetal to the stalk. When the dura is exposed, the surgeon can determine the relationship of the stalk to the torcular Herophili and the occipital sinus. Not uncommonly, the stalk that passes in a caudal direction as it penetrates deeper tissues will enter the midline dura by splitting the occipital sinus. In any event, the sinus can be obliterated as necessary to excise the stalk, although the latter should continue its passage through arachnoid and into the underlying cyst (Fig. 5–6A and B). All of this anatomic verification is much easier if there has not been a prior bout of complicating meningitis. The terminating dermoid tumor, if it exists, is usually nestled on the vermis or between the cerebellar tonsils and is easily circumscribed and dissected free. Should its contents spill during removal, the operative field can be irrigated with a long-lasting steroid compound, and dexamethasone should be administered intravenously.

The results of treatment of cranial dermal sinuses are determined by their location and the timing of treatment. One should not be satisfied with only an excision of the superficial stalk if it is known that intracranial extension exists. One's ability to remove the entire intradural component is greatly enhanced if the lesion is operated upon before any part of it has become infected. Having achieved total excision, the surgeon can expect the patient to be cured.

REFERENCES

1. Naidich TP, Altman NR, Braffman BH, McLone DG, Zimmerman RA: Cephaloceles and related malformations. AJNR 13:655, 1992.
2. Myrianthopoulos NC: Congenital malformations of the brain and skull. In Vinken PJ, Bruyn GW (eds): Handbook of Clinical Neurology. Vol. 30. Amsterdam, North-Holland Publishing Company, 1977, pp 139–171.
3. Lorber J: Prognosis of occipital encephalocele. Dev Med Child Neurol 9:75, 1967.
4. Davis CH, Alexander E, Jr.: Congenital nasofrontal encephalomeningoceles and teratomas. J Neurosurg 16:365, 1959.
5. James HE: Encephalocele, dermoid sinus and arachnoid cyst. In McLaurin RL, et al. (eds): Pediatric Neurosurgery: Surgery of the Developing Nervous System. Section of Pediatric Neurosurgery of the American Association of Neurological Surgeons. 2nd ed. Philadelphia, WB Saunders Co., 1989, pp 97–103.
6. Matson DD: Neurosurgery of Infancy and Childhood. 2nd ed. Springfield, Ill., Charles C Thomas, 1969, pp 61–75, 96–99.
7. Simpson DA, David DJ, White J: Cephaloceles: Treatment, outcome and antenatal diagnosis. Neurosurgery, 15:14, 1984.
8. Suwanwela C, Hongsaprabhas C: Fronto-ethmoidal encephalomeningocele. J Neurosurg 25:172, 1966.
9. Nager GT: Cephalocele. Laryngoscope, 97:77, 1987.
10. Yokota A, Kagiwara H, Kohchi M, et al.: Parietal cephalocele: Clinical importance of its atretic form and associated malformations. J Neurosurg 69:545, 1988.
11. Chapman PH, Swearingen B, Caviness VS: Subtorcular occipital encephaloceles, anatomical considerations relevant to operative management. J Neurosurg 71:375, 1989.
12. Von Recklinghausen G: Untersuchungen uber die Spina bifida. Part 2 (Uber die Art undie Entstenhun der spina bifida, ihre Beziehung zur Ruckenmarks und Darmspalte). Virchows Arch (A) 105:296, 1886.
13. Yokota A, Matsukado Y, Fuma I, et al.: Anterior basal encephalocele of the neonatal and infantile period. Neurosurgery 19:468, 1986.
14. Blackwood W, Corsellis JAN (eds): Greenfield's Neuropathology. 3rd ed. London, Arnold Publication, 1976, pp 377–380.
15. Weinstein P, Weinstein L, Dotters D, et al.: Prenatal diagnosis of occipital encephalocele by ultrasound scanning. Neurosurgery 12:680, 1983.
16. Guthkelch AN: Occipital cranium bifidum. Arch Dis Child 45:104, 1970.
17. Hoffman HJ: Editorial comment. Cephaloceles: Treatment, outcome, and antenatal diagnosis. Neurosurgery 15:21, 1984.
18. Emery JL, Kalhan SC: The pathology of exencephalus. Dev Med Child Neurol 22(Supp):51, 1970.
19. Mealey J, Jr., Dzenitis AJ, Hockey AA: The prognosis of encephaloceles. J Neurosurg 32:209, 1970.
20. McQuown SA, Smith JD, Gallo AE, Jr.: Intracranial extension of nasal dermoids. Neurosurgery 12:531, 1983.
21. Okuka Y, Oi S: Nasal dermal sinus and dermoid cyst with intrafalcial extension. Case report and review of the literature. Childs Nerv Syst 3:40, 1987.
22. Schijman E, Monges J, Cragnaz R: Congenital dermal sinuses, dermoid and epidermoid cysts of the posterior fossa. Childs Nerv Syst 2:83, 1986.
23. Flodmark O: Neuroradiology of selected disorders of the meninges, calvarium and venous sinuses. AJNR 13:483, 1992.

Chapter 6

ARACHNOID CYSTS

COREY RAFFEL, M.D., Ph.D., and J. GORDON McCOMB, M.D.

Primary or true arachnoid cysts are membrane-delimited collections of fluid that contain clear, colorless fluid indistinguishable from cerebrospinal fluid (CSF). The membrane consists of arachnoid cells and collagen fibers[1-3] and contains neither glia nor ependyma. The cyst wall is continuous with the surrounding normal arachnoid.[4] Secondary arachnoid cysts, occurring as a result of trauma, operation, or hemorrhage, will be discussed separately from congenital cysts in this chapter.

CONGENITAL ARACHNOID CYSTS

INCIDENCE

Arachnoid cysts account for about 1 per cent of intracranial space-occupying lesions and occur in about 0.5 per cent of autopsies as an incidental finding.[5, 6] The lesions are congenital, as evidenced by their predominant presentation in the first two decades of life.[7-12] The occurrence of cysts is rarely hereditary,[13] and more than one cyst occurs in the same patient in fewer than 10 per cent of cases.[13, 14] A recent report suggests that middle fossa cysts are more common in boys than in girls and occur more frequently on the left side.[15]

PATHOGENESIS

As the neural tube develops, it is surrounded by loose primitive mesenchyme. The outer compact layer of this mesenchyme develops into the dura mater and arachnoid; the loose inner layer develops into the pia. These two layers are separated by an extracellular ground substance. During the early development of the brain and ventricles, there is no CSF in the subarachnoid space. By 15 weeks of gestation, fluid can be detected in the subarachnoid space.[16] The normal subarachnoid space, present by birth, is formed as fluid replaces the loose extracellular ground substance of the endomeninx.[17] Arachnoid cysts most probably arise by anomalous splitting and duplication of the endomeninx during this critical period. Interestingly, arachnoid cysts are most frequently situated in the locations of normal arachnoid cisterns, indicating that the error in arachnoid splitting may occur most commonly during cistern formation.[2]

The mechanism by which arachnoid cysts enlarge is not known. The fluid inside the cyst has all of the characteristics of CSF. A minimally higher sodium or protein content would produce an osmotic gradient that could cause the cyst to expand, although such has never been shown. Arterial pulsations that force entry of fluid into the cyst via a flap valve mechanism that prevents subsequent fluid egress is another possible mechanism of cyst growth.[18] Fluid may be secreted directly into the cyst by the arachnoidal cells making up its wall. These cells have been shown to contain all of the organelles and enzymes of a secretory cell.[19, 20]

LOCATION

Two thirds of arachnoid cysts are supratentorial and one third are infratentorial.[12] Sylvian cistern/middle fossa cysts are the most common, accounting for about half of all cysts and three quarters of the supratentorial lesions (Fig. 6–1). Other supratentorial locations include suprasellar, interhemispheric, intraventricular, and over the cerebral convexities (Fig. 6–2). Infratentorial cysts are divided fairly evenly between lesions in the cerebellopontine angle, posterior to the vermis, and superior to the quadrigeminal plate (Fig. 6–3). Occasionally, arachnoid cysts occur anterior to the brainstem along the clivus.

Intracranial arachnoid cysts are rarely extradural in location. Case reports exist describing extradural cysts that have eroded the inner table of the skull and expanded the diploë.[21, 22] Extradural and intradiploic cysts always have a connection with the normal subarachnoid space through a small dural defect.[22]

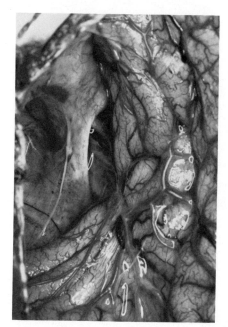

FIGURE 6–1. Intraoperative photograph of a sylvian fissure/middle fossa arachnoid cyst. This 12-year-old girl presented with seizures. The displacement of the temporal lobe and opening of the sylvian fissure is obvious. Medial to the free edge of the tentorium, the optic nerve and carotid artery are visible, and the third nerve is hidden by thickened arachnoid. Multiple wide openings were made into the basal cisterns after removing the arachnoid not adherent to the hemisphere. Postoperatively the patient has had no further seizure activity, and follow-up CT scans have shown progressive reduction in the size of the cyst.

SYMPTOMS AND SIGNS

Arachnoid cysts give rise to symptoms by compressing adjacent neural structures, increasing intracranial pressure by their own mass effect, and by obstructing CSF flow and causing hydrocephalus[7, 8, 23, 24] (Fig. 6–4).

The most common signs and symptoms relate to increased intracranial pressure, e.g., an abnormally enlarging head circumference and a full fontanelle in infants (Fig. 6–5) and headache, vomiting, and papilledema in older children. Symptoms and signs of neural compression include seizures, developmental delay, ataxia, cranial nerve palsies, nystagmus, and decreased visual acuity.

Children with suprasellar arachnoid cysts may present with a peculiar to-and-fro nodding of the head. This sign has been named the "bobble-headed doll syndrome"[25] and occurs in less than one in five children with cysts in this location.[26]

Sylvian cistern/middle fossa arachnoid cysts may present with acute intracranial hemorrhage following minor or no noted antecedent head trauma[7, 9, 18, 27–34] (Fig. 6–6). These hemorrhages are thought to result from the rupture of veins stretched by the cyst as they pass from the temporal lobe to the dural sinuses. The incidence of this presentation is difficult to determine. For this reason, arachnoid cyst should be considered in the differential diagnosis of any patient with an acute subdural hematoma after minor or no antecedent head trauma, especially if the patient is less than 20 years of age.[34] Expansion of the middle fossa on imaging studies may provide a clue that a pre-existing arachnoid cyst is present.

In the modern imaging era, arachnoid cysts are being discovered incidentally on computed tomography (CT) and magnetic resonance imaging (MRI) scans in patients who are totally asymptomatic from their cysts. Because these lesions are discovered in 0.5 per cent of autopsies, a large number of clinically silent cysts must exist. These asymptomatic patients require no treatment unless follow-up images show progressive enlargement of the cyst or symptoms develop. Asymptomatic patients well into the second decade of life rarely come to operation.

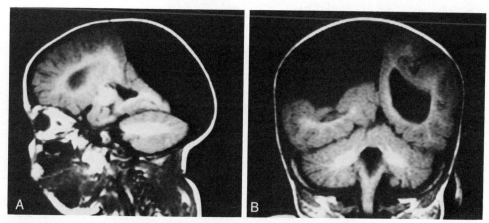

FIGURE 6–2. *A* and *B*, MRI study showing the presence of a convexity arachnoid cyst. This 8-month-old infant had an MRI study as part of a work-up for multiple congenital anomalies and developmental delay. At the time of surgery, it was noted that the cyst communicated with the right lateral ventricle. Histopathologic examination of the tissue removed revealed only arachnoid to be present. In addition to fenestration of the cyst, a choroid plexectomy was done. The CSF circulation remained normal. The patient's milestones continue to be severely delayed. Fenestration of the arachnoid cyst does not appear to have improved this patient's neurologic function, although the mass effect from the arachnoid cyst diminished.

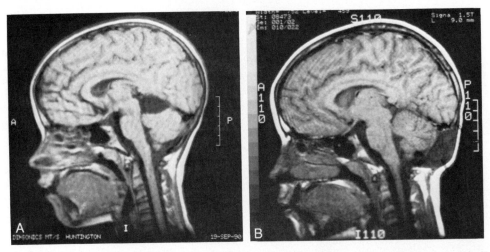

FIGURE 6–3. *A*, MRI study showing the presence of an arachnoid cyst compressing the superior cerebellar vermis and the quadrigeminal plate. This 9-year-old boy presented with an abnormal movement disorder that was thought to be a tic in nature and possibly even a component of Tourette's syndrome. Hydrocephalus was not a factor. *B*, MRI study approximately 1 year after fenestration of the cyst. The patient's abnormal movement disorder completely resolved. Neurologic examination was always normal.

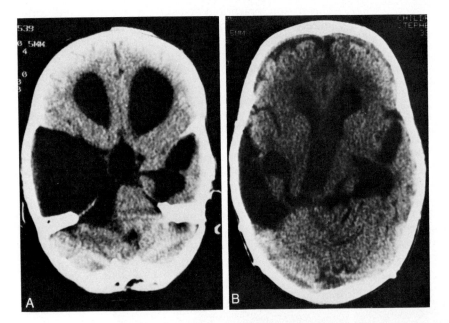

FIGURE 6–4. *A*, CT scan of a 21-month-old infant who presented with an abnormally large head showing the presence of a huge middle fossa arachnoid cyst and massive hydrocephalus. At the same operative procedure, the patient underwent fenestration of the arachnoid cyst and insertion of a ventriculoperitoneal shunt. Significant bilateral subdural fluid accumulation subsequently developed and was treated by placement of a separate subdural-peritoneal shunt. *B*, Follow-up CT scan 4 months later. Note the significant reduction in size of the arachnoid cyst and ventricles and elimination of the subdural fluid accumulation. With time, the patient's head circumference approached the 98th percentile as the cranial vault–brain disproportion lessened. This patient's development appears nearly normal at 6 years of age.

FIGURE 6–5. *A*, MRI study showing a posterior fossa arachnoid cyst and hydrocephalus. This patient was noted to have an abnormally increasing head circumference at 5 months of age. After having had a CT scan elsewhere, the patient was referred with a diagnosis of Dandy-Walker malformation. As the CT appearance was not typical of a Dandy-Walker malformation, an MRI study was done and confirmed the presence of a posterior fossa arachnoid cyst along with marked hydrocephalus. *B*, To control the hydrocephalus, a ventriculoperitoneal shunt was placed. Contrast introduced in the ventricles via the shunt did not communicate with the posterior fossa arachnoid cyst. Two weeks after shunt placement, the patient underwent fenestration of the arachnoid cyst. One month later, a proximal revision of the shunt was required. There has been no subsequent shunt malfunction in the past 3 years. The ventricles and cyst size are markedly reduced on follow-up imaging studies. At 3½ years of age, the patient's developmental milestones are normal.

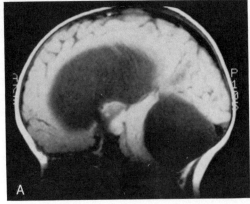

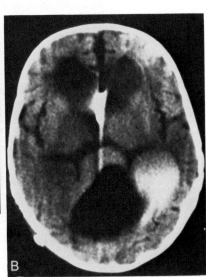

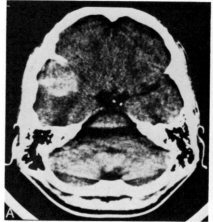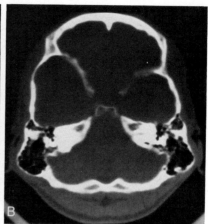

FIGURE 6–6. *A,* MRI study showing the presence of hemorrhage into a right middle fossa arachnoid cyst. A 13-year-old boy presented with headaches and a seizure. *B,* Bone windows show the asymmetry in the temporal regions. This patient underwent fenestration of the arachnoid cyst. The patient has had no subsequent seizure episodes. Follow-up CT studies showed progressive decrease in the amount of temporal lobe displacement.

IMAGING STUDIES

MRI scanning is the imaging modality of choice for visualizing arachnoid cysts.[35] The cyst is seen as a collection of fluid with the signal characteristics of CSF that compresses and displaces normal brain structures.[35] The signal characteristics of the fluid eliminate the differential possibility of a tumor-associated cyst or chronic hematoma cavity.[36] Arachnoid cysts are also seen well on CT scans, but the differential diagnoses of tumor and chronic hematoma are more difficult to exclude.

Arachnoid cysts differ in shape, depending on the location of the cyst.[25] Sylvian cistern/middle fossa cysts occupy the anterior middle fossa, displacing the temporal lobe posteriorly. When large, they splay open the sylvian fissure and are trapezoidal in shape with straight edges present where they abut the insula.[37] The middle fossa bony margins are expanded by the cyst. Large veins may be seen traversing the wall of the cyst on contrast-enhanced studies.

Suprasellar arachnoid cysts expand in all directions.[38] The cyst may bulge into and enlarge the sella turcica. The optic nerves and chiasm may be stretched over the anterior margin of the cyst. Large cysts expand upward, invaginating the floor of the third ventricle, and may obstruct both foramina of Munro, leading to hydrocephalus. In this case, a characteristic "Mickey Mouse" appearance of the cyst will be seen on axial images.

Symptomatic posterior fossa arachnoid cysts are large when diagnosed, two thirds having diameters greater than 5 cm.[5, 39] These cysts assume shapes according to the surrounding structures and thus are rarely round and can be lobulated.

TREATMENT

Arachnoid cysts may be treated either by fenestration of the cyst into the surrounding normal CSF spaces or by shunting the cyst to the peritoneal or pleural cavity. Both methods of treatment have their advocates and no consensus exists. In fact, authors of papers advocating shunting have been criticized by their reviewers for not fenestrating[40, 41] and vice versa.[42, 43] The advantage of shunting has been stated to be a smaller operation with fewer complications.[28, 44–47] However, shunting also has the major disadvantage of possible subsequent shunt complications, which have been reported to occur in up to 40 per cent of shunted cases.[17, 41, 46, 48, 49]

Successful fenestration renders a shunt unnecessary and solves the problem with a single operation. Although the procedure requires a craniotomy, complications are infrequent.[11, 14, 50] Unfortunately, fenestration is not always successful, and patients with recurrent accumulation of CSF at the cyst site require a subsequent shunt. Successful fenestration rates have varied from about three quarters to all cases in papers advocating fenestration.[9, 10, 14] Interestingly, the success rate for fenestration in papers advocating shunting is relatively low.[48] Initial successful fenestration of the cyst requires careful and fastidious removal of all cyst wall that is not adherent to adjacent neural structures and wide opening of any remaining cyst wall into all accessible, adjacent cisterns. Thus the success rate may reflect the extent of the fenestration. Those arachnoid cysts with recent or remote evidence of hemorrhage are more likely to require shunting after fenestration.

A particularly difficult problem is presented by patients with hydrocephalus and an arachnoid cyst. Data from the Children's Hospital of Los Angeles indicate that more than one half of patients with this condition will require a shunt when initially treated with fenestration.[14] In some, the fenestration is unsuccessful, and in others, the cyst decreases in size, but the hydrocephalus does not resolve.[6, 51, 52] For this reason, serious consideration should be given to simultaneous placement of a shunt catheter into the cyst and the ventricles,[44] or to shunting the ventricles as well as fenestrating the cyst. Stereotaxic, ultrasonographic, or ventriculoscopic guidance may be helpful when one is attempting to place a catheter into deeply located arachnoid cysts.

INTRASPINAL ARACHNOID CYSTS

Arachnoid cysts may also occur in the spinal canal. Just as with the intracranial lesions, intraspinal cysts

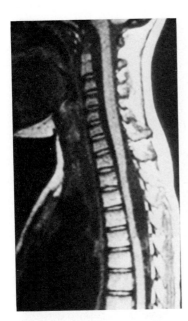

FIGURE 6–7. MRI study demonstrating an arachnoid cyst compressing the thoracic spinal cord. This patient's presenting symptoms were recurrent urinary tract infections and progressive constipation. The neurologic examination was normal. The child's symptoms resolved following fenestration of the arachnoid cyst. (From Rabb CH, McComb JG, Raffel C, Kennedy JG: Spinal arachnoid cysts in the pediatric age group: An association with neural tube defects. J Neurosurg 77:369, 1992.)

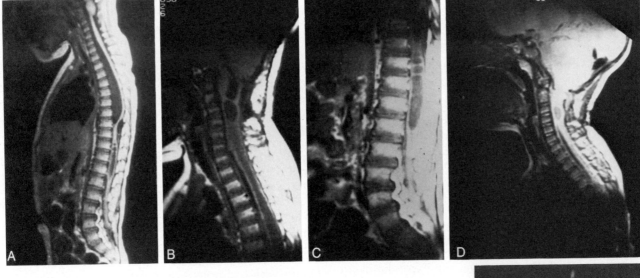

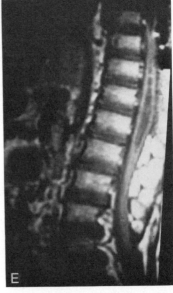

FIGURE 6–8. *A,* MRI study demonstrating a Chiari II malformation, anterior cervicothoracic arachnoid cyst, hydrosyringomyelia, and a low-lying tethered spinal cord in a 3-year-old child with a repaired myelomeningocele and shunted hydrocephalus. The patient had experienced multiple episodes of intermittent quadriparesis at the time of shunt malfunctions. The shunt was functioning normally when the child was first admitted. The initial treatment was a posterior fossa decompression and upper cervical laminectomy with no improvement on follow-up MRI studies or change in clinical status. The patient underwent a multilevel thoracic laminectomy with myelotomy of the spinal cord in the area of the syrinx and placement of the proximal end of a cyst-to-pleural space shunt through the spinal cord into the area of the arachnoid cyst. *B* and *C,* Follow-up MRI studies approximately 6 months after the operative procedure showing significant expansion of the hydrosyringomyelia. The patient's shunt was checked and found to be functioning normally. As the patient's neurologic condition had actually improved, nothing further was done. *D* and *E,* Follow-up MRI studies obtained approximately 1 year following the laminectomy and the placement of a cyst-pleural shunt. The anterior arachnoid cyst is collapsed. The hydrosyringomyelia has significantly diminished. The patient experienced a shunt malfunction at this point without suffering quadriparesis. (*A, D,* and *E* from Rabb CH, McComb JG, Raffel C, Kennedy JG: Spinal arachnoid cysts in the pediatric age group: An association with neural tube defects. J Neurosurg 77:369, 1992.)

may enlarge slowly over time and cause compression of the neural elements in the spinal canal (Fig. 6–7). Intraspinal arachnoid cysts can be either intradural or extradural in location; in children they occur with about equal frequency in each of these locations, as reported in older literature.[53] Intradural cysts are thought to have a pathogenesis similar to that of intracranial cysts, whereas extradural cysts arise from a dural defect that allows the arachnoid membrane to herniate through the dura into the extradural space. In addition, an association with congenital neural tube defects has been reported[53] (Fig. 6–8). This suggests that some of these lesions may be acquired, having developed as a result of abnormal CSF flow patterns and from the extensive arachnoidal adhesions that occur in many of these patients. There are, however, no reports of spinal arachnoid cysts following subarachnoid hemorrhage or meningitis, conditions expected to cause arachnoid scarring.

Just as with the intracranial cysts, spinal lesions are best visualized by MRI scanning. Intradural cysts appear as a widening of the subarachnoid space with compression of the spinal cord or nerve roots. Extradural cysts also have the signal characteristics of CSF

and compress the thecal sac or erode the surrounding bone from its extradural location.

The treatment of arachnoid cysts causing compression of the intraspinal neural structures is surgical. In most cases, the cyst is posterior to the neural elements and easily treated with fenestration via laminectomy. The cyst wall should be excised; a portion of the wall is frequently adherent to the spinal cord and can be safely left behind. For the rare anterior cysts, fenestration and partial wall removal should be attempted. If this procedure is not possible, the cyst can be shunted to the adjacent subarachnoid space or to the peritoneal/pleural cavity.

ACQUIRED OR SECONDARY ARACHNOID CYSTS

Rarely, CSF-filled cysts may appear after hemorrhage, trauma, or operation[5, 55] (Fig. 6–9). These CSF loculations are not limited by arachnoid cysts, but rather by a membrane containing collagen and hemosiderin. These cysts are differentiated from congenital arachnoid cysts only by their treatment. Because scar-

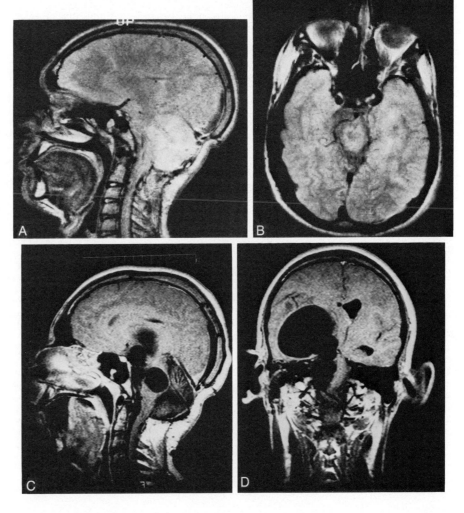

FIGURE 6–9. A and B, MRI study of a 17-year-old boy who, 10 years previously, had experienced an acute hemorrhage into the posterior fossa from an AVM of the cerebellum and brainstem. The patient has had several re-bleeding episodes from the residual inoperable segment of the AVM diffusely infiltrating the brainstem even after removal of all the subarachnoid portion of the malformation, and that extending into the cerebellum. A ventriculoperitoneal shunt was needed to treat impairment of CSF circulation. C and D, MRI study 5 years later demonstrating a huge acquired posterior fossa arachnoid cyst compressing the brainstem and herniating through the incisura to displace the temporal lobe. The patient had experienced a severe progressive neurologic impairment as a result of the cyst. The cyst was shunted, with some improvement in the patient's neurologic condition.

ring in the subarachnoid space is involved in the formation of these cysts, fenestration is much less successful, and shunting usually should be the initial treatment.

REFERENCES

1. Rengachary SS: Parasagittal arachnoid cyst: Case report. Neurosurgery 9:70, 1981.
2. Rengachary SS, Watanabe I: Ultrastructure and pathogenesis of intracranial arachnoid cysts. J Neuropathol Exp Neurol 40:61, 1981.
3. Rengachary SS, Watanabe I, Brackett CE: Pathogenesis of intracranial arachnoid cysts. Surg Neurol 9:139, 1978.
4. Schachenmayr W, Friede RL: Fine structure of arachnoid cysts. J Neuropathol Exp Neurol 38:434, 1979.
5. Matsuda M, Hirai O, Munemitsu H, et al.: Arachnoid cysts—report of two adult cases in the interhemispheric fissure and over the cerebral convexity. Neurol Med Chir, Tokyo 22:71, 1982.
6. Meche EGA van der, Braakman R: Arachnoid cysts in the middle cranial fossa: Cause and treatment of progressive and nonprogressive symptoms. J Neurol Neurosurg Psychiatry 46:1102, 1983.
7. Anderson FM, Segall HD, Caton WL: Use of computerized tomography scanning in supratentorial arachnoid cysts: A report on 20 children and four adults. J Neurosurg 50:333, 1979.
8. Bhandari YS: Non-communicating supratentorial subarachnoid cysts. J Neurol Neurosurg Psychiatry 35:763, 1972.
9. Gallassi E, Piazza G, Gaist G, Frank F: Arachnoid cysts of the middle cranial fossa: A clinical and radiological study of 25 cases treated surgically. Surg Neurol 14:211, 1980.
10. Hayashi T, Anegawa S, Honda E, et al.: Clinical analysis of arachnoid cysts in the middle fossa. Neurochirurgia (Stuttg) 22:201, 1979.
11. Menezes AH, Bell WE, Perret GE: Arachnoid cysts in children. Arch Neurol 37:168, 1980.
12. Robinson RG: Congenital cysts of the brain: Arachnoid malformations. Prog Neurol Surg 4:122, 1971.
13. Handa J, Okomato K, Sato M: Arachnoid cyst of the middle cranial fossa: Report of bilateral cysts in siblings. Surg Neurol 16:127, 1981.
14. Raffel C, McComb JG: To shunt or to fenestrate: Which is the best surgical treatment for arachnoid cysts in pediatric patients? Neurosurgery 23:338, 1988.
15. Webster K: Gender distribution and sidedness of middle fossa arachnoid cysts. A review of cases diagnosed with computerized imaging. Neurosurgery 31:940, 1992.
16. Pilu G, DePalma L, Romero R, et al.: The fetal subarachnoid cisterns: An ultrasound study with report of a case of congenital communicating hydrocephalus. J Ultrasound Med 5:365, 1986.
17. McLone DG: The subarachnoid space: A review. Childs Brain 6:113, 1980.
18. Smith RA, Smith WA: Arachnoid cysts of the middle cranial fossa. Surg Neurol 5:246, 1976.
19. Go KG, Houthoff HJ, Blaauw EH, et al.: Arachnoid cysts of the sylvian fissure: Evidence of fluid secretion. J Neurosurg 60:803, 1984.
20. Go KG, Houthoff HJ, Blaauw EH, et al.: Morphology and origin of arachnoid cysts: Scanning and transmission electron microscopy of three cases. Acta Neuropathol (Berl) 44:57, 1978.
21. Hande AM, Karapurkar AP: Hemorrhage into an intradiploic arachnoid cyst. J Neurosurg 75:969, 1991.
22. Weinand ME, Rengachary SS, McGregor DH, et al.: Intradiploic arachnoid cysts. J Neurosurg 70:954, 1989.
23. Plana JC, Clara JMC, Fernandez-Alvarez E: Quistes aracnoideos intracraneales en el nino: Revision de 34 observaciones. An Esp Pediatr 19:459, 1983.
24. Raimondi AJ, Simoji T, Gutierrez FA: Suprasellar cysts: Surgical treatment and results. Childs Brain 7:57, 1980.
25. Benton JW, Nellhaus G, Huttenlocher PR, et al.: The bobble-head doll syndrome. Report of a unique truncal tremor associated with third ventricular cyst and hydrocephalus in children. Neurology 16:725, 1966.
26. Pierre-Kahn A, Capelle L, Brauner R, et al.: Presentation and management of suprasellar arachnoid cysts. J Neurosurg 73:355, 1990.
27. Aicardi J, Bauman F: Supratentorial extracerebral cysts in infants and children. J Neurol Neurosurg Psychiatry 38:57, 1975.
28. Sprung C, Mauersberger W: Value of computed tomography for the diagnosis and assessment of surgical treatment. Acta Neurochir (Wien) 28(Suppl):619, 1979.
29. Auer LM, Gallhoper B, Ladurner G, et al.: Diagnosis and treatment of middle fossa arachnoid cysts and subdural hematomas. J Neurosurg 54:366, 1981.
30. Kadowaki H, Ide M, Takara E: A case of arachnoid cyst associated with chronic subdural hematoma. No Shinkei Geka 11:431, 1983.
31. Oliver LC: Primary arachnoid cysts. Br Med J 1:1147, 1958.
32. Robinson RG: The temporal lobe agenesis syndrome. Brain 87:87, 1964.
33. Varma TRK, Sedzimir CB, Miles JB: Post-traumatic complications of arachnoid cysts and temporal lobe agenesis. J Neurol Neurosurg Psychiatry 44:29, 1981.
34. Page AC, Mohan D, Paxton RM: Arachnoid cysts of the middle fossa predispose to subdural haematoma formation, fact or fiction? Acta Neurochir 42(Suppl):210, 1988.
35. Naidich TP, McLone DG, Radkowski MA: Intracranial arachnoid cysts. Pediatr Neurosci 12:112, 1985–1986.
36. Gandy SE, Heier LA: Clinical and magnetic resonance features of primary intracranial arachnoid cysts. Ann Neurol 21:342, 1987.
37. Banna M: Arachnoid cysts on computed tomography. Am J Roentgenol 127:979, 1976.
38. Krawchenko J, Collins GH: Pathology of an arachnoid cyst: Case report. J Neurosurg 50:224, 1979.
39. Little JR, Gomez MR, MacCarty CS: Infratentorial arachnoid cysts. J Neurosurg 39:380, 1973.
40. Hovind KH: Editorial comment. Childs Nerv Syst 3:124, 1987.
41. Locatelli D, Bonfanti N, Sfogliarini R, et al.: Arachnoid cysts: Diagnosis and treatment. Childs Nerv Syst 3:121, 1987.
42. Albright L: Treatment of bobble-head doll syndrome by transcallosal cystectomy. Neurosurgery 8:593, 1981.
43. Page LK: Comment. Neurosurgery 8:595, 1981.
44. Harsh GR IV, Edwards MSB, Wilson CB: Intracranial arachnoid cysts in children. J Neurosurg 64:835, 1986.
45. Kaplan BJ, Mickle JP, Parkhurst R: Cystoperitoneal shunting for congenital arachnoid cysts. Childs Brain 11:304, 1984.
46. Stein SC: Intracranial developmental cysts in children; Treatment by cystoperitoneal shunting. Neurosurgery 8:647, 1981.
47. Basauri L, Selman JM: Intracranial arachnoidal cysts. Childs Nerv Syst 8:101, 1992.
48. Ciricillo SF, Cogen PH, Harsh GR, et al.: Intracranial arachnoid cysts in children. J Neurosurg 74:230, 1991.
49. Pomeranz S, Wald U, Amir N, et al.: Arachnoid cysts: Unusual aspects and management. Neurochirurgia 31:25, 1988.
50. Little JR, Gomez MR, MacCarty CS: Infratentorial arachnoid cysts. J Neurosurg 39:380, 1973.
51. Hoffman HJ, Hendrick EB, Humphreys RP, et al.: Investigation and management of suprasellar arachnoid cysts. J Neurosurg 57:597, 1982.
52. Milhorat TH: Pediatric neurosurgery. Contemp Neurol Ser 16:192, 1978.
53. Rabb CH, McComb JG, Raffel C, Kennedy JG: Spinal arachnoid cysts in the pediatric age group: An association with neural tube defects. J Neurosurg 77:369, 1992.
54. Hyndman DR, Gerber WF: Spinal extradural cysts, congenital and acquired: Report of cases. J Neurosurg 3:474, 1946.
55. Schreiber F, Haddad B: Lumbar and sacral cysts causing pain. J Neurosurg 8:504, 1951.

Chapter 7

CRANIOSYNOSTOSIS

WILLIAM M. CHADDUCK, M.D.

Craniosynostosis, or premature closure of the cranial sutures, is a problem that is seen frequently in pediatric neurosurgical practice. The reported incidence of craniosynostosis varies but is conservatively estimated to be 0.4/1000.[1] Although most cases are sporadic, a familial incidence of 2 per cent in sagittal synostosis and 8 per cent in uncomplicated coronal synostosis has been reported.[2]

Cranial deformity occurs when one or more of the cranial sutures closes prematurely. Separation of the calvarial bones by the cranial sutures allows genetically determined shaping and progressive enlargement of the skull with growth of the brain. Measurements by Coppoleta and Wolbach indicate a 50 per cent increase in brain weight at age 2 months, 100 per cent at 6 months, and 200 per cent at 10 months.[3] This rapid brain growth is virtually complete at the end of the second year, and normally fusion of the sutures is completed by the age of 6 to 8 years. These data support the view that early correction of craniosynostosis is of great importance.[4, 5] When premature fusion of one or more sutures occurs, compensatory enlargement of the cranium must follow from the remaining open sutures, resulting in predictable patterns of skull deformity and, in some cases, compression of the underlying brain. Patterns of cranial deformity have long been recognized as the specific forms of craniosynostosis, named in reference to sutural involvement and the resulting head configuration. Sagittal synostosis (Fig. 7–1) results in scaphocephaly or dolichocephaly; coronal synostosis or lambdoid synostosis results in brachycephaly or plagiocephaly; metopic synostosis results in trigonocephaly. Less common forms—such as kleeblattschädel (or cloverleaf deformity as shown in Fig. 7–2), turribrachycephaly, acrocephaly, and oxycephaly—are all included in a spectrum of cranial deformities. Premature synostosis of the sagittal suture is the most common form, but coronal, unilateral or bilateral, lambdoidal, and metopic sutures are also frequently involved. Although Epstein once postulated that premature fusion of the sphenozygomatic suture could result in the deformities of plagiocephaly,[6] minor sutural involvement, such as squamosal, usually does not cause significant calvarial deformity. Reddy et al.[7] and others[8] have described the occurrence, though uncommon, of delayed multiple suture involvement following initial single suture disease. Although Gault and associates have shown that intracranial volume is often within normal limits in children with craniosynostosis,[9] increased intracranial pressure can occur in a variety of forms but is more common in multiple sutural and syndromal synostoses. Using epidural pressure monitors, Renier and St. Rose have reported an incidence of 33 per cent of obviously elevated intracranial pressure in patients with craniosynostosis,[10] its presence being least, 13 per cent, in those patients having the isolated sagittal variety. It is almost invariably present in cloverleaf deformities (kleeblattschädel). Lundar and Nornes have described a lumbar infusion test to delineate pathologic outflow resistance in some children,[11] indicating the need for decompressive surgery to ensure improved brain function as well as for cosmetic considerations.

In 1851, Virchow proposed that expansion of the skull in the face of premature sutural synostosis occurred perpendicular to the line of fusion.[12] Modern studies in rabbit models by Babler and associates,[13] as well as critical analyses of compensatory skull growth in patients with various forms of craniosynostosis by Delashaw and Persing,[14] indicate that the compensatory growth occurs primarily in sutures adjoining the one undergoing premature synostosis. Compensation results in growth only on the distal side of the involved suture, except in midline sutural synostosis, when the compensation occurs bilaterally. Studies by Persing et al. have also shown that experimentally induced calvarial suture synostosis can result in not only the cranial deformities but also deformities of the skull base and face.[15] These findings are in contrast to the theory of Moss,[16] who suggested that the primary abnormality occurs at the skull base, with transmission of forces through dural attachments resulting secondarily in synostosis. Studies of the subarachnoid spaces in patients

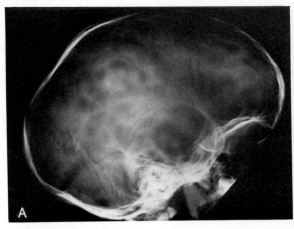

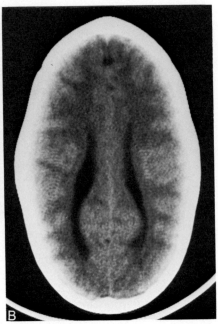

FIGURE 7–1. *A*, Lateral radiograph and *B*, CT scan of the head of a child with sagittal synostosis show the characteristic dolichocephaly.

with craniosynostosis in the first year of life have shown dilatations of the subarachnoid spaces beneath the areas of compensatory bone expansion, invoking a focal hydrodynamic factor in the progression of skull deformities.[17]

Although a number of mechanisms for early sutural fusion have been proposed, it is clear that multiple etiologies can be invoked. Metabolic conditions affecting bone formation, skull base abnormalities with transmission of forces by way of dural bands, intrauterine events and positioning, genetic determinants, positional molding, and syndromal conditions have all been shown to participate in the etiology of craniosynostosis.

Cohen has compiled extensive data on patients with craniosynostosis, carefully delineating the roles of genetics, associated anomalies and syndromes, metabolic disorders such as hyperthyroidism, hypercalcemia, and rickets, as well as mucopolysaccharide and hematologic disorders.[18] The roles of certain teratogens such as phenytoin, valproic acid, aminopterin, methotrexate, retinoic acid, and oxymetazoline have all been implicated. At least 50 syndromic conditions, including many with chromosomal abnormalities, have been reported in association with craniosynostosis. Knowledge of these conditions not only is important in understanding the heterogeneous etiologies of craniosynos-

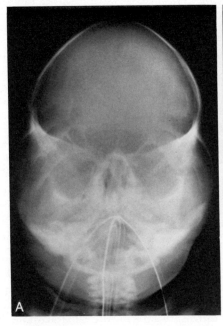

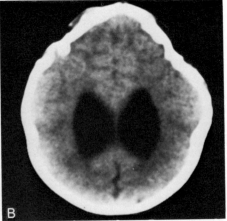

FIGURE 7–2. *A*, An anteroposterior radiograph of the skull shows the characteristic abnormalities of cloverleaf skull (kleeblattschädel). *B*, Axial view of the CT scan of a patient with cloverleaf skull shows shortened anteroposterior measurement, ventriculomegaly, and convolutional scalloping of the calvarium.

tosis but also is helpful in the preoperative evaluation of patients and the counseling of their families. Additional abnormalities associated with craniosynostosis are least common in the sagittal variety; however, underlying cerebral lesions can be found, including septooptic dysplasia, ventriculomegaly, and others.[19, 20] Well known are the syndromes associated with unilateral and bilateral coronal synostosis, such as Crouzon's disease and Apert's disease. In some of the syndromal synostoses, midface retrusion is common, altering the definitive surgical treatment. Associated orbital deformities occur with coronal and metopic synostoses, and hypertelorism or hypotelorism may occur with a number of forms of craniosynostosis. Thus, each form and variant of craniosynostosis may require individualized surgical treatment, depending upon the specific suture involved, multiplicity of sutures fused, age of the patient, and associated anomalies of orbital and facial structures.

CLINICAL ASSESSMENT

Recognition of the various skull deformities associated with craniosynostosis is apparent to the trained clinician. Ridges along the fused sutures can usually be palpated both by the physician and by the parents of the patient. With the widespread use of prenatal maternal ultrasonography, the diagnosis of craniosynostosis has been made and consultations arranged even prior to delivery of affected babies. Some argue that radiographic studies may be superfluous in patients having a classic presentation of craniosynostosis on physical examination. Nonetheless, the demonstration of a prematurely fused suture is helpful in establishing the diagnosis and can usually be appreciated on plain radiographs of the skull or CT scanning with bone windows. Skull radiographs may also show indentations of the inner table, suggesting raised intracranial pressure, and ventriculomegaly, if present, will be apparent on CT scanning. Utilization of CT scanning is helpful in ruling out underlying abnormalities of the brain, a reassuring finding when the study is normal, and useful information when abnormal in terms of surgical planning and family counseling. In view of the fact that in the majority of cases, surgical treatment is aimed at cosmetic improvement to prevent an appearance handicap, it is good to have the assurance, at least by imaging studies, of underlying normal brain anatomy. Moreover, it is imperative to know whether other conditions exist that may affect the long-term functional outcome for the patient. Imaging with three-dimensional reconstructions[21, 22] for some of the more complex craniofacial abnormalities greatly aids in surgical planning. In the past, increased activity at prematurely closing sutures, noted on isotope bone scans, has been considered helpful, especially in lambdoid synostosis.[23] Now, it is less commonly used in centers where surgical decisions regarding lambdoid deformities are based on the degree of cranial deformity, age of the patient, and response to nonsurgical treatments just as much as on the presence or absence of sutural fusion. The differentiation between microcephaly and multiple suture synostosis can readily be made by physical examination and neuroimaging studies, is not associated with raised intracranial pressure, and does not require surgical treatment (Fig. 7–3).

PATIENT AND FAMILY PREPARATION

Families should understand the primary reason for surgery for craniosynostosis. In single suture synostosis, cosmesis is, in reality, the only consideration. When brain compression and increased intracranial pressure are factors, especially in multiple suture synostoses, the need for surgery is imperative to preserve cerebral and visual function. Little evidence exists that seizures, mental retardation, and neurologic deficits are more common in the uncomplicated forms of craniosynostosis. If other abnormalities exist, however, especially in the syndromal conditions, they should be disclosed on an individual basis, especially with reference to whether synostosis surgery would be expected to alter the patient's neurologic outcome. Genetic counseling should be provided for the families of these patients.

The surgical mortality for treatment of craniosynostosis should be nil; therefore, the risk/benefit ratio justifies synostosis surgery for a cosmetic indication. For purposes of discussion, the role of surgery is to correct a congenital deformity, because of the common perception that cosmetic surgery per se is often unnecessary. The adverse psychological impact of allowing the child to compete in society with an appearance handicap is worthy of emphasis in family discussions.[24] Other than the expected morbidity of an extensive cranial procedure, complications should be few, but certain risks and expectations should be discussed thoroughly with the family. The proposed cosmetic result should be realistically described; the occasional need for secondary operations should be discussed, especially in the more complex forms of craniosynostosis, and the family should be made aware that they will notice minor cranial irregularities occurring during the healing process and bone reformation. Persistent defects may occur in as many as 5 per cent of patients, and some may require up to 2 years to close.[25]

In the postoperative period, expectations such as periorbital swelling, subgaleal blood collections, lowgrade fever, and general irritability of the child should be discussed with the family, making these consequences more acceptable to them after surgery. Infectious complications are uncommon but occur with a frequency requiring that this potential complication be disclosed. Antibiotic prophylaxis can be justified on the basis of wounds containing residual blood, free bone grafts, large dead spaces, and sometimes synthetic materials. When a subgaleal drain is used, the family should be prepared for its presence in the postoperative period. With more extensive procedures, blood trans-

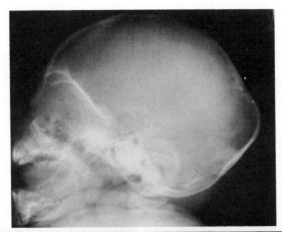

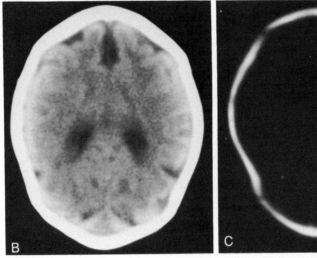

FIGURE 7–3. The features of microcephaly are shown by the characteristic appearance of *A,* the lateral radiograph, *B,* a CT scan showing no evidence of cerebral compression, and *C,* a CT scan with bone windows demonstrating the cranial sutures to be open.

fusion is almost inevitable to cover not only intraoperative blood loss but also the anticipated accumulation of blood beneath the scalp following surgery. However, rarely is more than a single unit of blood necessary. Because families are now aware of the risk of blood transfusion, especially acquired immunodeficiency syndrome (AIDS) transmission,[26] individual family members may wish to donor-direct blood for their child. It is important that a discussion of the local blood bank precautions and risks of disease transmission be provided to the child's family, and donor-directed blood should be encouraged. Postoperatively, careful attention to positioning of the child is necessary. The child having extensive craniectomies is vulnerable to positional molding of the skull until refusion occurs. Protective helmets and, occasionally, orthotic devices to maintain vertex compression[27] will enhance the surgical outcome. These can be applied as soon as postoperative swelling and discomfort have diminished.

TECHNICAL CONSIDERATIONS

POSITIONING OF THE PATIENT

Proper positioning for extensive exposure of the calvarium is most important in the surgery of craniosyn-

ostosis. If only frontal exposure is needed, the child can be positioned supine with moderate head flexion in a horseshoe head-holder without skull pins. When a sagittal strip craniectomy is anticipated, especially in young children with only minimal compensatory changes, the child's head may be positioned laterally with the vertex extending slightly beyond the head of the operating table. This allows adequate exposure of the sagittal suture by a midline incision. In most patients, however, when comprehensive cranial and facial reconstruction is anticipated, the modified prone or "seal" position described by Park et al. has been used to excellent advantage.[28] This position (Fig. 7–4) provides easy access to the entire calvarium, the orbits, and the face if necessary. The position utilizes a bean-bag support system that can be form-fitted to the child. The addition of egg-crate foam provides the necessary evenly distributed padding. The position takes advantage of mild chest and abdominal compression to counter the potential effect of the elevated position of the head with respect to the heart, thereby diminishing the risk of air embolism.[29] The application of the surgical drapes aids in holding the otherwise wobbly head in a stable, though intraoperatively movable, position. The degree of head extension is well tolerated, but in patients suspected of having craniovertebral anomalies such as Klippel-Feil syndrome, achondrodysplasia, or Down's

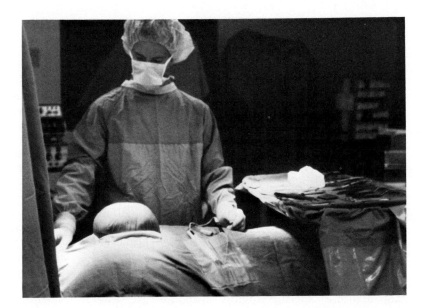

FIGURE 7–4. This operative photograph shows the modified prone position of a child used for excellent surgical exposure of the entire cranium.

syndrome, caution should be used in extending the head, and preoperative radiographs should be done to determine the anatomy of the craniovertebral junction.

INSTRUMENTATION

Cranial bone can best be removed and sculptured with the Midas Rex or an equivalent high-speed craniotome. Often, in young children, the thin calvarial bone can be cut easily with heavy scissors. Smooth dural elevators, small rongeurs, and tiny chisels are frequently helpful in the various reconstructive procedures. When necessary, bone fixation can be done with wires, miniplates, microplates, or various suture materials.[30] Caution should be employed in the use of rigid fixation devices, especially in younger children, in whom continued calvarial expansion with brain growth is anticipated. Opinion varies regarding the use of methacrylate for fixation or filling of cranial defects, especially in very young children. Free-floating bone grafts may be sutured to the dura with absorbable suture material, and occasionally the use of fibrin glue is helpful. Silastic interfacing at the craniectomy sites, especially in operative procedures for sagittal craniosynostosis, has worked well and has stood the test of time regarding any related complications. The same principle of Silastic interfacing may be applied to other reconstruction procedures attempting to delay bony union, such as orbital advancements.

MANAGEMENT OF THE DURA DURING CRANIOSYNOSTOSIS SURGERY

The surgical principle of maintaining the integrity of the dura mater is critical in craniosynostosis surgery. All dural openings should be meticulously closed, not only to prevent cerebrospinal fluid collections beneath the scalp but also to prevent the formation of leptomeningeal cysts and persistent bone defects caused by transmitted fluid pulsations. Opinion varies regarding the role of dural plication in craniosynostosis surgery. When compensatory bulging of the skull is associated with a dilated subarachnoid space beneath the expanded bone, dural plication aids in reforming normal dural contour for onlay bone replacements and theoretically dampens the CSF pulsations associated with bone expansion. Rarely is an enlargement duraplasty considered necessary; in cases of severe deformity such as cloverleaf skull, the dural configuration deforming the brain may need to be modified if the deformity persists after total calvarial removal. The dissection of the dura from convolutional indentations of the inner table of the calvarial bone when increased intracranial pressure is present requires meticulous care. Dissecting with dural elevators and manually operated instruments, rather than power-driven craniotomes, is preferred in these cases. With care, the rare incidence of dural and venous sinus entry is well worth the added surgical time.

SURGICAL PROCEDURES

SAGITTAL CRANIOSYNOSTOSIS

Isolated sagittal synostosis is by far the most common form of craniosynostosis, accounting for 50 per cent of the patients in the Arkansas Children's Hospital series. The scaphocephalic appearance of these patients is readily appreciated, as are the compensatory changes of frontal and occipital bossing. The original operative procedure for sagittal synostosis consisted of suturectomy,[31] but the numerous variations on the theme attest to shortcomings of this approach,[32] especially in older patients. It could be argued that almost any procedure works but that none is completely satisfactory. The excision of the sagittal suture, bilateral parasagittal craniectomies, with and without the application of polyethylene or Silastic, the use of larger and larger midline craniectomies, parietal morcellations, total vertex craniectomies, and variations on these approaches have all been done to improve what may have been frequently disappointing cosmetic results.[33–39] The application of caustic agents to the dura in an attempt to delay bone reformation is no longer acceptable.[40,41] Persistent dolichocephaly has been the most common shortcoming of operations directed at sagittal suturectomies, but if a direct approach to the midline suture can be accomplished early enough, within the first few weeks of life, a satisfactory cosmetic result may be expected,[25,32,36,38] and lateral movement of the parietal bones with brain growth has been documented. On the other hand, after significant compensatory cranial deformity has occurred, with frontal and occipital bossing, marked elongation of the anteroposterior measurement of the skull, and presence of a severe keel deformity, then deformity-specific surgical procedures are superior. Since most of the patients seen in the Arkansas Children's Hospital craniofacial program have already developed significant compensatory changes, strip craniectomies or variations thereof are less commonly used, and more extensive surgical procedures are the rule. The specific deformities of the skull are addressed on an individual basis, utilizing variations of the Pi pro-cedure described by Jane and associates.[42] The Pi procedure not only corrects specific deformities but also results in a biomechanical or squeeze effect, transmitted to the skull base and causing lateral movement of the parietal bones at the time of foreshortening of the skull. The standard Pi procedure (Fig. 7–5) is done by removing a large mass of cranial bone in the shape of the Greek letter Pi, the lateral arms extending along the coronal sutures, the posts being bilateral parasagittal bone struts, and the two halves being connected across the midline. The sagittal suture and residual bone are separated from the sagittal sinus and attached with wires or nonabsorbable sutures to the frontal bones. Thereby, the isthmus can safely be closed, foreshortening the anteroposterior distance of the skull 10 to 12 mm, without creating an increase in intracranial pressure. Barrel-stave osteotomies are then done to allow parietal contouring, and the midline hypertrophic keel is smoothed away with a high-speed burr. Larger craniectomies can be added across the lambdoid sutures if an extremely protuberant occipital eminence needs to be corrected. This maneuver is analogous to modifications of strip craniectomy proposed by Albright.[33] The bone fragments originally removed can then be trimmed, molded, and reapplied to the dura with absorbable suture material. As with other craniectomy procedures done in the very young infant, bone refor-

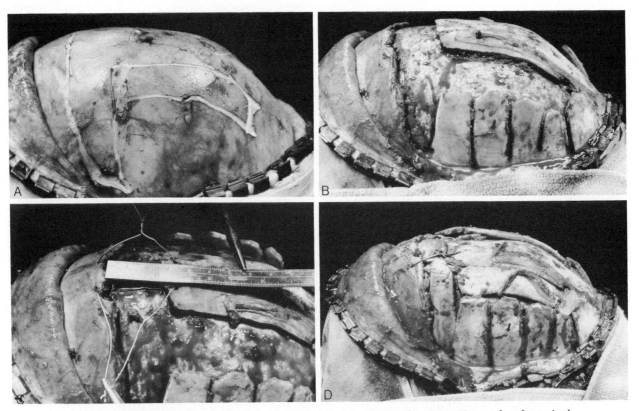

FIGURE 7–5. Intraoperative photographs of an 8-month-old patient undergoing a Pi procedure for sagittal craniosynostosis show: *A,* an outline of the planned bone removal; *B,* the Pi-shaped craniectomy and the barrel-stave osteotomies of the parietal bones; *C,* the skull foreshortening method using approximation of the sagittal strip to the frontal bones; and *D,* the onlay bone grafts used to complete the reconstruction of the calvarium.

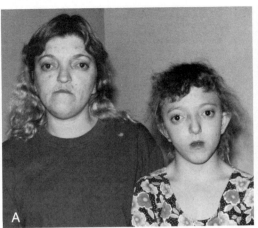
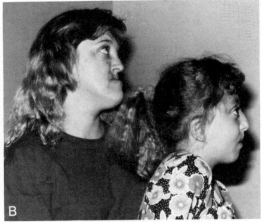

FIGURE 7–6. Frontal *(A)* and lateral *(B)* photographic views of a mother and her daughter, both with Crouzon's disease. The pictures emphasize the characteristic phenotypic findings, the genetic component of the disease, and the variations in midface retrusion seen to be severe in the mother and mild in the daughter.

mation is rarely a problem, and complete incorporation of the onlay bone grafts occurs rapidly. Marked frontal bossing may be treated by adding frontal craniotomies, dural plication, and medial movement of the lateral frontal exposures. When the most advanced changes are seen in the occipital region, a reverse of the standard Pi procedure may be more effective. Vollmer and co-workers have described the variants of sagittal craniosynostosis with surgical corrective measures, addressing each of the cranial deformities.[39] With these techniques, immediate correction of the cranial deformity has been the rule in sagittal craniosynostosis patients, and the satisfaction of the family with the surgical results has been gratifying. In children older than 12 to 18 months, more extensive cranial remodeling procedures such as those described by Marchac and Renier,[43] using multiple calvarial bone transpositions and segmental foreshortenings, may offer the best surgical option.

CORONAL SYNOSTOSIS

Coronal synostosis may be unilateral or bilateral and often occurs as part of a syndrome such as Crouzon's (Fig. 7–6) or Apert's. The characteristic deformity in unilateral coronal synostosis consists of ipsilateral frontal bone and orbital flattening (Fig. 7–7), the harlequin eye deformity seen on radiographs of the skull (Fig. 7–8), and contralateral frontal bossing. There is also an increased bitemporal diameter and a tendency for a towering configuration of the skull. A ridge of bone can be seen or palpated along the involved coronal suture. A distinction should be made between the plagiocephaly of coronal synostosis and that of lambdoid synostosis or positional molding. Both have unilateral frontal bossing, but with coronal synostosis it is contralateral, whereas with lambdoid pathology the frontal bossing is

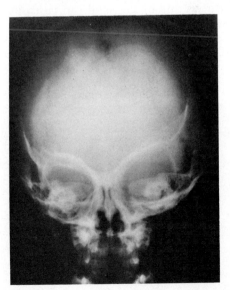

FIGURE 7–7. An oblique photograph of an infant with unilateral coronal synostosis shows the ridge of bone along the coronal suture and the flattened, retracted lateral orbit.

FIGURE 7–8. An anteroposterior view of the radiograph of a patient with unilateral coronal synostosis shows the harlequin eye deformity associated with elevation of the lateral sphenoid wing.

ipsilateral with associated forward displacement of the ipsilateral ear. With coronal synostosis, nasal deviation and midface asymmetry bespeak a problem requiring more complex craniofacial reconstruction. Treatment for unilateral coronal synostosis is more complex than for the sagittal forms. Strip craniectomy for coronal synostosis is rarely successful as a definitive procedure, even when done within the first weeks of life. Sometimes, with the more comprehensive surgical procedures, secondary operations may still be necessary despite early surgical correction. Orbital advancement is invariably required. Hoffman and Mohr described a canthal advancement procedure utilizing a strut graft from the orbital rim to the parietal bone.[44] Variations on the technique have evolved as a result of early fusion fixation of the strut graft; these include Silastic barriers, free-floating orbitotomies,[45] orbital ridge onlay grafts,[46] and various combinations.[47, 48] When possible, the periosteum of the orbital bandeau should be left intact to maintain its blood supply; delayed asymmetries due to failure of frontal sinus development may occur if the orbital bone is replaced unilaterally as a free bone graft.[49] Opinion varies as to the need for bilateral versus only unilateral frontal bone removal in the treatment of unilateral coronal synostosis. If severe asymmetry exists, both frontal bones may be removed, remodeled, reversed, and replaced using dural plication to obliterate the dilated subarachnoid space over the region of compensatory frontal bone expansion. Figure 7–9 shows the end result of treatment for unilateral coronal synostosis by bilateral frontal craniotomy, dural plication, and orbital advancement. Care must be taken to prevent the towering deformity that may occur in the posterior frontal region, when the anterior edges of the bone grafts are fixed to the orbital rims.

With bilateral coronal synostosis, other anomalies and syndromal conditions should be anticipated in a large percentage of cases. The characteristic brachycephalic appearance, bitemporal widening, ocular protrusion, and towering of the skull can be easily appreciated. Again, simple coronal suturectomy is not recommended as a definitive procedure even if done early. Attention to the orbital foreshortening and associated hypertelorism is often required. Orbital advance-ments and floating forehead operations are effective.[4, 50, 51] Decreasing the towering deformity of the head requires a circumferential craniectomy, with forward and downward replacement of the calvarium. The procedure must be done gradually, and intracranial pressure monitoring is advisable for this procedure. Midface retrusion, common in the syndromal forms, is neither prevented nor corrected by calvarial remodeling alone. Therefore, if these advanced compensatory changes and associated facial deformities have occurred, complex craniofacial procedures are required and are discussed further in Chapter 8.

LAMBDOID DEFORMITIES

True lambdoid synostosis is uncommon, and the reported incidence may sometimes include patients with positional lambdoid deformities unassociated with premature lambdoid suture fusion. These patients present with unilateral occipital flattening, frequently with focal alopecia in the flattened area of the skull. There is also protrusion of the ipsilateral frontal bone and forward displacement of the ipsilateral ear and petrous bone.[52] Even with positional deformities, fusion of the lambdoid suture may be evident on skull radiographs or CT scanning with bone windows, and if fusion is present, conservative measures utilizing positioning and helmets will not be effective. Since developmental delay may be one cause of positional molding, it is prudent to investigate prenatal and neonatal history, perform a careful neurologic examination, and consider preoperative neuro-imaging studies so as to be aware of any underlying cerebral pathology (Fig. 7–10). Congenital torticollis may be another cause of positional deformities and may require specific treatment.[53]

Surgical treatment consists of suturectomy in the very young patient having true lambdoid synostosis.[32] Procedures to obtain occipital symmetry by calvarial bone transfers have also been advocated[32] but do nothing to correct frontal asymmetry or ear displacement. Many patients with lambdoid deformities are referred with a diagnosis of coronal synostosis because of a prominent unilateral frontal bulge, obviously perceived

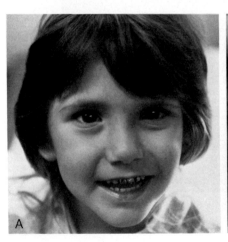
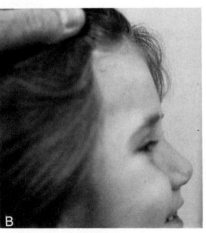

FIGURE 7–9. Frontal *(A)* and lateral *(B)* photographs of the child shown preoperatively in Figure 7–7, 5 years after correction of unilateral coronal synostosis, demonstrates asymmetry and normal forehead contouring.

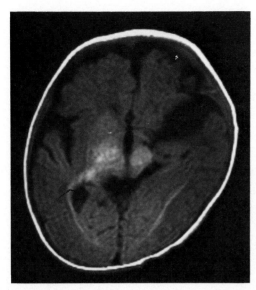

FIGURE 7–10. CT scan of a patient with positional lambdoid deformity shows an arachnoid cyst, gyral atrophy, and basal ganglial calcifications, suggesting primary cerebral pathology accounting for the child's motor delay.

as the most disabling cosmetic handicap. When surgical treatment is contemplated for cosmetic purposes, attention to the frontal deformity must be included in surgical planning. Frontal calvarial transfers may be used alone or in combination with procedures directed at the occiput.[54] Although opinion varies concerning the advisability of surgical treatment of lambdoid deformities other than true lambdoid synostosis, it is apparent that a comprehensive craniofacial approach must be used to correct the deforming compensatory changes distant from the site of the primary pathology.

METOPIC SYNOSTOSIS

Metopic synostosis or trigonocephaly is recognized easily by the pointed forehead and triangular shape of the patient's skull. Apparently, Mozart, the musical genius, had this condition.[55] Bilateral flattening of the lateral orbits is part of the deformity. Metopic suturectomy is not considered to be an effective treatment for this entity. The surgical procedure requires removal of the beaked frontal bones (Fig. 7–11), bilateral canthal advancement, and replacement of the frontal bone with a contoured free bone graft from the parietal bones. The frontal bones may be fragmented and the pieces used to cover the parietal donor sites. A number of variations of the approach have been described.[56–59]

MULTIPLE SUTURE SYNOSTOSES

When multiple suture synostoses occur, increased intracranial pressure must be anticipated and may be associated with papilledema and vision loss. Restoration

of a normal cranial vault/brain mass ratio is imperative to preserve neurologic function. As shown in Figure 7–12, severe brain constriction and deformation can occur with oxycephaly. In some instances, cerebrospinal fluid shunting procedures are necessary but may complicate cranioplastic efforts by collapsing the cerebral mantle. As an initial operation, total calvarial removal has been advocated for most forms of multiple suture fusion, including kleeblattschädel, acrocephaly, and oxycephaly. In the very young infant, prompt regeneration of the calvarial bone may be expected, but the quality of the new bone may be less than ideal. In older children, bone replacement is advocated by use of remodeling techniques for frontal deformities, canthal advancement, barrel-stave osteotomies carried to the skull base, and onlay grafts to the dura (Fig. 7–13). When these aggressive techniques are used, excellent cosmetic results and restoration of normal physiology can be expected (Fig. 7–14). Split-thickness calvarial grafts are employed when total coverage of the expanded surface areas is needed in older patients. When an enlargement of the skull has been accomplished, it may be difficult to close the scalp. The need for multiple operative procedures should be anticipated.

POST-SHUNTING DEFORMITIES

On occasion, shunting procedures, especially those done for extreme degrees of hydrocephalus, may result in overlapping and premature fusion of the calvarial bones. Marked deformity may occur when one parietal bone overlaps the other in the midline and deforms the sagittal sinus. In these instances correction of the deformity may be indicated not only for cosmetic purposes but also to prevent bone erosion through the scalp. Extreme caution should be exercised in the dissection of the region of bone fusion from the sagittal sinus.

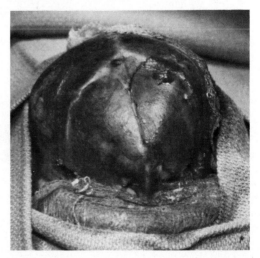

FIGURE 7–11. Intraoperative photograph of a child with trigonocephaly shows the beaked bony deformity associated with metopic synostosis.

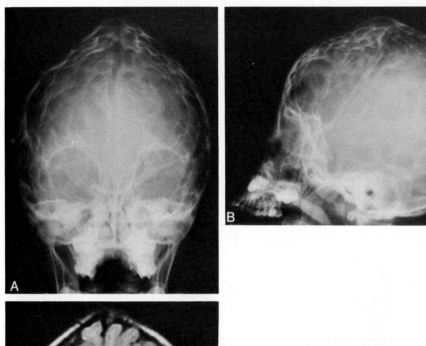

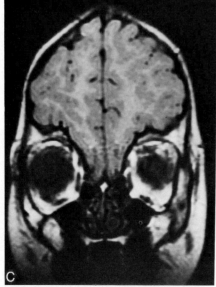

FIGURE 7–12. Anteroposterior *(A)* and lateral *(B)* views of the skull radiographs and a coronal section of an MRI scan *(C)* of a 3-year-old child with papilledema and cranial deformity show the acrocephalic configuration (oxycephaly), the marked convolutional indentations in the calvarium, and herniation of inferior frontal gyri into the skull base.

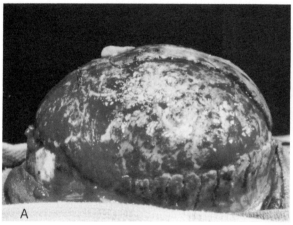

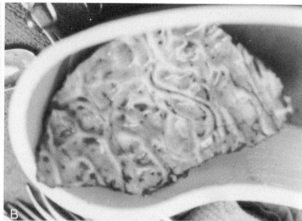

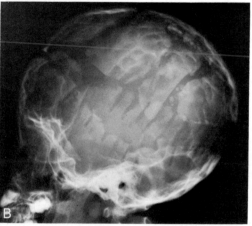

FIGURE 7–13. Operative photographs show the correction of a patient with the acrocephalic variety of multiple suture synostosis: *A,* removal of calvarial bone and barrel-stave osteotomies carried to the skull base to allow further release of the compressed brain. Dural plication has been done anteriorly. *B,* Marked convolutional indentations of the bone specimen. *C,* Replacement bone grafts. Rigid fixation devices were not used in this case to allow postoperative expansion.

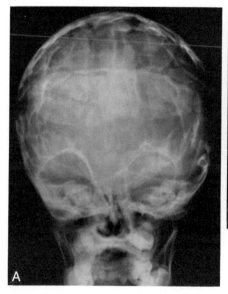

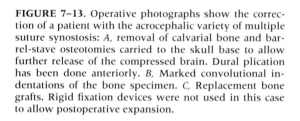

FIGURE 7–14. Postoperative radiographs of the child with oxycephaly. *A,* Anteroposterior view shows the normal calvarial contour. *B,* Lateral view shows the extensive cranial reconstruction. The patient's vision improved immediately postoperatively.

The scaphocephaly frequently seen in premature babies is but another example of positional molding and ordinarily does not require surgical treatment. However, there are extreme cases of scaphocephaly with biparietal narrowing producing enough deformity in these infants to justify cosmetic intervention. In these instances, suturectomy or strip craniectomy usually is not effective, and more complex cranial reconstructive procedures are necessary. Careful attention must be given to the position of the shunt and the possible deformation of the shunt trajectories with such procedures. Finally, evidence is accumulating to show that some children with effective shunts have early fusion of their cranial sutures and that overshunting may result in the creation of a smaller than normal cranial cavity. Even though the shunt may be effective in lowering intracranial pressure, there remains a disparity between the normal brain volume and the volume of the intracranial cavity. The efficacy of cranial expansion procedures in this form of craniostenosis is an area of current investigation in pediatric neurosurgery.

SUMMARY

In recent years, much progress has been made in the understanding and treatment of craniosynostosis. Although the etiology of craniosynostosis involves multiple factors and the mechanisms remain debatable, information is accumulating regarding both environmental and genetic factors important in the occurrence of the disease. Advances in surgical technique have resulted in more favorable cosmetic outcomes for the children, and the safety of the surgical procedures has improved. Utilization of a team approach is favored in many centers, taking advantage of the expertise of pediatric neurosurgeons, facial plastic surgeons, neuro-ophthalmologists, developmental pediatricians, and geneticists, as well as the dedicated pediatric anesthesiologists and intensivists, all of whom contribute significantly to the final management of these patients. There remain many areas for fruitful research in the complex but rewarding field of craniosynostosis.

REFERENCES

1. Hunter AGW, Rudd NL: Craniosynostosis I sagittal synostosis: its genetics and associated clinical findings in 214 patients who lacked involvement of the coronal suture(s). Teratology 14:185, 1976.
2. Hunter AGW, Rudd NL: Craniosynostosis II coronal synostosis: its familial characteristics and associated clinical findings in 109 patients lacking bilateral polysyndactyly or syndactyly. Teratology 15:301, 1977.
3. Coppoleta JM, Wolbach SB: Body length and organ weights of infants and children: a study of the body length and normal weights of the more important vital organs of the body between birth and twelve years of age. Am J Pathol 9:55, 1933.
4. Laurent JP, Balasubramaniam C, Stal S, Cheek WR: Early surgical management of coronal synostosis. Clin Plast Surg 17:183, 1990.
5. Persing J, Babler W, Winn HR, Jane J, Rodeheaver G: Age as a critical factor in the success of surgical correction of craniosynostosis. J Neurosurg 54:601, 1981.
6. Epstein FJ: Misguided concepts: the bases of scientific advancement. Childs Nerv Syst 7:239, 1991.
7. Reddy K, Hoffman H, Armstrong D: Delayed and progressive multiple suture craniosynostosis. Neurosurgery 26:442, 1990.
8. Norwood CW, Alexander E Jr., Davis CH, Kelly DL Jr: Recurrent and multiple suture closures after craniectomy for craniosynostosis. J Neurosurg 41:715, 1974.
9. Gault DT, Renier D, Marchac D, Ackland FM, Jones BM: Intracranial volume in children with craniosynostosis. J Craniofacial Surg 1:1, 1990.
10. Renier D, Sainte-Rose C, Marchac D, Hirsch J: Intracranial pressure in craniosynostosis. J Neurosurg 57:370, 1982.
11. Lundar T, Nornes H: Steady-state lumbar infusion tests in the management of children with craniosynostosis. Childs Nerv Syst 7:31, 1991.
12. Virchow R: Über den cretinismus, namentlich in franken, und über pathologische schädelformen. Verh Phys Med Ges (Wurzburg) 2:230, 1851/1852.
13. Babler WJ, Persing JA, Winn HR, Jane JA, Rodeheaver GT: Compensatory growth following premature closure of the coronal suture in rabbits. J Neurosurg 57:535, 1982.
14. Delashaw JB, Persing JA, Broaddus WC, Jane JA: Cranial vault growth in craniosynostosis. J Neurosurg 70:159, 1989.
15. Persing JA, Lettieri JT, Cronin AJ, Wolcott WP, Singh V, Morgan E: Craniofacial suture stenosis: morphologic effects. Plast Reconstr Surg 88:563, 1990.
16. Moss ML: The pathogenesis of premature cranial synostosis in man. Acta Anat 37:351, 1959.
17. Chadduck WM, Boop FA, Blankenship JB, Husain M: Meningioma and sagittal craniosynostosis in an infant: case report. Neurosurgery 30:441, 1992.
18. Cohen MM: The etiology of craniosynostosis. In Cohen MM (ed): Craniosynostosis, Diagnosis, Evaluation and Management. New York, Raven Press, 1986, pp 59–80.
19. Chadduck WM, Chadduck JB, Boop FA: The subarachnoid spaces in craniosynostosis. Neurosurgery 30:867, 1992.
20. Fishman MA, Hogan GR, Hodge PR: The concurrence of hydrocephalus and craniosynostosis. J Neurosurg 34:621, 1971.
21. Parisi M, Mehdizadeh HM, Hunter JC, Finch IJ: Evaluation of craniosynostosis with three-dimensional CT imaging. J Comp Assist Tomogr 13:1006, 1989.
22. Vannier MW, Hildebolt CF, Marsh JL, Pilgram TK, McAlister WH, Shackelford GD, Offutt CJ, Knapp RH: Craniosynostosis: diagnostic value of three-dimensional CT reconstruction. Radiology 173(3):669, 1989.
23. Muakkassa KF, Hoffman HJ, Hinton DR, Hendrick EB, Humphreys RP, Ash J: Lambdoid synostosis. Part 2: Review of cases managed at the Hospital for Sick Children 1972–1982. J Neurosurg 61:340, 1984.
24. Bentovim A: The impact of malformation in the emotional development of the child and his family. In Berry CL, Poswillo DE (eds): Teratology—Trends and Applications. Berlin, Springer-Verlag, 1975, pp 223–233.
25. Olds MV, Storrs B, Walker ML: Surgical treatment of sagittal synostosis. Neurosurgery 18:345, 1986.
26. Kearney RA, Rosales JK, Howes WJ: Craniosynostosis: an assessment of blood loss and transfusion practices. Can J Anesthesia 36(4):473, 1989.
27. Semmler CJ, Hunter JG: Early occupational therapy intervention: neonates to three years. Aspen Publications, Inc., Gaithersburg, MD, 1990, pp 340–352.
28. Park TS, Haworth CS, Jane JA, Bedford RB, Persing JA: Modified prone position for cranial remodeling procedures on children with craniofacial dysmorphism: A technical note. Neurosurgery 16:212, 1985.
29. Phillips RJL, Mulliken JB: Venous air embolism during a craniofacial procedure. Plast Reconstr Surg 82:155, 1986.
30. Sadove AM, Eppley BL: Microfixation techniques in pediatric craniomaxillofacial surgery. Ann Plast Surg 27:36, 1991.
31. Lane LC: Pioneer craniectomy for the relief of mental imbecility due to premature sutural closure and microcephalus. JAMA 18:49, 1892.

32. Laurent JP, Cheek WR: Craniosynostosis. *In* McLaurin RL, Scut L, Venes JL, Epstein F (eds): Pediatric Neurosurgery. 2nd ed. Philadelphia, WB Saunders Co., 1989, pp 107–119.

33. Albright AL: Operative normalization of skull shape in sagittal synostosis. Neurosurgery 17:329, 1985.

34. Duff TA, Mixter RC: Midline craniectomy for sagittal suture synostosis: comparative efficacy of two barriers to calvarial reclosure. Surg Neurol 35:350, 1991.

35. Epstein N, Epstein F, Newman G: Total vertex craniectomy for the treatment of scaphocephaly. Childs Brain 9:309, 1982.

36. Foltz EL, Loeser JD: Craniosynostosis. J Neurosurg 43:48, 1975.

37. Greene CS, Winston KR: Treatment of scaphocephaly with sagittal craniectomy and biparietal morcellation. Neurosurgery 23:196, 1988.

38. Stein C, Schut L: Management of scaphocephaly. Surg Neurol 7:153, 1977.

39. Vollmer DG, Jane JA, Park TS, Persing JA: Variants of sagittal synostosis: strategies for surgical correction. J Neurosurg 61:557, 1984.

40. McComb JG, Withers GT, Davis RL: Cortical damage from Zenker's solution applied to the dura mater. Neurosurgery 8:68, 1981.

41. Marlin AE, Brown WE Jr., Huntington HW, Epstein F: Effect of the dural application of Zenker's solution on the feline brain. Neurosurgery 6:45, 1980.

42. Jane JA, Edgerton MJ, Futrell JW, Park TS: Immediate correction of sagittal synostosis. J Neurosurg 49:705, 1978.

43. Marchac D, Renier D: Scaphocephaly. *In* Marchac D, Renier D (eds): Craniofacial Surgery for Craniosynostosis. Boston, Little, Brown, 1982, pp 88–92.

44. Hoffman HJ, Mohr G: Lateral canthal advancement of the supraorbital margin. A new corrective technique in the treatment of coronal synostosis. J Neurosurg 45:376, 1976.

45. Persing JA, Jane JA, Park TS, Edgerton MT, Delashaw JB: Floating C-shaped orbital osteotomy for orbital rim advancement in craniosynostosis: preliminary report. J Neurosurg 72:22, 1990.

46. Cohen SR, Kawamotto HK Jr., Burstein F, Peacock WJ: Advance-ment-onlay: an improved technique of fronto-orbital remodeling in craniosynostosis. Childs Nerv Syst 7:264, 1991.

47. Elisevich K, Bite U, Colcleugh RG: Orbital rim and malar advancement for unilateral coronal synostosis in the older pediatric age group. J Neurosurg 74:219, 1991.

48. Jane JA, Park TS, Zide BM, Lambruschi P, Persing JA, Edgerton MT: Alternative techniques in the treatment of unilateral coronal synostosis. J Neurosurg 61:550, 1984.

49. McCarthy JG, Karp NS, LaTrenta GS, Thorne CHM: The effect of early fronto-orbital advancement on frontal sinus development and forehead aesthetics. Plast Reconstr Surg 86:1078, 1990.

50. Marchac D, Renier D, Jones BM: Experience with the "floating forehead." Br J Plast Surg 41:1, 1987.

51. Persing JA, Jane JA, Delashaw JB: Treatment of bilateral coronal synostosis in infancy: a holistic approach. J Neurosurg 72(2):171, 1990.

52. Fernbach SK, Feinstein KA: The deformed petrous bone: a new plain film sign of premature lambdoid synostosis. Am J Roentgenol 156(6):1215, 1991.

53. Douglas MT: Wryneck in the ancient Hawaiians. Am J Phys Anthropol 84:261, 1991.

54. Persing JA, Delashaw JB, Jane JA, Edgerton MT: Lambdoid synostosis: surgical considerations. Plast Reconstr Surg 81:852, 1987.

55. Puech B, Puech PF, Tichy G, Dhellemmes P, Cianfarani F: Craniofacial dysmorphism in Mozart's skull. J Forensic Sci 34:487, 1989.

56. Di Rocco C, Marchese E, Velardi F: Metopic craniosynostosis. Surgical results in 35 surgically treated cases under 1 year of age. Minerva Pediatr 41:559, 1989.

57. Friede H, Alberius P, Lilja J, Lauritzen C: Trigonocephaly: clinical and cephalometric assessment of craniofacial morphology in operated and non-treated patients. Cleft Palate J 27:362, 1990.

58. Ousterhout DK, Eskenaki L, Golabi M, Edwards MS: Histologic evaluation of the coronal sutures in trigonocephaly. J Craniofacial Surg 1(1):15, 1990.

59. Sadove AM, Kalsbeck JE, Eppley BL, Javed T: Modifications in the surgical correction of trigonocephaly. Plast Reconstr Surg 85:853, 1989.

Chapter 8

CRANIOFACIAL SURGERY

HAROLD J. HOFFMAN, M.D., and JOHN R. W. KESTLE, M.D.

Craniofacial surgery is a new subspecialty that crosses the disciplines of neurosurgery, plastic surgery, and oral surgery. It deals with anomalies of the bony architecture of the cranial vault and/or facial skeleton. The modern era of craniofacial surgery began in 1967 when Tessier reported a two-stage intracranial and extracranial procedure to move the entire orbit for hypertelorism.[1] Tessier emphasized collaboration between specialists and demonstrated that large bony masses could be largely denuded of their blood supply, moved, and still survive.

The scope of disorders that craniofacial teams treat is continually evolving and includes congenital lesions, traumatic lesions, and neoplastic lesions. In the pediatric population, most of the procedures are for congenital malformations.

TIMING OF SURGERY

The timing of surgical intervention in craniofacial anomalies in children is based on their untreated natural history and on the fact that there is dramatic brain growth in the first year of life.[2] The volume of the brain almost triples in the first year of life, and by 2 years of age the cranial capacity is four times that at birth. Soon thereafter fibrous union of the sutures begins. The sutures are largely ossified by 8 years of age. If a skull suture closes prematurely, irregular growth of the skull occurs to make room for the growing brain. Virchow's law states that compensatory skull growth occurs in a direction perpendicular to the fused suture.

When premature suture closure is left uncorrected, severe abnormalities of the skull shape will result. There may also be other complications. Of male patients at the Royal Institute for the Blind in Copenhagen surveyed in 1913, 21 per cent had oxycephaly.[3] In another series of 171 patients with craniosynostosis, there were 26 patients with papilledema, 33 with optic atrophy, 85 with headaches, 39 with epilepsy, and 42

with below-average intelligence.[4] We believe that early recognition and prompt surgical management can prevent many of these disastrous complications and give excellent cosmetic results.

In order to take advantage of the skull-molding effects of the growing brain and to avoid the major deficits that may result, the repair of craniofacial anomalies is ideally undertaken early in life. By removing the pathologic suture and allowing the skull to reshape under the influence of the growing brain, good cosmetic results are achieved.

ASSOCIATED PROBLEMS

A number of specific syndromes are encountered in craniofacial surgery, each of which is associated with unique medical and surgical problems. However, some problems may be seen with any of the craniofacial anomalies, and a discussion of these follows.

INTRACRANIAL HYPERTENSION

This may be a major problem in premature suture fusion. It is seen when there is a disparity between brain growth and intracranial capacity and may occur in as many as half the children with synostosis of more than one suture. It can be identified by its clinical symptoms or by secondary changes on neuroradiologic investigations (Fig. 8–1).

OPHTHALMOLOGIC PROBLEMS

With chronic raised intracranial pressure, papilledema and optic atrophy may occur. Some of the syndromes include shallow orbits, and when exophthalmos is present, there is a risk of corneal abrasion and globe trauma. Orbital hypertelorism may compromise

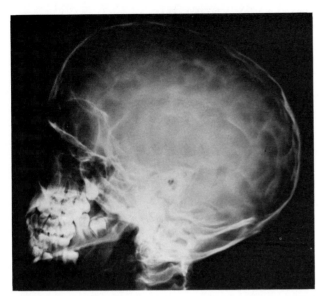

FIGURE 8–1. Lateral plain skull x-ray of a child with late multiple suture closure and a "beaten copper" skull secondary to raised intracranial pressure.

visual acuity and restrict binocular vision. With deformation of the orbit, dysconjugate vision (nonparalytic) may result.

HYDROCEPHALUS

This is seen in a variable proportion of patients with different craniofacial anomalies. It is particularly associated with Apert's syndrome, Crouzon's syndrome, and kleeblattschädel. The etiology of hydrocephalus in these syndromes is not clear. It has been proposed that it is secondary to involvement of the cranial base in the synostosis process, with impaired venous drainage and secondary venous hypertension.[5]

CLASSIFICATION OF CRANIOFACIAL ANOMALIES

A number of classification systems have been proposed for the craniofacial anomalies. As the understanding of the etiopathogenesis of most of these disorders is limited, the classification schemes are often descriptive based on the final appearance of the deformity. Many of the disorders are also named after the person who described them.

A classification system was proposed by the American Cleft Palate Association Committee on Craniofacial Disorders.[6] We have modified this, and it is outlined in Table 8–1.

SYNOSTOSIS

The synostoses are conveniently classified as nonsyndromic or syndromic. The nonsyndromic forms usually involve one or two sutures. Rarely are multiple sutures involved. Facial involvement, if present, is mild and probably secondary to the craniosynostosis. The syndromic forms of craniosynostosis are often referred to as craniofacial dysostoses. There is a deformity of the skull secondary to craniosynostosis, and there is a marked deformity of the face. Some of the syndromic forms are described in Table 8–2.

The clinical examination of a child with suspected craniosynostosis will often give the diagnosis. The common combinations of suture fusion cause characteristic changes in head shape. Invariably the parents will say that the changes in head shape have been present since birth. A bony ridge may be palpable along the fused suture. The presence of synostosis may be confirmed by plain skull films, and radionuclide bone scans may demonstrate decreased uptake along the closed suture. Computed tomography (CT) scanning is invaluable in the evaluation of patients with craniofacial disorders in general. In particular, the recently available software for production of highly detailed three-dimensional reconstructions has become an essential part of the surgical planning.[7, 8]

THE "NONSYNDROMIC" FORMS OF SYNOSTOSIS

Simple sagittal and lambdoid synostoses are discussed in other chapters in this text, and these will not be considered here.

Coronal Synostosis

Coronal synostosis is the second most common single-suture synostosis. It accounts for about a fifth of the cases of synostosis at The Hospital for Sick Children.[9]

Patients with unilateral coronal synostosis present with a characteristic appearance (Fig. 8–2). The forehead on the involved side is flattened, and the contralateral forehead bulges forward. The eye on the involved side is higher than its counterpart, and the lateral canthus is elevated (Fig. 8–3). The ipsilateral cheek is flattened, and the tip of the nose deviates away from the stenotic suture.

If both coronal sutures close prematurely, the forehead above both eyes is flattened. The anterior fossae are short and the midface is hypoplastic. The orbits are small and proptosis is the result. Bilateral coronal syn-

TABLE 8–1. A CLASSIFICATION SYSTEM FOR CRANIOFACIAL DISORDERS

Synostosis
Nonsyndromic
Syndromic
Clefts
Atrophy/Hypoplasia
Hyperplasia
Dysplasia
Neoplasia
Other

TABLE 8–2. SYNDROMES WITH CRANIOSYNOSTOSIS

SYNDROME	STRIKING FEATURE	FREQUENCY OF CRANIOSYNOSTOSIS	ETIOLOGY
Chromosomal Syndrome			
5p + syndrome	Variable CNS anomalies, dolichocephaly, craniosynostosis, mental deficiency, respiratory difficulties, renal or ureteral malformations, short first toes, phenotype not completely delineated at present	?	Trisomy for most of the short arm of chromosome 5
7p—syndrome	Craniosynostosis and variable anomalies, phenotype not completely delineated at present	Apparently common	Deletion of short arm of chromosome 7
13q—syndrome	Microcephaly, lobar holoprosencephaly, trigonocephaly, craniosynostosis, mental deficiency, microphthalmia, iris coloboma, retinoblastoma, malformed ears, micrognathia, hypoplastic thumbs, imperforate anus, hypospadias, cryptorchidism, congenital heart defects	8/11	Deletion of long arm of chromosome 13
Monogenic Syndromes			
Apert's syndrome	Craniosynostosis, proptosis, down-slanting palpebral fissures, strabismus, ocular hypertelorism, midface deficiency, highly arched palate, complete symmetric syndactyly of hands and feet minimally involving digits 2–4	Almost all cases	Autosomal dominant
Atimendares syndrome	Craniosynostosis, microcephaly, retinitis pigmentosa, ptosis of the eyelids, malformed ears, micrognathia, highly arched palate, clinodactyly, simian creases, short stature	Apparently common	Probably autosomal or X-linked recessive
Baller-Gerold syndrome	Craniosynostosis, radial aplasia, absent or hypoplastic carpal bones and preaxial digits	Apparently common	Probably autosomal recessive
Berant's syndrome	Craniosynostosis involving sagittal suture, radioulnar synostosis	Apparently common	Probably autosomal dominant
Carpenter's syndrome	Craniosynostosis, mental deficiency, preaxial polysyndactyly of the feet, variable soft-tissue syndactyly with brachymesophalangy of the hands, displacement of patellae, genua valga, congenital heart defects, short stature, obesity	All reported cases	Autosomal recessive
Christian's syndrome I	Craniosynostosis, microcephaly, ocular hypertelorism, down-slanting palpebral fissures, cleft palate, arthrogryposis	Apparently common	Autosomal recessive
Christian's syndrome II	Craniosynostosis involving metopic suture, ocular hypertelorism, epicanthal folds, down-slanting palpebral fissures, C2–3 fusion, hemivertebrae, anomalous ears, clinodactyly, simian creases, foot abduction, imperforate anus, short stature	Apparently common	X-linked semidominant
Craniofacial dyssynostosis	Craniosynostosis involving lambdoidal and posterior sagittal suture and variably the coronal suture, prominent forehead, ocular hypertelorism, frequent Spanish ancestry	All known cases	? Autosomal recessive
Crouzon's syndrome	Craniosynostosis, shallow orbits with proptosis, strabismus, midface deficiency	Almost all cases	Autosomal dominant
Elejalde's syndrome	Craniosynostosis, swollen face, epicanthal folds, ocular hypertelorism, hypoplastic nose, malformed ears, redundant neck tissue, gigantism at birth, short limbs, polydactyly, omphalocele, lung hypoplasia, cystic renal dysplasia, sponge kidney, redundant connective tissue in skin and many viscera, proliferation of perivascular nerve fibers	Apparently common	Autosomal recessive
FG syndrome	Variable growth problems, disproportionately large head circumference, mental deficiency, congenital hypotonia, high narrow palate, imperforate anus, sacral dimple, partial 2–3 syndactyly of feet, and various other findings including craniosynostosis and frontal bossing	Apparently uncommon	X-linked
Frontonasal dysplasia	Ocular hypotelorism, cranium bifidum occultum, widow's peak, broad nasal root, flat nasal up or bifid nose, notching or colobomas of nostrils, and median cleft lip in variable combinations; occurrence of many low-frequency anomalies including craniosynostosis	Uncommon	Biologically heterogeneous, probably representing many poorly delineated entities; some cases are consistent with autosomal-dominant inheritance

TABLE 8–2.   SYNDROMES WITH CRANIOSYNOSTOSIS *Continued*

SYNDROME	STRIKING FEATURE	FREQUENCY OF CRANIOSYNOSTOSIS	ETIOLOGY
Monogenic Syndromes *Continued*			
Gorlin-Chaudhry-Moss syndrome	Craniosynostosis, midface deficiency, hypertrichosis, down-slanting palpebral fissures, upper eyelid colobomas, patent ductus arteriosus, hypoplastic labia majora	Apparently common	Probably autosomal recessive
Hootnick-Holmes syndrome	Frontal bossing, dolichocephaly, craniosynostosis involving sagittal suture, ocular hypertelorism, strabismus, preaxial and postaxial polysyndactyly of hands, preaxial polysyndactyly of feet	?	Probably autosomal dominant
Lowry's syndrome	Craniosynostosis, prominent eyes, strabismus, highly arched or cleft palate, fibular aplasia, talipes equinovarus, simian creases	Apparently common	Probably autosomal recessive
Pfeiffer's syndrome	Craniosynostosis, proptosis strabismus, ocular hypertelorism, down-slanting palpebral fissures, midface deficiency, broad thumbs and great toes, mild cutaneous syndactyly of fingers and toes (variable)	All known cases	Autosomal dominant
Saethre-Chotzen syndrome	Craniosynostosis, facial asymmetry, low-set frontal hairline, ptosis of the eyelids, deviated nasal septum, variable brachydactyly and cutaneous syndactyly especially of the second and third fingers, normal thumbs and great toes	All known cases	Autosomal dominant
Summitt's syndrome	Craniosynostosis, strabismus, variable symmetrical syndactyly of hands and feet from partial to complete with clinodactyly, normal-sized thumbs and great toes, genua valga, obesity	Apparently common	Probably autosomal recessive
Washington's syndrome I	Craniosynostosis involving the sagittal suture, short fourth and fifth metacarpals	Apparently common	Probably autosomal recessive
Washington's syndrome II	Craniosynostosis, midface hypoplasia, lack of extension of the distal interphalangeal joints	Apparently common	Probably autosomal recessive
Weiss's syndrome	Craniosynostosis, medially deviated great toes, altered tarsal morphogenesis, mild syndactyly, wide variability of craniofacial involvement	Apparently common	Autosomal recessive
Teratogenically Induced Syndromes			
Aminopterin syndrome	Craniosynostosis, hypoplasia of cranial and facial bones, low-set ears, cleft palate, micrognathia, hypodactyly of feet, mild syndactyly of hands	Apparently common	Aminopterin or methotrexate during pregnancy
Sporadic, Incompletely Delineated Syndromes			
Andersen-Pindborg syndrome	Craniofacial dysostosis, ectodermal dysplasia, short stature	?	?
Antley-Bixler syndrome	Trapezoidocephaly, deformed ears and nose, elongated hands and feet, radiohumeral synostosis, digit contractures	?	?
Fairbanks's syndrome	Craniosynostosis, proptosis, short stature, brachydactyly, failure of tooth eruption	?	? (two sporadic cases known)
Hall's syndrome	Craniosynostosis and Turner-like phenotype	?	?
Hermann's syndrome I	Craniosynostosis, mental deficiency, hypoplastic supraorbital ridges, bitemporal flattening, ocular hypertelorism, ear anomalies, micrognathia, partial soft-tissue syndactyly of fingers 2–4, absent toes	?	?
Hermann's syndrome II	Craniosynostosis, microbrachycephaly, mental deficiency, anomalous ears, cleft lip and palate, symmetric limb reduction defects with absent fingers 4 and 5, short forearms, valgus positioning of the hands, ankylosis at knees, and varus positioning of feet	?	?
Idaho syndrome I	Craniosynostosis, scaphocephaly, strabismus, mental deficiency, congenital heart defect, umbilical hernia, complete anterior dislocation of tibia and fibula, talipes equinovarus, camptodactyly of fingers 2–5, deviation of fingers to ulnar side, proximally placed thumbs	?	?

Table continued on following page

TABLE 8–2.   SYNDROMES WITH CRANIOSYNOSTOSIS *Continued*

SYNDROME	STRIKING FEATURE	FREQUENCY OF CRANIOSYNOSTOSIS	ETIOLOGY
Sporadic, Incompletely Delineated Syndromes *Continued*			
Idaho syndrome II	Craniosynostosis, scaphocephaly, mental deficiency, down-slanting palpebral fissures, beaked nose, micrognathia, small low-set posteriorly angulated ears, preauricular tags, long neck, sloping shoulders, narrow thorax, pectus carinatum, winging of scapulae, cubitus valgus	?	?
Pederson's syndrome	Craniosynostosis, exostoses of the skull, premature exfoliation of deciduous teeth, linear verrucous nevi of neck, scaly patches on hands	?	?
Sakati's syndrome	Craniosynostosis, disproportionately small face, anomalous ears, patches of alopecia with atrophic skin, short limbs, polysyndactyly of feet, polydactyly of hands, congenital heart defect	?	?
Waardenburg's craniosynostosis syndrome	Craniosynostosis, hydrophthalmos, down-slanting palpebral fissures, cleft palate, micrognathia, low-set ears, malposed clavicles, contractures at elbows and knees, soft-tissue syndactyly of fingers 2–4, absent distal phalanx of thumb with absent nail, double nail with bifid terminal phalanx on second fingers, clinodactyly of fingers 4 and 5, hammertoes, ambiguous external genitalia, patent ductus arteriosus	?	?
Wisconsin syndrome	Craniosynostosis, mental deficiency, up-slanting palpebral fissures, microtia, short fourth metatarsals	?	? (two sporadic cases known)

From Cohen MM: Genetic perspectives on craniosynostosis and syndromes with craniosynostosis. J Neurosurg 47:886–898, 1977.

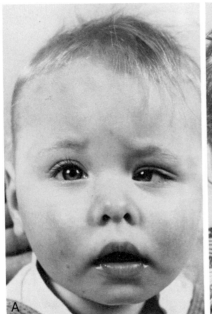 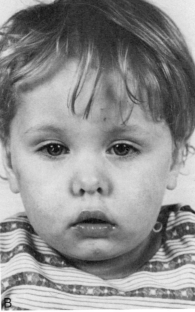

FIGURE 8–2. *A,* Nine-month-old girl with right unilateral coronal synostosis. *B,* Same patient 13 months after right lateral canthal advancement.

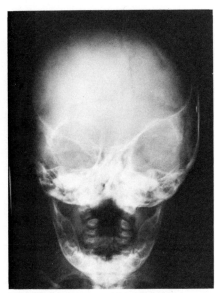

FIGURE 8–3. Skull x-ray of patient with left coronal synostosis showing harlequin orbit.

ostosis may be sporadic, but it is usually found in patients with one of the inherited craniofacial dysmorphic syndromes listed in Table 8–2.

SURGICAL REPAIR

Early in infancy the procedure of lateral canthal advancement adequately deals with both unilateral and bilateral coronal synostosis.[10] General endotracheal anaesthesia is induced, and a bifrontal subperiosteal scalp flap is reflected down to the orbit. A frontal bone flap is elevated and the pterion is removed. The orbital roof is exposed extradurally and incised along its junction with the frontal bone. The frontozygomatic process is also divided, and the supraorbital margin can then be broken by a greenstick fracture and advanced to align with the contralateral supraorbital margin (Fig. 8–4). The greatly thickened pterion, which is characteristic of this condition, is removed together with the lesser wing of the sphenoid ridge down to the superior orbital fissure. The free supraorbital margin is kept in place by a strut of bone taken from the frontal bone flap and wired to the lateral edge of the supraorbital rim anteriorly and to the parietal bone posteriorly. The parietal bone edge is covered with Silastic. The frontal bone is then divided and repositioned on the dura and held in place by the periosteal flap.

The results of lateral canthal advancement for unilateral coronal synostosis at The Hospital for Sick Children have recently been reviewed[11] (Fig. 8–5). Among the 39 patients treated with unilateral lateral canthal advancement between 1971 and 1989, there was an equal distribution of boys and girls. Sixty-one per cent were treated before the age of 6 months. The right coronal suture was affected in 26 patients and the left in 13. There was facial asymmetry in 13 patients. One patient had a family history of craniosynostosis (the mother had the same condition). No hydrocephalus or other major brain anomalies were present. Fifteen patients had other associated problems including myelomeningocele in one patient, torticollis in two, and strabismus in 12. One patient died and one patient was lost to follow-up. Of the remaining 37 patients, 35 of them were classified as having a good result as assessed by the surgeon and the family, and as confirmed by photographs and imaging studies. Two patients had sufficient deformity to require further surgery. The mean follow-up was 5 years.

In the case of bilateral coronal synostosis, bilateral lateral canthal advancement performed early in infancy allows for normal cranial and facial growth in more than half the patients[2] (Fig. 8–6). After the age of 6 months, more radical procedures are usually necessary. The older infant may be treated by the "floating forehead" technique of Marchac and Renier.[12] In this procedure, the entire supraorbital region is removed as a single supraorbital bar. The supraorbital bar is then fixed to the face only at the root of the nose and at the malar bones. It is believed that this technique allows the growing brain to continue to push the forehead forward. Although the floating forehead technique is an excellent technique in the older infant, it cannot be done before the metopic suture has fused sufficiently to allow removal of the entire supraorbital region as a single bar. Frequently, in the young neonate, the metopic suture is widely split and does not allow for this technique. In such situations, the procedure of lateral canthal advancement is preferable.

In the older child, who has not had an adequate repair in infancy, a radical craniofacial procedure is usually necessary (Fig. 8–7), as described by Tessier.[1] The procedure begins with a tracheotomy. If there is some degree of hydrocephalus, it is useful to insert a lumbar drain to allow escape of cerebrospinal fluid

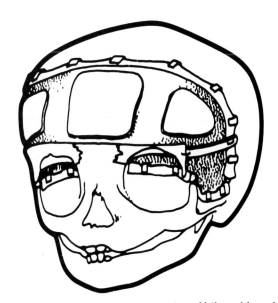

FIGURE 8–4. Diagrammatic representation of bilateral lateral canthal advancement procedure.

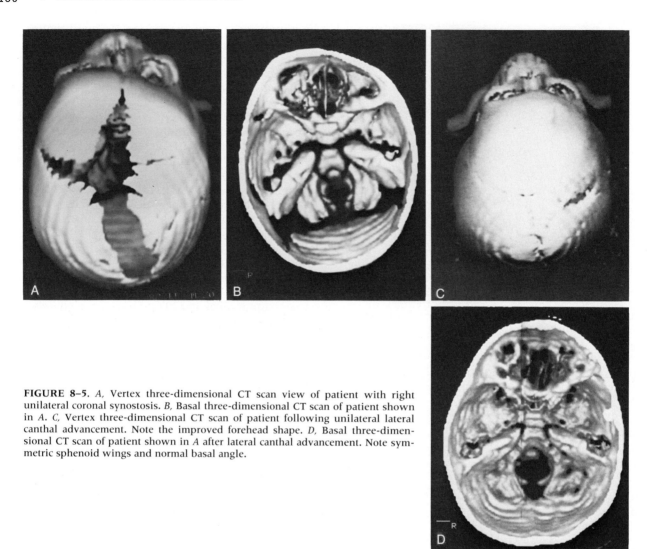

FIGURE 8–5. *A,* Vertex three-dimensional CT scan view of patient with right unilateral coronal synostosis. *B,* Basal three-dimensional CT scan of patient shown in *A. C,* Vertex three-dimensional CT scan of patient following unilateral lateral canthal advancement. Note the improved forehead shape. *D,* Basal three-dimensional CT scan of patient shown in *A* after lateral canthal advancement. Note symmetric sphenoid wings and normal basal angle.

(CSF). When the patient has an indwelling diversionary CSF shunt, this is not necessary. Mannitol, 20 per cent in a dose of 2 gm/kg, is given to provide adequate brain shrinkage. Blood and fluid loss are carefully monitored during the procedure, with adequate replacement being carried out.

A bicoronal scalp incision, well behind the coronal suture and extending down to the ears bilaterally, is used. The periosteum is incised and carried down into the orbits with the scalp flap. The lacrimal sac is identified and dissected free from the orbital wall. Then the periosteum is elevated from the lateral orbital wall, inferior orbital rim, and the zygoma.

The entire frontal bone, back to the coronal suture, is removed in one segment. The inferior frontal osteotomy is then extended horizontally to include the temporal bone and is continued in a step-by-step fashion inferiorly, toward the base of the skull. This outlines a posterior slot in the temporal bone, which guides the subsequent advancement of the supraorbital margin and allows maintenance of bony contact. Horizontally, the osteotomy extends into the lateral orbital wall, then continues through the orbital roof and across the na-

sion. Once this is done bilaterally, it is possible to remove the supraorbital bar in one piece.

At this point, one has an excellent view of the dura along the floor of the anterior fossa. Frequently, with craniofacial dysostosis, there are numerous stalactites of bone protruding up from the floor. Consequently, dural lacerations can occur during craniofacial repair. It is absolutely imperative that these dural tears be adequately sealed to avoid postoperative rhinorrhea, which is a dreaded complication.

The maxilla is advanced with a Le Fort 3 osteotomy. The root of the nose is sectioned horizontally into the medial orbital wall; the osteotomy is then continued along the medial wall behind the lacrimal sac to the inner third of the orbital floor. The lateral wall of the orbit is split in a sagittal plane, and the osteotomy is continued into the orbital floor. The osteotomy is then extended to the malar bone, and the maxilla is advanced and fixed in position by interdental wiring. For this procedure, the patient must be old enough to have primary dentition. If there are any abnormalities of the nasal structure, a rhinoplasty can be done. The advance of the forehead can be as much as 20 to 30 mm in these

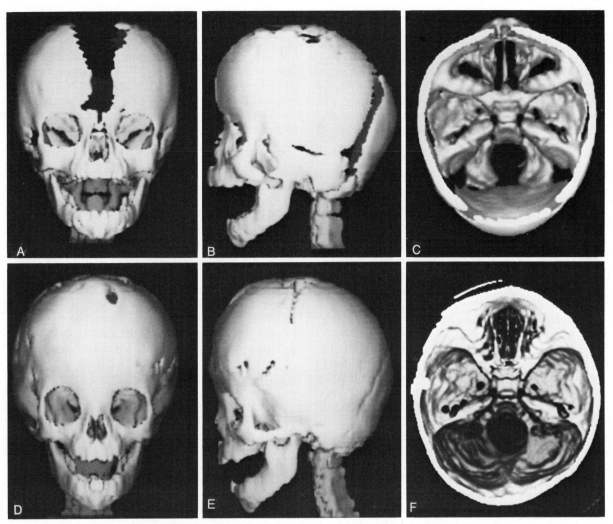

FIGURE 8–6. *A,* Coronal three-dimensional CT of infant with Crouzon's disease. Note open metopic suture. *B,* Lateral three-dimensional CT scan of patient shown in *6A.* Note closed coronal suture. *C,* Basal three-dimensional CT scan of patient shown in *6A.* Note short anterior fossa and obtuse basal angle. *D,* Coronal three-dimensional CT scan of patient shown in *5A* after bilateral lateral canthal advancement. Note normal shape of forehead. *E,* Lateral three-dimensional CT scan of patient shown in *6A* after bilateral lateral canthal advancement. Note expansion of forehead. *F,* Basal three-dimensional CT scan of patient shown in *5A.* Note expanded anterior fossa and change in basal angle to normal configuration.

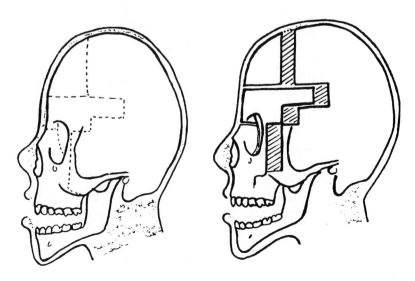

FIGURE 8–7. Diagrammatic representation of forehead and face advancement in older patient with craniofacial dysmorphism.

children, and consequently bone grafts (split skull) must be taken to fill in the defects created by the advancement. The frontal bone flap is then replaced.

Since this procedure allows free communication between cranial cavity, face, and mouth, there is significant risk of infection. Prophylactic antibiotics are used, and the wound is profusely irrigated with Betadine solution (10 per cent povidone-iodine; manufactured by The Purdue Frederick Co., 123 Sunrise Avenue, Toronto, Canada).

Trigonocephaly

Premature closure of the metopic suture results in a marked narrowing of the forehead, as if the frontotemporal region had been pinched in. When examined from above, the forehead appears wedge-shaped, and a vertical keel appears along the midline of the forehead. The lateral corners of the eyebrows tend to be elevated. The prominent medial epicanthal fold may make the eyes appear hyperteloric even though the orbits are in fact hypoteloric.[13] In more severe cases, the lateral supraorbital ridge is deficient.

The metopic suture is functional in the first 18 months of life and is completely obliterated by the age of 2 years. When closure occurs after birth, but before the age of 2 years, the abnormality is much less dramatic. Usually there is only a ridge along the metopic suture in its posterior portion, and the forehead has a normal shape. One or both of the parents may have the same finding. This form of synostosis does not require treatment.[2]

The incidence of metopic synostosis as a form of simple synostosis ranges between 10 and 16 per cent.[9] There is a male predominance in most series.[14] In our experience with uncomplicated trigonocephaly that is repaired early, the patients have normal intelligence, but metopic synostosis may be associated with underlying cerebral anomalies, and in such cases there is developmental delay. Mental retardation has been reported in six of 18 patients in one series.[15] There appears to be an association with holoprosencephaly, and in these cases there is usually a medium cleft lip as well.[16]

SURGICAL REPAIR

The entire frontal bone is removed from just above the supraorbital margin to the coronal suture. It is then fragmented, and the separate fragments are loosely applied to the dura and held there by a preserved sheet of frontal periosteum. The forehead then achieves a normal contour quickly, and with the passage of time, the orbits move out into a normal position (Fig. 8–8). In the more severe forms of trigonocephaly in which the forehead is markedly depressed above the orbits, a bilateral lateral canthal advancement may be required.

Others have advocated a procedure in which the frontal bones are removed, reshaped, and sutured to the supraorbital margins, which are advanced.[17]

Multiple Suture Synostosis

Multiple suture synostoses unassociated with craniofacial dysmorphism account for 7.6 per cent of cases of craniosynostosis in our series.[9] The head shape varies according to the sutures involved. A not infrequent combination is that of synostosis of the sagittal and both lambdoid sutures. Marked frontal bossing, ridging over the sagittal suture, and a narrow head from posterior to the coronal suture are the result. Occasionally,

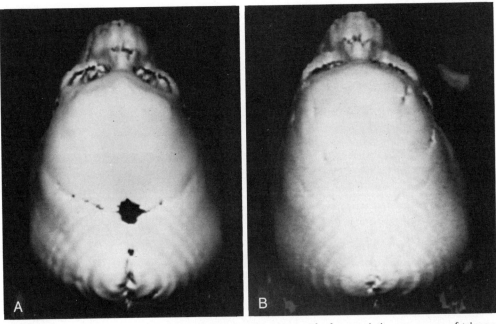

FIGURE 8–8. *A,* Vertex three-dimensional CT scan of patient with characteristic appearance of trigonocephaly. *B,* Vertex three-dimensional CT scan of same patient following repair of trigonocephaly.

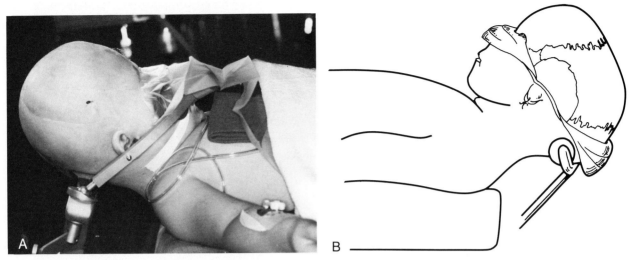

FIGURE 8–9. *A,* Patient in craniofacial headrest, which allows access to the entire calvarium. *B,* Diagrammatic representation of scalp reflection allowing access to the entire calvarium.

patients with Crouzon's syndrome initially present in this fashion, and only at a later stage do the coronal sutures fuse.

In the past, multiple suture synostoses were frequently treated in several stages. With the modern techniques of pediatric neuroanesthesia, it is possible to open all sutures simultaneously.[2] The head is supported by a special headrest applied to the cheeks and suboccipital region (Fig. 8–9A). A meisterschnitt incision is used so that the scalp can be reflected both anteriorly and posteriorly (Fig. 8–9B). Thus, it is possible to perform multiple linear craniectomies and, if necessary, a bilateral lateral canthal advancement all at the same time.

THE SYNDROMIC FORMS OF SYNOSTOSIS

Craniosynostosis occurs in the context of numerous congenital syndromes. In these patients there is often bilateral coronal synostosis and premature closure of the frontoethmoidal and frontosphenoidal suture (Fig. 8–10).[18] This combination results in premature closure of a ring around the anterior end of the skull resulting in a severe limitation of the anterior cranial fossa growth (see Fig. 8–10). The growth of the midface is determined by the growth of the floor of the anterior fossa to which it is attached, and therefore midface hypoplasia is a frequently associated finding in these syndromes. Shallow orbits and progressive proptosis also occur.

The most common syndromes encountered by the craniofacial surgeon are Crouzon's and Apert's. There are many others, and these are outlined in Table 8–2.

The most common of the craniofacial dysmorphic states is Crouzon's syndrome. It is characterized by multiple suture synostoses, maxillary hypoplasia, and shallow orbits with proptosis.[19] There is autosomal dominance inheritance. About two thirds of the cases are familial and one third are sporadic.[20] Penetrance is

either complete or extremely high. Mental deficiency occurs in about 10 per cent of untreated patients and is usually associated with hydrocephalus. This figure is lower in patients treated with early corrective surgery.[21] The most common skull abnormality is brachycephaly related to bilateral coronal synostosis with associated frontosphenoidal and frontoethmoidal closure. Other sutures may be involved.

Apert's syndrome is also characterized by multiple suture synostoses and midface hypoplasia.[22] There is symmetric syndactyly of hands and feet, and frequently there is proptosis. The facial anomalies may be asymmetric. The inheritance pattern is autosomal dominant, but most cases are sporadic. Familial cases with almost complete penetrance have been reported.[23] The syndactyly usually involves the second, third, and fourth digits of the hands and feet. Progressive calcification and fusion of the bone of the hands, feet, and cervical spine

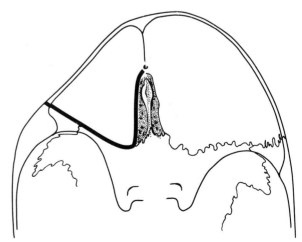

FIGURE 8–10. Diagram showing closure of frontosphenoidal and frontoethmoidal suture in patient with unilateral coronal synostosis.

occur with advancing age.[24] Mental retardation in hydrocephalus is seen more commonly in Apert's syndrome than in Crouzon's syndrome.

Pfeiffer's syndrome consists of craniosynostosis, broad thumbs and great toes, and variable partial soft tissue syndactyly of the hands and feet.[2] The inheritance pattern is autosomal dominant with high penetrance and variable expression. Associated mental retardation and hydrocephalus are rare.

Saethre-Chotzen syndrome is characterized by craniosynostosis, low-set frontal hairline, facial asymmetry, ptosis, deviated nasal septum, and variable brachydactyly and partial soft tissue syndactyly. The inheritance pattern is autosomal dominant with high penetrance and variable expression. Hydrocephalus and mental retardation are rare.[2]

Carpenter's syndrome includes craniosynostosis, preaxial polysyndactyly of the feet, brachydactyly, clinodactyly and variable soft tissue syndactyly of the hands, short stature, and obesity. The inheritance pattern is autosomal recessive. One third of patients have an associated congenital heart defect. Mental deficiency is common and is not clearly related to hydrocephalus.

Kleeblattschädel, or cloverleaf skull syndrome,[21, 25, 26] is a rare form of craniofacial dysostosis resulting in a characteristic trilobar skull configuration. This deformity can be seen in association with either Crouzon's syndrome or Apert's syndrome. In the past it was largely regarded as a curiosity, but modern craniofacial surgery may be carried out in early infancy and can restore these patients to a normal appearance with normal intellectual function.[26–28]

CLEFTS

Several failures of midline closure result in defects that come to the attention of the craniofacial surgeon.

ENCEPHALOCELE

Encephaloceles are discussed in detail elsewhere in this text. They may come to the attention of the craniofacial team when they are large, basal, or associated with other craniofacial anomalies.

Sincipital encephaloceles are divided into (1) nasofrontal lesions, which pass between nasal and frontal bone and produce a rounded, skin-covered mass in the midline of the root of the nose; (2) nasoethmoidal encephaloceles, which pass between ethmoidal, frontal, and nasal bones and appear on the side of the nose; and (3) naso-orbital encephaloceles, which pass between ethmoidal, frontal, and lacrimal bones into the anterior medial part of the orbit.[29]

The sincipital encephaloceles are associated with hypertelorism (Fig. 8–11), presumably produced by the protrusion of brain and meninges, which prevents the orbits from moving together during development. Furthermore, as the brain grows and if the encephalocele

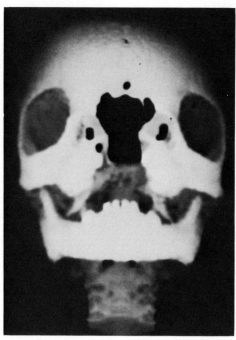

FIGURE 8–11. Three-dimensional coronal CT scan in patient with frontonasal encephalocele and hypertelorism showing defect through which the encephalocele emerged.

is not repaired, the continued pulsation of the encephalocele moves the orbits further apart.

The basal encephaloceles are associated with a split crista galli, and the encephalocele passes between the two halves of the crista galli into the nasal cavity, with no external evidence of the encephalocele.

HYPERTELORISM

Hypertelorism is a rare abnormality characterized by an increased distance between the eyes, occurring in 1 person in 60,000. Normally, during embryonic development, the eyes initially separate from the diencephalon as diverticula and migrate to a lateral position on the head as in lower animals. As the face matures, the eyes rotate forward, reducing the orbital angle from 180 degrees to 71 degrees by birth, and to 68 degrees by maturity. Therefore, hypertelorism may result not only from failure of this forward migration but also from its obstruction by congenital malformations such as encephaloceles.

In the median cleft face syndrome,[30] hypertelorism occurs in conjunction with one or more facial malformations, which include a V-shaped frontal hairline (widow's peak), cranium bifidum occultum, median cleft nose, and cleft lip and palate. Hypertelorism can also occur in association with the craniofacial dysmorphic states. Occasionally, hypertelorism is seen as a completely isolated event. In such instances, brain development and intellect are always normal.

Tessier[31] described hypertelorism according to the measured distance between the anterior lacrimal crests,

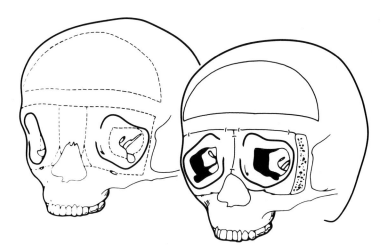

FIGURE 8–12. Diagrammatic representation of operative repair of hypertelorism.

as seen on skull x-ray films. This distance was called the intraorbital distance (IOD). IOD cannot be reliably measured on physical examination and must be differentiated from the medial intercanthal distance, which is used to diagnose telecanthus (a soft tissue problem). Age-related normal values for IOD have been published.[32]

SURGICAL REPAIR OF ENCEPHALOCELE AND HYPERTELORISM

Early attempts at treating hypertelorism consisted only of altering soft-tissue structures. In 1966, Schmid[33] described his experience with shifting the bony medial walls of the orbit. In 1967, Tessier and associates[34] described the now classic procedure for moving both orbits medially, resulting in total correction of hypertelorism.

Unlike most cranial anomalies, hypertelorism is best corrected in the older child. However, when it coexists with a frontonasal encephalocele, repair should be done early in childhood. Early in infancy, sincipital encephaloceles can be easily repaired, and surgery for the associated hypertelorism may be unnecessary.

Definitive repair of hypertelorism requires a bifrontal craniotomy, leaving a bar of bone 2.5 cm in height above the supraorbital margins[2] (Fig. 8–12). The floor of the anterior fossa is exposed back to and including the crista galli. The termination of the sagittal sinus at the foramen cecum must be divided, and the dura must be elevated off the crista galli. Where there is a fronto-nasal encephalocele, the crista galli is typically split, and the dural protrusion descends through this split. In such situations, the dura must be transected at the level of the crista galli and repaired. Through the coronal scalp incision, osteotomies can be made that free the anterior one third of the bony orbit from the skull and facial bones. Then, a carefully estimated central naso-frontal segment of bone is removed. A transverse bar of bone, 1.5 cm in height, is left intact just above the orbits, and this allows for correct horizontal and antero-posterior positioning of the orbits. The bony orbits are approximated to within a distance of 20 to 25 mm,

depending on the age of the patient. Bone grafts consisting of split ribs taken from the patient are wired into the lateral orbital walls, and the frontal bone flap is replaced. A bilateral medial canthopexy is done, and the nose is rebuilt from a bone graft. If necessary, excessive skin of the nose is removed.

ATROPHY/HYPOPLASIA

NEUROFIBROMATOSIS

In neurofibromatosis, there may be absence of the sphenoid wing. This allows contact between the temporal lobe and the soft tissues of the orbit, resulting in pulsatile exophthalmos[35] (Fig. 8–13). The dura is also deficient so that during the repair it is necessary to separate the temporal lobe from the orbital soft tissues and carry out a duroplasty. The sphenoid wing is then reconstructed from a split skull graft.

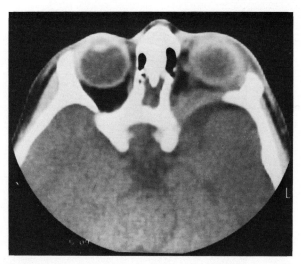

FIGURE 8–13. CT scan of patient with neurofibromatosis showing absence of left sphenoid wing with attendant exophthalmos.

HYPERPLASIA

Lymphangioma and hemangioma result in hyperplasia of adjacent tissues including skin, subcutaneous tissue, muscle, and underlying bone.[6] Primary hyperplastic disorders of bone are less common. An example is seen in Figure 8–14. This patient had thalassemia major and presented with visual loss. Investigations revealed severe hyperplastic changes of the marrow of her skull resulting in optic nerve compression.

Osteopetrosis is a hereditary disorder of bone characterized by diffuse sclerosis. Narrowing of the foramina of the skull base may lead to cranial nerve palsies, most commonly of cranial nerves II, III, and VI.[36]

DYSPLASIA

FIBROUS DYSPLASIA

Fibrous dysplasia is a disease of focal abnormal bone development of unknown etiology, in which cellular fibro-osseous tissue replaces normal bone in one or more locations. The abnormal lesions tend to expand during childhood and stabilize after puberty, although stabilization is not invariable.[37] The disease may be monostotic (limited to one bone) or polystotic (present in two or more bones) or may be associated with endocrine hyperfunction and pigmented skin lesion (Albright's syndrome). Cranial involvement occurs in 50 per cent of polystotic cases and 10 to 27 per cent of monostotic cases.[38–40] In the skull, the lesions tend to spread across sutures, but in the case of simple lesions, they are still classified as monostotic. Most commonly involved are the frontal, sphenoidal, and facial bones. Lesions are more frequent in the base of the skull than in the calvarium.

Gross enlargement of the involved bone is characteristic of fibrous dysplasia. The abnormal masses of tissue may be gritty and yellowish gray. Histologic examination reveals fibroblasts, collagen, scattered islands of cartilage, occasional giant cells, and woven bone. An ample blood supply is typical. Malignant transformation of fibrous dysplasia has been reported but is rare in cranial lesions.[12]

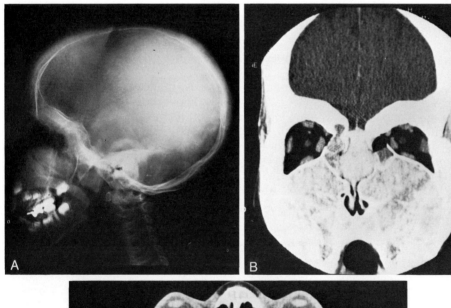

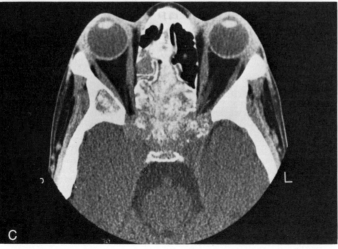

FIGURE 8–14. *A,* Lateral skull x-ray of patient with thalassemia major who presented with visual loss. Note thickening of cranial vault and base. *B,* Coronal CT scan of same patient showing thickening of the calvarium and base of skull and the hyperplastic bone in the area of the nasal sinuses. *C,* Basal CT scan of same patient showing hyperplastic bone replacing ethmoidal air cells and narrowing of optic foramina with attendant compression of optic nerves.

Radiographically, large lesions are seen as cystic or sclerotic masses expanding the bone. The affected areas may have a "ground-glass" appearance. In the skull, increased density of the base, thickening of the occiput, obliteration of the paranasal and nasal sinuses, and displacement of the orbit are typical findings.[39]

Children with fibrous dysplasia usually come to neurosurgical attention because of cranial nerve compression (most often optic or auditory) and craniofacial deformity.

Surgical management of fibrous dysplasia has three goals: (1) decompression of affected neural elements, (2) removal of all the abnormal bone, and (3) achievement of a pleasing cosmetic result. An attempt to remove all of the involved bone is necessary, as the lesion may recur and grow if a portion of dysplastic bone is left in place.

To achieve an adequate cosmetic result, we use split-thickness skull grafts to fill in the surgical bony defect. These grafts are harvested from calvarial bone not involved in the disease process. They can then be cut and molded to achieve an adequate facial appearance.[2]

CRANIOMETAPHYSEAL DYSPLASIA

Craniometaphyseal dysplasia is a skeletal abnormality characterized by bony overgrowth of the cranium and face. There is also metaphyseal widening of long and short tubular bones.[36] Cases of autosomal dominant and autosomal recessive transmission as well as sporadic cases have been recorded.

These patients appear normal at birth, but over the first year the nasal bridge begins to widen and they ultimately develop hypertelorism. The abnormality is due to a failure of resorption of the secondary spongiosa. This results in thickening and density of the cranial base, cranial vault, facial bones, and mandible (Fig.

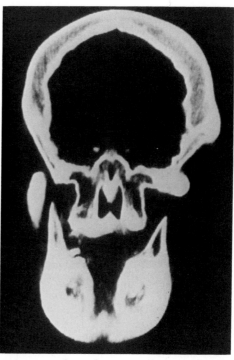

FIGURE 8–15. Coronal CT of patient with craniometaphyseal dysplasia. Note thickened cranial vault and thickened jaw in this patient.

8–15). This leads to obliteration of the paranasal sinuses and mastoid air cells. The hypertelorism is progressive, and the continued laying down of thick bone can produce a severe cosmetic deformity. Bony encroachment of the cranial foramina may lead to cranial nerve compression. Intelligence is usually unaffected.

In selected cases a craniofacial reconstructive procedure may be appropriate. Techniques similar to those described for the treatment of hypertelorism would be

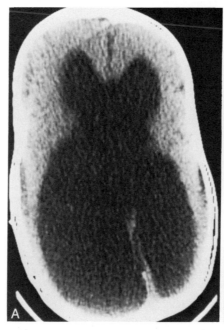
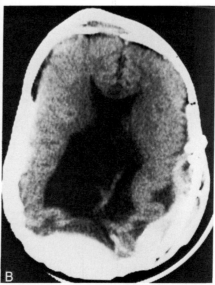

FIGURE 8–16. *A,* Axial CT scan of 2-year-old with gross hydrocephalus and craniomegaly. *B,* Axial CT scan of same patient following reduction of cranial vault and reduction of ventricular size.

incorporated. The skull is extremely thick in these cases and very hard so that high-speed drills and saws are necessary to perform the surgery.

NEOPLASIA

The craniofacial surgery team members are uniquely equipped to deal with tumors in the skull base, particularly when such tumors distort the patient's appearance. Following surgical resection of such tumors, large irregular bony defects may be created. The resection of dura beneath the involved bone may be necessary. Dural defects are repaired with cadaver freeze-dried dura. Bony defects in the base of the skull can then be reconstructed from split-thickness skull grafts.

HYDROCEPHALUS

In the poorly treated hydrocephalic patient with a markedly enlarged calvarium, the calvarium can be reduced to a relatively normal size, utilizing the existing skull for the reconstruction of the newer small calvarium (Fig. 8–16).

CONCLUSIONS

Craniofacial anomalies have become a focus of attention in recent years. Reasonable treatment is being provided at last to patients with these disorders. In the past, such patients were objects of ridicule and frequently were housed in circuses and amusement parks to be gawked at by idle crowds. Modern surgical techniques have made it possible for these patients to achieve a normal appearance and to lead a normal life.

REFERENCES

1. Tessier P: Osteotomies totales de la face, syndrome de Crouzon, syndrome d'Apert, oxycephalies, scaphocephalies, turricephales. Ann Chir Plast 12:273, 1967.
2. Hoffman HJ, Raffel C: Craniofacial surgery. In McLaurin R, Schut L, Venes J and Epstein F (eds): Pediatric Neurosurgery. Philadelphia, WB Saunders Co. 1989, pp 120–141.
3. Larsen H: DieSchadeideformat mit Augensymptomen. Klin Monatsbl Augenkeilkd 51:145, 1913.
4. Bertelsen TI: The premature synostosis of the cranial sutures. Acta Ophthalmol 63(Suppl):97, 1958.
5. Golobi M, Edwards M, Ousterhaut D: Craniosynostosis and hydrocephalus. Neurosurgery 21:63, 1987.
6. Whitaker L, Pashayan H, Reichman J: A proposed new classification of craniofacial deformities. Cleft Palate J 18:161, 1981.
7. Furuya Y, Edwards MSB, Alpers CE, et al.: Computerized tomography of cranial sutures. Part 2. Abnormalities of sutures and skull deformity in craniosynostosis. J Neurosurg 61:59, 1984.
8. Hemmy DC, David DJ, Herman GT: Three-dimensional reconstruction of craniofacial deformity using computed tomography. Neurosurgery 13:534, 1983.
9. Hoffman HJ: Congenital malformations of the spine and skull. In Goldsmith HS (ed): Practice of Surgery. New York, Harper and Row, 1980.
10. Hoffman HJ, Mohr G: Lateral canthal advancement of the supraorbital margin. A new corrective technique in the treatment of coronal synostosis. J Neurosurg 45:376, 1976.
11. Machade H, Hoffman HJ: Long-term results after lateral canthal advancement for unilateral coronal synostosis. J Neurosurg 76:401, 1992
12. Marchac D, Renier D: Le front flattant, traitement precoce de faciocraniostenoses. Ann Chir Plast 24:121, 1979.
13. Currarino G, Silverman F: Orbital hypotelorism, arhinencephaly, and trigonocephaly. Radiology 74:206, 1960.
14. David DJ, Poswillo DE, Simpson DA: The Craniosynostoses: Causes, History and Management. New York, Springer-Verlag, 1982, p 134.
15. Anderson FM, Gwinn JL, Todd JC: Trigonocephaly: Identity and surgical treatment. J Neurosurg 19:723, 1962.
16. Osaka K, Matsumoto S: Holoprosencephaly in neurosurgical practice. J Neurosurg 48:787, 1978.
17. Shaffrey M, Persing J, Delashaw J, Shaffrey C, Jane J: Surgical treatment of metopic synostosis. In Persing J, Jane J (eds): Craniofacial Disorders. Philadelphia, WB Saunders Co., 1991.
18. Seeger JF, Gabrielson TO: Premature closure of the fronto-sphenoidal suture in synostosis of the coronal suture. Radiology 101:631, 1971.
19. Crouzon O: Dystose cranio-faciale hereditaire. Bull Meme Soc Med Hop Paris 33:545, 1912.
20. Atkinson FRB: Hereditary cranio-facial dysostosis, or Crouzon's disease. Med Press Circular 195:118, 1937.
21. Holtermuller K, Wiedemann HR: Kleeblatschädel syndrome. Med Monatsschr 14:439, 1960.
22. Apert E: De l'Acrocephalosyndactylie. Bull Meme Soc Med Hop Paris 23:1310, 1906.
23. Cohen MM: Genetic perspectives on craniosynostosis and syndromes with craniosynostosis. J Neurosurg 47:886, 1977.
24. Schauerte EW, St-Aubin PM: Progressive synostosis in Apert's syndrome (acrocephalosyndactyly), with a description of roentgenographic changes in the feet. Am J Roentgenol 97:67, 1966.
25. Comings DE: The kleeblattschädel syndrome—a grotesque form of hydrocephalus. J Pediatr 67:126, 1965.
26. Muller PJ, Hoffman HJ: Cloverleaf skull syndrome. Case report. J Neurosurg 43:86, 1975.
27. Turner PT, Reynolds AF: Generous craniectomy for kleeblattschädel anomaly. Neurosurgery 6:555, 1980.
28. Zuleta A, Basauri L: Cloverleaf skull syndrome. Childs Brain 11:418, 1984.
29. Vincken PH, Bruyn GW: Handbook of Clinical Neurology. Vol. 39. Part 1, Congenital Malformations of the Brain and Skull. Amsterdam, Elsevier North-Holland, 1977, pp 219–225.
30. DeMyer W: The median cleft face syndrome. Differential diagnosis of cranium bifidum occultum, hypertelorism, and median cleft nose, lip, and palate. Neurology 17:961, 1967.
31. Tessier P: Experiences in the treatment of orbital hypertelorism. Plast Reconstr Surg 53:1, 1974.
32. Fearon J, Bartlett S, Whitaker L: The skeletal treatment of orbital hypertelorism. In Persing J, Jane J (eds): Craniofacial Disorders. Philadelphia, WB Saunders Co., 1991.
33. Schmid E: Surgical management of hypertelorism. In Longacre JJ (ed): Craniofacial Anomalies, Pathogenesis and Repair. Philadelphia, JB Lippincott Co., 1965, pp 155–161.
34. Tessier P, Guiot G, Rougerie J, et al.: Osteotomies cranio-naso-orbito-faciales. Hypertelorisme. Ann Chir Plast 12:103, 1967.
35. Hunt JC, Pugh DG: Skeletal lesions in neurofibromatosis. Radiology 76:1, 1961.
36. Kooh SW: Metabolic abnormalities of the skull and axial skeleton. In Hoffman HJ, Epstein F (eds): Disorders of the Developing Nervous System: Diagnosis and Treatment. Boston, Blackwell Scientific Publications, 1986.
37. Grabias SL, Campbell CJ: Fibrous dysplasia. Orthop Clin North Am 8:771, 1977.
38. Harris WH, Dudley HR, Jr, Barry RJ: The natural history of fibrous dysplasia: An orthopedic pathological and roentgenographic study. J Bone Joint Surg 44A:207, 1962.
39. Leeds N, Seaman WB: Fibrous dysplasia of the skull and its differential diagnosis. Radiology 78:570, 1962.
40. Windholz F: Cranial manifestations of fibrous dysplasia of bone. Their relation to leontiasis ossea and to simple bone cyst of the vault. Am J Roentgenol 58:51, 1947.

Chapter 9

ABNORMALITIES OF THE CRANIOCERVICAL JUNCTION

ARNOLD H. MENEZES, M.D., and TIMOTHY C. RYKEN, M.D.

The term "craniocervical junction" refers to the occipital bones surrounding the foramen magnum, the atlas, and the axis vertebrae. The funnel-shaped bony enclosure encompasses the medulla oblongata and the cervical spinal cord. Bony abnormalities affecting this complex can result in compression of the neural structures along the entire circumference. A constellation of congenital, developmental, and acquired lesions arises at the craniovertebral junction to produce changes that ultimately affect the neural structures.

Abnormalities of the craniocervical junction have been recognized since the late nineteenth century.[1-3] As their clinical implications became increasingly apparent, they were discussed more frequently. The clinical significance became appreciated after the classic radiographic studies on basilar invagination by Chamberlain in 1939.[4-9] The early classification of the atlantoaxial abnormalities was made by Greenberg.[10] Until then, the treatment of all bony lesions at the craniocervical junction consisted of a posterior decompression with enlargement of the foramen magnum and removal of the posterior arch of the atlas. At times, a fusion was combined with this procedure. The morbidity and mortality of such treatment with irreducible ventral lesions of the craniocervical junction were high owing to the cervicomedullary compression and its sequelae. Advances in neurodiagnostic imaging in the early 1970s and microsurgical instrumentation led to continued improvement in the treatment of such lesions.

In 1977, a physiologic approach to treatment of abnormalities of the craniocervical junction was implemented at the University of Iowa Hospitals and Clinics, based on a better understanding of the dynamics, the stability of the craniocervical region, the site of encroachment, and the associated neural abnormalities.[11] Since then, 1760 patients with neurologic symptoms and signs secondary to an abnormality of the craniocer-vical region have been investigated. Although these abnormalities may appear complex, they are easily understood and their treatment simplified if one has knowledge of the bony anatomy, biomechanics, and embryology.

ANATOMY

BONE-LIGAMENT COMPLEX

The occipital bone comprises the posterior portion of the skull and surrounds the foramen magnum. The sagittal diameter of the foramen magnum is approximately 35 mm ± 4 mm. The paired occipital condyles are located on the caudal aspect of the foramen magnum and are oval in configuration with a convexity pointing inferiorly. They are covered with cartilage and articulate with the superior facets of the atlas vertebra. The occipital condyles are partially everted and converge anteriorly. They are connected by a thin rim of bone fused to the basicranium called the condylus tertius or the third occipital condyle. A pit is situated behind each occipital condyle, which receives the posterior portion of the atlas superior articular facet when the head is extended.

The atlas vertebra (C1) is a washer between the skull and the cervical spine. It is an irregular ring and has two separate lateral masses, which form two fifths of the circumference. The superior articular facets are dorsal to the lateral atlantal masses and are oval, elongated, and deeply concave to adapt to the contour of the occipital condyles. The inferior articular facets are concave in the sagittal direction and slightly convex in the transverse plane.

The inferior and superior zygoapophysis of the atlas and the superior zygoapophysis of the axis are unique among the spinal vertebrae. This is because they are located ventral to the spinal nerve root exits. A groove for the vertebral artery is present at the rostral base of the posterior atlantal arch. The first spinal nerve runs parallel to the vertebral artery in this groove. A concave indentation on the posterior surface of the anterior atlantal arch is a site for odontoid articulation.

The odontoid process projects cephalad from the body of the axis, and its ventral surface is in contact with the anterior arch of the atlas. The atlantodental articulation is lined by synovial bursae that communicate with the bursae behind the odontoid process, thus making it a circumferential one.

The atlanto-occipital joint capsules are lax and provide poor stabilization.[12] The paired capsules are attached above the margin of the occipital condyle to attach caudal to the articular facets to the lateral masses. These capsules are reinforced laterally by the occipitoatlantal ligament passing from the transverse process to the jugular process.

The atlantoaxial complex is unique among the intervertebral joints in that it is horizontally oriented. The lateral facet joints are relatively flat and thus allow for a pivot motion at the atlantodental articulation, which is permitted by the special ligamentous support. The articular capsules of the lateral atlantoaxial facets surround the articular surfaces strengthened by atlantoaxial ligaments. There are oblique fibers that run from the tectorial membrane to reinforce this. The second cervical nerve exits from the cervical canal immediately adjacent and dorsal to the joint capsules.

The anterior occipitoatlantal and atlantoaxial ligaments are present anteriorly, and their counterparts present posteriorly.[13] The transverse atlantal ligament is 3 to 5 mm thick, originating as a band from the tubercles and the inner aspect of the atlas lateral masses. This ligament maintains close apposition to the odontoid and keeps it in proximity to the anterior arch of the atlas, permitting axial rotation. There are strong fascicles of vertical fibers that blend with the transverse ligament dorsally. The alar ligaments originate in the superior lateral aspect of the dens and insert to the medial aspect of each occipital condyle. These ligaments restrain, but do not prevent, the anterior dislocation of the atlas on the axis.[14]

The muscles that are attached to the craniovertebral complex assist in stabilization of the spine and initiate, as well as maintain, movements within the joints.[12]

Lymphatic Drainage

The lymphatic drainage of the occipitoatlantoaxial joint complex is primarily into the retropharyngeal lymph nodes and thence into the upper jugular deep cervical chain. The nodes also receive drainage from the nasopharynx, the retropharyngeal area, and the paranasal sinuses.[13] Thus, a retrograde infection may affect the synovial lining of the craniovertebral joint complex with resultant effusion, instability, and possible neurologic deficit, contributing to Grisel's syndrome.[15]

Blood Supply

There are two sources of blood supply around the craniovertebral bony complex.[16, 17] The vertebral arteries provide anterior and posterior ascending vessels, which pass both in front of and behind the bodies of the axis and the odontoid process. They anastomose in an apical arcade in the region of the alar ligament. These are the vessels that supply small perforating branches to the body of the axis and the odontoid process. The anterior ascending artery as well as the apical arcade receive contributions via the carotid and occipital arteries through the apical and alar ligaments.[18] This arrangement of blood supply has a developmental basis. The cartilaginous plates that represent the intervertebral disc between the base of the dens and the body of the axis effectively prevent the development of vascular communication between the axis and the odontoid process. This anatomic and embryologic basis of vascular supply to the axis—odontoid complex is important to our understanding of the etiology of os odontoideum and the formation of a sequestrum with a type II odontoid fracture.

Biomechanics of the Occipitoatlantoaxial Complex

The occipitoatlantoaxial complex serves as a transition zone between the vertebral joint structures and the completely different skull.[12, 14] It functions as a single unit, with the atlas serving as a "washer" between the skull and the spine. This is the most mobile portion of the axial skeleton.[19] Both the occipitoatlantal and the atlantoaxial articulations are involved with flexion and extension. Flexion is limited by the tectorial membrane and by contact between the dens and the occipital basion. Extension is restricted by the stretching of the tectorial membrane and by bony contact between the opisthion and the posterior arch of the atlas.[14, 20, 21] In a child, the amount of anterior-posterior translation that occurs between the dens and the anterior ring of the atlas is up to 5 mm. When the transverse component of the cruciate ligament has been disrupted, the alar ligaments are still intact; hence, the amount of displacement remains between 5 and 6 mm until the alar ligaments become incompetent. It is only when the alar ligaments and the transverse portion of the cruciate ligament are incompetent that a separation of more than 5 or 6 mm occurs.

The anatomic design of the occipitoatlantal articulation precludes rotation. The largest degree of rotation occurs at the atlantoaxial joint and is explained by the geometry of the articular surfaces, which is meant to allow maximum mobility. When rotation exceeds 40 to 50 degrees, an interlocking of the lateral inferior facet of the atlas over the superior articular facet of the axis vertebra occurs. If the transverse ligament becomes deficient, the anterior arch will sublux forward, producing a unilateral dislocation with an interlock at much less than 40 degrees (discussed in Chapter 23). Rotation of more than 30 to 35 degrees produces an angulation of the contralateral vertebral artery. With greater rotation, there is stretching of the vertebral artery, and at 45 degrees, the ipsilateral artery may demonstrate angulation and occlusion. This phenomenon has implications in wrestling and football injuries and in sudden rotation of a child's head, as with general anesthesia or with chiropractic manipulations. Usually, a large amount of the rotation of the atlantoaxial joint is shared by the remainder of the lower cervical spine.[22] This in vivo phenomenon is due to muscle contraction, which produces compressive forces across the cervical spine. The initial axial twist produces a threshold value that overcomes the "interlocking stiffening" of the subaxial segments, allowing for the completion of rotation.[12]

In vitro studies of the cranioverterbral junction have shown that application of small loads to the craniocervical complex results in significant rotation, flexion, and extension in comparison to the lower cervical spine. However, in vivo observation shows that this is not the case. Thus, the principal muscular action has to be held responsible for holding the head firmly to the neck and preventing abnormal excursions.[12] When the protective muscles are relaxed or inadequately developed, as in the case of a young child under general anesthesia, the craniocervical junction becomes inherently less stable than that in the adult. In children, this may also be due in part to the small occipital condyles and almost horizontal plane between the cranium and the atlas. The complete development of the occipital condyles with advancing age produces more vertical orientation of this joint space. As muscular development occurs, there is less tendency for instability at the craniocervical junction.

EMBRYOLOGY AND DEVELOPMENT OF THE CRANIOCERVICAL JUNCTION

Congenital anomalies at the base of the skull in the atlanto-occipital region involve both the osseous structures and the nervous system. The frequent occurrence of patterns with various combinations suggests an interrelationship, if not a common cause, of the origin and development. A review of the embryology outlining the developmental sequence and timing of events in this region is necessary and is simplified in Table 9–1.

Anomalies of the craniocervical junction appear to be the result of faulty development of the cartilaginous neurocranium and adjacent vertebral skeleton during the early embryonic weeks.[23] The mesoderm caudal to the basal plate condenses into four occipital somites. These are the precursors of the occipital sclerotomes. The occipital sclerotomes then fuse to form a single mass, which extends around the neural tube at the region of the foramen magnum. These sclerotomes correspond to the segmental nerves that group together to form the hypoglossal nerve, which passes through individual foramina through the bone. The first two occipital sclerotomes ultimately form the basiocciput. The third occipital sclerotome is responsible for the exoccip-

TABLE 9–1. EMBRYOLOGY AND DEVELOPMENT OF THE CRANIOCERVICAL JUNCTION (CCJ)

SCLEROTOMES	DIVISIONS	SUBDIVISIONS	FORMATIONS
Occipital 1st			
2nd			Basiocciput
3rd			Exoccipital centers (Jugular tubercles)
4th "Proatlas"	Hypocentrum		Anterior tubercle clivus
	Centrum		Apical ligament
			Apex of dens
	Neural arch	Ventral rostral	Occipital condyles, third cond.
			U-shape of foramen magnum
			Alar and cruciate ligaments
		Dorsal caudal	Posterior arch of atlas (C1)
			Lateral atlantal masses
Spinal 1st	Hypocentrum persists		Atlas anterior arch
	Centrum		Dens
	Neural arch		Posterior inferior atlas arch
Spinal 2nd	Hypocentrum disappears		
	Centrum		Body of axis
	Neural arch		Facets, posterior arch of axis

ital centers that form the jugular tubercles. The key to understanding craniocervical embryology is the "proatlas," which is the fourth occipital sclerotome.[24-26] The hypocentrum of the fourth occipital sclerotome forms the anterior tubercle of the clivus. The centrum itself, of the proatlas, forms the apical cap of the dens as well as the apical ligament. The neural arch component of the proatlas divides into ventral-rostral components and a dorsal-caudal portion. The anterior U-shaped margin of the foramen magnum is formed by the ventral-rostral component, which also forms the occipital condyles and the third condyle, which may be present in the midline. The alar and cruciate ligaments likewise are condensations of the lateral component of the proatlas. The dorsal-caudal division of the neural arch at the proatlas will form the lateral atlantal masses as well as the superior portion of the posterior arch of the atlas.

The major portion of the atlas vertebra is formed from the first spinal sclerotome and differs from the remaining spinal vertebrae in that the centrum is separated to fuse with the axis body, thus forming the midportion of the odontoid process. At an early stage a hypochondral bow is found in front of each vertebral segment and will subsequently disappear, except for the part that forms the anterior arch of the atlas. The neural arch of the first spinal sclerotome forms the posterior inferior portion of the atlas arch. The hypochondral bow of the proatlas itself may survive and joins with the anterior arch of the atlas to form a variant that, as such, may exist between the clivus or the anterior arch of the atlas and the apical segment of the odontoid process.

The hypocentrum of the second spinal sclerotome disappears in embryogenesis. The centrum forms the body of the axis vertebra, and the neural arch is developed into the facets and the posterior arch of the axis. Thus, the body of the dens arises from the first sclerotome, whereas the terminal portion of the odontoid arises from the proatlas. The inferior-most portion of the axis is formed by the second spinal sclerotome.[27]

At birth, the odontoid process is separated from the body of the axis vertebra by a cartilaginous band which represents a vestigial disc and is referred to as the neurocentral synchondrosis. This lies below the level of the superior facets of the axis and does not represent the anatomic base of the dens. The neurocentral synchondrosis is present in nearly all children below the age of 5 years and is absent after the age of 8 years. At birth, there should be a recognizable odontoid process, even though it is not fused to the base of the axis. The tip of the odontoid process is not ossified at birth and is represented by a small ossification center or ossiculum terminale, which is usually seen at 3 years of age. However, this fuses with the remainder of the dens by age 12 years.[28, 29] Should it fail to fuse with the odontoid process, it is called an ossiculum terminale persistens and is of little significance.

CLASSIFICATION OF ABNORMALITIES OF THE CRANIOCERVICAL JUNCTION

A wide variety of congenital, developmental, and acquired anomalies exist at the craniocervical junction and may occur singularly or as more than one anomaly in the same individual.[25, 29] The pathology of these abnormalities is extensive. Between 1977 and 1992, 1760 symptomatic patients with abnormalities of the craniocervical junction have been evaluated by the senior author. Seven hundred of these patients were treated at the University of Iowa Hospitals and Clinics. For purposes of understanding and discussing craniocervical abnormalities, these entities have been subdivided into separate categories under congenital, developmental, and acquired disorders (Table 9–2). It must be appreciated that there will be overlapping of etiologies with this classification.

NEURORADIOLOGIC INVESTIGATIONS OF CRANIOCERVICAL JUNCTION ABNORMALITIES

The diagnosis of craniocervical junction abnormality should be suspected when symptoms and signs referable to the brainstem, as well as the high cervical cord and cerebellum, are present.[6, 7, 27] The factors that influence treatment are (1) reducibility; (2) mechanics of compression; (3) etiology of the associated neural lesions such as syringohydromyelia, Chiari malformation, or associated vascular abnormalities; and (4) presence of abnormal ossification centers and epiphyseal growth plates with anomalous development.[27, 28] The term "reducible" refers to the ability to achieve reduction so as

TABLE 9–2. CLASSIFICATION OF CRANIOCERVICAL JUNCTION (CCJ) ABNORMALITIES

A. Congenital Anomalies and Malformations of the Craniocervical Junction
   I. Malformations of *occipital bone*
      A. Manifestations of occipital vertebra
         a. Clivus segmentations
         b. Remnants around foramen magnum
         c. Atlas variants
         d. Dens segmentation anomalies
      B. Basilar invagination
      C. Condylar hypoplasia
      D. Assimilation of atlas
   II. Malformations of *atlas*
      A. Assimilation of atlas
      B. Atlantoaxial fusion
      C. Aplasia of atlas arches
   III. Malformations of *axis*
      A. Irregular atlantoaxial segmentation
      B. Dens dysplasias
         a. Ossiculum terminale persistens
         b. Os odontoideum
         c. Hypoplasia-aplasia
      C. Segmentation failure of C2/C3
B. Developmental and Acquired Abnormalities of the Craniocervical Junction
   I. Abnormalities at *foramen magnum*
      A. Secondary basilar invagination, e.g., Paget's disease, osteomalacia, rheumatoid cranial settling, renal resistant rickets
      B. Foraminal stenosis, e.g., achondroplasia
   II. Atlantoaxial instability
      A. Errors of metabolism, e.g., Morquio's syndrome
      B. Down's syndrome
      C. Infections, e.g., Grisel's syndrome
      D. Inflammatory, e.g., rheumatoid arthritis
      E. Traumatic occipitoatlantal and atlantoaxial dislocation; os odontoideum.
      F. Tumors, e.g., neurofibromatosis, syringomyelia
      G. Miscellaneous, e.g., fetal warfarin syndrome, Conradi's syndrome

to have a normal osseous alignment, thereby relieving compression on the neural structures.[11] The direction of encroachment could be ventral, dorsal, or dorsal-ventral, as well as superior and lateral. An important association with neural abnormalities, such as the Chiari malformation and syringohydromyelia or vascular abnormalities, is taken into consideration in guiding the primary route of treatment.

The aforementioned factors are determined by plain radiographs, which must include a lateral view of the skull showing the cervical spine, the anterior-posterior or open-mouth view, and oblique views of the cervical spine. Supplementary views, such as Towne's view and the anterior-posterior projection of the foramen magnum, are done as necessary. Sophisticated pleuridirectional tomography allows the examiner to define more clearly and measure the craniocervical relationships and the dimensions. The relationships commonly visualized at the craniocervical border on the lateral projection are shown in Table 9–3.[4, 29–32] The slice thickness for polytomography is 1-mm thick sections, usually obtained with 5-mm separation to study the anterior-

TABLE 9–3.   TOMOGRAPHIC MEASUREMENTS OF CRANIOCERVICAL RELATIONSHIPS

SYNONYM	DEFINITION	NORMAL MEASUREMENTS	IMPLICATIONS
Chamberlain's palato-occipital line	Joins posterior tip of hard palate to posterior tip of foramen magnum	Tip of dens below this line ± 4 mm	In basilar invagination the odontoid process bisects the line
Wackenheim's clivus-canal line	Line drawn along clivus into cervical spinal canal	Odontoid is ventral to this line	Odontoid transects the line in basilar invagination
McRae's foramen magnum line	Joins anterior and posterior edges of foramen magnum	Tip of odontoid is below foramen magnum	When effective sagittal diameter of canal is less than 20 mm, neurologic symptoms occur
Bull's angle	Angle between Chamberlain's line and central plane of atlas	13 degrees or less	If the angle is more than 13 degrees, basilar impression is present owing to either hypoplastic clivus or occipital condyles

posterior as well as the lateral appearance of the craniocervical region. This is done in the flexed and extended positions to obtain an understanding of the biomechanics.[11] Lateral tomograms of the craniocervical region are obtained in this manner, starting from one atlas articular process and going to the other articular process. This gives an idea about the stability of the region.

Although plain tomography and computed tomography (CT) can outline the bony abnormality, cerebral spinal fluid enhancement with Iohexol utilizing the CT scan provides excellent anatomic detail of both the neural structure abnormality and the bony distortion.[27] Axial views provide confirmation in another dimension. Magnetic resonance imaging (MRI) is an ideal tool to use after plain radiographs are obtained.[33, 34] This identifies the neural abnormalities as well as the osseous compression. In the examination, flexion and extension views are required to obtain visualization in the parasagittal dimension utilizing the T1- and T2-weighted modes. The axial view supplements this. The effects of cervical traction also can be documented with MRI. Each of these techniques provides complementary information to define the craniocervical abnormality.

In all the techniques of investigation, dynamic flexion-extension studies are necessary to assess the stability and angular-osseous relationships to the neural structures to provide information regarding their reducibility and the position of fixation, should this be essential. The effects of cervical traction must be documented, not only with plain radiographs but also with MRI to confirm the relief of neural compromise and the restored relationships of the craniovertebral complex.

Vertebral angiography has been used in selected cases to identify a proven obstruction or one that occurs with dynamic changes of the craniocervical region (Fig. 9–1A through D). An unexplained neurologic sign or symptom that cannot be explained by the previously mentioned studies requires angiography. In basilar invagination with atlas assimilation and in rotational luxation of the atlas on the axis, vertebral artery distortion and occlusion are not uncommon. Information about the location of these vessels, as well as possible kinks that occur with changes in position, must be available to the treating physician before treatment is begun.

CLINICAL PRESENTATION OF CRANIOCERVICAL ABNORMALITIES

A constellation of symptoms and signs may occur as the result of compromise of the lower brainstem, cervical spinal cord, cranial nerves, cervical roots, and their vascular supply. Each step of the pathologic progression of hindbrain herniation syndromes, hydromyelia, and foramen magnum constriction due to basilar invagination presents with its own characteristic features. The list of pathologic states affecting the CCJ is extensive,[29] and these abnormalities may vary in the magnitude of neurologic dysfunction and in the pattern of association with abnormal findings exclusive of the nervous system.

The symptoms of craniocervical dysfunction may be insidious and, at times, may present with false localizing signs. In rare instances, a rapid neurologic progression is followed by sudden death. Frequently there is an antecedent history of minor trauma, which then sets off a pattern of symptoms and signs that progress at a galloping pace.[27, 35, 36] Thus, the most interesting feature of this region's pathology is the diverse presentation.[37]

Congenital abnormalities of the CCJ are often associated with an abnormal general physical appearance.[35] The head may be cocked to one side or the other, as in patients with rotary luxation of the atlas on the axis, or the classic triad of the Klippel-Feil syndrome—short neck, an abnormally low hairline posteriorly, and limitation of neck movement—may be noted.[36] In conjunction with this, there may be facial asymmetry and webbing of the neck. At times scoliosis is present. Sprengel's shoulder deformity and abnormal stature are seen in the spectrum of Klippel-Feil syndrome. It is not uncommon to see children with a small dysmorphic stature. At times, the Klippel-Feil syndrome is also associated with defects in the genitourinary, cardiopulmonary, skeletal, and nervous systems.[36, 38]

There is an increased incidence of craniocervical junction abnormalities with diseases such as achondroplasia, spondyloepiphyseal dysplasia, and the related diseases of dwarfism.[35, 39, 40]

The most common neurologic deficit, in our series of 1760 patients with craniocervical abnormalities, is myelopathy. The most common symptom is neck pain in

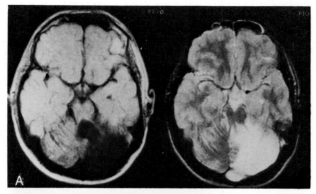

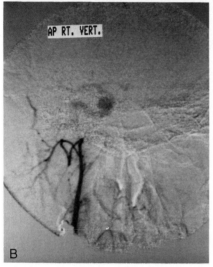
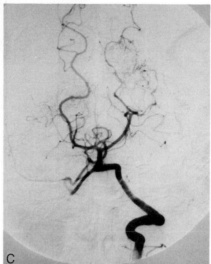
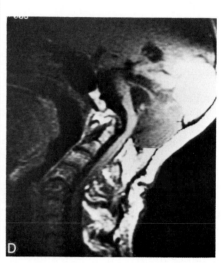

FIGURE 9–1. *A,* Composite of axial T1- (*left*) and T2- (*right*) weighted MRI through the rostral fourth ventricle. This 28-year-old male had undergone excision of a cerebellar hemispheric mass at age 10 years, which proved to be a hemorrhagic infarct. Note the residual porencephaly now. *B,* Frontal view of right vertebral angiogram. The artery stops at the C1–C2 articulation. *C,* Left vertebral angiogram with retrograde filling of the distal right vertebral artery. This stops just above the C1–C2 joint. *D,* Midsagittal T1-weighted MRI of CCJ. Note the ventral medullary compression by the odontoid invagination.

80 to 85 per cent of children, originating in the suboccipital area with radiation to the cranial vertex.

False localizing signs associated with abnormalities at the foramen magnum are usually motor and include monoparesis, hemiparesis, paraparesis, and quadriparesis. The "central cord syndrome" is often seen in children with basilar invagination in whom the myelopathy mimics a lower cervical disturbance. Taylor and Byrnes, in 1974, investigated this phenomenon and proved that the venous drainage of the central gray matter in the lower portion of the cervical cord is in an upward direction.[41] A separate venous drainage exists for the white and gray matter of the spinal cord. In compressive lesions at the cervicomedullary junction, there is a resultant venous stagnation that occurs in the lower cervical spinal cord resulting in hypoxia of the anterior horn cells, leading to a C6–C8 root dysfunction and lower cervical myelopathy.

The sensory abnormalities are usually manifested by neurologic deficits related to the posterior column dysfunction. Brainstem and cranial nerve deficits are evidenced by abnormalities such as sleep apnea and dysphagia. Not uncommonly, internuclear ophthalmoplegia is present, leading to a misdiagnosis of mesencephalic and upper pontine disturbance. Downbeat nystagmus is present in strictly compressive lesions of the craniocervical border with or without an associated Chiari malformation.

In our series, the most common cranial nerve dysfunction was a hearing loss in 20 to 25 per cent of patients. This had an increased incidence with the Klippel-Feil syndrome. A unilateral or bilateral paralysis or dysfunction of the soft palate and pharynx led to repeated bouts of aspiration pneumonia as well as poor feeding and inability to gain weight. The vascular symptoms, such as intermittent attacks of altered consciousness, confusion, and transient loss of visual fields, as well as vertigo, occurred in 15 to 25 per cent of children with abnormalities of the CCJ. At times, this was provoked by extension of the head or rotation, as with manipulation of the head and neck.

An extremely important symptom was "basilar migraine," which was not uncommon in children who had basilar invagination with atlas assimilation and compression of the medulla, as well as the vertebral basilar arterial tree. In these individuals, the symptoms completely regressed with surgical decompression of the area. The excessive mobility of an unstable occipitoatlantoaxial joint may cause repeated trauma to the anterior spinal artery as well as the perforating vessels of the medulla and upper cervical cord, leading to spasm or occlusion and the attendant neurologic deficit.

Children with nasopharyngeal infections and neck spasm or "torticollis" must be suspected of harboring craniocervical instability. This is because of effusion into the craniocervical joints and, at times, a rotary luxation of the occiput, C1, and C2.

TREATMENT OF CRANIOCERVICAL JUNCTION ABNORMALITIES

There is no single anterior or posterior operative procedure that can be used for children with craniocervical abnormalities. It is necessary to select the operation, or combination of procedures, for each patient based on a clear understanding of the pathophysiology and the functional anatomy. We now have an increased understanding of the associated craniocervical anomalies that occur with various syndromes, such as spondyloepiphyseal dysplasia, Morquio's syndrome, Down's syndrome, stippled-vertebra syndrome, and Goldenhar's syndrome. Thus, the diagnosis of these lesions in early infancy is becoming more common. The primary factor governing treatment is the ability to achieve reduction at the craniocervical junction.[11] In a reducible lesion, stabilization is paramount. Irreducible lesions require decompression in the manner in which encroachment has occurred. This treatment is further subdivided into a ventral and dorsal compression category. In the former, the operative approach is the transoral-transpharyngeal decompression or the lateral extrapharyngeal route. In the latter, posterior or posterolateral decompression is required. If instability is present after decompression, a posterior fixation is mandatory for stability.

An especially difficult problem is a very young infant with an unstable craniocervical junction, such as Goldenhar's syndrome, fetal warfarin syndrome, osteogenesis imperfecta, spondyloepiphyseal dysplasia, and allied conditions. It is essential in such situations to identify the potential for osseous development by recognizing the epiphyseal growth plates, which can be seen only on thin-section CT scanning.[27] In such infants, we have allowed growth to take place by supporting the occipitocervical region with custom-built braces, which are changed every few months according to the growth pattern. Periodically, the toddler or young child is re-evaluated with diagnostic procedures aimed at identifying the status of the craniocervical region and its neural compromise. Once adequate bone growth has been achieved, as with spondyloepiphyseal dysplasia or osteogenesis imperfecta, surgical therapy is then advanced. The operative procedure is selected as described in the previous paragraph.

Carl List (1941) was one of the earliest to recognize that both acute and chronic dislocations could be reduced—even years after the onset of symptoms.[5] Skull traction is best applied in the young child utilizing an MRI-compatible halo device. The youngest infant to tolerate a halo for traction was 8 months old. For children below the age of 2 years, it is recommended that 8- to 10-point fixation be used with finger tightening pressure. For those between the ages of 2 and 4 years, torque pressure applied is 1 to 2 pounds at the pin site. Traction is initiated at 3 to 4 pounds in the neutral position. This should not exceed the weight of the head. Reducible lesions that are the result of inflammatory states or recent trauma will respond to conservative treatment with external immobilization once reduction is achieved. Healing is usually ligamentous and, at times, may include bony reconstitution. However, if this does not occur, or if the condition is not the result of trauma or infection, a bony fixation is essential. This is best done via the posterior route.

Atlantoaxial osseous fusion requires a minimum of 3 months of immobilization. Halo immobilization for 5 to 6 months is necessary when the fusion extends to the occiput. The failure rate of this arthrodesis reaches 50 per cent when immobilization is inadequate. Wire fixation alone between the cervical vertebrae or between the skull and the cervical spine is to be avoided. Growth of the child will cause stress fatigue of the wire with resultant fracture and possible injury to the cord. There are situations in which bony fusion must be supplemented by internal stabilization. Such is the case with traumatic occipitoatlantal dislocation and with gross instability between the skull and the spine. Internal instrumentation, as with a contoured loop, must be supplemented with bone. Thus, bony fusions must be achieved at all times.

Foramen magnum stenosis and partially reducible instability are better handled from a dorsal route, where both a decompression and a fixation are possible with one procedure.

In the case of an irreducible ventral compression, the transoral-transpalatine route is utilized with the head extended and the child in traction. Thus the effect of the peg-like clivus odontoid abnormality is not exacerbated, as with the prone position. The offending pathology can be removed, including the granulation tissue. We believe that the transverse portion of the cruciate ligament should be left intact in a child. This will add to the stability of the atlantoaxial region. Craniocervical stability is tested at the end of a week. Pleuridirectional tomograms of the CCJ are obtained in the lateral planes—from facet to facet—in the flexed and extended positions. Should there be an offset of the facet joints, a fusion is made.

Results of such treatment have been encouraging. There has been no mortality or gross morbidity with the transoral, transpalatal, or extrapharyngeal route. Infection in the oropharyngeal wound is usually secondary to traumatic use of a Yankauer sucker or inadvertent placement of probes through the nares into the oral cavity. The surgical procedures utilized for this region are described elsewhere.[28, 33, 34, 42, 43]

SPECIFIC CONDITIONS AFFECTING THE CRANIOCERVICAL REGION IN CHILDREN

GRISEL'S SYNDROME

Grisel's syndrome is defined as a spontaneous subluxation of the atlantoaxial joint following parapharyngeal infection.[15] This unilateral or bilateral subluxation of the atlas on the axis vertebra is associated with an infectious process.[44] The pathology of inflammatory subluxation seen in this syndrome has been ascribed to metastatic inflammation causing ligamentous stretching and subluxation, muscle spasm, and regional hyperemia with decalcification of ligamentous structures.[45–47] More recently, Parke described a parapharyngeal-paravertebral venous complex that could provide a direct hematogenous route for inflammatory exudates to access the atlantoaxial articulations.[48] These draining venous complexes allow communication of the posterior-superior nasopharynx and lateral pharyngeal recesses with a periodontal venous plexus and upper cervical epidural sinuses. Some cases of Grisel's syndrome treated by us have been associated with tonsillitis, mastoiditis, retropharyngeal abscess, and otitis media. A review of the literature shows that the majority of patients affected are children below the age of 12 or 13 years. This may be explained by the greater ligamentous laxity and vascularity of the atlas in the pediatric population.[10, 27, 48] Wilson, in 1987, reviewed 62 cases of nontraumatic subluxation of the atlantoaxial articulation that fulfilled the otolaryngologic criteria of Grisel's syndrome.[49] This included 14 children following surgical procedures for tonsillectomy, adenoidectomy, mastoiditis, and resection of a pharyngeal rhabdomyosarcoma. Twelve children had symptoms of pharyngitis or cervical adenitis, seven had tonsillitis, and seven harbored cervical abscesses. There were five children who had acute rheumatic fever and four with acute mastoiditis. Several patients were assigned the diagnosis of nonspecific parapharyngeal infection. The neurologic deficit may range from paresthesias to quadriplegia, suggesting compression of the cervicomedullary junction or arterial compromise.

The treatment of such lesions consists of precise visualization of the area by means of MRI and elimination of the source of infection, once stabilization is achieved with either a sterno-occipitomandibular immobilizer (SOMI) brace or halo vest used for immobilization. In the acute stage, a Philadelphia collar can be applied to allow careful monitoring of respiratory function. Once the source of infection has been treated and there is no evidence of retropharyngeal swelling, further diagnostic procedures are indicated to obtain a definition of the instability and possible rotational abnormalities; these are corrected by traction, derotation, and immobilization. Rarely is it necessary to perform a fusion. This has not been necessary in any of the 16 children in our series.

KLIPPEL-FEIL SYNDROME

It is extremely important that the physician taking care of children with the Klippel-Feil syndrome be conversant with the entire spectrum of potential abnormalities, which should be monitored in the developing child. The classic triad of short neck, low posterior hairline, and limitation of neck movement occurs in approximately 50 per cent of patients.[35, 36, 38] Associated with this syndrome are segmentation anomalies of the spine such as fused vertebrae, hemivertebra, assimilation of the atlas, and spina bifida occulta. Atlas assimilation, associated with segmentation failures of the second and third cervical vertebrae, has a potential for atlantoaxial instability that may evolve into the much-feared basilar invagination. Scoliosis has been identified in approximately 50 per cent of reported cases.[50–52]

The other congenital abnormalities described with the Klippel-Feil syndrome include developmental anomalies of the head such as cleft face, deafness of mixed hearing type, lid ptosis, high-arch palate, Duane's contracture of the lateral rectus muscle, and facial palsies.[28, 53–57] The cardiovascular abnormalities include patent ductus arteriosis, ventricular septal defect, mitral valve disease, and coarctation of the aorta. Pulmonary abnormalities occur in approximately 18 to 20 per cent of individuals and include failure of lobe development and ectopic lungs secondary to deformed trunk and rib fusions. Abnormalities of the urogenital tract occur in 30 per cent of individuals, the most common being unilateral kidney, horseshoe kidney, and ectopic kidney. Other associated abnormalities include an elevation of the deformed scapula described as Sprengel's deformity, syndactyly, and (less commonly) an absent ulnar nerve.

The hearing loss is generally of a mixed type and may occur in 18 per cent of cases. A Mondini cleft has been reported in some children.

It is imperative that these abnormalities and their underlying state be recognized early to avoid sudden surprises once appropriate therapy has been initiated.

ASSIMILATION OF THE ATLAS

Defined as failure of segmentation between the fourth occipital sclerotome and the first spinal sclerotome,[27, 58–61] this anomaly occurs in 0.25 per cent of the population and may be bilateral, unilateral, segmental, or focal. In most instances it occurs in conjunction with other abnormalities such as basilar invagination and the Klippel-Feil syndrome. In the series published by McRae and Barnum in 1953, there was fusion between the second and third cervical vertebrae in 18 of 25 patients with atlas assimilation.[58] In our series, reviewed in 1988, 99 such patients were detected among 890 patients with craniocervical junction abnormalities.[27, 33] There were 32 segmentation failures between the second and third cervical vertebrae. In all these patients, a Chiari malformation existed (Fig. 9–2A through D). In addition, the Chiari malformation was seen in 42 of 99 patients with assimilation of the atlas. Paramesial invagination was present in 12 of 42 patients with Chiari malformation. A reducible atlantoaxial instability or reducible basilar invagination was present in 15 of 18 children below the age of 14 years. As age progressed, the lesion became irreducible. In partially reducible lesions, there was prolific granulation tissue around the dislocation. In those individuals in whom an irreducible lesion was present, the granu-

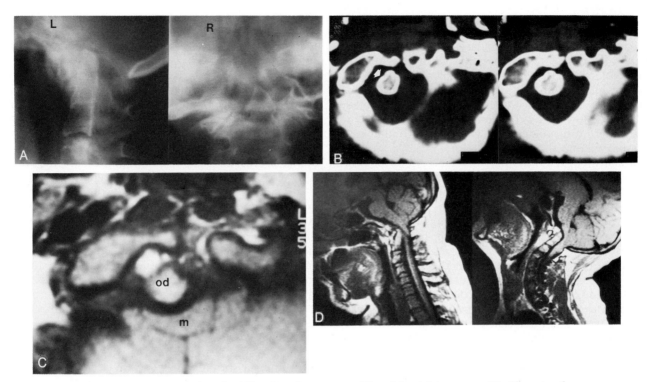

FIGURE 9–2. *A,* Composite of midline lateral tomogram (L) and frontal tomogram (R). There is atlas assimilation and odontoid invagination. This female always had nasal speech and recently complained of headaches, difficulty in swallowing, and hearing loss with weakness. *B,* Composite axial CT scan through foramen magnum. Note the odontoid invagination (*small arrow*) as well as the clefted clivus. *C,* T1-weighted axial MRI through posterior fossa. Note the compressed medulla (m) by the invaginated odontoid (od). *D,* Composite of flexion/extension midsagittal T2-weighted MRI. There is a hindbrain malformation. The MRI shows no change in the compression.

lation tissue was tough and fibrotic. The irreducible basilar invagination was associated with a horizontally oriented clivus and abnormal grooving behind the occipital condyle; the lateral masses of the axis vertebra fit into this groove. There is inability to move in a rostral-caudal dimension or in the sagittal plane.

In view of the findings described above, we strongly believe that assimilation of the atlas combined with segmentation failure between the second and third cervical vertebrae results in progressive laxity of the atlantodental joint and development of luxation between the atlas and the axis in childhood. Thus, a progressive proliferation of granulation tissue occurs secondary to the instability. Remodeling occurs at the inferior surface of the foramen magnum, which is composed of the occipital condyles, as well as the unsegmented atlas vertebra. This leads to an irreducible state with a newly formed socket attended to by the ball-like configuration of the superior facet of the axis vertebra placed in an abnormal position behind the occipital condyle and within the socket formed by the structures of the assimilated atlas. The odontoid invagination then combines with the abnormal clivus, leading to progressive neural compromise and thus causing these children to become symptomatic as adolescents. This finding has now been seen in 290 of the 1760 individuals whom we have evaluated for craniocervical anomalies.

Acute trauma (as with flexion-extension injuries) and chronic trauma (resulting from loads being carried on the head, as in developing countries) have been implicated in precipitating symptoms of atlantoaxial instability. This has been named "congenital atlantoaxial subluxation." Unfortunately, the stage had been set by the developmental abnormality, and the condition should be considered a developmental phenomenon rather than a congenital one.

Irregular segmentation of the atlas or the axis may be associated with assimilation or unilateral fusion between the axis and the atlas vertebrae. These fusions are not common and may be associated with other anomalies in the spine.

BASILAR INVAGINATION

This is a primary developmental defect implying prolapse of the vertebral column into the skull at the base.[25, 27] It is frequently associated with developmental bony anomalies of the region such as blocked vertebra, defects of fusion of the atlas, and occipitalization.[5–7, 25, 62, 63] The common manifestations of neurodysgenesis are the Chiari malformation and syringohydromyelia, which occur in 25 to 30 per cent of patients with basilar invagination.

The term "basilar invagination" was used by Chamberlain in 1939 as a synonym for platybasia. In addition, "basilar impression" has been used interchangeably with the latter. Basilar impression, an acquired form of basilar invagination secondary to softening of the skull,[28, 57] occurs in hyperparathyroidism, Paget's disease, osteogenesis imperfecta, rickets, Hurler's syndrome, and the Hajdu-Cheney syndrome.[64–71] Platybasia, on the other hand, refers to an abnormal obtuse basal angle formed by the clivus and the anterior skull base. There are no signs or symptoms attributable to platybasia alone.

Basilar invagination implies involvement of the basi-occiput and the exoccipital bones, as well as the squamous occipital bone. Thus, there are two types of basilar invagination. In the anterior or ventral variety, there is a shortening of the basiocciput so that the clivus is short. The clivus may be horizontally oriented, thus displacing the plane of the foramen magnum in an upward direction compared to the spinal column. This may be associated with platybasia. In this situation, the Bull's angle is more than 13 degrees. In the second type of basilar invagination, termed paramedian invagination, there is an associated hypoplasia of the exoccipital bones. Condylar hypoplasia may be present so that the clivus becomes dorsally displaced into the posterior fossa and may be of normal length. Unfortunately, the occipital hypoplasia may be unilateral, thus leading to torticollis. The clivus invagination is compensated for by an excessive downward curvature of the lateral squamous occipital bone. The distinction between these two types is not as clinically rigid as initially thought, since a mixture often occurs (Fig. 9–3A and B).

Basilar invagination should be suspected when the lateral atlantoaxial articulations cannot be visualized in the open-mouth projection cervical radiograph. The reference lines have been enumerated in Table 9–3.

In our series, if the effective sagittal diameter of the foramen magnum is less than 19 mm (normal 35 ± 4 mm), neurologic deficit is usually present. Basilar invagination is commonly associated with an abnormal odontoid process invaginating into the posterior fossa. However, of significance is the abnormal clivus odontoid articulation, which may occur with abnormalities of the hypochondral bow associated with the first spinal sclerotome. This resultant abnormal clivus canal angle is then less than 127 degrees (Fig. 9–3A). It produces an indentation on the pons or the medulla or the cervicomedullary junction in a ventral dimension. This is then irreducible. Symptomatic patients will require an attempt at cervical traction via the MRI-compatible halo ring. Basilar invagination associated with a Chiari malformation is not uncommon.[27, 72–74] Should a Chiari malformation be present with ventral compression of the cervicomedullary junction by a bony abnormality, a ventral decompression must be performed prior to the posterior surgical procedure. The ability to reduce the invagination is age related, as previously described under the atlas assimilation. The presence of a syringohydromyelia should not sway the treating neurosurgeon toward performing a posterior operative procedure. Most of the syringohydromyelia will disappear once the ventral abnormality has been corrected. This is due to the equalization of the abnormal craniospinal CSF dynamics whereby the CSF flow would now be restored to its normal values. In addition, the bony compression is reduced, leading to an improved neurologic state. If a posterior decompression is performed first, a significant number of these children will show

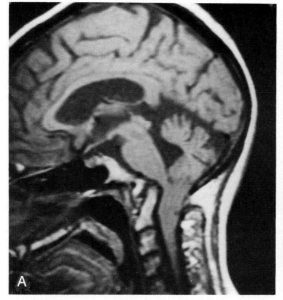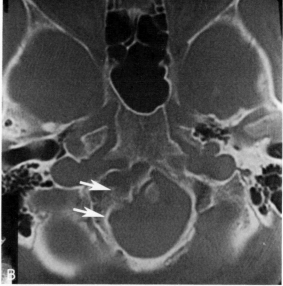

FIGURE 9–3. A, Midsagittal T1-weighted MRI in a 15-year-old girl with "basilar migraine" and tinnitus. She was weak in the arms and hyperreflexic. There is an acute angle between the clivus and odontoid with pontomedullary compression. The cerebellar tonsils and "medullary buckle" extend to the C2–C3 interspace. B, Axial CT through plane of foramen magnum with bone window imaging. Note the unilateral atlas assimilation (arrows) and paramesial invagination (narrow side to side). The clivus is short.

no improvement or a progressive deterioration of brainstem and high cervical cord function. Posterior decompression and rerouting of CSF pathways should be performed prior to a cervical fusion after the ventral pathology has been corrected.

Basilar impression is the consequence of disease leading to bone softening. This may result in steonosis of the foramen magnum and high cervical cord. In addition, fibrous bands may be present with dural adhesions of the dorsal cervicocranial junction. Treatment consists of recognition of the underlying pathology, relief of the compression, and prevention of further complications by fusion or bracing. Secondary basilar invagination, as occurs with early osteogenesis imperfecta or the Hajdu-Cheney syndrome with acro-osteolysis, re-

quires bracing as early as possible, preferably with a Minerva-style or custom-fitted brace. The youngest patient we have seen with this condition was a newborn.

The skeletal dysplasias deserve special mention and will be addressed separately.

ANOMALIES OF THE ODONTOID PROCESS

Aplasia-Hypoplasia of the Dens. This anomaly may be expressed in several degrees so that the rudimentary dens may be present or completely absent. The cruciate ligament is incompetent, leading to atlantoaxial instability (Fig. 9–4A through E). Extensive hypoplasia may be combined with developmental forms

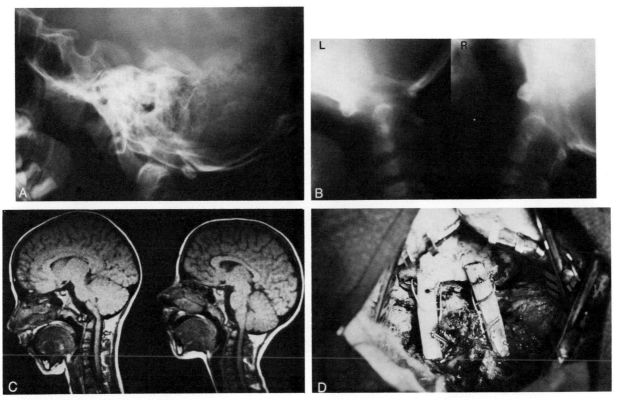

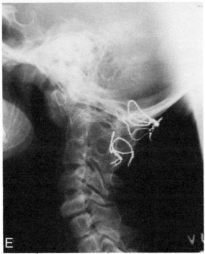

FIGURE 9–4. *A,* Lateral skull radiograph of an 8-year-old girl with occipital and neck pain. Note the atlantoaxial dislocation with a hypoplastic odontoid and atlas assimilation. *B,* Composite of lateral midline CCJ tomograms in the flexed (L) and extended (R) positions. Note the hypoplastic dens and the C1–C2 instability. *C,* Composite of midsagittal MRI of skull with cervical spine in flexion (L) and extension (R). There is less compression of the cervicomedullary junction in extension than in flexion. This reduced in traction. *D,* Operative photograph illustrating axial occipitocervical (O–C2) fusion using autologous rib grafts and wire. *E,* Lateral cervical spine radiograph made 6 months after O–C2 dorsal fusion.

of os odontoideum. Significant vascular compromise, from stretching and distortion of the vertebral arteries, has been seen with such lesions. Chronic atlantoaxial dislocation, in this situation, may result in the formation of granulation tissue at the site of the luxation, with compression of the cervicomedullary junction.[29, 43, 57]

Os Odontoideum. This term was first coined by Giacomini in 1886.[1] It refers to an independent bone, seen cranial to the axis, in place of the dens. It is not an isolated dens, but exists apart from a hypoplastic dens. Radiographically, the os odontoideum has rounded, smooth cortical borders that are separated by a variable gap from a small odontoid process. It is usually located in the position of the normal odontoid tip or near the basiocciput in the area of foramen magnum, where it may fuse with the clivus (Fig. 9–5A through C).[75] The gap between the free ossicle and the axis usually extends above the level of the axis superior facets. This leads to incompetence of the cruciate ligament and subsequent atlantoaxial instability. There are two varieties of os odontoideum, the orthotopic variety and the dystopic variety. In the orthotopic category, the ossicle lies in the position of the normal dens and moves in unison with the atlas and axis vertebrae. In the dystopic os odontoideum, the ossicle lies near the inferior end of the clivus and may fuse with the occipital bone; at times, it may move in unison with the clivus.

It may be difficult to distinguish radiologically between an os odontoideum and an old odontoid fracture. In the traumatic nonunion, the gap between the fracture fragments is charcteristically narrow and irregular and extends into the body of the axis below the level of the superior facets of the axis vertebra. The bone fragments appear to have no cortical margin or rounded appearance, and the fragments appear to "match."

The biomechanics of os odontoideum needs to be carefully studied, since it is varied.[27, 75] The movement of the os odontoideum is individual with each patient and cannot be extrapolated to others. In the dystopic os odontoideum, dorsal compromise of the spinal cord may occur by the ventral position of the posterior arch of the atlas in the flexed position, as well as ventral compromise by the odontoid ossicle (Fig. 9–6A and B).

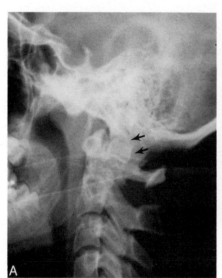

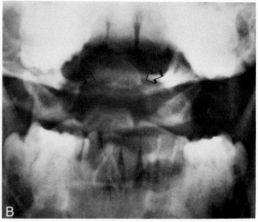

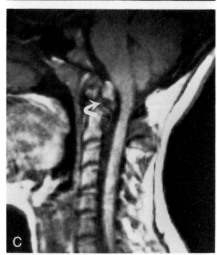

FIGURE 9–5. *A,* Lateral cervical spine radiograph. There is an os odontoideum present projecting below the clivus into the ventral spinal canal *(arrows). B,* Open-mouth view of odontoid process. There is a separate ossicle (os odontoideum) above an odontoid stub. *C,* Midsagittal T1-weighted MRI of CCJ. There is compression of the CMJ by the os odontoideum *(curved arrow).*

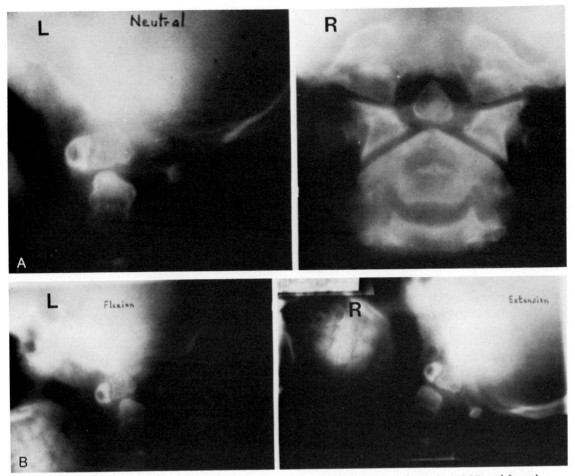

FIGURE 9–6. *A,* Composite of midline lateral tomogram (L) of craniocervical junction (CCJ) and frontal tomogram through the plane of the odontoid (R). There is a dystopic os odontoideum, with rounded borders attached to the C1 anterior arch. *B,* Composite of midline lateral CCJ tomograms in flexion (L) and extension (R). Note the abnormal motion and relationships of the entire CCJ complex.

The clivus, at times, may be displaced dorsally in extension and increase the ventral compromise. Thus, each case has to be carefully assessed by means of flexion-extension MRI and polytomography. In the orthotopic os odontoideum, the cruciate ligament appears to be functional since the transverse component can be brought into play.

Direct pathologic examination of the area at the time of ventral decompressive surgery has shown that an irreducible state may be caused by slippage of the transverse portion of the cruciate ligament beneath the ossicle and, at times, even in front of it. In addition, intense granulation proliferation may occur ventral to the bone defect owing to repeated luxations. This leads to an irreducible state. In severe chronic dislocation, this may become fixed over several years with severe basilar invagination. Os odontoideum, at its worst, has significant implications regarding the compression of the cervicomedullary junction. There is no question that in situations in which there are neurologic symptoms and signs, therapy is mandated. However, the most difficult question to answer is whether an asymptomatic child, recognized as having an os odontoideum

on a routine cervical spine radiograph after head trauma, should undergo treatment. It is not uncommon for children who are asymptomatic with os odontoideum to have severe neurologic deficit following minor trauma, as with dental work, sports activity, and gymnastics.[75, 76] The tenuous ligamentous stability becomes disrupted at this point. The patient then becomes symptomatic, and craniocervical dynamic studies show cervicomedullary compression due to the instability. We believe that all patients with recognizable instability at the craniocervical junction and associated os odontoideum should undergo stabilization. Evidence favors an unrecognized fracture in the region of the base of the odontoid as the most common cause of os odontoideum and less often a congenital origin.[75–82] Following fracture of the odontoid in early childhood or acute ligamentous injury, a separation takes place. With time and contracture of the alar ligaments, a distraction force pulls the odontoid fragments away from the centrum of the axis and toward the occipital bone. The blood supply of the odontoid is easily traumatized and may contribute to poor healing or callous formation that would now retard closure of the gap. The ossicle is then supplied through the proximal arterial arcade; and this could also account for the hypertrophy of the anterior atlantal arch, which shares the same blood supply. There is now increasing evidence that os odontoideum is more frequently associated with trauma, upper respiratory infections, bony abnormalities such as the spondyloepiphyseal dysplasia and Morquio's syndrome, and Down's syndrome.[83–90]

DOWN'S SYNDROME

In 1866, John Langdon Down published the first comprehensive review of the syndrome that has subsequently borne his name.[91] The phenotypic features of Down's syndrome are easily recognized and include characteristic facial features, hypotonia, ligamentous laxity, mental retardation, and transverse palmar creases. Associated manifestations and complications involve almost every organ system. This syndrome is the most common recognized chromosomal abnormality in man, the incidence being 1 in 700 live births. Craniovertebral instability in Down's syndrome has received increasing interest since the report by Spitzer of occipitoatlantal dislocation in 9 of 26 patients investigated with Down's syndrome.[92] However, atlantoaxial instability in Down's syndrome has been the most described after the initial publication by Tishler and Martel in 1965.[93]

Interest in the etiology of ligamentous laxity, radiographic assessment, and the natural history of atlantoaxial and occipitoatlantal instability in Down's syndrome led to the realization that atlantoaxial instability occurred in approximately 14 to 24 per cent of patients, although the incidence of symptomatic atlantoaxial instability was believed to be less than 1 per cent.[93–96] The prevalence of bony anomalies, such as os odontoideum, ossiculum terminale, hypoplastic odontoid process, and rotary atlantoaxial luxation, in patients with Down's syndrome has caused some concern regarding their participation in the Special Olympics. The Committee on Sports Medicine of the American Academy of Pediatrics recommended, in 1984, that operative stabilization of the cervical spine should be considered when the atlantodental space is greater than 4.5 mm.[97] Subsequently, several series reporting on the incidence of atlantoaxial instability and the extreme lack of attendant neurologic signs and symptoms have resulted in the unfortunate feeling that these children do not require surgical stabilization. To add to this misconception, there were pessimistic reports on the outcome of arthrodesis of the cervical spine in patients with Down's syndrome.[98, 99] This attitude has resulted in several unfortunate situations (Fig. 9–7A and B). We have reviewed our experience, between 1979 and 1991, with 18 symptomatic patients with Down's syndrome and cervicomedullary compromise. There were 11 males and seven females. A fixed atlantoaxial luxation was seen in eight patients, of whom five developed precipitous onset of cervicomedullary compression. Occipitoatlantal instability was present in nine, and an associated rotary luxation was present in nine. The average predental space was 8 mm in the neutral position in 18 individuals. Two adolescents had previously undergone atlantoaxial dorsal fusion with subsequent progressive basilar invagination due to unrecognized

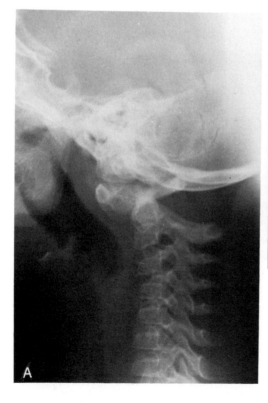

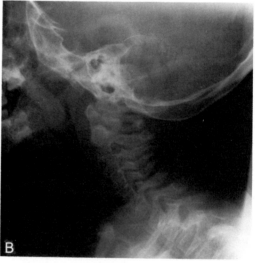

FIGURE 9–7. *A,* Severe atlantoaxial luxation (C1–C2) in a 4-year-old with Down's syndrome recognized at age 3 years. The patient awoke with quadriparesis after general anesthesia for myringotomies. *B,* The C1–C2 dislocation is reduced in extension.

occipitoatlantal instability. Os odontoideum was seen in three of 18 children. An irreducible invagination was present in two and was treated by anterior decompression followed by dorsal occipitocervical fixation. The occipitocervical fixation was utilized in ten individuals. Atlantoaxial dorsal fusion was made in seven, and two patients with acute rotary luxation of C1 and C2 were treated with immobilization alone. Halo immobilization in two individuals, following a dorsal occipitocervical fixation, produced anterior fusion at the craniovertebral complex, indicating active vertebral ligamentous pathology. The results of stabilization were felt to be excellent. The technique of occipitocervical fusion and atlantoaxial fixation has been described elsewhere.[11,26,29] Bilateral interlaminar fusion was accomplished utilizing full-thickness rib as donor bone, individually secured to the lateral portion of the laminae of C1 and C2 by transfixion of the donor bone graft with sublaminar wire, which allowed for spacing and prevention of flexion, extension, and lateral rotation. An extension of this procedure anchored the occipital squama when an occipitocervical fixation was mandated.

The immune system in Down's syndrome patients has been implicated in the increased prevalence of respiratory infections and of acute lymphocytic leukemia.[98, 99] Studies of the polymorphonuclear phagocytic system of patients who have Down's syndrome have shown impaired monocyte and neutrophil chemotaxis and a decreased ability to undergo phagocytosis. The T cell–dependent limb of the immune system has also been shown to have quantitative and qualitative deficiencies with decrease in the number of T lymphocytes. The functional capacity of the lymphocytes is also diminished by the decreased synthesis of lymphokines and the secretory products of these cells. It is believed that these products may affect the initial inflammatory stage of bone graft incorporation. The ultimate result is that the patient's ability to mount an effective initial inflammatory host response is impaired, and the bone graft ultimately does not become incorporated. This may be the reason these individuals have a high failure of fusion.

From review of the literature, as well as our own series, we strongly believe that the presence of cranial settling, reducible basilar invagination, and anterior-posterior or lateral cranial dislocation of the spine are indications for occipitocervical fixation. Atlantoaxial fusion is performed in individuals in whom the instability is limited to C1 and C2. Failure to maintain proper immobilization results in "nonunion, resorption of the graft, and progressive dislocation."

SKELETAL DYSPLASIAS

The practical approach to skeletal dysplasias in infancy was formulated by Dutton based on the international nomenclature of constitutional disease of the bone.[100] Many authors have attempted to clarify the older well-known titles of dysplasias, which now fall into the category of skeletal dysplasias. Skeletal dysplasias are divided into five large categories: (1) osteochondral dysplasia; (2) dysostosis; (3) idiopathic osteolysis; (4) chromosomal abberrations; and (5) primary metabolic abnormalities.[101–105]

The osteochondral dysplasias and dysostosis account for the largest and most complex entities. Each category is further subdivided into numerous subcategories and individual diagnoses. Osteochondral dysplasias are defined as abnormalities of cartilage or bone growth in development. This category includes achondrogenesis, thanatophoric dysplasia, chondrodysplasia punctata (Conradi-Hünermann syndrome), achondroplasia, dystrophic dysplasia, metatrophic dysplasia, spondyloepiphyseal dysplasia, Kniest dysplasia, cleidocranial dysplasia, and multiple epiphyseal dysplasias.

The dysostoses are defined as malformations of individual bones singly or in combination. This category may include Crouzon's, Apert's, and Carpenter's syndromes with vertebral defects. This category also will include Sprengel's deformity and Klippel-Feil syndrome.

The subcategory of idiopathic osteolysis includes the diagnosis of spondyloepiphyseal dysplasia tarda, fibrous dysplasia, neurofibromatosis, osteogenesis imperfecta, and multicentric forms such as the Hajdu-Cheney form.

The primary metabolic and chromosomal abnormalities are numerous. The metabolic abnormalities include problems with calcium or phosphorus metabolism, such as rickets and pseudohypoparathyroidism. Abnormalities of calcium and phosphorous metabolism will lead to bone softening and a secondary form of invagination. This may be paramesial, which is common, with achondroplasia in which the sagittal diameter of the foramen magnum is preserved while the transverse diameter is markedly reduced. In addition, an inward bending of the exoccipital bone results in further invagination and creation of a dural shelf, which compresses the dorsal cervicomedullary junction. Thus, in these syndromes, posterior decompression is necessary with a duraplasty (Fig. 9–8A through C). Upper cervical and spinal stenosis is a well-known entity with such syndromes as achondroplasia and Morquio's syndrome.

Atlantoaxial instability occurs with increasing incidence in the skeletal dysplasias.[105–113] In patients with achondroplasia, we have noted cervicomedullary compromise most frequently in those under the age of 3 years. Sleep apnea has been a major symptom, as well as progressive spastic quadriparesis. In this situation, CT myelography with Iohexol has permitted visualization of the compression at the foramen magnum as well as at C1 and C2. There is an inward bending of the posterior arch of the atlas, further compromising the stenosis. Prior to embarking on therapy, one must ascertain that proper attention has been given to hydrocephalus, should this be present.

Spondyloepiphyseal dysplasia is a complex disorder when atlantoaxial instability is encountered in infancy (Fig. 9–9A and B). Our approach has been to brace the infant with a custom-built orthosis until definitive surgical treatment can be performed some time between

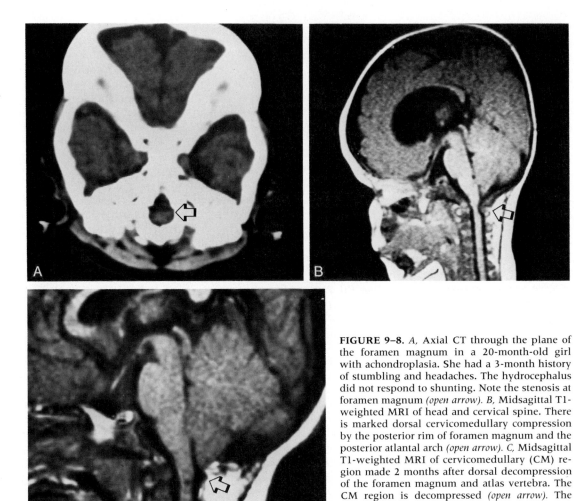

FIGURE 9–8. *A,* Axial CT through the plane of the foramen magnum in a 20-month-old girl with achondroplasia. She had a 3-month history of stumbling and headaches. The hydrocephalus did not respond to shunting. Note the stenosis at foramen magnum *(open arrow). B,* Midsagittal T1-weighted MRI of head and cervical spine. There is marked dorsal cervicomedullary compression by the posterior rim of foramen magnum and the posterior atlantal arch *(open arrow). C,* Midsagittal T1-weighted MRI of cervicomedullary (CM) region made 2 months after dorsal decompression of the foramen magnum and atlas vertebra. The CM region is decompressed *(open arrow).* The child had resumed walking.

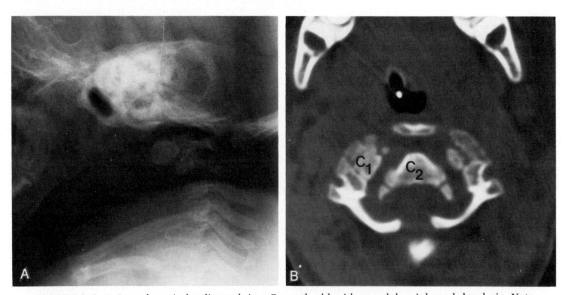

FIGURE 9–9. *A,* Lateral cervical radiograph in a 7-month-old with spondyloepiphyseal dysplasia. Note the abnormal atlas ossification and the anteriorly located C1 vertebra with occipitoatlantoaxial dislocation. She was treated with custom-fitted cervical bracing. *B,* Axial CT through atlas vertebra (C1). Note the abnormal ossifications of the lateral masses of C1 and the presence of the axis body within the atlas ring (C1–C2 dislocation). There is in-bending of the posterior arches of the atlas.

the ages of 2 and 4 years. In the individuals in whom this occurs at a later age, the treatment would be as previously outlined.

PAGET'S DISEASE

Paget's disease involving the craniovertebral junction results in basilar impression as originally described by Wycis.[114] There is a tendency to flatten the foramen magnum and diminish its anterior-posterior diameter. An axial invagination, with cranial upward migration, is the next progression and causes neural bony compression as well as changes in the CSF dynamics. It is thus not uncommon to see syringohydromyelia complicating the distorted brainstem and cervical cord. An important medical breakthrough has been the successful treatment of Paget's disease with calcitonin and diphosphate.[115-118] Although Paget's disease affects the middle-aged and elderly population with a greater prevalence in the older age group, the occasional adolescent has been seen with severe secondary basilar impression and pontomedullary dysfunction.

MUCOPOLYSACCHARIDOSIS

The mucopolysaccharidoses are primary metabolic abnormalities of complex carbohydrate metabolism. These are inheritable storage diseases often manifested by dwarfism, mental retardation, macrocephaly, corneal clouding, and skeletal dysplasia. Generalized ligamentous laxity is thought to contribute to atlantoaxial luxation described in a variety of mucopolysaccharidoses. In 1969, Blaw and Langer reviewed eight patients with Morquio-Brailford disease who had undergone neurologic follow-up.[119] All eight had roentgenographic evidence of hypoplasia or absence of the odontoid process and a thoracic gibbous formation. Four of these eight patients had evidence of cervical cord compression secondary to atlantoaxial dislocation or subluxation. Death commonly occurs from the Morquio's syndrome (mucopolysaccharidosis type IV) by age 7. This is secondary to cervical myelopathy as well as its effects on the respiratory system and resultant hypoxia. Holzgrene also described atlantoaxial instability in a review of 13 patients with type IV mucopolysaccharidosis.[120] In 1978, Brill first recognized failure of development of the dens as a cause of progressive spastic quadriparesis in Hurler's syndrome.[121] There was subluxation of the atlas on the axis, and the patient responded to traction and Minerva jacket with subsequent surgical stabilization.

Patients with type VI mucopolysaccharidosis or Maroteaux-Lamy syndrome with high cervical myelopathy have also been described.[122-124] The anesthetic complications obviously are great since a large number of these children require general anesthesia for numerous surgical procedures. A bright star on the horizon for mucopolysaccharidosis is the current success with bone marrow transplantation. This has been recognized as the treatment of choice for mucopolysaccharidoses, particularly for Hurler's syndrome. Early recognition, before the age of 3 years, has produced regression in the facial and organ features in these children with improvement also in their craniocervical anatomy. We have treated six patients who have responded to this therapy.

OSTEOGENESIS IMPERFECTA

The first description of osteogenesis imperfecta appeared in 1888, as a thesis on congenital osteomalacia by Eckman, a Swedish military surgeon (as quoted by Weil, 1981).[125] Osteogenesis imperfecta describes a group of inherited disorders characterized by excessive bone fragility with susceptibility to fracture. This syndrome has been subdivided into osteogenesis imperfecta congenita (characterized by fractures at birth or early infancy) and osteogenesis imperfecta tarda (onset of fractures in childhood). The fractures are attributed to deficiency in mineral and matrix content, decreased external volume of the bone itself, and reduction in tensile strength in each lamina of osteogenesis imperfecta bone. Impingement of the spinal cord is usually secondary to vertebral column collapse and severe kyphosis and kyphoscoliosis. Unfortunately, flattening of the vertex and prominence of the occiput with platybasia are evident because of the upward migration of the cervical spine. These changes result in an abnormal configuration of the brainstem and, in severe cases, may result in an acute flexion angulation between the midbrain and pons, and between the pons and medulla (Fig. 9–10A and B). A secondary aqueductal stenosis has been seen. The angulation of the superior cerebellar peduncles and the brachium conjunctivum leads to increased neurologic deficit.[124-130] Upper cervical cord compression as a cause of death in osteogenesis imperfecta type II has been documented by several authors.[126, 131] A variety of systemic treatments have been undertaken, including fluoride, vitamin D, calcitonin, and hormones. The incidence of osteogenesis imperfecta is 1 in 20,000 to 1 in 40,000 births.[129] Despite its apparent rarity, osteogenesis imperfecta remains the most serious form of lethal short-limbed dwarfism and crippling skeletal dysplasia. Suboccipital decompression, as described by Hunt and Decker in 1982, grants only temporary respite with subsequent full-blown brainstem dysfunction and death.[132] In such situations, it is imperative that a ventral decompression be first accomplished. This is extremely difficult via the simple transoral route and requires either a transpalatal approach, in addition, or a Le Fort I drop-down maxillotomy. Posterior decompression and occipitocervical fixation are mandatory. We have had the advantage of conducting a follow-up of two patients with osteogenesis imperfecta as they developed cranial settling. This was arrested with bracing and regression of the neurologic symptoms.

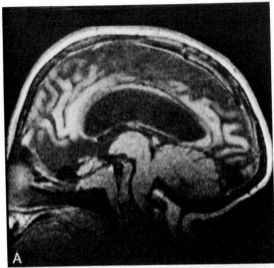

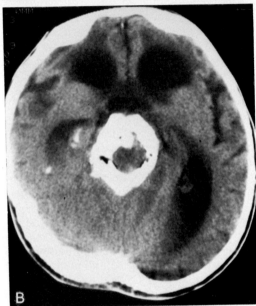

FIGURE 9–10. *A,* Midsagittal T1-weighted MRI of the head and CCJ. This 12-year-old has osteogenesis imperfecta with severe secondary basilar invagination. There is an upward in-bending of the skull base. The posterior fossa is grossly abnormal. A secondary hydrocephalus is noted. *B,* Axial CT scan of brain reveals hydrocephalus of the lateral ventricles and the third ventricle. The axis vertebra and odontoid tip are seen in this plane.

REFERENCES

1. Giacomini C: Sull' esistenza dell "os odontoideum" nell' nomo. G Accad Med Torino 49:24, 1886.
2. Macalister A: Notes on the development and variations of the atlas. J Anat Physiol 27:519, 1892–1893.
3. Gladsstone J, Erickson-Powell W: Manifestations of occipital vertebra and fusion of atlas with occipital bone. J Anat Physiol 49:190, 1915.
4. Chamberlain WE: Basilar impression (platybasia). Yale J Biol Med 11:487, 1938–1939.
5. List CF: Neurologic syndromes accompanying developmental anomalies of occipital bone, atlas and axis. Arch Neurol Psychiatry 45:577, 1941.
6. Mitchie I, Clark M: Neurological syndromes associated with cervical and craniocervical anomalies. Arch Neurol 18:241, 1968.
7. Spillane JD, Pallis C, Jones AM: Developmental abnormalities in the region of the foramen magnum. Brain 80:11, 1957.
8. Barucha EP, Dastur HM: Cranioverebral anomalies. Brain 87:469, 1964.
9. Wadia NH: Myelopathy complicating congenital atlanto-axial dislocation (a study of 28 cases). Brain 90:449, 1967.
10. Greenberg AD: Atlanto-axial dislocations. Brain 91:655, 1968.
11. Menezes AH, Graf CJ, Hibri N: Abnormalities of the craniovertebral junction with cervicomedullary compression. A rational approach to surgical treatment in children Childs Brain 7:15, 1980.
12. Goel VK, Clark CR, Gallaes K, et al.: Movement-rotation relationships of the ligamentous occipito-atlanto-axial complex. J Biomechanics 21(8):678, 1988.
13. Brasch JC: *In* Cunningham's Manual of Practical Anatomy, London, Oxford University Press, 1958, pp 258–295.
14. Werne S: Studies in spontaneous atlas dislocation. Acta Orthop Scand 23(suppl):1, 1957.
15. Grisel P: Enucleation des l'atlas et torticollis nasopharyngien. Presse Med 38:50, 1930.
16. Schiff DCM, Parke WW: The arterial blood supply of the odontoid process (dens). Anat Rec 172:399, 1972.
17. Althoff B, Goldie IF: The arterial supply of the odontoid process of the axis. Acta Orthop Scand 48:622, 1977.
18. Parke WW: The vascular relationships of the upper cervical vertebrae. Orthop Clin North Am 9:879, 1978.
19. White AA, III, Punjabi MM: The clinical biomechanics of the occipito-atlanto-axial complex. Orthop Clin North Am 9:867, 1978.
20. Jones MD: Cineradiographic studies of the normal cervical spine. Calif Med 93:293, 1960.
21. Jirout J: Changes in the atlas-axis relations on lateral flexion of the head and neck. Neuroradiology 6:215, 1973.
22. Selecki BR: The effects of rotation of the atlas on the axis: experimental work. Med J Aust 1:1012, 1969.
23. Bosma JF (ed): Symposium on Development of the Basicranium. Bethesda, US Department of Health, Education and Welfare, NIH, 1976, pp 700–710.
24. Ganguly DN, Roy KK: A study on the craniovertebral joint in the man. Anat Anz 114:433, 1964.
25. VonTorklus D, Gehle W: The upper cervical spine. Regional anatomy, pathology and traumatology. *In* Georg Thieme, Verlag (ed): Systemic Radiological Atlas and Textbook. New York, Grune & Stratton, 1972, pp 1–99.
26. VanGilder JC, Menezes AH: Craniovertebral abnormalities and their treatment. *In* Schmidek H, Sweet W (eds): Operative Neurosurgical Techniques. 2nd ed. New York, Grune & Stratton, 1988, Chapter 113, pp 1281–1293.
27. Menezes AH, VanGilder JC: Anomalies of the craniovertebral junction. *In* Youmans J (ed): Neurological Surgery. 3rd ed. Vol. 2, Philadelphia, WB Saunders Co., 1990, Chapter 45, pp 1359–1420.
28. Menezes AH: Normal and abnormal development of the craniocervical junction. *In* Hoff JT, Crockard A, Hayward R (eds): Neurosurgery—The Scientific Basis of Clinical Practice. 2nd ed. London, Blackwell Scientific Publishers, 1992, Chapter 10.
29. VanGilder JC, Menezes AH, Dolan K: Textbook of Craniovertebral Junction Abnormalities. Mount Kisco, New York, Futura Publishing Company, 1987, pp 1–255.
30. Wackenheim A: Radiologic diagnosis of congenital forms, intermittent forms and progressive forms of stenosis of the spinal canal of the level of the atlas. Acta Radiol (Diagn) (Stockh) 9:481, 1969.
31. McRae DL: The significance of abnormalities of the cervical spine. Am J Roentgenol 84:3, 1960.
32. Bull JWD, Nixon WLB, Pratt RTC: The radiological criteria and familial occurrence of primary basilar impression. Brain 78:229, 1955.
33. Menezes AH: Anterior approaches to the craniocervical junction. Clin Neurosurgery 37:756, 1991.
34. Menezes AH: Surgical approaches to the craniocervical junction. *In* Frymoyer J (ed): The Adult Spine: Principles and Practice. Vol. 2. New York, Raven Press, 1991, Chapter 46, pp 967–986.
35. Hensinger RN, Lang JE, MacEwen D: Klippel-Feil syndrome. A

constellation of associated anomalies. J Bone Joint Surg (Am) 6:1246, 1976.

36. Klippel M, Feil A: Un cas d'absence des vertebres cervicales avec cage thoracique remontant jusqu'a base du cranie. Nouv Icon Selpetriere 25:223, 1912.

37. Aring CE: Lesions about the junction of medulla and spinal cord. (Editorial) JAMA 229:1879, 1974.

38. MacEwen D: The Klippel-Feil syndrome. J Bone Joint Surg (Br) 57:261, 1975.

39. Perovic NM, Kopits SE, Thompson RC: Radiological evaluation of the spinal cord in congenital atlanto-axial dislocation. Radiology 109:713, 1973.

40. Kopits SE, Perovic MN, McKusick V, et al.: Congenital atlanto-axial dislocations in various forms of dwarfism. J Bone Joint Surg (Am) 54:1349, 1972.

41. Taylor AR, Byrnes DP: Foramen magnum and high cervical cord compression. Brain 97:473, 1974.

42. Menezes AH: The anterior midline approach to the craniocervical region in children. In McLone DG (ed): Concepts in Pediatric Neurosurgery. Basel, S Karger AG, 1992.

43. Menezes AH: Complications of surgery at the craniovertebral junction—avoidance and management. Pediatr Neurosurg 17(5):254, 1992.

44. Wetzel FT, LaRocca H: Grisel's syndrome. A review. Clin Orthop 240:141, 1989.

45. Grieg DM: Clinical Observations on the Surgical Pathology of Bone. London, Oliver & Boyd, 1931.

46. Watson-Jones R: Spontaneous dislocation of the atlas. Proc Roy Soc Med 25:785, 1932.

47. Lericke R, Policard H: Les problemes de la physiologic normale et pathologique de l'os. Paris, Mason et Cie, 1926.

48. Parke WW, Rothman RH, Brown MD: The pharyngovertebral veins. An anatomical rationale for Grisel's syndrome. J Bone Joint Surg (Am) 66:568, 1984.

49. Wilson BC, Jarvis BL, Handon RC: Nontraumatic subluxation of the atlantoaxial joint: Grisel's syndrome. Ann Otol Rhinol Laryngol 96:705, 1987.

50. Najib MG, Maxwell RE, Chou SN: Klippel-Feil syndrome in children: Clinical features and management. Childs Nerv Syst 1:255, 1985.

51. Baga N, Chusid EL, Miller A: Pulmonary disability in the Klippel-Feil syndrome. Clin Orthop 67:105, 1969.

52. Dyste GN, Menezes AH: Presentation and management of pediatric Chiari malformations without myelodysplasia. Neurosurgery 23:589, 1988.

53. Muhonen M, Menezes AH, Sawin P, et al.: Scoliosis in pediatric Chiari malformations without myelodysplasia. J Neurosurg 77:69, 1992.

54. Baird PA, Robinson GC, Buckler WSTJ: Klippel-Feil syndrome. A study of mirror movements detected by electromyelography. Am J Dis Child 113:546, 1962.

55. MacKlenburg RS, Krueger PM: Extensive genitourinary anomalies associated with Klippel-Feil syndrome. Am J Dis Child 128:92, 1974.

56. Palant DI, Carter BL: Klippel-Feil syndrome and deafness. Am J Dis Child 123:218, 1972.

57. Shapiro R, Robinson F: Anomalies of the craniovertebral border. Am J Roentgenol 127:281, 1976.

58. McRae DL, Barnum AS: Occipitalization of the atlas. Am J Roentgenol 70:23, 1953.

59. Lanier RR Jr: Anomalous cervico-occipital skeleton in man. Anat Rec 73:189, 1939.

60. Nicholson JT, Sherk HH: Anomalies of the occipitocervical articulation. J Bone Joint Surg (Am) 50:295, 1968.

61. Bystrow A: Assimilation des atlas und manifestation des proatlas. Ztschr Anat 95:210, 1931.

62. Tanzer A: Die basilare Impression. Radiol Clin 25:135, 1956.

63. Kalus E, Lehman W: Familiares vokomer bei basilarer impression. Acta Univ Palacki Olomuc Fac Med 46:115, 1967.

64. Shoenfeld Y, Fried A. Ehrenfeld NE: Osteogenesis imperfects. Review of the literature with presentation of 29 cases. Am J Dis Child 129:679, 1975.

65. Frank E, Berger T, Tew JM Jr: Basilar impression and platybasia in osteogenesis imperfecta tarda. Surg Neurol 17:116, 1982.

66. Rush PJ, Berbrayer D, Reilly BJ: Basilar impression and osteogenesis imperfecta in a 3 year old girl. CT and MRI. Pediatr Radiol 19:142, 1989.

67. Harkey HL, Crockard HA, Stevens JM, et al.: The operative management of basilar impression in osteogenesis imperfecta. Neurosurgery 27:782, 1990.

68. Kurimoto M, Ohara S, Takaku A: Basilar impression in osteogenesis imperfecta tarda. Case report. J Neurosurg 74:136, 1991.

69. Poppel MH, Jacobson HG, Duff BK: Basilar impression and platybasia in Paget's disease. Radiology 61:639, 1953.

70. Hajdu N, Kauntze R: Carnioskeletal dysplasia. Br J Radiol 21:42, 1948.

71. Cheney WD: Acro-osteolysis. Am J Roentgenol 94:595, 1965.

72. DiLorenzo N, Fortuna A, Guidetti B: Craniovertebral junction malformations—clinico-radiological findings, long-term results and surgical indication in 63 cases. Neurosurgery 57:603, 1982.

73. Driesen W, Oldenkott P, Rossi V: Results of surgical treatment of basilar impression. Acta Neurochir 15:83, 1966.

74. Gardner WJ, Goodall RJ: The surgical treatment of Arnold-Chiari malformation in adults. J Neurosurg 7:199, 1950.

75. Menezes AH: Os odontoideum—pathogenesis, dynamics and management. In Marlin AE (ed): Concepts in Pediatric Neurosurgery. Vol. 8, Basel, S Karger, 1988, pp 133–145.

76. Fielding JW, Hensinger RN, Hawkins RJ: Os odontoideum. J Bone Joint Surg (Am) 62:376, 1980.

77. Dyck P: Os Odontoideum in children: Neurological manifestations and surgical management. Neurosurgery 2:93, 1978.

78. Hawkins RJ, Fielding JW, Thompson WJ: Os odontoideum. Congenital or acquired. J Bone Joint Surg (Am) 58:413, 1976.

79. Hensinger RN: Osseous anomalies of the craniovertebral junction. Spine 11:323, 1986.

80. Hukuda S, Ota H, Norikazu O, et al.: Traumatic atlantoaxial dislocation causing os odontoideum in infants. Spine 5:207, 1980.

81. Lipson SJ: Dysplasia of the odontoid process in Morquio's syndrome causing quadriparesis. J Bone Joint Surg (Am) 59:340, 1977.

82. Riccardi JE, Kaufer H, Louis DS: Acquired os odontoideum following acute ligament injury. J Bone Joint Surg (Am) 58:410, 1976.

83. Blaw ME, Langer LO: Spinal cord compression in Morquio-Brailsford's syndrome. J Pediatr 74:593, 1969.

84. Curtis BH, Blank S, Fisher RL: Atlantoaxial dislocation in Down's syndrome. JAMA 205:464, 1968.

85. Dzenits AJ: Spontaneous atlantoaxial dislocation in a mongoloid child with spinal cord compression. Case report. J Neurosurg 25:456, 1966.

86. Finerman GA, Sakai D, Weingarten S: Atlantoaxial dislocation with spinal cord compression in a mongoloid child. J Bone Joint Surg (Am) 58:408, 1976.

87. Giblin PE, Mitchell LJ: The management of atlantoaxial subluxation with neurologic involvement in Down's syndrome. A report of two cases and review of the literature. Clin Orthop 140:66, 1979.

88. Goldberg MJ: Orthopedic aspects of bone dysplasias. Orthop Clin North Am 7:445, 1976.

89. Spranger JW, Langer LO: Spondyloepiphyseal dysplasia congenita. Radiology 94:313, 1970.

90. Menezes AH, Ryken TC: Craniovertebral abnormalities in Down's syndrome. Pediatr Neurosurg 18:24, 1992.

91. Herring JA: Cervical instability in Down's syndrome and juvenile rheumatoid arthritis. J Pediatr Orthop 2:205, 1982.

92. Spitzer R, Rabinowitch JY, Wybar KC: A study of the abnormalities of the skull, teeth and lenses in mongolism. Can Med Assoc J 84:567, 1961.

93. Tishler J, Martel W: Dislocation of the atlas in mongolism: Preliminary report. Radiology 84:904, 1965.

94. Martel W, Tishler JM: Observations on the spine in mongoloidism. Am J Roentgenol Rad Ther Nucl Med 97:630, 1966.

95. Michejda M, Menolascino FJ: Skull base abnormalities in Down's syndrome. Ment Retard 131:24, 1975.

96. Pueschel SM, Scola F: Atlantoaxial instability in individuals with Down's syndrome: Epidemiologic, radiographic and clinical studies. Pediatrics 80:555, 1987.

97. American Academy of Pediatrics Committee on Sports Medicine: Atlantoaxial instability in Down's syndrome. Pediatrics 74:152, 1984.

98. Segal LE, Drummond DS, Zanotti RM, et al.: Complications of posterior arthrodesis of the cervical spine in patients who have Down's syndrome. J Bone Joint Surg 73:1547, 1991.

99. Levin S: The immune system and susceptibility to infections in Down's syndrome. In McCoy EE, Epstein CJ (eds): Oncology and Immunology of Down's Syndrome, New York, Liss, 1987, pp 143–162.

100. Dutton RV: A practical radiologic approach to skeletal dysplasias in infancy. Radiol Clin North Am 25:1211, 1987.

101. Mackler B, Shepard TH: Human achondroplasia: Defective mitochondrial oxidative energy metabolism may produce the pathophysiology. Teratology 40:571, 1989.

102. Hecht JT, Horton WA, Butler IJ, et al.: Foramen magnum stenosis in homozygous achondroplasia. Eur J Pediatr 145:545, 1986.

103. Wynne-Davies R, Hall CM, Young ID: Pseudoachondroplasia: Clinical diagnosis at different ages and comparison of autosomal dominant and recessive types. A review of 32 patients (26 kindreds). J Med Genet 23:425, 1986.

104. Dubousset J: Cervical abnormalities in osteochondroplasia. Basic Life Sci 48:207, 1988.

105. Wong VC: Basilar impression in a child with hypochondroplasia. Pediatr Neurol 7:62, 1991.

106. Mayhew JF, Katz J, Miner M, et al.: Anesthesia for the achondroplastic dwarf. Can Anesth Soc J 33:216, 1986.

107. Scott RM: Foramen magnum decompression in infants with homozygous achondroplasia. (Letter) J Neurosurg 72:519, 1990; also Comment in J Neurosurg 70:126, 1989.

108. Reid CS, Pyeritz RE, Kopits SE, et al.: Cervicomedullary compression in young patients with achondroplasia: Value of comprehensive neurologic and respiratory evaluation. J Pediatr 110:522, 1987.

109. Shikata J, Yamamuro T, Idia H, et al.: Surgical treatment of achondroplastic dwarfs with paraplegia. Surg Neurol 29:125, 1988.

110. Hecht JT, Butler IJ: Neurologic morbidity associated with achondroplasia. J Child Neurol 5:84, 1990.

111. Aryanpur J, Hurko O, Francomano C, et al.: Craniocervical decompression for cervicomedullary compression in pediatric patients with achondroplasia. J Neurosurg 73:375, 1990.

112. Carson B, Winfield J, Wang H, et al.: Surgical management of cervicomedullary compression in achondroplastic patients. Basic Life Sci 48:207, 1988.

113. Kao SC, Waziri MH, Smith WL: MR imaging of the craniovertebral junction, cranium, and brain in children with achondroplasia. Am J Roentgenol 153:565, 1989.

114. Wycis HT: Basilar impression (platybasia). A case secondary to advanced Paget's disease with severe neurological manifestations: Successful surgical result. J Neurosurg 1:299, 1944.

115. Singer FR: Paget's disease of bone. In Avioli LV (ed): Topics in Bone and Mineral Disorders. New York, Plenum Medical Book Co., 1977, pp 121–150.

116. Melick RA, Ebeling P, Hjorth RJ: Improvement in paraplegia in vertebral Paget's disease treated with calcitonin. Br Med J 1:627, 1976.

117. Craig JB, Hodkinson MJ: Paraplegia in Paget's disease of the vertebral column. S Afr Med J 67:103, 1985.

118. Jawad AS, Berry H: Spinal cord compression in Paget's disease of bone treated medically. J Roy Soc Med 80:319, 1987.

119. Blaw ME, Langer LO: Spinal cord compression in Morquio-Brailsford's disease. J Pediatr 74:593, 1969.

120. Holzgrene W, Grope H, VonFigwrak E: Morquio syndrome. Clinical findings in 11 patients with mucopolysaccharidosis type IVA and two with mucopolysaccharidosis type IVP. Hum Genet 57:360, 1981.

121. Brill CB, Rose JS, Godmilow L, et al.: Spastic quadriparesis due to C1—C2 subluxation in Hurler's syndrome. J Pediatr 92:441, 1978.

122. Wald SL, Schmidek HH: Compressive myelopathy associated with type VI mucopolysaccharidosis (Maroteaux-Lamy syndrome). Neurosurgery 14:83, 1984.

123. Beighton P, Craig J: Atlantoaxial subluxation in the Morquio syndrome. A report of a case. J Bone Joint Surg 55:478, 1973.

124. Pizzutillo PD, Osterkamp JA, Scott CI, et al.: Atlantoaxial instability in mucopolysaccharidosis type VII. J Pediatr Ortho 9:76, 1989.

125. Weil VH: Osteogenesis imperfecta: Historical background. Clin Orthop 159:6, 1981.

126. Pozo JL, Crockard HA, Ransford AO: Basilar impression in osteogenesis imperfecta. A report of three cases in one family. J Bone Joint Surg (Br) 66:233, 1984.

127. Sillence DO, Senn AS, Danks DM: Genetic heterogeneity in osteogenesis imperfecta. J Med Genet 16:101, 1979.

128. Gertner JM, Root L: Osteogenesis imperfecta. Orthop Clin North Am 21:151, 1990.

129. Smith R: Osteogenesis imperfecta. Clin Rheumat Dis 12:655, 1986.

130. Frank E, Berger T, Tew JM: Basilar impression and platybasia in osteogenesis imperfecta tarda. Surg Neurol 17:116, 1982.

131. Pauli RM, Gilbert EF: Upper cervical cord compression as a cause of death in osteogenesis imperfecta type II. J Pediatr 108:579, 1986.

132. Hunt TE, Dekaban AS: Modified head-neck support for basilar invagination with brain stem compression. Can Med Assoc J 126:947, 1982.

Chapter 10

ETHICAL AND LEGAL CONSIDERATIONS IN DEVELOPMENTAL ANOMALIES OF THE NERVOUS SYSTEM

ROBERT L. McLAURIN, M.D., J.D.

A BRIEF HISTORY OF DECISION-MAKING ABOUT DEFECTIVE NEWBORNS

Current professional and public attitudes about dealing with children born with impairments have evolved in the past few decades largely in response to technical achievements since World War II. The noninterventionist philosophy that was prevalent in the early part of the century began to change as the technology, which had first been applied to adults, began to be used for newborns. These developments included such things as antibiotics, ventilatory control, artificial nutrition and hydration techniques, anesthesia methodology, monitoring devices, analysis of minute blood samples, and the like.

In the 1970s and early 1980s the debate concerning treatment of imperiled newborns, including premature infants and those with developmental abnormalities, had two dimensions: (1) Questions of substance: should all such babies be treated, and if not, which ones should not be treated? (2) Question of procedure: who should decide?

A few cases went to court, but the issue of nontreatment of defective newborns did not receive national attention until 1981, when the parents and the physician of conjoined Siamese twins decided not to resuscitate. They were charged with conspiracy to commit murder but were not convicted because of lack of testimony of witnesses. Interestingly, one of the twins is still alive after subsequent surgical separation, and to

this date, no parent or clinician has been successfully prosecuted criminally for withholding treatment from a defective newborn.

This brought us to the Baby Doe era, which was initiated by the birth in Bloomington, Indiana in 1982 of an infant with Down's syndrome and a surgically correctable gastrointestinal malformation. The parents and physician elected to refrain from surgical treatment because of the Down's syndrome. Shortly afterward, Baby Jane Doe was born in New York City with a neural tube defect, and after consultation with neurosurgeons and pediatricians, the parents declined surgical treatment. These cases resulted in intense public discussion and a deluge of governmental actions involving all branches of the federal government. "Baby Doe Directives" were issued from the Department of Health and Human Services. The U.S. Supreme Court invalidated these regulations, and Congress passed "compromise legislation" in 1984 in the form of amendments to the Child Abuse and Neglect Prevention and Treatment Act. The results of these actions will be discussed in more detail later in this chapter.

REVIEW OF MEDICAL ETHICS

There exists a body of substantive ethics that serve as bases for establishing social and legal doctrines concerning nontreatment of defective infants. It is good to be reminded that the flurry of interest in this entire matter of decision-making for imperiled newborns, including nontreatment options ("infanticide"), probably arose more from alterations in social consciousness than from the scientific progress that allows prolongation of life.

Infanticide has been practiced in various cultures throughout history. Moreno notes that infants have been put to death for a variety of reasons, including physical abnormalities, illegitimacy, population control, and undesirable sex.[1] Infanticide is referred to in the Bible (Isaiah 57:5), and Plato, in *The Republic,* supported the intentional exposure of sickly babies. Eskimos have only recently stopped physical exposure of infants for economic reasons, and China and India have practiced infanticide, especially of female infants, for population control.[1] Thus, awareness of the practices of other cultures may serve to increase our alertness and sensitivity to ethical standards. It is noteworthy, incidentally, that infanticide and infant euthanasia are not always distinguishable.

ETHICAL STANDARDS

The central ethical question concerns sanctity of life versus quality of life. Vitalists adopt the position that everything possible should be done to preserve life. There should be no discretion of parents, physicians, or courts regarding treatment decisions. Their position is the cornerstone of certain religious fundamentalists and the right-to-life movements. This position holds that therapy, even without cure, is an essential part of medicine if it contributes to care, despite the fact that the physician must sometimes suffer. Death of an unoperated infant is not an acceptable means of alleviating that suffering.

On the other hand, quality of life has many advocates despite the inherent difficulty in defining quality of life and the uncertainty as to who should make the judgment. Consideration may be given to the burden placed on the infant's family or on society. Estimations of the "relative value" of the infant's life as compared to a standard human being have been used. Noncomparative judgment may focus on the degree of physical and psychological illness, pain and suffering and the likelihood of achieving comfort.

The concept that has become termed "the best interest of the child" has been recently adopted and advocated by the President's Commission for the Study of Ethical Problems in Medicine and Biomedical and Behavioral Research.[2] Although in most circumstances there will be argument on whether a proposed course of therapy is in the infant's best interest, it is inevitable that conflicting opinions will arise in certain instances. Clearly, however, the "best interest" standard incorporates consideration of the quality of life.

The prevailing "best interest" notion presupposes that all infants have interests, but for some the burden of continued life can outweigh the benefits. In the more extreme view, the absence of pain is the only moral consideration regardless of whether the infant is doomed to a life of short duration and lacks the capacity for any distinct human development. This has led some ethicists to advocate the "relational potential" of the infant in the determination of "best interest."[3] This concept holds that an infant who lacks any potential for future human relationships can be said to have no interest at all except to be free of pain.

All ethical discussions of imperiled infants include the basic concepts outlined above, but other criteria have been proposed by some writers. For example, Rostain and Bhutani described an approach termed "objectivism."[4] This uses a purely statistical approach to determine which infants are likely to benefit from treatment, and only objective criteria are used in this approach (e.g., birth weight, gestational age, thickness of cerebral cortex). This method was recommended by Lorber in determining whether or not to surgically correct myelomeningoceles.[5] Based on the presence of certain physical deformities at birth, Lorber recommended a selection process that would exclude some infants from corrective surgery. One of the criteria used to justify this process was the existence of mental retardation, a factor that our present ethical and legal standards consider a handicap but certainly not an indication for infanticide.

Gostin has proposed a moral standard based on "personal interest,"[6] the criteria for which would indicate that there is "reasonable certainty that a competent individual would not choose to continue life in the circumstances presented." The specific criteria include: (1) the neonate is not conscious and sapient, (2) the potential for dealing with, and responding to, sensory information and experiencing thought is *de minimis*, or (3) the neonate is terminally ill and in the process of dying.

It is apparent that there is considerable overlap, as well as uncertainty, among the various ethical standards that have been proposed. The common denominator of all except *vitalism* appears to be the "best interest" concept, whether it be on a statistical foundation or based on certain criteria that often become subjective to the decision-maker. The courts also have not been immune to the subjectivity of judgment.

Phrased another way, the central question of decision-making involves the infant's "right to die." The bases for judgments as to the circumstances in which the right to die supersedes the right to live are frequently obscure and difficult to delineate. Goldworth recently attempted to define the circumstances as occurring ". . . when a failure to honor the infant's right to die results in the infant being deprived of the fundamental need *not* to suffer pain and *not* to be alienated from other human beings because of psychosocial deficits, and there is nothing in the infant's continued existence to adequately compensate it for the pain and alienation."[7] The author opined that to sustain such life medically constitutes a violation of the right to die.

MEDICAL CAPABILITIES AND THE UNCERTAINTY PROBLEM

Medicine is a probabilistic discipline with inherent unavoidable prognostic uncertainty. This results from the variability of the biologic response of any organism to a specific treatment. Thus, the risks and benefits of treatment are not entirely predictable. Ethical decisions, therefore, are necessarily made in the face of recognized diagnostic, therapeutic, and prognostic uncertainty.

The uncertainty problem has been accentuated by technologic advances. The ability to salvage 99 per cent of infants with nonlethal birth defects has led to long-term morbidity. Therefore, the uncertainty factor is concerned initially with survival but later, and more significantly, with the future quality of life. Decisions concerning treatment of imperiled infants must necessarily be based on two factors: the best available scientific data and the personal values one applies to the data.

The response to uncertainty has been explored by several authors.[3, 7, 8] The *statistical* approach requires the decision-maker to make an across-the-board statistical profile of the infant to determine the likelihood of response to treatment. If the chances of effectiveness fall below a certain cut-off point, aggressive measures will not be instituted. This is the basis of *objectivism*, described above, and was adopted by Lorber in his proposed management of neural tube defects.

A contrasting strategy is the *wait until certain* approach.[9] This includes treatment of every infant that is potentially viable until it is certain that the infant will not survive. This approach in generally accepted in the United States in the management of newborns with birth defects.

Each of these approaches has a built-in potential source of error: the unnecessarily prolonged and uncomfortable survival of some infants who are destined to die, and the possibility, however remote, of allowing a salvageable infant to die. The decision-making process, therefore, must include an evaluation of which type of mistake is least tolerable.

WHO SHALL DECIDE?

Closely related to the ethical principles on which decisions are based is the question that embraces social, medical, and legal consideration. The traditional mechanism by which treatment or nontreatment decisions have been made is consultation between physician and family, usually resulting in the family accepting the physician's recommendation. The ethical basis for the assumption of the family's authority over medical decisions is based on the traditional affection of parents for their offspring. The United States Supreme Court has, in several contexts, recognized the fundamental rights of parents to have decision-making power, not only in medical affairs but in other aspects of child care.

However, one can raise searching questions about the extent to which parental authority may be overridden. The most notable example concerns the right of parents to prohibit, on religious grounds, the use of blood transfusion which would be life-saving. The courts have said that parents are not free "to make martyrs of their children before they have reached the age of full and legal discretion when they can make that choice for themselves."[10]

In addition, there may be less clear, perhaps even subconscious, motivations behind certain decisions. Parents have often anticipated a healthy baby and are confronted with a deformed, ill infant. There may be a bias against a physically or mentally handicapped offspring, which is interpreted to reflect on the character of the parents.

An argument frequently used to support parental authority is that the parents must bear the responsibility for later care of the child. This, however, may lead to wrong decisions as viewed by our present sense of morality, which holds that even if parents sincerely believe themselves incapable of caring for a child with an impairment, such a belief is insufficient for allowing efficacious medical treatment to be withheld. Thus, the parents' decision in such circumstances does not reflect the "best interest" of the child.

The other player in the traditional decision-making process is the physician, who may face a dilemma of choosing between loyalty to the Hippocratic Oath, which favors "sanctity of life," or an obligation to third party (parents) wishes. If it is then recognized that parents are usually deferential to physicians' recommendations, the physician is in the position of practicing eugenics. Moreover, physicians, like all others, have variable views about the "best interest" criteria; there are differing opinions as to what constitutes an acceptable level of function, either physical or mental. Finally, the possibility exists that physicians may go beyond consideration of medical benefit in their enthusiasm to test new therapeutic approaches and innovative techniques.[11]

Such arguments or those described above suggest that there are certain situations that may require further mechanisms to participate in the decision-making. The President's Commission recognized that although in nearly all cases parents are best suited to collaborate with physicians in making decisions about an infant's care, there needs to be some method of ensuring appropriate review when there occurs physician/parent or physician/physician disagreement. To assist the resolution of such matters, a means of internal review was recommended, and this has evolved into our present ethics committees. Only as a last resort should the problems be submitted to judicial proceedings.

THE JUDICIAL POSTURE

The widely acknowledged stimulus for federal interest in the care of handicapped newborns was the birth of Baby Doe in 1982. The tracheoesophageal defect was surgically correctable but without correction was certain to be fatal within a short time. After discussion with their physician, the parents elected to refuse permission for surgery because of the presence of Down's syndrome. This event precipitated a brief but stormy sequence of judicial intervention.

Initially, the hospital brought action to overturn the parents' decision, but the court ruled in favor of the parents. This was upheld by the Indiana Supreme Court. The infant died six days after birth while efforts were made to appeal to the U.S. Supreme Court.

As a consequence of the widespread publicity and public debate generated by the case, President Reagan requested the Secretary of Health and Human Services to become involved. The result was the Baby Doe Regulations, which proscribed the withholding of medical or surgical treatment to correct life-threatening conditions if the withholding is based on the presence of a handicap that is not life-threatening. Hospitals were required to post notices in nurseries, and a toll-free "hot line" to the federal agency was established. These regulations were later struck down by the federal district court.

Meanwhile, the case of Baby Jane Doe was progressing through the courts. This infant, born in 1983, had multiple congenital anomalies including myelomeningocele, microcephaly, and latent hydrocephalus. After consultation with neurologists, nurses, neurosurgeons, social workers, and religious counselors, the parents refused to consent to surgery. This decision was challenged in the New York courts, and the Court of Appeals (the highest state court in New York) decided that the parents had made an informed decision based on medical consultation and had elected a conservative course of management, and their decision would be upheld.

Health and Human Services became involved also in the Baby Jane Doe litigation, and the two cases were combined and ultimately appealed through the federal courts to the U.S. Supreme Court.[12] The decision there was that no federal laws had been violated. Thus, essentially the traditional right of the parents to decide the course of treatment of defective newborns, after adequate consultation, was upheld. The present judicial posture, therefore, is that except under unusual circumstances, especially when there may be conflicting recommendations, the court should remain uninvolved in the decision-making process.

THE LEGISLATIVE POSTURE

The Supreme Court's decision did not foreclose further federal regulatory activity. While the judicial litigation was in progress, legislation was being introduced in Congress to amend the Child Abuse Prevention and Treatment Act of 1974. The original Act interpreted child abuse as "physical or mental injury, sexual abuse or exploitation, negligent treatment, or maltreatment of a child." In fashioning the amendments in 1984, Congress relied heavily on the report of the President's Commissions, which had made an exhaustive survey and report on the matter of handicapped infants. The Congressional Committee concluded that "where death is avoidable through surgical or other therapeutic means. . . . denial of such treatment is clearly abusive

to children."[13] Thus, Congress had focused on the imperiled infant for the first time in legislative history, and the withholding of medically indicated treatment was thereby included as a form of child abuse.

One section of the Child Abuse Amendments of 1984 is worth quoting as it defines the current federal mandates:

> [T]he term "withholding of medically indicated treatment" means the failure to respond to the infant's life-threatening conditions by providing treatment (including appropriate nutrition, hydration and medication) which in the treating physician's or physicians' reasonable medical judgment, will be most likely to be effective in ameliorating or correcting all such conditions, except that the term does not include the failure to provide treatment (other than appropriate nutrition, hydration, or medication) to an infant when, in the treating physician's or physicians' reasonable judgment, (A) the infant is chronically and irreversibly comatose; (B) the provision of such treatment would (i) merely prolong dying, (ii) not be effective in ameliorating or correcting all of the infant's life-threatening conditions, or (iii) otherwise be futile in terms of survival of the infant; or (C) the provision of such treatment would be virtually futile in terms of survival of the infant and the treatment itself under such circumstances would be inhumane.[14]

The amendments also specifically proscribed any discrimination on the basis of handicap, e.g., Down's syndrome or mental retardations. Additionally, the individual states must have procedures and programs within the state child protection services to respond to instances of withholding medical treatment from disabled infants. The law required that state protective agencies could initiate legal proceedings to prevent the withholding of indicated medical treatment.

Following passage of the Amendments, the Department of Health and Human Services published regulations that provided guidelines for health care providers to establish Infant Care Review Committees. Such review mechanisms had been recommended by the President's Commission. The regulations defined the role of ICRC in efforts to resolve physician/family disagreements in which the family recommends nontreatment. In certain circumstances, the ICRC was obligated to refer the matter to the appropriate child protective agency or court.

The noteworthy points made in the HHS regulations are: (1) Decisions to withhold medically indicated treatment may not be based on subjective opinions about the future "quality of life" of the retarded or disabled infant. (2) Even when the statute permits the withholding of medically indicated treatment, the infant must be provided appropriate nutrition, hydration, and medication. (3) The only circumstances in which treatment is not considered "medically indicated" are (a) irreversible coma, (b) treatment would be ineffective and merely prolong dying, and (c) treatment would be futile and inhumane.

Subsequent to publication of these regulations, each state has passed laws and regulations that are in conformity. No further major legislative or judicial decisions have occurred.

ANENCEPHALY: A UNIQUE PROBLEM

While the major focus of legal activity has been directed to problems such as treatable neural tube defects, the ethical and legal concerns relating to anencephaly have been based on a different issue. This issue concerns the criteria for brain death. Most states use a standard that requires total cessation of all brain functions, including those of the brainstem, to establish brain death. Recent interest in this condition has resulted from the increased success rate of organ transplantation and the very limited supply of infant organs for this purpose.

Most anencephalics die within a day or so of birth, but until that occurs there is persistence of some brainstem function. In 1987, Loma Linda University Medical Center adopted a plan that called for ventilator support from birth until all brain functions ceased. The infant was then considered as a donor. After one year the program was discontinued because only one infant achieved brain death in the 7-day period allowed by the protocol.

The only ethical issue involved under present legal constraints is whether an anencephalic newborn is, in fact, a being. The argument has been made that, given the lack of brain tissue by which any human relationship could be established, the question of whether it is live or dead is irrelevant.

The legal implications have been defined recently in a case heard in a Florida state court. The parents of an anencephalic offspring attempted to have the infant declared brain dead so that her organs could be harvested before they deteriorated. The request was denied since the statutory criteria of brain death were not present. The Florida Supreme Court refused to hear the arguments. Accordingly, the only way by which anencephalics would be available as organ donors would be through an alteration of the criteria of brain death or by making anencephalics a legal exception to the present standards. Ethicists are of the opinion that such maneuvers might actually harm the present organ-retrieval movement and that the possibility of abuse and the minimal yield would not justify that risk.

REFERENCES

1. Moreno JD: Ethical and legal issues in the care of the impaired newborn. Clin Perinatol 14:345, 1987.
2. President's Commission for the Study of Ethical Problems in Medicine and Biomedical and Behavioral Research. Deciding to Forego Life-Sustaining Treatment. U.S. Government Printing Office, 1983.
3. Caplan A, Cohen CB: Imperiled newborns; Standards of judgment for treatment. Hastings Cent Rep 17:13, 1987.
4. Rostain AR, Bhutani VK: Ethical dilemmas of neonatal perinatal surgery. Clin Perinatol 16:275, 1989.
5. Lorber J: Results of treatment of myelomeningocele. Dev Med Child Neurol 13:279, 1971.
6. Gostin L: A moment in human development: Legal protection, ethical standards and social policy on the selective nontreatment of handicapped neonates. Am J Law Med 11:31, 1985.
7. Goldworth A: Human rights and the omission or cessation of treatment for infants. J Perinatol 9:79, 1989.
8. Caplan A, Cohen CB: Imperiled newborns; The effect of new pediatric capabilities and the problem of uncertainty. Hastings Cent Rep 17:10, 1987.
9. Rhoden NK: Treating Baby Doe; the ethics of uncertainty. Hastings Cent Rep 16:34, 1986.
10. *People ex rel. Wallace v. Labrenz,* 411 Ill. 618, 104 NE2d 769 (1952).
11. Caplan A, Cohen CB: Imperiled newborns; Who shall decide? Hastings Cent Rep 17:17, 1987.
12. *Bowen v. American Hospital Association,* 106 S.Ct. 2101 (1986).
13. S. Rep. No. 246, 98th Cong., reprinted in U.S. Code Cong. and Admin. News, 2918 (1984).
14. *Child Abuse Amendments* of 1984, Pub. L. 98-457, Title I, Part B, Section 121(3).

PART

II

HYDROCEPHALUS

Chapter 11

CEREBROSPINAL FLUID AND THE BLOOD-BRAIN INTERFACE

J. GORDON McCOMB, M.D., and BERISLAV V. ZLOKOVIC, M.D., Ph.D.

Under normal physiologic conditions, most of the cerebrospinal fluid (CSF) is secreted by the choroid plexus and flows through the ventricular system to emerge from the fourth ventricle. The CSF then traverses the subarachnoid spaces (SAS) to drain from the central nervous system (CNS) through unidirectional open channels as a result of a hydrostatic pressure difference. This chapter reviews the clinical and experimental evidence for these conclusions as well as the alterations that occur in hydrocephalus. Also covered in this chapter is an overview of the blood-brain interface (BBI), an area that has seen the addition of much new knowledge and is an intregal part in CNS homeostasis and CSF physiology.

CHOROID PLEXUS

The choroid plexus, the major source of CSF, is found in the lateral, third, and fourth ventricles, with an extension of this tissue out the lateral foramina of Luschka into the cerebellopontine angles. In man, most of the choroid plexus resides in the lateral ventricles and is attached to the medial ventricular wall, where branches of the anterior and posterior choroidal arteries provide the vascular input. The remaining choroid plexus tissue hangs from the roof of the third and fourth ventricles and is supplied by branches of the medial posterior choroidal and posterior inferior cerebellar arteries, respectively. The choroidal veins drain mainly into the internal cerebral veins, which are part of the deep venous or galenic system.

During development, the choroid plexus forms lobules, which become fronds covered with villi. Each villus is lined with a single layer of cuboidal epithelium, which is a modified ependyma covering a stromal core derived from a layer of pia. Microvilli and a few cilia cover the apical or ventricular surface of these epithelial cells, while on the basal side, lateral infoldings interdigitate with neighboring cells. Tight junctions are present at the apical sides of the cells. The cells are affixed to a basement membrane beneath which is a stromal space containing collagen, fibroblast, and nerve fibers. A capillary, with the endothelium of the fenestrated type and devoid of tight junctions, is at the center of each villus (Fig. 11–1). A blood-CSF interface results from the presence of tight junctions at the apical end of the choroid epithelium, rather than at the capillary endothelium of the villus[1] (Fig. 11–2A). This is in contradistinction to the capillaries of the parenchyma, in which the tight junctions between the endothelial cells constitute the BBI (Figs. 11–2B and 11–3). The

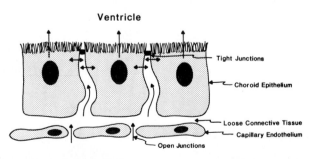

FIGURE 11–1. Diagrammatic representation of the choroid plexus. The capillary endothelium is of the attenuated fenestrated type that allows an ultrafiltrate of plasma to reach the basal side of the epithelial cells. Tight junctions at the apical or ventricular side of the epithelial cells restrict molecular movement and constitute the blood-CSF interface.

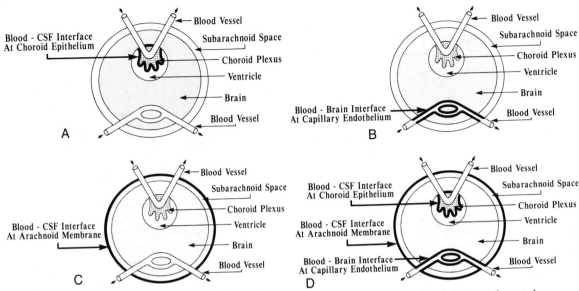

FIGURE 11–2. Diagrammatic representation of the central nervous system. *A,* Blood-CSF interface at the choroid epithelium. *B,* Blood-brain interface at the capillary endothelium. *C,* Blood-CSF interface at the arachnoid membrane. *D,* It is the three interfaces depicted in *A, B,* and *C* that provide the specialized environment of the central nervous system.

blood-CSF-brain interface complex is completed by the presence of tight junctions in the outer layers of the arachnoid membrane[2] (Fig. 11–2C). Together these barriers help to mitigate changes in the chemical composition of the CSF, thereby providing additional stability and consistency, which are essential to normal brain function (Fig. 11–2D).

FORMATION OF CSF

FORMATION SITES

It is generally agreed that most CSF is formed within the ventricular system. Possible sites of origin include the choroid plexus, the ependyma, and the paren-

chyma. A method has not been developed to separate the function of the ependyma from that of the remainder of the parenchyma; thus the roll of the ependyma in bulk CSF formation is not known, although from a morphologic standpoint its contribution is most likely to be insignificant. However, the choroidal epithelium has histologic features characteristic of epithelia specialized for transcellular transport of solutes and solvents.[3, 4] The discussion that follows will be limited solely to bulk secretion of CSF.

Results from isolated choroid plexus preparation would indicate that 80 per cent or more of CSF production is from this source alone.[5, 6] Perfusion of a portion of the ventricular system devoid of choroid plexus has demonstrated that 30 to 60 per cent of CSF is produced from a nonchoroidal source,[7, 8] which may explain the failure of choroid plexectomy in the clinical setting to

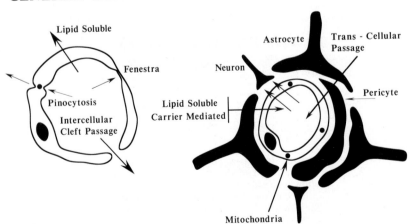

GENERAL CAPILLARY   BRAIN CAPILLARY

FIGURE 11–3. Diagrammatic representation of the differences between the general and brain capillaries. General capillaries allow all small molecules to diffuse through clefts between adjacent endothelial cells, i.e., extracellular. In contrast, the brain capillary permits exchanges only through the cells, i.e., transcellular. (From Oldendorf WH: Blood-brain barrier. *In* Bito LZ, Davson HM, Fenstermacher JD [eds]: The Ocular and Cerebrospinal Fluids. New York, Academic Press, 1977. Modified from Pardridge WM: Peptide Drug Delivery to the Brain. New York, Raven Press, 1991.)

adequately control progressive hydrocephalus.[7] It may be added that this operative procedure removes the choroid plexus only from the lateral ventricles, and not from the third or fourth ventricles. The contribution of the remaining intact choroid plexus to the formation of CSF is not clear, and whether or not it can compensate for that portion of the choroid plexus removed is not known.

The various lines of evidence showing the extracellular space (ECS) to be approximately 15 per cent of the brain volume have been summarized by Welsh.[9] The established presence of a substantial ECS, the lack of ependymal resistance to free exchange between the fluid in the ECS and the CSF, and the similar composition of ECF and CSF have a direct bearing on the possibility that the parenchyma may be the main source of nonchoroidal CSF formation.[1, 9–11] In summary, it appears that normally roughly 80 per cent of CSF secretion is derived from the choroid plexus, with the remaining portion probably originating from the parenchyma. The obvious candidate for the parenchymal source is the capillary endothelium (see Fig. 11–3), as its high content of mitochondria could provide the metabolic energy required for such a function.[12]

MECHANISMS OF CSF FORMATION

The first step in the formation of CSF is the passage of an ultrafiltrate of plasma through the non–tight-junctioned choroidal capillary endothelium by hydrostatic pressure into the surrounding connective tissue stroma beneath the epithelium of the villus. The ultrafiltrate is subsequently transformed into a secretion (namely, CSF) by an active metabolic process within the choroidal epithelium via a mechanism that is largely speculative (Fig. 11–4).[3, 9] Using the information available, a model has been constructed[13, 14] based upon the "standing gradient" hypothesis of Diamond and Bossert,[15] which assumes local osmotic forces within the cell to be responsible for the movement of water.

Sodium-potassium-adenosine triphosphatase (Na-K-ATPase) located in the microvilli on the apical surface extrudes sodium into the ventricle, followed by osmotic redrawn water. It has been speculated that various types of sodium carrier proteins are present at the basolateral side and provide facilitated diffusion of the sodium to the interior of the cell, including countertransport with hydrogen and/or potassium ions. Since the cells do not swell or shrink, the sum of the two processes must be in balance.[16] That water readily equilibrates in this process is indicated by the negligible difference in the osmolalities of plasma, plasma ultrafiltrate, and CSF.[17] Chloride may be coupled with this process or may enter the cell separately.[14] Carbonic anhydrase catalyzes the formation of bicarbonate inside the cell, with the hydrogen ion being fed back to the sodium transporter as a counterion with potassium.[18, 19]

FORMATION RATE

The earliest method used to estimate the rate of CSF formation simply entailed measuring the amount of fluid drained per unit of time or removing a known volume of CSF and noting the time required for opening pressure to be restored. The validity of the results obtained in this way can be criticized because CSF dynamic are changed by alterations in pressure. In spite of this objection, the volumes obtained by these methods are remarkably close to those determined by the more precise ventriculocisternal or ventriuclolumbar

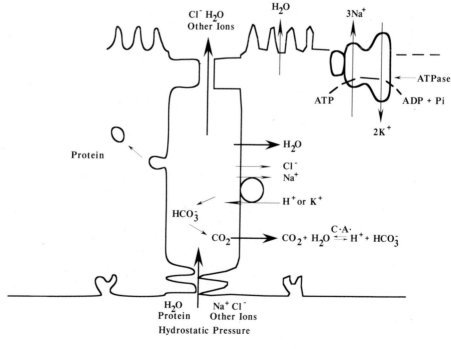

FIGURE 11–4. The postulated mechanism of CSF secretion by the choroid plexus. The presence of ion transporters has been documented, but the exact locations are still speculative. An ultrafiltrate of plasma enters the basal side of the cell whereupon it is modified by metabolic processes to produce a secretion at the apical or ventricular side. (From Segal MB, Pollay M: The secretion of cerebrospinal fluid. Exp Eye Res 25:127, 1977. [Modified])

perfusion technique introduced by Pappenheimer and associates.[20, 21] Although this method is used extensively in experimental models, its clinical use has been limited because the procedure is invasive. The protocol requires the infusion of artificial CSF containing a nondiffusible reference material (such as radioiodinated serum albumin: RISA), which moves only by bulk flow into the ventricles, while removing the artificial CSF diluted with the newly formed CSF from the cisterna magna or lumbar SAS at constant low pressure. By quantitating the volume of fluid in and out of the system and measuring the concentration difference of the reference marker in the two fluids, it is possible to evaluate the rate of CSF formation and absorption. Clinical studies have indicated a CSF formation rate of about 20 ml/hour or 500 ml/day.[22–24] Since the total volume of CSF in the ventricles and SAS in the adult averages approximately 150 ml, a threefold turnover of CSF occurs daily.

FORMATION RATE ALTERATIONS

Under normal physiologic conditions, CSF formation can be considered independent of pressure.[20, 22, 24] The process is pressure-responsive, but the effect is insignificant until the intraventricular pressure becomes markedly elevated. This elevated pressure diminishes the cerebral perfusion pressure[25] and probably interferes with the first step in CSF production by reducing the quantity of ultrafiltrate from the choroidal capillary.[9] The effect of temperature on CSF production in patients is not known and probably has little relevance except in marked hypothermia. Acute serum hyperosmolality in animal experiments has claimed to reduce CSF formation, whereas acute serum hypo-osmolality will increase the rate,[26, 27] but this appears to reflect movement of CSF into or out of the parenchyma.[28] Little doubt exists that a decrease in serum osmolality will increase the observed CSF volume flow secondary to movement of ECF within the parenchyma, but as none of the studies has dealt with an isolated choroid plexus preparation, no statement can be made regarding whether or not changes in serum osmolality in and of itself will alter CSF formation. The effect of change in serum osmolality, be it acute or chronic, on CSF production in the clinical setting is unknown as no data exist.

It has long been suspected that oversecretion of CSF occurs in cases of choroid plexus papilloma.[29] Unequivocal evidence for this has been documented by ventriculolumbar infusion studies on several occasions.[30, 31] Evidence for overproduction of CSF in the presence of "hypertrophy" of the choroid plexus has also been reported.[32] The clinical observation of what appears to be a temporary reduction in CSF production associated with ventriculitis is supported by two experimental studies.[33, 34] Through its presumed action on cyclic adenosine monophosphate, cholera toxin has been reported to double the flow of CSF,[35] a finding that has not been confirmed by another investigation.[36]

Drugs that reduce CSF formation do so by interfering with the entire cellular metabolic process or specific transport mechanisms. Dinitrophenol, an uncoupler of oxidative phosphorylation, is an example of the former, whereas cardiac glycosides, furosemide, acetazolamide, and an analog of diazepam[37] are examples of the latter. It is not clear whether glucocorticoids alter CSF formation, since some investigations show no change[38, 39] and others report a diminished production rate.[40, 41] Furosemide decreases CSF formation by what appears to be interference with chloride transport rather than any direct effect on carbonic anhydrase.[42] Acetazolamide (Diamox) decreases CSF production by interfering with the function of carbonic anhydrase and appears to significantly diminish CSF formation in man both acutely and chronically.[22, 24] Rapid intravenous injection of Diamox can also cause a transient elevation of intracranial pressure (ICP) consequent to the release of tissue carbon dioxide, with resultant increase in cerebral blood volume and cerebral blood flow. This could, theoretically, be hazardous in a clinical setting of marked ICP elevation. As Fishman has observed,[43] ICP is far more dependent upon cerebral hemodynamics than on the rate of CSF formation. The fact that total inhibition of CSF formation, be it choroidal or extrachoroidal, is not possible with a single agent indicates that several mechanisms are involved in the secretory process. Culter et al.[22] have noted that, owing to the nature of formation versus absorption curve, reduction of normal CSF production by one third would drop the ICP by only 1 torr. This helps to explain why Diamox, or other agents that reduce CSF formation, have not proved to be particularly useful in the control of hydrocephalus. The first report of CSF formation and absorption in humans by the ventriculolumbar perfusion technique was that of Rubin et al.,[24] who concluded that future studies into the pathogenesis of hydrocephalus should be focused on absorption and not on CSF formation.

ABSORPTION OF CEREBROSPINAL FLUID

The absorption of CSF and its constituents depends upon bulk flow in addition to passive or facilitated diffusion and active transport of specific solutes. This section will deal exclusively with bulk flow, the forces involved, and where it occurs.

ABSORPTIVE FORCES

That the rate of CSF absorption is pressure-dependent and relatively linear over a fairly wide physiologic range has been well established.[20, 22, 24, 44–46] The resistance to flow appears to diminish at higher than normal physiologic pressures[47, 48] and may relate to the opening of channels not available at lower pressures.

Weed[49] proposed an incremental colloid osmotic force in addition to hydrostatic force which would, by necessity, require the presence of a semipermeable membrane between the CSF and its site of absorption. Subsequent physiologic studies have shown that a colloid osmotic force does not exist; instead, Weed's prior observations are explained by particulate matter or an increase in viscosity occluding the absorptive sites, which slows bulk flow.[47, 50, 51] Studies have shown that the presence of pinocytotic vesicles in the arachnoid endothelial cells lining the venous sinuses is influenced by pressure.[52, 53] However, the process may not be metabolically dependent, as the absorption process is reported to be unaltered by the death of the animal.[54, 55] Thus, the only proven force responsible for bulk CSF absorption is that of a hydrostatic gradient.

ABSORPTION VIA THE ARACHNOID VILLUS

The arachnoid villus would seem to be ideally situated to drain CSF from the SAS into the major dural sinuses, as it consists of a cell cluster that projects from the SAS into the lacunae laterales adjacent to these venous structures. Electron microscopic studies have shown that the villi are covered by a layer of endothelium with tight junctions that are continuous with the inner surface of the venous sinuses.[56, 57] Those villi, also called "arachnoid granulations" or "pacchionian bodies," are grossly visible and are functionally similar to those that are not.[58] Key and Retzius,[59] and Weed[60] firmly established that these structures drain CSF. Welch and Friedman,[51] using a flux chamber containing a section of monkey superior sagittal sinus (SSS) with arachnoid villi, found unidirectional flow from the SSS to the venous sinuses when a critical opening pressure was exceeded.

A point of controversy regarding the structure of the arachnoid villus is the existence of open channels connecting the arachnoid side with the venous side, for the presence or absence of such channels would mean a basic physiologic difference in the manner in which CSF and its constituents drain. The open villus model would be solely pressure-responsive and would allow for passive escape of macromolecules, whereas a villus covered by a continuous tight-junctioned endothelial membrane would add the factors of osmosis and filtration, and macromolecules would require an active transport process to cross this barrier. The earlier anatomic studies were fairly evenly divided between these two possibilities; the more recent ones support the open-channel pathway. The discrepancy in findings may relate in part or whole to the manner in which the villus is prepared for histologic study: a zero pressure gradient between the arachnoid and venous side of the villus during fixation would allow for its collapse, and as a result open channels would not be apparent.[61]

Another possible mechanism that could bridge the gap between the open- versus closed-channel theory of CSF drainage has been proposed by Tripathi.[62] He reported the presence of a dynamic transendothelial vacuolization process that temporarily creates an open channel across the villus endothelium through which CSF and its constituents could flow from the SAS to the blood.[63] The effect of pressure on this mechanism was not investigated.

Attempts have been made to determine the size of the passageways in the arachnoid villus[64] and also to see if they are responsive to pressure, which they were not.[65] The size of the passageways in the arachnoid villus is only pertinent if this site is virtually the exclusive location for bulk egress of CSF into the blood stream. If a significant fraction of CSF and its constituents drains elsewhere, the size of the channels in the arachnoid villus is less relevant.

ABSORPTION INTO THE LYMPHATIC SYSTEM

The fact that CSF might drain at sites other than the arachnoid villus, under normal or abnormal physiologic conditions, has recently been given increasing consideration.

Weed's[60] work firmly established the arachnoid villus as a major site for bulk CSF outflow. It is rarely mentioned, though, that Weed acknowledged drainage of his injected solutions into the mucosa of the paranasal sinuses, nasal mucosa, cranial nerve root sheaths, and cervical lymph nodes; he thought that these routes were accessory. The idea that a portion of CSF could and did drain via the lymphatics was gradually relegated to obscurity, and for more than a generation, standard texts and teachings have limited CSF drainage solely to the arachnoid villus.

The concept of CSF drainage via the lymphatic system has been given additional support by a number of recent laboratory investigations that indicate that a significant quantity of CSF, and under certain circumstances even the majority, can drain via the lymphatic channels.[66–79] The infusion of substances with different molecular weights into the lateral ventricles can be found in the same concentration in the deep cervical lymph, indicating that the process of transport is by way of bulk flow.[66] Additional studies have shown that elevations of intraventricular pressure will increase the volume of CSF directed into the lymphatic pathways.[61, 75]

At present, no studies show to what extent lymphatic drainage of CSF exists in man, but some support for this concept comes from the clinical observation that occasionally parents of children with CSF-diverting shunts will report nasal congestion and periorbital or facial swelling when their child's shunt becomes obstructed.

ABSORPTION BY THE BRAIN

A question debated for some time is whether or not CSF can be absorbed by the brain. Penetration of substances into the periventricular region of the hydrocephalic animal has been well documented.[80–82] With the advent of computerized tomographic (CT) scanning, periventricular hypodensity may be noted in the presence of hydrocephalus and has been shown to be the result of CSF migrating into the area surrounding the ventricles in the face of increased intraventricular pressure.[83] Magnetic resonance imaging (MRI) has demonstrated this as well. CSF in the parenchyma, indicative of migration, however, does not necessarily equate with absorption. Bulk flow of CSF is usually measured via the clearance of various reference macromolecules, such as RISA, which by necessity would have to enter the lumen of the blood vessel and be removed by the systemic circulation. It has been shown that cerebral capillaries have a low permeability to RISA, and that most of any given quantity of RISA injected into the brain can be recovered from the lymph and CSF with little being lost to the blood.[67] Zervas et al.[84] have found that horseradish peroxidase (HRP), which has nearly the same molecular weight as albumin, could penetrate to the basal lamina of the capillary endothelium but not beyond. In addition to the impermeability of the capillaries to the various reference markers, clearance of which is the measure of CSF absorption, Welch[9] has pointed out that, as absorption occurs in response to a pressure drop, it would require a higher pressure outside the lumen of the capillary than inside, which obviously would lead to its collapse and preclude absorption. The ECS in the brain, which amounts to 15 per cent, readily allows fluid flow in the parenchyma. This flow of fluid within the parenchyma is present under normal physiologic conditions,[85] and its velocity and direction are responsive to changes in hydrostatic[86] and osmotic pressure gradients.[85, 87] Macromolecules injected into the CSF of the ventricles or SAS have been observed to readily penetrate the ECS of the parenchyma and vice versa.[10, 84, 88] Evidence thus supports the contention that the brain, rather than absorbing CSF, is acting as a conduit for fluid to move from the ventricles to the SAS.[79]

ABSORPTION VIA THE BLOOD VESSELS

As noted in the discussion of the absorption of CSF by the brain, there is no evidence to support CSF being absorbed by the capillary endothelium. However, this does not preclude net water changes when disequilibrium in the blood-brain osmotic gradient occurs because there is no barrier in this regard. One experimental study found that carbon black injected into the parenchyma could be later traced to the SAS, the walls of the cerebral blood vessels, the adventitia of the internal carotid artery outside the cranium, and the cervical lymph nodes.[88] Two newer studies are at variance with the observation that macromolecules travel extracranially in the adventitia of the major cerebral blood vessels for, in these studies, RISA injected into the brain or SAS stopped abruptly when the blood vessels exited the SAS.[67, 89] The parenchymal vessels appear to provide a passageway for macromolecules to reach the SAS, where absorption occurs via the arachnoid granulations or the lymphatic system from the cranial nerve root sleeves, particularly those sleeves surrounding the olfactory nerve roots.

ABSORPTION AT THE NERVE ROOT SLEEVES

Drainage of CSF into the nasal submucosa was first postulated by Schwalbe,[90] and this finding has been confirmed on many occasions since.[59, 60, 91–95] Yoffrey and Drinker noted that the best injections of the nasal submucosa were made by placing tracers in the cranial SAS.[95] The nasal submucosa has a dense network of lymphatic channels which subsequently drain into the deep cervical lymph nodes.[59, 60, 90, 91, 93, 95] The pathway of CSF into the nasal submucosa is via the extension of the SAS, which surrounds each olfactory filament as it passes through the lamina cribrosa, and can be blocked if the continuity of the space is disrupted.[68, 96] The pia-arachnoid layer progressively thins and blends into a perineural sheath as the olfactory filament passes through the cribriform plate. This perineural sheath becomes but a single cell layer in the submucosa. The perineural space between the filament and the sheath is reported to be in continuity with the SAS.[91, 95] A point of uncertainty has been whether or not open channels connect the perineural spaces (and thus the SAS) with the ECS of the submucosa. The presence or absence of open channels would mean a basic physiologic difference in the manner in which CSF and its constituents drain, just as with the arachnoid villus. A recent electron microscopic study indicates that a tight-junctioned endothelial membrane is not present, thus allowing the passive escape of macromolecules via bulk fluid flow on a pressure-responsive basis alone (Fig. 11–5).[70] Two additional studies found that the SAS surrounding the optic nerve divided into numerous tortuous channels to form an "arachnoid trabecular meshwork" containing "microcanals," which allow for passage of ferritin to reach the posterior intraorbital connective tissue. Once again the passageways were open and similar to that found in the olfactory region.[71, 77] A barrier that was present at the sclera prevented tracer entrance into the choroidal interstitium.

A physiologic study looking at CSF drainage from the spinal nerve roots indicates that the same physiologic processes operative at the cranial nerves occur in the spinal nerves as well.[97] CSF drainage from the spinal nerve root sleeves has yet to be studied from a morphologic standpoint, but evidence so far favors an open channel passageway similar to that found for the optic and olfactory nerves.

ABSORPTION FROM THE SUBARACHNOID SPACES

Experiments document CSF drainage from the SAS surrounding the cranial and spinal nerves, with entry into the lymphatic system, but the question of fluid egress from the membrane itself remains. Dandy and Blackfan[98] contended that CSF absorption was a diffuse process from the SAS, with the arachnoid villi accounting for only a small percentage of the fluid drained. Weed[58] found that under normal physiologic conditions the arachnoid membrane acted as a barrier but could be readily broached with cellular damage. Bowsher in-

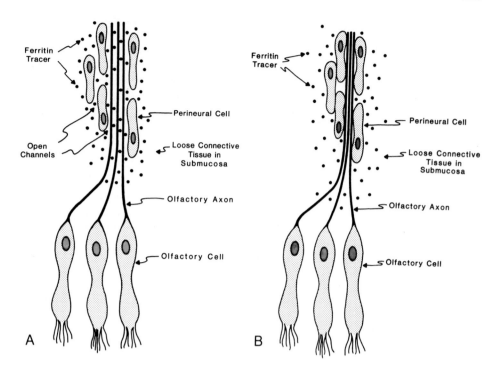

FIGURE 11–5. Schematic representation of the passage of macromolecules from the perineural space into the submucosal connective tissue. *A,* Positive hydrostatic gradient from the perineural space allows for passive drainage of cerebrospinal fluid and macromolecules. *B,* It is speculated that a negative hydrostatic gradient from the SAS to the nasal submucosa collapses the perineural space and acts as a one-way valve, preventing reflux into the SAS. (From Erlich SS, McComb JG, Hyman MS, Weiss MH: Ultrastructural morphology of the olfactory pathway for cerebrospinal fluid drainage in the rabbit. J Neurosurg 64:466, 1986.)

jected radioisotope-labeled protein into the SAS of cats and found an uptake at the arachnoid villi, around the blood vessels both on the surface and within the cortex, and along the cranial and spinal nerve root sheaths but no penetration through the arachnoid membrane, thus confirming the work of Weed.[99]

Electron microscopic studies have shown several layers of arachnoid cells between the SAS and dura; the cells in the outer portion of these layers exhibit tight junctions with occlusion of the intercellular clefts serving as an effective barrier to large molecules (i.e., they function as the blood-CSF interface in this location).[2] Butler[100] has noted that, contrary to the findings at normal pressure, the arachnoid barrier layer is disrupted at higher pressures, and HRP can penetrate through the arachnoid membrane to reach the ECS of the dura mater and dural lymphatic channels. Normally, it does not seem that much, if any, CSF drains through the arachnoid membrane, but at unphysiologically high pressures, disruption of this barrier may allow for significant bulk flow.

CIRCULATION OF CSF

CSF functions as a lymphatic system for the CNS. With the rapid turnover of CSF, it produces a concentration gradient or "sink" for the clearance of metabolic waste products to include macromolecules. The pressure gradient created between the newly secreted CSF and that at the sites of absorption produces the major force for bulk movement of CSF. Other factors that influence the circulation of CSF are the ciliary action of the ependyma and choroid plexus and the pulsations

induced by the arterial tree and respiration. The newly formed CSF has a protein content of approximately 10 mg/dl; that from lower spinal SAS is over 40 mg/dl. The difference reflects the rate of CSF turnover: the longer the CSF remains within the CNS, the more protein is added from the brain, spinal cord, and leakage from the blood-brain-CSF interface. That portion of CSF produced in the parenchyma travels via the ECS to reach the SAS or joins the CSF made by the choroid plexus within the ventricular system. The lower pressure at sites of absorption draws CSF from the brain and spinal cord surface.

ALTERATION OF CSF PHYSIOLOGY IN HYDROCEPHALUS

The observation that several laboratory animals and infants have arachnoid villi but no arachnoid granulations was cited by Dandy and Blackfan[98] as an argument against these structures having an important role in CSF absorption. Subsequent investigations have shown that the arachnoid villi and granulations are anatomically and functionally the same, the only difference being that the arachnoid villi are not visible to the unaided eye.[58, 101] If the arachnoid villi are the major site of CSF absorption, their numbers and individual structures should have some bearing on the development of hydrocephalus. That the number and size of arachnoid granulations increase with age need not have any implications, as there does not appear to be any relationship between those villi that are visible (namely, granulations) and their ability to absorb CSF. Few investigators have studied the villus in hydrocephalus. Those who have done so have mainly concentrated on the villi associated with the SSS, since the greatest concentration of these structures per volume of dural sinus exists in this region.[51, 101, 102] However, villi are present along all the other major sinuses, some of the major cerebral veins, and veins associated with the cranial and spinal nerves.[59, 64, 101, 103, 104]

Gilles and Davidson[102] examined only the SSS region for arachnoid villi at autopsy in an infant and a child, each with communicating hydrocephalus. In one case no villi were present, and in the other, only a few dysplastic villi were found. In a more thorough postmortem study, Gutierrez et al.[105] examined the superior sagittal, straight, and lateral sinuses of two children, searching for arachnoid villi. No villi were found in one child who had communicating hydrocephalus. In spite of the near or complete lack of observed villi, CSF was being absorbed somewhere, albeit inadequately in three of the four cases. Obviously CSF could have been absorbed via villi elsewhere at sites not studied or at locations without villi.

In the clinical setting, spontaneous subarachnoid hemorrhage can lead to hydrocephalus.[106–108] Experimental studies of the arachnoid villi following the introduction of blood into the SAS have shown a variable degree of villus distention and trapping of the red blood cells (RBCs) within.[56, 109] That RBCs can fill the villus following entry of blood into the SAS and can be associated with hydrocephalus does not necessarily imply that the villus is the sole or major site of CSF absorption, as the RBCs could affect all routes of drainage that have been previously considered.[110] The same argument holds true for those instances of hydrocephalus associated with elevated levels of protein within the CSF.[43]

The pressure relationships between the SSS and the SAS have been of some interest, since CSF drainage occurs in response to a hydrostatic difference and the greatest concentration of arachnoid villi are in this location. Under normal conditions, the pressure in the SAS is higher than in the SSS, an observation made by Weed and Hughson[111] and confirmed on a number of occasions since. Experimental models of congenital or kaolin-induced hydrocephalus found no pressure gradient present.[112, 113] Studies in human hydrocephalus have shown that the mean pressure in the SSS is often equal to or higher than that in the SAS.[114, 115] These observations indicate that little or no CSF absorption could be taking place in this region. CSF could certainly drain via villi in different areas where a hydrostatic gradient still remained or at locations other than the villus.

Experimental attempts to produce hydrocephalus by occlusion of the SSS,[116] torcular,[117] or vein of Galen[118] have not been successful.[119] Ventricular enlargement has not been reported following acute thrombosis of the dural sinuses in man.[120] Although hydrocephalus cannot be produced with venous obstruction intracranially, it appears to be possible to cause hydrocephalus with extracranial venous obstruction. Following ligation of all the major cephalic veins in the neck, Bering and Salibi[121] noted moderate ventricular dilatation. The clinical reports of hydrocephalus associated with impairment of venous drainage have revealed that obstructions are invariably extracranial.[122–126] One explanation could be that intracranial venous obstruction may not be sufficient to significantly raise the venous pressure throughout the intracranial venous bed. This is supported by Schlesinger,[127] who found that venous flow can be bidirectional, since no valves are present, and that the deep and superficial venous systems communicate with one another. Another suggestion is that the hydrocephalus did not result only from the impairment of cephalic venous drainage, but also from obstruction of the cervical lymphatic system.

With the single exception of CSF overproduction by excessive normally functioning choroid plexus tissue, hydrocephalus results from impaired CSF absorption.[23, 44, 128, 129] Production of CSF is only slightly pressure responsive[9] and does not diminish noticeably until cerebral perfusion pressure is markedly reduced.[25] Production of CSF in hydrocephalus is either normal or near normal.[23, 44, 128, 130] In compensated hydrocephalus, the rate of absorption must equal the rate of formation, approximately 500 ml/day, and in the noncompensated state only a small fraction of the total amount secreted is retained; thus the overwhelming majority of CSF output is still absorbed. As CSF formation is relatively constant, the change in resistance to absorption determines CSF pressure and whether or not the hydrocephalus is progressive.

Impairment of CSF absorption in communicating hydrocephalus could occur at some or all of the following sites: the arachnoid villus, the lymphatic channels associated with the cranial and spinal nerves, or the arachnoid membrane. If CSF outflow from the ventricles is blocked (noncommunicating hydrocephalus), fluid flow could still take place via the blood vessel adventitia and ECS of the cortical mantle to reach the SAS on the brain surface. Assuming a complete ventricular blockage, which is not always the case,[120, 131] additional ways for ECS to exit the ventricles would be via the dilated spinal cord central canal[132, 133] or through a fistulous opening created by a rupture of the ventricular system into the SAS at such a location as the lamina terminalis or suprapineal recess.[76]

Chronic hydrocephalus associated with neurologic abnormalities, especially in older patients in whom the measured CSF pressure is within physiologic limits, has been termed "normal-pressure hydrocephalus." Studies have shown that, in many cases, increased resistance to CSF drainage resulted in a rise in ICP that subsequently returned to normal levels with time.[107, 108, 110] However, the ventricles remained dilated as a result of a persistent transcortical pressure gradient.[134, 135] A problem with the older patient has been the proper selection of those who would benefit from CSF diversion. This difficulty is seldom encountered in the pediatric population as the ventricles usually continue to enlarge even though the ICP may not be significantly elevated.

Advances in imaging techniques have made possible

the visualization of CSF movement in normal and pathophysiologic states. Cisternography, the introduction of radiopharmaceuticals into the CSF compartment, was once thought to be the definitive study to determine which patients would benefit from shunting with normal-pressure hydrocephalus, but clinical experience has not borne this out.[136, 137] The recent development of phase image or cine MRI holds further promise in studying the dynamics of CSF circulation in normal and hydrocephalic conditions.[138–140]

THE BLOOD-BRAIN INTERFACE

HISTORY OF THE BLOOD-BRAIN BARRIER

The first studies that led to the concept of the blood-brain barrier (BBB) were performed at the beginning of this century. In 1885, Ehrlich[141] demonstrated that many dyes injected into the systemic circulation of laboratory animals stained virtually all organs in the body except the brain and spinal cord. Ehrlich's disciple, Goldmann,[142, 143] continued these experiments and, in 1909 and 1913, published two historical findings (Fig. 11–6). In his first paper he reported that intravenously administered trypan blue fails to stain the CNS and the CSF, although the choroid plexuses and meninges were stained. In the second paper, he demonstrated that intraventricularly injected trypan blue rapidly stains brain parenchyma. Thus it was concluded that there is a barrier between blood and brain, and that this barrier could be circumvented by direct injection of dyes into the CSF.

Electron microscopic cytochemical studies from the late 1960s duplicated Goldmann's first and second experiments.[10, 144] HRP injected intravenously was found in the lumen of brain microvessels, but no further movement of the label beyond the endothelial membrane was evident. When HRP was injected intraventricularly, it readily diffused across the ependyma and along the basement membrane of capillaries, but did not enter into the blood via endothelial membrane. These experiments have established the anatomic concept of the BBB, suggesting that the endothelial membrane restricts free exchanges of substances between blood and brain owing to the presence of tight junctions in the cerebral capillary endothelium. The sum of all the endothelial tight junctions forms a zipper-like continuous cellular membrane that exhibits high electrical resistance comparable with tight epithelial barriers.[145]

PRESENT ERA

During the last two decades, accumulating information has challenged the anatomic concept of an impermeable BBB, indicating that what is true for some vital dyes and HRP does not hold for many other biologically important molecules,[146, 147] or for the cells of the immune system. In addition, several classes of metabolic substrates, regulatory peptides, transport plasma proteins, steroid hormones, ions, and various groups of centrally active pharmacotherapeutics are able to utilize specialized shuttle services at the BBB. In fact, the concept of a BBB should be replaced by that of a blood-brain interface (BBI), as the endothelial layer in reality regulates the homeostasis of the neural milieu by numerous highly specific transport, enzymatic, receptor, and cell-mediated mechanisms, rather than simply impeding solute exchanges between blood and brain.

ANATOMY OF CEREBRAL MICROCIRCULATION

The brain contains a rich network of capillaries with an overall average density that is only somewhat less than in skeletal or cardiac muscle. However, there are considerable regional variations in cerebral capillary density, with gray matter containing about 2.5 times more capillaries than white matter. Since the cerebral

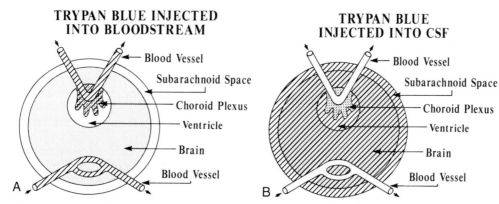

FIGURE 11–6. Diagrammatic representation of Goldman's experiments in which trypan blue was injected either into the blood stream (*A*) or into the CSF (*B*). The fact that the dye injected into the blood stream did not enter the CSF or brain while the dye injected into the CSF fully penetrated the brain gave rise to the first concept of a blood-brain barrier. In view of the extensive metabolic activity that occurs at the endothelial cell level between the blood and brain, this region is better described as an interface than simply as a barrier.

microcirculation supports the actions of brain cells, regional capillary density correlates well with the number of synapses, with oxygen consumption, and with glucose utilization.[148]

The tight junctions between endothelial cells are present in all brain regions except in some special areas known as circumventricular organs (CVO) or "windows" of the brain (see below). Cerebral endothelial junctions under the influence of astrocytes close the capillary pores that are found in the normally fenestrated endothelial interface of peripheral tissues.[145] The endothelial layer needs to be viewed as two separate membranes, one on the inside of the vessel (luminal) and that of the outside (abluminal) separated by 0.3- to 0.5-μm thick cytoplasm. The diameter of a capillary lumen is about 6 μm, and the capillaries are approximately 40 μm apart.[149]

The surface area of cerebral capillary endothelium is about 100 cm^2 per gram of brain tissue. In the adult human brain the total surface area of microvasculature is approximately 12 m^2, and the total length of the capillaries 650 km. The capillary volume represents 1 per cent of the total brain volume, with the volume of endothelial layer only one tenth that of the capillary volume. Thus, capillary endothelium in human brain occupies a surface area equal to the floor size of a small room, but its volume is only one fifth of a teaspoon. The endothelial cellular sheet, a phenomenally thin membrane spread over the brain surface, nevertheless acts as the primary homeostatic site for all molecular and cellular movements in and out of the CNS.

The surface capillary area available for blood-brain exchanges seems to be proportional to the local need for metabolic substrates (e.g., glucose, amino acids) and to exposure of receptors to their blood-borne ligands and/or cell-specific adhesion molecules. Large variations in capillary surface area are likely to be related to local metabolic activities and may include rapid or short-term changes, such as varying the number of perfused microvessels, or long-term regulations that involve remodeling of the capillary beds via angiogenesis.

REGULATION OF LOCAL CEREBRAL BLOOD FLOW

The cerebral capillary transit time is about one second. The normal cerebral angioarchitecture ensures almost instantaneous equilibration of solutes in brain ECF, once circulating molecules have been transported across the endothelial layer. It is well known that local cerebral blood flow (CBF) is adjusted to the metabolic needs of the brain. The CBF for the entire adult human brain is about 750 ml/min, or 15 per cent of the total resting cardiac output, giving average values between 50 and 60 ml per 100 gm of brain tissue.

There are normally marked differences in local CBF that can vary up to a 16-fold range.[150] Positron emission tomography (PET) studies in human cortex have revealed that local CBF in each individual segment of the brain changes within seconds in response to changes in surrounding neuronal activity. Simply making a fist of the hand results in immediate increase in local CBF in the areas of the appropriate motor cortex; or, reading a book increases local CBF in the occipital cortex and language areas of the temporal cortex. PET has also been shown to be useful in localizing the focus of epileptic attacks, since the local CBF acutely and markedly increases at the focal point of the attack at onset.

Local CBF is regulated by various metabolic factors such as P_{CO_2}, pH, and P_{O_2}. An increase in either P_{CO_2} or hydrogen ions causes an increase in local CBF, whereas it is a decrease in P_{O_2} that increases local CBF. Since a decrease in the pH of the brain tissue greatly depresses neuronal activity, an important function of the local microcirculation is to rapidly and efficiently remove the by-products of brain metabolism such as CO_2 and hydrogen ions.

The cerebral circulatory system also has a significant sympathetic innervation, but it appears that under normal physiologic conditions, the local CBF autoregulatory metabolic mechanisms are so powerful that they compensate almost entirely for any sympathetic stimulation. However, under certain pathologic conditions, for example, after subarachnoid hemorrhage following aneurysmal rupture, the sympathetic reflexes may cause vasospasm in intermediate and large arteries. Also, an increase in local CBF, brain metabolism, and endothelial permeability to a number of molecules by the administration of sympathomimetic drugs has been well documented.[151]

TRANSPORT BIOLOGY

Circulating molecules use a number of different mechanisms present at the BBI for transport, depending on their structure, and these include: (1) lipid-mediated transport for highly lipophilic drugs; (2) carrier-mediated transport for hydrophilic nutrients and their drug analogs; (3) plasma protein-mediated transport of drugs; (4) receptor- or absorptive-mediated transcytosis of peptides and proteins; and (5) bulk flow transcytosis.

Lipid-Mediated Transport. Lipophilic drugs with molecular weight less than 600 are assumed to readily enter the brain via diffusion into the lipid phase of the endothelial plasma membrane. The lipid solubility of the drugs can be assessed by determining their water/octanol partition coefficient and/or by computing the number of hydrogen bonds in the molecule. The increased lipid solubility and a smaller number of hydrogen bonds usually result in better brain penetrability of the drug. The relatively low lipid solubility of morphine is attributed to the two polar hydroxyl groups on the ring nucleus that may be masked by methylation or acetylation. Methylation of one of these hydroxyl groups converts morphine to codeine, with a transport ten times faster than that of morphine. Acetylation of both of the morphine hydroxyl groups transforms morphine to heroin and results in a transport 100 times faster than that of morphine.

Drugs form hydrogen bonds in water owing to the presence of polar functional groups on their molecules.

The total number of hydrogen bonds can be computed, according to the rules of Stein,[152] as: 3 for carboxyl, 2 for hydroxyl groups, amine and amide, 1 for carbonyls, aldehydes, or ketones, 0 for ether, and ½ for an ester group. A classic example of increasing numbers of hydrogen bonds resulting in reduced brain penetrability is the steroid hormone model. For six different steroids given in Figure 11–7, transport into the brain decreases by one log order of magnitude with the addition of each hydroxyl group on the parent molecule.[153] Thus, the decreasing order of brain transport of steroids is progesterone ≥ testosterone ≥ estradiol ≥ corticosterone ≥ aldosterone ≥ cortisol. A relatively low number of hydrogen bonds explains why some centrally active drugs such a diazepam (2 bonds) and phenytoin (5 bonds) are readily transported into the brain, whereas methotrexate (16 bonds) is poorly penetrable.

Although the partition coefficient and the number of hydrogen bonds may generally predict drug brain penetrability, there are exceptions of this rule. For instance, the immunosuppressive drug cyclosporine is transported into the brain at rates that are at least a two-log order of magnitude less than that predicted by its partition coefficient value.[154] Several mechanisms have been proposed to explain paradoxically low brain uptake of some highly lipophilic drugs. Some of these mechanisms are (1) steric hindrance for drugs with a molecular weight of more than 1000; (2) active efflux from the brain; (3) lack of rapid drug transfer from lipid endothelial phase into water ECF phase; and (4) molecular alteration at the BBI.

Carrier-Mediated Transport. Most circulating metabolic substrates are hydrophilic, and they traverse the BBI by specific carrier-mediated transport systems expressed at both the luminal and abluminal sides of the endothelial membrane. Eight different systems have been described in brain capillaries,[155–157] and these are specific for: (1) hexoses; (2) monocarboxylic acids; (3) neutral amino acids; (4) basic acids; (5) acidic amino acids; (6) amines; (7) nucleosides; and (8) purine bases. It is believed that these specific transport systems mediate the bidirectional movement of essential nutrients between plasma and brain ECF. Apart from the hexose

carrier, the biochemical and molecular identity of other transport systems have not yet been determined, but their presence at the BBI has been confirmed by physiologic methods.

It is believed that the carriers are enzyme-like proteins that are under genetic regulation. Each of the BBI nutrient transporters is able to act on a number of different nutrients if their structure is similar, but with a varying degree of affinity. For example, the hexose carrier in addition to glucose also transports 2-deoxyglucose, 3-0-methyl glucose, mannose, and galactose, and is sterospecific since the carrier does not recognize the L-isomers.[156] The monocarboxylic carrier also transports lactate, pyruvate, and acetate.[158] The neutral amino acid carrier transports L-phenylalanine and 12 other neutral L-amino acids,[156, 157, 159] but has a higher affinity for the large amino acids than for those that are small.

The possibility that nutrient carrier systems can be used for transport of centrally active hydrophilic drug analogs of metabolic substrates has been investigated. L-dopa and alpha-methyldopa, currently used in the treatment of Parkinson's disease and hypertension respectively, are transported into the brain by the neutral amino acid carrier.[160–164]

The purine nucleoside transporters[165] and more recently characterized pyrimidine transporters[166] at the BBI are of interest for the treatment of CNS viral diseases including acquired immunodeficiency syndrome (AIDS). These antiviral drugs are modified nucleosides, such as azidothymidine, dideoxycytidine, and dideoxyinosine. It seems inevitable that a host of new drugs with high affinity for other BBI carriers—such as those of glucose, choline, or monocarboxylic acid—will eventually be designed.

Molecular Characterization of Transporters. Three proteins with known transport functions at the BBI have been characterized by molecular techinques. Northern blot analysis has shown that the mRNA encoding glucose transporter, isoform GLUT-1, is enriched in brain microvessels,[167] and that the GLUT-1 gene is selectively expressed in brain capillary endothelium, with minimal or no expression in neurons or glial cells. GLUT-1 is a member of the sodium-independent glu-

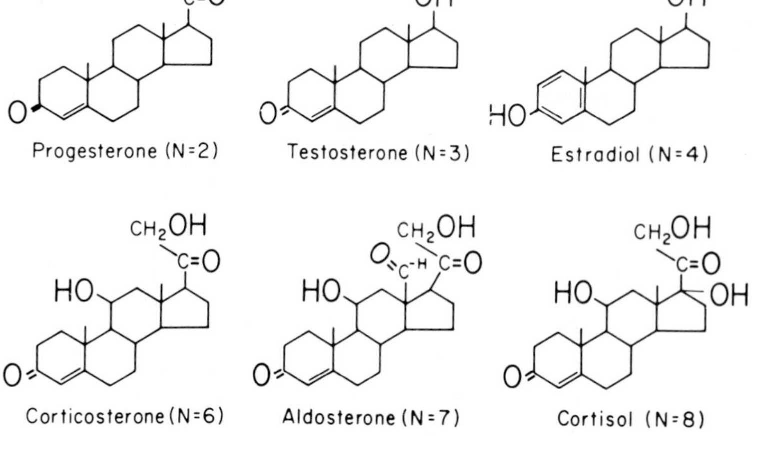

FIGURE 11–7. Molecular structures of steroid hormones emphasizing the polar functional groups (hydroxyls and carbonyls) that form the hydrogen bond with solvent water. The total number, N, of hydrogen bonds formed with solvent water are given in parentheses. (From Pardridge WM: Transport of protein-bound hormones into tissues in vivo. Endocr Rev 2:103, 1981.)

Progesterone (N=2)   Testosterone (N=3)   Estradiol (N=4)

Corticosterone (N=6)   Aldosterone (N=7)   Cortisol (N=8)

cose transporter supergene family. The selective localization of the GLUT-1 transporter isoform to brain capillary endothelium and to the basolateral membrane of choroid plexus epithelium has been confirmed by immunocytochemical studies in human brain, and by comparative Western blotting studies of brain capillary membranes and capillary-depleted synaptosomal membranes.[168]

Western blot studies have demonstrated that P-glycoprotein, the product of the multidrug resistance (MDR) gene, is present in brain microvessels.[169] P-glycoprotein extrudes many ligands from the cytoplasmic space in an ATP-dependent active efflux mechanism. The expression of this protein in many lines of cancer cells is associated with the development of resistance to a number of chemotherapeutic agents, such as vinblastin, actinomycin D, and Adriamycin. In addition, lipophilic amine drugs, calcium-channel blockers, and many steroid hormones also bind P-glycoprotein. Its exact role at the BBI remains unclear at present.

Recently, three alpha (alpha$_1$,alpha$_2$,alpha$_3$) and two beta (beta$_1$,beta$_2$) subunits of Na,K-ATPase have been detected in cerebral microvessels by Western blot analysis.[170, 171] The choroid plexus expresses only alpha$_1$, beta$_1$, and beta$_2$, as alpha$_2$, and alpha$_3$ were not found. The relative level of expression of alpha and beta subunit isoforms has also been determined and varies considerably as to site, reflecting different transport function (Fig. 11–8).

Plasma Protein–Mediated Transport. Acidic drugs and peptides are avidly bound to plasma albumin.[172] Recent physicochemical studies have revealed that the albumin molecule possesses at least six major binding sites for drugs. These sites correspond to the six primary alpha-helical subdomains on the albumin molecule and are distributed over the entire surface of the protein. Also, lipophilic amine drugs such as propranolol and bupivacaine are bound to an alpha$_1$-acid glycoprotein (globulin) called orosomucoid. Lipid-soluble peptides are bound to lipoproteins. The extent of

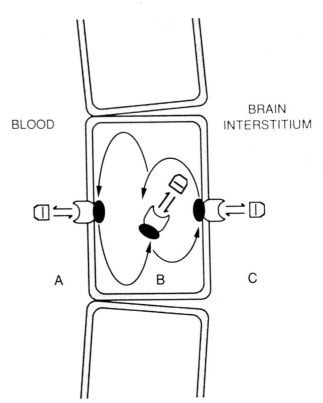

FIGURE 11–9. Receptor-mediated transcytosis model for large peptide and protein transfer across the blood-brain interface. *A,* Receptor-mediated endocytosis. *B,* Movement through the endothelial cytoplasm. *C,* Receptor-mediated exocytosis. (From Pardridge WM: Receptor-mediated peptide transport through the blood-brain barrier. Endocr Rev 7:314, 1986.)

plasma protein binding can be determined in vitro by equilibrium dialysis or ultrafiltration. According to free-hormone/drug hypothesis, the drug fraction that is freely (dialyzable or filtratable in vitro) should be identical to the fraction that is available for transport into the brain in vivo. However, recent studies have invalidated this hypothesis by demonstrating enhanced dissociation of ligand from the ligand-protein complex within cerebral microcirculation.[157] It is suggested that interactions between plasma proteins and the surface of brain capillary endothelium may induce transient conformational changes of drug-binding sites in protein molecule, resulting in enhanced dissociation of drugs.

Receptor-Mediated Transcytosis. Receptor-mediated transcytosis across cerebral capillaries has been observed for several proteins, such as insulin,[173] transferrin,[174] and insulin-like growth factors.[157] It is also suggested that some small neuroactive peptides, such as vasopressin[175, 176] or delta-sleep-inducing peptide,[177] are transported from blood into brain by a similar mechanism. The mechanim involves three steps: (1) receptor-mediated endocytosis at the luminal side of brain capillaries; (2) movement of the ligand-receptor complex through the endothelial cytoplasm; and (3) receptor-mediated exocytosis of the ligand into brain ECF at the abluminal side of brain capillaries[178] (Fig. 11–9). In contrast to rapid carrier-mediated transport of small nutrients, which occurs in milliseconds to sec-

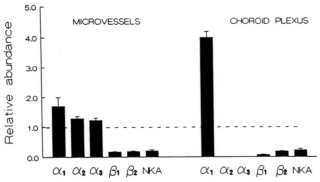

FIGURE 11–8. Distribution of sodium pump isoform subunits and Na,K-ATPase activity in rat cerebral microvessels and choroid plexus relative to capillary depleted brain homogenates as determined by Western blot quantitation. The values were normalized to a constant amount of protein in the studied samples. The dashed line is defined arbitrarily as one and indicates either a subunit abundance or paucity in relationship to a constant amount of protein. (From Zlokovic BV, et al.: Differential expression of Na,K-ATPase isoenzymes at the blood-brain barrier and the choroid plexus. J Biol Chem 268:8019, 1993.)

onds, receptor-mediated transcytosis takes place over a much longer time period, minutes to hours.

Absorptive-Mediated Transcytosis. Absorptive-mediated transcytosis at BBI is similar to receptor-mediated transcytosis, except that the first step at the luminal side of cerebral capillaries is accomplished by electrostatic or carbohydrate-mediated interactions, rather than by interaction with specific receptors. Polycationic proteins such as cationized IgG,[179] cationized albumin, or lectines[157] may use this mechanism. It is possible that antibodies with alkaline isoelectrical point undergo selective absorptive-mediated transcytosis at the BBI, as has been recently shown for IgG.[180]

Bulk-Flow Transcytosis. Fluid phase transcytosis indicates bulk movement of fluid and molecules across endothelial cells by pinocytosis and/or tubulocanalicular mechanism. Circulating molecules are endocytosed at a rate that is independent of their molecular weight. The trans-Golgi network is not involved. Bulk flow transcytosis at the BBI is minimal under normal physiologic conditions, but it may become significant under certain pathologic circumstances such as trauma, seizures, and acute hypertension wherein the BBI is damaged. Increased endothelial pinocytosis has also been observed in models of microwave radiation,[181] hyperbaric oxygen therapy,[182] hypothermia,[183] lymphostatic encephalopathy,[184] regeneration following brain trauma,[185] and during brain development.[186]

VIRUSES

Neurotropic viruses enter the brain by several different mechanisms. The polio virus first undergoes endocytosis by peripheral nerve endings and then is transported to spinal cord motor neurons by retrograde axonal transport. The HIV virus is believed to enter the brain by infecting monocytes and macrophages. More recent work has demonstrated that CD4 antigen, the receptor for endocytosis of free HIV, may be expressed in cerebral microvessels, suggesting that free HIV may undergo direct transport at the BBI.[187] There is evidence that some viruses express antigens that have affinity for various receptor-mediated or absorptive-mediated mechanisms within brain capillaries, such as the canine distemper virus[188] and possibly some reoviruses.[189]

IMMUNE CELLS

According to traditional concept, the CNS is regarded as an immunologically privileged site, but recent studies have shown that under pathologic conditions a large number of circulating immune cells can cross the endothelial barrier and enter the CNS. These immune cells contribute to or directly mediate neurologic damage. Lymphocytes and monocytes are the major infiltrating cells found in multiple sclerosis and experimental allergic encephalitis, whereas neutrophils predominate following head trauma and ischemia. The initial step of immune cell entry into the brain involves the attachment of circulating leukocytes to the luminal side of cerebral endothelium.

It has been demonstrated that antigen-activated T lymphocytes are able to cross into the brain, whereas unactivated lymphocytes do not.[190] Although the mechanisms that mediate blood-brain transfer of immune cells are not at present fully understood, it is believed that the expression of specific adhesion molecules on both the leukocytes and cerebral endothelial cells are required for these cellular interactions to occur. The expression of leukocyte adhesion molecules is found to be important for the attachment of lymphocytes and monocytes to the inflamed endothelium. The role of locally released cytokines from activated leukocytyes seems to mediate endothelial activation.

FOUR-CELL PARADIGM

A four-cell paradigm of the BBI describes the close anatomic proximity between cerebral endothelial cells, pericytes, astrocytes and neurons (see Fig. 11–3). Endothelial cells are separated from pericytes by a common basement membrane. Astrocytes send their foot processes to invest more than 90 per cent of the capillary surface. The neuronal endings may also directly innervate the endothelium.

Experiments with transplantation of embryonic tissues between chicks and quails[191] have provided strong evidence in support of the concept that the physiologic properties of the BBI arise from the expression of a unique set of genes within the capillary endothelium, and that this genetic expression is orchestrated by soluble factors secreted by the brain itself. For example, when embryonic quail brain was transplanted into embryonic chick gut, the quail brain became vascularized by chick gut vessels. These vessels expressed unique biochemical properties of brain capillaries such as tight junctions, gamma-glutamyl transpeptidase, and specialized transport processes. Conversely, when embryonic quail gut was transplanted into embryonic chick brain, the quail gut became vascularized by chick brain vessels that did not express any properties of brain capillaries.

Several subsequent studies have demonstrated the importance of astrocytes as the possible cellular source for the putative soluble factors that turn-on the BBI specific genes within brain capillary endothelium.[192] However, since these soluble factors have not been isolated yet, the contribution of neurons and pericytes cannot be excluded.

CIRCUMVENTRICULAR ORGANS

A number of areas in and around the ventricles are collectively called the CVOs. These regions have a fenestrated type of capillaries, comparable to capillaries in peripheral tissues[193] (Fig. 11–10). The CVOs include the posterior pituitary (neurohypophysis), pineal gland, subcomissural organ, subfornical organ (SFO), organum vasculosum laminae terminalis (OVLT), median

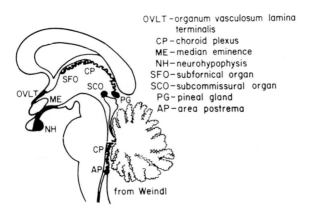

OVLT – organum vasculosum lamina
terminalis
CP – choroid plexus
ME – median eminence
NH – neurohypophysis
SFO – subfornical organ
SCO – subcommissural organ
PG – pineal gland
AP – area postrema

from Weindl

FIGURE 11–10. Circumventricular organs of the brain are tiny areas around the ventricles that lack the normal tight junctions found in the rest of the parenchyma. (From Weindl A: Neuroendocrine aspects of circumventricular organs. *In* Ganong WF, Martine L [eds]: Frontiers in Neuroendocrinology. New York, Oxford University Press, 1973.)

eminence (ME), and area postrema. The total volume and surface area of the CVOs is trivial compared to the total surface area of proper tight-junctioned cerebral microvessels, the difference being more than 5000 times.

The presence of the CVO in brain allows for the rapid uptake of circulating neuroendocrine substances at nerve endings. Thus, the SFO, OVLT, and ME may be regarded as a part of rapid signaling systems for neuroendocrine control, since the circulating substances may be transported from these CVO regions to neuronal cell bodies by axoplasmic flow. This in turn may have a direct effect on different neurovegetative functions of the CNS, such as regulation of water intake and/or blood pressure, as in the case of angiotensin II. Other CVOs, such as area postrema, act as a chemical triggering zone related to nausea and emesis.

STRATEGIES FOR DRUG DELIVERY

Several strategies are available for drug delivery to the brain and include those that are invasive, pharmacologic, physiologically based, and genetic.

Invasive Strategies. These procedures involve intraventricular or hyperosmotic carotid infusion methods. The intraventricular method requires implantation of a catheter, followed by infusion of drug by an implantable pump. This method may be useful for delivery of chemotherapeutic agents in diseases that have a predilection for the tissues adjacent to the ventricles or SAS, such as leukemic infiltration. However, the method is inefficient for drug delivery to the brain parenchyma because significant efflux of ECF and CSF from the ventricular compartment will keep the concentration in the parenchyma low. One variation of the intrathecal approach is administration of drugs by nasal spray, which may be directly taken up by the brain owing to a continuity of the subarachnoid space of the olfactory lobe and submucous space of the nose.[194]

Another invasive approach is administration of drugs preceded by hyperosmotic carotid infusion of mannitol and/or arabinose, which cause a transient shrinkage of cerebral endothelial cells and interruption of endothelial tight junctions. This approach has been applied in chemotherapy of brain tumors, but the toxicity of such a procedure is high, and the incidence of seizure may be as great as 20 per cent.[195] Little benefit has been derived from this technique to date.

Pharmacologic Strategies. The use of liposomes to transport drugs into the brain has so far proved inadequate since liposomes, although avidly taken up by the cells of the reticuloendothelial system of liver and spleen, are not measurably transported across cerebral endothelium.[196] A potentially more powerful approach is lipidization, which involves conversion of the functional group of the drug molecule from being water-soluble into one that is lipid-soluble. For example, coupling the carboxyl and amino groups of peptides results in a large increase in lipid solubility owing to the loss of several functional hydrogen bonds. Cyclised peptides such as thyroid-releasing hormone or oxytocin are more readily transported into the brain than are their parent analogs.

Physiologic Strategies. Formation of chimeric peptides represents an important application of physiologically based strategies.[178] The chimeric peptides are formed from a transportable peptide and a nontransportable peptide, preferably by using a cross-linking reagent that can be cleaved upon entering brain tissue. The chimeric peptides are then transported by a receptor-mediated mechanism at the BBI, existing for naturally transportable peptides such as insulin, transferrin, and cationized albumin. The classic example is B-endorphin/cationized-albumin chimer.

Genetic Strategies. Gene replacement therapy in the CNS has a potential to control genetically inherited diseases, brain tumors, and possibly some metabolic diseases. However, a number of problems must be resolved before this therapy can be adopted for clinical use. For example, direct injections of protein or recombinant virions, transplantation of genetically altered grafts, and bone marrow transplantation techniques have had limited success in treating CNS diseases. Another major obstacle is the delivery of specific proteins and/or recombinant genetic material across cerebral endothelium. To date, efforts have relied upon retroviral vectors to integrate recombinant DNA into host cells, a method that may be suitable for expressing toxic genes as a genetic approach to brain tumors, but such vectors are not suitable for replacement of necessary genes in neurons. Recent experimental work has shown that replication of defective recombinant herpes simplex virus in rats can lead to specific expression of foreign genetic material in brain neuronal cells.[196]

REFERENCES

1. Brightman MW: The intracerebral movement of proteins injected into blood and cerebrospinal fluid of mice. Prog Brain Res 29:19, 1968.

2. Nabeshima S, Reese TS, Landis DMD, et al.: Junctions in the meninges and marginal glia. J Comp Neurol 164:127, 1975.

3. Davson H, Welch K, Segal MB: Physiology and Pathophysiology of the Cerebrospinal Fluid. Edinburgh, Churchill Livingstone, 1987.

4. Dohrmann GJ: The choroid plexus in experimental hydrocephalus. A light and electron microscopic study in normal, hydrocephalic, and shunted hydrocephalic dogs. J Neurosurg 34:56, 1971.

5. Miner LC, Reed DJ: Composition of fluid obtained from choroid plexus tissue isolated in a chamber *in situ*. J Physiol (Lond) 227:127, 1972.

6. Welch K: Secretion of cerebrospinal fluid by the choroid plexus of the rabbit. Am J Physiol 205:617, 1963.

7. Milhorat TH: Hydrocephalus and the Cerebrospinal Fluid. Baltimore, Williams & Wilkins, 1972.

8. Pollay M, Curl F: Secretion of cerebrospinal fluid by the ventricular ependyma of the rabbit. Am J Physiol 213:1031, 1967.

9. Welch K: The principles of physiology of the cerebrospinal fluid in relation to hydrocephalus including normal pressure hydrocephalus. *In* Friedlander WJ (ed): Current Reviews. Advances in Neurology. Vol 13. New York, Raven Press, 1975, pp 247–332.

10. Brightman MW, Reese TS: Junctions between intimately opposed cell membranes in the vertebrate brain. J Cell Biol 40:648, 1969.

11. Rall DP: Transport through the ependymal linings. Prog Brain Res 29:159, 1968.

12. Oldendorf WH, Cornford ME, Brown WJ: The large apparent work capability of the blood-brain barrier: a study of the mitochondrial content of capillary endothelial cells in brain and other tissues of the rat. Ann Neurol 1:409, 1977.

13. Segal MB, Pollay M: The secretion of cerebrospinal fluid. Exp Eye Res 25(Suppl):127, 1977.

14. Wright EM: Active transport of iodide and other anions across the choroid plexus. J Physiol (Lond) 240:535, 1974.

15. Diamond JM, Bosert WH: Standing-gradient osmotic flow. A mechanism for coupling of water and solute transport in epithelia. J Gen Physiol 50:2061, 1967.

16. Segal MB, Burgess AMC: A combined physiological and morphological study of the secretory process in the rabbit choroid plexus. J Cell Sci 14:339, 1974.

17. Katzman R, Pappius HM: Brain Electrolytes and Fluid Metabolism. Baltimore, Williams & Wilkins, 1973.

18. Maren TH: Bicarbonate formation in cerebrospinal fluid: role in sodium transport and pH regulation. Am J Physiol 222:885, 1972.

19. Wright EM, Wiedner G, Rumrich G: Fluid secretion by the frog choroid plexus. Exp Eye Res 25(Suppl):149, 1977.

20. Heisey SR, Held D, Pappenheimer JR: Bulk flow and diffusion 203:775, 1962.

21. Pappenheimer JR, Heisey SR, Jordan EF, et al.: Perfusion of the cerebral ventricular system in unanesthetized goats. Am J Physiol 203:763, 1962.

22. Cutler RWP, Page L, Galicich J, et al.: Formation and absorption of cerebrospinal fluid in man. Brain 91:707, 1968.

23. Lorenzo AV, Page LK, Watters GV: Relationship between cerebrospinal fluid formation, absorption and pressure in human hydrocephalus. Brain 93:679, 1970.

24. Rubin RC, Henderson ES, Ommaya AK, et al.: The production of cerebrospinal fluid in man and its modification by acetazolamide. J Neurosurg 25:430, 1966.

25. Weiss MH, Wertman N: Modulation of CSF production by alterations in cerebral perfusion pressure. Arch Neurol 35:527, 1978.

26. Hochwald GM, Wald A, Malhan C: The sink action of cerebrospinal fluid volume flow. Effect on brain water content. Arch Neurol 33:339, 1976.

27. Stern J, Hochwald GM, Wald A, et al.: Visualization of brain interstitial fluid movement during osmotic disequilibrium. Exp Eye Res 25(Suppl):475, 1977.

28. Pullen RGL, DePasquale M, Cserr HF: Bulk flow of cerebrospinal fluid into brain in response to acute hyperosmolality. Am J Physiol, 253:F538, 1987.

29. Matson DD, Crofton FDL: Papillomas of the choroid plexus in childhood. J Neurosurg 17:1002, 1960.

30. Eisenberg HM, McComb JG, Lorenzo AV: Cerebrospinal fluid overproduction and hydrocephalus associated with choroid plexus papilloma. J Neurosurg 40:381, 1974.

31. Milhorat TH, Hammock MK, David DA, et al.: Choroid plexus papilloma. I. Proof of cerebrospinal fluid over-production. Childs Brain 2:273, 1976.

32. Welch K, Strand R, Bresnan M, et al.: Congenital hydrocephalus due to villous hypertrophy of the telencephalic choroid plexuses. J Neurosurg 59:172, 1983.

33. Breeze RE, McComb JH, Hyman S, et al.: Cerebrospinal fluid formation in acute ventriculitis. J Neurosurg 70:619, 1989.

34. Dacey RG, Welsh JE, Scheld WM, et al.: Alterations of cerebrospinal fluid outflow resistance in experimental bacterial meningitis. (Abstract) Ann Neurol 4:173, 1978.

35. Epstein MH, Feldman AM, Brusilow SW: Cerebrospinal fluid production: Stimulation by cholera toxin. Science 196:1012, 1977.

36. Hyman S, McComb JG, Megerdichian L, et al.: Blood-cerebrospinal fluid barrier alteration following intraventricularly administered cholera toxin. Brain Res 419:104, 1987.

37. Williams GL, Pollay M, Seale T, et al.: Benzodiazepine receptors and cerebrospinal fluid formation. J Neurosurg 72:759, 1990.

38. Martins AN, Ramirez A, Solomon LS, et al.: The effect of dexamethasone on the rate of formation of cerebrospinal fluid in the monkey. J Neurosurg 41:550, 1974.

39. Vela AR, Carey ME, Thompson BM: Further data on the acute effect of intravenous steroids on canine CSF secretion and absorption. J Neurosurg 50:477, 1979.

40. Sato O: The effect of dexamethasone on cerebrospinal fluid production rate in the dog. Brain Nerve 19:485, 1967.

41. Weiss MH, Nulsen FE: The effect of glucocorticoids on CSF flow in dogs. J Neurosurg 32:452, 1970.

42. McCarthy KD, Reed DJ: The effect of acetazalzmide and furosemide and cerebrospinal fluid production and choroid plexus carbonic anhydrase activity. J Pharmacol Exp Ther 189:194, 1974.

43. Fishman RA: Cerebrospinal Fluid in Diseases of the Nervous System. Philadelphia, WB Saunders Co., 1980.

44. Bering EA Jr, Sato O: Hydrocephalus: Changes in formation and absorption of cerebrospinal fluid within the cerebral ventricles. J Neurosurg 20:1050, 1963.

45. Katzman R, Hussey F: A simple constant-infusion manometric test for measurement of CSF absorption. I. Rationale and method. Neurology 20:534, 1970.

46. Mortensen OA, Weed LH: Absorption of isotonic fluids from the subarachnoid space. Am J Physiol 108:458, 1934.

47. Davson H, Hollingsworth G, Segal MB: The mechanism of drainage of the cerebrospinal fluid. Brain 93:665, 1970.

48. Mann JD, Butler AB, Johnson RN, et al.: Clearance of macromolecular and particulate substances from the cerebrospinal fluid system of the rat. J Neurosurg 50:343, 1979.

49. Weed LH: Forces concerned in the absorption of the cerebrospinal fluid. Am J Physiol 114:40, 1935.

50. Prockop LD, Schanker LS, Brodie BB: Passage of lipid-insoluble substance from the cerebrospinal fluid to blood. J Pharmacol Exper Ther 135:266, 1962.

51. Welch K, Friedman V: The cerebrospinal fluid valves. Brain 83:454, 1960.

52. Alksne JF, White Le Jr: Electron-microscope study of the effect of increased intracranial pressure on the arachnoid villus. J Neurosurg 22:481, 1965.

53. Gomez DG, Potts DG, Deonarine V, et al.: Effects of pressure gradient changes on the morphology of arachnoid villi and granulations of the monkey. Lab Invest 28:648, 1973.

54. Potts DG, Deonarine V, Welton W: Perfusion studies of the cerebrospinal fluid absorptive pathways in the dog. Radiology 104:321, 1972.

55. Wolfson LI, Katzman R: Infusion manometric test in experimental subarachnoid hemorrhage in cats. Neurology 22:856, 1972.

56. Alksne JF, Lovings ET: The role of the arachnoid villus in the

removal of red blood cells from the subarachnoid space. An electron microscope study in the dog. J Neurosurg 36:192, 1972.

57. Shabo AL, Maxwell DS: The morphology of the arachnoid villi: A light and electron microscopic study in the monkey. J Neurosurg 29:451, 1968.

58. Weed LH: The absorption of cerebrospinal fluid into the venous system. Am J Anat 31:191, 1923.

59. Key EAH, Retzius MG: Studien in der Antomie des Nervensystems und des Bindegewebes. Stockholm, Samson and Walin, 1875.

60. Weed LH: Studies on cerebrospinal fluid. No. III. The pathways of escape from the subarachnoid spaces with particular reference to the arachnoid villi. J Med Res 31:51, 1914.

61. Levine JE, Povlishock JT, Becker DP: The morphological correlates of primate cerebrospinal fluid absorption. Brain Res 241:31, 1982.

62. Tripathi RC: Ultrastructure of the arachnoid matter in relation to outflow of cerebrospinal fluid. A new concept. Lancet ii:8, 1973.

63. Tripathi BJ, Tripathi RC: Vacuolar transcellular channels as a drainage pathway for cerebrospinal fluid. J Physiol (Lond) 239:195, 1974.

64. Welch K, Pollay M: Perfusion of particles through arachnoid villi of the monkey. Am J Physiol 201:651, 1961.

65. James AE Jr, McComb JG, Christian J: The effect of cerebrospinal fluid pressure on the size of the drainage pathways. Neurology 26:659, 1976.

66. Bradbury MWB, Cole DF: The role of the lymphatic system in drainage of cerebrospinal fluid and aqueous humour. J Physiol (Lond) 299:353, 1980.

67. Bradbury MWB, Cserr HF, Westrop RJ: Drainage of cerebral interstitial fluid into deep cervical lymph of the rabbit. Am J Physiol 240:F329, 1981.

68. Bradbury MWB, Westrop RJ: Factors influencing exit of substances from cerebrospinal fluid into deep cervical lymph of the rabbit. J Physiol (Lond) 339:519, 1983.

69. Bradbury MWB, Westrop RJ: Lymphatics and the drainage of cerebrospinal fluid. In Shapiro K, Marmarou A, Portnoy H (eds): Hydrocephalus. New York, Raven Press, 1984, pp 69–82.

70. Erlich SS, McComb JH, Hyman S, et al.: Ultrastructural morphology of the olfactory pathway for CSF drainage in the rabbit. J Neurosurg 64:466, 1986.

71. Erlich SS, McComb JG, Hyman S, et al.: Ultrastructure of the orbital pathway for cerebrospinal fluid drainage in the rabbit. J Neurosurg 70:926, 1989.

72. Gomez DG, Fenstermacher JD, Manzo RP, et al.: Cerebrospinal fluid absorption in the rabbit: Olfactory pathways. Acta Otolaryngol 100:429, 1985.

73. Gomez DB, Manzo RP, Fenstermacher JD, et al.: Cerebrospinal fluid absorption in the rabbit. Graefe's Arch Clin Exp Ophthalmol 226:1, 1988.

74. Love JA, Leslie RA: The effects of raised ICP on lymph flow in the cervical lymphatic trunks in cats. J Neurosurg 60:577, 1984.

75. McComb JG, Davson H, Hyman S: Cerebrospinal fluid drainage as influenced by ventricular pressure in the rabbit. J Neurosurg 56:709, 1982.

76. McComb JG, Hyman S, Weiss MH: Lymphatic drainage of cerebrospinal fluid in the cat. In Shapiro K, Marmarou A, Portnoy H (eds): Hydrocephalus. New York, Raven Press, 1984, pp 83–98.

77. Shen JY, Kelly DE, et al.: Intraorbital cerebrospinal fluid outflow and the posterior uveal compartment of the hamster eye. Cell Tissue Res 240:77, 1985.

78. McComb JH, Hyman S: Lymphatic drainage of cerebrospinal fluid in the primate. In Johansson BB, Owman Ch, Widner H (eds): Pathophysiology of the Blood-Brain Barrier. Elsevier Science Publishers, 1990, pp 421–438.

79. Yamada S, DePasquale M, Patlak CS, et al.: Albumin outflow into deep cervical lymph from different regions of rabbit brain. Am J Physiol 261:H1197, 1991.

80. James AE Jr, Strecker EP, Sperber E, et al.: An alternative pathway of cerebrospinal fluid absorption in communicating hydrocephalus. Transependymal movement. Radiology 111:143, 1974.

81. Wislocki GB, Putnam TJ: Absorption from the ventricles in experimentally produced internal hydrocephalus. Am J Anat 29:313, 1921.

82. Tamaki N, Yamashita H, Kimura M, et al.: Changes in the components and content of biological water in the brain of experimental hydrocephalic rabbits. J Neurosurg 73:274, 1990.

83. Hiratsuka H, Tabata H, Tsurouka S, et al.: Evaluation of periventricular hypodensity in experimental hydrocephalus by metrizamide CT ventriculography. J Neurosurg 56:235, 1982.

84. Zervas NT, Liszczak TM, Mayberg MR, et al.: Cerebrospinal fluid may nourish cerebral vessels through pathways in the adventitia that may be analogous to systemic vasa vasorum. J Neurosurg 56:475, 1982.

85. Rosenberg GA, Kyner WT, Estrada E: Bulk flow of brain interstitial fluid under normal and hyperosmolar conditions. Am J Physiol 238:F42, 1980.

86. Reulen HJ, Tsuyumu M, Tack A, et al.: Clearance of edema fluid into cerebrospinal fluid. A mechanism for the resolution of vasogenic brain edema. J Neurosurg 48:754, 1978.

87. Ohata K, Marmarou A: Clearance of brain edema and macromolecules through the cortical extracellular space. J Neurosurg 77:387, 1992.

88. Casley-Smith R, Foldi-Borcsok E, Foldi M: The prelymphatic pathways of the brain as revealed by cervical lymphatic obstruction and the passages of particles. Br J Exp Pathol 57:179, 1976.

89. McComb JG, Song SH, Hyman S, et al.: The adventitia of the major cranial blood vessels does not provide a pathway for lymphatic drainage of cerebrospinal fluid. Presented at the American Association of Neurological Surgeons. San Francisco, California, April 11–16, 1992.

90. Schwalbe G: Der Arachnoidalraum ein Lymphraum und sein Zusammenhang mit den Perichoriodalraum. Zentralbl Med Wiss 7:465, 1869.

91. Brierley JB, Field EJ: The connections of the spinal subarachnoid space with the lymphatic system. J Anat 82:153, 1948.

92. DiChiro G, Stein SC, Harrington T: Spontaneous cerebrospinal fluid rhinorrhea in normal dogs. Radioisotope studies of an alternative pathway of CSF drainage. J Neuropathol Exp Neurol 31:447, 1972.

93. Faber FW: The nasal mucosa and the subarachnoid space. Am J Anat 62:121, 1937.

94. Schurr PH, McLaurin RL, Ingraham FD: Experimental studies on the circulation of the cerebrospinal fluid and methods of producing communicating hydrocephalus in the dog. J Neurosurg 10:515, 1953.

95. Yoffrey JM, Drinker CK: Some observations on the lymphatics of the nasal mucous membrane in the cat and monkey. J Anat 74:45, 1939.

96. Galkin WS: Uber die bedentung der 'nasenbahn' fur arbfluss aus subarachnoidal raum. Z Gesamte Exp Med 72:65, 1930.

97. McComb JG, Hyman S, Weiss MH: Contribution of the spinal compartment to cerebrospinal fluid drainage. Presented at the American Association of Neurological Surgeons, Pediatric Section. Salt Lake City, Utah, December 11–13, 1984.

98. Dandy WE, Blackfan KD: Internal hydrocephalus. An experimental, clinical and pathological study. Am J Dis Child 8:406, 1914.

99. Bowsher D: Pathways of absorption of protein from the cerebrospinal fluid fluid: an autoradiographic study in the cat. Anat Rec 128:23, 1957.

100. Butler A: Correlated physiologic and structural studies of CSF absorption. In Shapiro K, Marmarou A, Portnoy H (eds): Hydrocephalus. New York, Raven Press, 1984, pp 41–58.

101. Clark WEL: On the pacchionian bodies. J Anat 55:40, 1920.

102. Gilles FH, Davidson RI: Communicating hydrocephalus associated with deficient dysplastic parasagittal arachnoidal granulations. J Neurosurg 35:421, 1971.

103. McComb JG, Davson H, Hollingsworth JR: Attempted separation of blood-brain and blood-cerebrospinal fluid barriers in the rabbit. Exp Eye Res 25(Suppl):333, 1977.

104. Shantaveerappa TR, Bourne GH: Arachnoid villi in the optic nerve of man and monkey. Exp Eye Res 3:31, 1964.

105. Gutierrez Y, Friede RL, Kaliney WJ: Agenesis of arachnoid granulations and its relationship to communicating hydrocephalus. J Neurosurg 43:553, 1975.

106. Foltz EL, Ward AA, Jr: Communicating hydrocephalus from subarachnoid bleeding. J Neurosurg 13:546, 1956.
107. Gjerris F, Borgesen SE, Sorensen PS, et al.: Resistance to cerebrospinal fluid outflow and intracranial pressure in patients with hydrocephalus after subarachnoid hemorrhage. Acta Neurochir (Wien) 88:79, 1987.
108. Borgmann R: Natural course of intracranial pressure and drainage of CSF after recovery from subarachnoid hemorrhage. Acta Neurol Scand 81:300, 1990.
109. Ellington E, Margolis G: Block of arachnoid villus by subarachnoid hemorrhage. J Neurosurg 30:651, 1969.
110. Griebel RW, Black PM, Pile-Spellman J, et al.: The importance of "accessory" outflow pathways in hydrocephalus after experimental subarachnoid hemorrhage. Neurosurgery 24:187, 1989.
111. Weed LH, Hughson W: Intracranial venous pressure and cerebrospinal fluid pressure as affected by the intravenous injection of solutions of various concentrations. Am J Physiol 58:101, 1921.
112. Shulman K, Yarnell P, Ransohoff J: Dural sinus pressure in normal and hydrocephalic dogs. Arch Neurol 10:575, 1964.
113. Jones HC, Gratton JA: The drainage of cerebrospinal fluid in hydrocephalic rats. Z Kinderchir 44:14, 1989.
114. Norrell H, Wilson C, Howieson J, et al.: Venous factors in infantile hydrocephalus. J Neurosurg 31:561, 1969.
115. Shulman K, Ransohoff J: Sagittal sinus venous pressure in hydrocephalus. J Neurosurg 23:169, 1965.
116. Beck DJK, Russell DS: Experiments on thrombosis of the superior longitudinal sinus. J Neurosurg 3:337, 1946.
117. Guthrie TC, Dunbar HS, Karpell B: Ventricular size and chronic increased intracranial venous pressure in the dog. J Neurosurg 33:407, 1970.
118. Hammock MK, Milhorat TH, Earl K, et al.: Vein of Galen ligation in the primate. Angiographic, gross and light microscopic evaluation. J Neurosurg 34:77, 1971.
119. McComb JG: Is there risk to occlusion of the deep cerebral veins when removing pineal location tumors? Concepts Pediat Neurosurg 7:72, 1987.
120. Russel DS: Observations on the pathology of hydrocephalus. Medical Research Council Special Report Series No. 265. London. His Majesty's Stationary Office, 1949.
121. Bering EA Jr, Salibi B: Production of hydrocephalus by increased cephalic-venous pressure. Arch Neurol Psychiatry 81:693, 1959.
122. Haar FL, Miller CA: Hydrocephalus resulting from superior vena cava thrombosis in an infant. J Neurosurg 42:597, 1975.
123. Rosman NP, Shands KN: Hydrocephalus caused by increased intracranial venous pressure: A clinicopathologic study. Ann Neurol 3:445, 1978.
124. Sainte-Rose C, LaCombe J, Pierre-Kahn A, et al.: Intracranial venous sinus hypertension: Cause or consequence of hydrocephalus in infants? J Neurosurg 60:727, 1984.
125. Steinbok P, Hall J, Flodmark O: Hydrocephalus in achondroplasia: the possible role of intracranial venous hypertension. J Neurosurg 71:42, 1989.
126. Lundar T, Bakke SJ, Nornes H: Hydrocephalus in an achondroplastic child treated by venous decomposition at the jugular foramen: J Neurosurg 73:138, 1990.
127. Schlesinger B: The venous drainage of the brain, with special reference to the Galenic system. Brain 62:274, 1939.
128. Lorenzo AV, Bresnan MJ, Barlow CF: Cerebrospinal fluid absorption deficit in normal pressure hydrocephalus. Arch Neurol 30:387, 1974.
129. Sahar A, Hochwald GM, Sadik AR, et al.: Cerebrospinal fluid absorption in animals with experimental obstructive hydrocephalus. Arch Neurol 21:638, 1969.
130. Levin VA, Milhorat TH, Fenstermacher JD, et al.: Physiological studies on the development of obstructive hydrocephalus in the monkey. Neurology 21:238, 1971.
131. Milhorat TH, Hammock MK, Chandra RS: The subarachnoid space in congenital obstructive hydrocephalus. Part 2: Microscopic findings. J Neurosurg 35:7, 1971.
132. Murthy VS, Deshande DH: The central canal of the filum terminale in communicating hydrocephalus. J Neurosurg 53:528, 1980.
133. Welch K: Selected topics relating to hydrocephalus. Exp Eye Res 25(Suppl):345, 1977.
134. Ahearn EP, Randall KT, Charlton JD, et al.: Two-compartment model of the cerebrospinal fluid system for the study of hydrocephalus. Ann Biomed Eng 15:467, 1987.
135. Conner ES, Foley L, Black PM: Experimental normal-pressure hydrocephalus is accompanied by increased transmantle pressure. J Neurosurg 61:322, 1984.
136. Benzel EC, Pelletier AL, Levy PG: Communicating hydrocephalus in adults: Prediction of outcome after ventricular shunting procedures. Neurosurgery 26:655, 1990.
137. Vanneste J, Augustijn P, Davies GA, et al.: Normal-pressure hydrocephalus. Is cisternography still useful in selecting patients for a shunt? Arch Neurol 49:364, 1992.
138. James AE Jr: Evaluation of cerebrospinal fluid physiology by the new imaging modalities: A review using the development of communicating hydrocephalus for analysis. Invest Radiol (In press).
139. Levy LM, Di Chiro G: MR phase imaging and cerebrospinal fluid flow in the head and spine. Neuroradiology 32:399, 1990.
140. Quencer RM: Intracranial CSF flow in pediatric hydrocephalus: Evaluation with Cine-MR imaging. AJNR 13:601, 1992.
141. Ehrlich P: Das Sauerstoff-Bedurfnis des Organismus: eine farbenanalytische studie. Berlin, Hirschwald, 1885.
142. Goldmann EE: Die aussere ind innere sekretion des gesunden und kranken organismus im lichte der "vitalen farbung." Beitr Klin Chirurg 64:192, 1909.
143. Goldmann EE: Vitalfarbung am zentralnervensystem. Abh Preuss Akad Wiss Phys Math Kl 1:1, 1913.
144. Reese TS, Karnovsky MJ: Fine structural localization of a blood-brain barrier to exogenous peroxidase. J Cell Biol 34:207, 1967.
145. Crone C: The blood-brain barrier; a modified tight epithelium. In Suckling AJ, Rumsby MG, Bradbury MWB, Harwood VCH (eds): The Blood-Brain Barrier in Health and Disease. Chichester, Verlagsgesellschaft, 1986, pp 17–46.
146. Segal MB, Zlokovic BV: The Blood-Brain Barrier, Amino Acids and Peptides. Boston, Kluwer Academic Publisher, 1990.
147. Pardridge WM: Peptide Drug Delivery to the Brain. New York, Raven Press, 1991.
148. Sokoloff L: Relation between physiological function and energy metabolism in the central nervous system. J Neurochem 29:13, 1977.
149. Duvernoy H, Delon S, Vannson JL: The vascularization of the human cerebellar cortex. Brain Res Bull 11:419, 1983.
150. Fenstermacher J, Nakata H, Tajima A, et al.: In Segal MB (ed): Structural, Ultrastructural and Functional Correlations Among Local Capillary Systems Within the Brain. London, Macmillan, 1992, pp 59–72.
151. McCulloch J, Harper AM: Cerebral circulatory and metabolism changes following amphetamine administration. Brain Res 121:196, 1977.
152. Stein WD: The movement of molecules across cell membranes. New York, Academic Press, 1967.
153. Pardridge WM: Transport of protein-bound hormones into tissues in vivo. Endocr Rev 2:103, 1981.
154. Begley DJ, Squires LK, Zlokovic BV, et al.: Permeability of the blood-brain barrier to immunosuppressive cyclic peptide cyclosporin. J Neurochem 55:1222, 1990.
155. Oldendorf WH: Brain uptake of radio-labelled amino acids, amino acids, amines and hexoses after arterial injection. Am J Physiol 221:1629, 1971.
156. Oldendorf WH, Szabo J: Amino acid assignment to one of three blood-brain barrier amino acid carriers. Am J Physiol 230:94, 1976.
157. Pardridge WM: Recent advances in blood-brain barrier transport. Annu Rev Pharmacol Toxicol 28:25, 1988.
158. Oldendorf WH: The blood-brain barrier. In Bito LZ, Davson H, and Fenstermacher JD (eds): The Ocular and Cerebrospinal Fluids. London and New York, Academic Press, 1977, pp 177–190.
159. Smith QR, Momma S, Aoyagi M: Kinetics of neutral amino acid transport across the blood-brain barrier. J Neurochem 49:1651, 1987.
160. Nutt JG, Woodward WR, Hammerstad JP, et al.: The "on-off"

phenomenon in Parkinson's disease. Relation to levodopa absorption and transport. N Engl J Med 310:483, 1984.

161. Wade LA, Katzman R: Rat brain regional uptake and decarboxylation of L-dopa following carotid injection. Am J Physiol 228:352, 1975.

162. Markowitz DC, Fernstrom JD: Diet and uptake of Aldomet by the brain: Competition with natural large neutral amino acids. Science 197:1014, 1977.

163. Sved AF, Goldberg IM, Fernstrom JD: Dietary protein intake influences the antihypertensive potency of methyldopa in spontaneously hypertensive rats. J Pharmacol Exp Ther 214:147, 1980.

164. Smith QR, Takada Y, Greig N, et al.: Design of drugs with high affinity for the large neutral amino acid carrier of the blood-brain barrier. *In* Drewes L, Betz L (eds): Frontiers in Cerebral Vascular Biology: Transport and Its Regulation. New York, Plenum Press, 1992.

165. Cornford EM, Oldendorf WH: Independent blood-brain barrier transport systems for nucleic acid precursors. Biochim Biophys Acta 25:825, 1975.

166. Williams SA, Davson H, Segal: Thymidine transport into the guinea-pig brain and cerebrospinal fluid as measured using the in situ brain perfusion technique. J Physiol (London) (in press).

167. Boado RJ, Pardridge WM: The brain-type glucose transporter mRNA is specifically expressed at the blood-brain barrier. Biochem Biophys Res Commun 166:174, 1990.

168. Pardridge WM, Boado RJ, Farrell CR: Brain-type glucose transporter (GLUT-1) is selectively localized to the blood-brain barrier. Studies with quantitative Western blotting and in situ hybridization. J Biol Chem 265:18035, 1990.

169. Cordon-Cardo C, O'Brien JP, Casals D, et al.: Multidrug-resistance gene (P-glycoprotein) is expressed by endothelial cells at blood-brain barrier sites. Proc Natl Acad Sci USA 86:695, 1989.

170. Zlokovic BV, Mackic JB, Wang L, et al.: Differential expression of Na, K-ATPase isoenzymes at the blood-brain barrier and choroid plexus. J Biol Chem, 1992 (in press).

171. Zlokovic BV, Mackic JB, Magyar C, et al.: Experiment of Na, K-ATPase at the blood-brain interface. *In* Drewes L, Betz L (eds): Frontiers in Cerebral Vascular Biology: Transport and Its Regulation. New York, Plenum Press, 1992.

172. Carter DC, He X-M: Structure of human serum albumin. Science 249:302, 1990.

173. Pardridge WM, Eisenberg J, Yamada T: Human blood-brain barrier insulin receptor. J Neurochem 44:1771, 1985.

174. Pardridge WM, Eisenberg J, Yang J: Human blood-brain barrier transferrin receptor. Metabolism 36:892, 1987.

175. Zlokovic BV, Hyman S, McComb JG, et al.: Kinetics of vasopressin-arginine uptake at the blood-brain barrier. Biochim Biophys Acta 1025:191, 1990.

176. Zlokovic BV, Banks WA, ElKadi H, et al.: Transport, uptake, and metabolism of blood-borne vasopressin by the blood-brain barrier. Brain Res 590:213, 1992.

177. Zlokovic BV: In vivo approaches for studying peptide interactions at the blood-brain barrier. J Controlled Release 13:185, 1990.

178. Pardridge WM: Receptor-mediated peptide transport through the blood-brain barrier. Endocr Rev 7:314, 1986.

179. Triguero D, Buciak JB, Yang J, et al.: Blood-brain barrier transport of cationized immunoglobulin G. Enhanced delivery compared to native protein. Proc Natl Acad Sci USA 86:4761, 1989.

180. Zlokovic BV, Skundric DS, Segal MB, et al.: A saturable mechanism for transport of immunoglobulin G across the blood-brain barrier of the guinea-pig. Exp Neurol 107:263, 1990.

181. Albert EN, Kerns JM: Reversible microwave effects on the blood-brain barrier. Brain Res 230:153, 1981.

182. Lanse SB, Lee JC, Jacobs EA, et al.: Changes in the permeability of the blood-brain barrier under hyperbaric conditions. Aviat Space Environ Med 49:890, 1978.

183. Wells LA: Alteration of the blood-brain barrier system by hypothermia: Critical time period vs. critical temperature. Comp Biochem Physiol 44A:293, 1973.

184. Joo F, Zolton OT, Csillik B: Increased permeability of the blood-brain barrier in lymphostatic encephalopathy. Angiologica 6:318, 1969.

185. Trout JJ, Koenig H, Goldstone AD, et al.: Blood-brain barrier breakdown by cold injury. Lab Invest 55:622, 1986.

186. Lossinsky AS, Vorbrodt AW, Wisniewski HM: Characterization of endothelial cell transport in the developing mouse blood-brain barrier. Dev Neurosci 8:61, 1986.

187. Perry VH, Gordon S: Modulation of CD4 antigen on macrophages and microglia in rat brain. J Exp Med 166:1138, 1987.

188. Axthelm MD, Krakowka S: Canine distemper virus: the early blood-brain barrier lesion. Acta Neuropathol 75:27, 1987.

189. Sharpe AH, Fields BN: Pathogenesis of viral infections. N Engl J Med 312:486, 1985.

190. Wekerle H, Linington C, Lassmann H, et al.: Cellular immune reactivity within the CNS. Trends Neurosci 9:271, 1986.

191. Stewart PA, Wiley MJ: Developing nervous tissue induces formation of blood-brain barrier characteristics in invading endothelial cells: A study using quail-chick transplantation chimera. Dev Biol 84:183, 1981.

192. DeBault LE, Cancilla PA: Gamma-glutamyl transpeptidase in isolated brain endothelial cells: Induction by glial cells in vitro. Science 207:653, 1980.

193. Weindl A: Neuroendocrine aspects of circumventricular organs. *In* Ganong WF, Martini L (eds): Frontiers in Neuroendocrinology. New York, Oxford University Press, 1973, pp 3–32.

194. Neuwelt EA, Rapoport SI: Modification of the blood-brain barrier in the chemotherapy of malignant brain tumors. Fed Proc 43:214, 1984.

195. Patel HM: Liposomes: Bags of challenge. Biochem Soc Trans 12:333, 1984.

196. Neuwelt EA, Pagel MA, Geller A, et al.: Gene replacement therapy in the central nervous system. *In* Drewes L, Betz L (eds): Frontiers in Cerebral Vascular Biology: Transport and Its Regulation. New York, Plenum Press (in press).

Chapter 12

HYDROCEPHALUS: Etiology, Pathologic Effects, Diagnosis, and Natural History

CAROLYN MARIE CAREY, M.D., MICAM W. TULLOUS, M.D., and
MARION L. WALKER, M.D.

Hydrocephalus is a pathologic condition of relative ventricular enlargement and associated intracranial hypertension which arises from an imbalance between the production relative to the absorption of cerebrospinal fluid (CSF). This almost invariably results from a reduction in the flow of CSF due to an obstructive process. Discussion of numerous possible etiologies and variable clinical presentations will provide a basis for diagnosis. Current diagnostic modalities provide further insight into this condition and allow for early detection and institution of therapy. Although awareness of this entity has been present for centuries, current knowledge concerning the pathophysiology of hydrocephalus evolves from important findings recorded during this century.

HISTORY

Historical accounts about hydrocephalus date back to the era of Hippocrates and Galen. It is believed that these earliest accounts actually described the presence of extra-axial fluid collections, possibly subdural effusions. Vesalius is credited with the first accurate anatomic description of hydrocephalus in the sixteenth century. He made reference to it as a disease process with accumulation of fluid within an enlarged ventricular system. Descriptions by Morgagni during the eighteenth century noted that hydrocephalus was occasionally associated with involvement of the cerebellum, brainstem, and spinal cord. It is believed that this work makes reference to the first description of what later would be known as Arnold-Chiari malformation with myelomeningocele and hydrocephalus. In addition to anatomic descriptions of hydrocephalus recorded during the eighteenth century, writings also made reference to clinical findings. Robert Whytt's recordings are thought to describe cases of older children with increased intracranial pressure from hydrocephalus secondary to basilar meningitis.[1, 2]

Contributions during the nineteenth century include the work of Cheyne and West, early nineteenth century authors, who were thought to have presented the first classifications of hydrocephalus. Magendie and Luschka are credited with early work on CSF circulation during this period. Later during the same century, Key and Retzius correctly described ventricular and CSF pathways in their contributions to CSF physiology.[1, 2]

Early in the twentieth century, Dandy and Blackfan[3] produced obstructive hydrocephalus in a canine model by blocking the aqueduct of Sylvius. Dandy also occluded the foramen of Monro and this resulted in ventricular dilatation, confirming the lateral ventricle and, therefore, the choroid plexus as a site of CSF production. Subsequently, in an animal model, he removed the choroid plexus following occlusion of the foramen of Monro, and ventricular dilatation did not occur. These findings were the foundation for subsequent therapeutic maneuvers by Dandy.[1] Dandy also made contributions to diagnostic neuroradiology by the introduction of pneumoventriculography in 1918.[4] Also during this time, Wislocki and Putnam, and Nanagus used a dye marker to demonstrate transependymal movement of CSF into brain parenchyma in a hydrocephalic animal.[1]

Early treatment, as recommended by Galen and later

by Fantoni, was surgical release of fluid. However, this procedure frequently proved to be fatal. Because of the high risk of this form of intervention, nonsurgical approaches became more common. One direct form of therapy was cranial compression attempted with the use of muslin bandages, as reported by Riverius in 1656. Plaster replaced muslin in later head-wrapping procedures.[1] The utilization of lumbar puncture as a treatment for hydrocephalus was first described by Quinke in 1891.[2]

Removal of the source of CSF formation and diversion of CSF were both attempted early in the twentieth century. Dandy introduced choroid plexectomy in 1919 and later attempted endoscopic cauterization of the choroid plexus.[2, 5] These procedures were performed in several hundred individuals over the following 20 years, but were unsuccessful in providing consistent relief from this condition. The failure of choroid plexus extirpation to alleviate hydrocephalus was perplexing.[1, 2] An explanation was not available until 1967, when Pollay and Curl demonstrated extrachoroidal production of CSF by the ventricular surface.[1]

Early attempts at CSF diversion included both intra- and extracranial routes. Intracranial diversion included third ventriculostomy for noncommunicating hydrocephalus, in which initial attempts were via callososubarachnoidostomy performed in 1908. Alternate procedures included Dandy's subfrontal and subtemporal approaches.[2] Stookey and Scarf attempted a through-and-through ventriculostomy with fenestration of the third ventricle into the interpenduncular and chiasmatic cisterns.[6] Mixter described an endoscopic method for diversion of CSF by puncturing the floor of the third ventricle.[7] Diversion of CSF from the lateral ventricle to the cisterna magna, or ventriculocisternostomy, was described by Torkildsen[8] for obstruction of the aqueduct of Sylvius. Attempts were also made during this time to shunt fluid into the cranial venous sinuses.[2]

Extracranial diversion of CSF also originated in the early twentieth century. Shunting to the subgaleal space, vascular system, pleural and peritoneal cavities, and the lumbar subarachnoid space was attempted with little success. Heile described the first ureteral shunts in 1925. Later on, the technique of ureteral shunting was modified by Matson, who published his first case in 1949.[2, 5] This procedure was used in patients with documented communicating hydrocephalus. It required nephrectomy, with placement of a valveless polyethylene tube between the lumbar subarachnoid space and the ureter. This procedure became well established over the years following its introduction.[5]

The modern era in therapy began with the development of antireflux valves. Early steel and magnetically seated ball valves proved unsuccessful. In 1955, John Holter, a machine shop technician, became interested in shunts after his child was born with a lumbar myelomeningocele and hydrocephalus. He initially developed a one-way slit valve made of polyvinyl chloride tubing.[5] This was followed by models made of silicone that were placed into the internal jugular vein and into the right atrium. Concurrently, in California, Dr. Robert Pudenz

was experimenting with a similar system that would also be used as a ventriculoatrial shunt.[2, 5] Ventriculoatrial shunting became the standard practice of the 1960s. Early peritoneal diversions were attempted with polyethylene tubing. However, frequent revisions were necessary because of obstruction from intra-abdominal adhesions.[5] Ames, Raimondi and Matsumoto repopularized ventriculoperitoneal shunting when silicone devices became available. With improved materials and techniques, the peritoneal route became more popular in the 1970s. Simultaneously, the utilization of vascular shunts in the younger age group declined due to the frequent lengthening procedures necessitated by axial growth.[2]

Data obtained from many years of experience have provided a background of knowledge for development of improved diagnostic and therapeutic modalities. The effect of this experience on the development of improved devices for cerebrospinal fluid diversion allows for some measure of reliable compensation for this condition. Although system utilization and surgical technique vary, depending on the physician's preference and experience, the basic principle of ventriculoperitoneal diversion of CSF remains unchanged.

NATURAL HISTORY

A discussion of the outcome for individuals presenting with hydrocephalus prior to the advent of appropriate surgical therapy provides a basis for comparison to those now receiving this form of therapy. Reference to the natural history of this condition has appeared throughout the historical account in the preceding section. However, not until the latter half of this century was literature available on a larger series of untreated patients with this condition. The advent of standardized therapeutic modalities, particularly in reference to cerebrospinal fluid diversion, stimulated interest and provided expectations for improved survival and functional outcome for those suffering with this condition.

The earliest descriptions of hydrocephalus implied that it was an incurable illness, and a number of these case records included a postmortem description of the cranium and its contents. Representative of these writings is an intriguing case report by clinician and artist, Richard Bright, published in 1831.[9] He describes the case of James Cardinal who, following a hospital admission for seizures, died just prior to his thirtieth birthday from complications of a febrile respiratory illness. This report describes the patient's enormous head size and very thin cranium (Fig. 12–1). The author relates a description of cranial transillumination by sunlight or light from a burning candle until the patient was 14 years old. He states that closure of this patient's cranial sutures was accompanied by frequent headaches and occurred approximately 2 years prior to his death. In addition, he describes the development of an abscess in the patient's ear which drained intermittently and relieved his headaches. It is unknown whether this may have represented a CSF-cutaneous fistula. The post-

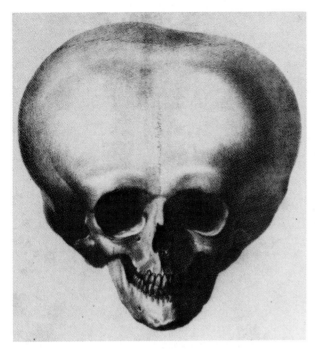

FIGURE 12–1. Untreated hydrocephalus in a 30-year-old man demonstrating abnormal formation of the cranium and enlarged head size.

mortem examination exhibited an enormous cranial as well as ventricular size (Fig. 12–2). It also demonstrated anatomic collapse of the cerebral hemispheres from presumed spontaneous rupture of the ventricular system into the subdural space via an opening on the lateral aspect of the corpus callosum. The author emphasizes that this case was remarkable for the length of time the patient survived.

Morgagni stated that successful outcome did not occur in chronic internal hydrocephalus. Early surgical treatment for this condition, which included ventricular puncture, almost always proved fatal. Owing to the

risk of surgical intervention and the promising results of medical management during the late eighteenth century, surgical approaches were abandoned. It is believed, however, that medical treatment was mainly symptomatic, and the cures that were described following treatment were early examples of "spontaneous arrest," as in the case described by A. Eason in 1795. Later, surgical management by early attempts at CSF diversion was associated with a high rate of infection and frequent shunt tube obstruction. These early shunt problems and the failure of plexectomy to control ventricular dilatation again led some practitioners toward medical management in the hope of effecting spontaneous arrest for their patients.[1]

During the early 1940s, most cases of hydrocephalus were considered hopeless; therefore, this condition was rarely treated. The cases that were treated were those not associated with myelodysplasia.[5] A 20-year review by Feeney and Barry,[10] in 1954, reported on 10 of 93 (11 per cent) live born infants with hydrocephalus who survived birth long enough to leave the hospital. In addition, Larson and Banner,[11] in their 30-year review to 1965, reported that of 35 infants with hydrocephalus, only 4 (11 per cent) survived long enough to undergo surgical therapy.

In 1962, Laurence and Coates published an analysis of 182 patients with hydrocephalus that had not received surgical intervention.[12] The data from this study were accumulated over a 20-year period. The patients were less than 13 years of age upon presentation. The 182 cases selected for review were from a total of 239 cases, 57 of which received surgical intervention. In the nonsurgical group, diagnosis of their condition was made by invasive techniques in 64 per cent, head measurements with or without skull radiographs in 33 per cent, and at postmortem examination in 3 per cent. In this group, the mortality at the end of the 20-year study was 49 per cent. Forty-six per cent were alive with arrested hydrocephalus and 5 per cent were alive with continued progressive hydrocephalus. Of the chil-

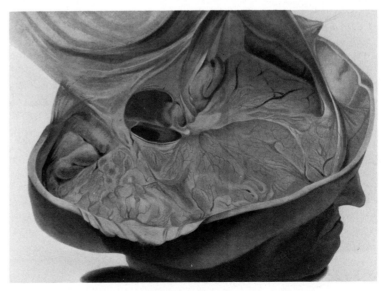

FIGURE 12–2. Postmortem examination of patient with untreated hydrocephalus (Fig. 12–1). A very thin cortical mantle is evident with large ventricular spaces.

dren who died, 52 per cent died from cardiorespiratory failure related to hydrocephalus, 18 per cent from infection, 25 per cent from related intraventricular hemorrhage, pneumonia, or tumor extension, 2 per cent from unrelated problems, and 3 per cent from unknown causes. Only 19 per cent of patients in the study group had associated myelomeningoceles, and this relatively low percentage was attributed to the large number who died before referral for treatment. Therefore, the study group was not representative of hydrocephalus in the general population because the severest cases were considered beyond help or died prior to being referred. Consequently, the mortality rate appeared relatively low because spina bifida cystica with hydrocephalus was reportedly the most common form of hydrocephalus in the community and carried a very high mortality rate, mainly from meningitis. The high mortality in the general population at an early age (0 to 3 months) was confirmed by comparing hospital deaths from hydrocephalus to deaths from hydrocephalus from the Registrar-General. Many newborn babies were not taken to the hospital and were allowed to die at home. Therefore, it was the opinion of the authors that hospital deaths from hydrocephalus became representative of the general population only after three months of age. Of survivors (81) in whom physical disability was recorded, 52 per cent were normal or only slightly handicapped, and 48 per cent were severely affected or incapacitated. Recording of the intelligence quotient demonstrated that 38 per cent had an IQ greater than 85, 35 per cent had an IQ between 50 and 85, and 27 per cent had an IQ less than 50. In addition, the author stated that no relation could be found between the thickness of the cortical mantle, as measured by air encephalography, and later intelligence quotients.

A follow-up study by Laurence and Coates,[13] published 6 years later, made reference to the 93 patients that had survived during the first study. This included the nine patients with progressive disease and the three patients who were initially lost to follow-up. It was determined that an additional five patients had succumbed from related illnesses, increasing the mortality rate from 49 to 55 per cent. Intelligence quotient testing demonstrated only minimal improvement over the follow-up period. There was little change in the percentage of children with either severe or incapacitating handicaps versus those who were normal or only slightly handicapped.

Yashon et al. published a study of long-term follow-up in 47 infants with severe untreated hydrocephalus.[14] The mortality in this study approached 49 per cent. It was also concluded, as in the study of Laurence and Coates, that cerebral mantle thickness could not be correlated with ultimate neurologic status.

Jette Jensen,[15] in 1985, published a report of 219 patients with proven and unproven hydrocephalus, without related spinal dysraphism. The diagnosis was made before the child reached 5 years of age. Follow-up of these patients was continued for 21 to 35 years. It should be noted that 54 of these patients were treated with various surgical techniques prior to improved survival with ventriculoatrial shunting, which, in the author's opinion, did not significantly alter the prognosis. It was felt that this group of patients represented untreated hydrocephalus as a whole. The overall mortality was reported at 45 per cent. The mortality in those 134 patients with proven hydrocephalus was 60 per cent, whereas only 21 per cent died with unproven hydrocephalus. The mortality in the 54 patients receiving some form of surgical intervention was 78 per cent. This high mortality was thought to be secondary to the degree of severity of hydrocephalus. The mortality for 165 who did not receive any form of surgical therapy was 34 per cent. This figure does not represent deaths in children with hydrocephalus and associated myelodysplasia.

Mealy et al.,[16] in 1973, supplied information on the prognosis of neonates presenting with hydrocephalus by reviewing the clinical records of 79 children. Cases were excluded if they were associated with known history of infection, megalencephaly, toxoplasmosis, or neoplasia. This series included 24 cases of hydrocephalus with associated myelodysplasia. In 51 of the other 55 cases not associated with myelodysplasia, the diagnosis of hydrocephalus was confirmed by means of pneumoencephalography or ventriculography. Five children in each of the surgical and nonsurgical groups were lost to follow-up. Twenty-seven of the 79 children who received supportive care only were available for follow-up. Only two (7 per cent) of these children were living at the time of the study. One of the two had an average level of intelligence; the other was reported as vegetative with a recorded occipitofrontal circumference of 83 cm. Of the 25 mortalities, 20 died during infancy, 5 thereafter. Forty-two cases that received surgical therapy were available for follow-up. Thirty-four patients received ventriculoatrial shunts, 5 had craniotomy or craniectomy for fenestration of cysts, one underwent a ventriculocisternostomy, another received a ventriculoparotid shunt, and the remaining patient had a choroid plexectomy. The mortality for the operative group was 26 of 42 (62 per cent). Five of the 16 survivors had normal IQs, five had moderate mental impairment, and the remaining six patients were markedly developmentally delayed. Fifteen (44 per cent) of the 34 children treated with ventriculoatrial shunts survived. Shunt complications accounted for 42 per cent of the 19 deaths. In conclusion, it was the author's opinion that early ventricular shunting should be performed to afford improved survival and functional outcome.

Extended survival (60 to 80 per cent) and improved functional outcome were achieved with the advent of more current methods of surgical therapy by CSF diversion through a one-way valve system.[17–19] This includes a report by Foltz,[17] in 1968, in which he demonstrated improved survival and a higher degree of intellectual capacity by surgical arrest of progressive ventriculomegaly utilizing ventriculoatrial shunts and close follow-up in a group of treated hydrocephalic children as compared to untreated children. His statistics include those 0 to 3 months of age, in contrast to the study of Lawrence and Coates,[12] which included only children who had survived longer than 3 months after birth. He found that those children who were treated surgically and whose thickness of cerebral mantle recovered promptly following surgery showed higher intellectual capacity in general than children who did not undergo surgery and in whom mantle thickness remained small.

CLASSIFICATION AND ETIOLOGY

Hydrocephalus can be classified as communicating and noncommunicating. Once that distinction is established, the etiology can be determined. Communicating hydrocephalus implies that CSF pathways are obstructed in the region of the basal cisterns, arachnoid villi, or subarachnoid spaces. Noncommunicating hydrocephalus would indicate a blockage of CSF pathways proximal to the foramina of the fourth ventricle. It also falls under the categories of congenital and acquired, and the etiologies are numerous. Once the diagnosis of hydrocephalus is made, one must determine whether this is progressive or arrested, and it must be distinguished from ventriculomegaly without increased pressure.

INCIDENCE

The overall incidence of hydrocephalus in the population is not known. The incidence of infantile hydrocephalus is approximately three to four per thousand live births. When a single congenital disorder is considered, this number drops to .9 to 1.5 per thousand live births. The incidence of hydrocephalus with myelomeningocele defects is 1.3 to 2.9 per thousand live births.[20, 21] Once acquired hydrocephalus is considered, the incidence increases, although the numbers again are not known.

ETIOLOGY

Hydrocephalus can be caused by obstruction of CSF pathways or overproduction of cerebrospinal fluid. These two basic causes can be precipitated by neoplasms, congenital malformations, or inflammatory processes (Table 12–1). The etiology of congenital hydrocephalus is not always apparent.[21] It is often associated with other malformations or syndromes[22] (Table 12–2).

DIAGNOSIS

It is important to establish a diagnosis of hydrocephalus versus other causes of macrocrania or increased intracranial pressure. A wide variety of safe and non-invasive diagnostic modalities are available to the clinician. The etiology of the hydrocephalus should be determined if possible. Good clinical judgment plays the most important role in deciding whether treatment is required and the timing of such treatment.

IMAGING

The three major techniques used for diagnosis and evaluation of hydrocephalus are computed tomography, ultrasonography, and magnetic resonance imaging.

Computed Tomography (CT). CT scanning continues to be the most commonly used radiologic technique for the diagnosis of hydrocephalus. It is the most rapid way to screen children with macrocrania or signs

TABLE 12–1. ANATOMIC-ETIOLOGIC CLASSIFICATION OF HYDROCEPHALUS

NONCOMMUNICATING	COMMUNICATING
Congenital	**Congenital**
Aqueductal obstruction	Arnold-Chiari malformation
Atresia of foramen of Monro	Dandy-Walker malformation
Arnold-Chiari malformation	Leptomeningeal inflammation
Dandy-Walker malformation	Incompetent arachnoid villi
Neoplasms	Encephalocele
Benign intracranial cysts	Benign cysts
Skull base anomalies	**Neoplastic Inflammatory**
Neoplastic Inflammatory	Infectious meningitis
Infectious ventriculitis	Subarachnoid hemorrhage
Intraventricular hemorrhage	(spontaneous, traumatic,
Chemical ventriculitis	surgical)
	Chemical arachnoiditis

TABLE 12–2. CONGENITAL HYDROCEPHALUS—ASSOCIATION WITH MALFORMATION SYNDROMES

Frequent Occurrence of Hydrocephalus
X-linked recessive hydrocephalus
Familial type of Dandy-Walker malformation
Spina bifida cystica
Albers-Schönberg disease (severe osteopetrosis)
Occasional Occurrence of Hydrocephalus
Achondroplasia
Acrodysostosis
Apert's disease
Basal cell nevus
Hurler's disease
Incontinentia pigmenti
Linear sebaceous nevus sequence
Meckel-Gruber syndrome
Oral-facial-digital syndrome
Osteogenesis imperfecta
Riley-Day syndrome
Thanatophoric dwarfism
Triploidy*
Trisomy 13*
Trisomy 18*

Adapted from Growth References from Conception to Adulthood, Suppl. 1. Clinton, SC, Jacobs Press, Inc., 1988, p. 128.
*Chromosomal anomalies.

of increased intracranial pressure, and it is accurate in imaging intracranial pathology.[23–25] When CT is coupled with contrast enhancement, tumors, as well as vascular malformations, may be better visualized. CT scanning also offers an efficient and accurate means of follow-up before and after treatment. Sedation is not required for this method of scanning except in rare cases. The amount of radiation now can be adjusted to a low level and, in spite of multiple scans, can have no apparent untoward effects. The cause and area of obstruction often can be identified on the CT scan.

Ultrasonography. Ultrasonography is particularly useful in evaluating the premature infant with suspected intraventricular hemorrhage, macrocrania, or signs of increased intracranial pressure (Fig. 12–3). The equipment is portable, involves no irradiation, and requires no sedation. It is also useful for follow-up screening of untreated and treated infants with hydrocephalus as long as an open anterior fontanelle is still present. Ultrasonography is less accurate in its ability to look at convexity lesions, posterior fossa anomalies, and vascular lesions. Congenital brain malformations and neoplasms may be noted, but for full evaluation another method of scanning is required, preferably MRI if available.

Magnetic Resonance Imaging (MRI). MRI has be-come more available over the last several years, and the quality and versatility of this method of scanning have also advanced significantly. Anatomic visualization is obtained in axial, coronal, and sagittal planes, providing excellent information as to the exact position and extent of lesions. More subtle findings, such as white matter pathology and dysmorphic anatomy, are more readily demonstrated. The aqueduct can be visualized, membranes and loculated ventricular systems often can be seen, and with the complement of gadolinium, neoplasms and vascular lesions are easily imaged. With the advent of MRA (magnetic resonance angiography), the vascular system can be visualized and vascular lesions easily defined. Once an atrioventricular malformation (AVM) is identified, traditional angiography should be undertaken prior to treatment. Phase-contrast cine magnetic resonance imaging technique can be used now to study CSF flow dynamics in normals as well as in communicating and noncommunicating hydrocephalus.[26, 27] The acquisition of flow information via the RACE-CE-FAST sequence takes only seconds and allows for real-time flow measurements.[27, 28] This technique appears to be useful in determining CSF flow following third ventriculostomy for treatment of hydrocephalus. Though relatively new, these imaging advances may have further

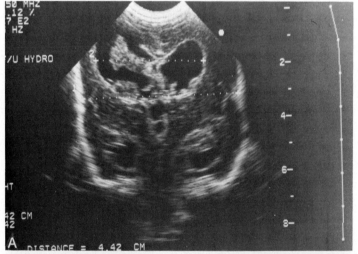

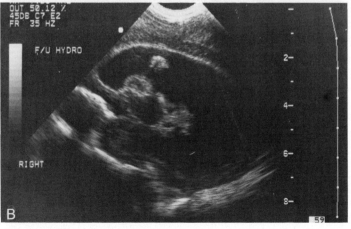

FIGURE 12–3. Ultrasound examination of preterm infant with posthemorrhagic hydrocephalus. Hemorrhagic clot is present within the ventricle. *A,* Axial view. *B,* Coronal view.

applications in evaluating CSF dynamics in hydrocephalus and, it is hoped, in determining shunt function in treated patients.

Ventriculography and Cisternography. Ventriculography is useful in evaluating patients with suspected loculations within the ventricular system as well as loculated fluid compartments outside the ventricular system, such as arachnoid cysts that may abut the ventricular structures. It is also a useful method of determining whether communication of loculated areas has occurred after ventriculoscopic procedures have been undertaken. Radionucleotide cisternography may also assist in confirming loculated ventricles or fluid compartments but is less helpful than other techniques mentioned and is now infrequently used.[29]

OTHER STUDIES

Once the diagnosis of hydrocephalus is made, other information may be needed prior to initiation of treatment. If the cause of the hydrocephalus is obstruction secondary to tumor or loculated cystic cavities, the course of treatment is relatively straightforward. If the child has experienced infection or hemorrhage, analysis of the CSF should be obtained prior to shunt placement. If the hydrocephalus is chronic or associated with other conditions that may cause ventriculomegaly, one would want to determine whether shunting would be helpful to that patient.

CSF Evaluation. If infection is suspected, it is important to determine cell counts and culture results prior to shunt placement. In children who have posthemorrhagic hydrocephalus, protein measurements and amount of blood product present should be determined. Fat-laden cells in the CSF have been associated with hydrocephalus, indicating brain damage in the postinfectious states. They provide prognostic data when levels are high.[30]

ICP Monitoring. The anterior fontanelle, when open, does provide a quantitative estimation of ICP. The level of a flat fontanelle is equivalent to the level of the top of a column of fluid in a manometer connected with the CSF.[31] This is a gross measurement of increased pressure, but more sophisticated methods can be used when questions arise whether pressures are elevated or sustained and in need of treatment. It has been demonstrated that ICP monitoring in term and premature infants had little predictive value regarding whether hydrocephalus was progressive, whereas in older children this is a more reliable factor. Intracranial pressure monitoring is useful in determining the need for shunting in normal pressure hydrocephalus and after intracranial surgery.[32] When evaluating normal pressure hydrocephalus, plateau waves were noted prior to treatment in children who demonstrated a favorable response to shunting.[33] These children also had episodic increases in intracranial pressure with REM sleep. These occurrences are thought to be the result of disturbances in cerebrovascular function.[34] Perfusion and infusion studies have been performed to evaluate chronic and progressive hydrocephalus.[35]

Neuropsychologic Evaluation. Neuropsychologic testing in the older child and developmental assessment in the infant and young child can provide useful information as to the progression of hydrocephalus in the untreated patient. Some insight as to the prognosis and outcome can also be projected.[36] Neuropsychologic evaluation can give us valuable information about the adequacy of shunt function when it is combined with scanning techniques to evaluate ventricular changes. The child with hydrocephalus can exhibit problems with learning[37] and development.[38–40] Subtle changes in school performance or behavior may indicate a progression of hydrocephalus or a deterioration in shunt function.

Cerebral Blood Flow and Doppler Studies. More work has been done in recent years to determine how cerebral blood flow is affected in hydrocephalus. Statistically significant correlations between intracranial pressure and resistive indices in the middle cerebral artery and anterior cerebral artery have been detected by the transcranial Doppler technique.[41] Transcranial Doppler flow studies in children with nonfunctioning shunts also demonstrated values outside the range of age-appropriate normal values.[42–44] Positron emission tomography (PET) scanning has also been used to evaluate cerebral blood flow in children with ventriculomegaly. It has been reported that cerebral blood flow and regional cerebral metabolic rate of oxygen ($rCMRO_2$) values were demonstrated in hydrocephalus before and after shunting. Although the $rCMRO_2$ values increased, little change was noted in the cerebral blood flow pattern, indicating decreased metabolic activity in the developing hydrocephalic brain.[45, 46] Changes in cerebral blood flow can also be recognized in normal pressure hydrocephalus.[47] Ventricular infusion and perfusion techniques are also used to evaluate treated and untreated hydrocephalus. In cases of normal-pressure hydrocephalus, valuable information acquired by means of these techniques will aid in the decision-making process regarding treatment.[35, 48]

EVALUATION OF HYDROCEPHALUS

The degree of hydrocephalus at presentation is variable and is based on the rate of CSF production, degree of flow obstruction, and the amount of compensatory absorption. Ventricular size is also variable and has many determinants. These include the time of initiation and the magnitude and duration of obstruction to CSF flow, the availability of compensatory CSF pathways, the presence or absence of an expansile cranium, and the volume and compliance of cerebral tissue.

PREMATURE INFANT

The most frequent cause of ventriculomegaly in the premature infant is intraventricular hemorrhage associated with germinal matrix bleeding. Ultrasonography is the method of choice for evaluating ventricular size in this age group. Measurement of head size, evaluation of the fontanelle, and sutural diastasis are also indicators of increased intracranial pressure in this population. The ventricular system does dilate before these signs become evident.[49] Reservoirs for serial tapping can be used prior to permanent shunt placement. These allow for clearing of blood products from the CSF. Approximately 30 per cent of children will respond to serial tapping and not require permanent shunt placement.[50] The possibility of infection should always be eliminated prior to placement of intracranial hardware.

INFANTS

Newborns who exhibit signs of increased intracranial pressure including large heads, full fontanelles, and sutural diastasis should be evaluated for hydrocephalus and/or other intracranial lesions. The CT scan has been the most widely used initial study to determine the cause of increased intracranial pressure. MRI is gaining increasing popularity. Its availability is increasing, and it is the study of choice once an intracranial lesion has been identified. Macrocrania in the child without signs of increased pressure may be familial. These children have normal CT scans and follow a normal curve. They do not cross percentage lines. The condition of benign extra-axial fluid of infancy is demonstrated in the slightly older infant. These children can cross several percentage lines while exhibiting no signs of increased intracranial pressure. Lumbar puncture studies have been done and normal pressures have been obtained in these children.[51] They often exhibit motor delay and have a typical CT scan appearance of a mildly dilated ventricular system and generous extra-axial fluid spaces. It is extremely rare for any treatment to be required. The child eventually returns to within the upper limits of the normal growth curve, and CT changes eventually are restored to normal.[52] It is important to distinguish this condition from chronic subdural hematomas secondary to nonaccidental trauma. If there is a question, an MRI can detect prior hemorrhages. Intrauterine infection, such as toxoplasma, rubella, cytomegalovirus, or herpes simplex virus, as well as neonatal meningitis can lead to hydrocephalus, and CSF evaluation should be undertaken before treatment is considered.

OLDER CHILDREN

The child who exhibits signs of increased intracranial pressure should be evaluated for hydrocephalus, and a cause for the hydrocephalus should be identified. CT or MRI scanning must be undertaken to evaluate ventricular size and rule out mass lesions. Neuropsychologic testing may be helpful in the older child to note signs of deterioration indicating progressive hydrocephalus.

DYSRAPHISM

The child with a myelomeningocele defect or an encephalocele should have imaging studies of the brain and should be evaluated for infection prior to shunt placement if progressive hydrocephalus is encountered. Cerebral imaging will also demonstrate other malformations present.

HYDROCEPHALIC SYNDROMES

CONGENITAL SYNDROMES

Congenital hydrocephalus is often associated with malformation syndromes (see Table 12–2). Aqueductal stenosis or malformation is a major finding in congenital hydrocephalus in the newborn.[53] This condition can present at a later age as well. Children born with a myelomeningocele defect also have a high incidence of associated hydrocephalus. Eighty to 85 per cent will require shunting procedures. Although ventriculomegaly can be present at birth, the need for treatment does not usually present itself until closure of the myelomeningocele sac.[54, 55] Once this potential reservoir is removed, the children develop signs of increased intracranial pressure. This also holds true in children with posterior encephaloceles.

The Dandy-Walker syndrome (Fig. 12–4), which involves failure of normal regressive changes in the posterior medullary velum and congenital absence of the cerebellar vermis leading to posterior fossa cyst formation, is also a congenital cause of hydrocephalus.[56] Other brain malformations can be associated with this entity. Outcome is poor in over 50 per cent of patients with Dandy-Walker malformation.[57, 58] This again may not present in early infancy. Symptoms may first be noted during the adolescent years. X-linked aqueductal stenosis in males is another reported cause of congenital hydrocephalus.[59–62]

Viral and Parasitic Causes. Viral infection has been

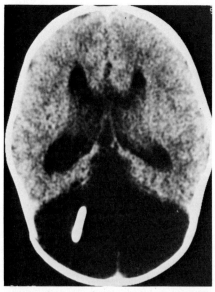

FIGURE 12–4. Dandy-Walker malformation. Note the large posterior fossa cyst with hypoplastic cerebellar structures. Shunt is in place.

recognized as a causative factor in the development of hydrocephalus. There is laboratory evidence that virus can cross placental membranes.[63, 64] Cytomegalovirus, rubella, mumps, varicella, and parainfluenza have been implicated in the development of hydrocephalus in the human. *Toxoplasma gondii*, a protozoan, is a cause of congenital infection and manifests itself with hydrocephalus, chorioretinitis, and intracranial calcification in the newborn.[65] This parasite also crosses placental membranes. Serologic data as well as CSF evaluation, coupled with radiologic and ophthalmologic studies, may confirm the diagnosis.

Arachnoid Cysts. Arachnoid cysts comprise approximately 1 per cent of all atraumatic mass lesions.[66, 67] The exact etiology is not often known, but it is believed that they are congenital expansions of the subarachnoid space which cause compression of cerebral tissue. Macrocrania, or increased intracranial pressure, is due to expansion of the cyst and/or development of hydrocephalus due to obstruction of CSF pathways.[42, 66] Ependymal cysts are believed to be aberrant nests of ependymal cells either in the subarachnoid space or in the intraventricular compartments. They may present later in life. Dilation of the ventricular atrium or unilateral ventricular dilation accompanied by headache may be the only clinical findings.[67, 68] Cavum vergae cysts rarely cause hydrocephalus by obstructing the aqueduct.[69] They can be communicated with a ventriculoscopic procedure.

Intracranial Neoplasms. Choroid plexus papilloma in infants and young children create an overproduction of CSF leading to ventriculomegaly and increased intracranial pressure.[70, 71] This may be coupled with obstructive components secondary to tumor position or size. Other tumors responsible for obstructive hydrocephalus are medulloblastomas, ependymomas, craniopharyngiomas, astrocytomas, and teratomas. Treatment of the lesions may obviate shunting.[72]

Vascular Causes. Vein of Galen aneurysms may obstruct CSF pathways and require shunt placement. Care should be taken in the treatment of hydrocephalus in these children since there is a 70 per cent complication rate reported.[73] Aneurysms of other vessels may also lead to obstructive hydrocephalus.[74, 75] Arteriovenous malformations have been responsible for obstructive hydrocephalus in some cases, depending on their location.[76]

Other Etiologic Factors. Various toxins as well as nutritional deficiencies have been implicated in the development of hydrocephalus. Hypervitaminosis A, vitamin A and B_{12} deficiencies, folic acid deficiency, azodyes, LSD, mescaline, triamcinolone acetamide, irradiation, and methyl mercury have all been implicated in the development of hydrocephalus.[77]

ACQUIRED HYDROCEPHALUS

Inflammatory Causes. Posthemorrhagic hydrocephalus is most commonly seen in the preterm infant.[78, 79] A germinal matrix hemorrhage is responsible for this presentation in the premature infant. In spite of aggressive treatment with serial tapping, drainage, and antifibrinolytic therapy, the overall percentage of children requiring permanent shunting remains around 70 per cent.[50, 80, 81] Hydrocephalus is secondary to obstruction by blood clot or aseptic meningitis as a result of the hemorrhage.[79] Plugging of arachnoid villi by small particulate matter has also been observed.[82] In the term infant or older child, subarachnoid or intraventricular hemorrhage may result from birth trauma, nonaccidental trauma, infection, tumors, vascular malformations, and intracranial injury. Again, drainage and fibrinolytic therapy are used in an attempt to avoid shunting and are somewhat more successful in the older age group than in the preterm infant.[83] A communicating hydrocephalus is usually found.[84] Intrauterine infection has been associated with congenital hydrocephalus. infection in the newborn period also can cause an adhesive arachnoiditis leading to communicating hydrocephalus.[85] This resulting hydrocephalus may occur within several days of the infection or may be a late sequela of the disease process.[86] In the younger infant, from birth to 3 months of age, the causative organisms tend to be *Escherichia coli*, *Staphylococcus aureus*, and other gram-negative enteric bacilli. In the 3-month to 3-year age group, *Haemophilus influenzae*, *Pneumococcus*, *Meningococcus*, and *Staphylococcus aureus* are more commonly seen. When the older child above 3-years of age is infected, the most common organisms are *Meningococcus*, *Pneumococcus*, *Streptococcus*, *Staphylococcus*, *Gonococcus*, and *Haemophilus influenzae*.[77] Acquired parasitic infections have led to the development of hydrocephalus. Cysticercosis is edemic in certain regions and can be found in children who travel to those regions as well. Intraventricular and cisternal involvement are due to the racemose form.[87, 88] Individual cysts may provide an obstructive component.

Loculations within the ventricular system can be found following infections involving the cerebrospinal fluid.[89] Unilateral or focal hydrocephalus can occur requiring treatment either with shunting or ventriculoscopic communication.[90] In the premature infant with posthemorrhagic hydrocephalus or the postinfectious hydrocephalic, the fourth ventricle may become trapped or loculated.[91, 92] If the child becomes symptomatic, shunting is required (Fig. 12–5).

Neoplasms. Tumors can cause obstructive hydrocephalus in the older child as well as in the neonate, and since onset is delayed, they fall in the category of acquired hydrocephalus[72] (Fig. 12–6). Choroid plexus tumors cause an overproduction of CSF and cause obstruction in some cases.[93, 94]

Venous Obstruction. There is no substantiating proof that hydrocephalus is an effect of venous sinus thrombosis. Sagittal sinus hypertension does not invariably accompany infantile hydrocephalus.[95] A correlation is possibly noted in the myelomeningocele population with an Arnold-Chiari malformation.[95] Ventriculomegaly is found in achondroplasia. Hydrocephalus in achondroplasia has been associated with venous outflow obstruction,[96, 97] but again no hard evidence supports this theory.

Other Causes. Posterior fossa hemorrhages, closed

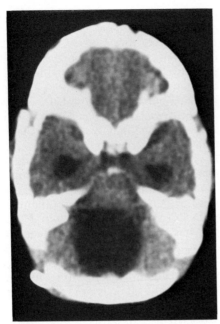

FIGURE 12–5. Loculated fourth ventricle in a preterm infant with treated posthemorrhagic hydrocephalus.

head injury, and traumatic brain injury as well as surgical intervention can also lead to hydrocephalus.

CLINICAL PRESENTATION

Hydrocephalus presents differently in the infant with an expansile cranium than in the older child with a fixed cranium. Because of the plasticity of the infant brain, ventriculomegaly can progress without obvious external signs of increased intracranial pressure.[49, 98] A slow-growing lesion can allow for pronounced ventriculomegaly even in the older child before symptoms are experienced. The presentation of hydrocephalus may be acute or chronic. The clinical presentation of this condition also varies, dependent upon the primary etiology, age of the patient, and associated intracranial and extracranial pathology.

NEWBORN AND INFANT

The young infant with hydrocephalus will typically exhibit macrocrania and a full, bulging fontanelle. The child may be a poor feeder or have episodes of vomiting. Lethargy or what is described as increased sleeping is also reported. The fontanelle should be examined with the child in the upright position or at a 45-degree incline. It is also important that the infant have serial head circumference measurements during the first year of life. If no signs of increased intracranial pressure are noted, but enlarging head size is encountered, CT scanning is warranted to rule out a slowly progressing hydrocephalus[99] or to confirm benign extra-axial fluid of infancy or familial macrocrania. Head shape may be altered by synostosis or positional molding, and other factors besides head circumference must be considered when determining when hydrocephalus is present.[100, 101] Other signs of hydrocephalus in the young infant include diastasis of sutures, scalp vein distention, and Parinaud's phenomenon, described as the sunsetting sign, caused by pressure on the tectal plate. Transcranial illumination is also illustrative of ventric-

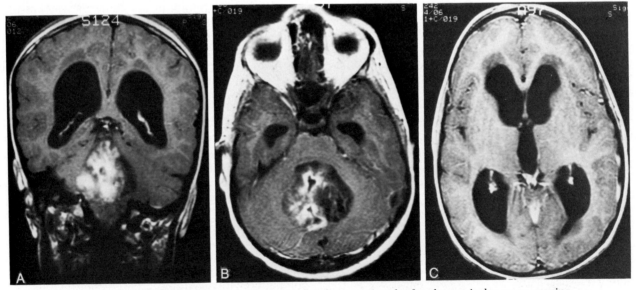

FIGURE 12–6. Medulloblastoma in a 6-year-old male occupying the fourth ventricular space, causing obstructive hydrocephalus. *A,* MRI demonstrating coronal view of medulloblastoma and dilated ventricular system. *B,* Axial MRI of the same patient with medulloblastoma, depicting dilatation of the temporal horns of the lateral ventricles. *C,* Axial MRI of supratentorial compartment with dilatation of lateral and third ventricles in the same patient with medulloblastoma.

ulomegaly in extreme hydrocephalus and hydranencephaly and can occasionally demonstrate intracranial cysts. Vascular lesions may be suspected if cranial bruits are audible. Other visual changes may be noted in the infant, such as tracking disorders or visual neglect.[102, 103] These may be due to stretching of frontal fibers by the anterior horns of the lateral ventricles or the optic radiations found occipitally when atrial enlargement is pronounced. If the head is large relative to body size, the infant often has difficulty with head control.

THE OLDER CHILD

Because of the inability of the cranium to expand, older children often have a more acute presentation. The triad of severe headache, vomiting, and lethargy is usually encountered. Children with colloid cysts (Fig. 12–7) or tumors obstructing the foramen of Monro may require emergent ventriculostomy. Papilledema, although uncommonly seen in infants, is found more often in the older child, particularly in those in whom chronic pressure due to slowly developing hydrocephalus is observed.[99] Chronic hydrocephalus is seen in children with slowly expanding lesions and gradual onset of hydrocephalus. Persistent headache, particularly awakening them from sleep or noted in the morning along with intermittent vomiting, is symptomatic of this condition. In children with headache and vomiting, a scan should be done to eliminate the possibility of an intracranial problem prior to assuming a gastrointestinal cause. If a mass lesion, such as a tumor or cyst, is the cause of chronic progressive hydrocephalus, the symptoms of hydrocephalus may present prior to other

neurologic deficits. If a careful neurologic examination is performed, these neurologic deficits, although previously unnoticed, might be elicited. Chronic hydrocephalus is also seen in cases of normal-pressure hydrocephalus or arrested hydrocephalus when ventriculomegaly is present, but the signs of pressure effects are subtle.[104–106] The typical triad of dementia, gait disturbance, and incontinence is not generally found in children. Delayed development, in both motor and cognitive function, can be encountered. Behavior changes are also a subtle finding. A slight spastic diplegia with positive Babinski can be elicited on examination.[107] These findings are responsive to shunting, and significant improvement can be obtained.[107, 108] Cerebral blood flow in normal-pressure hydrocephalus has been shown to increase in the white matter and cortex of frontotemporal, parietal, and occipital lobes, as well as in the thalamus following shunting.[47] Clinical improvement was also noted in these patients. SPECT scanning is used in some institutions to evaluate normal pressure hydrocephalus.[109] Intracranial pressure monitoring with infusion studies may be used to determine the need for treatment.[110] It is believed that the signs and symptoms found in normal pressure hydrocephalus are related to gradual stretching and deterioration of white matter fibers and metabolic changes due to chronic ventricular distention. MRI imaging to look at the periventricular edema is another means used to assist in determining the responsiveness of suspected normal-pressure hydrocephalus to shunting.[106] Intrauterine ultrasonography is now performed more often in the prenatal period. An intrauterine diagnosis of hydrocephalus can be made. The hydrocephalus may be associated with other anomalies, which are not well demonstrated by ultrasound.[111, 112] The sensitivity of ultrasound is more accurate than the specificity. To further elaborate the cause of hydrocephalus, fetal CT or MRI scanning can be done, but this is not the usual practice and specific diagnosis is not guaranteed. The presence of intrauterine hydrocephalus is valuable information for the parents. They can be prepared to deal with the problems surrounding infantile hydrocephalus once the child is born. Fetal surgery for treatment of hydrocephalus has been accomplished but is not in widespread use. There are complications associated with the procedure, and centers must be equipped to handle the surgery.[113, 114] It does offer hope for the child suffering from hydrocephalus in utero to obtain treatment before damage to cerebral tissues occurs, although it will not alter the congenital malformations present.

DIFFERENTIAL DIAGNOSIS

The cause of macrocrania in the infant (Table 12–3) must be determined before any treatment is initiated.[115] Besides familial macrocrania, the most common cause for increasing head circumference is benign extra-axial fluid of infancy. In this condition, the child's head size will often increase over several percentage lines and

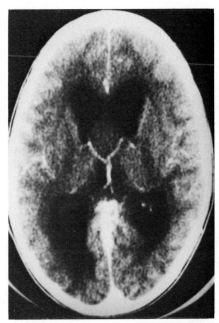

FIGURE 12–7. Colloid cyst at the foramen of Monro in a 10-year-old boy presenting with acute hydrocephalus. Bilateral ventriculostomies were placed on an emergency basis.

TABLE 12–3. MACROCRANIA

Hydrocephalus
Subdural fluid
  Hygroma
  Hematoma
  Effusion
Brian edema
  Toxic (e.g., lead
    encephalopathy)
  Endocrine (e.g.,
    hypoparathyroidism,
    galactosemia)
Thickened skull
  Anemia (e.g., thalassemia)
  Cranioskeletal dysplasia (e.g.,
    osteopetrosis, Russell's
    dwarf)

Megalencephaly
  Benign
    Familial or constitutional
      scaphocephaly
  Pathologic
    Gigantism
    Dwarfism
    Neurocutaneous syndrome
    Aminoaciduria
    Leukodystrophy (e.g.,
      Alexander's disease)
    Lysozymal disorders (e.g.,
      metachromatic
      leukodystrophy,
      mucopolysaccharidosis)

Adapted from DeMyer W: Megalencephaly in children. Neurology (Minn) 22:634, 1972.

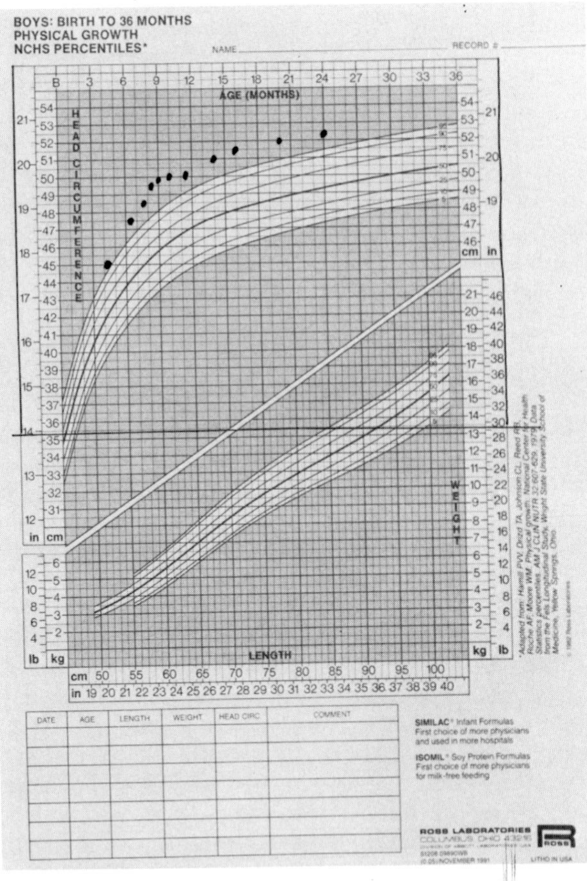

FIGURE 12–8. Growth chart demonstrating the typical appearance of orbital frontal circumference measurements in a child with benign extra-axial fluid of infancy. Head size begins to taper at 24 months.

remain elevated until approximately 18 to 24 months of age, when it begins to fall toward the upper percentiles of normal (Fig. 12–8). The CT scan demonstrates mild ventriculomegaly and pronounced extra-axial fluid spaces (Fig. 12–9). The condition resolves without intervention in almost every case.[51, 52] Hydranencephaly may also mimic hydrocephalus. In extreme or maximal hydrocephalus, there is reconstitution of the cerebral mantle once shunting is initiated (Fig. 12–10). In hydranencephaly there is only minimal occipital brain tissue (Fig. 12–11). There is no EEG cortical activity, and although shunting may be done to control head size, there is no re-expansion of the cortical mantle[116, 117] (Fig. 12–12).

PATHOPHYSIOLOGY

The effects of hydrocephalus on the developing brain are now known to involve the cerebral tissue surrounding the ventricular system as well as the cortex. Neurochemical alterations have also been demonstrated. In spite of shunting procedures leading to re-expansion of the cortical mantle, permanent changes

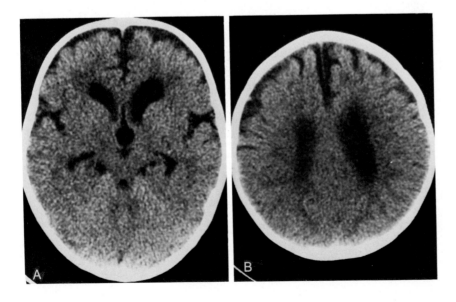

FIGURE 12–9. CT scan of benign extra-axial fluid of infancy. *A,* Note the mild ventriculomegaly and generous extra-axial fluid spaces. *B,* Gyral and sulcal patterns appear more pronounced owing to extra-axial fluid component.

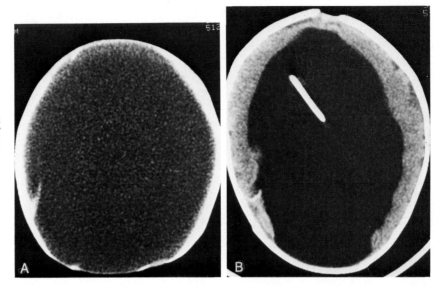

FIGURE 12–10. *A,* Maximal hydrocephalus prior to treatment. *B,* Initial reconstitution of cortical mantle in the same child several months after shunt placement.

may have taken place leading to the long-term sequelae of infantile hydrocephalus.

Studies have shown that ventriculomegaly causes cytoarchitectural and cytologic changes throughout the cerebral cortex and affects the periventricular white matter.[118] It had long been established that the ventricular ependyma and the periventricular white matter were affected in cases of hydrocephalus.[119–122] Following shunting there was re-expansion of these areas, but gliosis was believed to be the result of the prior ventriculomegaly.[84, 123–125] Some studies suggested involvement of cortical neurons. Abnormal proliferation, migration, and differentiation of neurons have been

observed in fetal cases of untreated preterm hydrocephalus.[86] There was an attempt to calculate cell number and size based on determination of amount of DNA, RNA, and protein in adult animal models. The DNA was noted to increase while the RNA/DNA ratio decreased, and it was concluded that neurons were not lost secondary to the hydrocephalus process.[126] A study performed on kittens with kaolin-induced hydrocephalus has demonstrated significant cytologic and cytoarchitectural changes within the cortical mantle. Cortical neurons exhibited edematous or dark and shrunken somata. These neurons were believed to be reactive (Fig. 12–13). Some pyknotic neurons were noted.

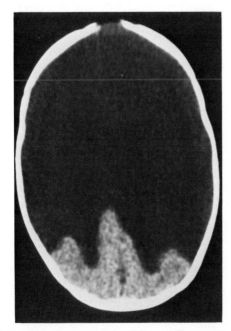

FIGURE 12–11. Hydranencephaly with a small amount of occipital cerebral tissue.

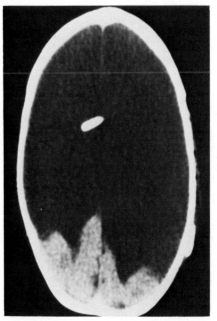

FIGURE 12–12. No reconstitution of cortical mantle noted in hydranencephaly in spite of shunt placement for control of head size.

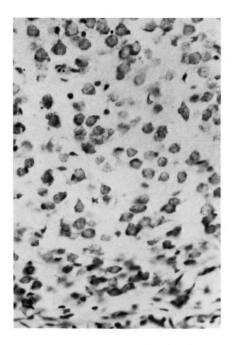

FIGURE 12–13. Cortical neurons in hydrocephalic neonatal kitten showing reactive, spongy, and pyknotic cells.

There was a disorientation in the laminae within the cortical mantle. Deeper cortical layers were more affected than the superficial laminae. When these animals were shunted, there was re-expansion of the cortical mantle and reorganization of the laminae (Fig. 12–14). Many of the neurons that were called reactive appeared to have the ability to recover.[127] The kittens, once shunted, made a good neurologic recovery, particularly where motor deficits were most obvious. These studies confirm that there is a significant degree of involvement of the cerebral cortex as well as the periventricular white matter and ependymal surface. These pertubations of neurons and their processes may be involved in the sequelae of treated hydrocephalus.[128, 129]

Alterations in CSF composition and neurotransmitters have been identified and probably contribute to the clinical changes as well as long-term sequelae observed with hydrocephalus.[130–132] Two phases have been demonstrated in laboratory-induced hydrocephalus: (1) an acute stage, in which high resistance and low compliance were observed, as well as ependymal damage and periventricular edema, and (2) a chronic phase, in which there was little resistance and normal compliance. Epithelial regeneration and subependymal gliosis

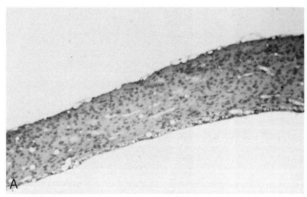

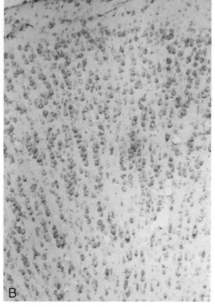

FIGURE 12–14. *A,* Cortical mantle and white matter compression in a neonatal kitten with severe hydrocephalus. Note the disorientation of laminae and ependymal disruption. *B,* Re-expansion of the cortical mantle following a shunting procedure in a neonatal kitten. Reorganization of laminae takes place, and neurons appear normal.

occurred during this phase. An increase in cerebral pulse pressure amplitude was observed in both phases.[133]

CONCLUSION

Even though this century has witnessed significant progress in the diagnosis and treatment of hydrocephalus, this condition continues to be a formidable problem in the area of pediatric neurosurgery. Extremely important is early recognition and institution of therapy. The application of improved diagnostic and therapeutic modalities will provide for prolonged survival and improved functional outcome.[134, 135]

REFERENCES

1. Torack RM: Historical aspects of normal and abnormal brain fluids. II. Hydrocephalus. Arch Neurol 39:276, 1982.
2. McCullough DC: A history of the treatment of hydrocephalus. Fetal Therapy 1:38, 1986.
3. Dandy WE, Blackfan KD: An experimental and clinical study of internal hydrocephalus. JAMA 61:2216, 1913.
4. Dandy WE: Ventriculostomy following the injection of air into the cerebral ventricles. Ann Surg 68:5, 1918.
5. Wallman LJ: Shunting for hydrocephalus: an oral history. Neurosurgery 11(2):308, 1982.
6. Stookey B, Scarff J: Occlusion of the aqueduct of Sylvius by neoplastic and non-neoplastic processes with a rational surgical treatment for relief of the resultant obstructive hydrocephalus. Bull Neurol Inst NY 5:348, 1936.
7. Mixter WJ: Ventriculostomy and puncture of the floor of the third ventricle. Boston Med Surg J 188:277, 1923.
8. Torkildsen A: A new palliative operation in cases of inoperable occlusion of the sylvian aqueduct. Acta Chir Scand 82:117, 1939.
9. Bright R: Hydrocephalus—the remarkable case of James Cardinal: From Reports of Medical Cases, Volume 11, 1831, by Richard Bright. Surg Neurol 27:4, 1987.
10. Feeney JK, Barry AP: Hydrocephaly as a cause of maternal mortality and morbidity: a clinical study of 304 cases. J Obstet Gynecol 61:652, 1954.
11. Larson SL, Banner EA: Hydrocephalus: a 30-year survey. Obstet Gynecol 28:571, 1966.
12. Laurence KM, Coates S: The natural history of hydrocephalus: Detailed analysis of 182 unoperated cases. Arch Dis Child 37:345, 1962.
13. Laurence KM, Coates S: Spontaneously arrested hydrocephalus: Results of the re-examination of 82 survivors from a series of 182 unoperated cases. Dev Med Child Neurol 13:4, 1967.
14. Yashon D, Janes JA, Sugar O: The course of severe untreated infantile hydrocephalus. J Neurosurg 23:509, 1965.
15. Jansen J: A retrospective analysis 21 to 35 years after birth of hydrocephalic patients born from 1946 to 1955. An overall description of the material and the criteria used. Acta Neurol Scand 71:436, 1985.
16. Mealey J Jr., Gilmor RL, Bubb MP: The prognosis of hydrocephalus overt at birth. J Neurosurg 39:348, 1973.
17. Foltz EL: Hydrocephalus: the value of treatment. South Med J 61:443, 1968.
18. Guthkelch AN, Riley NA: Influence of aetiology on prognosis in surgically treated infantile hydrocephalus. Arch Dis Child 44:29, 1969.
19. Lorber J, Zachary RB: Primary congenital hydrocephalus: long term results of a controlled therapeutic trial. Arch Dis Child 43:516, 1968.
20. Bamforth SJ, Baird PA: Spina bifida and hydrocephalus: a population study over a 35-year period. Am J Hum Genet 44:225, 1989.
21. Milhorat TH: Pediatric neurosurgery, 2nd ed. Philadelphia, F. A. Davis Co., 1979, p. 99.
22. Jansen J: Etiology and prognosis in hydrocephalus. Childs Nerv Syst 4:263, 1988.
23. Naidich TP, Epstein F, Lin JP, et al.: Evaluation of pediatric hydrocephalus by computed tomography. Radiology 119:337, 1976.
24. Centeno RS, Winter J, Bentison JR, et al.: CT evaluation of haemophilus influenzae meningitis with clinical and pathologic correlation. Comput Radiol 7:243, 1983.
25. Wikkelso C, Andersson H, Blomstrand C, et al.: Computed tomography of the brain in the diagnosis of and prognosis in normal pressure hydrocephalus. Neuroradiology 31:160, 1989.
26. Enzmann DR, Pelc NJ: Normal flow patterns of intracranial and spinal cerebrospinal fluid defined with phase-contrast cine MR imaging. Radiology 178:467, 1991.
27. Kahn T, Muller E, Lewin JS, et al.: MR measurement of spinal CSF flow with the RACE technique. J Comput Assist Tomogr 16 (1):54, 1992.
28. Nitz WR, Bradley WG Jr., Watanabe AS, et al.: Flow dynamics of cerebrospinal fluid: assessment with phase-contrast velocity MR imaging performed with retrospective cardiac gating. Radiology 183:395, 1992.
29. McCullough DC, Harbert JC, Miale A, et al.: Radioisotope cisternography in the evaluation of hydrocephalus in infancy and childhood. Radiology 102:645, 1972.
30. Chester DC, Emery JL, Penny SR: Fat-laden macrophages in cerebrospinal fluid as an indication of brain damage in children. J Clin Pathol 24:753, 1971.
31. Davson H, Welch K, Segal MB: The physiology and pathophysiology of the cerebrospinal fluid, 1st ed. Edinburgh, Churchill Livingstone, 1987, p 734.
32. McCullough DC: A critical evaluation of continuous intracranial pressure monitoring in pediatric hydrocephalus. Childs Brain 6:225, 1980.
33. Hammock MK, Milhorat TH, Baron IS: Normal pressure hydrocephalus in patients with myelomeningocele. Dev Med Child Neurol 18(suppl. 37):55, 1976.
34. Di Rocco C, McLone DG, Shimoji T, et al.: Continuous intraventricular cerebrospinal fluid pressure recording in hydrocephalus children during wakefulness and sleep. J Neurosurg 42:683, 1975.
35. Shapiro K, Fried A, Marmarou A: Biomechanical and hydrodynamic characterization of the hydrocephalic infant. J Neurosurg 63:69, 1985.
36. Donders J, Canady AI, Rourke BP: Psychometric intelligence after infantile hydrocephalus. A critical review and reinterpretation. Childs Nerv Syst 6:148, 1990.
37. Barnes MA, Dennis M: Reading in children and adolescents after early onset hydrocephalus and in normally developing age peers: phonological analysis, word recognition, word comprehension, and passage comprehension skill. J Pediatr Psychol 17:445, 1992.
38. Hanigan WC, Morgan AM, Anderson RJ, et al.: Incidence and neurodevelopmental outcome of periventricular hemorrhage and hydrocephalus in a regional population of very low birth weight infants. Neurosurgery 29:701, 1991.
39. Oi S, Matsumoto S, Katayama K, et al.: Pathophysiology and postnatal outcome of fetal hydrocephalus. Childs Nerv Syst 6:338, 1990.
40. Fernell E, Gillberg C, Von Wendt L: Autistic symptoms in children with infantile hydrocephalus. Acta Paediatr Scand 80:451, 1991.
41. Goh D, Minns RA, Hendry GM, et al.: Cerebrovascular resistive index assessed by duplex Doppler sonography and its relationship to intracranial pressure in infantile hydrocephalus. Pediatr Radiol 22:246, 1992.
42. Pople IK: Doppler flow velocities in children with controlled hydrocephalus: reference values for the diagnosis of blocked cerebrospinal fluid shunts. Childs Nerv Syst 8:124, 1992.
43. Sanker P, Richard KE, Weigl HC, et al.: Transcranial Doppler sonography and intracranial pressure monitoring in children

and juveniles with acute brain injuries or hydrocephalus. Childs Nerv Syst 7:391, 1991.

44. Norelle A, Fischer AQ, Flanner AM: Transcranial Doppler: a noninvasive method to monitor hydrocephalus. J Child Neurol 4(Suppl):S87, 1989.

45. Shirane R, Sato S, Sato K, et al.: Cerebral blood flow and oxygen metabolism in infants with hydrocephalus. Childs Nerv Syst 8:118, 1992.

46. George AE, de Leon MJ, Miller J, et al.: Positron emission tomography of hydrocephalus. Metabolic effects of shunt procedures. Acta Radiol 369(Suppl):435, 1986.

47. Kimura M, Tanaka A, Yoshinaga S: Significance of periventricular hemodynamics in normal pressure hydrocephalus. Neurosurgery 30:701, 1992.

48. Morgan MK, Johnston IH, Spittaler PJ: A ventricular infusion technique for the evaluation of treated and untreated hydrocephalus. Neurosurgery 29:832, 1991.

49. Volpe JJ, Pasternak JF, Allan WC: Ventricular dilation preceding rapid head growth following neonatal intracranial hemorrhage. Am J Dis Child 131:1212, 1977.

50. Brockmeyer DL, Wright LC, Walker ML, et al.: Management of posthemorrhagic hydrocephalus in the low-birth-weight preterm neonate. Pediatr Neurosci 15:302, 1989.

51. Hogueira GJ, Zaglul HF: Hypodense extracerebral images on computed tomography in children. External hydrocephalus: a misnomer? Childs Nerv Syst 7:336, 1991.

52. Shen WC, Yang CF, Chang T: Benign hydrocephalus in infants. A computed tomographic and clinical correlative study. Acta Radiol 369(Suppl):689, 1986.

53. Milhorat TH: Hydrocephalus and the Cerebrospinal Fluid, 1st ed. Baltimore, Williams & Wilkins, 1972, p 63.

54. Linder M, Nichols J, Sklar FH: Effect of meningomyelocele closure on the intracranial pulse pressure. Childs Brain 11:176, 1984.

55. Lorber J: Systematic ventriculographic studies in infants born with meningomyelocele and encephalocele. The incidence and development of hydrocephalus. Arch Dis Child 36:381, 1961.

56. Wilkins RH, Rengachary SS: Neurosurgery, Vol. III. New York, McGraw-Hill, 1985, p 2155.

57. Carmel PW, Antunes JL, Hilal SK, et al.: Dandy-Walker syndrome: Clinico-pathological features and re-evaluation of modes of treatment. Surg Neurol 8:132, 1977.

58. Sawaya R, McLaurin RL: Dandy-Walker syndrome: Clinical analysis of 23 cases. J Neurosurg 55:89, 1981.

59. Holmes LB, Nash A, ZuRhein GM, et al.: X-linked aqueductal stenosis: clinical and neuropathological findings in two families. Pediatrics 51:697, 1973.

60. Bickers DS, Adams RD: Hereditary stenosis of the aqueduct of sylvius as a cause of congenital hydrocephalus. Brain 72:246, 1949.

61. Schrander-Stumpel C, Fryns J, Cassiman JJ, et al.: MASA syndrome (a form of complicated spastic paraplegia) and X-linked hydrocephalus: variable expression of the same mutation at Xq28? J Med Genet 29:215, 1992.

62. Willems PJ, Vits L, Raeymaekers P, et al.: Further localization of X-linked hydrocephalus in the chromosomal region Xq28. Am J Hum Genet 51:307, 1992.

63. Takano T, Ohno M, Yamano T, et al.: Congenital hydrocephalus in suckling hamsters caused by transplacental infection with parainfluenza virus type 3. Brain Dev 13:371, 1991.

64. Davis LE: Communicating hydrocephalus in newborn hamsters and cats following vaccinia virus infection. J Neurosurg 54:767, 1981.

65. Martinovic J, Sibalic D, Djordjevic M, et al.: Frequency of toxoplasmosis in the appearance of congenital hydrocephalus. J Neurosurg 56:830, 1982.

66. Harsh GR IV, Edwards MSB, Wilson CB: Intracranial arachnoid cysts in children. J Neurosurg 64:835, 1986.

67. McCullough DC, Harbert JC, Manz HJ: Large arachnoid cysts at the cranial base. Neurosurgery 6:76, 1980.

68. Alvord EC: The pathology of hydrocephalus. In Fields WS, Desmond MM (eds): Disorders of the Developing Nervous System. Springfield, IL, Charles C Thomas, 1961, p 343.

69. Donauer E, Moringlane JR, Ostertag CB: Cavum vergae cyst as a cause of hydrocephalus, almost forgotten? Successful stereotactic treatment. Acta Neurochir 83:12, 1986.

70. Eisenberg HM, McComb JG, Lorenzo AV: Cerebrospinal fluid overproduction and hydrocephalus associated with choroid plexus papilloma. J Neurosurg 40:381, 1974.

71. Milhorat TH, Hammock MK, Davis DA, et al.: Choroid plexus papilloma. Childs Brain 2:273, 1976.

72. Rappaport ZH, Shalit MN: Perioperative external ventricular drainage in obstructive hydrocephalus secondary to infratentorial brain tumors. Acta Neurochir 96:118, 1989.

73. Schneider SJ, Wisoff JS, Epstein FJ: Complications of ventriculoperitoneal shunt procedures or hydrocephalus associated with vein of Galen malformations in childhood. Neurosurgery 30:706, 1992.

74. Osenbach RK: Giant aneurysm of the distal posterior inferior cerebellar artery in an 11-month-old child presenting with obstructive hydrocephalus. Pediatr Neurosci 15:309, 1989.

75. Morota N, Ohtsuka A, Kameyama S, et al.: Obstructive hydrocephalus due to a giant aneurysm of the internal carotid bifurcation. Surg Neurol 29:227, 1988.

76. Tien R, Harch GR IV, Dilon WP, et al.: Unilateral hydrocephalus caused by an intraventricular venous malformation obstructing the foramen of Monro. Neurosurgery 26:664, 1990.

77. Milhorat TH: Hydrocephalus and the Cerebrospinal Fluid, 1st ed. Baltimore, Williams & Wilkins, 1972, p 53.

78. Fernell E, Hagberg G, Hagberg B: Infantile hydrocephalus—the impact of enhanced preterm survival. Acta Paediatr Scand 79:1080, 1990.

79. Lorber J, Bhat US: Posthaemorrhagic hydrocephalus: diagnosis, differential diagnosis, treatment, and long-term results. Arch Dis Child 49:751, 1974.

80. Weninger M, Salzer HR, Pollak A, et al.: External ventricular drainage for treatment of rapidly progressive posthemorrhagic hydrocephalus. Neurosurgery 31:52, 1992.

81. Whitelaw A, Rivers RP, Creighton L, et al.: Low dose intraventricular fibrinolytic treatment to prevent posthaemorrhagic hydrocephalus. Arch Dis Child 67:12, 1992.

82. Hill A, Shackelford GD, Volpe JJ: A potential mechanism of pathogenesis for early posthemorrhagic hydrocephalus in the premature newborn. Pediatrics 73:19, 1984.

83. Hasan D, Lindsay KW, Vermeulen M: Treatment of acute hydrocephalus after subarachnoid hemorrhage with serial lumbar puncture. Stroke 22:190, 1991.

84. Ellington E, Margolis G: Block of arachnoid villus by subarachnoid hemorrhage. J Neurosurg 30:651, 1969.

85. Gelabert M, Castro-Gago M: Hydrocephalus and tuberculous meningitis in children. Report on 26 cases. Childs Nerv Syst 4:268, 1988.

86. Dodge PR, Swartz MN: Bacterial meningitis—a review of selected aspects. N Engl J Med 272:954, 1965.

87. Leblanc R, Knowles KF, Melanson D, et al.: Neurocysticercosis: Surgical and medical management with praziquantel. Neurosurgery 18:419, 1986.

88. Sotelo J, Marin C: Hydrocephalus secondary to cysticercotic arachnoiditis. A long-term follow-up review of 92 cases. J Neurosurg 66:686, 1987.

89. Kalsbeck JE, DeSousa AL, Kleiman MB, et al.: Compartmentalization of the cerebral ventricles as a sequela of neonatal meningitis. J Neurosurg 52:547, 1980.

90. Gaston BM, Jones BE: Perinatal unilateral hydrocephalus. Atresia of the foramen of Monro. Pediatr Radiol 19:328, 1989.

91. Scotti G, Musgrave MA, Fitz CR, et al.: The isolated fourth ventricle in children: CT and clinical review of 16 cases. AJNR 1:419, 1980.

92. Coker SB, Anderson CL: Occluded fourth ventricle after multiple shunt revisions for hydrocephalus. Pediatrics 83:981, 1989.

93. Dias MS, Albright AL: Management of hydrocephalus complicating childhood posterior fossa tumors. Pediatr Neurosci 15:283, 1989.

94. Bering EA Jr.: Circulation of the cerebrospinal fluid: demonstration of the choroid plexuses as the generator of the force for flow of fluid and ventricular enlargement. J Neurosurg 19:405, 1962.

95. Norrell H, Wilson C, Howieson J, et al.: Venous factors in infantile hydrocephalus. J Neurosurg 31:561, 1969.

96. Friedman WA, Mickle JP: Hydrocephalus in achondroplasia: a possible mechanism. Neurosurgery 7:150, 1980.

97. Steinbok P, Hall J, Flodmark O: Hydrocephalus in achondroplasia: the possible role of intracranial venous hypertension. J Neurosurg 71:42, 1989.

98. Korobkin R: The relationship between head circumference and the development of communicating hydrocephalus in infants following intraventricular hemorrhage. Pediatrics 56:74, 1975.

99. Kirkpatrick M, Engleman H, Minns RA: Symptoms and signs of progressive hydrocephalus. Arch Dis Child 64:124, 1989.

100. Collmann H, Sorensen N, Krauss J, et al.: Hydrocephalus in craniosynostosis. Childs Nerv Syst 4:279, 1988.

101. Hanieh A, Sheen R, David DJ: Hydrocephalus in Crouzon's syndrome. Childs Nerv Syst 5:188, 1989.

102. Tytla ME, Buncic JR: Recovery of spatial vision following shunting for hydrocephalus. Arch Ophthalmol 108:701, 1990.

103. Mankinen-Heikkinen A, Mustonen E: Ophthalmic changes in hydrocephalus. A follow-up examination of 50 patients treated with shunts. Acta Ophthalmol 65:81, 1987.

104. Schick RW, Matson DD: What is arrested hydrocephalus? J Pediatr 58:791, 1961.

105. Di Rocco C, Caldarelli M, Ceddia A: Occult hydrocephalus in children. Childs Nerv Syst 5:71, 1989.

106. Tamaki N, Shirakuni T, Ehara K, et al.: Characterization of periventricular edema in normal-pressure hydrocephalus by measurement of water proton relaxation times. J Neurosurg 73:864, 1990.

107. Hagberg B, Sjorgen I: The chronic brain syndrome of infantile hydrocephalus. Am J Dis Child 112:189, 1966.

108. Gordon N: Normal pressure hydrocephalus and arrested hydrocephalus. Dev Med Child Neurol 19:540, 1977.

109. Granado JM, Diaz F, Alday R: Evaluation of brain SPECT in the diagnosis and prognosis of the normal pressure hydrocephalus syndrome. Acta Neurochir 112:88, 1991.

110. Symon L, Dorsch NWC: Use of long-term intracranial pressure measurement to assess hydrocephalic patients prior to shunt surgery. J Neurosurg 42:258, 1975.

111. Hanigan WC, Gibson J, Kleopoulos NJ, et al.: Medical imaging of fetal ventriculomegaly. J Neurosurg 64:575, 1986.

112. Hill LM, Breckle R, Gehrking WC: The prenatal detection of congential malformations by ultrasonography. Mayo Clin Proc 58:805, 1983.

113. Clewell WH, Johnson ML, Meier PR, et al.: A surgical approach to the treatment of fetal hydrocephalus. N Engl J Med 306:1320, 1982.

114. Bannister CM: Fetal Neurosurgery—a new challenge on the horizon. Dev Med Child Neurol 26:822, 1984.

115. Strassburg HM: Macrocephaly is not always due to hydrocephalus. J Child Neurol 4(Suppl):S32, 1989.

116. Sutton LN, Bruce DA, Schut L: Hydranencephaly versus maximal hydrocephalus: an important clinical distinction. Neurosurgery 6:35, 1980.

117. Iinuma K, Handa I, Kojima A, et al.: Hydranencephaly and maximal hydrocephalus: usefulness of electrophysiological studies for their differentiation. J Child Neurol 4:114, 1989.

118. Glees P, Voth D: Clinical and ultrastructural observations of maturing human frontal cortex. I. Biopsy material of hydrocephalic infants. Neurosurg Rev 11:293, 1988.

119. Takei F, Shapiro K, Hirano A, et al.: Influence of the rate of ventricular enlargement on the ultrastructural morphology of the white matter in experimental hydrocephalus. Neurosurgery 21:645, 1987.

120. Takei F, Hirano A, Shapiro K, et al.: New ultrastructural changes of the ependyma in experimental hydrocephalus. Acta Neuropathol 73:400, 1987.

121. Rosenberg GA, Saland L, Kyner WT: Pathophysiology of periventricular tissue changes with raised CSF pressure in cats. J Neurosurg 59:606, 1983.

122. Takei F, Shapiro K, Kohn I: Influence of the rate of ventricular enlargement on the morphology of the white matter in experimental hydrocephalus. Neurosurgery 21:645, 1987.

123. Del Bigio MR, Bruni JE: Periventricular pathology in hydrocephalic rabbits before and after shunting. Acta Neuropathol 77:186, 1988.

124. Rubin RC, Hochwald GM, Tiell M, et al.: Hydrocephalus. III. Reconstitution of the cerebral cortical mantle following ventricular shunting. Surg Neurol 5:179, 1976.

125. Rubin RC, Hochwald GM, Tiell M, et al.: Hydrocephalus. I. Histological and ultrastructural changes in the pre-shunted cortical mantle. Surg Neurol 5:109, 1976.

126. Rubin RC, Hochwald GM, Tiell M, et al.: Hydrocephalus. II. Cell number and size, and myelin content of the preshunted cerebral cortical mantle. Surg Neurol 5:115, 1976.

127. Heiss WD, Rosner G: Functional recovery of cortical neurons as related to degree and duration of ischemia. Ann Neurol 14:294, 1983.

128. Wright LC, McAllister JP II, Katz SD, et al.: Cytological and cytoarchitectural changes in the feline cerebral cortex during experimental infantile hydrocephalus. Pediatr Neurosurg 16:139, 1991.

129. Hale PM, McAllister JP II, Katz SD, et al.: Improvement of cortical morphology in infantile hydrocephalic animals following ventriculoperitoneal shunt placement. Neurosurgery 31:1085, 1992.

130. Del Bigio MR: Hydrocephalus-induced changes in the composition of cerebrospinal fluid. Neurosurgery 25:416, 1989.

131. Lovely TJ, McAllister JP II, Miller DW, et al.: Effects of hydrocephalus and surgical decompression on cortical norepinephrine levels in neonatal cats. Neurosurgery 24:43, 1989.

132. Chovanes GI, McAllister JP II, Lamperti AA, et al.: Monoamine alterations during experimental hydrocephalus in neonatal rats. Neurosurgery 22:86, 1988.

133. Gonzalez-Darder J, Barbera J, Cerda-Nicolas M, et al.: Sequential morphological and functional changes in kaolin-induced hydrocephalus. J Neurosurg 61:918, 1984.

134. Renier D, Sainte-Rose C, Pierre-Kahn A, et al.: Prenatal hydrocephalus: outcome and prognosis. Childs Nerv Syst 4:213, 1988.

135. Fernell E, Uvebrant P, von Wendt L: Overt hydrocephalus at birth—origin and outcome. Childs Nerv Syst 3:350, 1987.

Chapter 13

TREATMENT OF HYDROCEPHALUS

HAROLD L. REKATE, M.D.

Hydrocephalus is not an "all or none" phenomenon. Although overproduction of cerebrospinal fluid (CSF) may account for hydrocephalus in a small number of choroid plexus papillomas, hydrocephalus in the overwhelming majority of cases is due to an obstruction of CSF flow between its point of production within the ventricular system and its normal point of absorption in the superior sagittal sinus. This obstruction of CSF outflow may be *complete*, as in aqueductal stenosis, or *partial*, as is the case following subarachnoid hemorrhage. When the obstruction is incomplete, the elevation in intracranial pressure (ICP) and the degree of ventriculomegaly may be mild before a new steady state is established. Nonetheless, the latter is hydrocephalus, even though no therapy is indicated. An important aspect of hydrocephalus management is to determine initially whether the patient indeed requires treatment.

PATIENT SELECTION

If there were no risks accompanying the performance of a shunting procedure, it would be recommended for all patients with the slightest degree of ventriculomegaly. However, shunting is not innocuous, and it is not clear whether ventriculomegaly results in a decrease in cognitive ability. Therefore, each child must be assessed individually, balancing the risks of shunting versus the risks of untreated hydrocephalus. A theoretical representation of the risks of shunting and the risks of hydrocephalus not treated with a shunt as a function of the depth of the cerebral mantle (thickness of the brain) can be seen in Figure 13–1.[1]

The risks involved in performing a shunt procedure are low and are independent of ventricular size, except when the ventricles are extremely small. Improved

techniques and instruments have greatly reduced the risks accompanying a shunt, but the possibility of shunt infection or malfunction is always present. Shunt infection is the most serious threat to life and intellectual function. It has been shown that when hydrocephalus is associated with the Arnold-Chiari malformation, shunt infection in the first 6 months of life can lead to intellectual downgrading.[2-4]

When considering the risks of hydrocephalus to the developing brain, there is much conflicting information. Certain patients tolerate ventriculomegaly better than others. A portion of this information is anecdotal, such as the intriguing discussion in *Science*, "Is the brain really necessary?" in which the computerized tomographic (CT) scan of a graduate student in mathematics shows a cerebral mantle of less than 1 cm.[5] Other patients attain a low level of intellectual functioning despite early aggressive and effective control of their hydrocephalus.

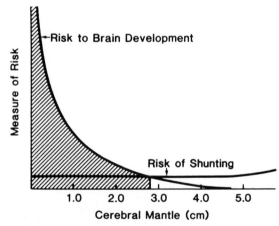

FIGURE 13–1. Theoretical representation of risk-benefit ratio of shunting versus ventriculomegaly in spina bifida patients. (From Rekate HL: To shunt or not to shunt. Clin Neurosurg 32:593, 1985.)

202

In trying to arrive at a rationale for patient selection, one of the most difficult tasks is to discern differences between the effects caused by the hydrocephalus itself and the underlying damage to neural function resulting from the cause of the hydrocephalus. The best information regarding the degree of hydrocephalus needed to cause intellectual downgrading was derived from the work of Young and colleagues.[6] Previous attempts to correlate outcome with severity of hydrocephalus with or without treatment had been unsuccessful.[7–9] Young and associates were able to correlate outcome with depth of the cerebral mantle following treatment. In their study, patients who had no associated central nervous system anomalies or perinatal asphyxia, but whose cerebral mantle remained less than 2.0 cm at the foramen of Monro, reached an intelligence quotient (IQ) as measured on the Wechsler Intelligence Scale for Children (WISC) or Stanford-Binet test of no better than 80. The IQ distribution became normal when the 2.8 cm level was reached. There did not seem to be an advantage in having a normal (i.e., 5 cm) cerebral mantle. This study also showed the time dependency of the treatment of hydrocephalus. After 5 months, the child with hydrocephalus was less likely to attain the stated goal of 3.5 cm than was the child treated earlier. The decision ''to shunt or not to shunt'' in infantile hydrocephalus should be made by five months of age.

The article by Young and associates includes patients with many different etiologies for their hydrocephalus.[6] The study was performed over a number of years, and the data on cerebral anatomy were based on pneumoventriculography. The end point of IQ has been challenged by neuropsychologists as too gross a measurement. Many people with normal IQ scores still have significant learning disabilities or ''holes'' in their cognitive abilities that limit severely their ability to compete successfully in society. This fact has been demonstrated definitively in patients with spina bifida and hydrocephalus related to the Arnold-Chiari malformation. These patients have normal or almost normal IQ scores but often have severe difficulty in learning mathematics.[10] Furthermore, since the development of sophisticated neuroimaging studies such as computed tomography (CT) and magnetic resonance imaging (MRI), the clinician has a better view of the intracranial anatomy than was available with ventriculography. By demonstrating associated developmental or acquired abnormalities of brain function, these imaging studies allow the clinician to understand why adequate treatment of the hydrocephalus does not always lead to a functional outcome.

The use of the article by Young and colleagues[6] to make treatment decisions has also been criticized specifically as it relates to the management of the premature neonate with posthemorrhagic hydrocephalus. In this case, the argument is that the primitive infant may somehow suffer more from the presence of ventriculomegaly, and intervention may be required at an earlier stage. Some experimental evidence supports this contention.[11, 12] I am unaware of a subsequent published work that correlates intellectual outcome to neurodiagnostic findings. This point is key in the discussion of the possibility of performing in utero shunting procedures, which are discussed below.

From the foregoing discussion and Figure 13–1, it is possible to make rational decisions regarding who is and who is not likely to benefit from a shunt. The neurosurgeon's goal for the infant with hydrocephalus should be to attain a 3.5-cm cerebral mantle by 5 months of age. The 3.5-cm mantle is chosen because the risk of shunting is not increased between 2.8 cm and 3.5 cm, and this higher number provides some added safety for the child. It does not seem to matter how this 3.5 cm-mantle is obtained (shunting, third ventriculostomy, nonsurgical measures, or close observation).

The one modifying factor is the neurologic and developmental status of the child. Although one cannot correlate results from the Denver Developmental Assessment (DDST) easily with later IQ, it is clear that poor performance on this test is likely to be associated with delayed intellectual development.[13] Accurate measurement by formal psychologic testing cannot be performed prior to age 3.[14] Because there is a minimum of data on very young children, it is difficult to determine whether the prognosis for a child (who is likely to be delayed intellectually) can be improved by shunting. It has been my policy to shunt developmentally delayed children with ventriculomegaly of almost any degree to assure both me and the family that all that could be done has been done.

Figure 13–2 represents my approach to the evaluation of the child who presents in infancy with enlarged ventricles and evidence of hydrocephalus. According to this format, only one child who had attained a cerebral mantle of 3.5 cm by 5 months subsequently needed shunting. All children, with or without shunting, should be observed by follow-up for the first 2 years with CT scans at 12 and 24 months and by assessment of school performance as they age.

NONSURGICAL MEASURES

Once an objective measurement of cerebral mantle is defined as a treatment goal, alternative methods of attaining those goals can be assessed. The wrapping of the infant's distensible head with a compressive dressing was evaluated by Epstein and colleagues[15]; in certain patients, it was effective in reversing progressive hydrocephalus. The theory underlying head wrapping was that in cases of moderate infantile hydrocephalus, the infant cranium could enlarge at relatively low pressures. Head wrapping led to a closed intracranial cavity as if the skull were fully formed and therefore not distensible. Higher pressures could then be generated, with a concomitant increase in CSF absorption and stabilization of ventricular size.[15]

Other mechanical measures have been advocated to prevent the need for shunting or to prevent shunt dependency. The use of an on-off valve with the shunt in

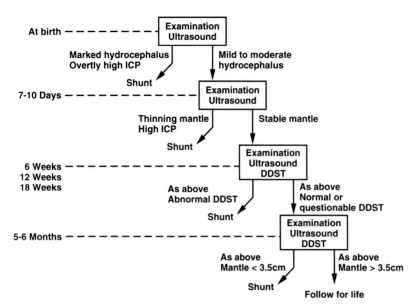

FIGURE 13–2. Algorithm for making treatment decisions in neonatal hydrocephalus (DDST = Denver Developmental Screening Test). (Modified from Rekate HL: To shunt or not to shunt. Clin Neurosurg 32:605, 1985.)

infants has been advocated to prevent shunt dependency. In the child with hydrocephalus, a shunt is placed with an on-off valve, and the shunt is opened to flow for only a short time each day. This technique may allow stabilization of head circumference and ventricular size and will avoid shunt dependency in certain cases.[16]

MANAGEMENT OF HYDROCEPHALUS SECONDARY TO NEONATAL INTRAVENTRICULAR HEMORRHAGE

In the special case of premature infants with hydrocephalus secondary to neonatal intraventricular hemorrhage, a number of nonsurgical measures have been employed that stabilize or improve ventricular size in critically low-birth-weight children. Various children subsequently need shunts, but some never require permanent shunts. For example, the use of intermittent lumbar punctures decreases ICP and helps to clear the CSF of toxic chemicals with the dissolution of the intraventricular hemorrhage.[17, 18] This procedure has been used in many premature neonates and has proved to be effective in preventing the need for shunting in some children. There are reports of resolution of hydrocephalus with this form of treatment alone, and there is one report of the resolution of progressive hydrocephalus after only one spinal tap.[18] This form of treatment does present some technical difficulties, however. To obtain adequate volumes of CSF to affect the intraventricular pressure and volume is often technically difficult. It requires prolonged periods of time with the spinal needle in place. These taps are usually done with the patient in an upright position, and for the duration of the tap, the infants are not in a closed Isolette. This poses a difficult dilemma for children who are on a respirator or are receiving high concentrations of oxygen. The amount of handling needed to perform such taps may be dangerous to these infants of fragile health

and could conceivably lead to an increased risk of further intraventricular hemorrhage. Although in some children intermittent spinal taps are effective in controlling hydrocephalus, great care must be used in selecting patients and performing these procedures.

Intermittent ventricular punctures serve a function similar to that of intermittent lumbar punctures. They can be performed in a shorter time and are more effective in removing large volumes of CSF. The risk of ventricular puncture in untreated hydrocephalus is the production of large porencephalic cysts ("needle porencephaly"). Because of this risk, the procedure has been abandoned as a prolonged temporizing measure.[19] The use of external ventricular drainage has a number of advantages in that large volumes of CSF can be removed under controlled circumstances. Except for the time of placement, the child may remain in the Isolette while CSF is withdrawn, and the drain can be used as an access to the ventricles for the purpose of removing toxic chemicals from the CSF by irrigation. The usefulness of external ventricular drainage is limited by the risk of infection, by highly viscous CSF, and by the propensity of the ventricular catheter to become encased in the blood clot. When employing this or any technique in which relatively large volumes of CSF are removed from small infants, the neurosurgeon and pediatrician must be constantly aware of the loss of volumes of CSF that are large relative to the circulating blood volume and contain ions and blood elements.[20] CSF should be replaced intravenously, cubic centimeter for cubic centimeter, with a fluid containing salt and electrolytes. Assessments of hemoglobin and albumin levels in peripheral blood should be performed routinely several times a week.

Manwaring and colleagues[21] have developed a technique called pulsed lumbar cisternostomy to manage children with hydrocephalus secondary to neonatal intraventricular hemorrhage. With a Touhy needle, polyethylene (PE) tubing is introduced into the spinal subarachnoid space (SSAS). Then, the PE tubing is connected to a special pump that applies a ''to and fro'' pulsation to the fluid in the tubing. Finally, a drainage bag is used, the height of which determines the pressure and flow characteristics of the system. The pulsations in the system effectively prevent blockage of the lumbar catheter and allow prolonged (weeks) treatment of the infants. The technique works well as a temporizing measure and prevents the need for shunting in some infants.

Several authors have advocated the use of a subcutaneous reservoir attached to a ventricular catheter. This technique allows the removal of large volumes of CSF on an intermittent basis. Because it is a closed system, it has a lower infection risk than does external ventricular drainage. As in other techniques mentioned in this section, ventricular size is assessed frequently using ultrasonography, by the amount of CSF withdrawn, and the frequency of its withdrawal (modified as needed). Using this technique, Marlin and colleagues reported that less than half the infants required eventual internal shunting. Some patients had subsequent stabilization of ventricular size, and a few died of other causes related to prematurity.[22, 23]

The use of a Broviac catheter with a long subcutaneous tunnel has recently been reported as a method for handling ventriculostomy.[24] This technique allows long-term drainage and potentially decreases the risk of infection. The procedure is performed in the operating room, and the catheter must be removed surgically. Side-to-side comparison of the safety and effectiveness of various techniques is not yet available.

One very exciting area of investigation involves the intraventricular instillation of agents that dissolve the intraventricular clot without damaging the brain or causing further bleeding. Pang and colleagues at the University of Pittsburgh have tested the efficiency of injecting urokinase intraventricularly in a canine model of intraventricular hemorrhage.[25–27] Urokinase was successful in accelerating clot lysis and preventing posthemorrhagic hydrocephalus, without any demonstrable effect on central nervous system tissue. A clinical trial in humans has been proposed by the researchers.[27] Kaufman,[28] in his comment on this work, points out that tissue plasminogen activator (Genentech, San Francisco, CA) may be superior to urokinase in this regard.

USE OF DRUGS TO CONTROL HYDROCEPHALUS

Many drugs that affect ICP and production of CSF have been used to treat hydrocephalus, with varying degrees of success. These drugs typically are categorized into two groups: (1) osmotic diuretics and (2) drugs that decrease CSF production at the choroid plexus level. Mannitol and urea, when administered intravenously, decrease ICP by removal of brain extracellular fluid, using an osmotic gradient with plasma. Since these drugs must be given intravenously, their use in the chronic management of hydrocephalus was not practical. Isosorbide is a dehydric alcohol derived from sorbitol that has been shown to lower effectively ICP in both laboratory animals and humans. The drug is effective when administered orally in doses of 2 to 3 gm per kg. However, the lowering of ICP is not associated with decreases in ventricular volume, since its mechanical function is to decrease brain extracellular fluid. Lorber reported gratifying results when using isosorbide in a large number of patients with myelomeningoceles, stating that the use of this drug obviated shunting in such children.[29] Other authors have not been able to duplicate his results from the use of this drug.[30] Isosorbide is not available in the United States for the treatment of hydrocephalus.

Approximately 50 per cent of CSF is produced by the choroid plexus in an energy-requiring process that is dependent on the enzyme carbonic anhydrase. The remainder of CSF production occurs as a result of bulk flow of CSF from brain extracellular fluid.[31] Acetazolamide, a potent inhibitor of carbonic anhydrase, has been shown to decrease CSF production by 49 per cent in rabbits[32] and 16 to 66 per cent in humans.[33] Several early reports of the use of acetazolamide showed the drug to be effective in up to one half of infants in whom it was tried.[33, 34] In one trial of 32 infants with myelomeningoceles, no effect could be seen with the drug.[35] Acetazolamide has proved to be effective as a temporizing measure in patients with transient CSF absorption defects and in patients with borderline shunt function.

In a study involving premature neonates with progressive hydrocephalus secondary to neonatal intraventricular hemorrhage, the combination of acetazolamide and furosemide was shown to be effective in preventing the need for shunting.[36] Furosemide is a diuretic that acts at the loop of Henle. The mechanism of decrease in ICP with this drug is unclear, but its action seems to be to decrease brain extracellular fluid. This combination seems a logical approach to the management of infantile hydrocephalus, but in my experience the treatment seems to involve the risk of severe dehydration of these fragile children. A multicentered study of this form of treatment seems indicated.

SURGICAL TREATMENT OF HYDROCEPHALUS

The modern era of the surgical treatment of hydrocephalus begins with the development of valve mechanisms for use in shunt systems.[37] For an excellent historical perspective on earlier management techniques in hydrocephalus, the reader is directed to the fine review article by Pudenz.[38] Only a brief view will be presented here. Whether shunts were from the ventricular or lumbar subarachnoid space to a variety of absorbing reservoirs, prior to the advent of valve-regulated shunting, they were largely unsuccessful for technical reasons. The lack of valves led to reflux of blood and coagulation, which resulted in blockage. Rapid overdrainage of massively enlarged ventricles led to fatal subdural hematomas. Finally, the materials available for implantation at that time characteristically excited an intense inflammatory response, which resulted in obstruction of the shunt systems. The lumboureteral shunt was the most effective form of treatment available prior to the early 1950s.[39] As originally conceived by Heile in 1927, the renal pelvis was sutured to the dura arachnoid.[38] Later, Matson performed a nephrectomy and inserted a piece of polyethylene tubing from the spinal subarachnoid space to the ureter.[39] Although the procedure was generally successful, a few patients experienced a profound hyponatremic dehydration resulting from CSF loss through the bladder.

In 1918, Dandy introduced the choroid plexectomy for the treatment of hydrocephalus, based on experiments performed by Blackfan and himself, which defined the choroid plexus as the site of CSF production.[40] Early experiences with this technique resulted in a high operative mortality. Later, this procedure was attempted by use of an endoscope with equivocal results.[41, 42] However, the procedure has been abandoned for the most part. It is now known that the choroid plexus is responsible for only one half of CSF production, and the beneficial results of choroid plexectomy usually were only temporary. Further, Milhorat has been able to show normal rates of CSF production 5 years after choroid plexectomy.[43, 44]

Procedures that bypassed the site of obstruction of CSF pathways were successful in a limited way, and some are employed today in specific situations. The earliest of these techniques involved fenestration of the ventricular system into the subarachnoid space, either at open surgery or using a ventriculoscopic technique.[45] Contemporary authors report encouraging results, using stereotactic techniques to create holes from the third ventricle to the cortical subarachnoid space (CSAS).[46-50] Sayers and Kosnick emphasized the need to demonstrate open subarachnoid pathways and intact absorptive mechanisms to ensure proper selection of patients.[51]

Advances in the development of endoscopes have led to a resurgence of interest in third ventriculostomy or ventriculocisternostomy as definitive treatment for hydrocephalus without shunting. The first report of this procedure was written by Vries, who in 1978 reported his experience with five patients, three of whom required subsequent shunting and two of whom had insufficient follow-up to determine its efficacy.[52] Jones and colleagues,[53] from Sydney, Australia, reported their results in 24 patients with hydrocephalus from different etiologies. In half the patients, shunts were removed, and in a third of the remaining patients, they were never inserted. Nonfunctional shunts were not revised. Therefore, two thirds of these patients are thought to have successful resolution of their hydrocephalus by treatment with endoscopic third ventriculostomy. They reported one patient with postoperative hemiplegia. In many of the patients who were treated successfully, the ventricles remained large. Whether large ventricles without overt intracranial hypertension indeed represent a ''success'' will require careful long-term follow-up of patients treated in this way, with supporting data from neuropsychologic assessment.

Ventriculocisternostomy, or the creation of a bypass channel between the lateral ventricle and the cisterna magna, was originally described by Torkildsen[54] and has been shown to be an effective procedure in patients with secondary obstructive hydrocephalus (e.g., from tumors). Enthusiasm for this procedure was dampened by the finding that it was not applicable in infantile hydrocephalus, presumably because of the lack of development of adequate absorptive mechanisms.[55]

TREATMENT OF HYDROCEPHALUS BY VALVE-REGULATED SHUNTS

A great majority of children with hydrocephalus are managed by valve-regulated shunting systems. All of these systems have common biologic and mechanical components, which will be discussed. All commercially available shunting systems are capable of managing hydrocephalus in most children.[56] Although some bias is unavoidable, I do not intend to advocate the use of one product over another. As experience with the idiosyncrasies of the individual systems is gained, the neurosurgeon becomes comfortable with one system and, except in specific circumstances, should abandon it only with great trepidation.

The Proximal Catheter

The first component of the shunting system is the proximal catheter. This plastic tube of multiple designs is placed within the CSF pathways proximal to the site of obstruction of CSF. Most commonly this means the placement of a catheter in the lateral ventricle. There is general agreement that it is technically advantageous to place the ventricular catheter anterior to the foramen of Monro to avoid the likelihood of having the holes in the catheter become occluded by the choroid plexus.[57, 58] A recent study of a large group of shunted children from Paris and Toronto concluded that the functioning of the ventricular catheter depended on the size of the ventricles and not on its relative position within the ventricular system. The authors concluded that the ventricular catheter should be placed where the ventricles are most enlarged.[59, 60]

There are two acceptable approaches to proper ventricular catheter placement in the frontal horn anterior to the foramen of Monro. These are (1) the placement of the ventricular catheter in the anterior horn of the lateral ventricle, by a parieto-occipital placement, and (2) the more direct approach through the frontal lobe at the area of the coronal sutures. Both procedures normally result in proper placement of the ventricular catheter in the frontal horn, anterior to the foramen of Monro.

With the anterior approach, the hole in the skull is made 3 cm lateral to the sagittal suture and just anterior or posterior to the coronal suture (Fig. 13–3). The catheter is directed perpendicular to the skull, aiming

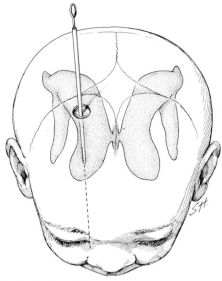

FIGURE 13–3. Anterior placement of ventricular catheter. (Courtesy of Barrow Neurological Institute.)

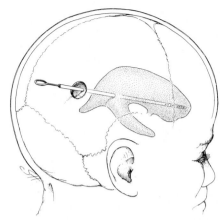

FIGURE 13–4. Posterior placement of ventricular catheter. (Courtesy of Barrow Neurological Institute.)

generally at the inner canthus of the ipsilateral eye unless the ventricular anatomy is distorted. In patients with small ventricles, particularly when replacing a ventricular catheter into a chronically shunted ventricle, it is often advantageous to drape the face (which is in a brow-up position), using sterile, transparent plastic so that these landmarks can be observed during the passage of the ventricular catheter. A tripod-shaped device has recently been introduced to make this pass easier. Conceptually, the device is logical, but I have had no experience with it.[61]

The anterior placement has an advantage in that the pass is a shorter distance through the brain and does not traverse eloquent areas of the brain. It is also more likely to lead to ventricular catheter placement in the proper position anterior to the choroid plexus. The disadvantage of the anterior placement relates to the distance the catheter must travel subgaleally. If this placement is used in infants, as the infant grows the external catheter under the scalp is fixed at each point by the dense adherence of scalp to periosteum. As the head grows, minimal or no sliding of this catheter is permitted, and a distracting force is slowly applied to the catheter end, often leading to disconnection or breakage of the catheter at points of stress. When used in the child older than 2 years of age or in adults, the rate of head growth is rarely fast enough to result in such problems.

Landmarks for the posterior approach to ventricular cannulation vary somewhat with the neurosurgeon and the purpose for which this approach was chosen. Positioning of patients and landmarks for the placement of ventricular catheters are strictly followed (Fig. 13–4). The patient is placed in a lateral decubitus position, with the hole 3 cm above and 3 cm behind the tip of the ear.[57] The catheter is aimed parallel to the sagittal suture in the direction of the ipsilateral eye. The length of the catheter should be approximately 1 cm longer than the distance from the hole to the coronal suture.

The advantage of this placement is that the catheter runs along the long axis of the ventricle, yielding a longer segment of the ventricular catheter containing drainage holes within the ventricular system itself (Fig. 13–5). It also has the advantage of the shorter subgaleal distance for the external tubing and therefore the smaller chance of disconnection. The disadvantage of this placement is the potential for harm to more eloquent areas of the brain, particularly the visual cortex. In infants, there is a selective dilation of the occipital horns of the lateral ventricles when the thickness of the brain in that location is less than 1 cm (Fig. 13–6). Ventricular catheter placement in the high parietal region traverses very little cortex.

At this time, the use of the anterior or posterior parietal approach should be considered a matter of personal preference. One retrospective study seemed to show a clear advantage to placement by the frontal approach.[62] Subsequently, there has been a prospective randomized study comparing anterior with posterior parietal placements, and no differences were noted in

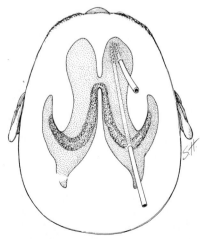

FIGURE 13–5. Relationship of ventricular catheters to Foramen of Monro and choroid plexus. (Courtesy of Barrow Neurological Institute.)

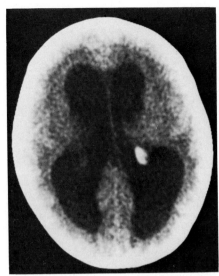

FIGURE 13–6. CT scan of infant with hydrocephalus, showing selective dilatation of occipital horns.

function, seizure frequency, or infection rates between the two appropriate approaches.[63]

A reservoir attached to the ventricular catheter is strongly recommended. Whether the neurosurgeon uses a separate reservoir (e.g., Rickham's reservoir) or one that is incorporated into the valve system is a matter of personal preference. The reservoir should allow the sampling of ventricular CSF and the measurement of intraventricular pressure.

In patients who have communicating hydrocephalus or, as Ransohoff and colleagues have described,[64] extraventricular obstructive hydrocephalus, the lumbar theca can be an excellent site of placement for the proximal catheter. The major advantage of this form of treatment is that it tends to maintain the integrity of the CSF pathways (e.g., will not lead to secondary obstruction of the aqueduct of Sylvius). Also, it does not lead to collapse of the ventricular wall around the catheter tip, resulting in obstruction. Although classically performed using a limited laminectomy and subarachnoid placement under direct vision, it is now possible to perform this procedure percutaneously using a Touhy needle.[65, 66] Reports of scoliosis and nerve root deficits in growing children have tended to result in a lesser use of this technique.[67]

Patients treated in infancy with lumboperitoneal shunts have a relatively high incidence of chronic tonsillar herniation (Chiari I malformation). It has been speculated that this results from cephalocranial disproportion.[65] Creation of a pressure gradient at the foramen magnum would also explain these findings. In some of these children, the development of syringomyelia or symptoms of brainstem compression have led to suboccipital decompression with success. The ability to perform lumboperitoneal shunts without the need to do a laminectomy in children over 2 years of age and the use of less irritating implantable materials (Silastic) make this procedure more attractive.

Testing the patency of lumboperitoneal shunts is difficult. If one attempts actually to follow the path of a radionuclide or radiopaque tracer through the shunt system, equivocal results are often obtained. If one remembers that for CSF to be absorbed by natural pathways it must ascend to the level of the sagittal sinus and that no absorption of CSF occurs at the level of the SSAS, a simple test of lumboperitoneal shunt potency can be derived. Radionuclide or radiopaque tracer introduced into the SSAS can be absorbed in one of two ways, either by normal absorptive pathways or via the shunt catheter. The peritoneal surface absorbs CSF quickly, but in the patient with partial obstruction of CSF pathways, CSF is slowly absorbed into the blood stream for clearance through the kidneys. If the shunt is patent, the tracer will be detectable in the bladder within one hour and could not have arrived there by natural pathways.

The Distal Catheter

In shunt systems, the distal catheter is a plastic tube that can be open on the end, can have a distal slit valve that adds a resistance element (to be discussed under valve systems), or can have holes in the sides to give multiple sites for release of CSF into the distal receptacle. The superiority of one form of tube over another has not been demonstrated. There remains some controversy as to the optimal receptacle for placement of the distal catheter. Since the development of Silastic materials, which do not usually incite walling off by the omentum, the peritoneal cavity has become the preferred site of distal catheters both for ventricular and lumbar shunt systems.[68, 69]

The Peritoneal Cavity. The peritoneum is an extremely efficient site of absorption of both fluids and drugs and, in many ways, is the ideal receptacle for the distal catheter of a shunt system. Attempts to use the peritoneum as a receptacle in the treatment of hydrocephalus date from Ferguson who in 1898 attempted to link the lumbar theca with the peritoneum using a silver wire.[70] Early ventriculoperitoneal (VP) shunts without valves led to overly rapid ventricular decompression, subdural hematoma, and death. The development of pressure-activated valve systems made the peritoneum a feasible receptacle for CSF diversion. However, valve-regulated VP shunts were unreliable because of a high incidence of distal obstruction resulting from the inflammatory response that they incited. Suprahepatic or intrapelvic placement was advocated, but the peritoneal placement was considered only a temporizing measure awaiting a permanent vascular placement.

With the development of Silastic tubing in 1968, the reliability of VP shunts increased greatly.[68, 69] VP shunts have two compelling advantages over vascular shunts and, at present, should be considered the shunt of choice in children. The performance of all shunts is associated with a risk of infection, with published incidences of 2 to 20 per cent per procedure.[71, 72] If a patient with a ventriculoatrial (VA) shunt develops an infection, there exists a potential for the life-threatening complications of septic endocarditis, septic pulmonary emboli, and immune complex glomerulonephritis. Conversely, infection in peritoneal shunts usually presents with distal obstruction from the local inflammatory process or may present as localized or generalized peritonitis, conditions that are rarely life-threatening.[73] The second major advantage of VP shunting has to do with the growth of the infant. VA shunts, to be reliable and safe, must be placed well proximal to the tricuspid valve and must extend at least into the large superior vena cava (usually at the level of the fourth thoracic vertebra).[57, 58] As the child grows, the distal catheter tends to pull out of this desired placement, and when it pulls into the jugular vein, the venous flow is often not great enough to prevent obstruction due to fibrosis at the end of the catheter. To maintain a working VA shunt usually requires several elective revisions with time. When the peritoneum is chosen, a nearly unlimited length of tubing can be placed within the peritoneal cavity that can uncoil as the child grows normally, resulting in fewer revisions during childhood. Figure 13–7 demonstrates the techniques available for the placement of the peritoneal catheter.

Occasionally, a child is found who will not tolerate peritoneal shunting, and an atrial or other distal receptacle will be required. There are three potential causes of this problem. The most common cause is unrecognized indolent infection of the shunt system. These cryptic infections may be due to anaerobic diphtheroids, the identification of which requires special culturing techniques and prolonged incubation.[74] The second cause is the chemical content of the CSF, which can be irritating to the peritoneal surface, particularly following intraventricular hemorrhage or with the extremely high protein levels seen in intraventricular tumors. Finally, some patients have a peritoneal surface that will not absorb CSF.

The Venous System. With the development of adequate valve systems, the right atrium became the preferred site of distal CSF diversion. Shunts inserted into the atrium were more reliable, and as long as they stayed, as seen radiographically, between T-7 and T-4, they remained patent for the most part.[58] Atrial shunts are a low-pressure system relative to intra-abdominal pressures, and because of the much shorter distance from the ventricle to the right atrium when the shunt is in the erect position, the effects of siphoning are minimized.

Maintaining VA shunts is often extremely difficult because of the limited number of points of access to the vascular tree. The first VA shunt placed into the right jugular vein, usually via the common facial vein, led to a direct path to the atrium with little difficulty. However, when this access point was not available, much difficulty in cannulating the right atrium was often encountered. With left jugular or subclavian cannulation, the tube tended to enter the right subclavian vein. Like-

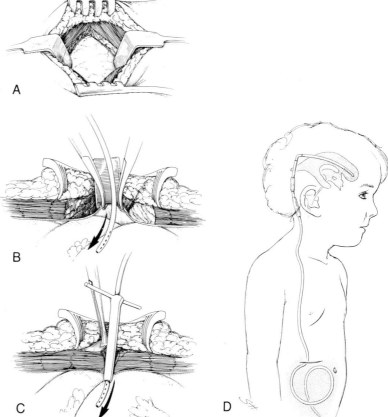
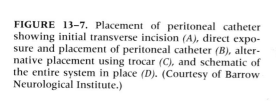

FIGURE 13–7. Placement of peritoneal catheter showing initial transverse incision *(A)*, direct exposure and placement of peritoneal catheter *(B)*, alternative placement using trocar *(C)*, and schematic of the entire system in place *(D)*. (Courtesy of Barrow Neurological Institute.)

wise, with right subclavian cannulation, the tubing tended to be directed to the left subclavian vein.

The difficulties of atrial cannulation could often be overcome by the use of fluoroscopy and Seldinger guide wires. Certain patients underwent right atrial cannulation by open thoracotomy, after multiple previous venous placements made cannulation difficult. Kaufman (Kaufman B, personal communication, 1977) developed a technique for placing right atrial catheters, using a transfemoral venous Seldinger technique. The catheter was passed through the right atrium into a vein in the neck, allowing the surgeon to palpate the wire in the neck, to prepare the area, and to cut down on the length of guide wire. The atrial catheter was placed over the guide wire and was drawn into the atrium. There it was disconnected with a quick tug, to remain in the proper position in the atrium, and then was connected to the rest of the shunt system in the neck (Fig. 13–8) (Kaufman B, personal communication, 1977).

The concept of siphoning and overdrainage of CSF is discussed in a later section on valve mechanisms. The natural CSF absorptive system involves the flow of CSF from the CSAS to the sagittal sinus across the arachnoid granulations. This process requires a pressure differential of 3 to 5 mm Hg between the CSF and the sagittal sinus. In contrast to valved shunts into the peritoneum or right atrium, the reference pressure for absorption remains constant in the normal individual regardless of the position of the body. Becker examined the sagittal sinus as a receptacle for CSF shunting and found that the sagittal sinus pressure was often greater than ventricular pressure.[75]

Theoretically, a ventriculosagittal sinus shunt would be ideal from a hydraulic perspective because of the constancy of the hydraulic relationship between the ventricles and sagittal sinus. El-Shafei and Hafez have developed a technique in which they perform a ventriculojugular shunt but direct the distal catheter cephalad toward the jugular bulb.[76] This technique approximates the normal physiologic situation closely as the ventricle and distal terminus of CSF absorption remain close together regardless of the patient's position. At this writing, El-Shafei has performed the procedure in 110 patients with a very low complication rate, excellent control of hydrocephalus, and no incidence of CSF overdrainage.

Other Sites of Distal Catheter Placement. Many sites for distal placement of shunt systems have been tried, with varying success. Most are used extremely rarely in contemporary practice. The use of the *stomach* and the *fallopian tube* has probably been abandoned altogether. The gallbladder continues to be used by various neurosurgeons when the difficulty in performing atrial shunts or the futility of performing peritoneal shunts justifies the risk of potential infection of the system.

The *pleural cavity* has been advocated for the treatment of hydrocephalus and does adequately absorb CSF in numerous patients.[77, 78] The length of time that the pleura retains its absorptive capacity varies from individual to individual. There have been cases in which the pleural cavity ceased to be an absorptive surface, and the patient presented with severe respiratory compromise with hydrothorax.

The *ureter* as a site of distal catheter placement is of special interest from a historical perspective. In 1925 Heile reported suturing of the renal pelvis to the lumbar subarachnoid space.[38] Matson,[39] who developed both lumbar and ventricular ureteral shunts, connected the CSF pathway to the ureter using PE tubing after performing a nephrectomy. As late as 1956, Matson considered ureterostomy to be the most reliable form of treatment for hydrocephalus. This procedure involved unique problems. CSF was released into the bladder and was irrevocably lost from the circulation.

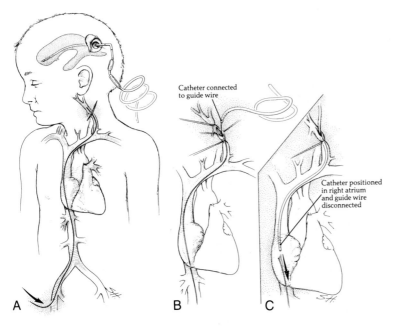

Catheter connected to guide wire

Catheter positioned in right atrium and guide wire disconnected

A   B   C

FIGURE 13–8. Performance of ventriculoatrial shunt revision using Seldinger's guidewire technique. (Courtesy of Barrow Neurological Institute.)

In certain instances in small children, this loss resulted in profound hyponatremic dehydration. It was also essential to prove that the ureterovesical junction was a competent valve that would prevent retrograde passage of urine and bacteria to the shunt system. Recently, ureterostomy has been modified by Smith and colleagues to preserve the kidney.[79] They perform a ureteroureterostomy in which both kidneys drain into one ureter, with the tubing being placed in the other ureter. This is an effective procedure in patients in whom it is difficult or unwise to place the catheter in the atrium or peritoneum, as in cases of chronic fungal meningitis or active neoplastic meningeal seeding.

THE VALVE SYSTEM

Although a few authors advocate the use of shunts without valves except in the specific case of posthemorrhagic hydrocephalus of premature infants, it was the development of the valve-regulated shunting systems that led to the expectation of successful treatment of hydrocephalus in the vast majority of cases.[37] Many different valve designs are marketed by nearly as many manufacturers, but they all share several important characteristics. The most important of these is that all valve systems marketed within the United States have been proved to control hydrocephalus successfully. This point is extremely important. The dogmatic stances taken by neurosurgeons that one system is always the best or that another does not adequately treat hydrocephalus are not justified by the available statistical information. Certain valve characteristics of opening or closing pressure or of valve resistance may or may not be more desirable in one or another clinical setting. The decision as to which valve system one should use depends to a great extent on the individual experiences of the neurosurgeon who does the implantation and who will perform patient follow-up.

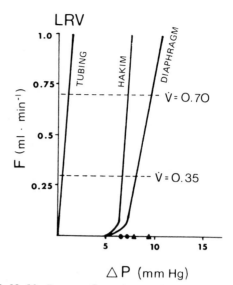

FIGURE 13–10. Pressure-flow characteristics of low-resistance shunts (i.e., Hakim and diaphragm valves). (From Portnoy HD: Treatment of hydrocephalus. *In* Pediatric Neurosurgery: Surgery of the Developing Nervous System. New York, Grune and Stratton, 1982, p 215.)

Minimal information is available relative to the rate of flow through shunts over a 24-hour period. Some evidence exists that there may be prolonged periods during the day when there is actually no, or extremely little, flow through shunt systems as well as other times when flow is extremely rapid.[80]

The resistance element in the shunt can be extremely simple (such as the inherent resistances to flow in a small-lumen tube or a distal slit-valve) or very complicated. Portnoy has divided shunt systems, according to their resistance-to-flow characteristics, into two categories, which he terms "high-pressure" shunts and "low-pressure" shunts.[81, 82] By "high-pressure" (high-resistance) shunts, he means that as the differential pressure across the valve decreases, the rate of flow becomes slower and slower (Fig. 13–9). These valves are mostly of the slit-valve type (Holter, Holter-Hausner, distal slit-valve). The low-pressure (low-resistance) valve shows a very low resistance to flow until the closing pressure of the valve is reached, at which time it stops flow abruptly (Fig. 13–10). All diaphragm valves (Pudenz, Pudenz-Shulte, LPV) are in this category, as well as the spring-loaded ball in a cup (Hakim).[81, 82] Both high-pressure and low-pressure shunt valves respond to differential pressures across the valve's resistance element and therefore are subject to the effects of siphoning. Siphoning occurs when fluid at one end of a closed system is higher than at the other end; therefore, gravity causes a pressure differential that would not be seen with the patient in a recumbent position (Fig. 13–11). This phenomenon can lead to ICPs in shunted patients that are markedly negative with respect to atmospheric pressure and possibly can collapse the ventricular system.[83, 84] In patients who are symptomatic from low ICP, the use of a valve system containing an antisiphon device often reverses

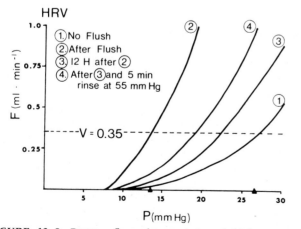

FIGURE 13–9. Pressure-flow characteristics of high-resistance shunts (i.e., slit valves). (From Portnoy HD: Treatment of hydrocephalus. *In* Pediatric Neurosurgery: Surgery of the Developing Nervous System. New York, Grune and Stratton, 1982, p 216.)

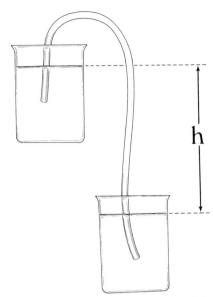

FIGURE 13–11. Representation of the concept of siphoning as it relates to CSF shunts. When a column of water is in an enclosed space, the hydrostatic pressure driving fluid flow is dependent only on the distances between the upper and lower reservoirs and not on the course that the fluid takes. In this equation, the driving pressure equals height times the mass of CSF times the acceleration of gravity. (Courtesy of Barrow Neurological Institute.)

the symptoms.[85] For mechanical reasons, Portnoy and associates recommend that antisiphon devices be used only with low-pressure shunt systems.[86]

At this writing, four devices marketed in the United States specifically address the problem of siphoning. The original antisiphon device, as developed by Portnoy and marketed by Baxter-V. Meuller (Chicago), is placed subcutaneously under freely movable skin. When the pressure inside the device is lower than atmospheric pressure, a diaphragm distorts and closes the mechanism to flow until the pressure inside the device is again positive.[87] Because it depends on an atmospheric pressure reference, scarring over the diaphragm may render it nonfunctional or may occlude it.[88]

The siphon control device marketed by P.S. Medical Corporation (Goleta, CA) works on a principle similar to that of the antisiphon device, except that it has two diaphragms that are normally closed (no flow). Upstream pressure forces the diaphragm to distend, allowing flow. The antisiphon and the siphon control devices differ in one important aspect that involves matching the upstream valve mechanism. The antisiphon device does not change the opening or closing pressure of the valve to which it is linked. In contrast, the siphon control device does have an intrinsic resistance yielding about a 30-mm H_2O increase in resistance. This has the effect of changing a low-pressure valve into a medium-pressure valve.

The Delta valve, also developed and marketed by P.S. Medical Corporation, incorporates a specially designed smaller version of the siphon control device with a diaphragm valve of the LPV type. This device comes in a performance level I (low pressure and siphon control device) and performance level II (medium pressure and siphon control device).

Sainte-Rose and colleagues have taken a novel approach to the overdrainage problem with the development of the Orbis-Sigma valve (Cordis Corp., Miami, FL).[59, 60] This device acts as a flow restrictor. Over a wide range of differential pressures between 80 and 350 mm H_2O, the flow through the valve remains constant between 20 and 30 ml per hour to (0.3 to 0.5 ml/min), approximating CSF production rates. At pressures higher than 350 mm H_2O, the valve opens to allow rapid egress of CSF.

Devices containing elements that retard siphoning or overdrainage are gaining popularity. At present, large series that compare the results of these devices relative to standard shunt devices or each other are not available.

Finally, two-valve systems have been developed that can be programmed externally to change the resistance characteristics in response to clinical or radiographic clues. These valves have magnetic devices that can allow the change from one setting to another without surgical intervention. At this writing, neither of these systems is marketed in the United States, and long-term efficacy studies are unavailable. These designs potentially offer significant benefit to patients when pressure needs to be controlled within a narrow range. Theoretically, they could also assist in preventing shunt dependency.[89, 90]

MANAGEMENT OF COMPARTMENTALIZED HYDROCEPHALUS

Often, neurosurgeons dealing with a large hydrocephalic population are confronted by shunt surgery complicated by the presence of CSF compartments that may or may not be drained by a ventricular shunting procedure. Managing these conditions is controversial. Each form of compartmentalization will be discussed separately.

THE DANDY-WALKER MALFORMATION

The Dandy-Walker malformation is a term used to describe several abnormalities of brain development that have posterior fossa cysts, hypoplasia of the cerebellar vermis, and hydrocephalus in common.[91, 92] The condition is associated with multiple other anomalies including agenesis of the corpus callosum, cleft palate, eye abnormalities, and subnormal intelligence in a significant percentage.[92] That this syndrome is not uniform pathologically is emphasized by the work of Entzian and colleagues,[93] who demonstrated two pathologically distinct cysts: one simply lined with ependyma and presenting after the perinatal period, and one that they thought represented a porencephaly of the cerebellar vermis presenting at or near delivery.

Therapy for this condition remains controversial. Direct surgical attack, as advocated by Matson, has been abandoned by contemporary authors as dangerous and futile.[92, 94–97] Carmel and colleagues point to the fact that free communication between the supratentorial ventricular system and the cyst can usually be demonstrated.[94] They advocate the shunting of lateral ventricles only. However, they do emphasize the potential change in the communicating nature of the cyst-ventricle relationship and recommend combined shunting of the cyst and the ventricle when free communication cannot be demonstrated.[94] In Hirsch's series of 25 patients treated primarily by shunting, 12 had VP shunts, and 13 had cyst-peritoneal shunts. One of his patients with a ventricular shunt subsequently required incorporation of the cyst into the system.[92] Bindal and colleagues reported their experience with the treatment of 50 patients with the Dandy-Walker syndrome.[98] Nine of their patients did not require a shunt, and 38 per cent of the patients who were initially shunted by a single-compartment shunt later required incorporation of the second compartment.

From the foregoing discussion, it follows that in the majority of cases the ventricles communicate with the cyst of the posterior fossa; therefore, shunting of either compartment is often successful. Raimondi,[96] Carmel,[94] Bindal,[98] and their co-workers have demonstrated that although communication can be shown early in the course, it does not necessarily remain patent throughout life. If mono-compartment shunting is selected, diligence must be maintained, or late deterioration will result from late ventricular isolation. Shunting of the lateral ventricles has resulted in upward herniation and prolonged apneic spells in a few patients.[96] In James' series, all six patients who were initially treated by only shunting the lateral ventricles subsequently required posterior fossa shunting.[97]

Because the incidence of late noncommunication between the supratentorial and infratentorial compartments is difficult to discern and because of the theoretical benefit of ensuring that a pressure gradient does not exist across the tentorial ring, I suggest that ventricular catheters be placed into the lateral ventricle and the posterior fossa cyst and that the tubing be spliced together proximal to the valve. On one occasion when such a procedure was attempted, the two leaves of the dura were found to be separated in multiple areas by a venous sinus of the entire posterior fossa. It was not possible to place a posterior fossa shunt. In this case, simply shunting the ventricle produced an excellent clinical outcome.

THE ISOLATED FOURTH VENTRICLE

Since the advent of CT scanning, the area of the posterior fossa has become easily visualized. Unexpectedly, dilatation of the fourth ventricle in chronically shunted patients (difficult to diagnose before CT scanning) is being recognized with increasing frequency. Foltz and Shurtleff recognized early the possibility that communicating hydrocephalus could be converted to aqueductal stenosis if the distending force (i.e., hydrocephalus) was removed by shunting, particularly with an inflammatory condition such as infection or hemorrhage.[87] Isolation of the fourth ventricle occurs under these circumstances. The sequence is described in Figure 13–12. Foltz and associates apparently recognized this condition in the era preceding CT scanning and

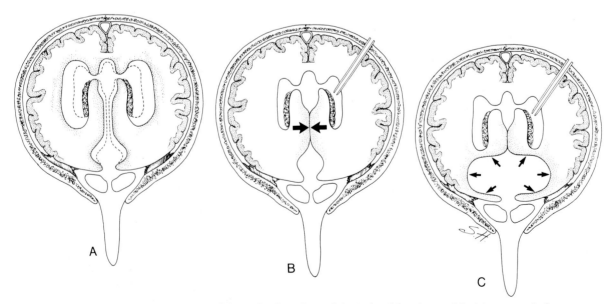

FIGURE 13–12. Representation of the pathophysiology of the isolated fourth ventricle (*A*) panventricular hydrocephalus with dilatation of the aqueduct of Sylvius and blockage of the basal cisterns (*B*). The shunting of the lateral ventricles leads to collapse of the aqueduct of Sylvius, which, with time, becomes irreversible (*C*). Since CSF is still being produced within the fourth ventricle and cannot be drained from above or below, it causes progressive dilatation of the fourth ventricle. (Courtesy of Barrow Neurological Institute.)

treated it by performing a Torkildsen shunt with a lateral ventricle shunt.[87, 99] In this situation, the original level of obstruction is at the basal meninges, theoretically creating a block to CSF passage between the SSAS and the CSAS. Alternatively, the blockage may occur at the level of the outlet foramina of the fourth ventricle. After shunting, the pressure distending the aqueduct of Sylvius is removed. The aqueduct, which has the form of a collapsible tube, then chronically assumes its collapsed position, with the walls abutting. Chronic apposition of these ependymally lined surfaces can lead to a scar that will eventually cause permanent stenosis of the aqueduct. During this time, CSF is still being produced within the fourth ventricle, which contains choroid plexus. Now that the aqueduct is closed, the CSF cannot be removed by flow through the shunt and is still obstructed from its normal absorption pathways, either by obstruction of the outlet foramina of the fourth ventricle or by a block of flow at the area of the basal cisterns. Pressure increases in the fourth ventricle are followed by distention of this compartment.

Signs and symptoms related to fourth ventricular or double-compartment hydrocephalus have been reported to include headache, ataxia, coma, cranial nerve palsies, anorexia, and vomiting.[99–105] In the course of routine surveillance of shunted hydrocephalic patients, dilatation of the fourth ventricle is occasionally found in patients without overt symptoms referable to posterior fossa mass lesions. In some of these, isolated fourth ventricular hydrocephalus leads to behavioral disturbances, short attention span, and deterioration in school performance. Such signs are difficult to interpret, but dramatic improvement in behavior and school performance may result from treating this condition.

It should be pointed out that the etiology of the hydrocephalus or subsequent complications of treatment play a significant role in the pathogenesis of the isolated fourth ventricle. The majority of patients reported to have this condition have had postmeningitic hydrocephalus or have suffered from multiple shunt infections.[99, 100, 102, 103] This condition seems to be frequently associated with fungal meningitis.[99, 101] This condition can also be encountered in patients whose hydrocephalus is a result of tumorous obstruction of CSF outflow, which in my experience includes one case of CSF seeding from medulloblastoma, one case of CSF obstruction at multiple sites in neurofibromatosis, and one case of subependymoma with blockage of the outlet foramina of the fourth ventricle.[106]

The treatment of this condition is controversial and often difficult. Foltz and Shurtleff[87] seem to advocate a direct surgical attack on the site of obstruction if it can be determined that this obstruction has a veil-like quality. Most authors recommend cannulating the cystlike fourth ventricle, usually creating a splice into the existing shunt system.[100–103] Cannulation of the fourth ventricle may be difficult, requiring multiple passes. Estimating the required length of the ventricular catheter may also be difficult. For this reason, I recommend placing the ventricular catheter under CT scan control. In my experience, it is best to trephine the posterior

fossa and incorporate the shunting system into the existing shunt in the operating room and to close the incisions not directly over the trephine. The patient is then transferred to the CT scanner, where the length and trajectory of the ventricular catheter can be accurately assessed (Fig. 13–13). Then, the wound is copiously irrigated with antibiotic solution and is closed. This allows accurate placement with minimum CT scan time and gives access to operating room equipment (for hemostasis) for the majority of the operative procedure.

Cannulation of the fourth ventricle is not without risk. The author has had two patients who had cannulation of a fourth ventricular cyst, in whom the catheter was found to be in an appropriate location postoperatively. These patients were asymptomatic at the time. Days to weeks later, one patient returned with a fifth nerve palsy, and the other had a seventh nerve palsy with some ataxia. Follow-up CT scans showed that as the fourth ventricle returned to its normal size, the ventricular catheter came to lie on the floor of the fourth ventricle, in the area of the appropriate cranial nerve nuclei (Fig. 13–14). Use of CT scan control may minimize the possibility of this complication.

If the site of obstruction is from the SSAS to the CSAS rather than involving the outlet foramina of the fourth ventricle, the risks and difficulties just described can be avoided by use of a lumboperitoneal shunt. Before performing such a procedure, it is essential to prove that the fourth ventricle is in communication with the lumbar theca. This is best accomplished by injecting iodinated contrast material into the lumbar thecal sac and tipping the head down to roll the dye into the posterior fossa. If the fourth ventricle fills with contrast material the patient is considered a candidate for the much easier and safer percutaneous lumboperitoneal shunt.[66, 107]

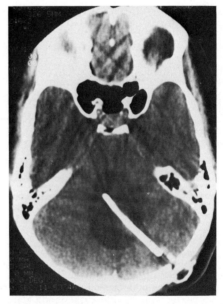

FIGURE 13–13. CT scan of the placement of a catheter in the fourth ventricle.

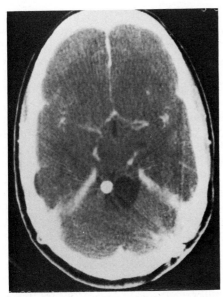

FIGURE 13–14. Catheter in the fourth ventricle. As the fourth ventricle became smaller, it came to lie within the brainstem, at the area of the cerebellar peduncle.

SUPRATENTORIAL CSF CYSTS

Intraventricular and other supratentorial cysts represent a broad spectrum of disease, and for the most part, their diagnosis and management lie outside this discussion. However, if they are seen in the context of hydrocephalus or as a complication of its treatment, three options are available to the neurosurgeon: (1) direct attack, with removal or fenestration into the ventricle; (2) cannulation of the cystic structure and incorporation of the new cyst shunt into the existing or newly placed ventricular shunt; or (3) endoscopic fenestration of the cyst with or without incorporation of the shunt system.[108–110] These cysts can be developmental, or they can result from the lifting off of ependymal surface from the ventricular wall as a result of infection.[111]

Occasionally, these cysts have firm capsules and tend to resist cannulation. The ventricular catheters may actually bounce off the cyst wall and fail to drain its contents. In this situation, these problems can be avoided by use of a ventriculoscope with fenestration under direct vision. Usually, the hole can be made simply by passing the ventriculoscope through the cyst wall. When the opening is not large enough, it has a tendency to reseal. It is essential to make the hole large enough to allow free flow of CSF among the various compartments. These can be made by means of direct puncture, electrocautery, a "saline torch,"[108] endoscopically linked laser system, or Fogarty catheter techniques. Figure 13–15 is the MRI of a child with posthemorrhagic hydrocephalus complicated by meningitis. The child has a large cyst at the level of the posterior third ventricle, leading to tonic deviation of her eyes in a downward position. Figure 13–16 shows the scan after endoscopic fenestration of the cyst into the ventricular system with placement of a left-sided VP shunt.

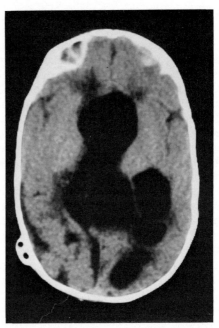

FIGURE 13–15. Magnetic resonance image of the brain in a premature neonate with posthemorrhagic hydrocephalus complicated by meningitis. The study shows an isolated cyst in the region of the posterior third ventricle.

In general, with the development of ventriculoscopic techniques, the management of loculated ventricles, or intraventricular cysts with hydrocephalus, I advocate ventriculoscopic inspection with attempts to fenestrate the cyst wall or septum pellucidum, leaving a single shunt behind.[109, 110] If this approach is unsuccessful, a second ventricular shunt joined to the existing shunt system proximal to the valve may be necessary.

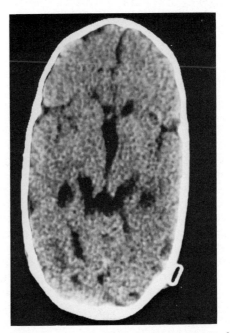

FIGURE 13–16. CT scan of the patient in Figure 13–15 after endoscopic fenestrations of the cyst wall and shunt revision.

MANAGEMENT OF HYDROCEPHALUS IN UTERO

Neurosurgeons are being called upon with progressively increasing frequency to render opinions on the treatment options available for the management of hydrocephalus that is diagnosed in the preterm infant. Assuming the mother has not elected to terminate the pregnancy or the fetus is near viability, most fetuses diagnosed with hydrocephalus have only moderate or slowly progressive hydrocephalus. These fetuses should be followed by serial ultrasonography examinations and delivered at term or after amniocentesis reveals the presence of sufficient lung maturity to ensure a reasonably smooth postnatal course if delivered early. As stated, even severe hydrocephalus treated within a few months of development will lead to the resolution of the ventriculomegaly and a good neurologic outcome in most patients.[6]

There have been reports of severe and rapidly progressive in utero hydrocephalus treated with percutaneous placement of a ventriculoamniotic shunt.[112, 113] Before this type of intervention is performed, a thorough diagnostic work-up is essential to exclude congenital anomalies and chromosomal disorders that would make the treatment of hydrocephalus futile.[114] The complication rate with percutaneous ventriculoamniotic shunts with dislodgment and inciting labor have limited enthusiasm for the use of these techniques.[105]

Open surgical approaches to in utero treatment of complex congenital anomalies is being pursued in laboratory animals. In these experiments, mothers are anesthetized and given hormonal treatment to prevent the onset of labor. The uterus is opened and a ventriculopleural or VA shunt is placed in hydrocephalic lambs and Rhesus monkeys. The uterus is then closed and the fetus is carried to term. The initial results of these studies have been encouraging, but more research is needed.[113, 115]

WHO CAN DO WITHOUT A SHUNT?

A discussion of the treatment of a disease process must always contain an evaluation of when such treatment may be discontinued. In a child or adult who is shunt-dependent, treatment must be continued throughout the life of the patient. Neurosurgical assessment of the child or adult to document the physical integrity of the shunt system should be performed at least once a year. The continuing higher cognitive functioning of the patient and the patient's neurologic functioning also should be assessed on at least a yearly basis. If a change occurs, the patient should be reassessed with CT scanning or MRI to determine ventricular size. Known shunt-dependent patients must have shunts repaired even if they do not have overt evidence of increased ICP. Within this category are shunts found to be disconnected or to be too short in the abdomen or jugular vein on x-ray film. The essential part of this discussion is who is and who is not dependent on shunting for life. An alternative way of stating this is who can do without a shunt?

The presence of a shunt, to some extent, creates a dependence on the shunt system. Flow of CSF is preferentially directed into the shunt system rather than through the partially obstructed and intrinsically higher-resistance natural pathways for CSF absorption. Abnormally low intraventricular pressures intrinsic to almost all shunt systems in the erect position may lead to collapse of the ventricular system, to the extent that the walls of the ventricles may collapse completely. When this occurs at the level of the aqueduct of Sylvius, a secondary aqueductal stenosis may occur that converts communicating (extraventricular obstructive) hydrocephalus to noncommunicating (intraventricular obstructive) hydrocephalus.[87] Especially in the presence of an inflammatory response, this process may be irreversible, and all chance for shunt independence is lost.

Hydrocephalus is "arrested" when the natural pathways of CSF absorption have been re-established, ICP has returned to normal, and ventricular volume has stabilized. This term implies that the patient is not being harmed by the process and would not be helped by the repair of a shunt or the placement of a new shunt. Hydrocephalus is "compensated" when ventricles have ceased to enlarge, and there are no overt signs of increased ICP. This term implies that, in subtle ways, the patient is being harmed by the condition and that intellectual, psychologic, or motor function would somehow be improved by the placement of a shunt.[116] Making this distinction is frequently difficult, but it is essential to the proper management of patients with hydrocephalus.[56] Views on this subject range from that of Foltz[117] and Hemmer,[118] who believe "Once a shunt—always a shunt," to that of Holzer and De-Lange,[119] who believe that shunt independence can be obtained in all forms of hydrocephalus.

Some guidelines are useful in making treatment decisions. Although this discussion is not intended to lead to decisions to remove shunts, neurosurgeons are frequently faced either with patients whose shunts are not working or with pediatric patients who have shunts that are barely functioning and who do not have signs of ICP. VA shunts have pulled into the jugular vein above the T-4 level. VP shunts have become disconnected or have been pulled up along the anterior chest wall. In these situations, the shunts either are not functioning or will soon be nonfunctioning, and a decision whether to fix the shunt must be made. The first decision to be made is the following: "Is this shunt functioning?" If, on CT scan or MRI, the ventricles are normal-sized or smaller than normal, the shunt is performing well.[56, 116] Hydrocephalus becomes arrested or compensated only when the ventricles are at least normal-sized and usually when they are larger than normal. Disconnected shunts may continue to function through fibrous tracts around the shunt. For the most part, a tenuously functioning shunt should be repaired.

If the ventricles are larger than normal, the shunt may not be adequate, and the next decision depends on the level of functioning of the patient. If there are any signs or symptoms of increased ICP, such as morning headaches, the shunt should be repaired. If there are any signs of decreases in higher cognitive functioning, the shunt should be repaired. Frequently, these problems are subtle and difficult to assess. Formal neuropsychologic evaluation may be necessary. A decrease in attention span or an increase in temper may indicate that the hydrocephalus is compensated rather than arrested. When there are emotional difficulties or poor school performance, it may be impossible to discern whether it is due to the hydrocephalus. Therefore, it may be necessary to re-establish the shunt to ensure possible benefit from its functioning. A common guideline is—"When in doubt, shunt."

The final step in determining whether it is essential to re-establish a shunt that may be malfunctioning is to determine the etiology of the hydrocephalus. Patients with noncommunicating hydrocephalus are extremely unlikely to have arrested hydrocephalus unless alternative pathways for CSF absorption are formed. Therefore, patients with aqueductal stenosis should be considered shunt-dependent for life unless a third ventriculostomy has been performed.

With few exceptions, children born with myelomeningoceles have the Arnold-Chiari malformation. In this anomaly, the posterior fossa is extremely small, and most of the medulla oblongata lies in the cervical canal and not in the posterior fossa. Syringomyelia is common in these children, and it seems that compensation for hydrocephalus occurs at the expense of dilatation of the central canal of the spinal cord. In this condition, syringomyelia can lead to weakness of shoulder and hand musculature as well as progressive scoliosis without overt signs of increased ICP.[120]

In a review of the concept of shunt independence from Case Western Reserve University in Cleveland, Ohio, four patients who had documented nonfunctioning shunts and spina bifida suffered respiratory arrest between 24 hours and 5 years after the shunt had been proved nonfunctional or removed for infection. Two of these patients died, and two suffered severe motor and intellectual downgrading. These patients were apparently asymptomatic before the incident.[121] Reigel presented a series of patients, the majority of whom had the Arnold-Chiari malformation, with massive ventriculomegaly and no overt signs of increased ICP.[122] Shunt repair led to rapid reconstitution of cerebral mantle and improvement in intellectual performance. Deterioration from hydrocephalus in the Arnold-Chiari malformation may be insidious, and generally, once children receive shunts for hydrocephalus with the Arnold-Chiari malformation, they should be considered shunt-dependent for life.

Communicating hydrocephalus resulting from obstruction of CSF flow from the SSAS through the CSAS to the sagittal sinus is not an "all-or-none" phenomenon, and when the cause (infection or hemorrhage) resolves, the increased resistance to CSF flow often resolves as well. It is in these patients that nonsurgical measures are often successful in preventing the need

for shunting in the first place. It is also these patients who have the potential to develop shunt independence. In the Case Western Reserve University study, 50 per cent of children with documented communicating hydrocephalus who were tested for shunt independence were found to have the capacity to be shunt-independent. This represented 25 per cent of cases in the series with this etiology. Long-term assessment of intellectual and neurologic performance failed to show any evidence of potential for late deterioration. In children with documented (by a form of dye study) communicating hydrocephalus, shunt independence is a realistic and valuable goal. If they have mild ventricular enlargement, stable intellectual functioning, and no new severe emotional disturbances, continued observation without shunt repair is indicated.[121]

SUMMARY: GOALS IN THE TREATMENT OF HYDROCEPHALUS

Although each child who presents to the neurosurgeon must be assessed as an individual, based on the previous discussion, it is possible to define a series of goals, some obvious and some subtle, that should link the treatment plans of most if not all patients. These goals include the following:

1. Decrease ICP to at least safe, if not normal, values.
2. Increase the volume of brain tissue (at least 3.5 cm of cortical mantle) to maximize the child's potential for intellectual, emotional, and motor development.
3. Minimize the frequency and severity of crises of ICP.
4. Minimize the likelihood of complications of treatment.
5. Maintain the integrity of CSF pathways, to prevent ventricular coaptation and to maximize the potential for life without shunt dependency.

Of these goals, the first two are met by most, if not all, shunt systems that are currently available. Failures are probably due to lack of careful follow-up of shunt function. Children who have been treated with or without shunting should be followed at 3-month intervals, at least, for the first year, with examinations including head-circumference measurements and ventricular-size determinations (ultrasound, CT, or MRI) when indicated, to make certain that the shunt performs as intended.

Goals 3 and 4 are outside the scope of this chapter and are discussed elsewhere in this volume.

Goal 5 is the most controversial. It has been claimed that collapsed or coapted ventricles should be an acceptable goal of shunting (Fried A, Walker M, personal communication, 1989).[123] In growing children, all shunt systems currently existing have been associated with the "slit-ventricle syndrome" or proximal shunt failure from ventricular collapse. Several authors have been successful in treating this condition by simply increasing valve resistance, whereas others have advocated subtemporal decompression.[124] In the series by Hyde-Rowan and colleagues,[85] the use of high-resistance valves with an antisiphon device has been shown to be effective in re-expanding previously collapsed ventricles, in preventing ventricular coaptation, and in treating the symptomatic slit-ventricle syndrome (small ventricles on CT, intermittent severe headaches lasting 10 to 90 minutes, and extreme slowness of valve refill).[85, 125]

To avoid these complications, which frequently interjfere with the lives of shunt-dependent children, requires hardware development, in the form of a variable-resistance or a variable-flow valve, or the performance of procedures that more closely mimic the natural state of ventricular-volume regulation. Examples are the performance of jugular shunts against the direction of flow, as advocated by El Shafei and Hafez,[76] or ventricular sagittal sinus shunts.[126] This is the technologic challenge remaining in the treatment of hydrocephalus.[89]

REFERENCES

1. Rekate HL: To shunt or not to shunt: Hydrocephalus and dysraphism. Clin Neurosurg 32:593, 1985.
2. McLone DG: Effect of complications on intellectual function in 173 children with myelomeningocele. (Abstract) Childs Brain 5:A561, 1979.
3. McLone DG, Czyzewski D, Raimondi AJ, et al.: Central nervous system infections as a limiting factor in the intelligence of children with myelomeningocele. Pediatrics 70:338, 1982.
4. Mapstone TB, Rekate HL, Nulsen FE, et al.: The relationship of CSF shunting and IQ in children with myelomeningocele: A retrospective analysis. Childs Brain 11:112, 1984.
5. Lewin R: Is your brain really necessary? Science 210:1232, 1980.
6. Young HF, Nulsen FE, Weiss MH, et al.: The relationship of intelligence and cerebral mantle in treated infantile hydrocephalus. IQ potential in hydrocephalic children. Pediatrics 52:38, 1973.
7. Foltz EL, Shurtleff DB: Five-year comparative study of hydrocephalus in children with and without operation (113) cases. J Neurosurg 20:1064, 1963.
8. Badell-Ribera A, Shulman K, Paddock N: The relationship of nonprogressive hydrocephalus to intellectual functioning in children with spina bifida cystica. Pediatrics 37:787, 1966.
9. Laurence KM: Neurological and intellectual sequelae of hydrocephalus. Arch Neurol 20:73, 1969.
10. Wills KE, Holmbeck GN, Dillon K, et al.: Intelligence and achievement in children with myelomeningocele. J Pediatr Psychol 15:161, 1990.
11. Miyazawa T, Sato K: Learning disability and impairment of synaptogenesis in HTX-rats with arrested shunt-dependent hydrocephalus. Childs Nerv Syst 7:121, 1991.
12. McAllister JP III, Cohen MI, O'Mara KA, et al.: Progression of experimental infantile hydrocephalus and effects of ventriculoperitoneal shunts: An analysis correlating magnetic resonance imaging with gross morphology. Neurosurgery 29:329, 1991.
13. Glascoe FP, Byrne KE, Ashford LG, et al.: Accuracy of the Denver-II in developmental screening. Pediatrics 89:1221, 1992.
14. Garrity L, Servos AB: Comparison of measures of adaptive behavior in preschool children. J Consult Clin Psychol 46:228, 1978.
15. Epstein F, Hochwald G, Ransohoff J: Neonatal hydrocephalus treated by compressive head wrapping. Lancet i:634, 1973.
16. Epstein FJ, Hochwald GM, Wald A, et al.: Avoidance of shunt dependency in hydrocephalus. Dev Med Child Neurol 17(535): (Suppl 135):71, 1975.

17. Goldstein GW, Chaplin ER, Maitland J, et al.: Transient hydrocephalus in premature infants: Treatment by lumbar punctures. Lancet i:512, 1976.
18. Blumenthal I, MacMillan M, Costalos C: Lumbar puncture in transient hydrocephalus. (Letter) Lancet i:756, 1976.
19. Salmon JH: Puncture porencephaly: Pathogenesis and prevention. J Dis Child 114:72, 1967.
20. Mori K, Raimondi AJ: An analysis of external ventricular drainage as a treatment for infected shunts. Child's Brain 1:243, 1975.
21. Manwaring KH, Pittman HW, Tarby TJ, et al.: New techniques in the investigation and management of post-hemorrhagic hydrocephalus. Barrow Neurological Institute Quarterly 1:24, 1985.
22. Marlin AE: Protection of the cortical mantle in premature infants with posthemorrhagic hydrocephalus. Neurosurgery 7:464, 1980.
23. McComb JG, Ramos AD, Platzker AC, et al.: Management of hydrocephalus secondary to intraventricular hemorrhage in the preterm infant with a subcutaneous ventricular catheter reservoir. Neurosurgery 13:295, 1983.
24. Chaparro MJ, Pritz MB, Yonemura KS: Broviac ventriculostomy for long-term external ventricular drainage. Pediatr Neurosurg 17:208, 1991–92.
25. Pang D, Sclabassi RR, Horton JA: Lysis of intraventricular blood clot with urokinase in a canine model. Part 1. Canine intraventricular blood cast model. Neurosurgery 19:540, 1986.
26. Pang D, Sclabassi R, Horton JA: Lysis of intraventricular blood clot with urokinase in a canine model. Part 2. In vivo safety study of intraventricular urokinase. Neurosurgery 19:547, 1986.
27. Pang D, Sclabassi R, Horton JA: Lysis of intraventricular blood clot with urokinase in a canine model. Part 3. Effects of intraventricular urokinase on clot lysis and posthemorrhagic hydrocephalus. Neurosurgery 19:553, 1986.
28. Kaufman HH: Comments. Neurosurgery 19:572, 1986.
29. Lorber J: Isosorbide in the medical treatment of infantile hydrocephalus. J Neurosurg 39:702, 1973.
30. Hayden PW, Foltz EL, Shurtleff DB: Effect of an oral osmotic agent on ventricular fluid pressure of hydrocephalic children. Pediatrics 41:955, 1968.
31. Milhorat TH, Hammock MK, Fenstermacher JD, et al.: Cerebrospinal fluid production by the choroid plexus and brain. Science 173:330, 1971.
32. Pollay M, Davson H: The passage of certain substances out of the cerebrospinal fluid. Brain 86:137, 1963.
33. Rubin RC, Henderson ES, Ommaya AK, et al.: The production of cerebrospinal fluid in man and its modification by acetazolamide. J Neurosurg 25:430, 1966.
34. Schain RJ: Carbonic anhydrase inhibitors in chronic infantile hydrocephalus. Am J Dis Child 117:621, 1969.
35. Mealey J Jr, Barker DT: Failure of oral acetazolamide to avert hydrocephalus in infants with myelomeningocele. J Pediatr 72:257, 1968.
36. Shinnar S, Gammon K, Bergman EW Jr, et al.: Management of hydrocephalus in infancy: Use of acetazolamide and furosemide to avoid cerebrospinal fluid shunts. J Pediatr 107:31, 1985.
37. Nulsen FE, Spitz EB: Treatment of hydrocephalus by direct shunt from ventricle to jugular vein. Surg Forum 2:399, 1952.
38. Pudenz RH: The surgical treatment of hydrocephalus—an historical review. Surg Neurol 15:15, 1981.
39. Matson DD: Current treatment of infantile hydrocephalus. N Engl J Med 255:933, 1956.
40. Dandy WE: Extirpation of the choroid plexus of the lateral ventricle in communicating hydrocephalus. Ann Surg 68:569, 1918.
41. Putnam TJ: Results of treatment of hydrocephalus by endoscopic coagulation of the choroid plexus. Arch Pediatr 52:676, 1935.
42. Scarff JE: The treatment of nonobstructive (communicating) hydrocephalus by endoscopic cauterization of the choroid plexuses. J Neurosurg 33:1, 1970.
43. Milhorat TH: Failure of choroid plexectomy as treatment for hydrocephalus. Surg Gynecol Obstet 139:505, 1974.
44. Milhorat TH, Hammock MK, Chien T, et al.: Normal rate of

cerebrospinal fluid production five years after bilateral choroid plexectomy. Case report. J Neurosurg 44:735, 1976.

45. Dandy WE: Diagnosis and treatment of strictures of aqueduct of Sylvius (causing hydrocephalus). Arch Surg 51:1, 1945.

46. Jaksche H, Loew F: Burr hole third ventriculo-cisternostomy. An unpopular but effective procedure for treatment of certain forms of occlusive hydrocephalus. Acta Neurochir 79:48, 1986.

47. Jack CR Jr, Kelly PJ: Stereotactic third ventriculostomy: Assessment of patency with MR imaging. AJNR 10:515, 1989.

48. Hoffman HJ, Harwood-Nash D, Gilday DL: Percutaneous third ventriculostomy in the management of noncommunicating hydrocephalus. Neurosurgery 7:313, 1980.

49. Hoffman HJ, Harwood-Nash D, Gilday DL, et al.: Percutaneous third ventriculostomy in the management of noncommunicating hydrocephalus. Concepts Pediatr Neurosurg I:87, 1981.

50. Hirsch J-F: Percutaneous ventriculocisternostomies in noncommunicating hydrocephalus. Monogr Neural Sci 8:170, 1982.

51. Sayers MP, Kosnick EJ: Percutaneous third ventriculostomy: experience and technique. Childs Brain 2:24, 1976.

52. Vries JK: An endoscopic technique for third ventriculostomy. Surg Neurol 9:165, 1978.

53. Jones RFC, Stening WA, Brydon M: Endoscopic third ventriculostomy. Neurosurgery 26:86, 1990.

54. Torkildson A: A new palliative operation in cases of inoperable occlusion of the sylvian aqueduct. Acta Chir Scand 82:117, 1939.

55. Matson DD: The treatment of hydrocephalus. Surg Clin North Am 34:1021, 1954.

56. Epstein FJ: How to keep shunts functioning, or "the impossible dream." Clin Neurosurg 32:608, 1985.

57. Nulsen FE, Becker DP: Control of hydrocephalus by valve-regulated shunt. J Neurosurg 26:362, 1967.

58. Nulsen FE, Becker DP: Control of hydrocephalus by valve-regulated shunt: Infections and their prevention. Clin Neurosurg 14:256, 1966.

59. Sainte-Rose C, Hoffman HJ, Hirsch JF: Shunt failure. Concepts Pediatr Neurosurg 9:7, 1989.

60. Sainte-Rose C, Piatt JH, Pierre-Kahn A, et al.: Mechanical complications in shunts. Pediatr Neurosurg 17:2, 1991–92.

61. Ghajar JB: A guide for ventricular catheter placement: Technical note. J Neurosurg 63:985, 1985.

62. Albright AL, Haines SJ, Taylor FH: Function of parietal and frontal shunts in childhood hydrocephalus. J Neurosurg 69:883, 1988.

63. Bierbrauer KS, Storrs BB, McLone DG, et al.: A prospective, randomized study of shunt function and infections as a function of shunt placement. Pediatr Neurosurg 16:287, 1990–91.

64. Ransohoff J, Shulman K, Fishman RA: Hydrocephalus. A review of etiology and treatment. J Pediatr 56:399, 1960.

65. Hoffman HJ, Hendrick EB, Humphreys RP: New lumboperitoneal shunt for communicating hydrocephalus. Technical Note. J Neurosurg 44:258, 1976.

66. Selman WR, Spetzler RF, Wilson CB, et al.: Percutaneous lumboperitoneal shunt: Review of 130 cases. Neurosurgery 6:255, 1980.

67. Kushner J, Alexander E Jr, Davis CH Jr, et al.: Kyphoscoliosis following lumbar subarachnoid shunts. J Neurosurg 34:783, 1971.

68. Braley S: The silicones as subdermal engineering materials. Ann NY Acad Sci 146:148, 1968.

69. Weiss SR, Raskind R: Twenty-two cases of hydrocephalus treated with a silastic ventriculoperitoneal shunt. Int Surg 51:13, 1969.

70. Davidson RI: Peritoneal bypass in the treatment of hydrocephalus: Historical review and abdominal complications. J Neurol Neurosurg Psychiatr 39:640, 1976.

71. Venes JL: Control of shunt infection: Report of 150 consecutive cases. J Neurosurg 45:311, 1976.

72. Schoenbaum SC, Gardner P, Shillito J: Infections of cerebrospinal fluid shunts: Epidemiology, clinical manifestations, and therapy. J Infect Dis 131:543, 1975.

73. Rekate HL, Yonas H, White RJ, et al.: The acute abdomen in patients with ventriculoperitoneal shunts. Surg Neurol 11:442, 1979.

74. Rekate HL, Ruch T, Nulsen FE: Diphtheroid infections of cerebrospinal fluid shunts: The changing pattern of shunt infection in Cleveland. J Neurosurg 52:553, 1980.

75. Becker DP, Jane JA, Nulsen FE: Investigation of sagittal sinus for venous shunt in hydrocephalus. Surg Forum 16:440, 1965.

76. El-Shafei I, Hafez MA: Ventriculojugular shunt against the direction of blood flow. IV. Technical modifications and policy for treatment. Childs Nerv Syst 7:197, 1991.

77. Ransohoff J: Ventriculo-pleural anastomosis in treatment of midline obstructional neoplasms. J Neurosurg 11:295, 1954.

78. Milhorat TH: Hydrocephalus and the Cerebrospinal Fluid. Baltimore, Williams and Wilkins, 1972, p 237.

79. Smith JA Jr, Lee RE, Middleton RG: Ventriculoureteral shunt for hydrocephalus without nephrectomy. J Urol 123:224, 1980.

80. Stein SC, Apfel S: A noninvasive approach to quantitative measurement of flow through CSF shunts: Technical note. J Neurosurg 54:556, 1981.

81. Portnoy HD, Tripp L, Croissant PD: Hydrodynamics of shunt valves. Child's Brain 2:242, 1976.

82. Portnoy HD: Treatment of hydrocephalus. In Pediatric Neurosurgery. Surgery of the Developing Nervous System. New York, Grune and Stratton, 1982, pp 211–227.

83. Nulsen FE, Rekate HL: Results of treatment for hydrocephalus as a guide to future management. In Pediatric Neurosurgery: Surgery of the Developing Nervous System. New York, Grune and Stratton, 1982, pp 229–241.

84. Nulsen FE, Fleming D, Rekate HL, et al.: Telemetry for intracranial pressure monitoring in children. Monogr Paediatr 15:17, 1982.

85. Hyde-Rowan MD, Rekate HL, Nulsen FE: Reexpansion of previously collapsed ventricles: The slit ventricle syndrome. J Neurosurg 56:536, 1982.

86. Portnoy HD, Schulte RR, Fox JL, et al.: Antisiphon and reversible occlusion valves for shunting in hydrocephalus and preventing post-shunt subdural hematomas. J Neurosurg 38:729, 1973.

87. Foltz EL, Shurtleff DB: Conversion of communicating hydrocephalus to stenosis or occlusion of the aqueduct during ventricular shunt. J Neurosurg 24:520, 1966.

88. Da Silva MC, Drake JM: Effect of subcutaneous implantation of antisiphon devices on CSF shunt function. Pediatr Neurosurg 16:197, 1990–91.

89. Rekate HL: Closed-loop control of intracranial pressure. Ann Biomed Eng 8:515, 1980.

90. Lumenta CB, Roosen N, Dietrich U: Clinical experience with a pressure-adjustable valve SOPHY in the management of hydrocephalus. Childs Nerv Syst 6:270, 1990.

91. Dandy WE, Blackfan KD: Internal hydrocephalus. An experimental, clinical and pathological study. Am J Dis Child 8:406, 1914.

92. Hirsch JF, Pierre-Kahn A, Renier D, et al.: The Dandy-Walker malformation: A review of 40 cases. J Neurosurg 61:515, 1984.

93. Entzian W, Szepan B, Wappenschmidt J, et al.: The so-called Dandy-Walker syndrome: Comments on morphologic, diagnostic and therapeutic problems. Monogr Neural Sci 8:215, 1982.

94. Carmel PW, Antunes JL, Hilal SK, et al.: Dandy-Walker syndrome: Clinico-pathological features and re-evaluation of modes of treatment. Surg Neurol 8:132, 1977.

95. Matson DD: Prenatal obstruction of the fourth ventricle. AJR 76:499, 1956.

96. Raimondi AJ, Samuelson G, Yarzagaray L, et al.: Atresia of the foramina of Luschka and Magendie: The Dandy-Walker cyst. J Neurosurg 31:202, 1969.

97. James HE, Kaiser G, Schut L, et al.: Problems of diagnosis and treatment in the Dandy-Walker syndrome. Childs Brain 5:24, 1979.

98. Bindal AK, Storrs BB, McLone DG: Management of the Dandy-Walker syndrome. Pediatr Neurosurg 16:163, 1990–91.

99. Foltz EL, DeFeo DR: Double compartment hydrocephalus—a new clinical entity. Neurosurgery 7:551, 1980.

100. Collada M Jr, Kott J, Kline DG: Documentation of fourth ventricle entrapment by metrizamide ventriculography with CT scanning: Report of two cases. J Neurosurg 55:838, 1981.

101. Harrison HR, Reynolds AF: Trapped fourth ventricle in coccidioidal meningitis. Surg Neurol 17:197, 1982.

102. Hawkins JC III, Hoffman HJ, Humphreys RP: Isolated fourth ventricle as a complication of ventricular shunting: Report of three cases. J Neurosurg 49:910, 1978.
103. Lourie H, Shende MC, Krawchenko J, et al.: Trapped fourth ventricle: A report of two unusual cases. Neurosurgery 7:279, 1980.
104. Clewell WH, Johnson ML, Meier PR, et al.: A surgical approach to the treatment of fetal hydrocephalus. N Engl J Med 306:1320, 1982.
105. Chervenak FA, Berkowitz RL, Tortora M, et al.: The management of fetal hydrocephalus. Am J Obstet Gynecol 151:933, 1985.
106. Azzarelli B, Rekate HL, Roessmann NW: Subependymoma: A case report with ultrastructural study. Acta Neuropathol 40:279, 1977.
107. Fedder SL, Richter HA: Double compartment hydrocephalus in an adult. Neurosurgery 28:746, 1991.
108. Heilman CB, Cohen AR: Endoscopic ventricular fenestration using a "saline torch." J Neurosurg 74:224, 1991.
109. Ciricillo SF, Cogen PH, Harsch GR, et al.: Intracranial arachnoid cysts in children. A comparison of the effects of fenestration and shunting. J Neurosurg 74:230, 1991.
110. Rekate HL: Multiloculated compartments of cerebrospinal fluid: Pathophysiology and management. Crit Rev Neurosurg 1:309, 1991.
111. McClone DA, Killion M, Yogev R, et al.: Ventriculitis of mice and men. Concepts Pediatr Neurosurg 2:112, 1982.
112. Frigoletto FD Jr, Birnholz JC, Green MF: Antenatal treatment of hydrocephalus by ventriculoamniotic shunting. JAMA 248:2496, 1982.
113. Glick PL, Harrison MR, Halks-Miller M, et al.: Correction of congenital hydrocephalus in utero II: Efficacy of in utero shunting. J Pediatr Surg 19:870, 1984.
114. Brodner RA: Antenatal diagnosis and treatment of hydrocephalus. In Wilkins RH, Rengachary SS (eds): Neurosurgery. New York, McGraw-Hill, 1985, pp 2156–2159.
115. Brodner RA, Markowitz RS, Latner HJ: Feasibility of intracranial surgery in the primate fetus. Model and surgical principles. J Neurosurg 66:276, 1987.
116. Epstein F: Diagnosis and management of arrested hydrocephalus. Monogr Neural Sci 8:105, 1982.
117. Foltz E: The first seven years of a hydrocephalus project. In Shulman K (ed): Workshop in Hydrocephalus. Children's Hospital of Philadelphia, 1965. Philadelphia, University of Pennsylvania, 1965, pp 79–114.
118. Hemmer R: Can a shunt be removed? Monogr Neural Sci 8:227, 1982.
119. Holtzer GJ, de Lange SA: Shunt-independent arrest of hydrocephalus. J Neurosurg 39:698, 1973.
120. Hall P, Lindseth R, Campbell R, et al.: Scoliosis and hydrocephalus in myelocele patients: The effects of ventricular shunting. J Neurosurg 50:174, 1979.
121. Rekate HL, Nulsen FE, Mack HL, et al.: Establishing the diagnosis of shunt independence. Monogr Neural Sci 8:223, 1982.
122. Reigel D: Changes in the subdural space following cerebrospinal fluid shunts. Concepts Pediatr Neurosurg 3:145, 1983.
123. Hirayama A: Slit ventricle—a reluctant goal of ventriculoperitoneal shunt. Monogr Neural Sci 8:108, 1982.
124. Epstein FJ, Fleischer AS, Hochwald GM, et al.: Subtemporal craniectomy for recurrent shunt obstruction secondary to small ventricles. J Neurosurg 41:29, 1974.
125. Gruber R: Should "normalisation" of the ventricles be the goal of hydrocephalus therapy. Z Kinderchir 38(Suppl II):80, 1983.
126. Wen HL: Ventriculo-superior sagittal sinus shunt for hydrocephalus. Surg Neurol 17:432, 1982.

Chapter 14

CEREBROSPINAL FLUID SHUNTS: Complications and Results

ARTHUR E. MARLIN, M.D., and SARAH J. GASKILL, M.D.

Shunt placement continues to be the primary treatment in the long-term management of hydrocephalus. The use of cerebrospinal fluid (CSF) shunts dates back to 1908 when Kausch first described a procedure for diverting CSF to the peritoneum.[1] Despite this long history, the use of shunts continues to be fraught with multiple complications. This chapter will outline these complications, discuss strategies for avoiding them, and review the management and outcome of various shunting mishaps.

Currently, multiple types of CSF shunts are employed. Ventriculoperitoneal shunts (VPS), ventriculoatrial shunts (VAS), and lumboperitoneal shunts (LPS) are the most commonly utilized shunts and will be the focus of this chapter.

MALFUNCTION

The leading cause of shunt malfunction is mechanical failure. This includes failure due to obstruction, disconnection, migration, and equipment failure. Malfunctions unique to the distal and proximal catheters will be discussed separately.

Obstruction occurs in a variety of settings and may develop at the proximal or distal end of the shunt, although obstruction of the ventricular catheter is most common. Obstruction may be due to brain parenchyma, choroid plexus, a protein plug, or tumor cells. Obstruction of the catheter with brain parenchyma may occur with suboptimal catheter placement. Preoperative measurements of the distance from the calvarium to optimal placement in the frontal horn should guide the length of catheter placed during surgery. In the setting of significant hydrocephalus, adequate catheter length is important to ensure continued shunt function with re-expansion of the cortical mantle. To avoid compromise of shunt function by choroid plexus, the ideal catheter placement is within the horn of the lateral ventricle anterior to the foramen of Monro, thus maximizing the distance of the tip of the catheter from the choroid plexus. The formation of a protein "plug" may result in catheter obstruction at the ventricular or distal end. Whenever a protein plug is noted at surgery, infection must be ruled out. Premature infants shunted in the setting of intraventricular hemorrhage (IVH) have a higher level of protein for several months after their initial hemorrhage and are predisposed to obstruction for this reason as well as others (e.g., low intracranial pressure [ICP]). One strategy for avoiding recurrent shunt malfunction in the premature infant is the use of a temporary drainage system such as a subgaleal shunt, external ventricular drainage, or subcutaneous ventricular reservoirs. This allows for management of the hydrocephalus while CSF protein diminishes prior to shunt placement. Shunts placed in the setting of a primary brain tumor may become obstructed by tumor cells, protein, and debris.

Preoperative evaluation may not specifically demonstrate catheter obstruction. Recently, fusiform swelling of the distal slit valve ("pantaloon sign") has been described in distal shunt obstructions in the setting of distal slit valves.[2] In some cases, computed tomography (CT) or magnetic resonance imaging (MRI) of the brain may show the ventricular catheter to be imbedded in parenchyma or choroid plexus (Fig. 14–1). When a shunt tap is being performed, the inability to aspirate from the ventricular catheter suggests a proximal obstruction. Similarly, irrigation of the distal catheter

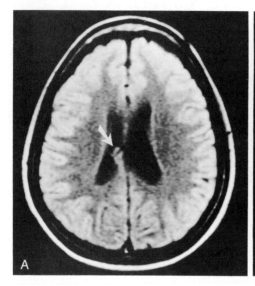
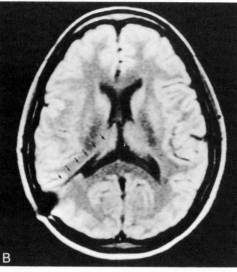

FIGURE 14–1. *A* and *B*, T1-weighted MRI showing imbedded ventricular catheter.

(taking care to occlude the proximal catheter) may be difficult or impossible, suggesting distal obstruction. Radiographic studies showing the peritoneal catheter tightly coiled in the abdomen suggest extraperitoneal placement, although this appearance may be seen in the setting of multiple abdominal adhesions.

DISCONNECTION

Disconnections may occur at any point in the system. Obviously sites of connection and mobility (i.e., the lateral neck) are at increased risk. Shunts that have been in place for some time often become fixed by the development of fibrous tissue around the catheter. The catheter itself undergoes mineralization and biodegradation.[3] The combination of fixation and mineralization contributes to catheter breakage with growth.

The continuity of a shunt can be assessed by palpation. However, the fibrous tract may feel and even act like tubing. In some cases a CSF collection develops over a shunt disconnection. Radiographic examination (AP/lateral skull, chest radiograph, and KUB) is definitive (Fig. 14–2). Note that some portions of the shunt system, such as the valve and connectors, may be ra-

diolucent and appear to represent disconnections. Comparison with postoperative radiographs and a working understanding of the various types of shunts in use should help one to avoid exploration of a "disconnected" (radiolucent) shunt.[4] The use of integral type shunts decreases the incidence of malfunction due to disconnection.

MIGRATION

Migration of the distal catheter may result in shunt malfunction. Migration to a wide variety of sites has been reported in the literature (Table 14–1).

With migration, shunt function may become compromised because of altered absorption of the CSF or blocking of the catheter by adjacent structures. With growth, the distal end of a vascular shunt may "migrate" from the atrium and become dysfunctional.

EQUIPMENT FAILURE

Equipment failures are rare, but should be considered in the appropriate setting. Valves come in a variety

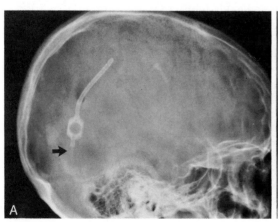
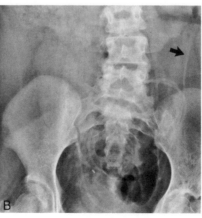

FIGURE 14–2. *A* and *B*, Plain radiographs of the skull and abdomen. The arrows demonstrate the ends of the fractured shunt.

TABLE 14–1. LOCATION OF SHUNT CATHETER MIGRATION

Scrotum[5, 6]
Internal jugular vein[7]
Umbilicus[8]
Intragastric[9]
Mouth[10]
Vagina[11]
Intestine[12]
Chest[13–15]
Intrahepatic[16]
Anus[17]
Coronary sinus[18]

of opening pressures (low: 5 to 50 mm H_2O; medium: 51 to 110 mm H_2O; high: 111 to 180 mm H_2O). They do not usually fail in and of themselves, but may result in shunt malfunction if an inappropriate pressure has been selected for a patient. A valve with too high an opening pressure may not relieve the symptoms of increased intracranial pressure. Similarly, a valve with too low an opening pressure may cause the development of subdural hematomas with overdrainage (see below). A variety of mechanical devices (antisiphon devices, variable-resistance shunts) are now available to prevent overdrainage.

DISTAL CATHETER MALFUNCTIONS

The distal catheter is associated with its own unique complications and malfunctions. Table 14–2 lists the wide variety of abdominal complications described in the literature.

Distal catheter malfunctions occur in a variety of settings. Abdominal procedures for appendicitis or urologic procedures can result in subsequent shunt malfunction due to infection or altered peritoneal absorption. In the setting of a perforated appendix with diffuse peritonitis or localized peritonitis in continuity with the shunt, the shunt should be externalized and replaced at a separate operation. Pseudocyst formation

TABLE 14–2. ABDOMINAL COMPLICATIONS

Acute abdomen[19]
Ascites[15]
CSF-enteric fistula[15]
Inflammatory pseudotumor of mesentery[20]
Inguinal hernia[21–23]
Intrahepatic abscess[24–26]
Omental cyst[6]
Perforation of bladder[21]
Perforation of bowel[21, 27–29]
Perforation of gallbladder[30]
Pseudocyst[6, 21, 31, 32]
Small bowel obstruction[33]
Umbilical fistula[32, 34]
Ureter obstruction[35]
Volvulus[21, 36]

may develop with infection (usually in the smaller cysts) or without infection (larger cysts) and impair CSF absorption.[31] Preperitoneal placement may present with sudden shunt malfunction.

PROXIMAL CATHETER MALFUNCTIONS

Intraoperative hemorrhage is an unusual but significant complication. If bleeding occurs at the time of placement, the shunt may malfunction in the perioperative period. Catheters removed after being in situ for some time may result in hemorrhage (Fig. 14–3). Intraventricular blood may cause subsequent obstruction and acute malfunction. Flanged catheters are particularly prone to this complication.

Pneumocephalus most often arises with resection of intracranial tumors. As air goes through the shunt tubing, an "air lock" can develop and cause subsequent shunt malfunction. Routine pumping of the shunt for several days may help to clear air from the system and encourage adequate shunt function.

Intrinsic ventricular anomalies may contribute to shunt malfunction. Loculated ventricles often develop in the setting of infection. Other causes include Dandy-Walker syndrome or severe IVH. Assessment of communication can be made with intraventricular injections of contrast material followed by delayed CT scanning. All symptomatic, isolated CSF collections that cause mass effect must be drained with separate catheters or be communicated with craniotomy or ventriculoscopy. Loculations in an otherwise routine case of hydrocephalus should raise concern for the possibility of infection.

There is debate about the long-term function of pa-

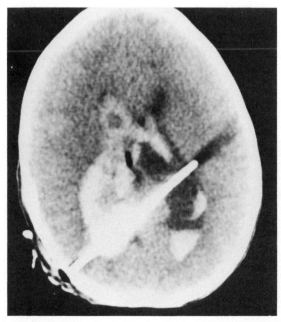

FIGURE 14–3. CT scan demonstrating intraventricular hemorrhage after removal of ventricular catheter at the time of shunt revision.

rietal versus frontal shunts.[37] It seems what is most important is placement of the catheter in front of the choroid plexus in the frontal horn. Whether this is done by a frontal or parietal approach is the surgeon's preference.

SURGICAL COMPLICATIONS

Several perioperative complications have been recognized. Retained fragments usually occur with revisions of systems that have been in place for some time. Catheters may adhere to the choroid plexus, making removal both difficult and dangerous. In these cases, it is usually preferable to leave the catheter behind. Fragments may fracture along the tract from the cranium to the abdomen, and rather than make numerous incisions for removal, one can leave these in situ. Peritoneal catheters that have become disconnected and are not easily accessible may also be left in place. These fragments are usually harmless, except in the setting of infection, in which case their removal is a prerequisite to clear the infection.

Bowel perforation may occur with peritoneal catheter placement. The use of the peritoneal trocar in selected patients (i.e., those without prior history of abdominal surgery or intra-abdominal processes such as necrotizing enterocolitis, peritonitis, or paralytic ileus) is not associated with an increased incidence of bowel perforation.[38] However, perforation of the bowel is associated with the development of gram-negative ventriculitis, and patients with this complication should be treated appropriately.[17, 28] Patients with prior abdominal procedures or processes, as described above, should undergo distal catheter placement under direct vision.

Bladder perforation can occur in patients who have undergone bladder augmentations, particularly patients with neurogenic bladders (Fig. 14–4). Again, in these

cases placement into the peritoneum should be done under direct vision.

INFECTION

Infections represent the second most common cause of shunt malfunction after mechanical failure. Shunt infection is a significant cause of morbidity associated with shunting and can lead to prolonged hospitalization, multiple operative procedures, diminished intelligence, and death. The incidence of shunt infection in published reviews varies dramatically from surgeon to surgeon and institution to institution, with a reported range of 2.6 to 38 per cent.[39–47] The rate of infection for ventriculoatrial shunts is about 15 per cent, generally higher than that seen with VPS.[48, 49] For patients requiring lifelong ventricular decompression, the per patient shunt infection rate is between 1.5 and 39 per cent, with a mean of 10 to 15 per cent.[45, 46, 50–54]

PREVENTION

The best management of shunt infection clearly lies in its prevention. A variety of antibiotic regimens and accessory equipment have been utilized; however, the most important factor contributing to the rate of shunt infections is surgical technique.

Surgical experience and meticulous technique from skin preparation to the dressing of the wound will have impact on the shunt infection rate. George reports that the surgeon is the single most important factor in the incidence of shunt infections; he noted a 25-fold variation in infection rate attributable to surgical technique.[43] Other authors confirm that inexperience leads to increased shunt infection rates.[55] Additionally, a longer duration of surgery has been shown to cause a higher rate of infection.[48]

The recommended operative technique includes: extensive skin preparation with antiseptic solution (Betadine or Hibiclens), meticulous draping of the operative field with Betadine-impregnated adhesive surgical drapes over the operative field, meticulous sterile operative technique, intraoperative antibiotic irrigation, minimal handling of the shunt system, soaking of the shunt system in antibiotic irrigant, and the use of talc-free gloves.

Adjunctive equipment designed to prevent shunt infection may be useful. Recently the use of a surgical isolation bubble system (SIBS) has become a feasible surgical adjunct. A large series of shunt procedures performed with and without the use of the SIBS reported the infection rate to be 5.8 per cent in the non-bubble group (N = 136) and 3.5 per cent (N = 144) in the bubble group. While the difference is not statistically significant, a detailed analysis of the infections suggested that the SIBS was effective in reducing infection rates.[56] Early attempts at impregnating shunt tubing made from Silastic impregnated with antimicrobial agents has

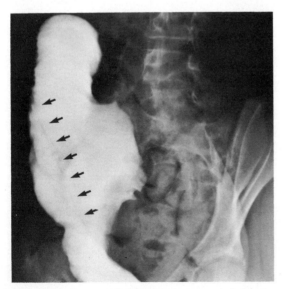

FIGURE 14–4. Cystogram demonstrating ventriculoperitoneal catheter within the bladder (*arrows*).

been used experimentally. Studies in animals have shown continued antibacterial activity with this method.[57, 58] It has also been suggested that there is a lower infection rate with the use of a simple one-piece shunt system rather than the more complicated three-piece systems.[59] These and other advances in surgical equipment may prove to be an effective means of diminishing shunt infections.

PROPHYLACTIC ANTIBIOTICS

The efficacy of prophylactic antibiotic regimens remains unanswered. Most reviews are retrospective, nonrandomized series that come from a variety of institutions and cover a large time span, making cross-comparison difficult.[40, 41, 43–47]

Only five prospective, randomized studies of antibiotic prophylaxis have been published.[47, 50, 51, 60, 61] None of these studies has found a statistically significant difference in the infection rate of patients who received prophylactic antibiotics versus those who did not. Only one study (not prospective or randomized) has shown a statistically significant reduction in shunt infection with the use of prophylactic antibiotics.[40] A multicenter, prospective, randomized study is needed to definitively determine the efficacy of prophylactic antibiotics in shunt surgery.

In spite of a lack of evidence that prophylactic antibiotics are effective, many centers continue to use them. If used, prophylactic antibiotics should be selected partly on the basis of infection patterns in the institution. The routes of administration are usually intravenous where available. Some centers advocate intraoperative antibiotic irrigation of the shunt system. Doses are usually based on weight; however, it has been shown that CSF levels of nafcillin are inversely proportional to the size of the ventricles, suggesting that the degree of ventriculomegaly might be important in dosing prophylactic antibiotics.[62] Prophylactic antibiotics should be started shortly before induction of anesthesia and be continued for 24 to 36 hours postoperatively.[45–47, 62] Earlier institution of therapy with prolonged administration for as long as 72 hours has been advocated by some authors.[43, 51]

When contemplating the use of prophylactic antibiotics, one should consider the increased cost and the potential for toxic side effects. The development of resistant strains with antibiotic prophylaxis has been observed.[45, 63] Also, an increase in gram-negative shunt infections has been reported in patients receiving prophylactic penicillinase-resistant penicillins.[45, 64] Another institution found that the epidemiology of infecting organisms shifted from *Staphylococcus epidermidis* to diphtheroids after the institution of intraoperative shunt irrigation with gentamicin.[64] These trends are a matter of concern and should be considered in the decision to use prophylactic antibiotics. Perhaps prophylactic antibiotics should be reserved for high-risk patients. Table 14–3 lists the most commonly utilized prophylactic antibiotics.

TABLE 14–3. PROPHYLACTIC ANTIBIOTICS

| AGENT | DOSE (mg/kg/day) Infants over 2 kilograms | |
	Age 0–7 Days	>7 Days
Intravenous		
Nafcillin	50 div q12h	75 div q6h
Vancomycin	10 div q12h	45 div q6h
Ceftriaxone	50–75 q24h	50–75 q24h
Cefotaxime	100 q12h	50–200 q4–6h
Oxacillin	50 div q12h	75 div q6h
Gentamicin	2.5 mg/kg/dose q12h	6–7.5 q8h
Methicillin	25–50 q6h	100–400 q4–6h
Oral		
Trimethoprim/ sulfamethoxazole (TMP-SMZ)		20 q6–8h (based on TMP)

RISK FACTORS

A number of underlying conditions are associated with increased infection rates including Dandy-Walker syndrome, aqueductal stenosis, and encephaloceles.[43] McCullough has reported a twofold increase in shunt infection rates in children with myelomeningocele compared with other etiologies of hydrocephalus.[62] Higher infection rates have been reported in children shunted in the first year of life, in particular the premature infants.[43, 59, 65] Successive shunt revisions have been noted to have progressively higher infection rates.[43, 46, 50]

CLINICAL PRESENTATION

Most shunt infections develop near the time of a prior shunt operation. Seventy per cent of infections are clinically apparent within 2 months of the procedure, and 80 per cent are manifested within 6 months.[43, 46, 53, 66] Cases presenting early are likely to be infected with *Staphylococcus aureus, Staphylococcus epidermidis*, or diphtheroids. Gram-negative enteric infections may present at any time. In general, the clinical presentation of shunt infection is nonspecific.[42, 65, 67] Fever (T >101° to 102°), irritability, and signs of shunt malfunction predominate.[42, 43, 65] Meningeal signs are present in a minority of patients (25 to 33 per cent).[42, 43, 46, 67] The most common signs and symptoms are fever, change in sensorium, irritability, shunt malfunction, emesis, abdominal pain, diarrhea, and peritonitis. Local signs of inflammation along the shunt tract are seen on occasion. Patients with ventriculoatrial shunts may present with signs and symptoms of shunt nephritis or septic emboli.[68]

DIAGNOSIS

The diagnosis of shunt infection is based on clinical presentation, CSF evaluation, and peripheral blood studies. In many cases there is radiographic evidence of shunt malfunction. A high index of clinical suspicion is imperative as the complications of infection increase with the duration of infection.[46, 69]

Evaluation of CSF is an essential part of the diagnosis.[69] CSF obtained by lumbar puncture is diagnostic in only 50 per cent of infected patients.[70] A shunt tap should be performed to assess for infection. Shunt infection is associated with an elevated leukocyte count (predominantly segmented cells), diminished glucose levels, and elevated protein levels. Infection with gram-positive organisms may yield low neutrophil counts and protein concentrations as they tend to cause only a mild inflammatory response.[70] The Gram stain of the fluid was positive in 82 per cent of cases of *Staphylococcus aureus* infection and 91 per cent of cases of gram-negative bacillary infection.[42] Bacteremia was noted to be present in 25 per cent of all ventriculoperitoneal shunt infections and in all cases of ventriculoatrial shunt infections.[42] Wound infection is most commonly associated with a *Staphylococcus aureus* infection.

Occult infections are being recognized with increasing frequency. Infections with indolent bacteria, such as diphtheroids, are difficult to diagnose. CSF cultures should be maintained for 14 days to ascertain the diagnosis of anaerobic infections.[63]

MICROBIOLOGY OF SHUNT INFECTIONS

The most common pathogens isolated from shunt infections are typical skin flora. *Staphylococcus epidermidis* (coagulase-negative staph) is the leading cause of infection in CSF shunts. The pathogenicity of *Staphylococcus epidermidis* is enhanced by the secretion of a mucoid substance that promotes adherence to foreign bodies.[71] This is in contrast to the inability of human neutrophils and monocytes to adhere to shunt catheters and phagocytose bacteria.[72] The use of bacitracin irrigation intraoperatively decreases the ability of the bacteria to adhere to the shunt catheter. The second most common pathogen is *Staphylococcus aureus* (coagulase-positive staph) accounting for 25 per cent of all shunt infections. A number of infections are due to gram-negative enteric bacteria such as *Klebsiella*, *Escherichia coli* and *Proteus*. The remainder of the infections are due to meningitis pathogens such as *Haemophilus influenzae*, *Streptococcus pneumoniae*, and *Neisseria meningitidis*. Delayed infection with anaerobic diphtheroids (*Propionibacterium* species), also part of the normal skin flora, has been reported.[73] Additional infections are seen with Actinobacter and *Streptococcus viridans*. Polymicrobial infections do occur, most commonly with the gram-negative enteric organisms.[66]

PATHOGENESIS OF SHUNT INFECTIONS

The three routes of shunt infection are direct inoculation at the time of surgery, hematogenous spread, and retrograde travel from a contaminated distal catheter.

Direct inoculation at the time of surgery does not necessarily imply a break in sterile technique. Bayston and Lari have suggested that, even with appropriate skin cleansing, normal skin flora remain in sweat and sebaceous glands and hair follicles, which are unaffected by antiseptic agents.[74] These organisms may gain access to the surgical wound and cause infection. Whether or not a wound becomes infected depends on the size of the inoculum, the virulence of the inoculating bacteria, and the ability of the host defense system to eradicate the infection.

Hematogenous spread is probably a rare cause of shunt infection. It is more common in current practice with ventriculovascular catheters. Holt observed that infected ventriculovascular shunts showed heavily contaminated vascular ends as compared to the valve or ventricular catheter.[75] He concluded that the one-way valve action could not prevent the backflow of organisms. Retrograde infection with enteric organisms in cases of bowel perforation have also been reported in the literature.[76]

MANAGEMENT OF SHUNT INFECTIONS

The management of shunt infections is a controversial issue. The debate revolves primarily around the need to remove hardware in order to effectively cure shunt infection versus sterilization of the shunt system in vivo.

Some authors contend that shunt infection can be cleared only through removal of the entire shunt system with the use of intravenous and intraventricular antibiotics.[46, 49] Historically, most authors have recommended complete shunt removal to manage infection, based primarily on the belief that there was bacterial colonization. This concept was initially introduced by Cohen et al. in their review of five colonized Spitz-Holter valves.[77] A series of articles subsequently confirmed the importance of shunt removal for the effective eradication of infection.[78–80] Evidence demonstrating that shunts, as foreign bodies, become colonized by bacteria[81], and more recent evidence that shunts actually inhibit the defense system,[72] support this treatment regimen.

At one time, only scattered cases of success in controlling shunt infections without removal were reported.[82] With reports of some successes with in vivo sterilization of shunt systems, some groups now advocate treatment without removal of the hardware in conjunction with intra-shunt and intravenous antibiotics.[41, 83, 84] As they are quick to point out, removal of shunts is not without risk, especially in cases of severe shunt dependency and in patients with closed sutures. This approach has been most successful with vascular shunts, having been effective in 50 to 75 per cent of cases.[52, 85] There is significant morbidity and mortality when treatment consists of antimicrobial therapy alone.[46]

Some groups take a middle of the road approach, recommending removal of the infected shunt, immediate replacement with a new shunt system and concomitant administration of intraventricular and intravenous antibiotics.[65, 68]

The following guidelines are recommended for the management of shunt infections. In patients who present with shunt malfunction and shunt infection, the shunt is removed. External ventricular drainage (EVD) is established in patients who require continuous drainage. Intravenous antibiotics are administered for 5 to 7 days, and then a new shunt system is inserted with continuation of antibiotics for another seven days. In patients without shunt malfunction, the shunt is left in place and intra-shunt and intravenous antibiotics are administered for 5 to 7 days followed by shunt removal and replacement.

In 1980 James et al. published a prospective, randomized study of the management of shunt infections.[86] Patients were randomly divided into three different treatment groups. In group 1 the shunt was removed, and EVD was instituted as necessary. Intraventricular and intravenous antibiotics were administered for a minimum of 7 days. Group 2 patients underwent shunt removal and replacement in one procedure, followed by 2 weeks of intra-shunt antibiotics and 3 weeks of intravenous antibiotics. In group 3 patients, the infected shunt was left in place and they were treated with the same antibiotic regimen as the second group. Group 1 patients had a 100 per cent cure rate with a mean hospital stay of 24 ± 17 days. Group 2 patients had a 90 per cent cure rate with a mean hospital stay of 33 ± 8 days. One failure in group 2 required treatment with shunt removal, EVD, and antibiotics (intraventricular and intravenous). Group 3 patients had a 30 per cent cure rate. Five of these patients with persistent infections were effectively cured with shunt removal, EVD, and antibiotics. Two patients died—one with a virulent *E. coli* and *Pseudomonas* infection, and one secondary to EVD disconnection. The conclusions from this study were that shunt infections should be treated by removal of the shunt with delayed or immediate replacement in conjunction with intravenous and intraventricular antibiotics. In vivo sterilization of an infected shunt system is rarely accomplished and is associated with an extended hospital stay and significant mortality, making it a poor treatment option in most cases.

ROUTE OF ANTIBIOTIC ADMINISTRATION

Most regimens that attempt to clear a shunt infection without the removal of hardware employ concurrent intra-shunt or intraventricular administration of antibiotics. The rationale behind this is that there is a known failure of antibiotics to penetrate the blood-CSF barrier except with meningeal inflammation. Shunt infections do not necessarily produce sufficient meningeal irritation to allow antibiotic penetrance. Therefore, systemic antibiotics alone cannot be relied upon to eradicate a shunt infection. Intraventricular antibiotics are essential for the treatment of ventriculitis, and these may be administered through ventricular puncture, EVD, or a shunt reservoir. Persistently higher and more uniform antibiotic levels are obtained with direct ventricular access.[87] Because there is tremendous variability in the concentration of intraventricular antibiotics within and between patients, it is essential to monitor intraventricular antibiotic concentration throughout the course of therapy and to adjust intraventricular antibiotic doses as necessary.[87, 88] Intravenous antibiotics eradicate tissue infection around the shunt apparatus and any blood-borne infection; they also improve CSF levels. Their role in the management of shunt infection should not be underestimated.

ANTIBIOTIC SELECTION

A wide variety of antibiotics with appropriate coverage and CSF penetration are available. Choices of antibiotics should be based in part on infection epidemiology within the institution. Once CSF is obtained for cultures, empiric therapy with a broad-spectrum antibiotic such as a third-generation cephalosporin should be initiated. If the CSF Gram stain suggests an infecting organism, more specific empiric therapy may be instituted (Table 14–4).

TABLE 14–4. TREATMENT OF SHUNT INFECTION BY ORGANISM

ORGANISM	INTRA-SHUNT	INTRAVENOUS
Staphylococcus epidermidis or *aureus*	Vancomycin	1. Vancomycin, or 2. Rifampin and TMP-SMZ
Enterococcus	Vancomycin and Gentamicin	Vancomycin
Other streptococci 1. PCN m.i.c. <=0.1 2. PCN m.i.c. >=0.2	Gentamicin Vancomycin and Gentamicin	Pen G (IV) Pen G (IV)
Aerobic gram-negative rods	Gentamicin	Cefotaxime
Diphtheroids	Vancomycin	1. Vancomycin, or 2. TMP-SMZ

PCN = penicillin; m.i.c. = minimum inhibitory concentration.

TABLE 14–5.   TREATMENT OF SHUNT INFECTION

ROUTE	<7 DAYS (mg/kg/24h)	>7 DAYS (mg/kg/24h)	PEAK LEVELS
Intravenous			*Serum*
Vancomycin	10 q12h	45 q6h	20–40 µg/ml
Gentamycin	2.5 mg/kg/dose q12h	6–7.5 q8h	5–10 µg/ml
Nafcillin	50 q12h	75 q6h	
Cefotaxime	100 q12h	50–200 q4–6h	70–100 µg/ml
Ceftazidime	60 q12h	90–150 q8h	
Ceftriaxone	50–75 q24h	50–75 q24h	
Penicillin G	50–150,000 U q8h	100–300,000 U q4–6h	
Oral			
Rifampin	10 q24h	20 q24h	
Trimethoprim/sulfamethoxazole (TMP-SMZ)		20 q6–8h (based on TMP)	
Intra-shunt			*CSF*
Vancomycin	5 mg qd	10 mg qd	10 µg/ml
Gentamicin	8 mg qd	8 mg qd	4 µg/ml

The antibiotic regimen should be adjusted as cultures and sensitivities become available. The importance of maintaining adequate doses without excessive peak levels is important, as the neurotoxicity of high levels of intraventricular antibiotics is well documented.[89, 90] The symptoms of antibiotic neurotoxicity include seizures, coma, myoclonus, fever, and CSF pleocytosis.[89, 90] Table 14–5 presents commonly used antibiotics with suggested doses.

EXTERNAL VENTRICULAR DRAINAGE

External ventricular drainage as an adjunct to the management of shunt infection provides a means of managing increased intracranial pressure and provides a route for intraventricular antibiotics. However, there are a number of concerns with EVD. These include the small but significant risk associated with ventriculostomy placement, and the management of fluids and electrolytes with chronic external cerebrospinal fluid drainage. Of most importance is the risk of superinfection with prolonged ventriculostomy drainage.[53, 91] However, this method is preferable to the risks associated with daily ventricular punctures.

PROGNOSIS

It has been demonstrated that children with a history of shunt infection have a significantly lower intelligence quotient (IQ) score (73 ± 26 SD) compared with shunted children who have not suffered a shunt infection (95 ± 19 SD).[92] The severity of the infection has not been correlated with the degree of IQ decline; however there is a trend for gram-negative infections to cause greater declines in intellectual function.[92, 93] Children who develop seizures with shunt infection are more likely to suffer further intellectual decline.[92]

The mortality associated with shunt infection has decreased from a high of 35 per cent in 1952 to 5 to 10 per cent in 1976 and is probably significantly lower now.[43, 46] The failure to obtain an early and effective eradication of shunt infection is associated with a higher mortality rate.[46, 49]

OTHER SHUNT COMPLICATIONS

SLIT-VENTRICLE SYNDROME

Slit-ventricle syndrome (SVS) is the association of episodic signs and symptoms of increased ICP (headache in particular) in patients with small or slit-like ventricular systems. This is an uncommon but problematic syndrome that develops in 0.9 to 3.3 per cent of shunted children.[94–96] A variety of mechanisms have been proposed to explain this syndrome including overdrainage of CSF, intermittent shunt malfunction with symptomatic mild increases in ventricular size, periventricular fibrosis, intracranial hypotension, and decreased intracranial compliance.[94–100] While none of these proposed mechanisms explains all cases of SVS, most cases are explained by one of the proposed mechanisms.

A variety of therapies have been introduced for the management of SVS, reflecting the variable etiology and difficulty in treating this syndrome. Medical options include therapy with furosemide (Lasix), acetazolamide (Diamox), and/or steroids. This therapy is effective in a significant number of cases. Antimigraine agents (propranolol, dihydroergotamine, amitriptyline and cyproheptadine) have recently been shown to be effective in all seven patients treated with one of these agents, suggesting that SVS may actually represent a form of "acquired" migraine in at least some shunt patients.[101]

Surgical options for treatment include shunt revision, in particular upgrading the pressure on the valve[100] or changing to a variable-resistance valve. Because of the rarity of the syndrome and a lack of large series, it is impossible to say how often shunt revision eliminates SVS. However, it must be noted that experience has shown that shunt revision may not eliminate or even alleviate SVS. Subtemporal decompression is a larger procedure, which has also been used in the management of SVS. Subtemporal decompression can provide a window to measure ICP, additional room to allow decompression of increased ICP, and further room for dilation of the ipsilateral ventricle, all of which are beneficial in the treatment and management of SVS. In a series of 22 patients presented by Holness et al., the frequency of shunt revision after subtemporal decompression was reduced in a majority of patients.[102] Other operations involving craniectomies and unroofing of the transverse sinus have been described.[103]

A recent study by Abbott et al. reported the monitoring of intracranial pressure in 12 patients with "slit-ventricle syndrome."[104] Of their 12 patients, three had headaches due to increased ICP, two had headaches due to decreased ICP, and seven had headaches that were unrelated to pressure. As the interventions would differ depending on the etiology of the headaches, pressure monitoring may become a useful adjunct, particularly in the management of recalcitrant cases of SVS.

It is important to recognize that the vast majority of patients with slit ventricles on CT scan do not develop SVS and will dilate their ventricles with shunt malfunction. Therefore, the prophylactic revision of a shunt to treat radiographically identified slit ventricles for the prevention of SVS is not recommended.

SEIZURES

Electroencephalogram (EEG) abnormalities have been noted in several series of shunted patients.[105, 106] Seizures occur at a rate of 5 to 48 per cent in children with shunts.[106, 107] One series reports the incidence of seizures with parietal shunts to be 6.6 per cent compared with a 54.5 per cent seizure rate with frontal shunts.[108] Hack et al. reported on a series of 346 children with myelomeningocele and shunted hydrocephalus.[109] They found that 9 per cent of shunt malfunctions presented with seizure. Ventriculitis has also been reported to increase the risk of seizures in the myelomeningocele population.[110] Therefore, shunt malfunction and/or infection should be ruled out when seizures occur in the shunted child. Once this has been ruled out, seizures should be managed with appropriate anticonvulsant therapy. Currently, routine seizure prophylaxis is not indicated in the management of shunted patients.

NEURO-OPHTHALMOLOGIC SEQUELAE

A variety of neuro-ophthalmologic sequelae related to shunts have been reported. Catheter misplacement has caused progressive visual loss and bitemporal field defects[111] and bitemporal hemianoptic scotoma.[112] Of course, shunt malfunction can be associated with a variety of ocular findings including third, fourth, or sixth nerve paresis, dorsal midbrain syndrome (paresis of up-gaze, light-near dissociation, convergence-retraction nystagmus), and visual loss secondary to recurrent or chronic papilledema.[113] A change in the baseline neuro-ophthalmologic examination suggests the possibility of shunt malfunction and necessitates a work-up in this regard.

TUMOR

The spread of tumor through shunts placed in the setting of primary brain tumors has been described rarely, but this remains a real concern. Medulloblastoma,[114] astrocytoma,[115] glioblastoma,[116] germinoma,[117] and endodermal sinus tumors[118] have all been reported to spread to the peritoneum via VPS. The risk of extraneural metastases due to VPS (or other types of shunts) has been addressed by two large series. The largest series (N=415) was reported by Berger et al. in 1991.[119] They found that eight of 415 patients developed extraneural metastases. All of these patients had medulloblastoma as their primary tumor. Five of the eight patients were not shunted and developed metastases to the bone, cervical lymph nodes, lung, or retroperitoneal space. The three patients with shunts (two VPS, one VA) had the shunts placed after their initial tumor resection. The sites of metastases for these patients were bone, retroperitoneal space, and abdominal cavity. A series of 282 patients with primary brain tumors and extraneural metastases was reported by Hoffman and Duffner.[120] They found that 114 (40.4 per cent) of these metastases occurred in the pediatric population. Nearly 30 per cent of the children had undergone some type of CSF diversionary procedure. The authors concluded that shunts contributed to the extraneural spread of tumor and recommended the use of the Millipore filter to diminish this risk. There remains significant debate about the effectiveness of Millipore filters as these frequently become occluded and may even be a site of seeding.

SUBDURAL COLLECTIONS

The development of subdural effusions and hematomas is a known complication of shunt placement in patients with a fixed cranium. In many cases this merely reflects the underlying problem of craniocerebral disproportion. In the majority of patients these collections are asymptomatic. With time and brain growth they frequently resolve. Symptomatic cases may require treatment with subdural catheter placement. This can be joined to the shunt distal to the valve.

CRANIOSYNOSTOSIS

Craniosynostosis has been described as an unusual complication of shunting.[121] This secondary synostosis is usually related to microcephaly or lack of cerebral growth. Secondary craniosynostosis with subsequent cerebellar and brainstem herniation into the upper spinal canal was reported by Hoffman and Tucker.[122] Six of the eight patients in that series were cases of communicating hydrocephalus treated with lumboperitoneal shunts. Posterior fossa decompression resulted in significant improvement in all cases.

PREGNANCY

Although pregnancy is not usually a pediatric topic per se, the incidence of teenage pregnancies has increased dramatically in recent years, and it seems appropriate to at least mention some of the complications associated with shunts in the setting of pregnancy. Three recent reports have addressed this issue and should be consulted for further detail.[123–125] The issues of concern include prenatal counseling (in the setting of a mother with a neural tube defect, the risk of having an affected offspring is about 3 per cent), shunt malfunction, shunt infection, and the management of seizures during pregnancy and lactation. These series have demonstrated that pregnancy can affect shunt function, but that these problems can be managed without damage to the mother or the fetus.

VENTRICULOATRIAL AND LUMBOPERITONEAL SHUNTS

Several studies have compared VPS and VA shunts.[126, 127] The revision rate is comparable for the two types of shunts, but the complications noted with VA shunts are more severe. Vascular shunts are associated with a number of unique complications including shunt nephritis, pulmonary embolism, cor pulmonale, septicemia, cardiac mural thrombus, endocarditis, septic emboli, cardiac arrhythmias, cardiac tamponade, pulmonary hypertension, detachment of a catheter segment into the vascular system, migration into the coronary sinus, and obstruction of the vena cava system.

Autopsy studies have shown that VA shunt catheters within the heart are surrounded by fibrinous material, which extends variable lengths into the atrium with associated fibrinous clots.[128] Nearly half (6/15) of the cases demonstrated vegetation within the wall of the right atrium, and all but one case showed evidence of pulmonary emboli within the pulmonary system.

Shunt nephritis results from an immunologic reaction between an antigen and immune complexes. The antigen-antibody complex is deposited in the kidney and can potentially cause renal damage. Clinically the symptoms may include nephrotic syndrome, hematuria, fever, proteinuria, anemia, nonthrombocytopenic purpura, and hypertension. Shunt nephritis at one time was believed to occur exclusively with VA shunts. However, it has been described in association with ventriculoperitoneal shunts.[129, 130]

Despite the serious complications that may occur with VA shunts, they are sometimes necessary. VA shunts may be required in particular in cases of abdominal infection or impaired abdominal absorption.

Lumboperitoneal shunts (LPS) are not frequently used in the pediatric population. In a retrospective study reviewing the efficacy of LPS compared with VPS, there were 28 pediatric patients (N = 207) with hydrocephalus of various etiologies.[131] Twenty-one per cent of the pediatric patients required revision of their LPS because of malfunction compared with 58 per cent in the VPS group. Two patients suffered acute neurologic decline after LPS, one with infantile hydrocephalus and one who, in retrospect, had an Arnold-Chiari malformation. They both improved after revision to a VPS. Complications of LPS (pediatric and adult) included radiculopathy (5 per cent), myelopathy (N = 1), acute neurologic decline (N = 2—both pediatric), infection (1 per cent), and acute subdural hematoma (1 per cent). This paper confirms the necessity of demonstrating true communicating hydrocephalus prior to placement of LPS, particularly in the pediatric population.

PROGNOSIS

The prognosis associated with the long-term management of hydrocephalus is difficult to assess because of wide variability within the population. Patient-related factors include the etiology and degree of hydrocephalus, number of shunt revisions, number and type of shunt infections, and environmental and parental influences. Additionally, the evolution of technical factors makes comparisons between patients difficult. Imaging techniques have markedly improved our ability to diagnose and treat shunt malfunctions. Shunt systems themselves have been improved to some extent, and experience with the use of shunts has diminished the morbidity and mortality associated with shunts. Attitudes about viability and prognosis have also evolved over the years. Patients who might not have had the benefit of treatment previously are treated early and aggressively.

All of these factors make it difficult to draw conclusions about the true prognosis of hydrocephalus in patients who are treated with current standards of therapy. Certainly, outcome is determined to some degree by the etiology and degree of hydrocephalus, the presence of associated anomalies, the timeliness of diagnosis and treatment, and the number and type of complications associated with treatment.

Older studies based on air encephalography attempted to correlate the width of cerebral mantle with outcome.[132, 133] In general these showed a trend toward poorer outcome with cerebral mantles less than 1 or 2 cm. However, these studies did not take into account the phenomenon of cortical reconstitution. There is some suggestion that a better prediction would be obtained if the width of mantle is measured after cortical reconstitution has taken place.[134]

One thing is obvious. Congenital hydrocephalus appears to have an excellent prognosis despite all of the mechanical problems related to shunting as long as adequate shunt function can be maintained and infection can be prevented.

REFERENCES

1. Kausch W: Die Behandlung des hydrocephalus der kleined kinder. Arch Klin Chir 7:709, 1908.
2. Le Roux P, Berger M, Benjamin D: Abdominal x-ray and pathological findings in distal unishunt obstruction. Neurosurgery 23:749, 1988.
3. Echizenya K, Satoh M, Murai H, Ueno H, Abe H, Komai T: Mineralization and biodegradation of CSF shunting systems. J Neurosurg 67:584, 1987.
4. Walker J, Cook RC, Cudmore R: "Disconnected" integral ventriculoperitoneal shunt systems. J Neurol Neurosurg Psychiatry 53(10):927, 1990.
5. Ramani PS: Extrusion of abdominal catheter of ventriculoperitoneal shunt into the scrotum: Case report. J Neurosurg 40:772, 1974.
6. Redman JF, Seibert JJ: Abdominal and genitourinary complications following ventriculoperitoneal shunts. J Urol 119:295, 1978.
7. Cowan MA, Allen MB: Retrograde migration of the venous catheter as a complication of ventriculoatrial shunts in adults: Case report. J Neurosurg 35:348, 1971.
8. Adeloye A: Spontaneous extrusion of the abdominal tube through the umbilicus complicating peritoneal shunt for hydrocephalus. J Neurosurg 38:758, 1973.
9. Oi S, Shose Y, Asano N, Oshio T, Matsumoto S: Intragastric migration of a ventriculoperitoneal shunt catheter. Neurosurgery 21:255, 1987.
10. Danismend N, Kuday C: Unusual complication of ventriculoperitoneal shunt. Neurosurgery 22:798, 1988.
11. Patel CD, Matloub H: Vaginal perforation as a complication of ventriculoperitoneal shunt. J Neurosurg 38:761, 1973.
12. Pierce KR, Loeser JD: Perforation of the intestine by a Raimondi peritoneal catheter. J Neurosurg 43:112, 1975.
13. Cooper JR: Migration of ventriculoperitoneal shunt into the chest. J Neurosurg 48:146, 1978.
14. Gaudio R, DeTommasi A, Ochiogrosso M, Vailati G: Respiratory distress caused by migration of ventriculoperitoneal shunt catheter into the chest cavity: Report of a case and review of the literature. Neurosurgery 23:768, 1988.
15. Agha FP. Amendola, MA, Shirazi KK, Amendola BE, Chandler WF: Unusual abdominal complications of ventriculoperitoneal shunts. Radiology 146:323, 1983.
16. Touho H, Nakauchi M, Tasawa T, Nakagawa J, Karasaw J: Intrahepatic migration of a peritoneal shunt catheter: Case report. Neurosurgery 21:258, 1987.
17. Schulof LA, Worth RM, Kalsbeck JE: Bowel perforation due to peritoneal shunt: A report of seven cases and a review of the literature. Surg Neurol 3:265, 1975.
18. Venes J: Personal communication.
19. Hubschmann OR, Countee RW: Acute abdomen in children with infected ventriculoperitoneal shunts. Arch Surg 115:305, 1980.
20. Keen PE, Weitzner S: Inflammatory pseudotumor of mesentery: A complication of ventriculoperitoneal shunt: Case report. J Neurosurg 38:371, 1973.
21. Grosfeld JL, Cooney DR, Smith J, Campbell RL: Intra-abdominal complications following ventriculoperitoneal shunt procedures. Pediatrics 54:791, 1974.
22. Grosfeld JL, Cooney DR: Inguinal hernia after ventriculoperitoneal shunt for hydrocephalus. J Pediatr Surg 9(30):311, 1974.
23. Moazam F, Glenn JD, Kaplan BJ, Talbert JL, Mickle JP: Inguinal hernias after ventriculoperitoneal shunt procedures in pediatric patients. Surg Gynecol Obstet 159:570, 1984.
24. Peterfy CG, Atri M: Intrahepatic abscess: A rare complication of ventriculoperitoneal shunt. AJR 155:894, 1990.
25. Fisher RA, Rodziewicz G, Selman WR, White RJ, Vibhakar SD: Liver abscess: Complication of a ventriculoperitoneal shunt. Neurosurgery 14:480, 1984.
26. Reddy SC: Subcapsular hepatic abscess: A rare complication of ventriculoperitoneal shunt. South Med J 80(10):1309, 1987.
27. Azimi F, Dinn WM, Naumann RA: Intestinal perforation: An infrequent complication of ventriculoperitoneal shunts. Radiology 12:701, 1976.
28. Rubin CR, Ghatak NR, Visudhipan P: Asymptomatic perforated viscus and gram-negative ventriculitis as a complication of valve-regulated ventriculoperitoneal shunts: Report of two cases. J Neurosurg 37:616, 1972.
29. Wilson CB, Bertan V: Perforation of the bowel complicating peritoneal shunt for hydrocephalus: Report of two cases. Am Surg 32:601, 1966.
30. Portnoy HD, Croissant PD: Two unusual complications of a ventriculoperitoneal shunt: Case report. J Neurosurg 39:775, 1973.
31. Gaskill SJ, Marlin AE: Pseudocysts of the abdomen associated with ventriculoperitoneal shunts: A report of twelve cases and a review of the literature. Pediatr Neurosci 15:23, 1989.
32. Bryant MS, Bremer AM, Tepas JJ, Mollitt DL, Nquyen TQ, Talbert JL: Abdominal complications of ventriculoperitoneal shunts: Case reports and review of the literature. Am Surg 54:50, 1988.
33. Hlavin ML, Mapstone TB, Gauderer MWL: Small bowel obstruction secondary to incomplete removal of a ventriculoperitoneal shunt: Case report. Neurosurgery 26:526, 1990.
34. Antunes ACM, Ribeiro TR: Spontaneous umbilical fistula from ventriculoperitoneal shunt drainage: Report of two cases. J Neurosurg 43:481, 1975.
35. Clarke CE, Pauls KS, Lye RH: Ventriculoperitoneal shunt procedure complicated by ureter obstruction: Case report. J Neurosurg 59:542, 1983.
36. Sakoda TH, Maxwell JA, Brackett CE: Intestinal volvulus secondary to a ventriculoperitoneal shunt. J Neurosurg 35:95, 1971.
37. Albright AL, Haines SJ, Taylor FH: Function of parietal and frontal shunts in childhood hydrocephalus. J Neurosurg 69:883, 1988.
38. Moss SD, Pattisapu JV, Walker ML: Use of peritoneal trocar in pediatric shunt procedures. In Marlin AE (ed): Concepts of Pediatric Neurosurgery. Volume 8:23, 1988.
39. Gardner P, Leipzig T, Phillips P: Infections of central nervous system shunts. Med Clin North Am 69:297, 1985.
40. McCullough DC, Kane JG, Presper JH, Wells M: Antibiotic prophylaxis in ventricular shunt surgery: I. Reduction of operative infection rates with methicillin. Child's Brain 7:182, 1980.
41. McLaurin RL: Infected cerebrospinal fluid shunts. Surg Neurol 1:191, 1973.
42. Odio C, McCracken GH, Nelson JD: CSF shunt infections in pediatrics: A seven-year experience. Am J Dis Child 138:1103, 1984.
43. George R, Leibrock L, Epstein M: Long-term analysis of cerebrospinal fluid shunt infections. J Neurosurg 51:804, 1979.
44. Rieder, MJ, Frewen TC, Del Maestro RF, Coyle A, Lovell, S: The effect of cephalothin prophylaxis on postoperative ventriculoperitoneal shunt infections. Can Med Asso J 136:935, 1987.
45. Venes JL: Control of shunt infection: Report of 150 consecutive cases. J Neurosurg 45:311, 1976.
46. Schoenbaum SC, Gardner P, Shillito J: Infections of cerebrospinal fluid shunt: Epidemiology, clinical manifestations, and therapy. J Infect Dis 131:543, 1975.
47. Wang EL, Prober CG, Hendrick BE, Hoffman HJ, Humphreys RP: Prophylactic sulfamethaxazole and trimethoprim in ventriculoperitoneal shunt surgery: A double-blind, randomized, placebo-controlled trial. JAMA 251:1174, 1984.
48. Forrest DM, Hole R, Wynne JM: Treatment of infantile hydrocephalus using the Holter valve: An analysis of 152 consecutive cases. Dev Med Child Neurol 11(Suppl):27, 1966.
49. Schurtleff DB, Christie D, Foltz EL: Ventriculoauriculostomy-associated infection: A 12-year study. J Neurosurg 35:686, 1970.
50. Ajir F, Levin AB, Duff TA: Effect of prophylactic methicillin in cerebrospinal fluid shunt infections in children. Neurosurgery 9:6, 1981.
51. Haines SJ, Taylor F: Prophylactic methicillin for shunt operations: Effects on incidence of shunt malfunction and infection. Child's Brain 9:10, 1982.
52. McLaurin RL: Treatment of infected ventricular shunts. Child's Brain 1:306, 1975.

53. Mori K, Raimondi AJ: An analysis of external ventricular drainage as a treatment for infected shunts. Child's Brain 1:243, 1975.
54. Overton MC, Snodgrass SR. Ventriculovenous shunts for infantile hydrocephalus: A review of five years' experience with this method. J Neurosurg 33:517, 1970.
55. Nelson JD: Cerebrospinal fluid shunt infections. Ped Infect Dis 3(Suppl 3):S30, 1984.
56. Marlin AE, Gaskill, SJ: The use of the surgical isolation bubble in the prevention of shunt infection. Concepts Pediatr Neurosurg 11:47, 1991.
57. Bayston R: Preliminary studies on the impregnation of Silastic elastomers with antimicrobial substances. Dev Med Child Neurol 18(Suppl 37):50, 1976.
58. Bayston R, Milner RDG: Antimicrobial activity of silicone rubber used in hydrocephalus shunts after impregnation with antimicrobial substances. J Clin Path 134:1057, 1981.
59. Raimondi AJ, Robinson JS, Kuwamura K: Complications of ventriculoperitoneal shunting and a critical comparison of the three-piece and one-piece systems. Child's Brain 3:321, 1977.
60. Weiss SR, Raskind R: Further experience with the ventriculoperitoneal shunt: Prophylactic antibiotics. Int Surg 53:300, 1970.
61. Bayston R: Antibiotic prophylaxis in shunt surgery. Dev Med Child Neurol 35(Suppl):99, 1975.
62. McCullough DC, Kane JG, Harleman G, Wells M: Antibiotic prophylaxis in ventricular shunt surgery: II. Antibiotic concentrations in cerebrospinal fluid. Child's Brain 7:190, 1980.
63. Rekate HL, Ruch T, Nulsen FE: Diphtheroid infections of cerebrospinal fluid shunts: The changing pattern of shunt infection in Cleveland. J Neurosurg 52:553, 1980.
64. Yu HC, Patterson RH: Prophylactic antimicrobial agents after ventriculoatriostomy for hydrocephalus. J Pediatr Surg 8:881, 1973.
65. O'Brien M, Parent A, Davis B: Management of ventricular shunt infections. Child's Brain 5:304, 1979.
66. Forward KR, Fewer HD, Stiver HG: Cerebrospinal fluid shunt infections: A review of 35 infections in 32 patients. J Neurosurg 59:389, 1983.
67. Yogev R, Davis AT: Neurosurgical shunt infections: A review. Child's Brain 6:74, 1980.
68. Perrin JCS, McLaurin RL: Infected ventriculoatrial shunts: A method of treatment. J Neurosurg 27:21, 1967.
69. Myers MG, Schoenbaum: Shunt fluid aspiration: An adjunct in the diagnosis of cerebrospinal fluid shunt infection. Am J Dis Child 129:220, 1975.
70. Bayston R: Hydrocephalus shunt infections and their treatment. J Antimicrob Chemother 15:259, 1985.
71. Bayston R, Penny SR: Excessive production of mucoid substance in Staphylococcus SIIA: A possible factor in colonisation of Holter shunts. Dev Med Child Neurol 14(Suppl 24):25, 1972.
72. Borges LF: Cerebrospinal fluid shunts interfere with host defenses. Neurosurgery 10:55, 1982.
73. Everett ED, Eickhoff TC, Simon RH: Cerebrospinal fluid shunt infections with anaerobic diphtheroids (Propionibacterium species). J Neurosurg 44:580, 1976.
74. Bayston R, Lari J: A study of the sources of infected colonised shunts: Dev Med Child Neurol 32(Suppl):16, 1974.
75. Holt RJ. Bacteriological studies on colonised ventriculoatrial shunts. Dev Med Child Neurol 22(Suppl):83, 1970.
76. Luthardt, T: Bacterial infections in ventriculoauricular shunt systems. Dev Med Child Neurol 22(Suppl):105, 1970.
77. Cohen SJ, Callaghan RP: A syndrome due to the bacterial colonization of Spitz-Holter valves: A review of five cases. Br Med J 5253:677, 1961.
78. Bruce AM, Lorber J, Shedden WIH, Zachary RB: Persistent bacteremia following ventriculocaval shunt operations for hydrocephalus in infants. Dev Med Child Neurol 5:461, 1963.
79. Nulsen FE, Becker DP: Control of hydrocephalus by valve-regulated shunt. J Neurosurg 26:362, 1967.
80. Nicholas JL, Kamal IM, Eckstein HB: Immediate shunt replacement in the treatment of bacterial colonization of Holter valves. Dev Med Child Neurol 22(Suppl):110, 1970.
81. Guevara JA, Zuccaro G, Trevisan A, Denoya CD: Bacterial adhesion to cerebrospinal fluid shunts. J Neurosurg 67:438, 1987.
82. Schimke RT, Black PH, Mark VH, Swartz MN: Indolent Staphylococcus albus or aureus bacteremia after ventriculoatriostomy. Role of foreign body in its initiation and perpetuation. N Engl J Med 264:264, 1961.
83. Wald SL, McLaurin RL: Cerebrospinal fluid antibiotic levels during treatment of shunt infections. J Neurosurg 52:41, 1980.
84. Mates S, Glaser J, Shapiro K: Treatment of cerebrospinal fluid shunt infections with medical therapy alone. Neurosurgery 11:781, 1982.
85. Frame PT, McLaurin RL: Treatment of CSF shunt infections with intrashunt plus oral antibiotic therapy. J Neurosurg 60:354, 1984.
86. James HE, Walsh JW, Wilson HD, Connor JD, Bean JR, Tibbs PA: Prospective randomized study of therapy in cerebrospinal fluid shunt infection. Neurosurgery 7:459, 1980.
87. James HE, Wilson HD, Connor JD, Walsh JW: Intraventricular cerebrospinal fluid antibiotic concentrations in patients with intraventricular infections. Neurosurgery 10:50, 1982.
88. Wilson HD, Bean JR, James HE, Pendley MM: Cerebrospinal fluid antibiotic concentrations in ventricular shunt infections. Child's Brain 4:74, 1978.
89. Weiss MH, Kurze T, Nulsen FE: Antibiotic neurotoxicity: Laboratory and clinical study. J Neurosurg 41:486, 1974.
90. Fossieck B Jr, Parker RH: Neurotoxicity during intravenous infusion of penicillin: A review. J Clin Pharmacol 14:504, 1974.
91. Scarff TB, Nelson PB, Reigel DH: External drainage for ventricular infection following cerebrospinal fluid shunts. Child's Brain 4:129, 1978.
92. McLone DG, Czyewski D, Raimondi AJ, Sommers RC: Central nervous system infections as a limiting factor in the intelligence of children with myelomeningocele. Pediatrics 70:338, 1982.
93. Venes J: Mental Retardation in Children with Myelomeningocele: An Acquired Disease? Presented at the American Association of Neurological Surgeons, Pediatric Section, New York, December, 1980.
94. Carteri A, Longatti PL, Gerosa M, et al.: Complications due to incongruous drainage of shunt operations. Adv Neurosurg 8:199, 1980.
95. Epstein F, Lapras C, Wisoff JH: Slit-ventricle syndrome: Etiology and treatment. Pediatr Neurosci 14:5, 1988.
96. Faulhauer K, Schmitz P: Overdrainage phenomena in shunt-treated hydrocephalus. Acta Neurochir (Wein) 45:89, 1978.
97. Collman H, Mauersberger W, Mohr G: Clinical observations and CSF absorption studies in the slit ventricle syndrome. Adv Neurosurg 8:183, 1980.
98. Epstein F, Marlin AE, Wald A: Chronic headaches in the shunt-dependent adolescent with near normal ventricular volume: Diagnosis and treatment. Neurosurgery 3:351, 1978.
99. Epstein F: Increased intracranial pressure in hydrocephalic children with functioning shunts: A complication of shunt dependency. Concepts Pediatr Neurosurg 4:119, 1983.
100. Hyde-Rowan MD, Rekate HL, Nulsen FE: Reexpansion of previously collapsed ventricles. The slit ventricle syndrome. J Neurosurg 56:536, 1982.
101. Obana WG, Raskin NH, Cogen PH, Szymanski JA, Edwards MSB: Antimigraine treatment for slit ventricle syndrome. Neurosurgery 27:760, 1990.
102. Holness RO, Hoffman HJ, Hendrick EB: Subtemporal decompression for the slit-ventricle syndrome after shunting in hydrocephalic children. Child's Brain 5:137, 1979.
103. Wisoff JH, Epstein FJ: Diagnosis and treatment of the slit ventricle syndrome. Concepts Pediatr Neurosurg 11:79, 1991.
104. Abbott R, Epstein FJ, Wisoff JH: Chronic headache associated with a functioning shunt: Usefulness of pressure monitoring. Neurosurgery 28:72, 1991.
105. Laws ER, Niedermyer E: EEG findings in hydrocephalic patients with shunt procedures. Electoenceph Clin Neurophysiol 29:325, 1970.
106. Graebner RW, Celsia CG: EEG findings in hydrocephalus and their relation to shunting procedures. Electroenceph Clin Neurophysiol 35:517, 1973.

107. DiRocco C, Iannelli A, Pallini R, et al.: Epilepsy and its correlation with cerebral ventricular shunting procedures in infantile hydrocephalus. J Pediatr Neurosci 1:255, 1985.

108. Dan NG, Wade MJ: The incidence of epilepsy after ventricular shunting procedures. J Neurosurg 65:19, 1986.

109. Hack CH, Enrile BG, Donat JF, Kosnik E: Seizures in relation to shunt dysfunction in children with myelomeningocele. J Pediatr 116:57, 1990.

110. Bartoshesky LE, Haller J, Scott RM, et al.: Seizures in children with myelomeningocele. Am J Dis Child 193:400, 1985.

111. Slavin ML, Rosenthal AD: Chiasmal compression caused by a catheter in the suprasellar cistern. Am J Ophthalmol 105:560, 1988.

112. Coppeto JR, Gahm NH: Bitemporal hemianoptic scotoma: A complication of intraventricular catheter. Surg Neurol 8:361, 1977.

113. Corbett JJ: Neuro-ophthalmologic complications of hydrocephalus and shunting procedures. Sem Neurol 6:111, 1986.

114. Hoffman HJ, Hendrick EB, Humphreys RP: Metastasis via ventriculoperitoneal shunt in patients with medulloblastoma. J Neurosurg 44:562, 1976.

115. Jimenez-Jimenez FJ, Gasrzo-Fernandez C, De Inovencio-Arocena J, Perez-Sotelo M, Castro-DeCastro P, Salinero-Paniagua E: Extraneural metastases from brainstem astrocytoma through ventriculoperitoneal shunt. J Neurol Neurosurg Psychiatry 54(3):281, 1991.

116. Wolf A, Cowen D, Stewart WB: Glioblastoma with extraneural metastases by way of a ventriculo-pleural anastamosis. Trans Am Neurol Assoc 79:140, 1954.

117. Triolo PJ, Schulz EE: Metastatic germinoma (pinealoma) via a ventriculoperitoneal shunt. AJR 135:854, 1980.

118. Kimura N, Namiki T, Wada T, Sasano N: Peritoneal implantation of endodermal sinus tumor of the pineal region via a ventriculoperitoneal shunt: Cytodiagosis with immunocytochemical demonstration of alpha-fetoprotein. Acta Cytol 28:143, 1984.

119. Berger MS, Baumeister B, Geyer JR, Milstein J, Kaney PM, LeRoux PD: The risks of metastases from shunting in children with primary central nervous system tumor. J Neurosurg 74:872, 1991.

120. Hoffman HJ, Duffner PK: Extraneural metastases of central nervous system tumors. Cancer 56:1778, 1985.

121. Anderson H: Craniosynostosis as a complication after operation for hydrocephalus. Acta Paediatr Scand 55:192, 1966.

122. Hoffman NJ, Tucker HJ: Cephalocranial disproportion. A complication of the treatment of hydrocephalus in children. Child's Brain 2:167, 1976.

123. Cuisimano MD, Meffe FM, Gentili F, Sermer M: Ventriculoperitoneal shunt malfunction during pregnancy. Neurosurgery 27:969, 1990.

124. Houston CS, Clein LJ: Ventriculoperitoneal shunt malfunction in a pregnant patient with myelomeningocele. Can Med Asso J 141:701, 1989.

125. Wisoff JH, Kratzert KJ, Handwerker SM, Epstein F, Young BK: Management of hydrocephalic women during pregnancy. Concepts Pediatr Neurosurg 11:60, 1991.

126. Ivan LP, Choo SH, Ventureyra ECG: Complications of ventriculoatrial and ventriculoperitoneal shunts in a new children's hospital. Can J Surg 23:566, 1980.

127. Little JR, Rhoton AL, Mellinger JF: Comparison of ventriculoperitoneal and ventriculoatrial shunts for hydrocephalus in children. Mayo Clin Proc 47:396, 1972.

128. Emery JL, Hilton HB: Lung and heart complications of the treatment of hydrocephalus by ventriculoauriculostomy. Surgery 50:309, 1966.

129. Horowitz NH, Rizzoli HV: Postoperative Complications of Intracranial Neurological Surgery. Baltimore, William & Wilkins, 1982, p 394.

130. Wald SL, McLaurin RL: Shunt-associated glomerulonephritis. Neurosurgery 3:146, 1978.

131. Aoki N: Lumboperitoneal shunt: Clinical applications, complications and comparison with ventriculoperitoneal shunt. Neurosurgery 26:998, 1990.

132. Nulsen FE, Rekate HL: Results of treatment for hydrocephalus as a guide to future management. In McLaurin RL, Schut L, Venes JL, Epstein F: Pediatric Neurosurgery. New York, Grune & Stratton, 1982, pp 229–241.

133. Young HF, Nulsen FE, Weiss MH, et al.: The relationship of intelligence and cerebral mantle in treated infantile hydrocephalus (IQ potential in hydrocephalic children). Pediatrics 52:38, 1973.

134. Oberbauer RW: The significance of morphological details for the developmental outcome in infantile hydrocephalus. Child's Nerv Syst 1:329, 1985.

Chapter 15

CONGENITAL CSF ANOMALIES OF THE POSTERIOR FOSSA

TIMOTHY B. MAPSTONE, M.D.

This chapter will focus on the diagnosis and management of posterior fossa CSF collections. These collections of fluid pose a stiff diagnostic and therapeutic challenge to any neurosurgeon. The restricted area of the posterior fossa with its many vital structures and often aberrant anatomy in the face of congenital anomalies makes it critical that the correct diagnosis be made. Once a diagnosis is in hand the best treatment, which may be no intervention, follows directly.

This chapter will cover arachnoid cysts and neuroepithelial cysts, the Dandy-Walker malformation, trapped fourth ventricle, pulsion diverticulum, mega cisterna magna, and ex vacuo states of the posterior fossa. Other chapters in this text will deal with other anomalies of the posterior fossa.

ARACHNOID AND NEUROEPITHELIAL CYSTS

Although a number of theories have been put forth postulating the etiology of arachnoid cysts, the most compelling suggest a congenital origin. Classically, arachnoid cysts are described as being formed by a splitting of the arachnoid membrane with layers comprised of thickened fibroconnective tissue. Rarely is there evidence of hemorrhage or inflammation. The normal trabeculation of the subarachnoid space is not present, and to date there is no good explanation why these cysts enlarge and cause mass effect.[1-4] At times neuroepithelial (glioependymal) cysts appear grossly as arachnoid cysts. However, neuroepithelial cysts are lined with a low cuboidal-to-columnar epithelium. This lining is heterogeneous and may have cilia, basement membrane, intercellular junctions, and, at times, underlying glial cells. In spite of a differing light microscopic appearance, there does not appear to be any difference in treatment or prognosis between arachnoid and neuroepithelial cysts.

Cysts arising in the posterior fossa represent 30 to 40 per cent of reported locations. It is believed that they are more likely to occur in infants and to be symptomatic than are the more common supratentorial cysts. However, as neuro-imaging has become more accessible and sophisticated, many lesions are found earlier, when asymptomatic or minimally symptomatic. Cysts of the posterior fossa generally present with signs and symptoms of increased intracranial pressure owing either to a secondary hydrocephalus or to mass effect from a large cyst.[5-8] Asymmetry of the skull may be present. Scalloping and thinning of the skull in the area of the cyst suggest locally elevated pressures. Cysts of the cerebellopontine angle often present with focal neurologic dysfunction, suggesting a tumor in that area[9] (Fig. 15-1). Cysts can also cause effects at a distance or very subtle abnormalities. A quadrigeminal plate area cyst has been known to cause tonsillar herniation leading to a cervical spinal cord syrinx, which resolved after the cyst was drained[10] (Fig. 15-2). The mechanism was thought to be the same as that seen with a Chiari I malformation. A giant prepontine cyst in a newborn caused prolongation of brainstem auditory evoked reponses (BAERs) which normalized when the cyst was drained[11] (Fig. 15-3). Thorough investigations need to be carried out if treatment is to be predicated upon the presence or absence of symptoms or the potential for abrupt or further deterioration.

Controversy over treatment arises in a child with a totally asymptomatic cyst. Although some neurosurgeons feel that these lesions may be more susceptible

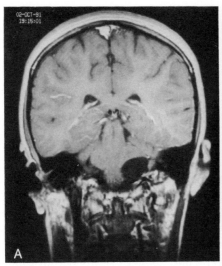

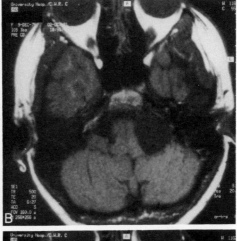

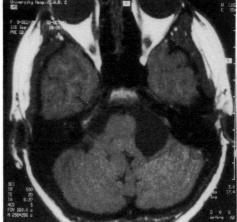

FIGURE 15–1. *A, B,* and *C,* MRI images of a large C-P angle cyst presenting with tinnitus and seventh nerve weakness.

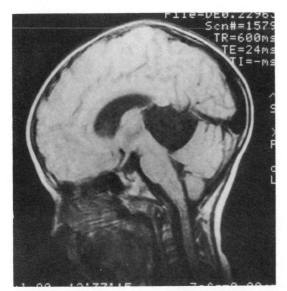

FIGURE 15–2. MRI of large supracerebellar cyst causing dysconjugate gaze. This type of cyst may cause syringomyelia if the tonsils are herniated as in a Chiari I malformation.

to hemorrhage from neurotrauma and thus should be treated expectantly, this posture seems overly aggressive. Currently we recommend careful follow-up, with surgery withheld until the cyst expands or the child becomes symptomatic. Surgery is warranted when there are neurologic symptoms and signs clearly referable to the cyst. Neuro-imaging findings suggesting local pressure phenomena such as scalloping or thinning of bone or significant compression of surrounding structures, even in the absence of findings on neurologic examination, may lead to surgical intervention.

The choice of the most appropriate surgical treatment for posterior fossa cysts is not clear-cut. A strong argument can be put forth that a cystoperitoneal shunt (usually with a low pressure valve) should be the initial procedure for a number of reasons. It is generally safe, it is reported to have a higher initial success rate than other surgical options, and even if the shunt eventually malfunctions, it may not need revision if the cyst has obliterated itself.[12] Proponents for cyst excision, which in reality is a wide connection of the cyst space to the subarachnoid space, argue that in the limited confines of the posterior fossa with its many important structures, a direct visual approach is safer. They also argue that the majority of the posterior fossa cysts do not obliterate when collapsed and that proximal shunt failure rate in posterior fossa cysts is high, necessitating multiple revisions.[13–16] Since most of the data on the effectiveness of cystoperitoneal shunts is related to the far more common temporal fossa cysts, there is not enough information to convincingly put the argument to rest. Our experience at Rainbow Babies and Chil-

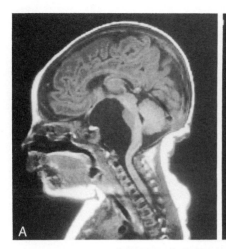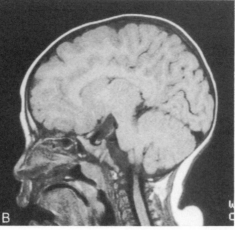

FIGURE 15–3. *A,* An MRI image of newborn with gigantic prepontine glial-ependymal cyst presenting with delayed conduction on BAER. *B,* MRI of same child one year after operation, showing resolution of cyst after craniotomy for fenestration. BAER is now normal.

drens Hospital has been that for posterior fossa arachnoid/neuroepithelial cysts, wide fenestration has been both safe and effective in the last eight patients. A much larger current data base is needed in order to resolve this issue.

DANDY-WALKER CYST

A relatively common posterior fossa cystic abnormality is seen with the Dandy-Walker syndrome or complex. The neuropathologic features of this syndrome are complete or incomplete agenesis of the vermis with the posterior vermis always involved. If vermian agenesis is incomplete, the remnant is rotated anteriorly. There is dilation of the fourth ventricle and enlarged posterior fossa classically with the torcula present in its fetal position at the skull vertex.[17] Although early characterizations required that the foramina of Luschka and Magendie be atretic, this does not happen to be the case in the majority of patients. The syndrome has a number of other associated anomalies such as hydro-

cephalus, agenesis of the corpus callosum, nuclear dysplasia of the brainstem, and other cerebral and cerebellar heterotopias (Fig. 15–4).

With the advent of MRI scanning, the diagnosis of Dandy-Walker cyst is generally straightforward. The presence of a large posterior fossa with an elevated torcula and complete or partial absence of the vermis is diagnostic. Cysts of the supracerebellar space can be confusing, but a sagittal image should indicate the floor of the Dandy-Walker cyst is the fourth ventricle while the floor of a supracerebellar cyst is the cerebellum. Other posterior fossa cysts can be excluded by careful review of multiple MRI images. Inferior-posterior cysts can elevate and rotate the vermis anteriorly and, on axial view, suggest a Dandy-Walker cyst with communication of the fourth ventricle. Sagittal images will almost always reveal the Dandy-Walker imposter.[18]

A number of authors, after careful review of MRI and autopsy studies of patients with posterior fossa cysts, have suggested an alternative classification based on the theory that Dandy-Walker malformations, Dandy-Walker variant, and mega cisterna magna represent embryologic abnormalities on a continuum and

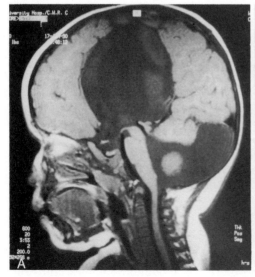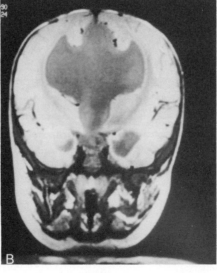

FIGURE 15–4. Sagittal *(A)* and axial *(B)* MRI showing large Dandy-Walker cyst with remaining vermis rotated anteriorly. Also note a partial agenesis of the corpus callosum.

should be considered part of a Dandy-Walker complex. This categorization depends upon the amount of cerebellar and vermian hypoplasia in the case of Dandy-Walker or cerebellar atrophy in the case of mega cisterna magna.[15, 19] Once the diagnosis is secured, consideration for treatment begins. A significant number (up to 20 per cent) of patients with Dandy-Walker cyst are asymptomatic from their cyst or hydrocephalus and consequently require no therapy.[20] More commonly, patients became symptomatic from an associated hydrocephalus, which requires treatment. Less often, the symptoms are related to the posterior fossa cyst and are usually seen in older children. Patients can present in infancy with increasing head size, bulging fontanelle, and delays in attaining milestones. There is currently no role for a direct surgical attack on the cyst with the goal of re-establishing normal CSF pathways. This has been tried since Dandy first described the entity and has met with virtually no success.

The main controversy surrounding treatment has to do with the placement of the proximal end of the shunt. Recent literature does not unequivocally support a single approach, but rather points out that about half the children requiring shunts do well with a single proximal catheter placed either in the lateral ventricle or in the posterior fossa cyst, while about half the shunted children require a combined ventriculocystoperitoneal shunt. It has been observed by a number of authors that in proximal shunt failure it is most likely to be the cyst catheter that occludes. If the decision is made to place a ventriculocystoperitoneal shunt either initially or in the case of secondary compartmentalization, the two compartments should be communicated via the shunt tubing and the valve placed distal to the "Y" connector. This measure will prevent intracranial pressure differentials should the shunt fail at the valve or distally.[21–24]

If the decision is made to shunt a single compartment, it should be kept firmly in mind that almost 40 per cent of individuals with a single shunt compartmentalize and require the other CSF space to be shunted (Fig. 15–5). There does not appear to be a clear preference as to which compartment to shunt initially, although there are isolated reports of third ventriculostomy being successful in patients with a cysto-peritoneal (C-P) shunt who eventually isolate their lateral ventricles. This may provide a rationale for initially shunting the cyst in anticipation of re-establishing CSF drainage from the lateral ventricles, if needed, by directly communicating them with the subarachnoid space.[25]

The failure rate of shunts in Dandy-Walker patients is comparable to that in other hydrocephalus syndromes. Outcome as measured by intelligence is variable due to other CNS anomalies associated with the malformation. Children with well-controlled hydrocephalus and no significant CNS anomalies can do very well. At our institution, over 50 per cent of Dandy-Walker patients are in the mainstream at school. We have two sets of twins, wherein one twin has Dandy-Walker syndrome and the other does not, and both twins are developing normally. This anecdotal evidence in conjunction with recent outcome studies suggests that aggressive control of CSF abnormalities in children with Dandy-Walker syndrome may have a salutary effect on outcome.[26–29]

ISOLATED FOURTH VENTRICLE

Analagous to the earlier discussion on Dandy-Walker cysts, a similar phenomenon can occur in isolated fourth ventricular hydrocephalus. Patients with hydrocephalus adequately treated by a ventriculoperitoneal shunt can develop a secondary aqueductal stenosis, presumably as a result of the diminished flow through the aqueduct of Sylvius. Generally this causes no problem when the CSF output of the fourth ventricle is handled in the subarachnoid space of the posterior

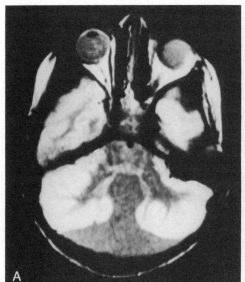
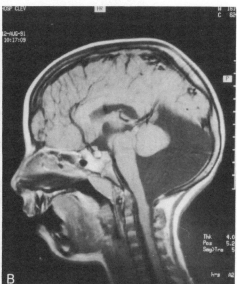

FIGURE 15–5. *A* and *B*, Axial *(A)* and sagittal *(B)* MRI showing Dandy-Walker cyst. Note the very narrow aqueduct of Sylvius. This child eventually required a V-C-P shunt after a VP shunt failed to relieve her occipital headaches.

fossa and spinal cord. There is a subset of patients, however, who develop a symptomatically enlarged fourth ventricle. The signs and symptoms of this are protean, but generally are those of a mass lesion in the posterior fossa with nystagmus, lower cranial nerve dysfunction, at times motor symptoms, and rarely cardiopulmonary arrest (Fig. 15–6). A detailed understanding of the pathophysiology leading to an isolated ventricle is lacking, and thus it is difficult to predict which patients are likely to develop this syndrome. Most reported cases occur in patients whose hydrocephalus is due to, or associated with, an inflammatory process of the meninges (e.g., hemorrhage, infection) or a Chiari II malformation. Presumably these not only are more likely to lead to secondary aqueductal stenosis

but, in addition, either prohibit CSF outflow from the fourth ventricle or prevent absorption once the CSF has exited the fourth ventricle.[30–34]

The obvious treatment is decompression of the fourth ventricle, generally by a ventriculostomy. This is especially dangerous in children with a Chiari II malformation and its small posterior fossa with aberrant anatomy of vital structures and venous sinuses. In this situation, cannulation of the fourth ventricle may need to be done as part of a Chiari decompression. Others have suggested that in the presence of a large tentorial notch, as seen in patients with Chiari II, a catheter can be passed, under ultrasound guidance, through the supratentorial compartment into the fourth ventricle.[35] Placement of a fourth ventricular cannula in the ab-

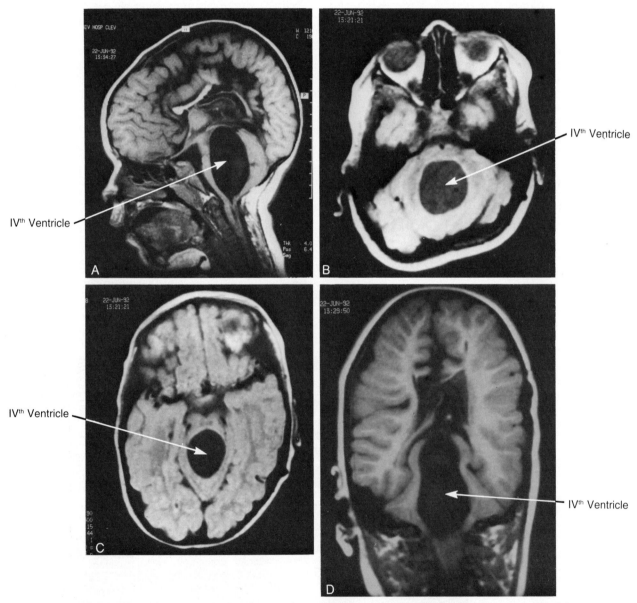

FIGURE 15–6. MRI of trapped fourth ventricle in a patient with spina bifida. She presented with left upper extremity monoparesis. *A,* Sagittal image–midline. *B,* Axial image at level of pons. *C,* Axial image at level of cerebral peduncle. *D,* Coronal image at level of posterior corpus callosum. IV Vent-fourth ventricle.

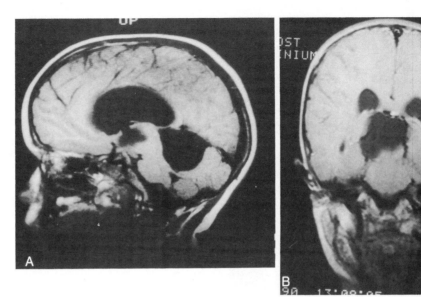

FIGURE 15–7. A and B, MRI of what appears to be a large supracerebellar cyst associated with hydrocephalus. This was believed to be a pulsion diverticulum of the right lateral ventricle, which resolved with a VP shunt.

sence of the Chiari malformation, while technically less demanding, can still lead to complications. It is difficult to devise a trajectory and catheter length which, once the ventricle has been drained, will not leave the patient with an overly long or short catheter. A catheter that is too short will malfunction, and one that is too long may cause neurologic dysfunction by compression or irritation of surrounding brainstem structures. Some have proposed placing this catheter under CT guidance to minimize such problems.[24] When not faced with shunting an isolated fourth ventricle in a Chiari II setting, it is possible at times to utilize a lumboperitoneal shunt once it has been proved that the fourth ventricle communicates with the lumbar subarachnoid space. This approach needs to be considered in the light of recent reports outlining a higher than previously expected complication rate for lumboperitoneal shunts, especially with respect to inducing tonsillar herniation. It is possible that an isolated fourth ventricle, when compounded by iatrogenic tonsillar herniation and arachnoidal adhesions further limiting CSF outflow, could lead to development of syringomyelia.

PULSION DIVERTICULUM

This is a rare cause of a posterior fossa cyst which occurs in relatively advanced hydrocephalus. As ventricular dilation progresses, the thinned ventricular wall may dehisce into the adjacent subarachnoid space, albeit separated from it by its intact pial membrane (Fig. 15–7). These diverticula occur commonly in the inferomedial wall of the atria, the suprapineal recess, and the area of the superior posterior fossa through the incisura, causing downward displacement of the cerebellum. This entity may be confused with a true supracerebellar cyst, which may also occur in the presence of hydrocephalus. Although the predominant clinical

picture is that of hydrocephalus, cerebellar signs may also be present, further confusing the diagnosis. The treatment of this entity is different from that of a true supracerebellar cyst since, in the case of a pulsion diverticulum of the lateral ventricle, a ventriculoperitoneal shunt will decompress not only the hydrocephalus but the posterior fossa cyst as well. Although contrast ventriculography will usually determine the presence of a pulsion diverticulum, other noninvasive neuroimaging means are useful. As mentioned earlier, the hydrocephalus is usually severe. High-resolution CT or detailed MRI may allow one to identify the breach in the medial ventricular wall. In addition, others have found that the addition of an ipsilateral shortening of the tentorial band as seen axially, a focal defect in the tentorial band seen coronally, dropping of the ventric-

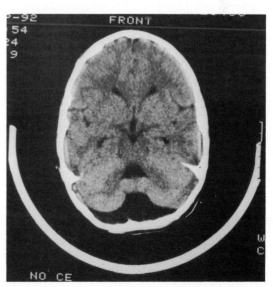

FIGURE 15–8. Axial CT showing typical appearance of enlarged cisterna magna.

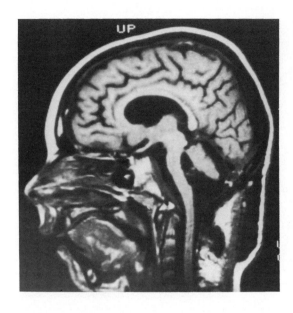

FIGURE 15–9. Large posterior fossa cyst in a developmentally delayed child with deterioration suggesting brainstem compression. This turned out to be due to an unnamed cerebellopontomedullary degeneration syndrome.

ular wall over the tentorium with CSF continuity, septa separating the diverticulum from surrounding CSF, and displacement of the deep structures of the third ventricular area further confirm the diagnosis.[35–39]

MEGA CISTERNA MAGNA, EX VACUO CYSTS

This final section deals with commonly seen posterior fossa CSF collections that do not require treatment since they are due to tissue absence and do not cause compression. These collections can range from a mildly enlarged cisterna magna (Fig. 15–8) to a picture suggesting severe cerebellar aplasia reminiscent of a Dandy-Walker cyst. This phenomenon can usually be differentiated from cysts requiring treatment by the relative paucity of symptoms and/or the absence of neuroimaging findings suggesting CNS compression or locally increased intracranial pressure, all of which are usually present in patients requiring therapy. In patients with primary cerebellar deterioration causing a severe loss of tissue and active neurologic deterioration, diagnosis of a nontreatable entity can be difficult, especially in the face of a concerned family with a worsening child (Fig. 15–9). In those circumstances, more invasive studies such as ventriculography or ICP measurements from the posterior fossa may put the issue to rest if careful review of high-quality MRI and CT images are unable to do so.[15, 40]

SUMMARY

Although symptomatic posterior fossa cysts have been described in detail since the beginnings of neurosurgery, we have benefited greatly in the understanding and treatment of these lesions as a result of vastly improved neuro-imaging and surgical therapies. These lesions are not an extremely common part of a neurosurgeon's practice. Nonetheless, an early accurate diagnosis leading to appropriate therapy, be it surgical treatment or observation, will often lead to a rewarding outcome. Controversies continue regarding the etiology and best surgical treatment of this diverse group of pathologies, and the thoughtful neurosurgeon is in a unique position to help resolve these issues.

REFERENCES

1. Friede RL: Developmental Neuropathology, 2nd ed. New York, Springer-Verlag, 1989, pp 209–213.
2. James HE: Encephalocele, dermoid sinus, and arachnoid cyst. *In* McLaurin RL, et al.: Pediatric Neurosurgery, 2nd ed. Philadelphia, WB Saunders, 1989, pp 103–106.
3. DiRocco C, DiTrapania G, et al.: Infratentorial arachnoid cysts in children. Child's Brain 8:119, 1981.
4. Rengachary SS, Watanabe I: Ultrastructure and pathogenesis of intracranial arachnoid cysts. J Neuropathol Exp Neurol 40:61, 1981.
5. Little JR, Gomez MR, MacCarty CS: Infratentorial arachnoid cysts. J Neurosurg 39:380, 1973.
6. Basauri L, Selman JM: Intracranial arachnoid cysts. Child's Nerv Syst 8:101, 1992.
7. Arai H, Kiuoshi S: Posterior fossa cyst: Clinical, neuroradiological and surgical features. Child's Nerv Syst 7:156, 1991.
8. Iacono RP, Labadie EL, Johnstone SJ, Bendt TK: Symptomatic arachnoid cyst at the clivus drained stereotactically through the vertex. Neurosurgery 27(1):130, 1990.
9. Krisht AF, O'Brien MS: Acquired mirror-image cerebellopontine angle arachnoid cysts: Case report. Neurosurgery 30(5):798, 1992.
10. Banna M: Syringomyelia associated with posterior fossa cysts. Am J Neuroradiol 9(5):867, 1988.
11. Warf BC, Mapstone TB: Ventral brainstem compression from a subarachnoid ependymal cyst. Child's Nerv Syst 6:255, 1990.
12. Harsh GR, IV, Edwards MSB, Wilson CB: Intracranial arachnoid cysts in children. J Neurosurg 64:835, 1986.
13. McLone DSG, Naidich TP, Cunningham T: Posterior fossa cysts: Management and outcome. Concepts Pediatr Neurosurg 7:134, 1987.
14. Bindal AK, Stoors BB, McLone DG: Occipital meningoceles in patients with the Dandy-Walker syndrome. Neurosurgery 28(6):844, 1991.

15. Barkovich AJ, Kjos BO, Norman D, Edwards MS: Revised classification of posterior fossa cysts and cystlike malformations based on the results of multiplanar MR imaging. Am J Roentgenol 153:1289, 1989.
16. Oberbauer RW, Haase J, Pucher R: Arachnoid cysts in children: A European cooperative study. Child's Nerv Syst 8:281, 1992.
17. Friede RL: Developmental Neuropathology, 2nd ed. New York, Springer-Verlag, 1989, pp 347–348.
18. Wolpert SM, Scott RM, Runge VM, Kwan ES: Difficulties in diagnosing congenital posterior fossa fluid collections after shunting procedures. Am J Neuroradiol 8(4):653, 1987.
19. Altman NR, Naidich TP, Braffman BH: Posterior fossa malformations. Am J Neuroradiol 13(2):691, 1992.
20. Bindal AK, Storrs BB, McLone DG: Management of the Dandy-Walker syndrome. Pediatr Neurosci 16(3):163, 1990–91.
21. Pascual-Castroviejo I, Velez A, Pascual-Pascual SI, Roche MC, Villarejo F: Dandy-Walker malformation: Analysis of 38 cases. Child's Nerv Syst 7(2):88, 1991.
22. Naidich TP, McLone DG: Radiographic classification and gross morphologic features of hydrocephalus. In Hoffman HJ, Epstein F (eds): Disorders of the Developing Nervous System: Diagnosis and Treatment. Boston, Blackwell Scientific Publications, 1986, pp 529–530.
23. Carmel PW, Antunes JL, Hilal SK, et al.: Dandy-Walker syndrome: Clinico-pathological features and re-evaluation of modes of treatment. Surg Neurol 8:132, 1977.
24. Rekate HL: Treatment of hydrocephalus. In McLaurin RL, et al.: Pediatric Neurosurgery, 2nd ed. Philadelphia, WB Saunders, 1989, pp 211–213.
25. Asai A, Hoffman HJ, Hendrick EB, Humphreys RP: Dandy-Walker syndrome: Experience at the Hospital for Sick Children, Toronto. Pediatr Neurosci 15(2):66, 1989.
26. Sawaya R, McLaurin RL: Dandy-Walker syndrome. Clinical analysis of 23 cases. J Neurosurg 55:89, 1981.
27. Hirsch J-F, Pierre-Kahn A, Renier D, Sainte-Rose C, Hoppe-Hirsch E: The Dandy-Walker malformation. A review of 40 cases. J Neurosurg 61:515, 1984.
28. Golden JA, Rourke LB, Bruce DA: Dandy-Walker syndrome and associated anomalies. Pediatr Neurosci 13:38, 1987.
29. Maria BL, Zinreich SJ, Carson BC, Rosenbaum AE, Freeman JM: Dandy-Walker syndrome revisited. Pediatr Neurosci 13:45, 1987.
30. Hawkins JC III, Hoffman HJ, Humphreys RP: Isolated fourth ventricle as a complication of ventricular shunting. Report of three cases. J Neurosurg 49(6):910, 1978.
31. Oi S, Matsumoto S: Pathophysiology of aqueductal obstruction in isolated IV ventricle after shunting. Child's Nerv Syst 2(6):282, 1986.
32. James HE: Spectrum of the syndrome of the isolated fourth ventricle in posthemorrhagic hydrocephalus of the premature infant. Pediatr Neurosurg 16(6):305, 1990–91.
33. Foltz EL, Shurtleff DB: Conversion of communicating hydrocephalus to stenosis or occlusion of the aqueduct during ventricular shunt. J Neurosurg 24:520, 1966.
34. Scotti G, Musgrave MA, Fitz CR, Harwood-Nash DC: The isolated fourth ventricle in children: A CT and clinical review of sixteen cases. AJNR 1:419, 1980.
35. Ruge JR, Dauser RC, Storrs BB: Posterior fossa cysts: supratentorial shunt placement with ultrasound guidance, Child's Nerv Syst 7:165, 1991.
36. Wakai S, et al: Diverticulum of the lateral ventricle causing cerebellar ataxia. Case report. J Neurosurg 59:895, 1983.
37. Wakai S, Narita J, Hashimoto K, Nagai M: Diverticulum of the lateral ventricle causing cerebellar ataxia. J Neurosurg 59:895, 1983.
38. Gilles FH, Gilles EE: Hydrocephalus in neonate, infant and child. In Hoffman HJ, Epstein F (eds): Disorders of the Developing Nervous System: Diagnosis and Treatment. Boston, Blackwell Scientific Publications, 1986, pp 560–561.
39. Naidich TP, McLone DG, Hahn YS, et al.: Atrial diverticula in severe hydrocephalus. AJNR 3:257, 1982.
40. Adam R, Greenberg JO: The mega cisterna magna. J Neurosurg 48:190, 1978.

Chapter 16

POSTHEMORRHAGIC HYDROCEPHALUS IN THE PREMATURE INFANT

CHARLES C. DUNCAN, M.D., and LAURA R. MENT, M.D.

Intraventricular hemorrhage (IVH), or hemorrhage into the germinal matrix tissues of the developing brain with possible rupture into the ventricular system and parenchyma, remains a major problem of preterm neonates.[1-3] IVH is believed to be attributable to alterations in cerebral blood flow to a damaged germinal matrix capillary bed.[4-7] Since the germinal matrix begins to involute following 34 weeks of gestation, germinal matrix and intraventricular hemorrhages (GMH/IVH) are lesions of preterm infants, and a recent study of 2928 neonates of <1500 gm birth weight demonstrated an incidence of GMH/IVH greater than 45 per cent.[1] Infants with GMH/IVH are more likely to develop seizures and hydrocephalus than their gestational age–matched peers without hemorrhage. Mortality rates are also higher for infants with GMH/IVH than for those without, and although the long-term neurodevelopmental outcome for infants with lower grades of hemorrhage remains unclear, most observers agree that infants with parenchymal hemorrhage are at higher risk for neurodevelopmental handicap.[2, 4, 7-9] Finally, neonates with GMH/IVH are at greater risk for associated periventricular leukomalacia, or infarction of the preterm brain, and the possibility that IVH represents a marker for cerebral insults of varying types must be considered.

The germinal matrix and the adjacent ventricular germinal zone are the site of proliferation of neuronal and glial precursors in the developing nervous system. During the late second and early third trimesters, they give rise to macroglia and microneurons by in situ mitosis.[10, 11] The germinal matrix is relatively large through 34 weeks of gestation, but almost completely involutes by 40 weeks. The capillary bed of the germinal matrix is composed of large irregular vessels with little evidence of basement membrane proteins or glial supporting structures.[12] These vessels represent the "watershed zone" of the ventriculofugal and ventriculopedal vessels of the developing brain and are not readily distinguishable as arterioles, venules, or capillaries.[13] In addition, Grunnet[12] has reported that the luminal areas of these vessels are significantly greater than those of cortical vessels of fetuses of the same gestational age. She hypothesized that the greater diameter of these vessels may permit greater pressure to be exerted on their walls, and thus they may be more susceptible to rupture.

Pathologically, germinal matrix hemorrhages and their associated intraventricular hemorrhages originate in the periventricular matrix zone located between the caudate nucleus and the thalamus at the level of, or slightly posterior to, the foramina of Monro.[4, 14] Neonates of less than 28 weeks of gestational age have been noted to experience hemorrhage in the germinal matrix overlying the body of the caudate nucleus, whereas neonates of greater gestational ages are more likely to experience hemorrhage in the germinal matrix at the head of the caudate nucleus at the level of the foramen of Monro. A small percentage of intraventricular hemorrhages in the preterm infant may also originate from the choroid plexus, a second cerebral region believed unable to autoregulate blood flow; in contrast, the choroid plexus is the most common site of intraventricular hemorrhage in full-term neonates.[15]

The neuropathologic consequences of IVH include germinal matrix destruction, periventricular hemorrhagic infarction, and posthemorrhagic hydrocephalus.[4, 16, 17] Germinal matrix destruction with secondary cystic formation is a common and expected feature of

Supported in part by NIH-NS 27116

GMH. In addition, 10 to 20 per cent of patients with GMH/IVH will suffer periventricular hemorrhagic infarction, also frequently called "hemorrhagic intracerebral involvement." Some investigators believe that the parenchymal involvement of insult readily visible by cranial ultrasonography represents a direct extension of hemorrhage from either the ventricular system or germinal matrix hemorrhage; others believe that these lesions represent venous infarction of the periventricular white matter. Both proposed mechanisms are dependent on increased intracranial, particularly intraventricular, pressure as a primary event. Distinguishing between the two lesions in vivo remains extremely difficult at this time, and it is likely that parenchymal lesions secondary to both mechanisms occur.

Posthemorrhagic hydrocephalus (PHH) has classically been described as secondary to a fibrous thickening of the meninges, particularly in the posterior fossa, with an obliterative arachnoiditis and obstruction of CSF flow through the normal subarachnoid pathways. This chemical arachnoiditis has been ascribed to the presence of blood and cellular debris in the ventricular CSF. Additionally, the shedding of cellular debris and red cells has been found to obstruct the aqueduct, resulting in an acquired aqueductal obstruction.

Periventricular leukomalacia (PVL) is a frequent neuropathologic accompaniment of GMH/IVH, but apparently is not caused by it. PVL is the generally symmetric injury of the periventricular white matter that is readily demonstrated as cystic lesions by cranial ultrasonography and at postmortem examination.[18] Frequently associated in risk factor studies with apneic, hypotensive, and other ischemic events, it has been reported in 25 to 50 per cent of infants with GMH/IVH and is believed to represent nonhemorrhagic infarction of the periventricular white matter watershed zone.[19, 20] The clinical correlate of PVL is spastic diplegia, although some infants with extensive cystic PVL may experience more generalized changes in tone.

The incidence of GMH/IVH increases as gestational age decreases, and as many as 50 per cent of infants of less than 25 to 26 weeks of gestation suffer GMH/IVH.[1, 21] In addition, although the incidence has been reported to vary from 20 to 45 per cent in large cohorts of infants of less than 34 weeks of gestational age, high-grade hemorrhages are more commonly found in very-low-birth-weight neonates.[22]

Hemorrhages have been reported within the first postnatal hour, and a significant number of hemorrhages occur by the sixth hour. Approximately half of all preterm infants who will ever develop GMH/IVH do so on the first postnatal day, and less than 5 per cent will experience hemorrhage after the fourth to fifth postnatal days (see Table 16–2).[9, 23–27] This risk period for GMH/IVH appears to be independent of gestational age.[21] Finally, some infants, and especially those with the earliest onset of GMH/IVH, will experience extension of hemorrhage over the first several postnatal days; this progression has been linked to clinical events such as pneumothoraces and seizures known to increase cerebral blood flow.[9, 23–27]

The risk factors for GMH/IVH appear to include both perinatal and postnatal events,[9, 28–30] and several authors have speculated that the pathophysiology of early-onset GMH/IVH in the first 8 to 12 postnatal hours may differ from that of later postnatal onset.[28, 31] Clinical events associated with GMH/IVH include respiratory distress syndrome, vigorous resuscitation, rapid volume re-expansion, hypoxemia, hypercarbia, acidosis, and the administration of sodium bicarbonate. In addition, bedside echoencephalography has permitted the demonstration of GMH/IVH after seizures and pneumothoraces in infants who were previously known to have no evidence of hemorrhage.[30, 32–34]

Perinatal risk factor studies for hemorrhage of very early onset in the first hours of life are less clear.[28, 31–38] Although some authors have suggested that vaginal delivery, labor, and intrapartum asphyxia may be related to the presence of early-onset GMH/IVH, these studies require further investigation.

The relationship between surfactant, respiratory distress syndrome, and the development of GMH/IVH must also be mentioned.[39] Although surfactant has been demonstrated to cause transient increases in cerebral blood flow,[40] most clinical studies have not noted an increase in GMH/IVH associated with its use.[39] In addition, because surfactant may diminish the acute hypoxemia and hypercarbia associated with respiratory distress syndrome, it may in fact contribute to the lower incidence of GMH/IVH which some centers are now reporting. Of equal concern, and perhaps more important for the neurodevelopmental outcome of these infants, is the observation of markedly diminished cerebral blood flow (CBF) after GMH/IVH. Both ^{133}Xe techniques for determining CBF[9, 41] and positron emission tomography[42] have demonstrated prolonged ischemia beyond the first postnatal week in preterm neonates with IVH.

Cranial ultrasonography, or echoencephalography, is now the method of choice for diagnosis of GMH/IVH in newborn special care units. A standard grading system, which was originally applied to the CT scan, has been adapted to cranial ultrasonographs.[43] Grade I or GMH describes blood in the germinal matrix only; grade II describes blood filling the lateral ventricles without distention; grade III describes blood filling and distending the ventricular system; and grade IV describes hemorrhages with parenchymal involvement. The most common site for parenchymal involvement with hemorrhage is the frontal region; many hemorrhages occur bilaterally. Less commonly, the caudate nuclei and occipital periventricular white matter regions are involved.

In most newborn intensive care units, echoencephalography is performed on postnatal days 2 to 3 and then repeated during the second postnatal week to routinely screen preterm neonates of 1500 gm or less or 34 weeks of gestational age for GMH/IVH and ventricular enlargement.

The clinical manifestations of GMH/IVH are varied.[44] In a significant percentage of cases, GMH/IVH is believed to be clinically silent, although infants with major hemorrhages may experience coma, seizures, abnormal eye findings, including dilated pupils and loss of eye movements, and changes in tone and reflexes. Persistent bradycardia and apneic spells may be secondary to increased intracranial pressure or alterations in cerebral blood flow to brainstem respiratory centers. Infants may be found to have significantly elevated values of blood glucose and evidence of inappropriate secretion of antidiuretic hormone. Finally, patients with large parenchymal hemorrhages frequently experience a persistent metabolic acidosis that is unresponsive to alkali therapy or pressor agents.

Infants with GMH/IVH are at risk for the development of posthemorrhagic hydrocephalus (PHH) and are known to have higher incidences of neonatal seizures and periventricular leukomalacia than do infants without hemorrhage. Mortality is clearly higher in groups of infants with hemorrhage, as compared with normal infants matched for birth weight or gestational age. Finally, most investigators agree that infants with parenchymal involvement of GMH/IVH are at high risk for neurodevelopmental handicap.[2, 4, 7–9]

Posthemorrhagic hydrocephalus[45] is the combination of ventriculomegaly, diagnosed by serial echoencephalographic studies, and increased intracranial pressure (defined as an opening pressure greater than 140 mm H_2O on either lumbar puncture or, if indicated, cerebral ventricular tap). Posthemorrhagic hydrocephalus is generally a communicating hydrocephalus with a block at the level of the arachnoid villi or, less commonly, at the foramina of Luschka and Magendie in the posterior fossa. Hydrocephalus results when the blood and protein in the CSF produce a chemical arachnoiditis, which may be transient or, less likely, permanent. A small percentage of infants with IVH will develop a noncommunicating hydrocephalus with a block at the level of the aqueduct secondary to an ependymal reaction similar to that of the arachnoid. Infants with the latter type of hydrocephalus will require neurosurgical intervention, whereas the treatment for neonates with communicating PHH is, at least initially, medical.

All infants with intraventricular blood require close ultrasonographic monitoring of ventricular size. These patients should undergo frequent head circumference measurements and cranial ultrasonography for determination of ventricular size. Since prolonged increased intracranial pressure may result in apnea, vomiting, lethargy, and ultimate optic atrophy, the intracranial pressure of infants with head circumferences crossing the expected growth curves and evidence for increasing

TABLE 16–2. TREATMENT ALTERNATIVES FOR COMMUNICATING POSTHEMORRHAGIC HYDROCEPHALUS

Serial lumbar punctures
Acetazolamide (25–100 mg/kg/day) and furosemide (2 mg/kg/day)
Ventriculostomy
Reservoir system
Valveless shunts
Standard shunt system

ventricular size should be checked. Once the diagnosis has been confirmed, treatment should be provided. Table 16–1 lists common signs and symptoms of posthemorrhagic hydrocephalus in the premature infant.

Several approaches to treatment for those infants with communicating hydrocephalus (Table 16–2) have been advocated. These include lumbar punctures with removal of cerebral spinal fluid to normalize intracranial pressure and frequent ultrasonographic checks of ventricular size. Acetazolamide (25 to 100 mg/kg/day) and furosemide (1 mg/kg/day) to decrease CSF production have been utilized as a temporizing measure. The side effects of acetazolamide include vomiting, lethargy, and electrolyte abnormalities, and infants treated with this medication should undergo frequent assessment of their metabolic status with serum electrolytes and bicarbonate measurements. Early operative strategies included ventriculostomy, reservoir systems, valveless shunts, and standard shunt systems. The presumed chemical meningitis causing PHH may resolve and represent a transient phenomenon. Serial lumbar punctures have been reported to resolve PHH in selected cases in 1 to 6 weeks. Persistent PHH clearly requires shunting. Probably related to the immune status of the preterm infant, shunt infection is a greater problem than in older individuals, with infection rates approaching 20 to 25 per cent in some series. Additionally, necrotizing enterocolitis may present difficulties in the distal location of the shunt system, necessitating an alternative location from the peritoneal cavity, such as the pleural space or vascular system.

For infants with evidence of noncommunicating hydrocephalus or intraparenchymal involvement of hemorrhage and shift of the cerebral midline, ventricular taps or the insertion of ventricular catheters with reservoirs are indicated early, and the placement of a ventriculoperitoneal shunt may ultimately be required (Table 16–3). The necessity for repeated ventricular taps suggests an associated porencephaly, but early shunt systems have frequently occluded because of high CSF protein and cellular debris. For this reason, several cen-

TABLE 16–1. SIGNS AND SYMPTOMS OF POSTHEMORRHAGIC HYDROCEPHALUS

Increasing occipital-to-frontal circumference
Tense anterior fontanelle
Pulse dips/bradycardia
Respirator dependence
Oxygen desaturations
Poor feeding
Lethargy

TABLE 16–3. TREATMENT ALTERNATIVES FOR NONCOMMUNICATING POSTHEMORRHAGIC HYDROCEPHALUS

Ventricular taps
Reservoir system
Early shunting

ters advocate reservoirs that may be regularly tapped and then later converted to functioning shunts.

The recent advent of flexible ventriculoscopes with capabilities for suction, irrigation, cautery, and assorted forceps offers the prospect of a wider range of early interventions: intraventricular protein may be lowered through irrigation, intraventricular septations fenestrated, and hemorrhages evacuated. Whether these approaches will lower the incidence of shunt dependency remains to be determined.

Figure 16–1 shows a series of head ultrasonograms on a female born at 28 weeks of gestation and weighing 1200 gm. This infant had an early, bilateral grade I hemorrhage which had extended to grade IV by 36 hours. She developed ventriculomegaly by day 5, and this progressed despite serial lumbar punctures. A res-

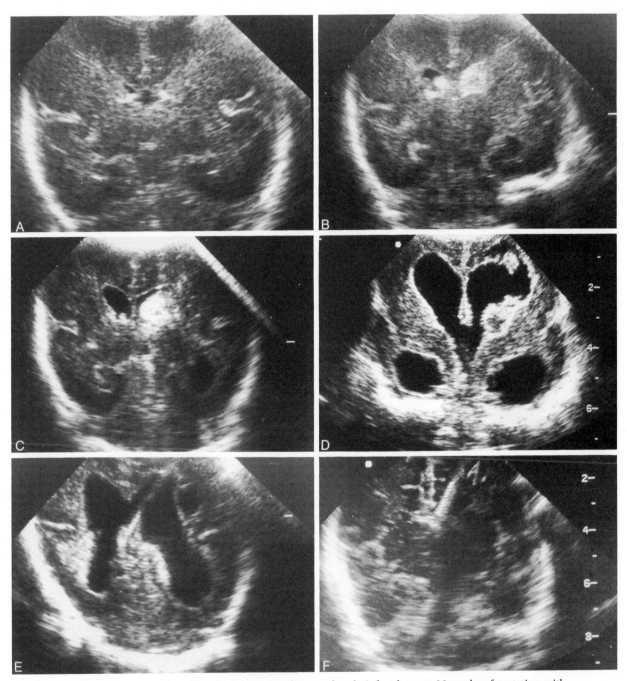

FIGURE 16–1. A series of head ultrasonographs on a female infant born at 28 weeks of gestation with birth weight of 1200 gm. *A*, At age 9 hours, this infant had an early hemorrhage, which was bilateral grade I. *B*, At age 36 hours, the hemorrhage had extended to grade IV. *C*, At age 5 days, ventriculomegaly. *D*, At age 24 days, progressive ventriculomegaly despite serial lumbar punctures. *E*, At age 36 days, reduction in ventricular size with reservoir system. *F*, At age 4 months, small ventricular size following shunt.

ervoir system was placed, since the protein ranged between 1 and 2 gm, and this partially controlled ICP and ventricular size. Once the protein decreased, she underwent ventriculoperitoneal shunting at 60 days with a resulting small ventricular size by 4 months. Ventriculoscopy at the time of shunt placement revealed complete resolution of the hemorrhage and cellular debris. At 4 months she had a normal neurologic examination for age and had a normal head size.

In many large series of preterm neonates, the incidence of motor handicaps appears to be low.[46–48] These abnormalities include spastic diplegia, hemiparesis, and, rarely, spastic quadriparesis. Most infants with spastic diplegia have neuro-imaging evidence of periventricular leukomalacia, but in general have normal head circumferences, no evidence of seizures, and cognitive scores within the normal range. Although many investigators believe that there are no differences in the developmental outcome of infants with grades I, II, or III IVH when compared with those with no known evidence of hemorrhage in the neonatal period, with or without PHH, recent data suggest that the rate of cognitive deficits may increase as the grade of IVH increases in this patient population.[2] Infants with parenchymal involvement of hemorrhage, or grade IV IVH, experience a wide range of outcomes; approximately 50 per cent of all neonates with grade IV IVH will experience motor and cognitive handicaps.[2, 44] For many of these neonates, the development of a porencephalic cyst follows the parenchymal blood resolution, and this can be easily demonstrated on CT scan and ultrasonogram. Finally, children with PHH are more likely to become shunt-independent over time than those with other forms of hydrocephalus presenting in the newborn period.

REFERENCES

1. Shankraran S, Bauer C, Bandstra E, Poland R, Edwards W, Onstad L, Wright E, Malloy M, Wright L: Intracranial hemorrhage (ICH) in 2928 <1500 g neonates. Pediatric Res 29:266A, 1991.
2. Leonard CH, Clyman RI, Piecuch RE, Juster RP, Ballard RA, Behle MB: Effect of medical and social risk factors on outcome of prematurity and very low birth weight. J Pediatr 116:620, 1990.
3. van de Bor M, Verloove-Vanhorick SP, Brand R, Keirse MJNC, Ruys JH: Incidence and prediction of periventricular-intraventricular hemorrhage in very preterm infants. J Perinat Med 15:333, 1987.
4. Volpe JJ: Intraventricular hemorrhage in the premature infant—current concepts. Part I. Ann Neurol 25:3, 1989.
5. Goddard J, Lewis RM, Alcala H, Zeller RS: Intraventricular hemorrhage—an animal model. Biol Neonate 37:39, 1980.
6. Ment LR, Stewart WB, Duncan CC, Scott DT, Lambrecht RL: Beagle puppy model of intraventricular hemorrhage: Effect of indomethacin on cerebral blood flow. J Neurosurg 58:857, 1983.
7. Perlman JM, Volpe JJ: Cerebral blood flow velocity in relation to intraventricular hemorrhage in the premature newborn infant. J Pediatr 100:956, 1982.
8. Krishnamoorthy KS, Kuban KCK, Leviton A, Brown ER, Sullivan KR, Allred EN: Periventricular-intraventricular hemorrhage. Sonographic localization, phenobarbital, and motor abnormalities in low-birth-weight infants. Pediatrics 85:1027, 1990.
9. Ment LR, Duncan CC, Ehrenkranz RA, et al.: Intraventricular hemorrhage of the preterm neonate: Timing and cerebral blood flow changes. J Pediatr 104:419, 1984.
10. Fujita S, Kitamura T: Origin of brain macrophages and the nature of the microglia. In Zimmerman H (ed): Progress in Neuropathology, vol III. New York, Grune & Stratton, 1976, pp 1–50.
11. Smart IHM: A pilot study of cell production by the ganglionic eminences of the developing mouse brain. J Anat 121:71, 1976.
12. Grunnet MRL: Morphometry of blood vessels in the cortex and germinal plate of premature neonates. Pediatr Neurol 5:12, 1989.
13. DeReuch J: The human periventricular arterial blood supply and the anatomy of cerebral infarctions. Eur Neurol 5:321, 1971.
14. Rorke LB: Pathology of Perinatal Brain Injury. New York, Raven Press, 1982, pp 13–18.
15. Donat JE, Okazaki H, Kleinberg F, et al.: Intraventricular hemorrhages in full-term and premature infants. Mayo Clin Proc 53:437, 1978.
16. Del Toro J, Louis PT, Goddard-Finegold J: Cerebrovascular regulation and neonatal brain injury. Pediatr Neurol 7:3, 1991.
17. Leech RW, Kohnen P: Subependymal and intraventricular hemorrhages in the newborn. Am J Pathol 77:465, 1974.
18. Armstrong DL, Saulas CD, Goddard-Finegold J: Neuropathologic findings in short term survivors of intraventricular hemorrhage. Am J Dis Child 141:617, 1987.
19. Rushton DI, Preston PR, Durbin GM: Structure and evolution of echo dense lesions in the neonatal brain. Arch Dis child 60:798, 1985.
20. Takashima S, Mito T, Ando Y: Pathogenesis of periventricular white matter hemorrhages in preterm infants. Brain Dev 8:25, 1986.
21. Ment LR, Oh W, Ehrenkranz, et al.: Risk factors for early intraventricular hemorrhage in low birth weight infants. J Pediatr 121:776, 1992.
22. Philip AGS, Allan WC, Tito AM, Wheeler LR: Intraventricular hemorrhage in preterm infants: Declining incidence in the 1980s. Pediatrics 84:797, 1989.
23. deCrespigny LC, Mackay R, Murton LJ, Roy RND, Robinson PH: Timing of neonatal cerebroventricular hemorrhage with ultrasound. Arch Dis Child 57:231, 1982.
24. Perlman JM, Volpe JJ: Cerebral blood flow velocity in relation to intraventricular hemorrhage in the premature newborn infant. J Pediatr 100:656, 1982.
25. Dolfin T, Skidmore MB, Fong KW, Hoskins EM, Shennan AT: Incidence, severity, and timing of subependymal and intraventricular hemorrhages in preterm infants born in a perinatal unit as detected by serial real-time ultrasound. Pediatrics 71:541, 1983.
26. McDonald MM, Koops BL, Johnson ML, Guggenheim MA, Rumack CM, Mitchell SA, Hathaway WE: Timing and antecedents of intracranial hemorrhage in the newborn. Pediatrics 74:32, 1984.
27. Beverley DW, Chance GW, Coates CF: Intraventricular haemorrhage—timing of occurrence and relationship to perinatal events. Br J Obstet Gynaec 91:1007, 1984.
28. Meidell R, Marinelli P, Pettett G: Perinatal factors associated with early-onset intracranial hemorrhage in premature infants. Am J Dis Child 139:160, 1985.
29. Clark CE, Clyman RI, Roth RS, et al.: Risk factor analysis of intraventricular hemorrhage in low-birth-weight infants. J Pediatr 99:625, 1981.
30. Cooke RWI, Rolfe P, Howart P: Apparent cerebral blood flow in newborns with respiratory disease. Dev Med Child Neurol 21:154, 1979.
31. Ment LR, Oh W, Philip AGS, Ehrkenranz RA: Risk factors for early neonatal germinal matrix/intraventricular hemorrhage (GMH/IVH). Pediatr Res 33:212a, 1992.
32. Milligan DWA: Failure of autoregulation and intraventricular haemorrhage in preterm infants. Lancet 1:896, 1980.
33. Hill A, Perlman MB, Volpe JJ: Relationship of pneumothorax to occurrence of intraventricular hemorrhage in the premature newborn. Pediatrics 69:144, 1982.
34. Hill A, Volpe JJ: Seizures, hypoxic-ischemic brain injury and intraventricular hemorrhage in the newborn. Ann Neurol 10:109, 1981.
35. Tejani N, Rebold B, Tuck S, et al.: Obstetric factors in the causation of early periventricular-intraventricular hemorrhage. Obstet Gynecol 64:510, 1984.

36. Anderson GD, Bada HS, Sibai BM, et al.: The relationship between labor and route of delivery in the preterm infant. Am J Obstet Gynecol 158:1382, 1988.

37. Horbar JD, Pasnick M, McAuliffe TL, Lucey JF: Obstetric events and risk of periventricular hemorrhage in premature infants. Am J Dis Child 137:678, 1983.

38. Leviton AL, Pagon M, Kuban KCK: Etiologic heterogeneity of intracranial hemorrhages in preterm newborns. Pediatr Neurol 4:274, 1988.

39. Leviton A, van Marter L, Kuban KCK: Respiratory distress syndrome and intracranial hemorrhage: Cause or association? Inferences from surfactant clinical trials. Pediatrics 84:915, 1989.

40. van de Bor M, Ma EJ, Walther FJ: Cerebral blood flow velocity after surfactant instillation in preterm infants. J Pediatr 118:285, 1991.

41. Lou HC, Lassen NA, Friis-Hansen B: Impaired autoregulation of cerebral blood flow in the distressed newborn infant. J Pediatr 94:118, 1979.

42. Volpe JJ, Herscovitch P, Perlman JM, et al.: Positron emission tomography in the newborn: Extensive impairment of regional cerebral blood flow with intraventricular hemorrhage and hemorrhagic intracerebral involvement. Pediatrics 72:589, 1983.

43. Papile LS, Burstein J, Burstein R, et al.: Incidence and evolution of the subependymal intraventricular hemorrhage: A study of infants with weights less than 1500 grams. J Pediatr 92:529, 1978.

44. Volpe JJ: Intraventricular hemorrhage in the premature infant—current concepts. Part II. Ann Neurol 25:109, 1989.

45. Ment LR, Duncan CC, Scott DT, et al.: Posthemorrhagic hydrocephalus. J Neurosurg 60:343, 1983.

46. Grogaard JB, Lindstrom DP, Parker RA, Culley B, Stahlman MT: Increased survival rate in very-low-birth-weight infants (1500 grams or less): No association with increased incidence of handicaps. J Pediatr 117:139, 1990.

47. Hack M, Fanaroff AA: Outcomes of extremely-low-birth-weight infants between 1982 and 1988. N Engl J Med 321:1642, 1989.

48. Kilbride HW, Daily DK, Claflin K, Hall RT, Maulik Dev, Grundy HO: Improved survival and neurodevelopmental outcome for infants less than 801 grams birth weight. Am J Perinatol 7:160, 1990.

PART III

TRAUMA

Chapter 17

MANAGEMENT OF SCALP INJURIES

JAMES T. GOODRICH, M.D., Ph.D.

The management of scalp injuries is as old as man. One can imagine that prehistoric man, upon dropping his child, learned very rapidly that early treatment was key to the child's survival. The principles that our ancestors learned for managing scalp injuries have remained the same throughout history: débridement, hemostasis, and primary closure. Review of the early medical literature from the Greco-Roman era shows an excellent understanding of the management of the scalp-injured patient. Many of the principles reviewed in this chapter take their origin in this early literature.

Scalp injuries can result from any number of diverse causes. Injuries can range from simple abrasions requiring minimal care to extensive scalping injuries with total scalp loss. Since the advent of the industrial revolution, society has become inventive in discovering new ways to injure the head and scalp. Each of the major types of injury can require its own management regimen. It is the purpose of this chapter to discuss the techniques available to the neurosurgeon (often in cooperation with colleagues in plastic surgery) for the care and management of scalp injury in the pediatric population.

ANATOMY OF THE SCALP

An understanding of the anatomy of the scalp is a prerequisite for repair of scalp lacerations of any type. A simple mnemonic still used by medical students—SCALP—is helpful in recalling some of the salient points of that anatomy (Fig. 17–1):

1. *S*kin: the outer hair-bearing portion of the scalp containing the dermis and epidermis—esthetically the most important structure in any repair.
2. *C*onnective tissue subcutaneum: a thick layer of fat and connective tissue which attaches the skin to the underlying galea. Contained within this layer are nerves, arteries, veins, and the lymphatic system, all linked in a key network of anastomoses.
3. *A*poneurotic: also called the epicranium or galeal layer, this is the fascial plane connecting the frontal and occipital muscles.
4. *L*oose connective tissue: a layer of tissue that lies between the aponeurotic layer and the pericranium. Its importance derives from the mobility it gives the scalp and from the fact that it is largely avascular, making it a useful plane for dissection and elevation of scalp flaps.
5. *P*ericranium: also called the periosteum of the skull, this layer is densely adherent to the cranial bones and contains their vascular supply. This layer of tissue is anatomically crucial in many of the repairs to be

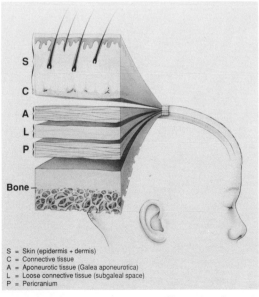

S = Skin (epidermis + dermis)
C = Connective tissue
A = Aponeurotic tissue (Galea aponeurotica)
L = Loose connective tissue (subgaleal space)
P = Pericranium

FIGURE 17–1. Anatomic representation illustrating the various anatomic layers of the scalp, using the mnemonic SCALP.

described. It figures importantly in repairs or reconstructions involving the face and anterior fossa and forms the foundation for skin grafts.[1-7]

VASCULAR ANATOMY OF THE SCALP

The scalp is essentially an end vessel in the vascular system. Twenty per cent of the cardiac output is supplied to the head and neck. As a result, bleeding associated with scalp lacerations and facial trauma can be massive and rapidly lethal if not controlled. The scalp vascular system is a rich arcade with a large overlapping anastomotic network. This system is so efficient that even a unilateral injury can be fed by the bilateral arterial network leading to rapid blood loss.

The blood supply to the scalp is outlined in Figure 17–2. The extent of the network and the multiplicity of its anastomoses are evident. The main vessels are outlined; they include the superficial temporal (with two branches, frontal and parietal), the supraorbital, the frontal, the posterior auricular, and the occipital arteries. This network is anatomically constructed in a ring-like fashion at the base of the skull to supply the head and scalp. An appreciation of the general anatomy of the main trunks is key to understanding the basis of any successful flap rotation or repair of scalp lacerations.

GENERAL PRINCIPLES IN THE MANAGEMENT OF SCALP INJURIES

It is beyond the scope of this chapter to consider injuries that are often associated with scalp lacerations. Skull, facial, and cervical injuries frequently accompany scalp injuries and should be evaluated as part of the initial examination.

The basic principles of wound care are outlined as follows:

1. *Hemostasis*
2. *Examination of skull*
3. *Débridement*
4. *Skin closure without tension*
5. *Antibiotics*
6. *Tetanus prophylaxis*

The mnemonic device is HEDSAT. Since scalp injuries as noted can hemorrhage extensively, early control of bleeding is essential. In the emergency situation, this is easily accomplished by application of pressure to the wound edges. Once hemostasis has been obtained, débridement and cleaning of the wound are necessary to reduce the risk of bacterial contamination (a useful rule of thumb is a bacterial count less than 10^5 per gram of tissue).[5] With a gloved finger the skull is examined for a defect or skull fracture.

Once cleaned and débrided, the wound is closed following one of the cardinal principles of wound care—closure without tension. Wounds closed under tension have a high risk of breakdown, and undesirable scars can form secondary to wound separation. Techniques to reduce wound tension are discussed in a later section of this chapter.

In children up to age 10, with up-to-date immunizations, tetanus prophylaxis given with their DPT shots provides adequate protection. In the older child, after age 10, a tetanus booster will be needed if the wound is believed to be contaminated. Antibiotics are often given to children with contaminated wounds; simple clean lacerations usually do not require antibiotic therapy. Potentially the most serious wounds are typically seen in the abused child afflicted with a human bite.

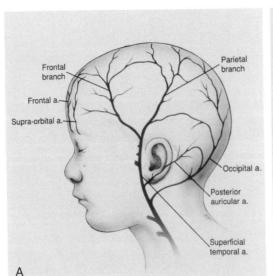
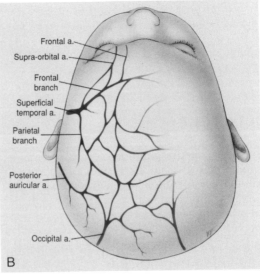

FIGURE 17–2. *A* and *B, Vascular anatomy* of the scalp showing the key feeding vessels and their general anatomic patterns within the scalp.

Animal bites are often seen in emergency rooms and also require treatment with antibiotics.

Most injuries seen in the pediatric emergency room can be managed with local anesthesia. For extensive scalp injuries, it is more reasonable to use general anesthesia.

MANAGEMENT OF SPECIFIC TYPES OF COMMON SCALP INJURY

SKIN ABRASIONS

The skin abrasion is the most common injury, but it is in most instances cared for by the emergency room staff and rarely called to the attention of the neurosurgeon. If the dermis is intact and only abraded, local wound care is provided. It is most important to remove any in-driven dirt or particles that can later tattoo the skin. Occasionally dermabrasion or coarse brushing of the dermis will be necessary; it is usually done with the patient under general anesthesia. Potential tattooing on the forehead can be a significant esthetic problem if not treated early; in the hair-bearing areas, such tattooing tends to be less important.

SKIN LACERATIONS

Simple skin lacerations are managed by achieving hemostasis, performing routine débridement, and aligning the skin edges. Two-layer closures are rarely necessary in children except in the instance of the forehead and periorbital region, where skin sutures are removed early to reduce scarring; two-layer closure allows early removal. On our service we routinely make a two-layer closure using undyed sutures in the subgaleal layer (dyed sutures can tattoo the very young child's skin) and a fine nylon suture (5.0 or 6.0) for skin closure; the nylon sutures are removed in 5 days. Suture placement must be meticulous and approximation of the skin edges perfect. Inadequate attention to detail makes for poor wound closure (resulting in a higher rate of infection) and disgruntled parents. Staples should never be used on the face or forehead region.

Scalp lacerations are often accompanied by injuries to esthetically important parts of the face and ears. It is particularly important to line up the helical rim of the ears and grey line of the eyelid so as to restore correct anatomic relationships; if this is done inadequately, the esthetic outcome can be dismal. At the same time, attention must always be paid to the potential skin stretching that can distort adjacent structures. For example, in a patient with a forehead laceration that causes tissue loss, stretching the scalp to close the wound can distort the face to an unacceptable degree. In children, as opposed to adults, there is less excess skin to mobilize.

In any laceration, the primary goals should always be

hemostasis, débridement, and a wound closure that restores normal anatomic relationships.

CONTAMINATED SCALP LACERATIONS

In a patient with heavily contaminated scalp lacerations, the surgical team should consider delayed secondary closure. Bites inflicted by humans or animals and wounds contaminated with dirt, as in farm machinery injuries and motor vehicle accidents (where the child is thrown from the car), are included in this category. In these situations it is often better to leave the wound open and apply frequent wound care for approximately 48 hours. Bacterial contamination should then be reduced to a level that allows a primary closure (i.e., a bacterial count less than 10^5 per gram of tissue). A swab wipe of the wound suffices to enable a bacteriology laboratory to obtain the desired organism count.

MANAGEMENT OF SCALP INJURIES WITH LOSS OF TISSUE

In the repair of scalp injuries involving a loss of tissue, a number of general principles must be applied: (1) Esthetic considerations always have to be taken into account in any tissue mobilization. (2) If possible, hair-bearing scalp is mobilized and used in the repair. (3) Whenever a flap is rotated, especially a split-thickness skin graft, the rotation must be from pericranium to pericranium. (4) Preservation of circulation in the design of the flap is critically important. Always include a major feeding vessel in any large flap rotation. (5) Never use the electrocautery, as heat or burn injury to hair-bearing cells can result in alopecia.

PARTIAL-THICKNESS AVULSION LOSS OF SCALP

Partial-thickness scalp loss can be treated in various ways. The particular technique that is chosen depends on the surface area of scalp that is lost and the extent of the injury.

Advancement Flap

In a partial avulsion of tissue with the pericranium intact, a simple technique is to elevate a flap of full-thickness scalp adjacent to the injury and then make radial cuts in the galeal layer, permitting the scalp to be "stretched" to cover the defect (Fig. 17–3).

Transposition and Rotation Flaps

A common scalp injury in a child is illustrated in Figure 17–4. It is easily managed by one of the flap transposition techniques. A relaxing incision is made on the side opposite the injury, and the tissue is undermined with Metzenbaum scissors, following the subga-

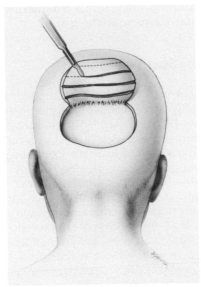

FIGURE 17–3. *Advancement flap.* A useful technique for providing "relaxation" to full-thickness scalp. By making linear incisions in the galea, one can stretch the flap to cover an adjacent defect.

SCALP REPAIRS WITH FREE FLAPS: SIMPLE TO COMPLEX

PARTIAL-THICKNESS SCALP LOSS

In combination with plastic surgery, a number of repairs that make use of flaps and skin grafts can be executed to accomplish closure of large scalp injuries. These techniques are reserved for cases in which full-thickness advancement, rotation, or transposition scalp grafts are not possible.

Skin grafts are classified in two categories according to their thickness: split-thickness or full-thickness. Split-thickness grafts are harvested to include the epidermis and only a portion of the dermis. Full-thickness skin grafts include both layers to their full extent. The advantages and disadvantages of each type dictate the choice of the one or the other for a given scalp repair.

Thin skin grafts do not transport hair follicles and sebaceous glands. However, these grafts can be meshed and thereby stretched to cover large areas; they also conform more easily to the underlying surfaces. Full-thickness grafts encompass the entire skin thickness and hence are more bulky than thin grafts. They are less conforming and, more importantly, take longer to vascularize; hence they are associated with a greater risk of sloughing. When they do take, the esthetic outcomes are better because they more closely resemble normal skin.

In partial avulsion injuries that leave the pericranium intact (thereby providing a vascular surface), it is possible to harvest and place split-thickness skin grafts. Such grafts will not survive on skull bone without pericranium, which is relatively avascular and unable to nurture the graft. Two areas useful for harvesting split-

leal plane. With wide mobilization of the skin, the initial defect can be closed primarily with little tension (Fig. 17–4B). If the extent of transposition is large, it may be necessary to place a split-thickness graft over the donor site to minimize tension at the wound. If such a skin graft is necessary, it can be applied over the well-vascularized pericranium, giving a better take.

Complicated flap techniques can be used to close large defects. These should be done in collaboration with a plastic surgeon.

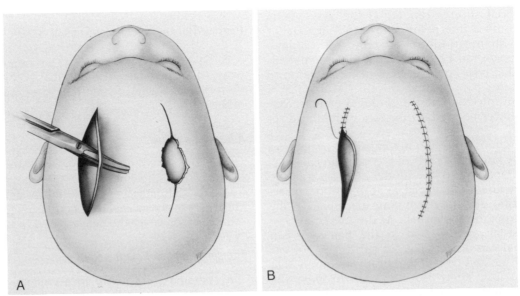

FIGURE 17–4. *Transposition flap.* To close a defect, a parallel incision is made 4 to 6 cm from the injury site (*A*). With wide undermining, the injury site can be closed first and then the lateral site closed secondarily (*B*).

thickness skin grafts are the buttocks and thighs. In choosing a donor site, particularly for full-thickness grafts, one must ascertain that such graft characteristics as color, texture, and hair-bearing qualities are appropriate to the recipient site. Except for color, these criteria are not as rigid in split-thickness grafts. Split-thickness grafts are harvested in thicknesses of ten thousandths to twelve thousandths of an inch and then meshed. These grafts are then anchored and sutured to the surrounding scalp. Bolsters are placed over the grafts to hold them securely in place for 7 to 10 days. As the grafts heal, their surfaces contract, decreasing the hair-bearing areas. This process usually takes 6 to 8 months. Flap rotations of hair-bearing skin can then be done later to cover the hairless areas.

PEDICLED FLAPS

Flaps harvested with a vascular supply are useful for covering large scalp defects over the calvarium. Such flaps can be harvested from a number of locations on the body; the limiting factors are the effect of graft excision on the donor site and the availability of a vascular supply for the graft. The harvesting and transposition of such flaps require a knowledge of flap vascular anatomy and microsurgical techniques. On our service, these flaps are routinely constructed by our plastic surgery colleagues. It is important for the neurosurgeon to appreciate what flaps are available and to play a role in designing and managing them.[1, 8, 9]

CUTANEOUS FLAP

The simplest of the flaps, the cutaneous flap is essentially full-thickness skin harvested with an arterial pedicle for blood supply.

MYOCUTANEOUS FLAP

These flaps anatomically incorporate a muscle unit with overlying skin, along with an easily harvested arterial pedicle. They are useful for covering large defects, particularly those in irradiated scalp areas. The flap is named after the vascular pedicle that supplies it and the muscle and skin overlying it. Examples of myocutaneous flaps include those harvested from the *latissimus dorsi, trapezius,* and *pectoralis* muscle groups. The trapezius and pectoralis myocutaneous flaps are probably the ones most commonly used in neurosurgical cases. They offer the surgical team a large volume of vascularized full-thickness skin and muscle covering.[10, 11]

OMENTAL FLAPS

Omental flaps were popular years ago because they were easy to harvest with a good vascular supply. However, an abdominal exposure is required, with the increased morbidity it entails, this technique, for the most part, has been replaced by the myocutaneous flaps.[12]

TISSUE EXPANSION TECHNIQUES

In recent years the use of tissue expanders has revolutionized esthetic approaches to scalp repair. A tissue expander is a Silicone prosthesis that is placed into a pocket of tissue following the subgaleal plane. There are a number of advantages to using this technique. With tissue expansion, one is able to develop available skin that has the same texture, color, and hair-bearing qualities as the recipient site. For esthetic purposes, none of these qualities can be overestimated, particularly the hair-bearing qualities. Normal scalp can be expanded to at least twice its normal interfollicular distance without showing any obvious changes in the hair-bearing areas.[13–15]

SUMMARY

As plastic surgeons and neurosurgeons have come to interact over the last decade, the potential for repair of complex scalp defects has greatly increased. Many repairs can be performed by the neurosurgical team that understands the relevant anatomy and principles underlying the various rotations. However, myocutaneous vascular flaps and split-thickness skin grafts should always be done in collaboration with the plastic surgery team. Careful attention to esthetic considerations can make the patients and their families much happier and less socially stigmatized.

REFERENCES

1. Goldstein RD, Strauch B: Plastic surgery wound coverage for the neurosurgery patient. *In* Goodrich JT, Post KD, Argamaso RD (eds): Plastic Techniques in Neurosurgery. New York, Thieme Medical Publishers, 1991.
2. Argenta LC, Adson MH: Management of scalp injuries. *In* McLaurin RL, et al. (eds): Pediatric Neurosurgery. Surgery of the Developing Nervous System. 2nd ed. Philadelphia, WB Saunders, 1989.
3. Janecka IP: Principles of wound healing. *In* Goodrich JT, Post KD, Argamaso RD (eds): Plastic Techniques in Neurosurgery. New York, Thieme Medical Publishers, 1991.
4. Peacock EE: Wound healing and wound care. *In* Schwartz SI (ed): Principles of Surgery. New York, McGraw-Hill Book Company, 1969.
5. Robson MC, Heggeis JP: Delayed wound closure based on bacterial counts. J Surg Oncol 2:379, 1970.
6. Coit DG, Sclafani L: Care of the Surgical Wound. *In* Wilmore DW, et al (eds): American College of Surgeons Care of the Surgical Patient. New York, Scientific American, Inc., 1988–91.
7. Lawrence WT, Bevin AG, Sheldon GF: Acute wound care. *In* Wilmore DW, et al. (eds): American College of Surgeons Care of the Surgical Patient. New York, Scientific American, Inc., 1988–91.
8. Juri C, Juri J, Colnago A: Monopedicled transposition flaps for

treatment of traumatic scalp alopecias. Ann Plast Surg 4:349, 1980.

9. Brent B: Experience with the temporoparietal fascial free flap. Plast Reconstr Surg 76:177, 1985.

10. Mathes SJ, Nahai F (eds): Clinical Applications for Muscle and Musculocutaneous Flaps. St. Louis, C.V. Mosby, 1982.

11. Vasconez L, Mathes SJ, Gant TD: Musculocutaneous flaps in reconstructive surgery. Contemp Surg 14:15, 1976.

12. Ikuta Y: Autotransplant of omentum to cover large denudation of the scalp. Plast Reconstr Surg 55:490, 1975.

13. Manders EK, Graham WP, Schenden MJ, et al.: Skin expansion to eliminate large scalp defects. Ann Plast Surg 2:305, 1984.

14. Austad ED, Thomas S, Pasyk KA: Tissue expansion: Dividend or loss. Plast Reconstr Surg 78:63, 1986.

15. Argenta LC, Austad ED: Tissue expansion. Clin Ann Plast Surg 14:3, 1987.

ACKNOWLEDGMENTS: The author would like to acknowledge the wonderful cooperation of his plastic surgery colleagues in the conceptual development of this chapter. These people include Ravelo D. Argamaso, Robert Goldstein, Craig Hall, and Berish Strauch—all of whom over the years have contributed immensely to our neurosurgical practice. In addition, special thanks to Vaughn Hatch, our medical illustrator who was able to conceptualize, and present in illustration form, some rather difficult concepts.

Chapter 18

SKULL FRACTURES

COREY RAFFEL, M.D., Ph.D., and N. SCOTT LITOFSKY, M.D.

In children, the head is frequently involved in traumatic injuries. The skull provides protection for the underlying brain and absorbs some of the force of the impact. If sufficient force is applied, fractures of the skull will result. This chapter focuses on pediatric skull fractures; it describes the major classes of fractures, their variants particular to children, their complications, and their treatment.

LINEAR FRACTURES

Linear skull fractures, in which no depression of the inner table occurs, are the most common type of fracture in children, occurring in about one fifth of childhood head injuries and representing almost three quarters of all skull fractures. Most often, the parietal bone is involved, followed by the occipital then frontal bones. The fracture may cross suture lines and may cross the midline and underlying sagittal sinus.[1] The diagnosis is suspected when significant scalp swelling is present. In children with neurologic deficits, computed tomographic scans of the head may reveal the fracture. Isolated linear skull fractures are treated by observation only. Scalp lacerations, if present, should be meticulously débrided and sutured. Admission to the hospital may not be necessary if the child has no neurologic deficits and can be adequately observed at home.

The significance of linear skull fracture has long been debated. By itself, linear skull fracture is believed to be of no great clinical significance.[2] The presence of the fracture simply indicates that the skull has been subjected to sufficient traumatic stress to cause the fracture. On the other hand, the presence of a linear fracture may increase the risk of intracranial complications.[3–5] If patients of all ages are considered, an increased risk of intracranial complications does exist in those with fractures. Conversely, if neurologic findings are normal on initial evaluation, the risk of intracranial complications is not significantly altered by the presence of a fracture.[2, 5, 6]

Diastatic sutural fractures, in which the suture is disrupted and becomes widely separated, are a special case of linear skull fracture (Fig. 18–1A). They occur primarily in infants and usually require no treatment. Widely separated fractures through bone may also occur in infants. These diastatic fractures are believed to be the result of incomplete calcification and lack of tensile strength in the infant's skull. In children past the age of 2 or 3 years, linear fractures become more like those of adults.[7]

Complications of linear skull fracture do occur. Perhaps the most significant is intracranial hematoma. Although the fracture may not cause the hematoma directly, impact severe enough to fracture the skull may disrupt intracranial vascular structures and cause hemorrhage. Patients with hematomas usually have neurologic abnormalities in addition to the fracture. Less than 5 per cent of patients with fractures will have a surgically significant hematoma and a normal neurologic examination.[4] As a corollary, most intracranial hematomas occur without evidence of fracture.[1, 6] An exception is the epidural hematoma, which is often found in conjunction with fractures across the groove of the middle meningeal artery or across venous sinuses.

Subgaleal hematoma complicating linear skull fracture is of no clinical significance in most children. However, children less than 1 year old may become anemic from blood loss under the scalp.[8, 9] Infants with large subgaleal hematomas should be admitted to the hospital and closely observed for hemodynamic instability. Serial hematocrits should be drawn to monitor further blood loss.

Subpericranial hematoma, or cephalohematoma, is a collection of cerebrospinal fluid and blood under the periosteum after linear skull fracture. The majority of patients with this complication are less than one year old. Typically, the collection is a soft, fluctuant swelling in the parieto-occipital area. Treatment consists of observation only, as the collection almost always resolves spontaneously.[10] On rare occasions, the collection may calcify, requiring surgical extirpation to restore a normal skull contour.

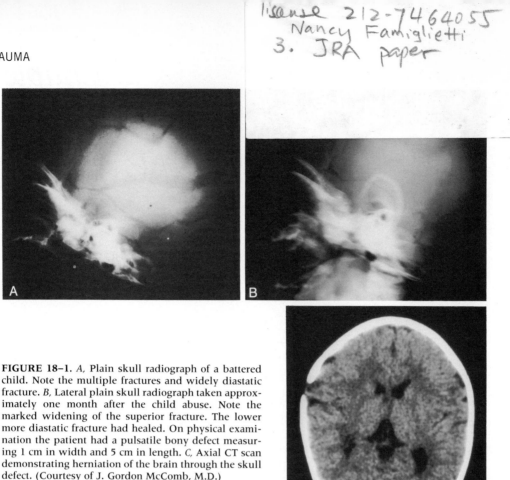

FIGURE 18–1. *A,* Plain skull radiograph of a battered child. Note the multiple fractures and widely diastatic fracture. *B,* Lateral plain skull radiograph taken approximately one month after the child abuse. Note the marked widening of the superior fracture. The lower more diastatic fracture had healed. On physical examination the patient had a pulsatile bony defect measuring 1 cm in width and 5 cm in length. *C,* Axial CT scan demonstrating herniation of the brain through the skull defect. (Courtesy of J. Gordon McComb, M.D.)

An uncommon complication of linear skull fracture in children is a "growing skull fracture," also known as a "leptomeningeal cyst" (Fig. 18–1*B*). In this lesion, a dural tear occurs with a linear fracture because the dura is adherent to the bone in young children. A brain injury deep to the site of the fracture is also usually present.[11, 12] Because the gliotic cortex adheres to the edges of the dural lacerations, the dura does not heal[13] (Fig. 18–1*C*). Continued pulsation of brain and arachnoid is thought to enlarge the fracture over time.[12, 14, 15] In many cases the ventricle communicates with the underlying encephalomalacia.[14] More than half of these injuries are seen in children less than 1 year old, and almost all occur in children under 3 years of age.[11, 12, 14]

Leptomeningeal cysts are rare, occurring in less than 1 per cent of all pediatric linear fractures.[14, 16, 17] Most growing fractures are parietal in location.[12, 15, 16] On radiographs, the edges of the fracture are scalloped and irregular. Areas of surrounding sclerosis suggest bone resorption and deposition.[12, 14, 15] Serial radiographs show progressive enlargement of the fracture.[18] Most children should have a surgical repair[11, 12, 14–16, 19] (Fig. 18–2*A*). Principles of surgery include (1) reconstruction of the dura, (2) reconstruction of the skull, and (3) excision of excessive scalp.[14] A dural graft is necessary for closure, as the edges of dura retract under the edges of the fracture. Split-thickness skull graft can be used to reconstruct the skull. In patients who also have

ventricular enlargement, a ventriculoperitoneal shunt may be necessary to achieve adequate decompression.[16, 20] Although some authors have advocated early surgery for widely diastatic fractures associated with scalp swelling and contralateral neurologic deficits, in the hope of preventing growing skull fractures,[9] the rarity of the lesion should deter the surgeon from early surgery.

A rare complication of linear skull fracture is traumatic cerebral aneurysm (Fig. 18–2*B*). Although such aneurysms are more commonly associated with depressed fractures or basilar skull fractures,[21–23] a small number of cases associated with linear skull fracture in children have been described.[21, 22] If the dura is disrupted, a cortical artery can be injured by the overlying fracture, leading to development of the aneurysm.

DEPRESSED SKULL FRACTURE

A depressed skull fracture usually occurs when an object with a small surface area, such as a hammer or the corner of a table, impacts the skull with high kinetic force.[6] Approximately one half of depressed skull fractures occur in the pediatric population, with one third in children under the age of 5 years.[24–26] These fractures are most commonly found in the parietal and frontal

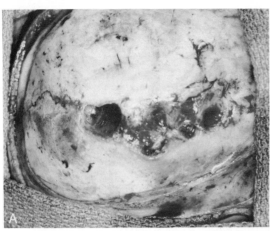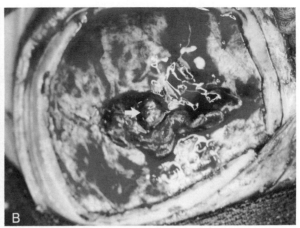

FIGURE 18–2. *A,* Intraoperative photograph of a leptomeningeal cyst. Note the wide bony defect filled with glial scar. *B,* After a craniotomy was performed, the edge of the dura could be identified. Under the bone a dural patch graft was placed, and the bone was reconfigured so that the area was covered with solid bone. Note the small traumatic aneurysm present in the field (*arrow*). This was excised before closure.

bones.[24, 27] Depressed skull fractures can be grouped into closed or open fractures; their management is significantly different.

About one third of depressed skull fractures are closed,[1, 24, 28] occurring more commonly in younger children[28] (Fig. 18–3). Contamination of the intracranial contents is not an issue.[28] Surgery for simple depressed fractures is recommended for children with cosmetic deficits present after the scalp swelling subsides and for children with neurologic deficits.[2, 24, 28] The incidence of post-traumatic seizure is unlikely to be changed by surgery.[2]

Treatment of compound depressed skull fractures is more complicated, because dural lacerations and associated cortical injury are common.[27, 29] Initial examination includes careful palpation of any scalp laceration with a gloved finger to search for an underlying fracture. If a fracture is identified, computed tomography can delineate the extent of bony injury and will reveal any unsuspected cerebral injury. Infection is a major risk of injury; thus, surgical exploration should be performed promptly.[2, 24, 30] Principles of surgery include (1) débridement of the skin edges, (2) elevation of the bone fragments, (3) inspection of the dura and repair of any defects, (4) treatment of the underlying cerebral injury, (5) reconstruction of the skull, and (6) closure of the skin (Fig. 18–4*A* and *B*). In most instances, the fractured bone fragments can be placed back into the wound after they have been soaked in povidone-iodine (Betadine). No increase in the infection rate has been observed with primary replacement of fragments.[27, 29–31] Of particular importance in children is replacement of the superior orbital ridge, which is difficult to repair by subsequent cranioplasty. If the fracture and laceration are posterior to the hairline, the laceration can be extended into an "S" to provide adequate exposure.[2] Frontal fractures are best exposed by bicoronal incisions.[27] The dura can be closed primarily after débridement of its edges; in more severe cases, a pericranial graft may be necessary. Conservative management should be contemplated if the fracture is juxtaposed to a venous sinus.[24, 26] Removal of a fragment piercing the sinus can lead to brisk and catastrophic hemorrhage.[2, 32]

The major complications of depressed skull fracture are intracranial hematoma, neurologic deficit, seizure, and infection. Intracranial hematomas occur in few cases; intracerebral hematomas are most common. Mortality and neurologic deficit are increased in cases with hemorrhage.[24, 26] Neurologic deficit is observed in about 10 per cent of cases, most commonly with parietal and temporal fractures.[24, 28]

Seizures occur more frequently after depressed skull fracture than after other fractures. Ten per cent of patients of all ages with depressed skull fractures have

FIGURE 18–3. Axial CT scan demonstrating a comminuted depressed skull fracture in the left parietal region. Although the fracture is depressed more than the full thickness of the bone, there was no associated intracranial injury visible on the scan. The child had normal findings on neurologic examination, and the fracture was not elevated.

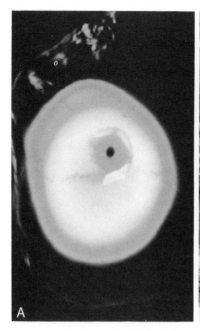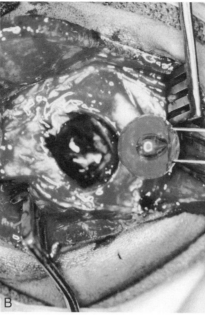

FIGURE 18–4. *A,* Axial CT scan of a 5-year-old child who fell backward off a swing and had an open depressed skull fracture. The CT scan demonstrates the fracture and also an air bubble in the fracture. *B,* Intraoperative photograph of the same case. At the time of operation a plastic ball was found in the fracture. This had been used to secure the child's hair into a ponytail. The ball was removed, and the fragments of bone removed from the brain. Necrotic brain was débrided. A dural patch graft was fashioned. The bony fragments were replaced. The patient made an uneventful recovery.

early seizures (within the first 7 days), whereas 15 per cent suffer from late epilepsy (after 7 days), as compared with 4 and 3 per cent respectively for patients with other fractures.[25] The increased incidence of seizure probably reflects the cortical injury that results from the depressed fragments.

Infection can be markedly decreased by prompt surgical intervention. Postoperative infection rates are commonly reported at about 5 per cent.[24, 30, 31] If surgery is delayed beyond 48 hours after injury, the infection rate increases. Patients with infection have increased incidence of neurologic deficits, seizures, and death.[30]

A special variant of depressed skull fracture, known as the "ping-pong" fracture or congenital molding depression, may be found in the neonate, occurring in utero, during birth, or soon thereafter[32–36] (Fig. 18–5). Neurologic signs and symptoms, resulting from associated hemorrhage, are uncommon.[34] Treatment of these fractures is controversial. Many surgeons have recommended elevation of the depression, either by an open procedure or by externally applied suction.[33, 34, 36–38] On the other hand, spontaneous elevation occurs in most cases.[34, 39] For this reason, surgery should be reserved for the following indications: (1) radiographic evidence of bone fragments in the cerebrum, (2) associated neurologic deficits, (3) signs of increased intracranial pressure, (4) signs of cerebrospinal fluid deep to the galea, and (5) difficulty with long-term follow-up.[39]

BASILAR SKULL FRACTURE

Basilar skull fractures occur in about 5 per cent of pediatric head trauma cases; they are less common than in adult patients.[1, 40] This difference may be due in part to the greater pliability of the skull of the infant and

small child.[41] Signs of the fracture will depend upon its site. For instance, fractures of the floor of the anterior fossa may present with anosmia, periorbital ecchymosis, or rhinorrhea, whereas children with fractures of the petrous pyramid may have hemotympanum, decreased hearing, facial paresis, otorrhea, or Battle's sign.[2, 42] Diagnosis of basilar skull fracture is made on clinical grounds. Computed tomography can be helpful, but a significant number of fractures will be missed. In most instances, treatment requires only observation of the patient. Antibiotics are of no proven value; some evidence exists that prophylactic antibiotic use changes the nasopharyngeal flora to one of more invasive organisms.[40, 43] The importance of recognizing basilar

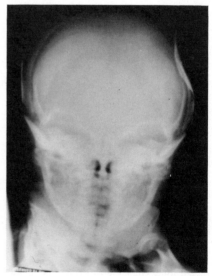

FIGURE 18–5. Plain radiograph of a newborn with a typical depressed skull fracture of the "ping-pong" type, which occurred at the time of delivery. (Courtesy of J. Gordon McComb, M.D.)

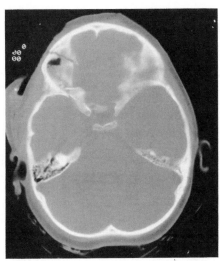

FIGURE 18–6. Axial CT scan using expanded windows to demonstrate basilar skull fracture. The fracture extends through the roof of the orbit and involves the greater wing of the sphenoid bone. Intracranial air is also noted.

skull fracture is to identify those patients at risk for its major complications—cerebrospinal fluid fistula and attendant meningitis, and cranial nerve deficits.

Fractures of the orbital roof, which are generally uncommon isolated injuries, are fairly common in young children[44] (Fig. 18–6). Because young children do not have a pneumatized frontal sinus, forces from blows to their brow are transmitted to the orbital roof rather than being absorbed by the sinus. These fractures may be linear or comminuted; they are classified as nondisplaced, inferiorly displaced, or superiorly displaced. The majority of patients present with periorbital ecchymosis, orbital dystopia, and exophthalmos. A significant number have associated intracranial injuries. Computed tomography has increased the diagnosis of these lesions. While the majority of these fractures do not require surgery, some children with inferior displacement of bone fragments may develop orbital encephaloceles.[44, 45] An intracranial and extracranial surgical approach is necessary to reduce the inferiorly displaced fractures to prevent this complication. Split calvarial bone grafting may also be necessary.[45]

Children may occasionally suffer from fractures of the petrous pyramid. Even with signs or symptoms of such injuries, the fracture usually is not seen radiographically. The most common signs are hemotympanum, cerebrospinal otorrhea, and peripheral facial nerve paresis.[42] Longitudinal fractures of the petrous bone, caused by laterally directed impacts, are associated with cerebrospinal fluid leak, ossicular disruption, and injury to the facial nerve in the horizontal portion of its course. The tympanic membrane is often torn. In children, most of the fractures are longitudinal.[42] The rarer transverse fracture, usually emanating from an occipital blow, may result in injury to the seventh and eighth cranial nerves.[7, 42, 46] The ataxia and vertigo that follow such an injury usually resolve, the dizziness is

tolerated, but tinnitus and hearing loss are permanent.[46]

CEREBROSPINAL FLUID FISTULAS

Cerebrospinal fluid fistulas are a major, but uncommon, complication of basilar skull fracture. They occur with almost equal frequency from the nose or ear.[1] The absence of pneumatized sinuses in infancy and the cartilaginous, less rigid nature of the base of the skull reduce the likelihood of fracture with communication to the outside environment. By the age of 3, however, the risk of cerebrospinal fluid fistula equals that in the adult.[41, 47]

Diagnosis of a cerebrospinal fluid fistula is usually made on physical examination. The child will have clear, watery fluid spontaneously draining from the nose or ear. In most patients, drainage will occur within 48 hours after injury.[47, 48] The nature of the fluid can be deduced by determining its glucose and chloride concentrations. Glucose in cerebrospinal fluid will be approximately one half of the serum value; this value will exceed that of discharge from the nasal mucosa. Results obtained from the use of glucose test strips may be misleading as some glucose is normally present in mucosal drainage.[49] Chloride will exceed serum values; this test should be used to establish the diagnosis. If the diagnosis is not suspected at the time of injury, the patient may present with a delayed leak. Alternatively, he may develop meningitis, sometimes multiple episodes. This complication is the major risk of cerebrospinal fluid fistula.[19, 47, 50, 51] Prophylactic antibiotics provide no assistance in preventing these infectious complications.[52]

In most instances, the leak will spontaneously subside.[48, 53] On occasion, however, drainage persists for more than 3 days. Conservative measures should be taken first. The patient's head should be elevated at all times to decrease the cerebrospinal fluid pressure. Serial lumbar punctures with a large-bore needle and multiple dural perforations will create a fistula into the paraspinal tissues to decrease the flow through the cranial fistula. A spinal drain, which may be less traumatic to the child, but more difficult to maintain, may be placed.[2] If these measures do not stop the leak, a surgical approach will be necessary.

A computed tomography scan of the head with thin cuts of the base of the skull, especially in the coronal plain, can reveal the fracture that marks the location of the cerebrospinal fluid leak. Although some have recommended radionuclide studies to identify the leak, the best study to establish the site of an active CSF leak is metrizamide computed tomographic cisternography.[54–56] In most cases of cerebrospinal fluid rhinorrhea, the source of the leak is a fracture in the floor of the anterior fossa. Leakage into the sphenoid sinus occurs in up to 15 per cent of cases.[2] A small percentage of patients can have rhinorrhea from petrous fractures without tympanic membrane perforation. In these cases the fluid will escape down the eustachian tube.[57] Appropriate diagnostic studies will help to define the source.

For most anterior fossa lesions, a bicoronal incision should be used. A unilateral craniotomy on the side of the lesion can provide exposure. An intradural dissection to identify the tear is recommended in order to avoid making other dural defects. One centimeter of normal dura surrounding the defect should be identified. Primary closure of the dural defect is often not possible. Therefore, a pericranial, temporalis fascia or tensor fascia lata graft is necessary. The graft should be laid over the defect so that a rim of dura surrounding the defect is covered by the graft.[2, 48] Sutures can be used to secure the graft in place, but this maneuver is often difficult. Some authors advocate the use of tissue adhesives to fix the graft in position and seal the leak.[58, 59] Postoperative drainage of cerebrospinal fluid via lumbar punctures or a spinal drain helps to promote healing by reducing flow through the defect.

Fistulas from sella or parasellar sites, including sphenoid sinus fractures, are probably best approached from a trans-sphenoidal approach.[2, 19] A fat graft in the sphenoid sinus can help to eliminate the fistula by obliterating the sinus as well as the pterygoid recesses.[19]

Repair of petrous fractures resulting in cerebrospinal otorrhea is similar to anterior fossa repairs. The key to treatment is determining whether the fistula is in the middle fossa or the posterior fossa.[2]

CRANIAL NERVE INJURIES

Cranial nerve injuries may occur with basilar skull fracture. Although fractures may be associated with cranial nerve deficits, one cannot always determine whether the fracture is the cause of the injury.

The olfactory is the cranial nerve most commonly injured in head injury.[60, 61] Over one third of anterior fossa fractures in patients of all ages have associated olfactory injury.[51] Additional patients may have postoperative anosmia from surgical repairs of anterior fossa cerebrospinal fluid fistulas.[48] About one third of patients with anosmia will have recovery of olfactory function, most within 3 months, but recovery has been observed as late as 5 years after injury.[60]

Visual loss from optic nerve injury occurs rarely. Direct injury to the nerve from a fracture in the optic canal or of the anterior clinoid process occurs in a small percentage of cases.[61–64] In the majority of instances, the deficit is believed to be from contusion of the nerve or injury to the vascular supply.[62, 64–66] Thus, surgical decompression is of little value in cases of acute visual loss after head trauma.[62, 66] If visual loss occurs in a delayed fashion, an intracranial approach to decompress the optic canal may be of some benefit, especially if CT scanning reveals a narrow canal or an intracanalicular bone spicule.[63, 66]

Oculomotor, trochlear, and abducens nerve palsies are found uncommonly in head injury.[1, 61] Differentiation of which deficits are due to brainstem injury and which are due to cranial nerve injury may be difficult. Oblique and transverse fractures of the clivus have been shown to have a high incidence of associated injury to these cranial nerves.[67] Fracture of the superior orbital fissure may also cause such injuries.[68] Abducens injury has also been shown to occur in crushing injuries of the skull in children, when the nerve is stretched by the opening of the spheno-occipital synchondrosis.[69]

Injury to the trigeminal nerve usually occurs as it exits from the skull through the supraorbital and infraorbital foramina.[66] More proximal injury is much less common.[61] Trigeminal nerve injury has been observed in clivus fractures and in crushing head injuries; displacement of the brainstem is believed to be the major factor.[67–69]

Facial nerve paresis occurs in association with petrous fractures. Birth injuries, primarily from forceps, account for nearly half of these.[42] In transverse fractures, the nerve is either lacerated or sectioned in the internal auditory meatus or the horizontal portion of the fallopian canal. Cranial nerve dysfunction is usually immediate. Longitudinal fractures may injure the facial nerve by causing stretching, swelling, contusion, or compression of the nerve.[66, 70] If the patient suffers immediate facial nerve palsy without recovery, several authors recommend surgical decompression after 3 weeks.[66, 71] In the majority of cases of longitudinal fracture, recovery will be spontaneous and begin within this time frame.[70] If neither spontaneous nor surgical recovery occurs, nerve grafting may be an option. When delayed onset of paresis occurs, surgical decompression is indicated immediately.[66]

Auditory nerve dysfunction can result from fractures involving the otic capsule. Facial nerve paresis often accompanies this injury.[66] Usually, these injuries occur with transverse petrous fractures. Hearing loss, with tinnitus, is permanent. Vestibular deficits improve or are tolerated. In longitudinal petrous fractures, ossicular disruption causes hearing loss. Tympanoplasty may be necessary for improvement.[46]

Lower cranial nerve injuries are exceedingly rare after head injury.[1, 61] In an experimental model, oblique crushing injuries have been observed to cause fractures through the jugular foramen.[68] The glossopharyngeal, vagus, and accessory nerves could be injured by this mechanism.

PENETRATING INJURIES

Skull fractures from penetrating trauma account for only a small fraction of head injuries in children.[1] However, the frequency may be increasing, as several more recent studies have accumulated larger numbers of these injuries in shorter periods of time.[72–74] Gunshot wounds to the head in children now represent about one fifth of such injuries.[73, 75] Children of all ages are victims of craniocerebral gunshot wounds. Mortality is at least 50 per cent for the pediatric population; it is higher in older children, reflecting the increased incidence of suicide attempts in this group.[73]

Treatment of gunshot wounds to the head in children is minimally different from that in adults. Perhaps the major difference in therapy is the determination of surgical candidates. While this point is still being debated, the consensus for the management of adult patients appears to be that surgical débridement should be performed on those patients with Glasgow Coma Scale scores greater or equal to 6 after resuscitation who do not have transventricular passage of the missile; outcome in other patients is poor.[76–78] Abnormal posturing in children does not necessarily predict a poor outcome. Therefore, all children save those who have Glasgow Coma Scale scores of 3, bilaterally dilated and unreactive pupils, and absent oculocephalic reflexes, those who are hemodynamically unstable, or those with coagulopathy should undergo surgery.[73] Ad-

ditionally, surgery is not indicated in children who are moribund with bilateral transventricular injuries.

The purpose of surgical débridement is to remove hemorrhagic mass lesions, débride necrotic and devitalized tissue, repair the dura, restore the integrity of the skull, and close the skin. The primary goal is to prevent infection. Computed tomography of the head will identify the injuries to the brain and skull and define any intracranial bone and missile fragments. Prior to surgery, coagulation and hemodynamic status should be normalized. Although the entrance wound can be enlarged for exposure, a scalp flap will sometimes permit better skin closure. A craniotomy, with the entrance site centered in the bone flap, will usually obviate craniectomy and subsequent cranioplasty. The tract of the missile should be débrided of necrotic tissue, hair, and bone fragments. Copious irrigation is a must. Bone chips frequently create a second tract.[75] If fragments are

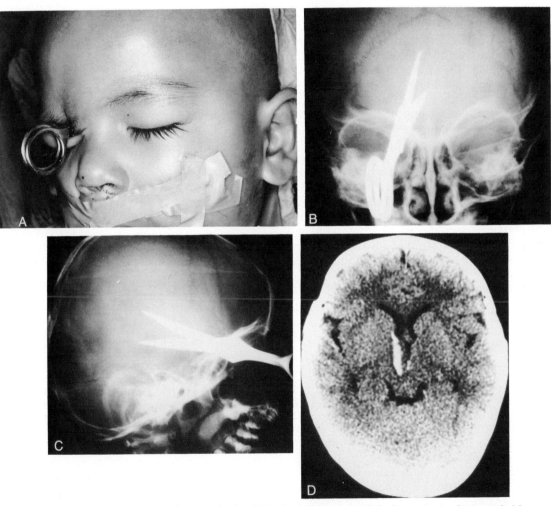

FIGURE 18–7. A, Preoperative photograph of a child who fell from a bunk-bed onto a pair of scissors held by his sister. B, Anterior-posterior plain skull radiograph demonstrating the intracranial course of the scissors. C, A lateral plain skull radiograph demonstrating the intracranial course of the scissors. The patient underwent an operation consisting of a frontal craniotomy and dural opening. The scissors were then removed, and since there was no bleeding after removal of the scissors, the wound was simply closed after reconstruction of the roof of the orbit. D, Postoperative axial CT scan demonstrating the course of the scissors through the hypothalamus, as outline by a small hematoma. The patient has made a complete neurologic recovery.

deep within the substance of the brain or in eloquent sites, they can be allowed to remain there since they pose relatively little risk of subsequent infection.[79, 80] After débridement of its edges, the dura can be closed primarily in some cases, but usually a pericranial or temporalis fascia graft is necessary. The continuity of the skull should be re-established. Large fragments should be secured in place. The entrance site should be débrided and closed in two layers if at all possible. Intracranial pressure monitoring is indicated in patients with Glasgow Coma Scale scores of 7 and less.

Complications of gunshot wounds are common, and the mortality rate is high.[73] Intracranial hematomas are found frequently.[75, 76] Up to 10 per cent of patients have post-traumatic seizures.[73, 76, 81] This frequency is not much different from that for depressed skull fracture, despite the impression that seizures are more common after penetrating trauma.[25] Infection is the most common complication in both adults and children.[73, 76–78, 81–83] Cerebrospinal fluid leak is the major cause of infection, substantiating the need for a good dural closure.[82] Unfortunately, basilar skull fractures cause a significant number of fistulas that are discontinuous with the fracture at entry or exit of the missile, especially if the missile crosses midline. The incidence of infection with otorrhea or rhinorrhea from these basilar skull fractures is over 40 per cent in patients of all ages.[84]

An unusual type of penetrating injury seen in children results from transorbital penetration of sharp objects, such as sticks or pencils (Fig. 18–7). Such an injury can occur when a child falls while carrying an instrument. The orbital roof is the usual site of penetration. Intracranial complications frequently accompany such injuries. Those children with acute neurologic signs often harbor intracranial hematomas. In others, the injury is not suspected, and the child presents in a delayed fashion with an intracranial abscess or meningitis or carotid–cavernous sinus fistula. An intracranial approach is necessary to repair the dura and manage any intracranial complication.[85]

SKULL FRACTURE IN THE BATTERED CHILD SYNDROME

A discussion of skull fracture in children would not be complete without discussing its association with the battered child syndrome. The skull radiograph is generally part of the radiographic evaluation of children in whom battering is suspected, even though skull fracture is uncommon.[86, 87] Most of these fractures are linear and occur in the parieto-occipital area. Comminuted, depressed, and diastatic fractures are common. If a fracture is present, an associated intracranial hematoma occurs in about half the cases. Multiple skull fractures and acute and healing fractures suggest child abuse.[87] The neurosurgeon must be alert to the features of this syndrome. An increased awareness of this syndrome as a possible diagnosis will lead to prevention of recurrent battering.

REFERENCES

1. Hendrick EB, Harwood-Nash DCF, Hudson AR: Head injuries in children; a survey of 4465 consecutive cases at the Hospital for Sick Children, Toronto, Canada. Clin Neurosurg 11:46, 1964.
2. Cooper PR: Skull fracture and traumatic cerebrospinal fluid fistulas. In Cooper PR (ed): Head Injury. Baltimore, Williams & Wilkins, 1982, pp 65–82.
3. Galbraith S, Smith J: Acute traumatic intracranial hematoma without skull fracture. Lancet i:501, 1976.
4. Mendelow AD, Teasdale G, Jennett B, et al.: Risks of intracranial hematoma in head-injured adults. Br Med J, 287:1173, 1983.
5. Thornbury JR, Campbell JA, Masters SJ, et al.: Skull fracture and the low risk of intracranial sequelae in minor head trauma. AJR 143:661, 1984.
6. Cooper PR, Ho V: Role of emergency skull x-ray films in the evaluation of the head-injured patients: a retrospective study. Neurosurgery 13:136, 1983.
7. Thomas LM: Skull fractures. In Wilkins RH, Rengachary SS (eds): Neurosurgery. New York, McGraw-Hill, 1985, pp 1623–1626.
8. Bruce DA, Schut L, Sutton LN: Cephalohematoma and subgaleal hematoma. In Wilkins RH, Rengachary SS (eds): Neurosurgery. New York, McGraw-Hill, Inc., 1985, pp 1622–1623.
9. Thompson JB, Mason TH, Haines GL, et al.: Surgical management of diastatic linear skull fractures in infants. J Neurosurg 39:493, 1973.
10. Epstein JA, Epstein BA, Small M: Subepicranial hygroma. A complication of head injuries in infants and children. J Pediatr 59:562, 1961.
11. Kingsley D, Till K, Hoark R: Growing fractures of the skull. J Neurol Neurosurg Psychiatry 41:312, 1978.
12. Lende RA, Erickson TC: Growing skull fractures of childhood. J Neurosurg 10:479, 1953.
13. Stein BM, Tenner MS: Enlargement of skull fracture in childhood due to cerebral herniation. Arch Neurol 26:137, 1972.
14. Arseni C, Ciurea AV: Clinicotherapeutic aspects in the growing skull fracture. A review of the literature. Child's Brain 8:161, 1981.
15. Taveras JM, Ransohoff J: Leptomeningeal cysts of the brain following trauma with erosion of the skull. A study of seven cases treated by surgery. J Neurosurg 10:233, 1953.
16. Locatelli D, Messina AL, Bonfanti N, et al.: Growing fractures: An unusual complication of head injuries in pediatric patients. Neurochirurgia 32:101, 1989.
17. Ramamurthi B, Kalyanaraman S: Rationale for surgery in growing fractures of the skull. J Neurosurg 32:427, 1970.
18. Nalls G, Lightfoot J, Lee A, et al.: Leptomeningeal cyst: Nonenhanced and enhanced computed tomography findings. Am J Emerg Med 8:34, 1990.
19. Spetzler RF, Wilson CB: Management of recurrent CSF rhinorrhea of the middle and posterior fossa. J Neurosurg 49:393, 1978.
20. Kashiwagi S, Abiko S, Aoki H. Growing skull fracture in childhood. A recurrent case treated by shunt operation. Surg Neurol 26:63, 1986.
21. Buckingham MJ, Crone KR, Ball WS, Tomsick TA, Berger TS, Tew JM: Traumatic intracranial aneurysms in childhood: Two cases and a review of the literature. Neurosurgery 22:398, 1988.
22. Burton C, Velasco F, Dorman J: Traumatic aneurysm of a peripheral cerebral artery: Review and case report. J Neurosurg 28:468, 1968.
23. Hahn YS, McLone DG: Traumatic bilateral ophthalmic artery aneurysms: a case report. Neurosurgery 21:86, 1987.
24. Braakman R: Depressed skull fracture: data, treatment and follow-up in 225 consecutive cases. J Neurol Neurosurg Psychiatry 35:395, 1972.
25. Jennett B, Miller JD, Braakman R: Epilepsy after non-missile depressed skull fracture. J Neurosurg 41:208, 1979.
26. Miller JD, Jennett WB: Complications of depressed skull fractures. Lancet ii:991, 1968.
27. Nadell J, Kline DG: Primary reconstruction of depressed frontal skull fractures including those involving the sinus, orbit and cribriform plate. J Neurosurg 41:200, 1974.
28. Steinbok P, Flodmark O, Martens D, et al.: Management of simple depressed skull fractures in children. J Neurosurg 66:506, 1987.

29. Carrington KW, Taren JA, Kahn EA: Primary repair of compound skull fractures in children. Surg Gynecol Obstet 110:203, 1960.

30. Jennett B, Miller JD: Infection after depressed fracture of skull. Implications for management of non-missile injuries. J Neurosurg 36:333, 1972.

31. Kriss FC, Taren JA, Kahn EA: Primary repair of compound skull fractures by replacement of bone fragments. J Neurosurg 30:698, 1969.

32. Schneider RC: Head injuries in infancy and childhood. Surg Clin North Am 41:1255, 1961.

33. Alexander E, Davis CH: Intrauterine fractures of the infant's skull. J Neurosurg 30:446, 1969.

34. Axton JHM, Levy LF: Congenital moulding depressions of the skull. Br Med J 1:1644, 1965.

35. Garza-Mercado R: Intrauterine depressed skull fractures of the newborn. Neurosurgery 10:694, 1982.

36. Saunders BS, Laxoritz S, McArtor RD, et al.: Depressed skull fracture in the neonate. Report of three cases. J Neurosurg 50:512, 1979.

37. Raynor R, Parsa M: Nonsurgical elevation of depressed skull fracture in an infant. J Pediatr 72:262, 1968.

38. Schrager GO: Elevation of depressed skull fracture with a breast pump. J Pediatr 77:300, 1970.

39. Loeser JD, Kilburn HL, Jolley T: Management of depressed skull fracture in the newborn. J Neurosurg 44:62, 1976.

40. Einhorn A, Mizrahi EM: Basilar skull fractures in children. The incidence of CNS infection and the use of antibiotics. Am J Dis Child 132:1121, 1978.

41. Caldicott WJH, North JB, Simpson DA: Traumatic cerebrospinal fluid fistulas in children. J Neurosurg 38:1, 1973.

42. Harwood-Nash DC: Fractures of the petrous and tympanic parts of the temporal bone in children. A study of 1187 patients. Am J Roentgenol Rad Ther Nucl Med 110:598, 1970.

43. Igneczi RS, Vanderark GD: Analysis of the treatment of basilar skull fracture with and without antibiotics. J Neurosurg 43:721, 1975.

44. Greenwald MJ, Boston D, Pensler JM, et al.: Orbital roof fractures in childhood. Ophthalmology 96:491, 1989.

45. Messinger A, Radkowski MA, Greenwald MJ, et al.: Orbital roof fractures in the pediatric population. Plast Reconstr Surg 84:213, 1989.

46. Barber HO: The diagnosis and treatment of auditory and vestibular disorders after head injury. Clin Neurosurg 19:355, 1972.

47. Park J, Strelzow VV, Friedman WH: Current management of cerebrospinal fluid rhinorrhea. Laryngoscope 93:1294, 1983.

48. Lewin W: Cerebrospinal fluid rhinorrhea in non-missile head injuries. Clin Neurosurg 12:237, 1966.

49. Hull HF, Morrow G: Glucorrhea revisited. Prolonged promulgation of another plastic pearl. JAMA 234:1052, 1975.

50. Jamieson KG, Telland JON: Surgical repair of the anterior fossa because of rhinorrhea, aerocele, or meningitis. J Neurosurg 39:328, 1973.

51. Jefferson A, Reilly G: Fractures of the floor of the anterior cranial fossa. The selection of patients for dural repair. Br J Surg 59:585, 1972.

52. Klastersky J, Sadeghi M, Brihaye J: Antimicrobial prophylaxis in patients with rhinorrhea or otorrhea: a double-blind study. Surg Neurol 6:111, 1979.

53. Brawley RW, Kelly WA: Treatment of basal skull fracture with and without cerebrospinal fluid fistulae. J Neurosurg 26:57, 61, 1967.

54. Allen MB, Gammal TE, Ihnen M, et al.: Fistula detection in cerebrospinal fluid leakage. J Neurol Neurosurg Psychiatry 35:664, 1972.

55. Curnes JT, Vincent LM, Kowaksky RJ, et al.: CSF rhinorrhea: detection and localization using overpressure cisternography with Te-99M-DTPA. Radiology 154:795, 1985.

56. Ahmadi J, Weiss MH, Segal HD, et al.: Evaluation of cerebrospinal fluid rhinorrhea by metrizamide computed tomography cisternography. Neurosurgery 16:54, 1985.

57. Ecker A: Cerebrospinal fluid rhinorrhea by way of the eustachian tube. Report of cases with the dural defect in the middle or posterior fossa. J Neurosurg 4:177, 1947.

58. Lehman RAW, Hayes GJ, Martus AN: The use of adhesive and lyophilized dura in the treatment of cerebrospinal rhinorrhea. Technical note. J Neurosurg 26:92, 1967.

59. Maxwell JA, Goldware SI: Use of tissue adhesive in the surgical treatment of cerebrospinal fluid leaks. Experience with isobutyl 2-cyanocrylate in 12 cases. J Neurosurg 39:333, 1973.

60. Sumner D: Post-traumatic anosmia. Brain 87:107, 1964.

61. Turner JWA: Indirect injuries of the optic nerve. Brain 66:140, 1943.

62. Edmund J, Godtfredsen E: Unilateral optic atrophy following head injury. Acta Ophthalmol 41:693, 1963.

63. Hughes B: Indirect injury of the optic nerves and chiasm. Johns Hopkins Hosp Bull 111:98, 1962.

64. Anderson RL, Panse WR, Gross CE: Optic nerve blindness following blunt forehead trauma. Ophthalmology 89:445, 1982.

65. Laursen AB: Traumatic bitemporal hemianopsia. Survey of the literature and report of a case. Acta Ophthalmol 49:134, 1971.

66. Rovit RL, Murali R: Injuries of the cranial nerves. In Cooper PR (ed): Head injury. Baltimore, Williams & Wilkins, 1982, pp 99–114.

67. Corradino G, Wolf AL, Mirvis S, et al.: Fractures of the clivus: Classification and clinical features. Neurosurgery 27:592, 1990.

68. Russell WR, Schiller F. Crushing injuries to the skull: Clinical and experimental observations. J Neurol Neurosurg Psychiatry 12:52, 1949.

69. Sumners CG, Wirtschafter JD: Bilateral trigeminal and abducens neuropathies following low-velocity, crushing head injury. Case report. J Neurosurg 50:508, 1979.

70. McHugh HE: Facial paralysis in birth injury and skull fractures. Arch Otolaryng 78:443, 1963.

71. Fisch U: Management of intratemporal facial nerve injuries. J Laryngol Otol 94:129, 1980.

72. Barlow B, Niemirska M, Gandhi RP: Ten years experience with pediatric gunshot wounds. J Pediatr Surg 17:927, 1982.

73. Miner ME, Ewing-Cobbs L, Kopaniky DR, et al.: The results of treatment of gunshot wounds to the brain in children. Neurosurgery 26:20, 1990.

74. Valentine J, Blocker S, Chang JHT: Gunshot injuries in children. J Trauma 24:952, 1987.

75. Kirkpatrick JB, Dimaio U: Civilian gunshot wounds of the brain. J Neurosurg 49:185, 1978.

76. Clark WC, Muhlbauer MS, Watridge CB, et al.: Analysis of 76 civilian craniocerebral gunshot wounds. J Neurosurg 65:9, 1976.

77. Graham TW, Williams FC, Harrington T, et al.: Civilian gunshot wounds to the head: A prospective study. Neurosurgery 27:696, 1990.

78. Hubschmann O, Shapiro K, Baden M, et al.: Craniocerebral gunshot injuries in civilian practice—prognostic criteria and surgical management; experience with 82 cases. J Trauma 19:6, 1979.

79. Aarabi B: Comparative study of bacteriological contamination between primary and secondary exploration of missile head wounds. Neurosurgery 20:610, 1987.

80. Pitlyk PJ, Tolchin S, Stewart W: The experimental significance of retained bone fragments. J Neurosurg 33:19, 1970.

81. Nagib MG, Rockswold GL, Sherman RS, et al.: Civilian gunshot wounds to the brain: Prognosis and management. Neurosurgery 18:533, 1986.

82. Aarabi B: Causes of infections in penetrating head wounds in the Iran-Iraq war. Neurosurgery 25:923, 1989.

83. Carey ME, Young HF, Rish BL, et al.: Follow-up of 103 American soldiers who sustained a brain wound in Vietnam. J Neurosurg 41:542, 1974.

84. Meirowsky AM, Caveness WF, Dillon JF, et al.: Cerebrospinal fluid fistulas complicating missile wounds of the brain. J Neurosurg 54:44, 1981.

85. Duffy GP, Bhandar YS: Intracranial complications following transorbital penetrating injuries. Br J Surg 56:685, 1969.

86. James HE, Schut L: The neurosurgeon and the battered child. Surg Neurol 2:415, 1974.

87. Merten DF, Osborne DRS, Radkowski MA, et al.: Craniocerebral trauma in the child abuse syndrome: Radiological observations. Pediatr Radiol 14:272, 1984.

Chapter 19

ACUTE TRAUMATIC CEREBRAL INJURIES

THOMAS G. LUERSSEN, M.D.

A major element of concern regarding any injury to the head is whether there has been a significant injury imparted to the brain. The presence of a brain injury generally determines the initial clinical presentation of the head-injured patient, and the magnitude of the brain injury plays a pivotal role in determining the ultimate outcome for that individual. At the most elementary level, it is the concurrent alteration of neuronal function either by hypoactivity (i.e., loss of consciousness or neurologic deficit) or hyperactivity (i.e., seizures) that calls most nonpenetrating cranial injuries to medical attention.

Even though the degree of cerebral injury rapidly becomes the focus of attention for the families and the physicians of head-injured children, in the very early stages after the traumatic event, there is frequently little that differentiates a life-threatening brain injury from a mild one. Although as time goes on, this particular distinction becomes progressively clearer, the process that is occurring is extremely complex. For instance, in the absence of demonstrable neuronal disruption, the absolute physiologic events that result in ongoing neuronal dysfunction and, perhaps more important, in the dynamic recovery from neuronal injury are just being identified. Clinical and basic research efforts, including modern neuro-imaging such as magnetic resonance imaging (MRI) and spectroscopy, positron emission tomography, detailed clinical studies of cerebral blood flow and metabolism after head injury and during various therapies, neuropathologic studies in human autopsy material, as well as some very elegant work in the laboratory, have resulted in a major advance in our knowledge about traumatic cerebral injury. This increase in understanding has allowed the development of a variety of clinically relevant classifications of head injury and a better understanding of the treatment paradigms for human brain injury. This chapter will attempt to provide an overview of the spectrum of direct cerebral injury, concentrating on the clinical presentations and the management issues commonly seen in the pediatric age group.

PRIMARY VERSUS SECONDARY BRAIN INJURY

An extremely useful classification of brain injury was propounded by Miller et al. over 25 years ago,[1] whereby traumatic brain injury could be better understood if divided into primary and secondary types. Primary injury represents the immediate and/or irreversible effects of energy dissipation in the substance of the brain. The vast majority of these phenomena occur within milliseconds of impact or penetration. Primary injuries include direct neuronal and glial disruptions, vascular injuries, shearing injuries, and brain lacerations due to penetrations or missile injuries. Stalhammar has further categorized the primary injury by mechanism and by the attendant immediate complications (Fig. 19–1), thereby providing a useful link to the important clinicopathologic classifications of focal and diffuse brain injuries.[2] There is strong evidence that some of the primary injury can occur in a delayed fashion, perhaps over hours to days.[3] These phenomena have been referred to as "delayed primary injuries," "irreversible nondisruptive axonal damage," or "secondary axonotomy." Regardless of whether neuronal and supporting structures are injured immediately or in a delayed fashion, at the clinical level, the unifying properties of the primary injury are that it is self-limited, mechanism-dependent, and theoretically irreversible.

Immediately after the primary insult, an array of reactive events begins, some of which cause acceleration or augmentation of the initial cellular injury and some of which cause "new" injuries. This complex cascade of events constitutes the secondary brain injury (Fig. 19–2). Secondary brain injuries can be categorized in several ways. Extracranial events, such as hypoxia and

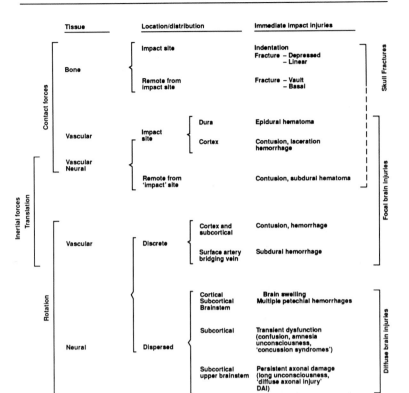

FIGURE 19–1. The relationships of cranial impacts or inertial forces and the development of either focal or diffuse primary brain injuries and their immediate cerebral effects. (From Stålhammar DA: The mechanism of primary brain injuries. *In* Braakman R [ed]: The Handbook of Clinical Neurology, Vol 13 [57]: Head Injury. New York, Elsevier Science Publishing, 1990, p 32, with the kind permission of Professor Daniel Stalhammar.)

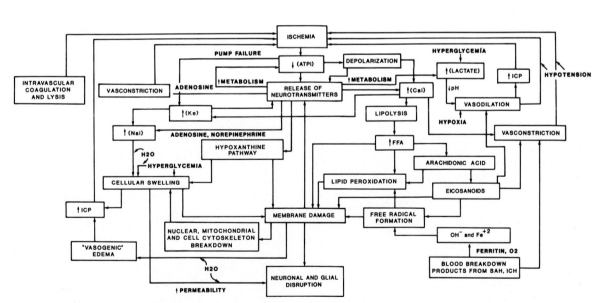

FIGURE 19–2. Schematic representation of the major biochemical cascades acting to cause the secondary brain injury. The diagram indicates areas where medical complications such as hypoxia, hypotension, or fluid disturbances can aggravate the secondary injury. Despite the complexity of interactions involved in the secondary injury, one can see areas whereby the development of new pharmacologic agents may be useful in blocking or reversing some harmful cascades. Also illustrated is the importance of brain ischemia as the major primary process instituting those cascades and aggravated by their products. (ATP_i) = intracellular adenosine triphosphate; (Ca_i) = intracellular calcium; (K_e) = extracellular potassium; (Na_i) = intracellular sodium. (From Luerssen TG, Marshall LF: The medical management of head injury. *In* Braakman R [ed]: The Handbook of Clinical Neurology, Vol 13 [57]: Head Injury. New York, Elsevier Science Publishing, 1990, p 209.)

hypotension, may occur as a result of the primary injury or may be due to systemic trauma, aspiration, or even misguided resuscitative efforts. Furthermore, metabolic alterations, fluid or electrolyte imbalances, or local or systemic infection can aggravate a traumatic injury. At the cellular level, biochemical reactions occur which can result in the death of partially injured or even initially uninjured cells.

Unlike the primary brain injury, the systemic and biochemical processes that constitute the secondary brain injury should be amenable to a variety of interventions or pharmacologic therapies. Despite this, the overall focus of the clinical care of brain injury is currently directed toward accomplishing three major goals: (1) preventing brain ischemia, specifically by controlling intracranial pressure, removing symptomatic focal masses, and maintaining normal systemic blood pressure; (2) providing appropriate physiologic substrates for cellular energy maintenance (i.e., oxygen and glucose); and (3) preventing the complications of systemic or local infection, metabolic disruptions, or other insults that might result in a further injury to the brain. It is important to remember that most permanent brain damage from nonpenetrating injuries is due to local or diffuse ischemia.[4, 5] Management of the secondary brain injury rarely involves complicated surgical procedures. Instead, most therapy of cerebral injuries involves aggressive and time-consuming medical management aimed at anticipating and recognizing the variety of direct and indirect responses to a primary brain injury and manipulating, directly or pharmacologically, the various body systems in order to prevent further injury and facilitate all possible neuronal recovery.

FOCAL AND DIFFUSE BRAIN INJURIES

Another useful way to conceptualize cerebral injury is as either focal or diffuse.[6] Focal injuries include contusions, lacerations, traumatic hematomas, and localized damage due to expanding masses, shifts, and distortions of the brain. The less common direct brainstem shearing injuries, avulsions of the pituitary stalk, avulsions of the cranial nerves, and localized infections are also considered to be focal brain injuries. Diffuse injuries include the spectrum of diffuse axonal injury, global ischemia, systemic hypoxia, diffuse brain swelling, and diffuse vascular injury. Focal injuries are usually immediately apparent on the admitting computed tomographic (CT) scans, but may be otherwise asymptomatic. In contrast, diffuse injuries may show much less striking changes on early neuro-imaging studies, even though the patient may exhibit profound alterations in consciousness and neurologic function.

FOCAL CEREBRAL INJURIES

Contusions

Contusions are mainly impact-related lesions that occur directly at the site of impact injury, i.e., underneath a skull fracture, or as a result of rotational forces that cause the brain to glide in relation to surrounding supportive structures or adjacent irregular bony surfaces of the skull.[7] *Fracture contusions* occur underneath skull fractures and are related to the forces generated by the fracture of the bone. They tend to occur over the convexities or along the base of the temporal lobe when there is a petrous bone fracture. These injuries are most commonly seen as a result of falls.[8] *Coup contusions* are localized at the site of an impact to the brain and may occur in the absence of a skull fracture. These contusions are generally related to direct blows to the stationary head.[8] *Contrecoup contusions* occur directly opposite the point of an impact injury and are produced by a deceleration of the head (Fig. 19–3). *Gliding contusions*, which are related to rotational or translational

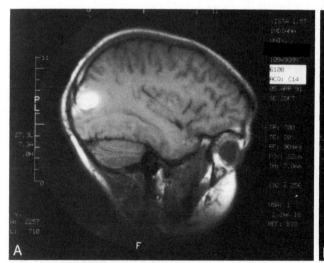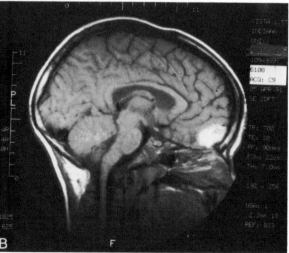

FIGURE 19–3. Contusions. MRI (TR = 700 msec, TE = 20 msec) of a 4-year-old boy who was injured in a pedestrian–motor vehicle accident. Although combative at the scene, he rapidly improved and was neurologically normal. He had swelling of the occipital scalp, but no skull fracture. CT showed an occipital contusion. *A,* The ''coup'' injury at the site of impact in the left occipital region. *B,* The ''contrecoup'' and asymptomatic right frontal contusion due to deceleration of the head.

decelerations of the head, are generally more symmetrical, tend to be bilateral, and tend to occur in the frontotemporal or parasagittal regions.[6, 9]

Cerebral contusion is the hallmark of brain injury, and the structural damage from cerebral contusion is evident long after the injury. Acutely, contusions are characterized by areas of hemorrhage and by tears in the cortical layers and subcortical white matter. The clinical presentation of cerebral contusions depends mostly upon the extent of the initial injury, the amount of associated hemorrhage resulting in mass effect, and the location of the contusion in the brain. Even though cerebral contusions may develop localized swelling, isolated lesions are not generally life threatening. Many cerebral contusions are asymptomatic, discovered on admitting CT scan underlying a skull fracture. When these injuries are symptomatic, they usually cause focal neurologic deficit. Seizures are thought to occur commonly in adults with acute cerebral contusions.[10, 11] However, the incidence of seizures for children with parenchymal contusions appears to be no greater than for those children with either normal CT scans or epidural hematomas.[12]

Traumatic Intracerebral Hematomas

These are unusual lesions in the pediatric age group. The pathogenesis of these hemorrhages is unclear, but it seems likely to be related to disruption of central blood vessels. Traumatic intracerebral hematomas are distinguished from hemorrhagic contusions by their lack of contact with the surface of the brain.[6] They are occasionally large enough to require surgical intervention.

Nonmissile Penetrating Injuries

The penetrating injuries of childhood result in focal contusions, lacerations, focal hemorrhage, and infections. Children are predisposed to cranial penetrations, which occur as the result of a fall onto or being struck by a sharp object. Generally, the offending agents are nails, pencils, sharp sticks, or lawn toys. The anterior penetrations of the skull frequently occur transorbitally, by penetrating the thin bone of the orbital roof (Fig. 19–4). One of the major dangers of these particular injuries lies in the initial clinical presentation. If the penetrating object is not embedded or retained in position, the entrance wound can appear to be relatively minor, or even trivial. Careful radiologic studies are called for when transcranial penetration is suspected. Even so, wood, glass, and residual bits of debris may be difficult to detect on CT scans.[13] Because of this, the diagnosis may be delayed, heralded only by the subsequent development of infection.

Missile Injuries

It is distressing that 12 per cent of all the deaths occurring in children aged 1 to 19 years are related to firearms.[14] The majority of unintentional firearm deaths occur in children less than 16 years of age.[15] Older children and adolescents commonly use firearms to attempt suicide.[16] Even low-velocity guns such as BB guns or air pellet rifles are more commonly used by children than by adults and pose a hazard for cranial injuries.[17] Other than the circumstances of the injury (i.e., being accidental), the clinical presentations and management issues associated with gunshot wounds to the head are similar for adults and children.[18, 19]

DIFFUSE CEREBRAL INJURIES

Diffuse brain injuries are characterized by general disturbances of neuronal function that begin immediately at the time of injury, the lack of a surgical mass lesion, and the lack of evidence of major structural change on the admitting neuro-imaging studies. These injuries exist on a continuum from extremely mild to

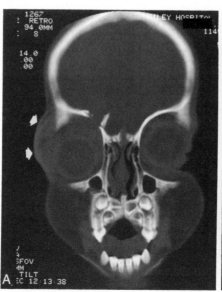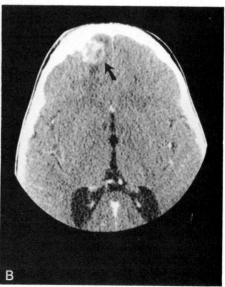

FIGURE 19–4. Penetrating injury. CT scans obtained several days after this 22-month-old female fell into a recently trimmed decorative bush. There was a small and apparently insignificant laceration of the eyelid that was cleaned and sutured. She developed a progressively worsening orbital cellulitis. A, Bone windows show a penetration of the orbital roof. Note the intense orbital cellulitis (arrows). B, A small and asymptomatic hemorrhagic contusion of the frontal lobe. The orbit and the anterior fossa were explored to drain the infection, and small bits of vegetable matter were removed at surgery.

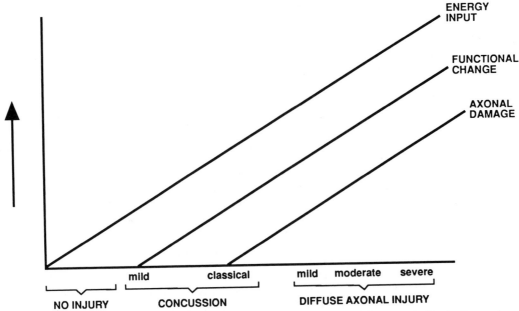

FIGURE 19–5. The clinical spectrum of diffuse brain injuries is presented diagramatically. As the acceleration input increases, the severity of the cerebral injury increases from no injury to severe diffuse axonal injury (DAI), and the attendant amount of axonal damage increases. The relationships are depicted as linear only for illustrative purposes, since quantitative correlations are not yet available. (From Gennarelli TA, Adams JH, Graham DI: Diffuse axonal injury—A new conceptual approach to an old problem. *In* Baethmann A, Go KG, Unterberg A [eds]: Mechanisms of Secondary Brain Damage. New York, Plenum Press, 1986, p 17, with the kind permission of Doctor Thomas Gennarelli.)

immediately fatal and include, in the mild range, the classic cerebral concussion (Fig. 19–5). As the amount of axonal disruption increases, the depth and duration of coma increases, and the neurologic outcome worsens. Frequently, the different types of diffuse brain injury occur together and can act synergistically to affect the neurologic presentation and the outcome.

Cerebral Concussion

Historically, concussion was defined as a reversible general neurologic disturbance without any evidence of pathology. This simplistic definition failed to explain the variety of clinical syndromes seen after "mild" brain injuries. The work of Ommaya and Gennarelli has resulted in the development of a clinically relevant theory of concussion. In their view, concussive brain injuries are caused by mechanically induced centrifugal strains acting on the brain that result in a *graded set of clinical syndromes showing increasing disturbances of the level and content of consciousness.*[20, 21] This definition allows the inclusion of specific post-traumatic disturbances commonly seen in children after "mild" head injuries: confusion without amnesia (the clinical appearance of being "stunned"); confusion associated with amnesia of varying depths and duration; and the classic loss of consciousness, with and without sensorimotor paralysis and disturbances of respiration or circulation. Furthermore, at some point fairly early in the clinical spectrum of concussion, permanent axonal disruption becomes apparent at the microscopic level.[3, 22, 23]

Transient disturbances of neurologic function are common after head injury in childhood, but the clinical presentations are somewhat age dependent. For instance, even though head-injured infants may suffer a skull fracture or large subgaleal hematoma, a history of unconsciousness is unusual. At best, one might obtain a history of a brief period of wide-eyed immobility followed by crying. Older children tend to show the more classic signs of cerebral concussion, including a clear-cut period of unconsciousness and a more prolonged recovery phase.

Children tend to show certain postconcussion symptoms that are much less commonly seen in adults. One of the most common is postconcussion emesis. As many as half the children suffering a minor head injury will vomit at least once.[24] Post-traumatic emesis in adults is usually a sign of elevated intracranial pressure or an expanding mass lesion. In children, vomiting is more frequent after a mild head injury than after a severe head injury, and it is rarely associated with elevated intracranial pressure. Protracted vomiting is an indication for a CT scan (in all ages of patients) and occasionally requires intravenous hydration until it ceases.

Early seizures are common after mild head injury in childhood. These have been termed "impact seizures," and they are not apparently associated with intracranial masses (as in adults) or with the development of post-traumatic epilepsy. For the most part, early post-traumatic seizures are self-limited and require no further therapy. However, multiple seizures or seizures that occur longer than a few hours after the injury are associated with both intradural hemorrhages and the development of true post-traumatic epilepsy. A CT scan is warranted for all children with post-traumatic seizures.

A syndrome of neurologic dysfunction that seems to be unique to young children has been called the *pediatric concussion syndrome*. Shortly after an impact injury, and usually after a period of apparent recovery, a young child may exhibit the acute appearance of pallor, diaphoresis, and varying levels of diminished responsiveness. This event is extremely frightening to caretakers when it occurs, but it seems to clear rapidly and without any specific therapy. The underlying mechanism of this phenomenon is unknown although it has been suggested that it may be a variation of early post-traumatic epilepsy.[25]

Other much more rarely occurring transient neurologic disturbances that seem to be focal in nature have been reported after concussive injuries in childhood. The most common of these syndromes is transient cortical blindness.[26, 27] Other disturbances include speech arrest, ataxia, receptive dysphasia, and prolonged disorientation. CT scans are (by definition) normal, and the symptoms seem to clear over minutes to hours. As with the other postconcussion syndromes, the etiology of these phenomena is not clear.

Diffuse Axonal Injury

It is now clear that a major cause of prolonged coma after head injury (in the absence of a mass, or hypoxia or ischemia) is diffuse axonal injury (DAI). This injury has a characteristic neuropathology that includes focal lesions in the corpus callosum and upper brainstem, and diffuse microscopic damage to axons.[6, 23]

Patients who have suffered DAI are unconscious from the time of injury and remain so for a prolonged period.[28] Not infrequently there are pupillary changes, skew gaze, and decerebration. This constellation of symptoms had been called "brainstem contusion" in the era prior to MRI, and although isolated brainstem contusion can certainly occur, it is extremely rare. Instead, most patients in coma who show brainstem dysfunction have suffered DAI.

The findings on initial CT scanning depend upon the severity of the injury and the degree of associated hemorrhages (Fig. 19–6). In some cases the initial CT scan may be normal. Subsequently, the characteristic lesions may be discovered on MRI, with the yield dependent upon how hard one searches. The characteristic CT scan appearance of DAI consists of multiple petechial hemorrhages in the deep white matter and central structures. However, the finding of intraventricular hemorrhage or subarachnoid hemorrhage specifically located in the prepontine cistern is strongly suggestive of DAI.

Hypoxic and Ischemic Injuries

It has been clear for some time that the presence of systemic hypoxia and/or hypotension significantly worsens the outcome from all types of brain injury. Both of these entities can occur as an immediate effect of the primary brain injury.[1, 29] Significant cerebral impact is frequently accompanied by a period of apnea, which is occasionally prolonged.[7, 30, 31] Furthermore, it is now clear that systemic hypotension can occur solely as the result of a head injury. Recent analyses of the Traumatic Coma Data Bank[32] indicate that as many as 10 per cent of purely head-injured patients show profound systemic hypotension in the prehospital phase of treatment.[33] Of these two early insults, it appears that hypotension is more likely to have a permanent deleterious effect on the brain. The initial CT scans can be completely normal despite the severe neurologic disturbance. Later, the characteristic global changes of hypoxic/ischemic encephalopathy appear on the scan, which distinguish the pure hypoxic or ischemic injuries from DAI.

Diffuse Brain Swelling

Diffuse brain swelling is a vasoreactive post-traumatic phenomenon that occurs within hours of a head injury. These patients have significant intracranial hypertension that is apparently due to a marked increase in cerebral blood volume. The appearance of the CT scans and the rapidity of onset separate diffuse cerebral swelling from the post-traumatic brain swelling that occurs later as a result of vasogenic or cytotoxic cerebral edema.[34, 35] The increased cerebral blood volume is apparently due to cerebrovascular congestion and not to a loss of normal autoregulation.[36]

Diffuse brain swelling occurs more commonly in children than in adults. Furthermore, it has been suggested that this phenomenon may be completely reversible with early and aggressive therapy.[34, 37] However, the severity of this process is underscored by a recent multicenter study, which found that the mortality associated with this process in severely head-injured children was over 50 per cent.[38]

This syndrome can appear after an apparently mild head injury. There is frequently a lucid interval prior to the onset of a rapid deterioration in consciousness and the associated intracranial hypertension. Patients at risk for this phenomenon almost always show compression of the perimesencephalic cisterns on the admitting CT scan. These changes may be subtle, but should not be ignored just because the patient seems to be clinically well (Fig. 19–7). Aggressive therapy, instituted prior to deterioration and guided by early monitoring of intracranial pressure, appears to control the swelling and results in improved outcome.[37, 39]

The Shaken/Impact Syndrome of Infancy

This particular injury was described over 20 years ago[40] and may be the most common cause of severe brain injury in very young children.[41–43] Most of what is known about this injury comes from neuropathologic studies and the burgeoning information obtained from CT and MRI. It is notable that the clinical syndrome associated with this particular injury is virtually never seen after accidental injury or in older children. Bio-

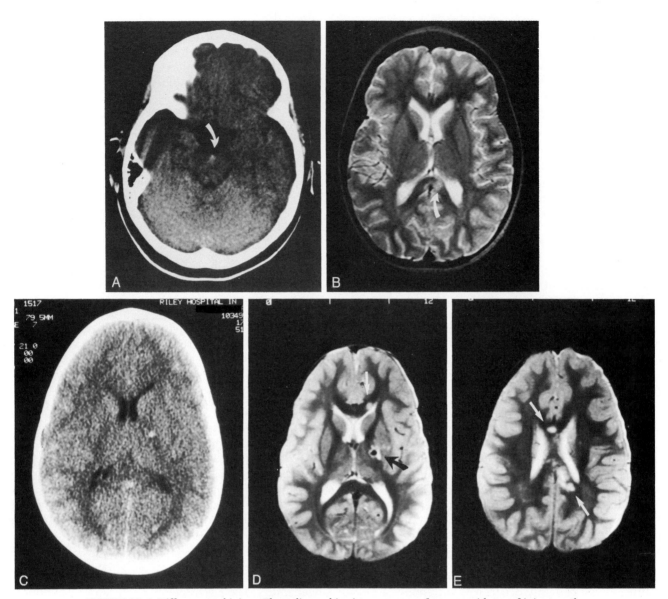

FIGURE 19–6. Diffuse axonal injury. The radiographic picture can vary from no evidence of injury on the CT scan to widespread abnormalities. *A,* The findings may be as subtle as a small amount of subarachnoid blood in the prepontine cistern, as found on this acute CT scan of the brain of a 6-year-old boy who was struck by an automobile. He was unconscious for more than a week, but ICP was not elevated. *B,* The MRI (TR = 2500 msec, TE = 80 msec) shows a nonhemorrhagic shear in the splenium of the corpus callosum. *C,* The "characteristic" CT appearance of acute DAI is shown in the scan of this 5-year-old boy who was a passenger involved in a high-speed motor vehicle collision. There are small hemorrhages in the deep white matter and central structures, along with intraventricular and subarachnoid hemorrhage. *D* and *E,* MRI (TR = 2500 msec, TE = 80 msec) shows widespread hemorrhagic *(black arrow)* and nonhemorrhagic *(white arrows)* shear.

mechanical models of this injury have indicated that an impact of the head is a necessary component of the primary injury, but that this impact can occur on a padded surface, which would reduce the degree of external injury.[44] This mechanism explains the pathologic findings of a mixture of focal brain injuries due to impact and the diffuse brain injuries due to angular and rotational decelerations of the cranium. Skull fractures, cerebral contusions, subdural hemorrhages, deep white matter and corpus callosum shears, with and without massive brain swelling, and with and without evidence

of hypoxia or ischemia have all been described in infants who have been shaken.[44–46]

This injury must be suspected whenever an infant not involved in a motor vehicle collision presents with a severe brain injury. Frequently, no history of an injury is forthcoming, and these children may initially be suspected of having meningitis. Less often, a history of a short fall or being struck by another child is put forth.[43] The child may be irritable, or in the throes of status epilepticus, or in deep coma. The fontanelle is full. It is interesting that many of these children present

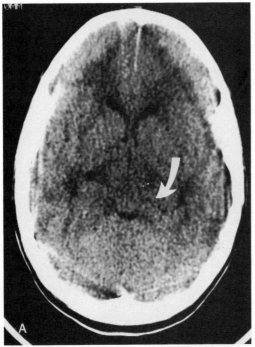

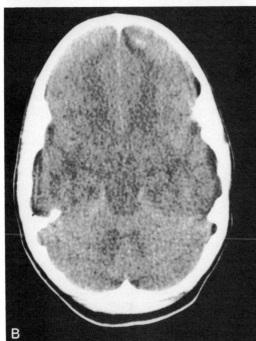

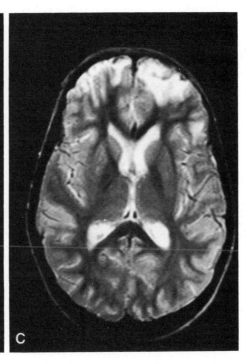

FIGURE 19–7. Diffuse brain swelling. A series of images of the brain of a 9-year-old female who was struck by a slow-moving automobile. She was briefly unconscious and persistently disoriented during transport to the hospital. She was assigned a coma score of 14, suggesting a "mild" head injury. *A,* The acute CT scan shows effacement of the peri-mesencephalic cistern, which indicates early swelling. *B,* A CT scan about 6 hours after injury showing diffuse swelling and the appearance of increased density of the brain, consistent with cerebrovascular congestion. The ICP responses indicated poor compliance, and intensive therapy was needed to control the swelling. *C,* MRI (TR = 2500 msec, TE = 80 msec) shows bilateral frontal "gliding contusions."

with an enlarged head circumference,[47] suggesting a more chronic repetitive nature to the injury. Retinal hemorrhages are detectable in the vast majority of children who are shaken.[42, 44] Subarachnoid and/or subdural hemorrhages, the latter characteristically interhemispheric in location (Fig. 19–8), are detectable on CT scans and MRI.[48, 49] As mentioned, skull fractures need not be present, but the finding of acute or healing long bone or rib fractures in children with this constellation of neurologic findings is pathognomonic for nonaccidental injury.[43, 50]

CLINICAL CLASSIFICATIONS AND OUTCOMES

The value of a clinical classification for brain injury is that it allows one to characterize the severity of injury in order to direct immediate therapy. Implicit in this strategy is the expectation that a classification scheme should be predictive of the ultimate outcome of the injury. A basic tenet of management has been that the outcome from traumatic brain injury is generally related to the magnitude of the initial neurologic dysfunction. A variety of scoring systems have been used

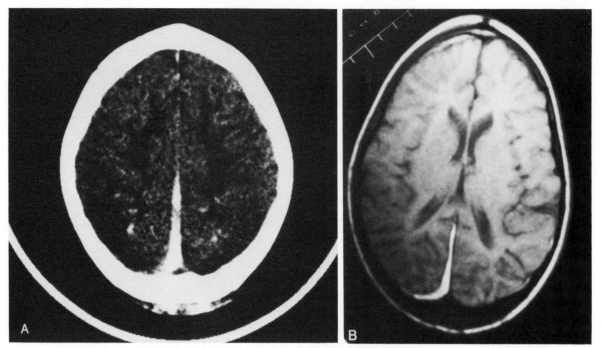

FIGURE 19–8. The characteristic CT and MRI appearance of the shaking/impact injury of infancy. The subdural hemorrhage is frequently interhemispheric *(A)*. MRI (TR = 800 msec, TE = 25 msec) invariably shows more of the extent of the hemorrhage including subdural hemorrhage over the convexity *(B),* and will also demonstrate injuries to the brain parenchyma.

to quantify the neurologic disturbances seen after head injury, and each of the many systems has advantages and disadvantages, especially relating to the evaluation of head-injured children. The most widely used and studied coma scoring system for head-injured patients is the Glasgow Coma Scale (GCS) score.[51] This scale is a numeric descriptor of the level of consciousness of a brain-injured patient. Other coma scoring systems add parts of the neurologic examination, most frequently some indication of brainstem function, and this additional information adds some predictive power to the scale.[52–55]

The GCS has been criticized as inaccurate for very young children, because of a perceived inability to characterize accurately the true level of eye opening or speech function in a young child. However, rather than abandon the most widely used and studied coma scoring system for head-injured patients, most centers have successfully modified the scale to allow for the examination of a young child (Table 19–1). The eye and verbal portions of the scale will always be somewhat examiner dependent and occasionally difficult to assign, but these two elements are also the least important part of the scale. For head-injured patients of all ages, the motor score is most predictive of the ultimate outcome and is also the most reproducibly assigned portion of the scale.[56]

The major problem with all the described brain injury scaling systems is the lack of standardization in applying any one scale.[53, 57] This lack of uniformity hinders the comparison of groups of head-injured patients. Although it is almost impossible to standardize the clinical examination,[56] the uniform timing of the examination and the correction of mitigating factors will add much to increasing the reliability of a clinical scoring system. For instance, early work with the Glasgow scale used scores assigned to patients at a 6-hour interval after the injury. With improved transport and triage, most head-injured patients are already undergoing treatment at this time after the injury. Furthermore, head-injured patients with systemic hypotension or hypoxia will show an artificially depressed coma score because of

TABLE 19–1.   GLASGOW COMA SCALE SCORE FOR ADULTS AND CHILDREN

Function	Adults	Infants and Children	Score
Eye opening	Spontaneous to command	Spontaneous	4
		To sound	3
	To pain	To pain	2
	None	None	1
Verbalization	Oriented	Appropriate for age Fixes and follows Social smile	5
	Disoriented	Cries but consolable	4
	Inappropriate	Persistently irritable	3
	Incomprehensible	Restless, lethargic	2
	None	None	1
Motor	Obeys commands	Spontaneous	6
	Localizes pain	Same	5
	Withdraws	Same	4
	Reflex flexion	Same	3
	Reflex extension	Same	2
	None	Same	1
Total score			15

these alterations. Recognition of these findings has caused most head injury centers to perform the relevant scoring examinations as soon after the injury as possible, but also after all the systemic parameters have been normalized with fluids, blood, or ventilation. This allows the most accurate determination of the initial degree of neurologic dysfunction.

Brain-injured patients are generally categorized clinically as having sustained a mild, moderate, or severe brain injury, based mostly on the GCS. Using this scheme, severe brain injury in children (i.e., GCS sum score of 3 to 8, or a motor score of 4 or less) occurs at a rate roughly equal to that in adults and with an attendant mortality of roughly half of that in adults.[57] Moderate injury (i.e., GCS sum score of 9 to 12) occurs at about the same rate in children and adults, but carries an extremely low mortality in childhood. Accordingly, most brain injuries in childhood are clinically graded as mild injuries, although there is clearly a group of mildly or moderately head-injured children who appear to be at risk for deterioration and death.[58, 59]

The identification of the head-injured patient who appears "clinically" well but is nevertheless truly at risk for deterioration has spurred the study and development of systems aimed at classifying brain-injured patients by their radiographic findings. It has long been known that the finding of a skull fracture in a head-injured patient is a significant indicator of a traumatic intracranial hematoma.[60, 61] The presence of a skull fracture, especially in a child, although a definite indicator of increased risk, is still relatively nonspecific. In contrast, the CT scan is a relatively specific indicator of the degree of cerebral injury. Certain findings on the admitting CT scan are clearly associated with more severe injuries, elevated intracranial pressure (ICP), and poor outcome,[62–64] regardless of the clinical grade of the patient. Furthermore, it appears that the findings on the initial CT scan can be as predictive of outcome, including the very important aspect of being able to identify a head-injured patient at risk for deterioration, as the clinical examination.[65, 66] The identification of compressed or absent cisterns, intraventricular hemorrhage, significant or perimesencephalic subarachnoid hemorrhage, or a shift of the midline structures is a strong indicator of a patient at risk to deteriorate neurologically due to significant and life-threatening elevations of intracranial pressure or the subsequent development of an intracranial mass lesion. This radiographic indicator of the degree of brain injury removes concern about examiner error in the clinical scoring systems discussed previously and may be the study that identifies accurately those patients who may "talk and die."[39] This appears to be most relevant for the patients who have suffered DAI, which includes most children with severe brain injuries. As shown in Table 19–2, the more structural alterations seen on the admitting CT scan, the worse the outcome, even with aggressive management in experienced head injury centers.

When this general scheme is applied to a series of head-injured children, who underwent early CT scan-

TABLE 19–2. PERCENTAGE OF PATIENTS IN THE TRAUMATIC COMA DATA BANK ACHIEVING THE DESCRIBED NEUROLOGIC OUTCOME AT DISCHARGE USING A RADIOGRAPHIC CHARACTERIZATION OF DIFFUSE CEREBRAL INJURIES

OUTCOME*	DIFFUSE BRAIN INJURY			
	I	II	III	IV
Good	27	8.5	3.3	3.1
Moderate	34.6	26	13.1	3.1
Severe	19.2	40.7	26.8	18.8
Vegetative	9.6	11.3	22.9	18.8
Dead	9.6	13.5	34.0	56.2

*At discharge utilizing the Glasgow Outcome Scale.[67]

Diffuse Injury I = No visible pathology seen on CT scan (patient in coma); *Diffuse Injury II* = Cisterns present, midline shift less than 5 mm, with or without parenchymal hemorrhages less than 25 cc; *Diffuse Injury III* = Swelling; cisterns compressed or absent, midline shift less than 5 mm, with or without parenchymal hemorrhages less than 25 cc; *Diffuse Injury IV* = Shift; midline shift of over 5 mm, with or without parenchymal hemorrhages less than 25 cc.

Modified from Marshall LF, Marshall SB, Klauber MR, et al.: A new classification of head injury based on computerized tomography. J Neurosurg 75(suppl):S14, 1991.

ning, the findings are similar, but the results are shifted toward better outcomes (as is true for almost all aspects of brain injury). The finding of a normal CT scan in a head-injured child appears to be associated with a mortality of less than 1 per cent, whereas the presence of swelling and shift carries a mortality of 40 per cent.[66]

MANAGEMENT ISSUES

Most, if not all, penetrating injuries are best treated by surgical débridement and dural repair. A notable exception may be certain BB gun injuries,[17] in which case there is little to be gained by trying to find any except the most superficial BB. Broad-spectrum antibiotics that penetrate well into the CSF are probably advisable in most cases. Most authors recommend the use of prophylactic anticonvulsants for patients suffering gunshot wounds to the brain,[19] but the value of anticonvulsants for the other types of penetrating injuries is not clear.

With the exception of the penetrating injuries, the role of surgery in the management of direct cerebral injury in childhood is a limited one. As previously discussed, surgically significant hemorrhagic contusions or parenchymal hematomas (which represent approximately 10 per cent of the post-traumatic lesions encountered in severely head-injured adults) are an unusual occurrence in the pediatric age group. However, a polar or accessible hemorrhage or contusion that is causing mass effect or is contributing to elevations of intracranial pressure should be removed. The location of the contusion must also be considered when surgery is contemplated. Contusions of the temporal lobe are notorious for causing compression of the brainstem at relatively low intracranial pressures.[68, 69] Patients harboring these lesions who show pupillary changes or a shift on the CT scan, regardless of the ICP, generally benefit from early surgery.

The main treatment of most direct cerebral injuries is medical. Assuming that (by definition) the primary brain injury is not reversible, the objective of current medical therapy is to create a milieu that permits the recovery of cerebral tissues not already irreversibly damaged and to prevent or even reverse as much of the secondary brain injury as is possible.[70] Despite the variety of secondary injury cascades shown in Figure 19–2, almost all of the acute therapeutic effort is directed toward the prevention of global or localized cerebral ischemia, mainly by preventing intracranial hypertension and correcting or preventing mismatches in cerebral perfusion and metabolism, particularly those due to repeated seizures. Accordingly, the mainstay of directed therapy involves the early and accurate measurement of intracranial pressure. Whenever a head-injured patient presents in coma or whenever the admitting CT scan indicates that a head-injured patient is at risk for elevations of intracranial pressure, a monitor is inserted and therapy is instituted as necessary.

Isolated focal injuries of the brain are rarely associated with elevations in intracranial pressure. However, if there is a mass large enough to cause effacement of the cistern or shift of the midline structures, or if the child has a coma score indicating a moderate or severe brain injury, intracranial pressure monitoring is warranted, especially if the mass is not considered surgically accessible. For the spectrum of diffuse axonal injuries, it appears that abnormal elevations in intracranial pressure occur in less than 25 per cent of patients.[71] However, it is now clear that the more severe the radiographic appearance of DAI, the more likely are elevations in intracranial pressure.[65] Children with diffuse injuries who show any indication of swelling or shift on the CT scan, even if they are not in coma, are candidates for intracranial pressure monitoring. If intracranial hypertension is not seen over the course of 48 hours, assuming that the only therapy administered has been supportive, and that follow-up CT scanning does not show the development of a mass, shift, or cisternal effacement, the monitor may be removed.

At the time of this writing, there is no direct medical therapy for cerebral injury. Historically, corticosteroids have been recommended for brain-injured patients. However, when the effect of steroid administration was examined critically in both retrospective and randomized prospective studies, no demonstrable beneficial effect could be found for these drugs.[72–74] However, recent work studying the effect of a brief course of extremely high doses of methylprednisolone in acute traumatic spinal cord injury has apparently shown some effect in improving the outcome from this particular injury.[75] This unexpected effect of corticosteroids on the outcome of spinal cord injury is interesting, but until these types of studies are performed in brain-injured patients, and in view of their known deleterious effects on the immune response and on metabolism, steroids are not currently recommended for the therapy of traumatic cerebral injury. In summary, other than the administration of anticonvulsants when indicated, the basic medical management of acute brain injury is aimed at the detection and management of intracranial hypertension (which is discussed elsewhere in this volume) and the prevention of cerebral and systemic complications.

ANTICIPATED DEVELOPMENTS

New medical therapies for head injury are sure to be developed, and each new approach will benefit a select group of patients. At present, it is now possible to identify certain groups of patients who will respond to specific therapies for elevated ICP.[76] With improved technology and more sophisticated monitors of brain function, it will become possible for the dynamic pathology of traumatic brain injury to be monitored in real time. This will allow therapy to be much more individualized than it is now.

As this chapter is being prepared, several new pharmacologic agents are in various stages of clinical trial in both North America and Europe. Because of improved understanding of the secondary injury cycles, drugs could be developed with the aim of interrupting or reversing some of the deleterious biochemical processes that occur after brain injury. Traumatic brain injury is such a heterogeneous process that it is unlikely that any one drug will have the major impact on the management of brain injury that was seen with the advent of, for instance, CT scanning or ICP monitoring. Instead, these new drugs are likely to benefit individual patients, perhaps at specific times, or with specific types of brain injury.

At all times, we must continue to focus on a logical and systematic approach to traumatic brain injury in order to continue to improve the outcome. Further organization of trauma systems, which include guidelines for the care of injured children, should improve outcomes. Within the current systems, there should be increased emphasis on an approach that identifies the less severely injured patient who is at risk for deterioration or complication and treating that patient as aggressively as those who are immediately severely injured. It seems clear that that particular group of patients, having suffered less from the primary injury, are more likely to recover more rapidly and more completely than the severely injured patients. All children will benefit from increased efforts at injury prevention, including continued emphasis on proper use of restraint in motor vehicles, proper helmeting for bicycling and sporting activities, improved education regarding the dangers of firearms around children, and enforcement of appropriate regulations on these weapons, as well as continued efforts aimed at identifying the causes and prevention of child abuse.

REFERENCES

1. Miller JD, Sweet RC, Narayan R, Becker DP: Early insults to the injured brain. JAMA 240:439, 1978.
2. Stalhammar DA: The mechanism of brain injuries. *In* Braakman R (ed): The Handbook of Clinical Neurology, Vol 13 (57): Head Injury. New York, Elsevier Science Publishing, 1990, pp 17–41.
3. Povlishock JT, Becker DP, Cheng CLY, Vaughn GW: Axonal change in minor head injury. J Neuropathol Exp Neurol 42:225, 1983.
4. Adams JH, Graham DI, Scott G, et al: Brain damage in fatal non-missile head injury. J Clin Pathol 33:1132, 1980.
5. Graham DI, Ford I, Adams JH, et al: Ischaemic brain damage is still common in fatal non-missile head injury. J Neurol Neurosurg Psychiatry 52:346, 1989.
6. Adams JH: Brain damage in fatal non-missile head injury in man. *In* Braakman R (ed): The Handbook of Clinical Neurology, Vol 13 (57): Head Injury. New York, Elsevier Science Publishing, 1990, pp 43–63.
7. Gennarelli TA, Segawa H, Wald V, et al.: Physiological response to angular acceleration of the head. *In* Grossman RG, Gildenberg PL (eds): Head Injury: Basic and Clinical Aspects. New York, Raven Press, 1982, p 129–140.
8. Lindenberg R: Trauma of meninges and brain. *In* Minckler J (ed): Pathology of the Nervous System. New York, McGraw-Hill, 1971, pp 1705–1765.
9. Gennarelli TA, Abel JM, Adams H, Graham D: Differential tolerance of frontal lobes to contusion induced by angular acceleration. In Proceedings of the 23rd Stapp Car Crash Conference, October 17–19, San Diego, California. Warrendale, Pennsylvania, The Society of Automotive Engineers, 1979, pp 563–586.
10. Caveness WF, Meirowsky AM, Rish BL, et al.: The nature of post-traumatic epilepsy. J Neurosurg 50:545, 1979.
11. DeSantis A, Capprecci E, Granata G: Early post-traumatic seizures in adults: Study of 84 cases. J Neurosurg Sci 23:207, 1979.
12. Hahn YS, Fuchs S, Flannery AM, et al: Factors influencing post-traumatic seizures in children. Neurosurgery 22:864, 1988.
13. Hansen JE, Guedeman SK, Holgate RC, Saunders RA: Penetrating intracranial wood wounds: Clinical limitations of computed tomography. J Neurosurg 68:752, 1988.
14. Fingerhut LA, Kleinman JC, Godfrey E, Rosenberg H: Firearm mortality among children, youth, and young adults 1 to 34 years of age. Trends and current status: United States, 1979–88. Monthly Vital Statistics Report, Vol 39, No 11 (suppl), 1991, pp 1–16.
15. Wintemute GJ, Teret SP, Kraus JF, et al.: When children shoot children. JAMA 258:3107, 1987.
16. Bolt JH, Moscicki EK: Firearms and youth suicide. Am J Public Health 76:1240, 1986.
17. Miner ME, Cabrera JA, Ford E, et al.: Intracranial penetration due to BB air rifle injuries. Neurosurgery 19:952, 1986.
18. Miner ME, Ewing-Cobbs L, Kopaniky DR, et al.: The results of treatment of gunshot wounds to the brain in children. Neurosurgery 26:20, 1990.
19. Kaufman HH: Treatment of civilian gunshot wound to the head. Neurosurg Clin North Am 2:387, 1991.
20. Ommaya AK, Gennarelli TA: Cerebral concussion and traumatic unconsciousness: Correlation of experimental and clinical observations on blunt head injuries. Brain 97:633, 1974.
21. Ommaya AK: Biomechanics of head injury: Experimental aspects. *In* Nahum AM, Melvin J (eds): The Biomechanics of Trauma. Norwalk, CN, Appleton-Century-Crofts, 1985, pp 245–269.
22. Pilz P: Axonal injury and head injury. Acta Neurochir (Suppl) 32:119, 1983.
23. Adams JH, Mitchell DE, Graham DI, Doyle D: Diffuse brain damage of the immediate impact type. Brain 100:489, 1977.
24. Hugenholtz H, Izukawa D, Shear P, et al.: Vomiting in children following head injury. Childs Nerv Syst 3:266, 1987.
25. Ryan CA, Edmonds J: Seizure activity mimicking brain stem herniation in children following head injuries. Crit Care Med 16:812, 1988.
26. Kaye EM, Herskowitz, J: Transient post-traumatic cortical blindness: Brief vs. prolonged syndromes in childhood. J Child Neurol 1:206, 1986.
27. Yamamoto LG, Bart RD: Transient blindness following mild head trauma. Clin Pediatr 27:479, 1988.
28. Gennarelli TA, Adams JH, Graham DI: Diffuse axonal injury—A new conceptual approach to an old problem. *In* Baethmann A, Go KG, Unterberg A (eds): Mechanisms of Secondary Brain Damage. New York, Plenum Press, 1986, pp 15–28.
29. Eisenberg HM, Cayard C, Papanicolaou A, et al.: The effects of three potentially preventable complications on outcome after severe closed head injury. *In* Ishii S, Nagai H, Brock M (eds): Intracranial Pressure V. New York, Springer-Verlag, 1983, pp 549–553.
30. Levine JE, Becker D: Reversal of incipient brain death from head injury: Apnea at the scene of accidents. N Engl J Med 301:109, 1979.
31. Ishige N, Pitts L, Pogliani L, et al.: The effect of hypoxia on traumatic brain injury in rats. I. Changes in neurological function, electroencephalograms and histopathology. Neurosurgery 20:848, 1987.
32. Foulkes MA, Eisenberg HM, Jane JA, et al.: The traumatic coma data bank: Design, methods, and baseline characteristics. J Neurosurg 75(Suppl):S8, 1991.
33. Chesnut RM, Gautille T, Blunt B, Marshall LF: Neurogenic shock in the Traumatic Coma Data Bank. Proceedings of the 60th Meeting of the American Association of Neurological Surgeons, San Francisco, California, 1992, pp 357–358.
34. Bruce DA, Alavi A, Bilaniuk L, et al.: Diffuse cerebral swelling following head injuries in children: The syndrome of "malignant brain edema." J Neurosurg 54:170, 1981.
35. Zimmerman RA, Bilaniuk LT, Bruce D, et al.: Computed tomography of pediatric head trauma: Acute general cerebral swelling. Radiology 126:403, 1978.
36. Muizelaar JP, Ward JD, Marmarou A, et al.: Cerebral blood flow and metabolism in severely head injured children. Part 2: Autoregulation. J Neurosurg 71:72, 1989.
37. Bruce DA, Raphaely RC, Goldberg AI, et al.: Pathophysiology, treatment and outcome following severe head injury in children. Childs Brain 5:174, 1979.
38. Aldrich EF, Eisenberg HM, Saydjari C, et al.: Diffuse brain swelling in severely head injured children. J Neurosurg 76:450, 1992.
39. Luerssen TG, Hults K, Klauber M, et al.: Improved outcome as a result of recognition of absent and compressed cisterns on initial CT scans. *In* Hoff JT, Betz AL (eds): Intracranial Pressure VII. New York, Springer-Verlag, 1989, pp 598–602.
40. Caffey J: On the theory and practice of shaking infants. Am J Dis Child 124:161, 1972.
41. Duhaime AC, Alario AJ, Lewander WJ, et al.: Head injury in very young children: Mechanisms, injury types and ophthalmologic findings in 100 hospitalized patients younger than 2 years of age. Pediatrics 90:179, 1992.
42. Luerssen TG, Huang JC, McLone DG, et al.: Retinal hemorrhages, seizures and intracranial hemorrhages: Relationships and outcomes in children suffering traumatic brain injury. *In* Marlin AE (ed): Concepts in Pediatric Neurosurgery XI. Basel, Karger, 1991, pp 87–94.
43. Rivera FP, Kamitsuka MD, Quan L: Injuries to children younger than 1 year of age. Pediatrics 81:93, 1988.
44. Duhaime AC, Gennarelli TA, Thibault LE, et al.: The shaken baby syndrome: A clinical, pathological, and biomechanical study. J Neurosurg 66:409, 1987.
45. Hadley MN, Sonntag VKH, Rekate HL, Murphy A: The infant whiplash-shake injury syndrome: A clinical and pathological study. Neurosurgery 24:536, 1989.
46. Calder IM, Hill I, Scholtz CL: Primary brain trauma in non-accidental injury. J Clin Pathol 37:1095, 1984.
47. Ludwig S, Warman M: Shaken baby syndrome: A review of 20 cases. Ann Emerg Med 13:104, 1984.
48. Zimmerman, RA, Bilaniuk LT, Bruce D: Computed tomography of craniocerebral injury in the abused child. Radiology 130:687, 1979.
49. Sato Y, Yuh WTC, Smith WL, et al.: Head injury in child abuse: Evaluation with MR imaging. Radiology 173:653, 1989.

50. Billmire ME, Myers PA: Serious head injury in infants: Accident or abuse? Pediatrics 75:340, 1985.
51. Teasdale G, Jennett, B: Assessment of coma and impaired consciousness. Lancet 11:81, 1974.
52. Born JD, Albert A, Hans P, Bonnal J: Relative prognostic value of best motor response and brain stem reflexes in patients with severe head injury. Neurosurgery 16:595, 1985.
53. Starmark JE, Holmgren E, Stalhammar D: Current reporting of responsiveness in acute cerebral disorders. J Neurosurg 69:692, 1988.
54. Braakman R, Gelpke GJ, Habbema JDF, et al.: Systematic selection of prognostic features in patients with severe head injury. Neurosurgery 16:362, 1980.
55. Klauber MR, Marshall LF, Luerssen TG, et al.: Determinants of head injury mortality: Importance of the low risk patient. Neurosurgery 24:31, 1989.
56. Teasdale G, Knill-Jones R, Van der Sande J: Observer variability in assessing impaired consciousness and coma. J Neurol Neurosurg Psychiatry 41:603, 1978.
57. Luerssen TG, Klauber MR, Marshall LF: Outcome from head injury related to patient's age. J Neurosurg 68:409, 1988.
58. Humphreys RP, Hendrick EB, Hoffman HJ: The head injured child who "talks and dies": A report of four cases. Childs Nerv Syst 3:139, 1990.
59. Snoek JW, Minderhoud JM, Wilmink JT: Delayed deterioration following minor head injury in children. Brain 80:1505, 1987.
60. Mendelow AD, Teasdale G, Jennett B, et al.: Risk of intracranial hematoma in head injured adults. Br Med J 287:1173, 1983.
61. Teasdale GM, Murray G, Anderson E, et al.: Risks of acute traumatic intracranial haematoma in children and adults: Implications for managing head injuries. Br Med J 300:363, 1990.
62. Gennarelli TA, Speilman GM, Langfitt TW, et al.: Influence of the type of intracranial lesion on outcome from severe head injury. J Neurosurg 56:26, 1982.
63. Eisenberg HM, Gary HE Jr, Aldrich EF, et al.: Initial CT findings in 753 patients with severe head injury. A report from the NIH Traumatic Coma Data Bank. J Neurosurg 73:688, 1990.
64. Toutant SM, Klauber MR, Marshall LF, et al.: Absent or compressed basal cisterns on first CT scan: Ominous predictors of outcome in severe head injury. J Neurosurg 61:691, 1984.
65. Marshall LF, Marshall SB, Klauber MR, et al.: A new classification of head injury based on computerized tomography. J Neurosurg 75(suppl):S14, 1991.
66. Luerssen TG, Huang JT, McLone DG, et al.: CT scan findings in a population of head injured children. Incidence and outcome. Childs Nerv Syst 6:298, 1990.
67. Jennett B, Bond M, Assessment of outcome after severe brain damage. A practical scale. Lancet i:480, 1975.
68. Andrews BT, Chiles BW, Olsen WL, et al.: The effect of intracerebral hematoma location on the risk of brainstem compression and on clinical outcome. J Neurosurg 69:518, 1988.
69. Marshall LF, Barba D. Toole BM. Bowers SA: The oval pupil: Clinical significance and relationship to intracranial hypertension. J Neurosurg 58:566, 1983.
70. Luerssen TG, Marshall LF: The medical management of head injury. In Braakman R (ed): The Handbook of Clinical Neurology, Vol 13 (57): Head Injury. New York, Elsevier Science Publishing, 1990, pp 207–247.
71. Levi L, Guilburd JN, Lemberger A, et al.: Diffuse axonal injury: Analysis of 100 patients with radiological signs. Neurosurgery 27:429, 1990.
72. Saul TG, Ducker TB, Salcman M, Carro E: Steroids in severe head injury: A randomized clinical trial. J Neurosurg 54:596, 1981.
73. Braakman R, Schoutern HJ: Megadose steroids in severe head injury: Results of a prospective double blind clinical trial. J Neurosurg 58:326, 1983.
74. Dearden NM, Gibson JS, McDowall DG, et al.: Effect of high-dose dexamethasone on outcome from severe head injury. J Neurosurg 64:81, 1986.
75. Bracken MB, Shepard MJ, Collins WF, et al.: A randomized, controlled trial of methylprednisolone or naloxone in the treatment of acute spinal cord injury. Results of the Second National Acute Spinal Cord Injury Study. N Engl J Med 322:1405, 1990.
76. Dearden, NM, Miller JD: Paired comparison of hypnotic and osmotic therapy in the reduction of raised intracranial pressure (ICP) after severe head injury. In Hoff JT (ed): Intracranial Pressure VII. New York, Springer-Verlag, 1989, pp 474–481.

Chapter 20

POST-TRAUMATIC HEMATOMAS

KEITH E. ARONYK, M.D.

Head injuries in the pediatric age group (less than 15 years of age) have many features that distinguish them from head injuries in the adult age group.[1-3] The pediatric skull and brain change rapidly during development, and the clinical profile of head injury changes accordingly. While head trauma is common among infants, children, and adolescents, most injuries are minor and few are complicated by intracranial hemorrhage.[1-5] The neonatal head injury differs greatly from the adolescent head injury.[6] However, in all age groups, head trauma can be complicated by intracranial hemorrhage, and it is the purpose of this chapter to discuss the common patterns of post-traumatic intracranial hemorrhage and outline management principles within each subgroup. In all of these groups, almost all post-traumatic intracranial hematomas are extra-axial and are readily accessible to the surgeon. As a general rule, post-traumatic intracranial hematomas in infants, children, and adolescents may lead to secondary cerebral insults, and surgical evacuation must always be a leading consideration among management options.

Points that deserve emphasis are as follows:

1. Of all post-traumatic intracranial hematomas in children, extradural hematomas are the most common and often follow relatively minor head injuries.

2. Occipital blows are always worrisome. If a child is not improving rapidly, especially if an occipital skull fracture is present, radiologic studies must be carried out in search of an intracranial hemorrhage.

3. Significant intracerebral/cerebellar hematomas are uncommon in all pediatric age groups.

4. Any child with a head injury who has an alteration in consciousness, headache, persistent vomiting, skull fracture, or seizure should have a computed tomographic (CT) scan in search of an intracranial hematoma. A high index of suspicion is also required in children with congenital cerebral malformations, cerebrospinal fluid (CSF) shunts, or coagulation disorders.

The skull, brain, and cervical spine represent a steadily developing unit that responds in a different way to trauma at each stage during development.

During the birth process, the cranial bones move in relation to one another as the head molds. The occipital bone hinges at the basal-squamosal junction, and the base of the skull flexes slightly as the cranial vault "towers" until the coronal and lambdoidal sutures lock to prevent excessive narrowing of the biparietal diameter.[7] The head and the cervical spine are subjected to traumatic forces during the birth process, but it is usually the difficult birth (often aided by forceps or vacuum extraction) that distorts the skull, brain, and dural reflections enough to injure the brain or cause intracranial hemorrhage.

The neonatal skull is a loose aggregate of thin pliable bone plates which are hardly protective; the brain is remarkably fragile, easily torn, and very large in relation to the rest of the body. The neck is weak, is unable to support the large head, and will permit an unphysiologic range of motion if stressed.

During infancy and early childhood, cranial sutures approximate each other, fontanelles close, and strong protective bone develops as the skull becomes a solid unit. The cerebral vasculature matures, and the brain becomes less fragile as myelination proceeds and water content decreases. Somewhere between the first and second years, the skull loses many of its resilient properties and becomes more solid. As this occurs, the high incidence of acute subdural hematoma falls as if sutural closure in some way protects against formation of subdural hematomas.[8] As an infant becomes a toddler, the overall incidence of intracranial hemorrhage falls, and extradural hematomas become more common.

The infant, before the ambulatory stage, is completely dependent and totally vulnerable. The infant brain is particularly prone to serious injury from the excessive forces experienced by the infant as passenger in a motor vehicle accident.[9, 10] During the first few months of life, high-speed acceleration-deceleration injuries result in unusually severe cerebral injuries, especially if the infant is unrestrained. However, in infants, many severe cerebral injuries involving intracranial hemorrhage are the result of nonaccidental trauma,[6] and subdural hematomas figure prominently.[8, 11] Post-traumatic intracranial hemorrhage in infants usually occurs close to the surface in the subdural or subarachnoid spaces, but it is what lies beneath the surface that is important. Whereas the subdural collections may be minor, the forces are often major, and the brain injury may be severe. With severe injuries the young brain is particularly prone to early, diffuse swelling (malignant edema or cerebral hyperemia[6, 12–14]), as the cerebral vasculature is still maturing. Early aggressive intervention is important as the young brain has less pressure-volume reserve than the older brain; intracranial pressure rises rapidly. It is the brain's response to injury that leads to this increasing intracranial pressure as cerebral autoregulation is lost, vasogenic and cytotoxic edema spread, and the blood-brain barrier fails.

The older child is ambulatory and adventurous and feels independent. Head injuries often occur when limits are tested, especially with falls from heights or from bicycles or with pedestrian traffic accidents. Intracranial bleeding is again usually close to the surface near the area of impact. Now, extradural hematomas outnumber subdural hematomas,[11] but diffuse cerebral swelling still represents a common secondary insult.

The adolescent brain seems well protected within the confines of the skull, but the adolescent is so difficult to rigidly confine. The skull and brain are no match for the forces they must absorb from various motorized vehicles, projectiles, or combat-like recreational activities. Major forces disrupt the delicate circuitry of the brain, alter the vascular properties of the brain, and often result in prolonged brain swelling and edema. The pattern approximates that seen in young adults, in whom intracranial hematomas represent one of the few reversible factors in a prolonged battle with a swollen decompensated brain.

Post-traumatic intracranial hematomas can collect in the extradural space or the subdural space or within the brain and its CSF spaces. From a practical pediatric point of view, post-traumatic hematomas often follow common clinical patterns and can best be discussed from this clinical orientation. These patterns are (1) posterior fossa hemorrhage in the neonatal period, (2) acute and chronic subdural collections in infancy, (3) extradural hematomas, and (4) intracerebral hematomas. Before the discussion can begin, however, several practical surgical points must be made:

1. Cervical spinal injuries are difficult to document in the pediatric age group, and more caution is required, as spinal cord injury does occur without obvious spinal fracture or subluxation.

2. Incision lines often cross open fontanelles or open sutures, and all skull defects must be kept in mind. Blood loss is always a concern, and scalp bleeding must be carefully controlled.

3. Surgery in the neonate is difficult, as blood loss rapidly reaches excessive levels and the neonate has a unique set of problems related to hemostasis and blood transfusions.

COAGULATION CONCERNS

It is at this point that coagulation concerns in the neonate should be addressed, as it is the experience of many surgeons that the coagulation cascade performs poorly in the premature and term neonate.[15, 16] Surgery that involves major bleeding within the first few days of life must be approached with great caution. Intracranial hemorrhage in a premature neonate is just one of the many factors that makes these infants extremely ill. It is in this setting that disseminated intravascular coagulation (DIC) is common (shock, sepsis, acidosis, hypoxia, hypothermia, abruptio placentae, retention of dead twin fetus) so that the platelet count, prothrombin time (PT), and partial thromboplastin time (PTT) must be known before any surgical procedure can be performed on a seriously ill premature infant. DIC is characterized by prolonged PT and PTT with a low platelet count, low serum fibrinogen level, and increased fibrin split products. DIC should be treated initially with platelet transfusion (1 unit every 12 to 24 hours) and fresh frozen plasma (10 ml per kg every 12 hours). If a coagulopathy occurs in a healthy term neonate, one must have vitamin K deficiency and hemophilia in mind. Occasionally, the presence of large cutaneous angiomas can result in a coagulopathy.[17]

Vitamin K deficiency results in hemorrhagic disease of the newborn. The normal newborn has almost no vitamin K stores to support hepatic elaboration of coagulation proteins. Vitamin K must be supplied by dietary intake and later by intestinal bacterial synthesis. Human milk is deficient in vitamin K, and it is possible that exclusively breast-fed infants who are not given vitamin K at birth may have a coagulopathy due to vitamin K deficiency. It is also possible that maternal drugs such as phenytoin, phenobarbital, isoniazid, or rifampin can affect the neonatal liver and result in a similar decrease in coagulation proteins. Babies of epileptic mothers or mothers being treated for tuberculosis may have a coagulopathy that becomes evident within the first 24 hours of life. In the neonatal unit, these early forms of hemorrhagic disease of the newborn (drug related or vitamin K deficiency) can be recognized by abnormal bleeding in the setting of a normal platelet count and prolonged PT and PTT studies. Vitamin K administration (vitamin K_1 oxide, 0.5 to 1.0 mg IM) will allow the liver to elaborate the necessary coagulation proteins within approximately 4 hours. However, rapid correction may be required, and vitamin K (1 mg) must be administered intravenously along with fresh frozen plasma (10 ml per kg). The fresh frozen plasma may have to be repeated in 12 hours.

It is worth repeating that vitamin K is obtained by

dietary intake and must be absorbed via the gastrointestinal tract. Neonates who have chronic gastrointestinal disorders or prolonged diarrhea absorb vitamin K poorly and may be predisposed to a vitamin K deficiency coagulopathy. It is the recommendation of the American Academy of Pediatrics that infants with prolonged diarrhea (over 1 week in duration) receive at least one intramuscular injection of vitamin K (0.5 to 1.0 mg) during the illness. Infants not receiving vitamin K at birth, as is routine in most nurseries, may be predisposed to a late coagulopathy (1 to 12 months), especially if they are primarily breast-fed. This must be kept in mind if a healthy neonate/infant presents with an intracranial hemorrhage (subarachnoid/subdural) with other evidence of excessive bleeding. At first sight, the clinical picture may suggest child abuse. Hemophilia can present with intracranial bleeding in the neonatal period, but in this case the platelets and PT are normal; PTT is markedly abnormal. This coagulopathy is reversed by administration of fresh frozen plasma or specific factor VIII preparations.

POSTERIOR FOSSA HEMORRHAGE IN THE NEONATAL PERIOD

Intracranial hemorrhage in a neonatal unit is a relatively common problem. However, most hemorrhages cannot be classified as post-traumatic as they are related to prematurity and hypoxic/ischemic insults. Periventricular-intraventricular hemorrhages usually occur in premature neonates of less than 32 weeks' gestation. A combination of hypoxic and hemodynamic factors results in hemorrhage within the highly cellular germinal matrix, which has poorly supported vessels draining into veins that seem predisposed to thrombosis.[18] It is important to recognize the infant with this type of intracranial hemorrhage in the neonatal intensive care unit (ICU), as these babies do sometimes have posterior fossa (cerebellar) hemorrhages as a component of their periventricular-intraventricular hemorrhage pattern, and the prognosis, with or without surgical intervention, is poor. However, there is a subset of infants in the neonatal intensive care unit who do have post-traumatic hemorrhage, often in the posterior fossa, and do respond favorably to surgical intervention.

Even though there are coagulation concerns and anesthesia is difficult, emergency craniotomy for intracranial bleeding is sometimes required. Intraparenchymal hemorrhages (especially cerebellar) in the term neonate may reach surgical significance and are not as ominous as those that occur in the premature infant.[18–20] In term neonates, most cerebellar hemorrhages are post-traumatic and most involve the superior vermis (Fig. 20–1). These are thought to result from the trauma of the birth process as prolonged labor, major cranial molding, and breech presentation are all etiologic factors. The occipital bone is "hinged" where the squamosal portion meets the basal portion near the occipital condyles. It is possible that this synchondrosis separates during a difficult delivery (occipital osteodiastasis) and that the squamous portion of the occipital bone thrusts inward, forcing the cerebellum up through the tentorial incisura. In a similar way, the superior vermis may be injured with excessive vertical skull molding, which also may tear the tentorium and enclosed venous sinuses. Many cerebellar hemorrhages in otherwise healthy term neonates can be managed nonsurgically, or at most with temporary CSF drainage. However, permanent CSF diversion will be required in at least one third of these infants. Similar etiologic mechanisms are thought to be operative in acute subdural hematomas of the posterior fossa in neonates, and these two entities are often considered together.[19–23] The distinction between acute subdural and intracerebellar hematomas is somewhat blurred in many cases, but it is clear that the acute subdural hematoma is a lesion that responds favorably to surgical intervention. In term neonates, it is the acute subdural hematoma, rather than the cerebellar hematoma, that usually involves the neurosurgeon. The same traumatic forces involved in delivery are implicated with posterior fossa subdural hematomas, and these otherwise healthy term neonates also present with lethargy, irritability, bulging anterior fontanelle, nuchal rigidity, increased extensor tone, respiratory irregularities, lower cranial nerve palsies, and finally respiratory arrest.[23] This pattern develops within the first few days of life when a high index of suspicion is required to detect this posterior fossa hematoma, which may only be seen with careful coronal CT scan or magnetic resonance images. Often, the hematoma accumulates along the tentorial surface of the cerebellum and does represent a significant mass lesion. The more massive hematomas occurring as a result of a major tentorial or venous sinus tear may be rapidly fatal. Whereas the cerebellar hematoma in the term neonate can be managed nonsurgically, the acute subdural hematoma is best managed surgically. Again, careful preoperative preparation and planning are required.

Traumatic forces during birth, especially with excessive vertical molding, can also result in acute subdural hematomas over the cerebral convexities. The clinical presentation still involves an irritable, lethargic infant with a bulging fontanelle, but now seizures are more common and a focal neurologic deficit may be noted. Convexity subdural hematomas are prominent over the temporal lobes and may be associated with cerebral contusions or lacerations. Some are silent, but most present with neonatal seizures and focal neurologic deficits. Coagulation disorders must again be considered. Convexity hematomas are managed initially by subdural tapping, but craniotomy may be necessary if subdural tapping is ineffective and a mass lesion remains. It is possible, although not proven, that neonatal acute subdural hematomas may be the cause of chronic subdural hematomas noted later in infancy.[22]

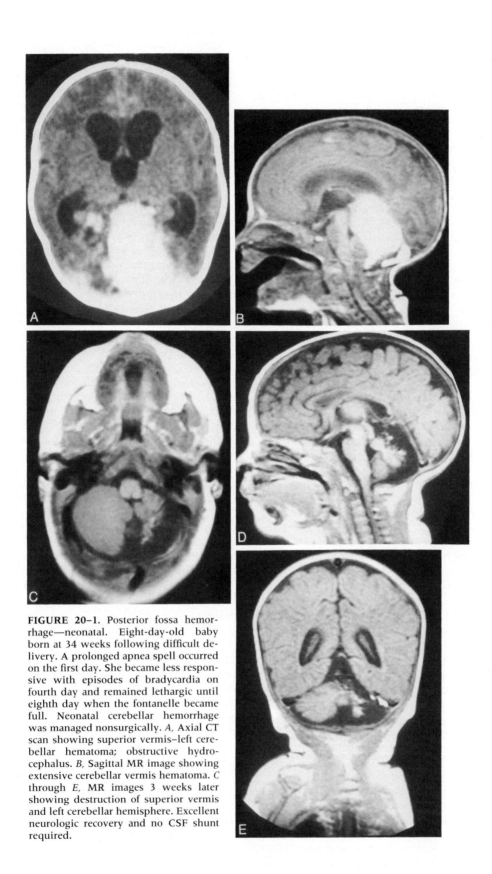

FIGURE 20–1. Posterior fossa hemorrhage—neonatal. Eight-day-old baby born at 34 weeks following difficult delivery. A prolonged apnea spell occurred on the first day. She became less responsive with episodes of bradycardia on fourth day and remained lethargic until eighth day when the fontanelle became full. Neonatal cerebellar hemorrhage was managed nonsurgically. *A,* Axial CT scan showing superior vermis–left cerebellar hematoma; obstructive hydrocephalus. *B,* Sagittal MR image showing extensive cerebellar vermis hematoma. *C* through *E,* MR images 3 weeks later showing destruction of superior vermis and left cerebellar hemisphere. Excellent neurologic recovery and no CSF shunt required.

ACUTE AND CHRONIC SUBDURAL COLLECTIONS OF INFANTS

The main surgical issues to be discussed here involve management of intracranial hemorrhages in child abuse and management of chronic subdural collections of infancy. Both require close surgical supervision as well as sound surgical judgment. Although there is often some doubt about the traumatic nature of chronic subdural collections in infancy, there is usually no doubt about the traumatic nature of acute subdural hematomas.

ACUTE SUBDURAL HEMATOMA

Acute hemorrhage in the subdural space in infants and children is considered to be traumatic in nature, although one must always consider the possibility of subdural abscess or leptomeningeal tumor presenting as a subdural collection. For practical purposes, however, acute subdural hematomas in infants and children represent recent trauma, and in fact nonaccidental injury (child abuse) should be the first consideration. In the spectrum of pediatric head trauma, acute subdural hematoma is most common in young infants, less common in toddlers and older children, then more common in adolescents as brain injury patterns approximate those seen in young adults.[8, 11, 24] In the subset of older infants and toddlers, however, chronic subdural hematoma is far more common than acute subdural hematoma. The exact relationship between acute and chronic subdural hematomas is unclear as many chronic subdural hematomas present with no history of

trauma. Both acute and chronic subdural hematomas in infants should raise the suspicion of child abuse, although a coagulopathy must be considered and vitamin K deficiency ruled out (Fig. 20–2).[25, 26]

Acute subdural hematoma in infants or older children usually presents in dramatic fashion, whereas chronic subdural hematoma is much less dramatic. Infants and children with acute subdural hematoma are seriously ill, and surgical intervention is often required urgently.

Occasionally an infant will be dropped or an older child will fall, and an acute subdural hematoma will result from a tear of a convexity bridging vein. As the hematoma collects slowly, the brain is compressed and shifted; seizures, focal neurologic signs, and finally a deteriorating level of consciousness follows. The CT scan makes the diagnosis, and immediate craniotomy is successful in relieving the compression and distortion; the brain recovers.[27] More commonly, however, the acute subdural hematoma reflects a much more severe cerebral injury,[28, 29] and the surgical evacuation is a minor component of the long therapeutic struggle to control brain swelling and intracranial hypertension. In infants and children, the hematoma usually arises from parietal-occipital parasagittal bridging veins rather than from extensive orbital-frontal or temporal tip contusions/lacerations as occurs with adult acute subdural hematomas. The cerebrum in infants and children is definitely not spared, however. The parietal-occipital tentorial/interhemispheric subdural hematoma may be minor, but the cerebral injury is not. Such injuries may occur when the child is involved in a motor vehicle accident as an occupant or falls from a great height, but most severe cerebral injuries in infants are the result of

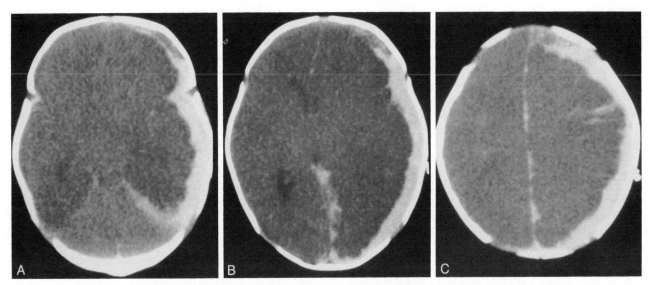

FIGURE 20–2. Hemorrhagic disease of the newborn. Five-week-old baby admitted in moribund condition. Two-day history beginning with irritability and vomiting, then respiratory irregularities and seizures. Rapid decompensation just prior to admission to hospital. Hemoglobin, 0.9 gm/dl; hematocrit, 3.0 per cent; platelets, 103,000. No retinal hemorrhages or evidence of previous trauma. Baby was born by home delivery and exclusively breast-fed. Baby bleeding from all puncture sites, old and new, and diagnosis of hemorrhagic disease of the newborn made. Axial CT images show large left acute subdural hematoma with associated subarachnoid hemorrhage and midline shift.

nonaccidental trauma (child abuse). Acute subdural hematoma in the setting of child abuse is the prime example of pediatric acute subdural hematoma, and most pertinent points will be covered by a discussion of this entity.

Acute Subdural Hematoma in Child Abuse

The peak incidence of child abuse resulting in intracranial hemorrhage is at age 6 months, and almost all cases occur before the age of 2 years. Difficult family social circumstances breed anger and frustration in caregivers, and the defenseless infant is often the target of this anger. Unfortunately, the head and face bare the brunt of the attacks, and the infant head is ill-equipped to withstand this attack. The infant head is large and poorly supported by the weak neck musculature; the cerebrum is fragile because of its high water content and poor myelination, and the subarachnoid space is relatively large—all making the brain relatively "mobile." The exact mechanism of cerebral injury is controversial as it has not been firmly established whether or not a violent shake of the head alone can result in the severe cerebral injuries observed.[29–33] Some evidence suggests that the rapid deceleration of an impact is required to cause the injury forces necessary to result in this degree of cerebral injury.[30] Children with acute subdural hematoma are usually seriously ill at presentation, but trauma is not always obvious. The infant who is obtunded or unconscious with a bulging fontanelle and a history of respiratory arrest or seizures must be considered as a possible child abuse victim. An urgent brain CT scan and a careful ophthalmologic assessment (for retinal hemorrhages) must be arranged. Cerebral trauma belongs in the differential diagnosis of meningitis, encephalitis, status epilepticus, and intoxication. The presence of retinal hemorrhages is extremely significant, and a formal ophthalmologic assessment is necessary as the characteristics of the retinal hemorrhages (traumatic retinoschisis, preretinal hemorrhages) are virtually diagnostic of the violently shaken infant.[34–41] Retinal hemorrhages rarely occur following severe accidental trauma,[41] spontaneous intracranial hemorrhage,[42] or vigorous cardiopulmonary resuscitation.[43, 44] For all practical purposes, however, retinal hemorrhages in infants mean acute subdural bleeding, and the combination of retinal hemorrhages and acute subdural bleeding means violent shaking with or without impact. A diagnosis of child abuse rests on supportive medical evidence such as CT scan[45, 46] as well as plain x-ray and bone scan abnormalities,[47] but it also relies on social/legal evidence obtained by interviews with caregivers and close examination of the home setting.

The cerebral injury resulting from this acceleration-deceleration force is a remarkably severe injury. A combination of factors must certainly be involved as the intracranial hemorrhages are often relatively minor, whereas the ultimate cerebral destruction is major and widespread. Often, at initial presentation, there is a description of an arrest or apneic event. An ischemic or hypoxic insult may be added to the primary shake injury. In this setting, it is known that severe cerebral injuries may be associated with injuries to brainstem regions important for respiratory function at the cranial-cervical junction.[32] The physical cerebral injury results in cerebral white matter tears, cerebral cortical contusions, and intracranial hemorrhage.[46, 48] The hemorrhages usually arise from disrupted bridging veins, leading to posterior interhemispheric and tentorial subdural hematomas. Cerebral arteries may also be injured. Subarachnoid hemorrhage is common, and vasospasm may be a factor leading to further cerebral ischemia. As the brain swells or is compressed by the intracranial hematoma, the intracranial pressure increases and cerebral perfusion pressure falls, again contributing to widespread ischemia. Also, as intracranial pressure rises, cerebral herniations and shifts occur, compressing arteries on the cerebral surface as well as in the tentorial incisura, leading to hemorrhagic necrosis in arterial distributions. This complicated chain of events results in acute subdural hematomas, cerebral white matter tears/clefts, subarachnoid hemorrhage, and widespread cerebral cortical necrosis (Fig. 20–3).

The cerebral injury therefore is severe even if the subdural hematoma is relatively small. Occasionally, a large acute subdural hematoma will require craniotomy for removal; only rarely is a subdural tap useful in the setting of acute subdural hemorrhage. More commonly, neurosurgical involvement is limited to intracranial pressure monitoring and possibly CSF drainage (ventriculostomy catheter) as the severe ischemic-hypoxic insult must be managed medically in an intensive care setting until the cerebral swelling subsides. It is at this time that surgical intervention may again be required as cerebral destruction may be widespread and brain bulk greatly diminished. The subarachnoid and ventricular spaces enlarge as do the subdural spaces, and occasionally the subdural spaces require long-term drainage (subdural-peritoneal shunt).

Acute subdural hematoma in infants is always serious, and the prognosis in cases of child abuse is poor. The mortality rate is approximately 20 per cent and the morbidity rate 50 per cent in most series.[31, 33, 49]

CHRONIC SUBDURAL HEMATOMA

Whereas acute subdural hematoma in an infant or child presents a dramatic clinical picture with a severe brain injury, chronic subdural hematoma of infancy often presents simply as megalencephaly. The differential diagnosis includes hydrocephalus, benign enlargement of the subarachnoid space, and brain tumor.

Chronic subdural collections are common problems during infancy, and as with other post-traumatic hemorrhages, males are affected more commonly than females. Chronic subdural collections are regarded as post-traumatic lesions in the great majority of cases. Birth trauma is sometimes implicated, but this is unlikely. Rather, it seems that minor injuries during infancy or even more violent injuries such as infant shak-

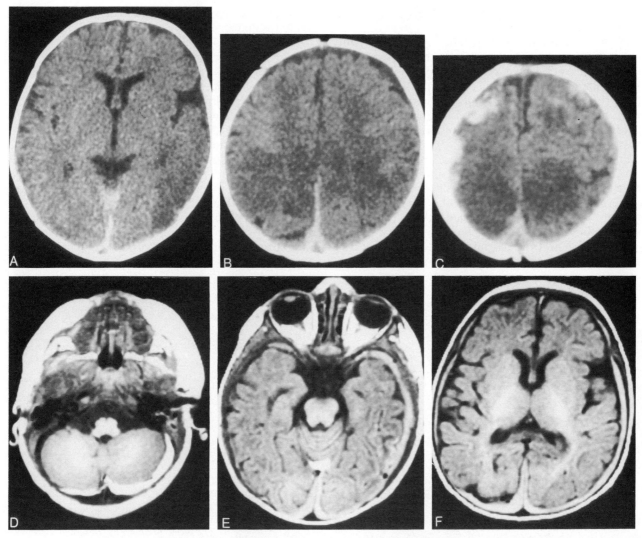

FIGURE 20–3. Child abuse—intracranial hemorrhage. Two-month-old infant presenting with one day history of lethargy, seizures, and irritability. Bilateral retinal hemorrhages were noted. Diagnosis: child abuse. *A, B,* and *C,* Axial CT images showing acute subdural hematoma in the parietal-occipital and interhemispheric regions. Multiple areas of infarction in both occipital regions. *D, E,* and *F,* MRI images showing subdural collections in the parietal occipital and even posterior fossa regions.

ing and/or cranial impact are the inciting events. In many cases a clear history of injury is not forthcoming, but there should always be a suspicion of trauma, and the opportunity should be seized to investigate the child and the social setting at least in a screening fashion (social service interview, skeletal survey, bone scan, and ophthalmologic assessment). Congenital cerebral anomalies, such as arachnoid cysts,[50, 51] may predispose toward subdural hematoma formation.[52] Occasionally, subdural collections do follow meningitis[53, 54] (*Haemophilus influenzae, Streptococcus pneumoniae*) or appear as a complication of a known coagulopathy (vitamin K deficiency, leukemia). On a neurosurgical service, another common cause of subdural fluid accumulation is cranial-cerebral disproportion resulting from CSF shunting. This may result in large accumulations of subdural fluid as the cerebrum collapses ("over-shunting"), but it is the feeling of many that these represent a relatively benign form of subdural accumulations. These accumulations seem less likely to enlarge, and thick restrictive membranes rarely develop. Post-traumatic subdural hematomas are different in that many do progress. As a reaction to the opening of the potential subdural space, the inner surface of the dura mounts an inflammatory and neovascular response that makes it resemble granulation tissue.[55–58] As a result of recurrent hemorrhage from this fragile, leaky, vascular membrane, subdural collections tend to increase in stacatto fashion and often appear multilayered on CT or MRI images. Over time, there is a tendency for the reactive appearance of the inner membrane to gradually resolve as recurrent hemorrhages cease and the subdural fluid disappears.

The important points are that subdural collections in infants should be considered as traumatic lesions and that they do have a tendency to increase in size. These lesions, which are almost always bilateral, are best managed surgically.

The clinical presentation is usually subtle, and one is often relieved to discover subdural fluid collections in a child thought to possibly have hydrocephalus or a brain tumor. Bilateral subdural collections must be differentiated from benign enlargement of the subarachnoid space,[59] but the diagnosis can be made on the basis of CT scans with contrast or, even better, MRI studies with coronal images.

Clinically, these are usually infants or toddlers less than 2 years of age who may have a history of moderate irritability and vomiting. The head size is just above the normal range, and the anterior fontanelle is still open and large. The history of generalized seizures is common, and in fact, this is a common presenting feature. There are no truly diagnostic signs and few physical signs. It is uncommon to find papilledema, sun-

setting of the eyes, or prominent frontal bossing with dilated scalp veins as are seen in hydrocephalus. A careful search should be made for retinal changes, which may reflect the underlying traumatic nature of the inciting event.

The combination of CT and MRI images is usually diagnostic, demonstrating the bilateral extra-axial collections that are distinct from the underlying subarachnoid space (Fig. 20–4). It is of note that the subarachnoid space is usually widened rather than compressed. The subdural space is also wide except for the area where the subdural space meets the subarachnoid space in the parasagittal (superior sagittal sinus) region. Although subdural collections can extend into the interhemispheric fissure, they often are limited by the adherence of the arachnoid to the dura in the region of CSF absorption near the superior sagittal sinus. It may be the distortion of this region by the subdural collec-

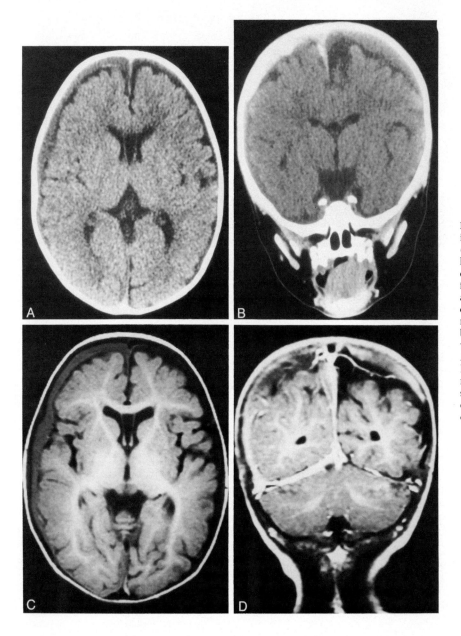

FIGURE 20–4. Chronic subdural hematoma in infancy. Thirty-three-month-old triplet (32-week premature) presented with minor head injury from a fall. His head circumference was above the 95th percentile; anterior fontanelle was open and full. Neurologic examination normal except for minor nonspecific retinal hemorrhages. Skeletal survey was normal; bone scan was normal. Images reveal bilateral subdural collections of varying ages with dilated subarachnoid space. *A* and *B,* Axial and coronal CT cuts to demonstrate bilateral subdural collections with right more recent than left. *C* and *D,* MRI images clearly showing wide subarachnoid space and subdural collections of different ages. No evidence of cerebral parenchymal injury.

tion that impairs CSF absorption and results in the widening of the subarachnoid space. This situation is significantly different from that seen in adults, in whom the subarachnoid spaces and cerebral ventricles are compressed by bilateral chronic subdural collections. Chronic subdural collections also occur in the posterior fossa, and similar mechanisms are implicated (Fig. 20–5).

The management of chronic subdural collections of infancy is surgical. There remains some controversy in this area, but removal of the subdural fluid and avoidance of intracranial hypertension are the most important considerations. Craniotomy for excision of membranes is no longer advocated as a primary approach, but occasionally this is still required when all else fails. The major area of controversy centers around subdural tapping; some believe that the procedure carried out at the bedside is dangerous (hemorrhage, infection) and is not as effective as shunting procedures. The techniques for subdural tapping have been well described,[60, 61] and it is the experience of many neurosurgeons that serial subdural tapping alone can successfully manage bilateral subdural collections in some cases. Taps should be carried out 3 cm from midline through the anterior fontanelle or coronal suture, and subdural fluid should drain spontaneously. Fluid should be drained until the fontanelle sinks, but as a rule, caution is advised after removal of 25 ml from one side. The tap can always be repeated. Multiple taps are required in most cases, and the progress of the subdural collections must be followed closely by repeated CT scans. Most now feel that the optimal management of subdural collections of infancy is a form of shunting, and usually the subdural-peritoneal shunt system with little resistance to flow is the method of choice. Even bilateral collections can usually be drained with a unilateral shunting procedure.[62, 63] Again, the shunt system should have little resistance to flow. This form of management works best when a normal brain is growing rapidly because within 2 to 3 months the subdural space is obliterated by the combination of fluid drainage and brain growth. If there is underlying brain injury or atrophy, or if a ventricular shunt is in place, the subdural spaces persist longer and are more difficult to manage. In this situation, a more long-term shunt is required, and occasionally a combination of a ventricular and subdural shunt is required. The resistance to flow through the ventricular shunt should be greater than that through the subdural shunt. Most infants progress well following drainage of the subdural collections (approximately 75 per cent develop normally), but all too often there is significant underlying cerebral trauma that limits the potential of these children.

Subdural hygroma refers to collections of CSF in the subdural space, and these are considered in much the same light as subdural hematomas. They are best considered as post-traumatic lesions. The same forces that tear bridging veins may tear the arachnoid where it attaches to the parasagittal dura, and both CSF and blood can collect in the subdural space. The clinical presentation is similar as is the management strategy, except that there is less urgency. Subdural membranes are not well formed, and rebleeding is not such a concern. Subdural tapping or burr hole drainage seems to be more successful in the setting of subdural hygroma, although again a shunt system may be required.

EXTRADURAL HEMATOMA

Extradural hematomas deserve emphasis in a chapter on pediatric post-traumatic intracranial hematomas. They may not be common complications of pediatric head injuries (2 to 3 per cent of all head injury admissions[64–67]), but they constitute the major post-traumatic intracranial hematoma occurring after infancy and before the high-velocity injuries of adolescents and young adults. Even though the surgical management is straightforward, the timing is critical and judgment

FIGURE 20–5. Chronic subdural hematoma—posterior fossa. Nine-month-old male presented with 1-week history of nausea, vomiting, and irritability. He had lost the ability to sit or stand and had become more somnolent. Negative birth history. Head circumference—95th percentile; anterior fontanelle closed. A, Axial CT scan showing posterior fossa chronic subdural collections. B, MRI demonstrating right chronic subdural collection with marked dilatation of temporal horns.

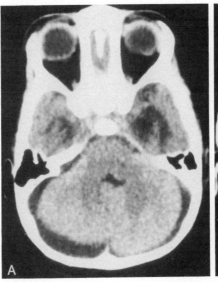
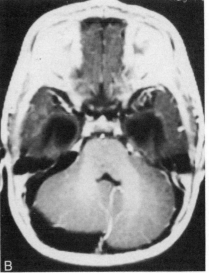

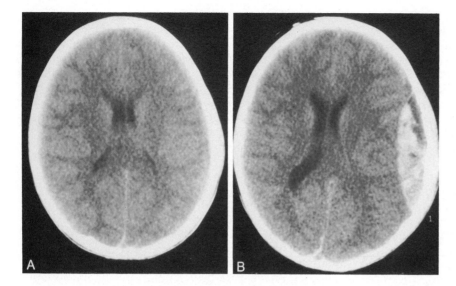

FIGURE 20–6. Delayed extradural hematoma. A 6-year-old boy fell 20 feet, striking his head. Following a short loss of consciousness, he awakened and seemed to be intact until he had a generalized seizure in the Emergency Room. *A,* Initial CT scan at 1935 hours. *B,* Follow-up CT scan when intracranial pressure began to rise at 0336 hours (8 hours later).

more difficult now that some extradural hematomas are thought to be suitable for nonsurgical management. The main points are:

1. Extradural hematoma usually follows a relatively mild head injury in children. Skull fractures are common but not invariable. An extradural hematoma must be considered in any child whose condition does not improve rapidly following a relatively mild head injury.

2. Extradural hematoma can enlarge while the child is under supervision. If an extradural hematoma is found on the same day as the injury, begin arranging for surgical evacuation of the mass lesion.

3. It is not rare for extradural hematomas to develop and present in a delayed fashion (Fig. 20–6). Even if the first CT/MRI images are normal, repeat the studies if the child is not improving. This is especially true if some form of treatment has begun, such as hemodynamic resuscitation from shock or the institution of therapy to decrease intracranial pressure. Even if the craniotomy has already been carried out to remove a

mass lesion, one must always think of a second hematoma (delayed extradural hematoma) appearing at another site if the child is not improving steadily. If the condition of a child with a CSF leak deteriorates while under supervision, consider a delayed extradural hematoma as a possible cause.

4. Occipital blows in children deserve special consideration, especially if there is a fracture and especially if the child's condition is not improving. Posterior fossa extradural hematomas, although rare, do occur, and many present 1 or 2 days following the injury. Deterioration can be rapid and catastrophic, and the mortality rate is still too high. A high degree of suspicion is required, and special attention to posterior fossa imaging techniques is important.

The reported incidence of extradural hematomas in pediatric head injury series is between 2 and 3 per cent, but they certainly seem much more common in surgical series.[64, 65] Although extradural hematomas can occur in any pediatric age group, they are least com-

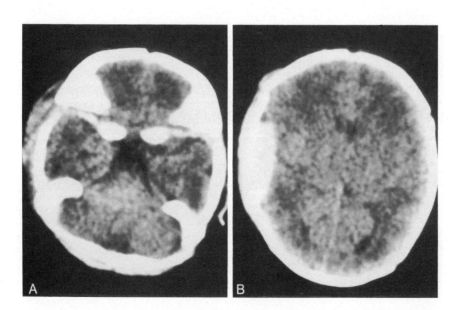

FIGURE 20–7. Extradural hematoma in infancy. Two-day-old baby born at 37 weeks by cesarean section. Accidental head trauma resulted in diastasis of right squamosal suture. Small extradural hematoma increased over 2 days. Subperiosteal hematoma communicated with extradural space. *A,* Right temporal subperiosteal hematoma. *B,* Right temporal parietal extradural hematoma.

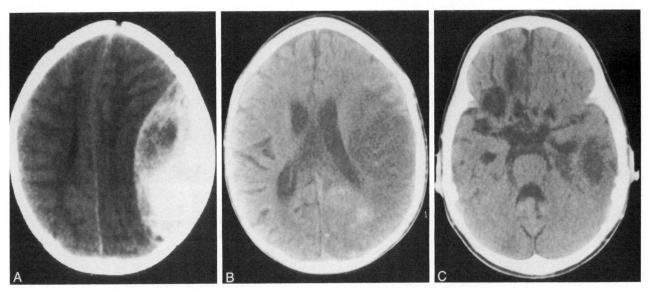

FIGURE 20–8. Extradural hematoma caused by child abuse. Eleven-month-old male, a victim of child abuse. Sustained a direct blow to the left parietal region and was unconscious on admission. After a prolonged hospital course, he recovered with mild right hemiparesis. *A,* CT scan on admission shows large left parietal extradural hematoma. *B,* CT scan 10 days after injury. *C,* CT scan 3 weeks after injury showing signs of a more diffuse cerebral injury.

monly encountered in neonates and infants (Fig. 20–7). Child abuse must still be considered (Fig. 20–8). They are largely a disorder of the older, adventuresome child who is prone to fall, and they are best considered a low-velocity "impact" injury. Pediatric extradural hematomas have been reviewed,[66–70] and several general points can be made. Most extradural hematomas are located in the temporal or parietal region, and only rarely are the frontal or posterior fossa regions involved. Even though the posterior fossa location is uncommon, it is a perilous lesion that must be recognized early and treated immediately.

Extradural hematomas usually result from a localized skull injury, often as a result of a fall.[66] Localized skull trauma is a prerequisite, but the skull of a child is relatively "elastic" and a skull fracture is not invariable (60 to 75 per cent of children will have skull fractures).

Almost all skull fractures are linear fractures, and most cross either a middle meningeal arterial branch or a venous sinus. Blood may collect on either side of the skull fracture. Whenever an epicranial hematoma collects overlying a skull fracture in an infant, a CT scan must be carried out to rule out a similar intracranial collection (Fig. 20–9). Extradural hematomas form in a space that has been split open as a result of a skull impact. The skull is deflected inward and rebounds outward, thereby stripping the dura from the underside of the bone. It is known that both the dura on the inside and the periosteum on the outside of growing bone are attached by multiple fibrovascular attachments that are even more plentiful in the rapidly expanding infant skull.[70] As an infant skull grows, the vascularity of the dura decreases, and the density of the fibrovascular attachments also decreases. Also with growth, large

FIGURE 20–9. Extradural hematoma in infancy. Three-week-old infant was dropped by sibling. No retinal hemorrhages; no skeletal injuries. CT images show right parietal subperiosteal hematoma, which communicated through diastatic fracture with extradural hematoma. Excellent outcome.

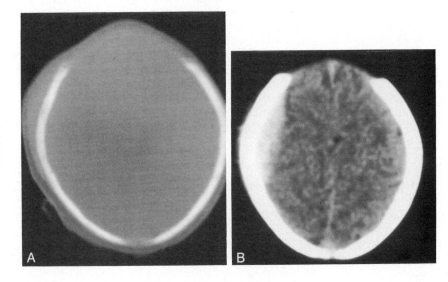

bone plates such as the parietal bone continue to grow rapidly near suture lines, but much less rapidly near the center of the bone plate where resorption and remodeling are taking place. The dura is less adherent in the regions of bone resorption/remodeling and more adherent in the regions of suture lines, where osteoblastic activity is greatest. When the dura is stripped from the underside of bone, blood can accumulate from torn arterial (middle meningeal) branches, from multiple small bleeding points on the dural surface, or from emissary venous channels in the bone. Impact injuries in the occipital region can detach dura bearing large venous sinuses, and again, extradural collections can occur.

Clinically, there is no typical presentation, but the point must be made that a child who has sustained a relatively minor head injury should steadily improve over the 24 to 48 hours following the injury. If a child is deteriorating in any way, especially if there is a skull fracture, an extradural hematoma must be considered. Clinical signs in neonates and infants are particularly nonspecific as large hematomas can collect with few clinical signs. Deterioration may be rapid, but there is usually a history of irritability and vomiting before the deteriorating level of consciousness.

Management is straightforward in the majority of cases. The child should be prepared for urgent craniotomy, and either a free bone flap or osteoplastic bone flap should be used to evacuate the hematoma and suture the dura both to the periphery of the craniotomy and to the center of the craniotomy flap. Many pediatric neurosurgeons prefer an osteoplastic bone flap, but these bone flaps remain highly vascular, and special care must be taken to control all significant bone bleeding from the underside of the bone flap and to secure the dura to the bone flap with at least one suture. The dura in a child is usually thin enough so that one can appreciate the presence of a subdural hematoma or significant contusion without opening the dura widely. If the child was unconscious preoperatively or has another intracranial injury, it is wise to monitor intracranial pressure during the postoperative period.

Management of extradural hematoma is gratifying. The outcome is excellent if the hematoma is removed before the child lapses into coma. The mortality rate for management of uncomplicated extradural hematomas in children should approach zero. Unfortunately, extradural hematomas are sometimes only a component of a more severe intracranial injury, and the diagnosis is still delayed in some extradural hematomas so that the mortality in most series is still approximately 10 per cent.[64, 67–69] In all series, the younger the child the better the outcome.

POSTERIOR FOSSA EXTRADURAL HEMATOMAS

Extradural hematomas of the posterior fossa,[65, 71–75] although rare, usually occur in the pediatric age group. They are the most common post-traumatic mass lesions occurring in the posterior fossa. Almost all are complications of occipital blows, and occipital skull fractures are noted in approximately 80 per cent of cases. The mechanism of injury is usually a fall on the occiput, and invariably there is soft tissue evidence of an occipital injury. The skull fracture usually crosses a venous sinus and extends down toward the foramen magnum. In most cases, the hemorrhage is venous rather than arterial and therefore accumulates slowly. The hematoma is usually unilateral and may extend above the transverse sinus into the occipital region. A discrete source of hemorrhage may not be found. The diagnosis is made by CT scan, but special attention must be paid to the posterior fossa and a high level of suspicion is required. Often, the hematoma presents in subacute fashion and the lesion may be isodense (CT scan) with brain; the significance of an effaced or slightly shifted fourth ventricle must be appreciated (Fig. 20–10). Clinically, there are no absolutely typical features, but it is not uncommon for a child to present several days after an occipital injury with persistent headaches, vomiting, and possibly some unsteadiness. The most important clinical point is that a child can deteriorate in rapid catastrophic fashion after having been stable for several days. The management is surgical in all patients with posterior fossa extradural hematomas, and even the smallest extradural collection must be removed if another surgical procedure that will decrease intracranial pressure (ventriculostomy for CSF drainage, evacuation of supratentorial hematoma) is to be carried out. The suboccipital craniotomy is performed with the child in the prone or park bench position, and provisions must be made for extensions into the occipital region. Usually, a paramedian incision is made and a small bone opening suffices. The craniotomy must be planned carefully to avoid disturbing the venous sinuses, especially if a depressed fracture is present over a major venous sinus. The depressed fragments should be removed only after the surrounding dura has been widely exposed. The patient may have to be placed in the head-up position rapidly if major bleeding is encountered, but air embolism must be kept in mind. Posterior fossa extradural hematomas are perilous lesions and, although rare, must be recognized early and treated with a sense of urgency.

DELAYED EXTRADURAL HEMATOMA

Extradural hematomas may present after some delay,[76–79] as an extradural hematoma does not always achieve its maximum size within minutes of injury. Any fracture site is a possible site for the accumulation of an extradural hematoma. Even if a hematoma is not initially visible, it may form if measures are taken to decrease intracranial pressure (surgical evacuation of previous hematoma, CSF traumatic fistulas, medical measures to decrease intracranial pressures). Delayed extradural hematomas usually occur in the setting of a severe head injury when it is particularly difficult to follow the neurologic status of the child. Intracranial pressure monitoring is especially valuable when the

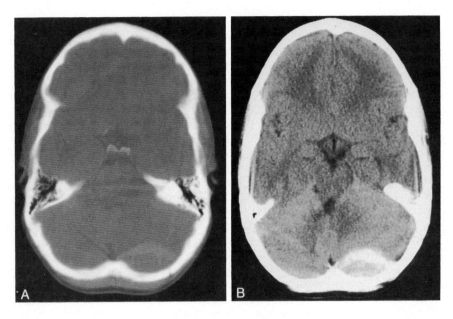

FIGURE 20–10. Posterior fossa extradural hematoma. Eleven-year-old boy presented with persistent vomiting and lethargy 2 days after having fallen backward, striking his occiput. Headache was mild; child was neurologically intact. *A,* CT scan (bone windows) documenting left occipital skull fracture. *B,* Posterior fossa extradural hematoma.

neurologic status is in question, and whenever the intracranial pressure becomes difficult to control, a CT scan is indicated to look for a delayed intracranial hematoma.

NONSURGICAL MANAGEMENT OF EXTRADURAL HEMATOMA

There is an emerging group of patients with extradural hematoma that can be managed nonsurgically, but it is a small group. It must be emphasized that this form of management should only be undertaken where children are cared for in a specialized neurosurgical unit with 24-hour supervision by neurosurgical personnel with 24-hour access to CT scanners. Multiple publications have helped to define the natural history of small extradural hematomas and to delineate a subpopulation of patients that can be managed nonsurgically.[80–90] The suitable patient is a child who arrives at least 24 hours after an injury and is completely lucid with normal findings on neurologic examination and minimal or no headache. The discovery of an extradural hematoma is a surprise, and the extradural hematoma is small (less than 1.5 cm in maximal dimension; 40 ml or less volume). The hematoma should not be located in the posterior fossa or near the base of the middle cranial fossa. There should be no significant midline shift, and the fracture line should not cross a main middle meningeal arterial branch or a major venous sinus. There should be no associated intradural lesions. Even with these restrictions, there are patients who present just in this manner and can be managed without craniotomy. However, it must be stressed that it is not acceptable to await neurologic deterioration in the acute setting if an extradural hematoma is thought to be "small." Remember, it is only those who have begun to deteriorate neurologically who fare poorly. Children with small extradural hematomas who present later than 24 hours after injury and are steadily improving can be considered for nonsurgical management if they are closely observed on an experienced neurosurgical unit with ready access to a CT scanner.

POST-TRAUMATIC INTRACEREBRAL HEMATOMA

In pediatric age groups, most post-traumatic hemorrhages occur in the extradural, subdural, or subarachnoid space; intraparenchymal bleeding is not common. Intraparenchymal hemorrhages follow typical patterns, and most can be managed without surgical intervention. The important points are as follows:

1. Most hematomas represent confluent cerebral cortical contusions, either beneath the site of impact or directly opposite the site of impact. Occasionally, deeper vessels are disrupted by more diffuse rotational forces and deep intracerebral hematomas result. The edema is worse with confluent contusions than it is with intracerebral hematomas.[91]

2. Parenchymal hemorrhages may represent significant mass lesions and, as such, are considered reversible factors in intracranial pressure management. Judgment is required, but removal of a hematoma or massive contusion may facilitate management of intracranial hypertension.[92, 93]

3. Delayed intracerebral hemorrhage does exist in children, and serial CT scans are important if intracranial pressure becomes difficult to manage or new symptoms develop even weeks after head injury.

4. If the characteristics of the hematoma are unusual or difficult to correlate with the traumatic event, consider the possibility of a vascular malformation and arrange appropriate imaging studies.

5. There is a higher incidence of post-traumatic seizures with hemorrhagic contusions, and prophylactic anticonvulsants are important in the acute phase.

Intraparenchymal hemorrhages are not common in any pediatric age group[64, 94] until late adolescence and early adulthood, at which time falls give way to high-speed motor vehicle accidents as major etiologic factors. Traumatic intraparenchymal hemorrhage occurs both in the form of small, scattered, superficial contusions and as larger, deep, discrete white matter hematomas. The patterns may coexist, but usually one predominates. Frontal and temporal lobes are by far most frequently involved, and distinct patterns of hemorrhage are discernible. The cerebral parenchyma, and its vasculature, may be injured by direct blunt or penetrating forces or may be injured indirectly by forces transmitted through the brain. A blunt direct blow may result in a depressed fracture and a surface cortical contusion beneath the impact site. A direct penetrating blow will pierce the dura and brain parenchyma, carrying air and debris inward as cerebral vessels are disrupted along the way. Whenever an intracerebral hematoma is discovered in a child, penetrating injuries must be considered. The site of penetration may not be obvious (ear, nose, eye, or small scalp wound), but the implications regarding vascular injuries (traumatic aneurysms, carotid-cavernous fistulas), CSF fistulas, or infections (meningitis, brain abscess) are obvious.

Instead of damaging the brain directly, impact may send reverberating waves of force through the parenchyma, setting up violent swirls and shear strains within the brain. Axonal pathways, dendritic circuitry, and penetrating vessels are all disrupted, leading to diffuse axonal injury patterns,[15, 95, 96] intracerebral hemorrhages,[94] and sometimes deep cerebral infarctions.[97] Multiple surface contusions occur particularly in the orbital-frontal and temporal tip regions as the reverberating brain is traumatized by the sphenoid wing and uneven anterior cranial fossa floor (Fig. 20–11). The actual mechanism of hemorrhage probably differs between surface contusions and deep, discrete intracerebral hematomas. Surface contusions occur in necrotic, hemorrhagic cortex, and vessels may be directly disrupted or indirectly affected as the surrounding necrotic cerebral tissue releases vasoactive substances. Local loss of autoregulation may lead to regional increases in blood flow in damaged vessels, and hemorrhage may result. This hemorrhagic process may not be immediate, but damaged vessels may fail and small contusions may coalesce over several days, leading to delayed intracerebral hemorrhages.[94, 98–101] Surface hemorrhages may also lead to vasospasm and secondary ischemic lesions. Larger vessels may be damaged as well. Injuries

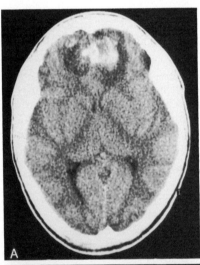
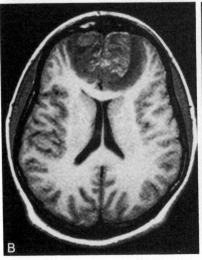
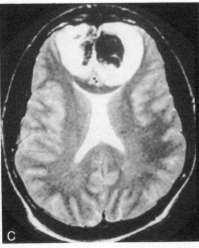
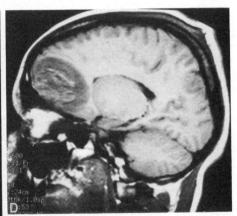

FIGURE 20–11. Intracranial hematoma—contre coup. Fifteen-year-old male fell backward from a ladder, striking occipital region. He was agitated and confused and complained of headaches for 10 days. Discharged home. A, CT scan (axial image) demonstrating bifrontal cerebral contusions (contre coup). B, C, and D, MRI images demonstrating extent of bifrontal contusion hematomas resulting from occipital impact.

to large arteries may lead to traumatic aneurysms that rupture even weeks later. Any child with an unexplained recurring intracerebral hemorrhage in the setting of recent trauma must have a cerebral angiogram. Traumatic aneurysms usually involve the pericallosal artery or distal middle cerebral branches.[102, 103] Injuries to larger veins or venous sinuses may lead to venous hypertension or sinus thrombosis. Thrombosis of the superior sagittal sinus must always be considered in the case of unexplained parasagittal hemorrhages and seizures.

Deep discrete hematomas are thought to result from disruption of penetrating vessels by reverberating forces swirling violently through the brain as a result of sudden, rotational forces. Discrete hematomas develop deep within the white matter, and some may be large enough to severely compress and distort surrounding brain structures or CSF pathways. Rarely are these hematomas large enough to require surgical removal, and the edema surrounding these deep hematomas seems less severe than that associated with extensive cortical contusions.

Clinically, intracerebral hematomas are relatively silent and are often completely overshadowed by the diffuse cerebral injury or extra-axial hematoma. The head injury usually is not minor and the child looks unwell. One is expecting an intracranial hemorrhage, but seizures and focal neurologic deficits lead one to suspect an intracerebral hematoma rather than an extra-axial hemorrhage. Even days after the injury, the child may deteriorate or intracranial pressure may become difficult to control, and a delayed intracerebral hemorrhage must be suspected.

Management of intracerebral hemorrhage is largely nonsurgical. Most hematomas will resolve over 2 to 3 weeks, although the rare hematoma may persist or even expand and be confused with a cerebral abscess or tumor.[52] Brain swelling and edema must be controlled and intracranial pressure should be monitored if the CT scan suggests raised intracranial pressure. Surgical intervention is a consideration for large intracerebral hematomas or extensive frontal-temporal contusions, but intracranial pressure monitoring should help to guide this decision.

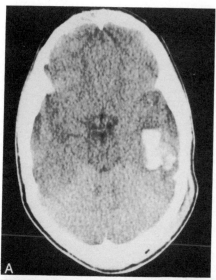
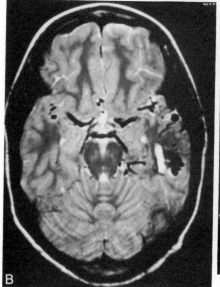
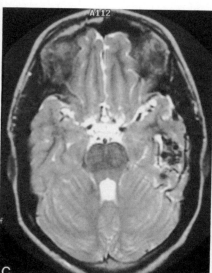
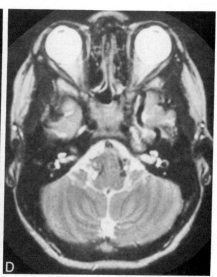

FIGURE 20–12. Intracerebral hematoma with arteriovenous malformation. Eleven-year-old boy, struck by an automobile while riding a bicycle, was combative at the scene but obtunded on arrival at hospital. He required intubation and ventilation but steadily improved. Excellent outcome. *A,* Initial CT scan with left temporal lobe hematoma near impact site. *B, C,* and *D,* MRI images showing vascular malformation associated with intraparenchymal hematoma.

A cerebral angiogram is advised if the hematoma is not well explained by the traumatic event (Fig. 20–12). Blood must be available for transfusion, and the hematoma can be evacuated by open craniotomy or stereotactic aspiration. In most cases, the hematoma dissects close to the cortical surface and is best managed by open craniotomy. Surgical hematomas are often located in the orbital-frontal or temporal tip regions, and resections can be wider than in areas of more eloquent cortex. Removal of necrotic or severely contused cortex may help to decrease the overall mass effect of the hematoma. Prophylactic anticonvulsants are important in the acute phase, and serum electrolytes must be carefully controlled to avoid hyponatremia. Long-term anticonvulsant therapy may be required, but usually prophylactic anticonvulsants can be discontinued within three months of the injury.

SUMMARY

Post-traumatic intracranial hematomas occur in all pediatric age groups, and sound surgical judgment is important at all stages. The pediatric brain and skull are ever-changing, and at each pediatric stage, intracranial hematomas are characterized differently. Knowledge of neonatal coagulation peculiarities and of the characteristics of acute and chronic subdural hemorrhage is fundamental to the management of intracranial hematomas in infants. The significance of skull fractures in children must be appreciated so that extradural hematomas can be discovered before neurologic deterioration occurs. In older children, the significance of occipital blows and occipital skull fractures in relation to posterior fossa extradural hematoma must be kept in mind to allow early detection and early surgical intervention. Post-traumatic intracranial hematomas are reversible lesions, but the characteristics of each hematoma pattern must be known to allow the benefits of surgery to be weighed against the risks.

REFERENCES

1. Luerssen TG: Head injuries in children. Neurosurg Clin North Am 2:399, 1991.
2. Kraus JT, Mayer TA, Storrs BB, Hylton PD: Brain injuries among infants, children, adolescents, and young adults. Am J Dis Child 144:684, 1990.
3. Walker ML, Mayer TA, Storrs BB, Hylton PD: Pediatric head injury—factors which influence outcome. Concepts Pediat Neurosurg 6:84, 1985.
4. Kraus JF, Fife D, Cox P, Ramstein K, Conroy C: Incidence, severity, and external causes of pediatric brain injury. Am J Dis Child 140:687, 1986.
5. Chan KH, Yue CP, Mann KS: The risk of intracranial complications in pediatric head injury. Childs Nerv Sys 6:27, 1990.
6. Duncan CC, Ment LR, Ogle E: Traumatic injury to the developing brain. Concepts Pediatri Neurosurg 9:211, 1989.
7. Moloy HC: Studies on head molding during labor. Am J Obstet Gynecol 44:762, 1942.
8. Raimondi AJ, Hirschauer J: Head injury in the infant and toddler. Childs Brain 11:12, 1984.
9. Baker SP: Motor vehicle occupant deaths in young children. Pediatrics 64:860, 1979

10. Kraus JF, Fife D, Cox P, Ramstein K, et al.: Incidence, severity, and external causes of pediatric brain injury. Am J Dis Child 140:687, 1986.
11. Hahn YS, Chyung C, Barthel MJ, Bailes J, Flannery AJ, McLone DG: Head injuries in children under 36 months of age. Childs Nerv Syst 4:34, 1988.
12. Bruce DA, Alavi A, Bilaniuk L, Dolinskas C, et al.: Diffuse cerebral swelling following head injuries in children: The syndrome of "malignant brain edema." J Neurosurg 54:170, 1981.
13. Aldrich EF, Eisenberg HM, Saydjari C, Luerssen TG, et al.: Diffuse brain swelling in severely head injured child. J Neurosurg 76:450, 1992.
14. Sganzerla EP, Tomei G, Guerra P, Tiberio F, et al.: Clinicoradiological and therapeutic considerations in severe diffuse traumatic brain injury in children. Childs Nerv Syst 5:168, 1989.
15. Glader BE, Amylon MD: Hemostatic disorders in the newborn. Hematol Syst 84:777, 1991.
16. Buchanan GR: Coagulation disorders in the neonate. Pediatr Clin North Am 33:203, 1986.
17. Kontras SB, Green OC, King L, Doran RJ: Giant hemangioma with thrombocytopenia; Case report with survival and sequestration studies of platelets labeled with chromium-51. Am J Dis Child 105:188, 1963.
18. Volpe JJ: Neonatal intracranial hemorrhage. Clin Perinatol 4:77, 1977.
19. Cheek WR, Fishman MA, Speer ME, Williamson WD, et al.: Cerebellar hemorrhage in the term neonate. Concepts Pediatr Neurosurg 5:48, 1985.
20. Menezes AH, Smith DE, Bell WE: Posterior fossa hemorrhage in the term neonate. Neurosurgery 13:452, 1983.
21. Takagi T, Fukuoka H, Wakabayashi S, Nagai H, et al.: Posterior fossa subdural hemorrhage in the newborn as a result of birth trauma. Childs Brain 9:102, 1982.
22. Hovind KH: Traumatic birth injuries. In Raimondi AJ, Choux M, DiRocco C (eds): Head Injuries in the Newborn and Infant. New York, Springer-Verlag Inc, 1986, pp 87–109.
23. Serfontein GL, Rom S, Stein S: Posterior fossa subdural hemorrhage in the newborn. Pediatrics 65:40, 1980.
24. DiRocco C, Velardi F: Epidemiology and etiology of craniocerebral trauma in the first two years of life. In Raimondi AJ, Choux M, DiRocco C (eds): Head Injuries in the Newborn and Infant. New York, Springer-Verlag Inc, 1986, pp 125–139.
25. Lane PA, Hathaway WE, Githens JH, Krugman RD, et al.: Fatal intracranial hemorrhage in a normal infant secondary to vitamin K deficiency. Pediatrics 72:562, 1983.
26. Chaou WT, Chou ML, Eitzman DV: Intracranial hemorrhage and vitamin K deficiency in early infancy. J Pediatr 105:880, 1984.
27. Aoki N, Masuzawa H: Infantile acute subdural hematoma. J Neurosurg 6:273, 1984.
28. Gutierrez FA, Raimondi AJ: Acute subdural hematoma in infancy and childhood. Childs Brain 1:269, 1975.
29. Yashon D, Jange JA, White RJ, Sugar O: Traumatic subdural hematoma. Arch Neurol 18:370, 1968.
30. Duhaime AC, Gennarelli TA, Thibault LE, Bruce DA: The shaken baby syndrome. J Neurosurg 66:409, 1987.
31. Ludwig S, Warman M: Shaken baby syndrome. Ann Emerg Med 13:104, 1984.
32. Hadley MN, Sonntag K, Rekate HL, Murphy A: The infant whiplash-shake injury syndrome: A clinical and pathological study. Neurosurgery 24:536, 1989.
33. Alexander R, Sato Y, Smith W, Bennett T: Incidence of impact trauma with cranial injuries ascribed to shaking. Am J Dis Child 144:724, 1990.
34. Greenwald M: The shaken baby syndrome. Semin Ophthalmol 5:202, 1990.
35. Greenwald M, Weiss A, Oesterle CS, Friendly DS: Traumatic retinoschisis in battered babies. Ophthalmology 93:618, 1986.
36. Harcourt B, Hopkins D: Ophthalmic manifestations of the battered-baby syndrome. Br Med J 3:398, 1971.
37. Harley RD: Ocular manifestations of child abuse. J Pediatr Ophthalmol Strabismus, 17:5, 1980.
38. Lambert SR, Johnson TE, Hoyt CS: Optic nerve sheath and retinal hemorrhages associated with the shaken baby syndrome. Arch Ophthalmol 104:1509, 1986.

39. Eisenbrey AB: Retinal hemorrhage in the battered child. Childs Brain 5:40, 1979.
40. Wilkinson WS, Han DP, Rappley MD, Owings CL: Retinal hemorrhage predicts neurologic injury in the shaken baby syndrome. Arch Ophthalmol 107:1472, 1989.
41. Luerssen TG, Huang JC, McLone DG, Walker ML, Hahn YS, et al.: Retinal hemorrhages, seizures, and intracranial hemorrhages: Relationships and outcomes in children suffering traumatic brain injury. Concepts Pediatr Neurosurg 11:87, 1991.
42. Mclellan NJ, Prasad R, Punt J: Spontaneous subhyaloid and retinal hemorrhages in an infant. Arch Dis Child 61:1130, 1986.
43. Kanter RK: Retinal hemorrhage after cardiopulmonary resuscitation or child abuse. J Pediatr 108:430, 1986.
44. Goetting MG, Sowa B: Retinal hemorrhage after cardiopulmonary resuscitation in children: An etiologic reevaluation. Pediatrics 85:585, 1990.
45. Zimmerman RA, Bilaniuk LT, Bruce D, Uzzell B, et al.: Interhemispheric acute subdural hematoma: A computed tomographic manifestation. Neuroradiology 16:39, 1978.
46. Ordia IJ, Strand R, Gilles F, Welch K: Computerized tomography of contusional clefts in the white matter in infants. J Neurosurg 54:696, 1981.
47. Merten DF, Carpenter BL: Radiologic imaging of inflicted injury in the child abuse syndrome. Pediatr Clin North Am 37:815, 1990.
48. Lindenberg R, Freytag E: Morphology of brain lesions from blunt trauma in early infancy. Arch Pathol 87:298, 1969.
49. Hahn YS, Raimondi AJ, McLone DG, Yamanouchi Y: Traumatic mechanisms of head injury in child abuse. Childs Brain 10:229, 1983.
50. Page A, Paxton RM, Mohan D: A reappraisal of the relationship between arachnoid cysts of the middle fossa and chronic subdural hematoma. J Neurol Neurosurg Psychiatry 50:1001, 1987.
51. Cappelen J, Unsgaard G: Arachnoid cysts of the middle cranial fossa and traumatic complications. Childs Nerv Syst 2:225, 1986.
52. Pozzati E, Giuliani G, Gaist G, Piazza G, et al.: Chronic expanding intracerebral hematoma. J Neurosurg 65:611, 1986.
53. Goodman JM, Mealey J: Postmeningitic subdural effusions: The syndrome and its management. J Neurosurg 30:658, 1969.
54. Rabe EF, Flynn RE, Dodge PR: A study of subdural effusions in an infant. Neurology 12:79, 1961.
55. McLone DG, Gutierrez FA, Raimondi AJ, Wiederhold M: Ultrastructure of subdural membranes of children. Concepts Pediatr Neurosurg 1:174, 1981.
56. Markwalder TM: Chronic subdural hematomas: A review. J Neurosurg 54:637, 1981.
57. Labadie EL, Glover D: Physiopathogenesis of subdural hematomas. J Neurosurg 45:382, 1976.
58. Glover D, Labadie EL: Physiopathogenesis of subdural hematomas. J Neurosurg 45:393, 1976.
59. Ment LR, Duncan CC, Geehr R: Benign enlargement of the subarachnoid spaces in the infant. J Neurosurg 54:504, 1981.
60. Aoki N: Chronic subdural hematoma in infancy. J Neurosurg 73:201, 1990.
61. McLaurin RL: Subdural hematomas and effusions in children, developmental anomalies, and neurosurgical disease of childhood. In Wilkins RH, Rengachary SS (eds): Neurosurgery, Vol 3. New York, McGraw-Hill, 1984, pp 2211–2215.
62. Aoki N, Masuzawa H: Bilateral chronic subdural hematoma without communication between the hematoma cavities: Treatment with unilateral subdural-peritoneal shunt. Neurosurgery 22:911, 1988.
63. Aoki N, Mizutani H, Masuzawa H: Unilateral subdural-peritoneal shunting for bilateral chronic subdural hematomas in infancy. J Neurosurg 63:134, 1985.
64. Choux M, Lena G, Genitori L: Intracranial hematomas. In Raimondi A, Choux M, DiRocco C (eds): Head Injuries in the Newborn and Infant. New York, Springer-Verlag Inc, 1986, pp 204–216.
65. Obana WG, Pitts LH: Extracerebral lesions. Neurosurg Clin North Am 2:351, 1991.
66. Gutierrez FA, McLone DG, Raimondi AJ: Epidural hematomas in infancy and childhood. Concepts Pediatr Neurosurg 1:188, 1981.
67. Dhellemmes P, Lejeune JP, Christiaens JL, Combelles G: Traumatic extradural hematomas in infancy and childhood. J Neurosurg 62:861, 1985.
68. Choux M, Grisol F, Pergut T: Extradural hematomas in children—104 cases. Childs Brain 1:337, 1975.
69. Jamieson KC, Yelland JDN: Extradural hematoma—Report of 167 cases. J Neurosurg 29:13, 1968.
70. Campbell JB, Cohen J: Epidural hemorrhage and the skull of children. Surg Gynecol Obstetr 92:257, 1951.
71. Wojak J, Cooper PR: Traumatic lesions of the posterior cranial fossa. Contemp Neurosurg 8:1, 1986.
72. Zuccarello M, Pardatscher K, Andrioli GC, Fiore DL, et al.: Epidural hematomas of the posterior cranial fossa. Neurosurgery 8:434, 1981.
73. Garza-Mercado R: Extradural hematoma of the posterior cranial fossa. J Neurosurg 59:664, 1983.
74. Ammirati M, Tomita T: Posterior fossa epidural hematoma during childhood. Neurosurgery 14:541, 1984.
75. Wright RL: Traumatic hematomas of the posterior cranial fossa. J Neurosurg 25:402, 1966.
76. Borovich B, Braun J, Guilburd JN, Zaaroor M, et al.: Delayed onset of traumatic extradural hematoma. J Neurosurg 63:30, 1985.
77. Piepmeier JM, Wagner FC: Delayed post-traumatic extracerebral hematomas. J Trauma 22:455, 1982.
78. Feuerman T, Wackym PA, Gade GF, Lanmann T, et al.: Intraoperative development of contralateral epidural hematoma during evacuation of traumatic extraaxial hematoma. Neurosurgery 23:480, 1988.
79. Bullock R, Hannemann CO, Murray L, Teasdale GM: Recurrent hematomas following craniotomy for traumatic intracranial mass. J Neurosurg 72:9, 1990.
80. Weaver D, Poberskin L, Jane JA: Spontaneous resolution of epidural hematomas: Report of two cases. J Neurosurg 54:248, 1981.
81. Pang D, Horton JA, Herron JM, Wilberger JE, et al.: Nonsurgical management of extradural hematomas in children. J Neurosurg 59:958, 1983.
82. Illingworth R, Shawdon H: Conservative management of intracranial extradural hematoma presenting late. J Neurol Neurosurg Psychiatry 46:558, 1983.
83. Tochio H, Waga S, Tashiro H, Takeuchi T, et al.: Spontaneous resolution of chronic epidural hematomas: Report of three cases. Neurosurgery 15:96, 1984.
84. Bullock R, Smith RM, van Dellen JR: Nonoperative management of extradural hematoma. Neurosurgery 15:602, 1985.
85. Pozzati E, Tognetti F: Spontaneous healing of acute extradural hematomas: Study of twenty-two cases. Neurosurgery 18:696, 1986.
86. Knuckey NW, Gelbard S, Epstein MH: The management of ''asymptomatic'' epidural hematomas. J Neurosurg 70:392, 1989.
87. Servadei F, Staffa G, Morichetti A, Burzi M, et al.: Asymptomatic acute bilateral epidural hematoma: Results of broader indications for computed tomographic scanning of patients with minor head injuries. Neurosurgery 23:41, 1988.
88. Rivas JJ, Lobato RD, Sarabia R, Cordobes F, et al.: Extradural hematoma: Analysis of factors influencing the courses of 161 patients. Neurosurgery 23:44, 1988.
89. Aoki N: Rapid resolution of acute epidural hematoma: Report of two cases. J Neurosurg 68:149, 1988.
90. Sakai H, Takagi H, Ohtaka H, Tanabe T: Serial changes in acute extradural hematoma size and associated changes in level of consciousness and intracranial pressure. J Neurosurg 68:566, 1988.
91. Statham PFX, Todd NV: Intracerebral hematoma: Aetiology and hematoma volume determine the amount and progression of brain oedema. Acta Neurochirurg 51:289, 1990.
92. Aldrich EF: Surgical management of traumatic intracerebral hematomas. Neurosurg Clin North Am 2:373, 1991.

93. Bullock R, Golek J, Blake G: Traumatic intracerebral hematoma: Which patients should undergo surgical evacuation? CT Scan Features and ICP Monitoring as a Basis for Decision Making. Surg Neurol 32:181, 1989.

94. Kang JK, Park CK, Kim MC, Kim DS: Traumatic isolated intracerebral hemorrhage in children. Childs Nerv Syst 5:303, 1989.

95. Levi L, Guilburd JN, Lemberger A, Soustiel JF: Diffuse axonal injury: Analysis of 100 patients with radiological signs. Neurosurgery 27:429, 1990.

96. Takenaka N, Mine T, Suga S, Tamura K, et al.: Interpeduncular high-density spot in severe shearing injury. Surg Neurol 34:30, 1990.

97. Maki Y, Akimoto H, Enomoto T: Injuries of basal ganglia following head trauma in children. Childs Brain 7:113, 1980.

98. Broderick JP, Brott TG, Tomsick T, Barsan W, et al.: Ultra-early evaluation of intracerebral hemorrhage. J Neurosurg 72:195, 1990.

99. Brown FD, Mullan S, Duda EE: Delayed traumatic intracerebral hematomas. J Neurosurg 48:1019, 1978.

100. Atlura V, Epstein LG, Zilka A: Delayed traumatic intracerebral hemorrhage in children. Pediatr Neurol 2:297, 1986.

101. Jaimovich R, Monges JA: Delayed post-traumatic intracranial lesions in children. Pediatr Neurosurg 17:25, 1991–92.

102. Smith KR, Bardenheier JA: Aneurysm of the pericallosal artery caused by closed cranial trauma. J Neurosurg 29:551, 1968.

103. Buckingham MJ, Crone KR, Ball WS, Tomsick TA, et al.: Traumatic intracranial aneurysms in childhood: Two cases and a review of the literature. Neurosurgery 22:398, 1988.

Chapter 21

LATE COMPLICATIONS OF HEAD INJURY

THOMAS G. LUERSSEN, M.D., HOWARD M. EISENBERG, M.D.,
and HARVEY S. LEVIN, Ph.D.

In many cases, the ability of a child to reach full potential after a serious head injury depends upon the development and management of late or chronic sequelae of the injury. These added problems can occur at any time after the injury. Some complications occur relatively soon, for instance cerebrospinal fluid (CSF) fistulas, cranial nerve palsies, pneumonia, acute infections, and delayed traumatic hematomas. These more "acute" complications are discussed in other chapters. This chapter will focus on the delayed or more chronic disorders that complicate pediatric head injury such as skull defects, hydrocephalus, endocrine disorders, vascular disorders, epilepsy, and neurologic and neurobehavioral dysfunction.

COMPLICATIONS RELATED TO THE SKULL AND DURA

GROWING SKULL FRACTURE

Although skull fractures are common in childhood, this particular complication is actually quite rare. The "growing" fracture is really a post-traumatic cranial erosion that includes a clinical syndrome that becomes evident even prior to the acquisition of the confirmatory radiographic studies. The affected children are almost universally infants and have a history of a head injury (if radiographic studies were obtained) that resulted in a skull fracture. At some time, usually weeks to months, after the injury, they develop a progressively enlarging pulsatile mass or an enlarging and sunken palpable cranial defect, usually accompanied by the development of a neurologic deficit and/or a seizure disorder.

There are several extensive reviews of this complication, and it is clear from clinical studies[1-5] and from studies in laboratory animals[6,7] that the essential elements required for the development of a "growing fracture" are: (1) a dural tear and (2) an outward driving force, such as the normally growing brain, hydrocephalus, an arachnoid cyst, or a progressive porencephaly.[8-10] This latter requirement explains the predominance of this complication in very young children.[1,2,11] Most series have demonstrated that up to 75 per cent of the patients with growing fractures are less than 1 year old, and reports of growing fractures in children over the age of 3 years are rare. The laceration of the dura results in the loss of the normal tensile forces of the dura, and the ongoing growth of the brain results in expansion of the dural defect. At some point, a true cerebral herniation occurs and the bone edges are absorbed (Fig. 21–1). Frequently, there is a severe underlying brain injury, which explains the neurologic symptoms commonly associated with growing fractures. However, it is not clear whether the cerebral injury is acquired in conjunction with the skull defect or whether an underlying cerebral injury aggravates the process. Not all patients have evidence of a structural injury to the brain,[5] and therefore cerebral injury is not an essential element of the syndrome.

The most common presenting symptom is a scalp mass or a palpable cranial defect. Other symptoms are related to the underlying brain injury, most commonly seizures or focal weakness. The radiologic picture is characteristic (Fig. 21–2). On plain skull radiographs there is an irregular, elliptical skull defect. The inner table is frequently eroded, and the edges of the defect can be everted and sclerotic. If skull radiographs taken at the time of the initial injury are available, they will universally demonstrate a diastatic fracture, with the edges separated by more than 3 mm.[4] Most commonly, the parietal bone is involved, although growing fractures can occur anywhere on the calvarium, and growing fractures have been shown to cross suture lines.[8]

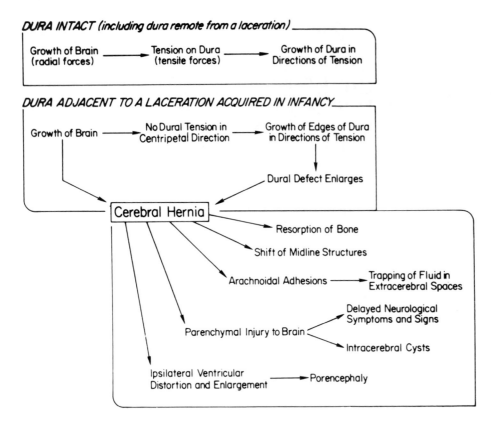

FIGURE 21–1. Summary of the mechanisms involved in expanding dural defects. The dural defect "grows" larger as a result of misdirected normal processes. Since dura grows in response to tension and in the direction of tension, a disruption of the dural envelope alters the tension on the dura in the region of the defect. There is continued growth of the dura along the edges of the defect and diminished growth in the centripetal direction (i.e., there is no tension and hence no growth toward the defect itself). A hernia can occur only if there is an outward driving force such as normally growing brain, an expansion due to pathologic processes, or both. (From Winston K, Beatty RM, Fischer EG: Consequences of dural defects acquired in infancy. J Neurosurg 59:839, 1983.)

Images of the brain also show characteristic findings. Almost every patient will show unilateral ventricular enlargement and a shift toward the skull defect.[1,4] The cause of the unilateral ventricular enlargement is uncertain. It has been postulated that it may be related to pressure in the ventricle unopposed by the resistance of normal dura.[9] However, it is more likely that this enlargement is seen because of brain atrophy or because an underlying structural injury has occurred. Support for this idea is provided by the frequent demonstration of a porencephaly, cystic encephalomalacia, or gliosis directly under the skull defect.

The natural history of this complication has not been defined. It appears that there is an early rapid progression of the cranial defect, which is followed by a period of slower progression. Patients have been described in whom the skull defect has stabilized and no new neurologic findings have occurred over long periods.[7] However, in most series, the majority of cases have shown a progressively worsening neurologic deficit over time. Pathologic studies of the brains of patients undergoing repair of the defect have documented evidence of progressive brain damage.[3] There is no indication that the condition ever improves spontaneously. Therefore, when this complication is discovered, the child should be treated immediately.

The surgical repair of these lesions is frequently more involved than might be imagined by viewing the skull films or the computed tomographic (CT) scan. The main goal of the surgery is the structural repair of the dura, and the dural defect usually extends for some distance away from the edges of the bony defect. Fur-

thermore, the bone edges can be involved with intense glial scarring, and there is frequently an underlying cyst that must be fenestrated. The dura must be completely identified and closed, preferably with autograft. We prefer to perform the cranioplasty immediately, utilizing split or transposed cranial bone, but the repair of the skull defect can be performed later if necessary. Frequently, very young children will require only the dural repair, which will allow the skull defect to heal spontaneously.

IATROGENIC CRANIAL DEFECTS

Operative removal of the calvarium either for the treatment of depressed skull fractures or to treat brain swelling should be avoided in the pediatric age group. With the current medical management of elevated intracranial pressure, there seems to be little enthusiasm for treating any severe head injury with cranial decompression. Furthermore, with the advent of microfixation plating, most compound skull fractures can be successfully reconstructed in the acute phase, even when they are extremely complex and widely open.

However, occasions do arise whereby a child is left with a residual cranial defect. Skull defects in very young children will usually heal spontaneously as long as the underlying dura is intact and the brain is growing normally. Children older than the age of 2 years can be expected to heal small skull defects. However, large skull defects occurring in the face of structural loss of the brain or hydrocephalus (Fig. 21–3), or in older chil-

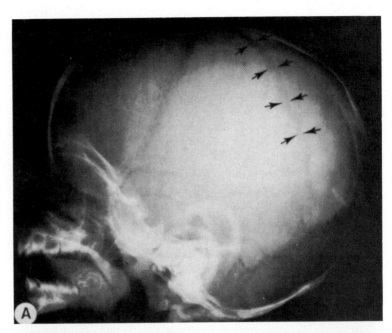

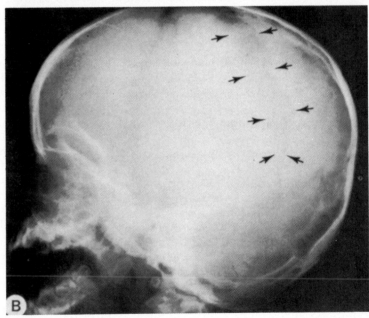

FIGURE 21–2. Evolution of a growing skull fracture. *A,* Diastatic parietal skull fracture in an 8-month-old girl. *B,* Enlargement of the cranial defect demonstrated 5 months later.

dren, will usually require a cranial reconstruction. These defects must be treated not only to improve the cosmetic appearance, but also to protect the brain and improve neurologic function.

Ideally, the skull should be reconstructed with autogenous bone, which will serve as a scaffold for the infiltration of osteoblasts and will result in the development of normally growing bone. We prefer to use grafts of cranial bone whenever possible. In older children, whose skull is thick enough to be split, large amounts of bone can be obtained and shaped to repair almost every region of the cranium. In younger children, whose skull defects involve the frontal bone or the fronto-orbital region, full-thickness skull can be obtained from areas behind the hairline for use in the cosmetically important region, and rib or iliac grafts,

which result in a less pleasing cosmetic result, are used to fill the donor sites.

A variety of synthetic materials are available for the purpose of reconstructing the skull. These materials are less suitable for use in the growing skull and have the added complications of all implanted foreign bodies, most notably infection. In appropriate circumstances, however, the use of synthetic materials as filler, implants, or onlays are extremely useful for structural or cosmetic reconstructions. Because of the risk of infection, synthetic material probably should be avoided when one is reconstructing compound fractures. Furthermore, when synthetic material is being considered for implantation in a formerly contaminated wound, a delay of the surgery for several months is usually recommended, and a diligent search should be made for

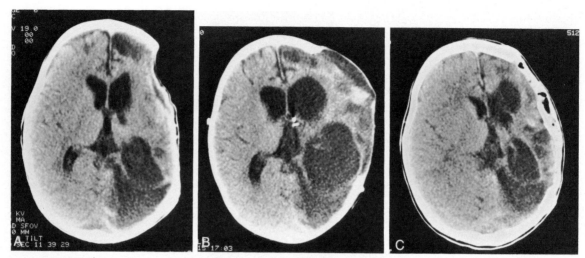

FIGURE 21–3. A series of CT scans of the brain of a 15-month-old child with a severe head injury treated in a community hospital by decompressive craniectomy. The cranial flap was not saved, and the child was left with a large calvarial defect. She had a ventriculoperitoneal shunt placed for post-traumatic hydrocephalus. *A*, With the shunt functioning, the child was lethargic and exhibited a pronounced sunken area over the defect, which placed a great deal of tension on the skin at the edges of the craniectomy. *B*, With the shunt obstructed, the brain herniated out of the defect. *C*, After repair of the dura, cranial reconstruction, and revision of the shunt, the child improved neurologically and has a normal cosmetic appearance to the skull.

any sign of smoldering osteomyelitis in the region of the calvarial defect.

CEREBROVASCULAR COMPLICATIONS

TRAUMATIC ANEURYSMS

Traumatic intracranial aneurysms are extremely rare occurrences in head-injured patients of all ages. However, it appears that about one fifth of all post-traumatic aneurysms occur in children,[12] which means that, in relative terms, these lesions are much more common in children than in adults. Buckingham et al. have recently reviewed the literature regarding traumatic aneurysms in children.[13] The majority of children presented with an intracranial hemorrhage a few days to a few weeks after a head injury. Although most of the children suffered a severe closed head injury, those with penetrating injuries, especially with sharp objects, are also prone to this complication. The diagnosis of a traumatic aneurysm begins with a high index of suspicion. Early angiography or magnetic resonance angiography should be considered for all head-injured children who show evidence of intracranial hemorrhage suggestive of a vascular lesion on the initial CT scan, or who have suffered a penetrating injury, especially stab injuries. A diagnostic angiogram should be obtained for any head-injured child who exhibits a delayed intracerebral or subarachnoid hemorrhage, recurrent epistaxis, or a progressive cranial nerve palsy.

CAROTID-CAVERNOUS FISTULA

Carotid-cavernous sinus fistulas are rare complications of head injury and are extremely uncommon in children. Although few pediatric cases have been reported,[14–16] it is likely that the clinical presentations and natural history of this lesion are the same for children and adults. This lesion is usually the result of a direct injury to the carotid artery. It is seen in relation to a fracture of the sphenoid bone whereby the carotid artery is sheared or suffers an intimal tear. The subsequent dissection or pseudoaneurysm ruptures into the cavernous sinus.[17] The treatment of choice is endovascular obliteration of the fistula, with direct surgical repair being reserved for those few cases in which endovascular techniques cannot be used or have failed.

POST-TRAUMATIC HYDROCEPHALUS

It appears from limited studies that the overall incidence of symptomatic hydrocephalus following head injury in childhood is about 4 per cent.[18, 19] It is important to make a distinction between chronic progressive hydrocephalus and the temporary disturbance of CSF absorption that can occur in the early recovery phases of the brain injury. In these cases, the patients who were improving neurologically show a rather abrupt change in their course. If intracranial pressure is still being monitored, a low-grade intracranial hypertension returns. The CT scan shows mild ventricular enlargement along with enlargement of the subarachnoid spaces, consistent with a communicating hydrocephalus. This early "hydrocephalus" is frequently transient and therefore can be managed by a short course of ventricular drainage, intermittent lumbar punctures, or continuous spinal drainage.

When the ventricular enlargement is more dramatic or persistent, the patient should undergo CSF shunting. Occasionally it is difficult to distinguish between active hydrocephalus and cortical atrophy, especially if the patient is still showing neurologic compromise. Nevertheless, a shunt will improve neurologic functioning in the vast majority of patients with post-traumatic hydrocephalus. Patients with post-traumatic hydrocephalus will show a decrease in their ventricular dimensions after shunting (assuming that the shunt is functional), unless the ventriculomegaly is due entirely to cerebral atrophy.

NEUROLOGIC AND SYSTEMIC COMPLICATIONS

PERSISTENT NEUROLOGIC DEFICITS

The vast majority of head-injured children, even severely head-injured children, survive their injury.[20] Despite this, relatively little is known about the biology of neurologic recovery from traumatic brain injury. Furthermore, the ultimate functional outcome of a patient who has suffered a brain injury is dependent upon the presence of any persistent neurologic deficit along with the presence of and relationship to any cognitive or behavioral disturbance. The most widely used scale describing the neurologic outcome from brain injury is the Glasgow Outcome Scale (GOS).[21] The functional descriptions used at the higher levels of recovery in this scale and in its expanded version[22] are aimed more at the adult age group. For example, the determination of moderate disability and good recovery includes some description of the patient's capacity to return to work, which is really not applicable to pediatric patients. Nevertheless, this scale has been used to describe the outcomes from childhood brain injuries, and it does provide a useful marker to scale the recovery. However, much more work needs to be done to try to accurately characterize the true outcome for head injury occurring in children.

It is clear that the age of the patient at the time of injury is an extremely important factor influencing the overall neurologic outcome. There is a much higher rate of poor outcomes (i.e., severe disability, vegetative survival, and delayed death) for children less than 5 years of age than for older children or adults with similar injury severities. In contrast, children aged 5 through 10 years seem to show a remarkable capability for neurologic recovery over the first year after injury, with over 60 per cent of the surviving children in this age range achieving a "good" outcome by GOS criteria.[22] However, as suggested earlier, these findings must be viewed as tentative, and perhaps excessively optimistic, because of our inability to accurately characterize a truly "good" outcome for a patient who has yet to exhibit his or her neurologic and intellectual potential.

It has been generally accepted that focal neurologic deficits related to isolated cortical injuries recover more fully in younger patients.[23, 24] Furthermore, the "physical" recovery from childhood brain injury occurs earlier and more rapidly than does the neurobehavioral or cognitive recovery.[25] Thus, most reports that separate the neurologic (i.e., physical) recovery from the cognitive recovery show that far more children suffering traumatic brain injury will be left with long-standing neurobehavioral sequelae than with neurologic deficits.[26]

THE VEGETATIVE STATE

Prolonged vegetative survival is extremely rare in head-injured children. Although as many as 13 per cent of severely head-injured children may be in coma at the time of discharge from the acute care hospital, less than half are still in coma one year later.[22, 25] As mentioned above, it appears that very young children who are vegetative have an extremely high mortality, whereas older children tend to improve to much better levels of function.[22] This recovery happens early, generally within the first 3 months after injury. In contrast, most children who are still in coma 6 months after the injury will remain in a persistent vegetative state.[25]

POST-TRAUMATIC SEIZURES

Despite the relatively common occurrence of seizures after head injury in children, there are profound limitations in our understanding of the natural history and the management of patients who might be at risk for the development of these seizures. Temkin et al. have recently reviewed the current understanding of this complicated entity as it relates to all head-injured patients.[27] Few studies have addressed this issue exclusively in the pediatric age group.[28, 29]

A distinction must be made between early and usually isolated post-traumatic seizures and a chronic epilepsy imparted by a traumatic brain injury. Early seizures, as defined by Jennett,[30] include the immediate and "impact" types of seizures that occur within minutes to hours after the injury and the more "delayed" early seizures that can occur up to 1 week after the injury. These types of seizure are considered to be acute reactions to the brain injury. Unlike the early seizures occurring in adults, early post-traumatic seizures in children are not necessarily associated with a significant brain injury.[28, 29, 31] Post-traumatic seizures that occur after the first week are termed "late" seizures and are much more likely to be part of a chronic and recurring seizure disorder, which would appropriately be called post-traumatic epilepsy.[27, 30] Late post-traumatic seizures have been reported in 2 to 3 per cent of all closed head injuries and up to 50 per cent of all penetrating head injuries.[32] However, in the series of children reported by Hahn et al., although about 10 per cent of head-injured children experienced a post-traumatic seizure, only 2 per cent of those children (i.e., 0.2 per cent of the whole population of head-injured children) experienced a seizure after the first week.[28]

Ideally, one would wish to identify patients at risk for seizures after head injury and prevent their occurrence, although the means of accomplishing both of these desires is not at all clear. Hahn et al. found that the more severe the brain injury, either by GCS criteria or by the radiographic findings of acute subdural hematoma or cerebral swelling, the higher the incidence of seizures, generally following what had been shown previously in adults.[28, 30] This finding must be reconciled with the demonstration, in the same study, that over half of all the seizures that occurred in head-injured children occurred in patients with mild head injuries by GCS criteria and in patients with normal CT scans. Another multicenter study of acute head injuries found almost identical distributions of acute seizures and that the vast majority of patients experiencing acute seizures achieved a good or moderate outcome at discharge from the hospital.[29] Although prevention of early seizures would be desirable, most of the seizures occur around the time of the injury, well before therapeutic levels of anticonvulsants could be achieved. Furthermore, most of these seizures are isolated and self-limiting events. In contrast, the occurrence of a "late" seizure is strongly associated with a high chance of recurrence. Once a patient has experienced a "late" post-traumatic seizure, the risk for a subsequent seizure is about 45 per cent, and therapy aimed at preventing seizures could be considered.[33]

Unfortunately, the most rigorous study of the effectiveness of anticonvulsant medication on post-traumatic epilepsy did not demonstrate any long-term beneficial effect for the treated patient group.[34] In that study, phenytoin therapy (no other currently available drug has been shown to be better than phenytoin for the prevention of traumatic seizures) was effective in reducing seizures in the "early" period after injury, but had no beneficial effect after the first week. Previous studies of phenytoin prophylaxis on early post-traumatic seizures had failed to demonstrate a positive effect.[35] These findings are generally consistent with several previous studies of post-traumatic epilepsy that demonstrated not only a clear lack of effectiveness for prophylactic phenytoin, but also a strong suggestion that the risk of seizures is actually *increased* in patients receiving the "prophylactic" anticonvulsant.[27] Finally, it appears that the natural history of post-traumatic epilepsy is one of improvement. There is a significant rate of remission in this seizure disorder, with up to 50 per cent of patients becoming free of seizures without medication.[33] This information, added to the not insignificant risks and side effects of anticonvulsant administration, makes it difficult to recommend the "routine" administration of prophylactic anticonvulsants for post-traumatic seizures. Some patients will require anticonvulsant administration early after the head injury to control recurrent seizures. Temkin et al. have indicated that current data support the use of phenytoin therapy for the short term.[27] A decision to use long-term prophylaxis, and with what drug, and for what length of time, must be balanced against the likely benefits (or the lack thereof) and the risks of the medication selected.

ENDOCRINE DISTURBANCES

The complication of central precocious puberty after diffuse (nontraumatic) brain injuries has been well described.[36] With the advances in critical care, more severely head-injured children are surviving, and reports of precocious puberty following closed head injury are becoming more common.[37–39] The early recognition of this complication is important because, if untreated, precocious puberty results in the rapid progression of the secondary sexual characteristics, acceleration of skeletal growth, and early fusion of the skeletal epiphyses. In addition to the psychosocial implications, these children stop growing much earlier and achieve much smaller than normal adult stature. The process is not reversible, but if recognized early, it can be blocked by the administration of long-acting luteinizing-releasing-hormone-agonist analogues.[40]

Other than the complication of precocious puberty, there are very few reports of persistent anterior pituitary dysfunction after traumatic brain injury in childhood, and even fewer reports of persistent posterior pituitary dysfunction.[41, 42] Unlike the early onset of secondary sexual characteristics, the clinical manifestations of the other anterior pituitary endocrine deficiencies, especially in the absence of diabetes insipidus, may be extremely subtle in children. It is likely that this complication is under-reported because it is under-diagnosed.

HETEROTOPIC OSSIFICATION

Periarticular soft tissue calcification is an entity that occurs in as many as 20 per cent of children who have sustained a severe brain injury, especially if there has been prolonged coma.[43] This complication can markedly inhibit the rehabilitation process. Pain, swelling, and limited joint movement, most commonly in the elbow, hip, and knee, generally appear a few months after the injury. Children at risk for this complication tend to be somewhat older and are likely to have suffered other injuries, most frequently multiple long bone fractures. Although the cause is unknown, it appears that local tissue injury may be the instigating factor. This process is usually noted well after the joint or tissue has begun to ossify, at which point it is difficult to reverse. Therefore, the importance of prevention, initiated as early as possible after the head injury, has been emphasized.[44]

NEUROBEHAVIORAL SEQUELAE

POST-TRAUMATIC AMNESIA

Post-traumatic amnesia (PTA) refers to the early period after recovery of consciousness during which the patient is unable to store information about ongoing events. The clinical relevance of PTA derives from the relationship between its duration and the long-term outcome of head injury. However, the traditional approach to assessing PTA by questioning the patient retrospectively about the return of memory has been criticized because of doubtful reliability. Daily assessment of PTA during the initial hospitalization, which involves direct measurement of orientation and memory for information familiar to children (e.g., a Sesame Street character) rather than retrospective estimates is more useful for monitoring recovery. The Children's Orientation and Amnesia Test[45] evaluates orientation to person, place, and time using questions and material that are appropriate for the child's age. Plotting daily scores yields a recovery curve that can be useful for planning hospital discharge as well as for clinical studies that require a reproducible measure of early outcome. Support for the prognostic usefulness of this measure of PTA duration was provided by Ewing-Cobbs et al. who found that it was more strongly related than the Glasgow Coma Scale (GCS) score[46] to tests of verbal and nonverbal memory administered 6 months later.[45]

INTELLECTUAL FUNCTION

Intellectual ability after head injury has been studied most extensively using the age-appropriate Wechsler Scale. As early as 1970, Brink and her co-workers found that intellectual impairment 1 to 7 years after injury was directly related to the duration of coma.[47] Two thirds of the patients had evidence of intellectual deficit, according to the criterion of an intellectual quotient (IQ) that fell two or more standard deviations below the mean (i.e., an IQ of 70 or lower). Contrary to a generalized interpretation of cerebral plasticity, the children who were younger than 10 years at the time of injury exhibited more severe intellectual impairment than older children who had similar durations of coma. Subsequent studies,[48-53] which have used the GCS or the duration of PTA to classify their patients, have confirmed the relationship between severity of injury and intellectual deficit. Qualitative features of intellectual impairment have been studied primarily by comparing the relative sensitivity of the Verbal and Performance Scales of the Wechsler Intelligence Test. In general, the Performance Scale (Fig. 21–4) demonstrates a clearer recovery pattern over time and a stronger relationship to the severity of injury.[48, 50] Speeded tasks (e.g., motor speed) are more sensitive to severity of injury than untimed performance measures.

Consistent with the results reported earlier by Brink et al., Levin and co-workers found that intellectual deficit was more frequent in children who were younger than 12 years at the time of injury.[52] The investigation of long-term intellectual outcome of head injury was extended to infants and preschoolers by Ewing-Cobbs et al., who employed the Bayley Scales of Infant Development and the McCarthy Scales of Children's Ability.[54] Consistent with studies of older children, intellectual impairment was directly related to severity of head injury as measured by the GCS score. The motor component of the Bayley Scale was more sensitive to severity of injury than the mental portion of this test, a finding that parallels the vulnerability of the Performance Scale of the Wechsler test in older children. Ongoing studies of head-injured children utilize tasks of problem solving, planning, and conceptualization of se-

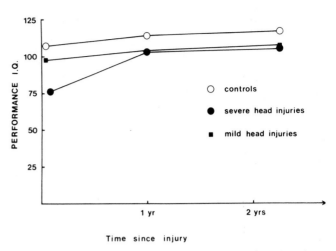

FIGURE 21–4. Recovery of performance IQ over time plotted according to severity of head injury in children. Note the pattern consistent with recovery in the severely injured patients, whereas the mildly injured patients show minimal change over time and have a slope that is similar to that of children who sustained orthopedic injuries. (From Chadwick O, Rutter M, Brown G, et al.: A prospective study of children with head injuries: II. Cognitive sequelae. Psychol Med 11:49, 1981.)

mantic relationships derived from cognitive psychology.[55]

MEMORY IN RELATION TO SEVERITY OF HEAD INJURY

In contrast to the acquisition and overlearning of essential information by adults prior to sustaining a head injury, children and adolescents are challenged at school by demands for learning and retaining new information. Studies of memory in head-injured children have typically employed tests of recalling word lists and retention of visually presented material such as reproducing designs and recognizing pictures of familiar animals and plants.[52, 53, 56, 57] The pattern of findings indicates that children sustaining severe head injury typically exhibit a residual impairment of memory in both verbal and nonverbal measures. Figure 21–5 reflects the persistence of this memory deficit on tests of recalling word lists and recognizing recurring pictures of familiar living things over one year after injury. In contrast, the initial memory disturbance found in pediatric patients following mild to moderate head injury tends to resolve over the first year.

LANGUAGE

The clinical features of post-traumatic aphasia in children reflect the predominance of expressive deficit (i.e., anomia, diminished fluency), which is frequently present in head-injured adults.[54] However, Levin and Eisenberg found that comprehension of complex commands on the token test was frequently impaired in head-injured children.[56, 57] Initial mutism is common during the early stage of aphasia following head injury in children, whereas long-term sequelae include diffi-

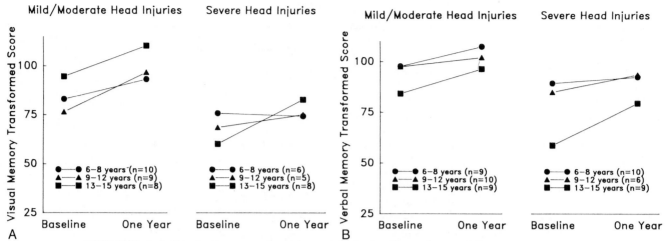

FIGURE 21–5. *A,* Visual memory transformed scores on the baseline and 1-year follow-up examinations, plotted separately according to age at injury and severity of injury according to the GCS score. The transformed scores are based on normative data collected from 83 children and adolescents in the Galveston community. The mean score for each age group is equal to 100 with a standard deviation of 10. *B,* Verbal memory transformed scores (total retrieval) summed across trials on the baseline and 1-year follow-up examinations, plotted separately according to age at injury and GCS score. Note the greater impairment of verbal learning and memory in adolescents in relation to expectation for their age. The transformed scores are based on normative data collected from 83 children and adolescents in the Galveston community. The mean score for each age group is equal to 100 with a standard deviation of 10. (From Levin HS, High WM, Ewing-Cobbs L, Fletcher JM, et al.: Memory functioning during the first year after closed head injury in children and adolescents. Neurosurgery 22:1043, 1988.)

culty in naming, reduced fluency, and problems in spelling and arithmetic. Investigators have recently acknowledged that linguistic measures at the word or sentence level are insufficient to characterize the reduced communication skills of head-injured children.[58] Studies of discourse have disclosed that coherent ties are frequently reduced in number or are absent, thus conveying the impression of fragmented stories produced by severely injured children. The patients tended to omit much of the gist information of the stories presented to them. Analysis of other tests administered in the same session disclosed that a primary memory deficit of loss of verbal ability (as reflected by range of vocabulary) was not sufficient to explain the impoverished discourse.

BEHAVIORAL DISTURBANCE AND PSYCHOSOCIAL MALADJUSTMENT

Behavioral problems tend to be common in children at risk for head injury, thus complicating the assessment of sequelae.[59, 60] To circumvent this confounding, Rutter and co-workers assessed new behavioral problems which developed after head injury. As shown in Figure 21–6, new behavioral problems increased in frequency during the 2 years after severe head injury, whereas the rate of new behavioral disturbance after mild head injury was comparable to the finding obtained in children sustaining orthopedic injuries.[60] Converging evidence for the manifestation of behavioral and psychosocial sequelae of severe head injury in children was reported by Fletcher et al., who used standardized questionnaires completed by the parent to char-

acterize the post-injury changes.[61] Comparison of the follow-up findings to baseline data that characterized pre-injury adjustment revealed that the severity of head injury was directly related to post-traumatic behavioral disturbance and immature patterns of psychosocial adjustment.

AGE AT INJURY

Extrapolation of evidence from ablation experiments in nonhuman primates leads to the prediction that

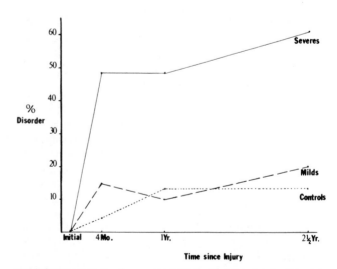

FIGURE 21–6. Rate of new psychiatric disorder developing since the date of injury plotted separately for groups of children who sustained severe head injury, mild head injury, or orthopedic injuries (controls). (From Rutter M: Developmental neuropsychiatry: Concepts, issues, and prospects. J Clin Neuropsychol 4:91, 1982.)

young children recover more fully from head injury than older children and adolescents. However, the effects of diffuse axonal injury on subsequent cognitive development do not parallel findings obtained with focal brain lesions. Comparison of neurobehavioral outcome in relation to age at injury is complicated by differences in the cause of head trauma (e.g., falls are more common in young children), and the neurobehavioral measures are often different. Notwithstanding these caveats, studies that have compared the outcome of different age groups indicate that the long-term consequences of severe head injury are at least as devastating to young children as to older children and adolescents.[47, 52, 53]

MILD HEAD INJURY

The neurobehavioral consequences of mild head injury have been more controversial than the outcome of severe injury. Sequelae such as reading disability and attentional disturbance have been implicated by several investigations.[62, 63] However, Brown and co-workers documented that behavioral problems were frequently present in these children before they sustained a mild head injury.[59] Differences in the definition of mild head injury also contribute to discrepancies in the literature. A recent English study involving a large cohort of children who sustained a mild head injury failed to find any excess in post-traumatic behavioral disturbance relative to a comparison group of children.[64] Other studies have underscored the exacerbation of sequelae due to parental anxiety,[65] a complication that is potentially mitigated by educating the family on the time course of recovery (1 to 3 months) and the prevention of further injuries, which may have cumulative effects.

CONCLUSIONS AND RECOMMENDATIONS

Severe head injury has persistent adverse effects on memory, cognition, communication skills, and psychosocial adaptation. Although there is a strong relationship between the initial GCS score and neurobehavioral outcome, direct assessment of PTA duration can contribute useful information. Baseline and at least one year follow-up neuropsychologic examinations can assess the sequelae and identify the need for rehabilitation and remedial education. Although initial neuropsychologic deficits are also common after moderate head injury, the clinical course is characterized by substantial recovery over one year. Psychosocial adaptation is also an important domain for follow-up assessment.

ACKNOWLEDGMENT: The authors are indebted to Ora H. Pescovitz, M.D. (Indiana University), and Joseph J. Sockalosky, M.D. (University of Minnesota), for their help and advice regarding the section on post-traumatic endocrinopathies.

REFERENCES

1. Ito H, Tetsuro M, Onodra Y: Growing skull fracture of childhood. Childs Brain 3:116, 1977.
2. Pezzotta S, Silvani V, Gaetani P, et al.: Growing skull fractures of childhood. J Neurosurg Sci 29:129, 1985.
3. Roy S, Sarkar C, Tandon PN, Banerji AK: Cranio-cerebral erosion (growing fracture of the skull in children). Part I. Pathology. Acta Neurochir (Wien) 87:112, 1987.
4. Tandon PN, Banerji AK, Bhatia R, Goulatia RK: Cranio-cerebral erosion (growing fracture of the skull in children). Part II. Clinical and radiological observations. Acta Neurochir (Wien) 88:1, 1987.
5. Winston K, Beatty RM, Fischer EG: Consequences of dural defects acquired in infancy. J Neurosurg 59:839, 1983.
6. Goldstein F, Sakoda T, Kepes JJ, et al: Enlarging skull fractures: An experimental study. J Neurosurg 27:541, 1967.
7. Ramamurthi B, Kalyanaraman S: Rationale for surgery in growing fractures of the skull. J Neurosurg 32:427, 1970.
8. Kingsley D, Till K, Hoare R: Growing fractures of the skull. J Neurol Neurosurg Psychiatry 41:312, 1978.
9. Sato O, Tsugane R, Kageyama N: Growing skull fractures of childhood. Possible mechanisms of its focal ventricular dilatation. Childs Brain 1:148, 1975.
10. Stein BM, Tenner MS: Enlargement of skull fracture in childhood due to cerebral herniation. Arch Neurol 26:137, 1972.
11. Lende RA: Enlarging skull fractures of childhood. Neuroradiology 7:119, 1974.
12. Fox JL: Traumatic intracranial aneurysms. In Fox, JL (ed): Intracranial Aneurysms. New York, Springer-Verlag, 1983, pp 1453–1463.
13. Buckingham MJ, Crone KR, Ball WS, et al.: Traumatic intracranial aneurysms in childhood: Two cases and a review of the literature. Neurosurgery 22:398, 1988.
14. Agnetti V, Pav A, Pinna L, et al.: Cerebral pseudo-angiomatous pattern in a case of carotid-cavernous fistula. J Neurosurg Sci 18:75, 1974.
15. Arseni C, Horvath L, Caurea V, et al.: Carotid-cavernous fistula in the child. Rev Roum Med Neurol Psychiatr 16:29, 1978.
16. Broughton WL, Gee W, Doppman J, et al.: Nonpulsatile exophthalmos in carotid-cavernous sinus fistula. J Pediatr Ophthalmol 14:221, 1977.
17. Bonafe A, Manelfe C: Traumatic carotid-cavernous fistulas. In Braakman R (ed): The Handbook of Clinical Neurology, Vol 13 (57): Head Injury. New York, Elsevier Science Publishing, 1990, pp 345–366.
18. Luerssen TG, Sutton LN, Bruce DA, Schut L: Posttraumatic hydrocephalus in the neonate and infant. In Raimondi AJ, Choux M, DiRocco C (eds): Head Injuries in the Newborn and Infant. New York, Springer-Verlag, 1986, pp 241–256.
19. Oi S, Matsumoto S: Post-traumatic hydrocephalus in children. Pathophysiology and classification. J Pediatric Neurosciences 3:133, 1987.
20. Luerssen TG, Klauber MR, Marshall LF: Outcome from head injury related to patient's age. J Neurosurg 68:409, 1988.
21. Jennett B, Bond M: Assessment of outcome after severe brain damage: A practical scale. Lancet i:480, 1975.
22. Jennett B, Snoek J, Bond MR, Brooks N: Disability after severe head injury: Observations on the use of the Glasgow Outcome Scale. J Neurol Neurosurg Psychiatry 44:285, 1981.
22. Levin HS, Aldrich EF, Saydjari C, et al.: Severe head injury in children: Experience of the Traumatic Coma Data Bank. Neurosurgery 31:435, 1992.
23. Loonen MCB, van Dongen HR: Acquired childhood aphasia. Arch Neurol 47:1324, 1990.
24. Shapiro K: Head injury in children. In Becker DP, Povlishock JT (eds): Central Nervous System Trauma Status Report 1985. Bethesda, National Institutes of Health, 1985, pp 243–253.
25. Boyer MG, Edwards P: Outcome 1 to 3 years after severe traumatic brain injury in children and adolescents. Injury 22:315, 1991.
26. Mahoney WJ, D'Souza BJ, Haller JA, et al.: Long-term outcome of children with severe head trauma and prolonged coma. Pediatrics 71:756, 1983.

27. Temkin NR, Dikmen SS, Winn HR: Post-traumatic seizures. Neurosurg Clin North Am 2:425, 1991.

28. Hahn YS, Fuchs S, Flannery AM, et al.: Factors influencing post-traumatic seizures in children. Neurosurgery 22:864, 1988.

29. Luerssen TG, Huang JC, McLone DG, et al.: Retinal hemorrhages, seizures, and intracranial hemorrhages: Relationships and outcomes in children suffering traumatic brain injury. *In* Marlin AE (ed): Concepts in Pediatric Neurosurgery, Vol. 11. Basel, Karger, 1991, pp 87–94.

30. Jennett B: Post-traumatic epilepsy. *In* Vinken PJ, Bruyn GW (eds): Handbook of Clinical Neurology, Vol 24: Injuries of the Brain and Skull Part II. New York, American Elselvier Publishing Co. Inc., 1976, pp 445–454.

31. Jennett B, Teasdale G: Management of Head Injuries. Philadelphia, F. A. Davis & Co., 1981, p 237.

32. Bricolo AP, Turella GS: Electrophysiology of head injury. *In* Braakman R (ed): Handbook of Clinical Neurology, Vol 13 (57): Head Injury. New York, Elsevier Science Publishers, 1990, pp 181–206.

33. Hauser, WA: Post-traumatic epilepsy in children. *In* Shapiro K (ed): Pediatric Head Trauma. Mount Kisco, New York, Futura Publishing Co., 1983, pp 271–287.

34. Temkin NR, Dikmen SS, Wilensky AJ, et al.: A randomized, double-blind study of phenytoin for the prevention of post-traumatic seizures. N Engl J Med 323:497, 1990.

35. Young B, Rapp RP, Norton JA, et al.: Failure of prophylactically administered phenytoin to prevent early post-traumatic seizures. J Neurosurg 58:231, 1983.

36. Balagura S, Shulman K, Sobel EH: Precocious puberty of cerebral origin. Surg Neurol 11:315, 1979.

37. Blendonohy PM, Puliyodil PA: Precocious puberty in children after traumatic brain injury. Brain Injury 5:63, 1991.

38. Maxwell M, Karacostas D, Ellenbogen RG, et al.: Precocious puberty following head injury. J Neurosurg 73:123, 1990.

39. Sockalosky JJ, Kriel RL, Krach LE, Sheehan M: Precocious puberty after traumatic brain injury. J Pediatr 110:373, 1987.

40. Pescovitz OH, Cutler GB, Loriaux DL: Management of precocious puberty. J Pediatr Endocrinol 1:85, 1985.

41. Edwards OM, Clark JDA: Post-traumatic hypopituitarism. Medicine 65:281, 1986.

42. Paxson CL, Brown DR: Post-traumatic anterior hypopituitarism. Pediatrics 57:893, 1976.

43. Hurvitz EA, Mandac BR, Davidoff G, et al.: Risk factors for heterotopic ossification in children and adolescents with severe traumatic brain injury. Arch Phys Med Rehabil 73:459, 1992.

44. Rogers RC: Heterotpic calcification in severe head injury: A preventive programme. Brain Injury 2:169, 1988.

45. Ewing-Cobbs L, Levin HS, Fletcher JM, et al.: The Children's Orientation and Amnesia Test: Relationship to severity of acute head injury and to recovery of memory. Neurosurgery 27:683, 1990.

46. Teasdale G, Jennett B: Assessment of coma and impaired consciousness: A practical scale. Lancet ii:81, 1974.

47. Brink JD, Garrett AL, Hale WR, Woo-Sam J, Nickel VL: Recovery of motor and intellectual function in children sustaining severe head injuries. Dev Med Child Neurol 12:565, 1970.

48. Bawden HN, Knights RM, Winogron HW: Speeded performance following head injury in children. J Clin Exp Neuropsych 7:39, 1985.

49. Chadwick O, Rutter M, Brown G, et al.: A prospective study of children with head injuries: II. Cognitive sequelae. Psychol Med 11:49, 1981a.

50. Chadwick O, Rutter M, Shaffer D, Shrout PE: A prospective study of children with head injuries: IV. Specific cognitive deficits. J Clin Neuropsychol 3:101, 1981b.

51. Chadwick O, Rutter M, Thompson J, Shaffer D: Intellectual performance and reading skills after localized head injury in childhood. J Clin Psychol Psychiatry 22:117, 1981c.

52. Levin HS, Eisenberg HM, Wigg NR, Kobayashi K: Memory and intellectual ability after head injury in children and adolescents. Neurosurgery 11:668, 1982.

53. Levin HS, High WM, Ewing-Cobbs L, Fletcher JM, et al.: Memory functioning during the first year after closed head injury in children and adolescents. Neurosurgery 22:1043, 1988.

54. Ewing-Cobbs L, Miner ME, Fletcher JM, Levin HS: Intellectual, motor, and language sequelae following closed head injury in infants and preschoolers. J Pediatr Psychol 14:531, 1989.

55. Levin HS, Culhane KA, Hartmann J, et al.: Developmental changes in performance on tests of purported frontal lobe functioning. Dev Neuropsychol 7:377, 1991.

56. Levin HS, Eisenberg HM: Neuropsychological impairment after closed head injury in children and adolescents. J Pediatr Psychol 4:389, 1979a.

57. Levin HS, Eisenberg HM: Neuropsychological outcome of closed head injury in children and adolescents. Childs Brain 5:281, 1979b.

58. Dennis M, Barnes MA: Knowing the meaning, getting the point, bridging the gap, and carrying the message: Aspects of discourse following closed head injury in childhood and adolescence. Brain Lang 39:428, 1990.

59. Brown G, Chadwick O, Shaffer O, Rutter M, Traub M: A prospective study of children with head injuries: III. Psychiatric sequelae. Psychol Med 11:63, 1981.

60. Rutter M: Developmental neuropsychiatry: Concepts, issues, and prospects. J Clin Neuropsychol 4:91, 1982.

61. Fletcher JM, Ewing-Cobbs L, Miner ME, et al.: Behavioral changes after closed head injury in children. J Consult Clin Psychol 58:93, 1990.

62. Gulbrandsen GB: Neuropsychological sequelae and light head injuries in older children 6 months after trauma. J Clin Neuropsychol 6:257, 1984.

63. Shaffer D, Bijur P, Chadwick O, Rutter M: Head injury and later reading disability. J Am Child Psychiatry 19:592, 1980.

64. Bijur PE, Haslum M, Golding J: Cognitive and behavioral sequelae of mild head injury in children. Pediatrics 86:337, 1990.

65. Casey R, Ludwig S, McCormick MC: Morbidity following minor head trauma in children. Pediatrics 78:497, 1986.

Chapter 22

INTRACRANIAL HYPERTENSION:
Mechanisms and Management

KENNETH SHAPIRO, M.D., WILLIAM J. MORRIS, M.D.,
and CHARLES TEO, M.D.

"The control of intracranial pressure is perhaps the principal task in the neurosurgical care of infants."[1] This statement may be extended to all children because many of the medical and surgical diseases encountered in children are accompanied by intracranial hypertension. Widely differing conditions including congenital lesions, neoplasms, metabolic and infectious syndromes, and trauma require evaluation and treatment for elevated intracranial pressure (ICP). Because intracranial hypertension frequently accompanies disease processes in children, an understanding of its mechanisms and treatment is of paramount importance to the neurosurgeon.

One must be cautious in applying to children the concepts of intracranial hypertension derived from experience with adults. Although many of the clinical manifestations are similar in both age groups, distinct differences exist. Children may harbor an intracranial mass for some time without overt signs of increased ICP, only to deteriorate rapidly and dramatically to an unsalvageable state. Often, intracranial masses may be accompanied by phenomena not encountered in adults, such as failure to reach developmental milestones or accelerated growth of the head. Unique properties of the immature brain and its container affect the brain's response to changes in ICP. The following discussion integrates the mechanisms that lead to raised ICP with the properties of the immature nervous system and presents in detail the treatment of intracranial hypertension in children.

NORMAL INTRACRANIAL PRESSURE

The upper limit of normal ICP in adults and older children is usually given as 15 mm Hg. Transient changes resulting from coughing, sneezing, or straining often produce pressures exceeding 30 to 50 mm Hg, but ICP returns rapidly to baseline levels. Measurements of ICP in younger children and infants by spinal puncture using manometers have been criticized because of the poor cooperation from the child and the displacement of fluid into the manometric device. Given these practical difficulties, published norms for children range from 3 to 7.4 mm Hg and for infants from 1.5 to 5.9 mm Hg.[1-3]

All reported values for the ICP of younger children are lower than those reported for adults but are probably reasonable approximations of the actual level of ICP. A teleologic explanation might account for this relatively low normal ICP in children. In adults, the ability to perfuse the brain effectively depends on the maintenance of a cerebral perfusion pressure (CPP) greater than 50 mm Hg.[4] The critical CPP of the immature brain has not been determined. Since the mean arterial blood pressure (MAP) of infants and children is considerably lower than that of adults, a lower normal ICP may be a mechanism for maintaining adequate CPP.

Measurements of ICP using low-volume displacement transducers to interface with the CSF pathways yield considerably more information than an absolute pressure that exceeds atmospheric pressure by 4 to 8 mm Hg. The pulsatile ICP wave-form can be divided into three major components (Fig. 22–1). The *baseline*, or diastolic, level is commonly referred to as the ICP, while rhythmic components are associated with cardiac and respiratory activity. In order to completely describe ICP, one should specify the magnitude of the baseline, or "steady state," level and the amplitude and periodicity of the pulsatile components. Although some workers report ICP as a mean pressure, paralleling the con-

307

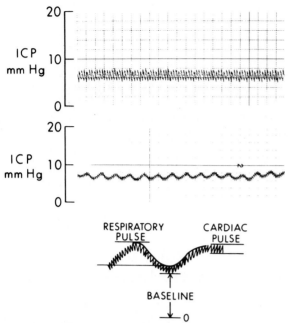

FIGURE 22–1. The intracranial pressure (ICP) wave-form consists of respiratory and cardiac variations superimposed upon a steady state level that is usually above atmospheric pressure. The upper panel displays the ICP at fast chart speed to accentuate the cardiac pulsations. Specification of ICP should include a measure of both baseline level and amplitude of pulsatile components.

vention used in systemic blood pressure, this has not been universally adopted. Many eliminate the pulsatile components and specify diastolic pressure as the ICP.

STEADY STATE DYNAMICS

In the physiologic steady state, baseline ICP remains constant despite a variety of transient perturbations. Since ICP depends on relative constancy of volume, any change in the volume of one of the normal intracranial components must occur at the expense of the other two:

$$V_{CSF} + V_{BLOOD} + V_{BRAIN} + V_{OTHER} = V_{INTRACRANIAL\ SPACE}$$
$$= (constant)$$

Explanation of this interaction between volume and pressure is based on the Monro-Kellie doctrine, which states that for ICP to remain normal, intracranial volume must remain nearly constant because the skull, after closure of the fontanelle and sutures, forms a rigid container.[5–7] Presence of an abnormal component such as a tumor or hematoma demands reciprocal changes in the volumes of brain, blood, or CSF to maintain ICP at physiologic levels. Even the physiologic state is far from static. Constant changes induced by the heart beat as well as systemic blood pressure, fluid status, and intrathoracic pressure require dynamic changes within the intracranial compartment to maintain the steady state.

GENERAL SYSTEMIC PHYSIOLOGY

In the condition of physiologic equilibrium, both the baseline ICP and the amplitude of the pulsatile components of ICP remain constant. Pulse pressure, which is reflected in the amplitude of the ICP wave form, is dependent on cardiac output and systemic arterial resistance. Children differ from adults in that cardiac output is governed by heart rate more than by myocardial contractility. Also, peripheral vascular resistance in children is often inefficient at physiologic extremes. Pulmonary function is different in that pulmonary blood flow is more subject to the effect of gravity. Other organ systems may also contribute to these contrasts between adults and children. Although the overall effect of these physiologic variables can lead to more erratic fluctuations in ICP in children compared to adults, steady state baseline values are usually maintained.[8]

CEREBRAL BLOOD FLOW (CBF)

From the time of delivery to adulthood CBF increases from 40 ml/100gm/min to the normal adult value of 53 ml/100gm/min. CBF is determined by cerebral perfusion pressure and vascular resistance. The low flows in the healthy newborn can be attributed to the resistance of cerebral vessels, which are in a state of relative vasoconstriction. This is due to a combination of factors including (1) an autoregulatory response to a greater MAP than that experienced in utero and (2) a relatively low concentration of vasodilating metabolites produced by the low cerebral metabolic rate.[9] Between the ages of 1 and 9 years, CBF is higher than in adulthood, averaging 65 to 106 ml/100gm/min.[9] Although ICP is low in this age group, the MAP is proportionally lower still, thereby creating a state of relative luxury perfusion.[10] The combination of higher CPP and a steady degree of resistance results in a higher CBF. Once the child reaches puberty, CBF attains its normal value of 53 ml/100gm/min.[11]

Autoregulation is essentially the same in children and adults. This capability maintains adequate CBF in response to changes in systemic arterial pressure as long as $PaCO_2$ is between 20 and 70 mm Hg and MAP between 50 and 160 mm Hg. One difference is that CO_2 responsivity appears to be greater in children.[12]

CEREBROSPINAL FLUID (CSF) DYNAMICS

In the adult, approximately 80 per cent of the intracranial space is occupied by the brain, leaving 10 per cent for CSF and 10 per cent for blood. In the child, although total ratios of CSF to brain may be similar, the relative amount of CSF within the intracranial cavity is probably less, as demonstrated by CT and MRI, which show small ventricles and subarachnoid spaces in children.

The interactions of these volumes can be addressed using a mathematical model that analyzes the physiologic mechanisms of: (1) CSF formation, (2) volume storage, or compliance and (3) fluid absorption (Fig. 22–2).[13]

Conceptually, the formation of CSF can be depicted as a pump that continuously introduces fluid into the CSF spaces of the neural axis. The rate of formation of fluid (I_f) is considered constant and independent of the pressure head seen by the pump mechanism, in accordance with observations that the rate of CSF formation is affected minimally, if at all, by changes in the ICP. The fluid enters a compliant storage space, which can expand to accommodate the added volume, or proceeds via outflow pathways and is absorbed across the arachnoid villi into the dural venous sinuses. The compliance mechanism is represented by an element (C), which decreases its contractility with increasing volume, much like the resistance offered by a rubber balloon at maximum inflation. Both the resistance of the CSF channels leading to the arachnoid villi and the resistance of the villi to fluid flow are combined into a single resistance element (R_o). This component represents the total resistance to the outflow of the CSF which, under normal conditions, remains fixed and independent of ICP. The final element of this model is the dural sinus pressure (P_d). Fluid crossing the arachnoid villi must overcome the P_d, so that the exit pressure of CSF is determined by P_d.

From this conceptual framework a theory has been developed to describe the interaction of the formation, storage, and absorptive elements in the steady state. First, both pressure and volume are in equilibrium, and there can be no net increase or decrease in the total volume of the CSF spaces. The CSF formed must pass through the absorptive elements so that no net fluid is stored, and the total volume within the CSF spaces remains constant.

Since all fluid formed passes through the resistive element (R_o), a pressure gradient will be developed across the absorptive element that is equal to the product of fluid flow (I_f) and the fluid resistance (R_o). The greater the magnitude of flow or resistance, the greater the pressure gradient ($I_f \times R_o$). As long as a condition of equilibrium is imposed upon the system, the pressure of the CSF spaces must be of sufficient magnitude to force all newly formed fluid through the arachnoid villi. This requires that the CSF pressure (ICP) be equal to the sum of the pressure gradient developed by the absorptive element ($I_f \times R_o$) and the exit pressure. The equation

$$ICP = (I_f \times R_o) + P_d$$

shows that the steady state ICP is proportional to three parameters: (1) the rate of CSF formation, (2) the resistance to CSF absorption, and (3) the dural sinus pressure. When these parameters remain constant, ICP is unchanged and the compliance element does not participate actively.

This dynamic equilibrium is altered in cases of raised ICP, which can result from an increase in CSF formation, outflow resistance, or venous pressure at the site of fluid absorption. Computer studies show that the contribution of the product of CSF formation rate and outflow resistance ($I_f \times R_o$) is approximately 10 per cent of the total ICP.[14] The remainder is attributed to the magnitude of the dural sinus pressure (P_d). With this distribution, the outflow resistance would have to increase markedly to cause a significant rise in the ICP. However, elevations of sagittal sinus pressure caused by venous sinus obstruction would be transmitted directly to the CSF system, resulting in an increase in resting ICP. Since the increase in P_d equals the change in ICP, the gradient across the arachnoid villi is not altered, CSF absorption remains constant, and the equilibrium shift to a higher ICP level is sustained. This concept is supported by the work of Johnston, who demonstrated normal CSF resistance in the presence of raised ICP induced by venous obstruction; it is also supported by observations in children with anomalous venous return.[4, 15] In both conditions, there is no net storage of CSF volume and presumably no change in the compliance element.

NON–STEADY STATE DYNAMICS

Unlike the physiologic steady state, pathologic conditions are usually associated with net changes in volume of the intracranial components. Changes of volume that occur rapidly or exceed the ability for reciprocal volume reductions to occur require more descriptors than the steady state. Changes in volume-pressure relationships can be depicted by graphing the response of ICP to volume added to the neural axis (Fig. 22–3). As shown by Ryder et al., this relationship describes a hyperbolic curve.[16]

Along the flat portion of the curve, increases in volume affect ICP minimally since compensatory mecha-

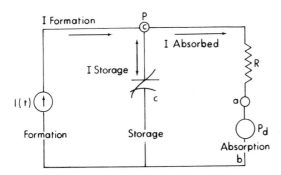

FIGURE 22–2. The CSF system was depicted by an equivalent electric circuit that distributed the CSF parameters among three fundamental mechanisms: formation, represented by a constant-current generator; storage, represented by a nonlinear capacitance (C); and absorption, represented by a resistance element (R). The venous outflow site (dural sinus) was represented by a constant pressure source P_d. The system equations were derived from this configuration.

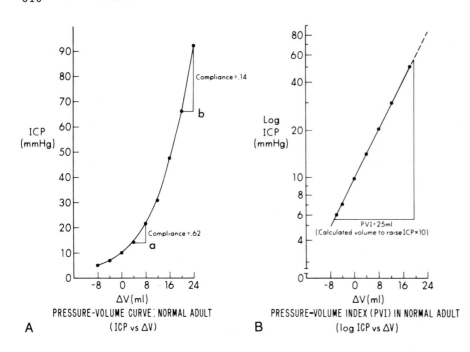

A
PRESSURE-VOLUME CURVE: NORMAL ADULT
(ICP vs ΔV)

B
PRESSURE-VOLUME INDEX (PVI) IN NORMAL ADULT
(log ICP vs ΔV)

FIGURE 22–3. A, Neural axis pressure-volume curve obtained by measuring the immediate cerebrospinal fluid pressure response to successive bolus injections (+ ΔV) or withdrawals (− ΔV) of CSF in a normal adult. Compliance (ΔV/ΔP) is measured at two points on this curve: at point a compliance is greater than at point b. The differences in compliance at these points are a normal function of CSF pressure. B, The same pressure volume curve has been transformed to a linear function by plotting the response of CSF pressure on a logarithmic scale. Only two points are needed to define this linear function. The pressure-volume index (PVI) is the calculated volume (ml) needed to raise CSF pressure by a factor of 10.

nisms can effectively maintain the physiologic state. The slope of the curve (ΔV/ΔP) represents compliance and is maximal at this portion of the curve. As increments of volume are added, relative increases in ICP become greater, and compliance lessens.

Another method of expressing information about compliance is to plot ICP logarithmically against volume. This gives a straight line called the pressure-volume index (PVI).[17] Its slope is the calculated volume (ml) needed to raise ICP by a factor of 10 (Figs. 22–3 and 22–4). In normal adults, PVI is approximately 25 ml.[18] When compliance is reduced by some mass or injury, PVI diminishes. Values less than 13 ml are considered clearly abnormal.[19] In children, PVI varies in proportion to estimated neural axis volume. Normal infants have PVIs below 10 ml, and the adult PVI of 25 ml is reached at around 14 years of age. As a consequence, the slope of a normal infant's pressure-volume curve is steeper than that of a normal teenager (Fig. 22–5). A 10-ml volume added to the neural axis of a teenager may produce modest elevations in ICP, but the same increment can be lethal in an infant.[18]

The compensatory abilities of brain, blood, and CSF at any given point along the pressure-volume curve depend on their respective volumes, their ease of egress from the skull, and the level of ICP at which these interactions occur. As previously mentioned, brain fills 80 per cent of the intracranial space, blood and CSF about 10 per cent each. The large space occupied by brain would seem to offer much compensatory volume, but this ability is realized only when incursions are small and applied slowly over time. In the short term, brain shifts or herniations offer the only form of compensation. Although blood and CSF provide less total volume for compensation, what they offer can be utilized more rapidly, for example, by vasoconstriction caused by hyperventilation, or by displacing CSF into the spinal subarachnoid space or increasing absorption through arachnoid villi.[20]

The preceding discussion assumes a rigid container of

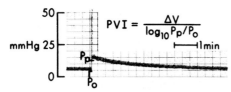

$$PVI = \frac{\Delta V}{\log_{10} P_p/P_o}$$

FIGURE 22–4. This strip chart recording shows the ICP response to a bolus injection of CSF into the cisterna magna of a child. Following injection, the baseline pressure P_o is immediately raised to P_p, the peak pressure response to the injection. Pressure then begins to return toward P_o as CSF is absorbed. The PVI can be calculated from the formula (inset), using data derived from the bolus injection.

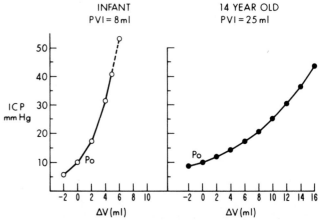

FIGURE 22–5. The pressure-volume curves shown were generated by injecting and withdrawing CSF from a normal infant (left) and a normal teenager (right). The slope of the infant's pressure-volume curve is steeper than that of the teenager, resulting in less ability to buffer equal increments of volume.

the brain. In hydrocephalic infants with open sutures, increases in intracranial volume can be accommodated by expansion of the cranial vault without elevating ICP. It is believed that the steeper pressure volume curve found in infants exists until pressure causes separation at the sutures. Once this occurs, the immature brain can accommodate volume more readily than the rigidly enclosed adult brain.[21, 22]

These concepts become more complex, as do most models, when applied to clinical practice. While movement along a single pressure-volume curve occurs during the treatment of a patient, changing intracranial dynamics can create a new pressure-volume curve (Fig. 22–6). Increases in cerebral blood volume and cerebral edema as well as changes in biomechanical properties of the brain due to treatment are also likely to play a role in producing these dynamic pressure-volume interactions.[23] Thus, knowledge of both the absolute pressure coupled with some expression of the steepness of the intracranial pressure volume curve at any time provide more complete descriptors of the stability or precariousness of intracranial dynamics.

INTRACRANIAL PRESSURE MONITORING

Since knowledge of the actual ICP is fundamental to many clinical decisions in the care of patients, an accurate and safe method of obtaining these data is essential. Besides the technical aspects of measurement, clinical judgment must be exercised in determining which patients should undergo monitoring and what pressures constitute critical levels.

Initial work on direct monitoring of ICP by ventricular puncture was performed by Guillaume and Janny (1951) and by Lundberg (1960).[24, 25] In Lundberg's classic report, he described three basic patterns of ICP: A waves (plateau waves), B waves, and C waves. A waves are characterized by increases of ICP that are sustained for several minutes and then return spontaneously to a new baseline, which is usually slightly higher than the preceding one. Plateau waves identify ICP dynamics exceeding the limits of compensatory reserves. B waves are short elevations of a modest nature (10 to 20 mm Hg) related to respiration and are believed to reflect increased ICP in a qualitative manner. Both A waves and B waves have been attributed to increases in intracranial blood volume. C waves are produced by intracranial transmission of arterial pulse waves, possibly reflecting decreased compliance, again in a qualitative way.

The ventriculostomy coupled with an electrical pressure transducer remains the standard for monitoring ICP because of accuracy and ease of calibration. Access to CSF for dynamic testing and drainage to control ICP are additional benefits. Catheter placement can be difficult when ventricles are small or shifted from the midline. Infections may occur in ventriculostomies left in place more than 3 or 4 days, although this risk is lessened by tunneling the catheter under the skin.

Alternative methods of monitoring ICP include the subarachnoid bolt, epidural transducer, and fiberoptic catheter-transducer. The bolt and epidural devices are useful, but are prone to inaccuracy due to their physical characteristics.[26–28] Although fiberoptic catheter-transducers cannot be recalibrated externally, their accuracy in practice has proved excellent.[29] The extreme ease and safety with which this intraparenchymal monitor can be placed has made it attractive for both adult and pediatric applications.

The decision to monitor a patient's ICP is premised on the assumption that intracranial hypertension is detrimental and that knowledge of the ICP will assist in appropriate management and be reflected in improved outcome. Early controversy regarding whether ICP elevations are detrimental has largely been laid to rest. Intracranial hypertension is found in 40 to 60 per cent

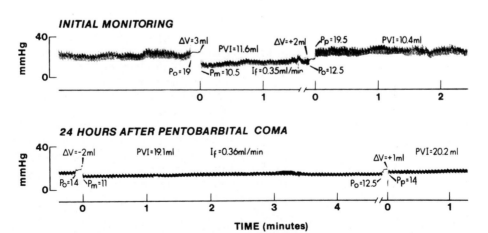

FIGURE 22–6. The strip chart recordings shown were obtained through a ventricular catheter placed in a child with severe closed head injury. The upper tracing shows that PVI was markedly reduced from the predicted normal value (23 ml) for this child and was manifested by dramatic elevations of intracranial pressure. The lower tracing shows a PVI determination performed after barbiturate coma was induced in this child. The increased PVI of 19 ml represents an improvement in the slope of this child's pressure-volume curve and was associated with normalization of intracranial pressure.

of severe head injuries and is a major factor in the deaths of 50 per cent of patients who die.[30] That information gained from ICP monitoring leads to better patient outcomes has been more difficult to establish. Data recently published from the Traumatic Coma Data Bank has shown that the proportion of hourly ICP recordings greater than 20 mm Hg is highly significant in predicting outcome.[31] The role of ICP monitoring in nontraumatic settings depends on the nature and severity of the disease process. Management of intracranial hypertension may be required in Reye's syndrome or other causes of hepatic failure, in large cerebral infarctions, in diffuse cerebritis, or after intracranial operations.

In general, most would monitor head-injured children with GCS ≤8 and CT evidence of brain abnormality or those with GCS ≤8 and normal CT who are in shock or exhibit decorticate or decerebrate motor posturing. Patients with higher GCS may be candidates if CT scans demonstrate significant mass lesions or if surgical or intensive respiratory treatment is required for associated injuries.

There is no uniform agreement about the critical level of ICP beyond which treatment is mandatory. In adults, ICPs above 20 mm Hg are usually treated. Saul and Ducker demonstrated benefits by treating ICP above 15 mm Hg when compared to a group of patients treated for ICP above 25 mm Hg.[32] In view of the 5 to 10 mm Hg normal ICP of infants or young children, the threshold for treatment is usually 15 mm Hg in children.

MANAGEMENT OF ELEVATED INTRACRANIAL PRESSURE

Whenever possible, the therapy of intracranial hypertension should be directed toward the underlying cause. The equation:

$$V_{CSF} + V_{BLOOD} + V_{BRAIN} + V_{OTHER} = V_{INTRACRANIAL\ SPACE}$$

provides a conceptual framework for examining the components of intracranial volume responsible for non–steady state situations and allows treatment to be directed in a focused manner.

V_{CSF}

When hydrocephalus causes intracranial hypertension and its etiology cannot be eradicated in some manner, temporary or permanent CSF diversion may be necessary. When obstruction of the CSF pathways by a tumor or other mass causes the hydrocephalus, it is usually possible, and indeed preferable, to treat the obstruction in an effort to open the CSF pathways.

If CSF diversion is required, options exist which permit either temporary external drainage (ventriculostomy), temporary internal drainage (ventriculosubgaleal shunt), or permanent internal drainage (VPS or third ventriculostomy). Advantages and disadvantages of external ventriculostomy as a method of monitoring ICP have been mentioned earlier in the chapter. Its value as a method for measuring and controlling ICP in the preoperative or immediate postoperative period is well known and is especially helpful when deciding whether a permanent shunt will be necessary. In these situations a rational method for managing and interpreting CSF drainage should be clear in the surgeon's mind and should be communicated plainly to all involved in the patient's care. One approach includes CSF drainage against minimal resistance early on with eventual elevation of the drip chamber to a level commensurate with physiologic ICP. Pressure is monitored continuously, and CSF is allowed to escape when threshold ICP levels are exceeded. Maintenance of normal ICP and minimal volumes of CSF drainage usually indicate that a permanent shunt will not be needed. The entire process just described can normally be accomplished within 48 to 72 hours.

Ventriculosubgaleal shunt (VSGS) provides a closed, temporary method for continuous CSF diversion. It involves placement of a ventricular catheter attached to a reservoir (with or without a valve mechanism) with a short side arm opening into a subgaleal space, which is dissected at the time of surgery. We have used this mainly in premature infants following IVH, but it could be performed in other situations as well. VSGS provides continuous ventricular decompression for several weeks to months without the need for percutaneous aspirations of the reservoir.

Permanent internal CSF diversion by VPS carries a full array of indications, technical considerations, and risks which are addressed elsewhere in this volume. Third ventriculostomy using both stereotactic and endoscopic techniques has been repopularized recently.[33, 34] This technique offers an alternative in certain situations without the potential risks inherent in standard ventriculoperitoneal shunting.

When mechanical methods of CSF diversion are not possible or desirable, adjunctive therapy using medications such as acetazolamide, furosemide, and corticosteroids can transiently decrease CSF production. Acetazolamide, which inhibits carbonic anhydrase–mediated CSF production is used most frequently. Reductions of CSF production by 16 to 66 per cent have been achieved in up to one half of the infants treated with acetazolamide for posthemorrhagic hydrocephalus.[35] Synergy has been reported when acetazolamide is combined with furosemide.[36] Acetazolamide also has a cerebral vasodilator effect, which may transiently worsen intracranial hypertension, and so its use is contraindicated in patients with closed head injury.[37]

V_{BLOOD}

The second component of volume is blood contained within the cerebral vasculature. While most of the cerebral blood volume resides within the pial vessels and veins, the precapillary arterioles control cerebral blood flow. The parameters that reflect the status of the cerebral vasculature are summarized in Table 22–1. Relationships among the various factors are complex and vary depending on the timing of measurements, degree of injury, presence or absence of hypoxia or ischemia, systemic blood pressure, ICP, cerebral metabolic rate, and arterial blood gases.

Extremes of CBF, both low and high, have been seen in patients with poor outcome after head injury.[38–41] Bouma et al. showed that measurements of CBF performed within 6 hours of severe head trauma (GCS ≤ 8) are reduced (22.5 ± 5.2 cc/100gm/min) and correlate well with Glasgow motor score and eventual outcome.[42] These findings are more common in patients with bilateral diffuse injuries than in patients with mass lesions, who tend to have higher global CBF in the hemisphere of the mass lesion. Between 45 and 65 per cent of head injury victims, probably more so in children, will exhibit hyperemia in the 12 to 24 hours after injury.[43–47] The increase in CBF is presumably accompanied by increased CBV, which can cause intracranial hypertension. Increased CBF and CBV are seen in the acute encephalopathy of Reye's syndrome as well. CBF tends to normalize by 36 to 48 hours after injury, that is, it increases in patients with initially low values and decreases in those with initial or subsequent hyperemia.[38, 40, 45, 48]

The association between CBF, Cerebral Metabolic Rate of O_2 ($CMRO_2$), Arteriovenous Oxygen Difference ($AVDO_2$) and what is observed clinically (ICP, GCS, and outcome) is more easily documented by multivariate analysis than it is explained in terms of physiologic cause and effect. With increases in ICP, $AVDO_2$ usually increases due to reductions in VO_2 caused by greater extraction of oxygen as blood flow is reduced. CBV increases with vasodilatation in response to lowered CPP, pressure autoregulation, or a rise in $PaCO_2$. Hyperventilation decreases total intracranial blood volume as vasoconstriction squeezes blood from the pial circulation to the veins and sinuses. Reductions of $CMRO_2$

TABLE 22–1. NEUROPHYSIOLOGY CONCEPTS

TERM	DEFINITION	NORMAL AND ABNORMAL VALUES	VARIABLES AFFECTING VALUES
Cerebral metabolic rate of O_2 ($CMRO_2$)	Measurement of brain metabolism ($CMRO_2 = CBF \times AVDO_2$)	Normal: 3.0–3.5 ml/100 gm/min Value <1.4 ml/100 gm/min in patient with coma usually incompatible with regaining consciousness	CBF $AVDO_2$

Cerebral perfusion pressure (CPP)	Pressure which circulates blood through the brain: ($CPP = MAP - ICP$)	Adults:
		  Normal ≈ 80 mm Hg
		  Acceptable ≥50 mm Hg
		Children (Normals):
		  Infants ≈ 70–73 mm Hg
		  Children ≈ 73–77 mm Hg
			MAP
			ICP
			Integrity of autoregulation

$PaCO_2$ responsivity	Vasodilatation/vasoconstriction occurring with changes in $PaCO_2$	Normal: 35–40 mm Hg	Max vasodilatation seen at ≈ 60 mm Hg $PaCO_2$ Max vasoconstriction seen at ≈ 20 mm Hg $PaCO_2$
PaO_2	Measurement of partial pressure of O_2 in the blood	Normal: 95–100 mm Hg	Cerebral vasodilation occurs when PaO_2 <50 mm Hg
Cerebral blood flow (CBF)	Volume of blood circulating through a volume of brain in a given moment of time; usually expressed as cc/100 gm tissue/min	Normal ≈ 40 ml/100 gm/min (age <1 yr) ≈ 65–106 ml/100 gm/min (age 1–9 yr) ≈ 53 ml/100 gm/min (age >10 yr) Infarction threshold <18 ml/100 gm/min Reduced flow <32.9 ml/100 gm/min	Systemic blood pressure ICP and CPP Vascular resistance ABGs Metabolic demand of brain Viscosity $PaCO_2$ usually corrected to 34 torr
Cerebral blood-volume (CBV)	Volume of blood in intravascular compartment at a given time	Gray matter ≈ 5 ml/100 gm White matter ≈ 3.5 ml/100 gm	Vasodilation Venous return Vascular resistance ICP
Arteriovenous oxygen difference ($AVDO_2$)	Measures cerebral oxygen extraction from circulting blood by difference in O_2 content between arterial blood (AO_2) and venous blood (VO_2); expressed as vol %: ($AVDO_2 = [AO_2 - VO_2]$) Also expressed in relation to $CMRO_2$: ($AVDO_2 = CMRO_2/CBF$)	Normal: 5–7.5 vol % Relative ischemia >7.5 vol % Threshold for advent of ischemia: >9.0 vol % Relative hyperemia <5 vol %, i.e., blood flow available exceeds metabolic requirements	$CMRO_2$ CBF

are seen after trauma, but these reductions may not reflect the energy demands of the injured brain. Some have attributed these reductions to mitochondrial incapacities or enzymatic deficits, which render the neuron incapable of utilizing oxygen.[42, 49]

Applications of this information as well as replication have been hampered by methodology of CBF measurements. Global CBF obtained by the Kety-Schmidt method includes the white matter, but regional CBF determined by the [133]Xenon inhalation ignores the contribution of the white matter.[11] Focal areas of ischemia can be missed if surrounded by zones of relatively high flow.[50] Although stable Xenon/CT technique can determine CBF of individual lobes, basal ganglia, and brainstem, flows in these areas often differ by 25 per cent or more from global averages. Diminished CBF of the brainstem does not always correlate with clinical estimates of brainstem function.[51]

Although some success has been reported with drug therapy for CBV,[52, 53] clinical treatment can be best accomplished by hyperventilation and elevation of the head. Hyperventilation (HV) causes constriction of pial vessels with intact CO_2 responsivity. CO_2 responsivity can be preserved despite loss of pressure autoregulation. The alkalosis induced by HV can buffer the intracellular and CSF lactic acidosis often found after severe head injury.[54] This potential advantage may only last about 24 hours and can be offset by extreme HV, which can cause vasoconstriction sufficient to produce cerebral ischemia.[55, 56] Attempts to improve and prolong the buffering effect of HV have led to the use of tromethamine (THAM), a systemic and intracellular alkanizing agent that crosses the blood-brain barrier and raises cellular pH to a level where aerobic metabolism can continue. In a randomized, prospective trial, Muizelaar showed that HV to a $PaCO_2$ of 25 ± 2 in patients with Glasgow motor scale of 4 or 5 resulted in Glasgow Outcome Scores significantly worse than in controls or in patients treated with THAM.[57]

Some have advanced the concept of "inverse steal" to call attention to the risk of HV-induced ischemia. In patients with intact or supersensitive CO_2 responsivity, hypocapnia can lead to shunting of blood from high-resistance, maximally constricted vessels to low-resistance, dilated vessels which lack CO_2 responsivity.[58] When possible, these investigators recommend that $AVDO_2$ and CBF be monitored along with ICP, and that HV be performed cautiously in patients with evidence of cerebral ischemia.[59]

Since CBF monitoring is not available in many clinical settings, less stringent criteria for use of HV must be used. Bruce described effective control of ICP in children using HV to lower $PaCO_2$ below the 20 mm Hg threshold believed to represent the limit of responsiveness in adults.[12] Although he recommended monitoring of $AVDO_2$ when lowering $PaCO_2$ below 20 mm Hg, he doubted that cerebral ischemia would be produced by HV because metabolites accumulate as CBF decreases, producing local vasodilatation. Metabolic studies by MacMillan and Seisjo demonstrated that energy poten-tial did not change until CO_2 was decreased below 10 mm Hg.[60]

While laboratory studies suggest otherwise, most clinical observations indicate that sustained reductions of ICP can be maintained for several days by using HV. When HV is discontinued, it should be tapered over 24 to 48 hours. Abrupt discontinuation can cause vasodilatation as extracellular pH falls, resulting in ICP elevations.[61, 62]

Elevation of the head to 30 degrees decreases ICP by encouraging venous return. This degree of elevation does not alter cerebral perfusion pressure.[63] Transmission of elevated intrathoracic pressure to the intracranial veins can be avoided by using sedation and limiting the inspiratory phase of the respirator.[64] Positive end-expiratory pressure (PEEP) could theoretically raise central venous and intracranial venous pressures, but this does not seem to be the case in clinical practice.[65] The reduced pulmonary compliance that necessitates PEEP in the first place probably dampens retrograde transmission of pressure.[66]

Although the inexperienced might attempt to decrease CBV by reducing systemic blood pressure, lowering CPP results in arteriolar vasodilatation and subsequently increases both CBV and ICP. This effect is seen in systemic hypotension, in which CBF is reduced, but CBV and ICP are increased because of vasodilatation related to hypercapnea, anoxia, or acidosis.

V$_{BRAIN}$

The third component is the volume occupied by brain tissue (V_{BRAIN}). Increases in V_{BRAIN} occur most frequently as a result of cerebral edema, which is a nonspecific reaction to a variety of processes. Cerebral edema is defined as an increase in water content of the brain and can be broadly categorized as vasogenic or cytotoxic.[67] Vasogenic refers to leakage of protein-rich fluid across the capillary membrane into the extracellular space of the white matter. Vasogenic edema can produce local or generalized mass effects, which result in increased ICP. Cytotoxic edema is caused by expansion of the intracellular fluid compartment due to cellular toxins or injury. This occurs preferentially in astrocytes of the gray matter. Cytotoxic edema also contributes to injury by impairing cellular pump mechanisms.

Conceptually, treatment of increased ICP due to brain edema is directed toward removing the cause of edema, controlling its propagation, and enhancing its clearance. Further efforts to decrease the formation of vasogenic edema include prevention of cerebrovascular hypertension, preservation of an adequate CPP, and appropriate choice of fluid resuscitation.

Control of systemic and cerebrovascular hypertension is especially important when intracranial hypertension exists or when cerebral autoregulation is impaired. The choice of antihypertensive drugs in patients with increased ICP is important. Hirose et al. and others have shown that nifedipine, chlorpromazine, and reserpine all decreased mean arterial pressure (MAP) and increased ICP, thereby reducing CPP.[68-70] These findings were more pronounced when ICP exceeded 40 mm Hg. Thiopental decreased MAP and ICP leaving CPP unchanged but caused respiratory depression, necessitating intubation and mechanical ventilation. In a laboratory study using inflated balloons to produce intracranial hypertension, sodium nitroprusside, nitroglycerine, and trimetaphan were used to reduce MAP by 20 per cent. All three drugs reduced regional CBF and CO_2 responsivity, leading the authors to recommend caution in their use for blood pressure control in patients with increased ICP. Propranolol has been shown to be superior to hydralazine for control of hypertension in head-injured patients because propranolol decreases both cardiac demands and serum levels of epinephrine and norepinephrine.[71] Clonidine has also been reported to decrease plasma catecholamines.[72]

The choice of intravenous fluids for resuscitation is important because 10 to 15 per cent of head-injured patients are hypotensive due to associated injuries. Aggressive correction of shock improves survival and clinical outcome. Isotonic fluids—e.g., D5 1/2 NS, NS, and lactated Ringer's—are all acceptable, but hypotonic solutions, such as D5W, which lower serum osmolality as they are metabolized, will increase cerebral edema. Controversy exists as to whether colloids (mw>8000) are more beneficial than crystalloids for fluid resuscitation. Some authors have found no difference,[73] whereas Tranmer showed a definite advantage using the colloid hetastarch.[74] In a laboratory model of vasogenic edema, treatment with colloid for 2 hours after injury produced no change of ICP, whereas normal saline and D5W infusions led to elevations of ICP of 91 per cent and 141 per cent, respectively.

In the case of cytotoxic injury, efforts to decrease formation of edema center around correction of the etiology of disordered cell function. With toxins this would involve treatment directed toward the causative agent. When anoxia or ischemia exist, reversal of causative factors may bring improvement if the duration of anoxia and ischemia has not been prolonged.

The second goal in treating cerebral edema is to improve neuronal/axonal function. Although a variety of agents have been tried to improve neuronal-axonal function,[75-83] steroids and barbiturates are most generally employed for treating both vasogenic and cytotoxic forms of edema. Steroids are of unquestionable value in the treatment of patients with brain tumors, but no definite benefits have been shown when they are used in patients with head injury.[84-89] Corticosteroids have been shown to inhibit membrane lipid hydrolysis and decrease free radical–induced lipid peroxidation, the principal molecular basis for post-traumatic neuronal degeneration.[90-93] The ability to inhibit lipid peroxidation can be quantitated as the lipid antioxidant capacity. Among commonly used corticosteroids, methylprednisolone has the highest lipid antioxidant capacity whereas prednisolone is efficacious in vitro but only half as potent. Even in high doses, hydrocortisone has no antioxidant activity; dexamethasone is slightly less effective than methylprednisolone or prednisolone.[94] Interestingly, excessive doses may possibly be deleterious and exacerbate lipid peroxidation.[94] Under investigation are newer configurations of steroids, Lazeroids, of which U-74006F (tirilazad mesylate) is an example.[95-98] These are potent antioxidants without associated glucocorticoid effects. The inhibition of membrane lipid hydrolysis by steroid reduces formation of vasoactive substances called eicosanoids, e.g., prostaglandin F_{2a} and thromboxane A_2. Cerebral production of thromboxane A_2 was shown to be increased by the combination of shock and intracranial hypertension in one laboratory study.[99]

Dexamethasone (0.4 to 1 mg/kg/day in divided doses) is especially effective in patients with tumors. In larger children, the usual adult dosage of 4 mg every 6 hours can be used. Use of steroids in subarachnoid hemorrhage has no proven benefit, but angiographically demonstrable vasospasm can be decreased by their use.[100] In cases of cerebral ischemia, steroids worsen outcome either by means of a direct glucocorticoid toxicity or as a consequence of elevated serum glucose levels, which exacerbate ischemic lactic acidosis.[101, 102]

Barbiturates are the second group of agents used to improve neuronal/axonal function in the presence of edema. Their benefit appears to accrue from reducing ICP (improving CPP), reducing cerebral blood flow (lowering end-capillary pressure and limiting edema formation), and decreasing $CMRO_2$ (permitting tolerance of a degree of ischemia/anoxia not otherwise acceptable on the cellular level). Cerebral vasoconstriction probably plays a role in barbiturate effect, but whether this results from reduction in $CMRO_2$ or is a direct vascular effect is unknown. Barbiturates seem to have maximum effect in situations in which CBF is greater than metabolism (hyperemia).[12] Additionally, Messeter et al. have shown that preservation of cerebral CO_2 responsivity can predict the response of ICP to iatrogenic barbiturate coma.[103] When CO_2 responsivity was normal, barbiturates reduced CBF and normalized ICP in 75 per cent of patients. When this response was reduced or absent, CBF was unchanged or increased, and ICP was reduced in only 20 per cent. Pentobarbital has proved more effective at controlling ICP than phenobarbital or thiopental sodium.

First used to control ICP in 1937, barbiturates are effective in reducing ICP but do not improve outcome in many studies.[12, 104, 105] Even prophylactic use of barbiturates has not improved outcome or led to easier control of ICP.[106] Considering the risks of high-dose barbiturates, their application is most appropriate for patients in whom conventional measures to control ICP have failed. Usually a bolus of pentobarbital (5 to 10 mg/kg) is administered over 30 minutes followed by a continuous hourly maintenance infusion of 1 to 5 mg/kg to achieve a serum concentration of 3.5 to 4.5 mg/100 ml[107] or burst suppression monitored by bedside EEG monitoring.

Barbiturate coma should only be used in an intensive care setting where ongoing monitoring of MAP, ICP, cardiac index (3.5 to 5 liters/min/m²), oxygen delivery/consumption (delivery: 500 to 600 ml O_2/min/m²; consumption normally ≈25 per cent), pulmonary capillary wedge pressure (lowest necessary to maintain cardiac index), and drug levels is available. Despite maintenance of normal blood volume and cardiac output, hypotension occurs in 50 per cent of cases and is probably due to decreased peripheral vascular resistance. Volume expansion in addition to dopamine or levarterenol may be necessary to restore systemic blood pressure. Other potential complications related to high-dose barbiturates include hyponatremia, pneumonia, and cardiac depression, which often responds to dobutamine.

Finally, V_{BRAIN} can be reduced by increasing the clearance of edema. Both osmotic and loop diuretics are widely used and can treat both vasogenic and cytotoxic edema.

Osmotic agents increase serum osmolarity and create an osmotic gradient between the serum and brain. This effect draws free water from the brain into the intravascular compartment along the osmotic gradient. The drugs used most commonly for increasing intravascular osmolarity are mannitol, urea, and glycerol. Mannitol (20 per cent solution) is usually the agent of choice. It has been shown that water is removed from normal brain rather than edematous brain, since the barrier is intact in all but the area of edema formation.[108–110] Osmotic agents also reduce blood viscosity, resulting in vasoconstriction and lowering of ICP.[111] However, osmotic agents transiently increase CBF independent of their effect on ICP, and so their use in the presence of hyperemia and increased CBV may be contraindicated. Since some head injured children exhibit hyperemia, lack of responsiveness to mannitol may prompt use of barbiturates earlier in the treatment of severe intracranial hypertension.

The dose of mannitol is .25 to 1 gm/kg, and this can be given as a repeated bolus or, in smaller doses, as a continuous infusion. Complications with osmotic therapy are dehydration, electrolyte imbalance, and, with extreme hyperosmolarity, renal failure. Fluid replacement is aimed at preserving isovolemia while increasing serum osmolality. Osmolarity should not exceed 320 mOsm/kg because the renal tubule can be injured as osmolarity exceeds this level. Maintenance of high serum mannitol levels can lead to penetration of mannitol into injured brain,[112] reversing the blood-brain osmotic gradient and causing rebound intracranial hypertension.

Mannitol is used more commonly than urea (30 per cent solution) and glycerol (10 per cent solution) because plasma and brain concentrations tend to equilibrate more rapidly with urea and glycerol than with mannitol. Glycerol can also cause hemolysis and renal failure when administered parenterally.[113] Because glycerol is metabolized, sustained hyperosmolarity is less than with mannitol. In one study comparing mannitol and glycerol, glycerol was less effective in reducing ICP, but there was no rebound of ICP as seen with the mannitol group.[114] Also, MAP was more stable with glycerol and increases in CBF were more gradual. An-

other study compared doses and infusion rates of mannitol and glycerol.[115] Slower infusion rates of equal doses produced more sustained reductions of ICP for both drugs. Rebound phenomena were seen in 12 per cent of the mannitol group and 34 per cent of the glycerol patients, but the authors believed that this reflected their method of infusion.[115]

Loop diuretics such as furosemide and ethacrynic acid can be used in conjunction with mannitol to control ICP associated with edema.[116, 117] Furosemide works synergistically with mannitol to remove free water and is most appropriate in patients with fluid overload. The addition of furosemide increases the likelihood of dehydration and loss of potassium.[37] Although furosemide decreases CSF production, this effect probably does not contribute greatly to lowering ICP in the acute setting.

V_{OTHER}

The most effective treatment of ICP consists of removing volumes not normally found within the intracranial compartment; these include tumors, abscesses, and hematomas. When a definable, abnormal mass is responsible for intracranial hypertension, the mass should be removed. The modalities discussed above should be considered adjunctive and supportive therapy in these settings.

In addition to intracranial masses, it is useful to consider conditions in which the skull limits the expansion of the brain. In a few settings, cranial expansion has reduced intracranial hypertension in children. Examples would include multisutural craniosynostosis, slit ventricle syndrome, and even large depressed skull fractures (Fig. 22–7). This concept has been extended to some acute settings of severe refractory ICP elevations. While limited usefulness of decompressive craniectomy can be found in a decreased incidence of transtenorial herniation, formation of edema is enhanced, residual brain injury is severe, and, at least in Reye's syndrome, reductions in ICP are rarely significant.[12] Clearly this procedure has an extremely limited role.

PRACTICAL ISSUES

In many clinical settings, the conceptual approach to the treatment of intracranial hypertension outlined above cannot be followed for a variety of reasons. First, the decision to monitor the ICP of a child initiates a cascade of events which blurs the distinctions made above. The initiation of ICP monitoring and treatment of intracranial hypertension are begun simultaneously. Except in unusual settings, it is impossible to obtain a consistent and reliable tracing of the child's ICP without intubation and pharmacologic paralysis of the child. These maneuvers, along with elevation of the head, will effectively control ICP in many children. Moderate hyperventilation using volume respirators and lowering the $PaCO_2$ to 25 to 28 torr can be added as needed.

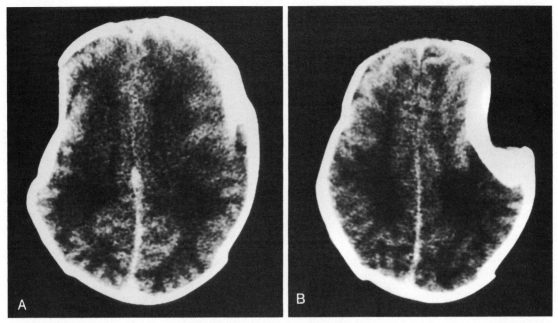

FIGURE 22–7. *A* and *B,* CT scan showing bilateral depressed skull fractures due to use of forceps during vaginal delivery.

If these initial measures are not adequate, treatment advances in a stepwise fashion. If a ventricular catheter has been inserted to monitor ICP, CSF can be removed to lower pressure. The ventricles of head-injured children are usually small, so that only 1 to 2 ml of CSF can be withdrawn at a time. However, removing even this small volume will often lower the ICP markedly because of the steep pressure–volume curve found in these children. If this maneuver has to be repeated frequently to control ICP, the next step should be directed toward reducing the bulk of the brain by removing extracellular fluid using osmotic diuretics. Serum osmolarity should be measured frequently, especially when mannitol is given more often than every 6 to 8 hours. In the majority of children, intracranial hypertension will be successfully managed by the steps outlined above. However, 10 to 15 per cent of children will require additional treatment, and therapy should be advanced to barbiturates. Once stability of ICP has been maintained for 24 to 48 hours, therapies are withdrawn starting with the last added.

REFERENCES

1. Welch K: The intracranial pressure in infants. J Neurosurg 52:693, 1980.
2. Munro D: Cerebrospinal fluid pressure in the newborn. JAMA 90:1688, 1928.
3. Salmon JH, Hajjar W, Bada HS: The fontogram: A noninvasive intracranial pressure monitor. Pediatrics 60:721, 1977.
4. Johnston I: Reduced CSF absorption syndrome. Lancet ii:418, 1973.
5. Cushing H: Studies in Intracranial Physiology and Surgery. London, Oxford University Press, 1926, pp 19–23.
6. Kellie G: An account of the appearances observed in the dissection . . . with some reflections on the pathology of the brain. Trans Med Chir Sci Edinb 1:84, 1824.
7. Monro A: Observations on the Structure and Function of the Nervous System. Edinburgh, Creech and Johnston, 1783, pp 5–6.
8. Pollock LJ, Boshes B: Cerebrospinal fluid pressure. Arch Neurol Psychiatry 36:931, 1936.
9. Kennedy C, Sokoloff L: An adaptation of the nitrous oxide method to the study of the cerebral circulation in children: Normal values for cerebral blood flow and cerebral metabolic rate in childhood. J Clin Invest 36:1130, 1957.
10. Chiron C: Changes in regional cerebral blood flow during brain maturation in children and adolescents. J Nucl Med 33:696, 1992.
11. Kety SS, Schmidt CF: The nitrous oxide method for the quantitative determination of cerebral blood flow in man: Theory, procedures, and normal values. J Clin Invest 27:476, 1948.
12. Bruce DA: Treatment of intracranial hypertension. *In* McLaurin RL et al. (eds): Pediatric Neurosurgery, 2d ed. Philadelphia, WB Saunders, 1989, pp 245–254.
13. Marmarou A: A Theoretical and Experimental Evaluation of the Cerebrospinal Fluid System. PhD Thesis, Drexel University, 1973.
14. Marmarou A, Shulman K, Rosende R: A nonlinear analysis of the cerebrospinal fluid system and intracranial pressure dynamics. J Neurosurg 48:332, 1978.
15. Shapiro K, Shulman K: Facial nevi associated with anomalous venous return and hydrocephalus. J Neurosurg 45:20, 1976.
16. Ryder HW, Espey FF, Kimbell FD, et al.: The mechanism of the change in cerebrospinal fluid pressure following an induced change in the volume of the fluid space. J Lab Clin Med 41:428, 1953.
17. Marmarou A, Shulman K: Pressure-volume relationships—basic aspects. *In* McLaurin RL (ed): Head Injuries. New York, Grune and Stratton, 1976, pp 233–236.
18. Shapiro K, Marmarou A, Shulman K: Characterization of clinical CSF dynamics and neural axis compliance using the pressure-volume index. 1. The normal pressure-volume index. Ann Neurol 7:508, 1980.
19. Maset AL, Marmarou A, Work JD, et al.: Pressure-volume index in head injury. J Neurosurg 67:832, 1987.
20. Welch K, Friedman V: The cerebrospinal fluid values. Brain 83:454, 1961.
21. Shapiro K, Fried A, Takei F, et al.: Effect of the skull and dura on neural axis pressure-volume relationships and CSF hydrodynamics. J Neurosurg 63:76, 1985.

22. Weed LH: Some limitations on the Monro-Kellie hypothesis. Arch Surg 18:1049, 1929.

23. Shapiro K, Marmarou A: Clinical applications of the pressure-volume index in treatment of pediatric head injuries. J Neurosurg 56:819, 1982.

24. Guillaume J, Janny P: Manometric intracranienne continue interet de la methode et premeiers resultats. Rev Neurol (Paris) 84:131, 1951.

25. Lundberg N: Continuous recording and control of ventricular fluid pressure in neurosurgical practice. Acta Psychiatr Neurol Scand 36:1, 1960.

26. Mendelow DA, Rowan JO, Murray L, et al.: A clinical comparison of subdural screw pressure measurements with ventricular pressure. J Neurosurg 58:45, 1983.

27. Miller JD, Bobo H, Kapp JP: Inaccurate pressure readings for subarachnoid bolts. Neurosurgery 19:253, 1986.

28. North B, Reilly P: Comparison among three methods of intracranial pressure recording. Neurosurgery 18:730, 1986.

29. Crutchfield JS, Narayan RK, Robertson CS, et al.: Evaluation of a fiberoptic intracranial pressure monitor. J Neurosurg 72:482, 1990.

30. Narayan RK, Kishore PRS, Becker DP, et al.: Intracranial pressure: To monitor or not to monitor? A review of our experience with severe head injury. J Neurosurg 56:650, 1982.

31. Marmarou A, Anderson RL, Ward JD, et al.: Impact of ICP instability and hypotension on outcome in patients with severe head trauma. J Neurosurg 75:559, 1991.

32. Saul TG, Ducker TB: Effect of intracranial pressure monitoring and aggressive treatment on mortality in severe head injury. J Neurosurg 56:498, 1982.

33. Kelly P, Goerss S, Kall B, et al.: Computed tomography based stereotactic third ventriculostomy: Technical note. Neurosurgery 18:791, 1986.

34. Teo C, Jones R, Stening W, et al.: Neuroendoscopic third ventriculostomy. Proceedings of the International Symposium on Hydrocephalus, July 1990.

35. Rubin RC, Henderson ES, Ommaya AK, et al.: The production of cerebrospinal fluid in man and its modification by acetozolamide. J Neurosurg 25:430, 1966.

36. Shinner S, Gammon K, Bergman EW, et al.: Management of head injury in infancy: Use of acetazolamide and furosemide to avoid cerebrospinal fluid shunts. J Pediatrics 107:31, 1985.

37. Chestnut RM, Marshall LF: Treatment of abnormal intracranial pressure. Neurosurg Clin North Am 2:267, 1991.

38. Fieschi C, Battistini N, Beduschi A, et al.: Regional cerebral blood flow and intraventricular pressure in acute head injuries. J Neurol Neurosurg Psychiatry 37:1378, 1974.

39. Jaggi JL, Obrist WD, Gennarelli TA, et al.: Relationship of early cerebral blood flow and metabolism to outcome in acute head injury. J Neurosurg 72:176, 1990.

40. Overgaard J, Tweed WA: Cerebral circulation after head injury. Part 1: Cerebral blood flow and its regulation after closed head injury with emphasis on clinical correlation. J Neurosurg 41:531, 1974.

41. Uzell BP, Obrist WD, Dolinskas CA, et al.: Relationship of acute CBF and ICP findings to neuropsychological outcome in severe head injury. J Neurosurg 65:630, 1986.

42. Bouma GJ, Muizelaar P, Choi SC, et al.: Cerebral circulation and metabolism after severe traumatic brain injury: The elusive role of ischemia. J Neurosurg 75:685, 1991.

43. Bruce DA, Alavi A, Bilaniuk L, et al.: Diffuse cerebral swelling following head injuries in children: The syndrome of "malignant brain edema." J Neurosurg 54:170, 1981.

44. Bruce DA, Raphaely RC, Goldberg AI, et al.: Pathophysiology, treatment and outcome following severe head injury in children. Childs Brain 5:174, 1979.

45. Langfitt TW, Obrist WD, Gennarelli TA, et al.: Correlation of cerebral blood flow with outcome in head-injured patients. Ann Surg 186:411, 1977.

46. Muizelaar JP, Marmarou A, DeSalles AAF, et al.: Cerebral blood flow and metabolism in severely head-injured children. Part 1: Relationship with GCS score, outcome, ICP and PVI. J Neurosurg 71:632, 1989.

47. Obrist WD, Langfitt TW, Jaggi JL, et al.: Cerebral blood flow and metabolism in comatose patients with acute head injury: Relationship to intracranial hypertension. J Neurosurg 61:241, 1984.

48. Gobiet G, Grote W, Bock WJ: The relationship between intracranial pressure and cerebral blood flow in patients with severe head injury. Acta Neurochir (Wein) 32:13, 1975.

49. Sutton LN, McLaughlin AL, Dante S, et al.: Cerebral venous oxygen content as a measure of brain energy metabolism with increased intracranial pressure and hyperventilation. J Neurosurg 73:927, 1990.

50. Hanson EJ Jr., Anderson RE, Sundt TMJ: Comparison of ^{85}krypton and ^{133}xenon cerebral blood flow measurements before, during, and following focal, incomplete ischemia in the squirrel monkey. Circ Res 36:18, 1974.

51. Marion DW, Darby J, Yonas H: Acute regional cerebral blood flow changes caused by severe head injuries. J Neurosurg 74:407, 1991.

52. Grande PO: The effects of dihydroergotamine in patients with head injury and raised intracranial pressure. Intensive Care Medicine 15 (8):523, 1989.

53. Jennett B: Epilepsy After Nonmissile Injuries, 2d ed. Chicago, Year Book Medical Publishers Inc., 1975.

54. Becker DP: Brain acidosis in head injury: A clinical trial. In Becker DP, Povlishock JT (eds): Central Nervous System Trauma Status Report—1985. Richmond, Byrd Press, 1985, p 229.

55. Muizelaar JP, van der Poel HG, Li ZC, et al.: Pial arteriolar vessel diameter and CO_2 reactivity during prolonged hyperventilation in the rabbit. J Neurosurg 69:923, 1988.

56. van der Poel H: Cerebral vasoconstriction is not maintained with prolonged hyperventilation. In Hoff JT, Betz AL (eds): Intracranial Pressure VII. Berlin, Springer-Verlag, 1989.

57. Muizelaar JP, Marmarou A, Ward JD, et al.: Adverse effects of prolonged hyperventilation in patients with severe head injury: A randomized clinical trial. J Neurosurg 75:731, 1991.

58. Paulson OB: Regional cerebral blood flow in apoplexy due to occlusion of the middle cerebral artery. Neurology 20:63, 1970.

59. Sharples PM, Stuart AG: A practical method of serial bedside measurement of cerebral blood flow and metabolism during neurointensive care. Arch Dis Child 66:1326, 1991.

60. MacMillan V, Seisjö BK: The influence of hypocapnia upon intracellular pH and upon some carbohydrate substrates, amino acids, and organic phosphates in the brain. J Neurochem 21:1283, 1973.

61. Hayes GJ, Slocum HC: The achievement of optimal brain relaxation by hyperventilation technics of anesthesia. J Neurosurg 10:65, 1961.

62. James HE, Langfitt TW, Kumar VS: Analysis of the response to therapeutic measures to reduce intracranial pressure in head injured patients. J Trauma 16:437, 1976.

63. Rosner MJ, Coley IB: Cerebral perfusion pressure, intracranial pressure, and head elevation. J Neurosurg 60:636, 1986.

64. Ersson U, Carlson H, Mellstrom A, et al.: Observations on intracranial dynamics during respiratory physiotherapy in unconscious neurosurgical patients. Acta Anaesthesiol Scand 34 (2):99, 1990.

65. Frost EAM: Effects of positive end-expiratory pressure on intracranial pressure and compliance in brain-injured patients. J Neurosurg 47:195, 1977.

66. Shapiro HM, Marshall LF: Intracranial pressure responses to PEEP in head-injured patients. J Trauma 18:254, 1978.

67. Klatzo I: Neuropathological aspects of brain edema. J Neuropathol Exp Neurol 26:1, 1967.

68. Hayashi M, Kobayashi H, Kawano H: Treatment of systemic hypertension in cases of brain hemorrhage. Stroke 19:314, 1988.

69. Hirose S, Handa Y, Kobayashi H: Effects of antihypertensive drugs on intracranial hypertension. Zentralbl Neurochir 52 (2) 69, 1991.

70. Tateishi A, Sano T, Takeshita H: Effects of nifedipine on intracranial pressure in neurosurgical patients with arterial hypertension. J Neurosurg 69:213, 1988.

71. Robertson CS, Clifton GL, Taylor AA, et al.: Treatment of hypertension associated with head injury. J Neurosurg 59:455, 1983.

72. Payen D, Quintin L, Plaisance P, et al.: Head injury: Clonidine decreases plasma catecholamines. Crit Care Med 18:392, 1990.

73. Lowe RJ, Moss GS, Jilek J, et al: Crystalloid versus colloid in the etiology of pulmonary failure after trauma—a randomized trial in man. Crit Care Med 7:107, 1979.

74. Tranmer BI, Iacobacci RI, Kindt GW: Effects of crystalloid and colloid infusions on intracranial pressure and computerized electroencephalographic data in dogs with vasogenic brain edema. Neurosurgery 25:173, 1989.

75. Albers GW, Goldberg MP, Choi DW: N-methyl-D-aspartate antagonists: Ready for clinical trial in brain ischemia?. Ann Neurol 25:398, 1989.

76. Astrup J, Sørensen PM, Sørensen HR: Inhibition of cerebral oxygen and glucose consumption in the dog by hypothermia, pentobarbital, and lidocaine. Anesthesiology 55:263, 1981.

77. Bedford RF, Persing JA, Pobereskin L, et al.: Lidocaine or thiopental for rapid control of intracranial hypertension. Anesthesiology 59:435, 1980.

78. Benveniste H, Drejer J, Schousboe A, et al.: Elevation of the extracellular concentrations of glutamate and aspartate in rat hippocampus during transient cerebral ischemia monitored by intracerebral microdialysis. J Neurochem 43:1369, 1984.

79. Choi DW: Calcium-mediated neurotoxicity: Relationship to specific channel types and role in ischemic damage. Trends Neurosci 11:465, 1988.

80. Choi DW: Cerebral hypoxia: Some new approaches and unanswered questions. J Neurosci 10:2493, 1990.

81. Donegan MF, Bedford RF: Intravenously administered lidocaine prevents intracranial hypertension during endotracheal suctioning. Anesthesiology 52:516, 1980.

82. Plangger CA: Effect of gammahydroxybutyrate on intracranial pressure in systemic arterial pressure and cerebral perfusion pressure in experimentally induced brain edema of the rat. Acta Neurochir 51 (Suppl):404, 1990.

83. Rasool N, Faroqui M, Rubinstein EH: Lidocaine accelerates neuroelectrical recovery after incomplete global ischemia in rabbits. Stroke 21:929, 1990.

84. Braakman R, Schouten HJA, Blaauw-van Dishoeck M, et al.: Megadose steroids in severe head injury. Results of a prospective double-blind clinical trial. J Neurosurg 58:326, 1983.

85. Cooper P, Moody S, Clark W, et al.: Dexamethasone and severe head injury. A prospective double blind study. J Neurosurg 51:307, 1979.

86. Deardon NM, Gibson JS, McDowal DG, et al.: Effect of high-dose dexamethasone on outcome from severe head injury. J Neurosurg 64:81, 1986.

87. Giannotta SL, Weiss MH, Apuzzo MJ, et al.: High dose glucocorticoids in the management of severe head injury. Neurosurgery 15:497, 1984.

88. Gudeman S, Miller J, Becker DP: Failure of high-dose steroid therapy to influence intracranial pressure in patients with severe head injury. J Neurosurg 51:301, 1979.

89. Saul TG, Ducker TB, Salcman M, et al.: Steroids in severe head injury. A prospective, randomized clinical trial. J Neurosurg 54:596, 1981.

90. Anderson DK, Saunders RD, Demediuk P, et al.: Lipid hydrolysis and peroxidation in injured spinal cord: Partial protection with methyl prednisolone or vitamin E and selenium. Cent Nerv Syst Trauma 2:257, 1985.

91. Braughler JM, Hall ED: Correlation of methylprednisolone levels in cat spinal cord with its effects on (Na+ + K+)-ATPase, lipid peroxidation and alpha motor neuron function. J Neurosurg 56:838, 1982.

92. Caron MJ, Hovda DA, Becker DP: Changes in the treatment of head injury. Neurosurg Clin North Am 2:483, 1991.

93. Hall ED, Braughler JM: Effects of intravenous methylprednisolone on spinal cord lipid peroxidation and (Na++K+)-ATPase activity. Dose response analysis during 1st hour after contusion injury in the cat. J Neurosurg 57:247, 1982.

94. Hall ED: The neuroprotective pharmacology of methylprednisolone. J Neurosurg 76:13, 1992.

95. Anderson DK, Braughler JM, Hall ED, et al.: Effects of treatment with U-74006F on neurologic outcome following experimental spinal cord injury. J Neurosurg 69:562, 1988.

96. Braughler JM, Chase RL, Neff GL, et al.: A new 21-aminosteroid antioxidant lacking glucocorticoid activity stimulates adrenocorticotropin secretion and blocks arachidonic acid release from mouse pituitary tumor (AtT-20) cells. J Pharmacol Exp Ther 244:423, 1988.

97. Hall ED, Pazara KE, Braughler JM: 21-Aminosteroid lipid peroxidation inhibitor U74006F protects against cerebral ischemia in gerbils. Stroke 19:997, 1988.

98. Zuccarello M, Marsch JT, Schmitt G, et al.: Effect of the 21 aminosteroid U-74006F on cerebral vasospasm following subarachnoid hemorrhage. J Neurosurg 71:98, 1989.

99. Kong DL, Prough DS, Whitley JM, et al.: Hemorrhage and intracranial hypertension in combination increase production of thromboxane A2. Crit Care Med 19:532, 1991.

100. Chyatte D, Fode NC, Nichols DA, et al.: Preliminary report: Effects of high dose methylprednisolone on delayed cerebral ischemia in patients at high risk for vasospasm after aneurysmal subarachnoid hemorrhage. Neurosurgery 21:157, 1987.

101. Koide T, Wieloch T, Seisjö BK: Chronic dexamethasone pretreatment aggravates ischemic brain damage by inducing hyperglycemia. J Cereb Blood Flow Metab 5 (Suppl 1):251, 1985.

102. Sapolsky RM, Pulsinelli WA: Glucocorticoids potentiate ischemic injury to neurons: Therapeutic implications. Science 229:1397, 1985.

103. Messeter K, Nordstrom CH, Sundbarg G, et al.: Cerebral hemodynamics in patients with acute severe head trauma. J Neurosurg 64:231, 1986.

104. Brain Resuscitation Clinical Trial Study Group: A randomized clinical trial of barbiturate loading in cardiac arrest survivors. In Wirth FP, Ratcheson RA (eds): Neurosurgical Critical Care. Baltimore, Williams & Wilkins, 1987, p. 204.

105. Horsley JG: Intracranial pressure during barbital narcosis. Lancet i:141, 1937.

106. Ward JD, Becker DP, Miller JD, et al.: Failure of prophylactic barbiturate coma in the treatment of severe head injury. J Neurosurg 62:383, 1985.

107. Eisenberg H, Frankowski R, Contant C, et al.: High-dose barbiturate control of elevated intracranial pressure in patients with severe head injury. J Neurosurg 69:15, 1988.

108. Bell BA, Smith MA, Kean CM, et al.: Brain water measured by magnetic reasonance imaging. Lancet i:66, 1987.

109. Millson C, James HE, Shapiro HM, et al.: Intracranial hypertension and brain edema in albino rabbits. Part II. Effects of acute therapy with diuretics. Acta Neurochir 56:167, 1981.

110. Nath F, Galbraith S: The effect of mannitol on cerebral white matter content. J Neurosurg 65:41, 1986.

111. Muizelaar JP, Wei EP, Kontos HA, et al.: Mannitol causes compensatory cerebral vasoconstriction and vasodilation in response to blood viscosity changes. J Neurosurg 59:822, 1983.

112. Wise B, Perkins R, Stevenson E, et al.: Penetration of ^{14}C-labelled mannitol from serum into cerebral spinal fluid and brain. Exp Neurol 10:264, 1964.

113. Feldman Z, Narayan RK, Robertson CS: Secondary insults associated with severe closed head injury. Contemp Neurosurg 14:1, 1992.

114. Garcia-Sola R, Pulido P, Capilla P: The immediate and long-term effects of mannitol and glycerol. A comparative experimental study. Acta Neurochir 109(3–4):114, 1991.

115. Node Y, Nakazawa S: Clinical study of mannitol and glycerol on raised intracranial pressure and on their rebound phenomenon. Adv Neurol 52:359, 1990.

116. Pollay M, Fullenwider C, Roberts PA, et al.: Effect of mannitol and furosemide on blood-brain osmotic gradient and intracranial pressure. J Neurosurg 59:945, 1983.

117. Wilkinson HA, Rosenfeld SR: Furosemide and mannitol in the treatment of acute experimental intracranial hypertension. Neurosurgery 12:405, 1983.

Chapter 23

SPINAL CORD INJURY

ARNOLD H. MENEZES, M.D., and RICHARD K. OSENBACH, M.D.

Spinal cord injury resulting in neurologic deficit is a devastating affliction. Fortunately, injury to the spinal column and spinal cord is relatively infrequent in the pediatric population. The unique biomechanical features of the pediatric spine make the injury patterns differ considerably from those in teenagers and adults. In addition, children have substantial growth potential, and hence the risk of post-traumatic spinal deformity is much greater than that in adults. The management of specific pediatric injuries differs from that in adults in both the surgical approach and the method of external immobilization.

INCIDENCE OF PEDIATRIC SPINAL INJURY

The incidence of hospitalization for acute spinal cord injury in the United States (1970–1977) for individuals 19 years of age or younger was 21.2 per million, whereas the highest incidence was in those 20 to 24 years of age, being 68.0 per million.[1–3] This does not take into account the large number of patients who die at the scene of the accident or prior to admission. Kewalramani and colleagues, in a population survey in northern California, reported 58 children younger than 15 years of age who suffered a spinal cord injury during a 1-year span. Twenty-eight of these died at the scene of the accident or prior to hospitalization. Autopsies revealed severe spinal cord injury in the majority and associated multisystem trauma. Most series reporting on pediatric spinal cord and spinal column injuries discuss only the incidence of hospitalization rather than the true incidence of injuries. Accurate estimates of the true incidence of pediatric spinal injury are thus difficult to determine. This is compounded by the variation in the ages included as "pediatric" cases. Birth injuries, as well as injuries occurring in children with congenital abnormalities of the vertebral column, have been excluded from some reports.[4, 5]

The anatomy and biomechanics of the spine change from birth through adolescence. This produces alterations in the bony and ligamentous relationships and leads to variations in the etiology and the pathophysiology of the injury.[6–12] When taken as a whole, motor vehicle accidents account for 45 per cent of pediatric spinal injuries; diving injuries, 23 per cent; falls, 12 per cent; gymnastics, 7 per cent; football and other sports, 5 per cent; and miscellaneous, 8 per cent.[13] Between 20 and 25 per cent suffer from multisystem injuries.[2, 4, 11, 14–20]

As with the adult population, a large portion of spinal fractures result in no neurologic deficits. Of 74 cervical spine fractures encountered in children under 18 years of age, only 27 were accompanied by a neurologic deficit.[13] In the study by Hadley et al., 48 per cent had no neurologic deficit.[4] Pedestrian injuries were ten times greater in children under 9 years of age than in teenagers.

Anderson and Schutt reviewed the Mayo Clinic experience with all children who were under 14 years of age when admitted with spinal column and spinal cord injuries.[14] There were 156 children treated between 1950 and 1978. Forty-four of these had a neurologic deficit. The neurologic deficit was complete in 16, and 11 of these died. None of the patients with complete injuries showed any recovery. Of the 28 patients with incomplete spinal cord injuries, two died. Within this series, lesions above the fourth cervical level occurred in 39 of 156 (25 per cent), and half of these had a neurologic deficit. Twenty-two children (14 per cent) had a lesion between the fourth and seventh cervical segments, and seven had neurologic dysfunction. Cervical injuries accounted for 39 per cent of patients in this series. In 15 children, the injury was between T1 and T5; in 42 children, it was between T6 and T12. Twenty-seven children had localization of their injury between L1 and L4, and in nine it was below this level. McPhee reported on 42 children under 15 years of age with fractures or dislocations of the spine admitted to the Royal Brisbane Hospital complex.[18] Males accounted for 68 per cent of patients with these injuries.

Half of the injuries occurred in the cervical spine, and injuries at more than one level occurred in 35 per cent of the patients. Spinal cord injuries occurred in 14 per cent of these patients. Lesoin and co-workers had a similar experience, with 50 per cent of injuries being in the cervical spine.[21]

Spinal cord injury without radiographic abnormality (SCIWORA) was identified in five of the 97 patients in the series by Kewalramani and Tori.[22] Osenbach and Menezes reported a 19 per cent incidence of SCIWORA.[23] Similarly, the incidence of SCIWORA in the series by Ruge was 21 per cent,[5] and Hadley et al.[4] reported a 16 per cent incidence of SCIWORA. Various authors have thus stressed the frequent occurrence of spinal cord injury without evidence of radiographic abnormality in the pediatric population.[2, 4, 5, 15, 17, 23–25] Burke reviewed the cases of 29 infants and children under 13 years of age who were admitted over an 18-year span with spinal cord injury.[16] Five were due to birth injuries (four were breech delivery), and in 16 no fracture was visualized. Melzak, in researching the Stoke-Mandivelle Hospital series of the National Spinal Injury Center in Buckinghamshire, found 29 patients who were admitted with spinal cord injuries and only 16 had fractures.[26] At the Hospital for Sick Children in Toronto, 95 children were admitted with spinal cord injuries over a 15-year period.[27] No radiographic evidence of injury was found in 39 patients, and eight of these 39 had traumatic infarction of the spinal cord.

Thus it is evident that certain areas of the pediatric spine and spinal cord are more susceptible than others to injury, and this varies with age. Injuries to the upper cervical spine and the cervicothoracic junction are common with trauma.[28–35] Subsequent to the neonatal period, 75 per cent of injuries sustained by children between infancy and 8 years of age occur in the cervical spine, with a predilection for the upper cervical spine.[8, 13, 14, 24, 36–42] Between the ages of 8 and 14 years, 60 per cent of injuries occur in the cervical spine, 20 per cent in the thoracic region, and the remainder in the thoracolumbar junction and the lumbar spine. In adolescents 14 to 16 years of age, the pattern of injuries parallels that of the adult population.

PECULIAR FEATURES OF THE PEDIATRIC SPINE

The normal cervical spine in children differs considerably from that in adults. By the age of 8 to 10 years, most spines have achieved an adult configuration. When injury occurs in childhood, fractures and dislocations of the upper cervical spine occur with relatively greater incidence than in other locations. The youngest patients with these lesions have been newborns, in whom autopsies have revealed atlanto-occipital and atlantoaxial dislocation, fracture of the odontoid, and transection of the spinal cord.[20, 28, 29, 35]

The newborn spine is elastic, and the supporting ligamentous structures allow longitudinal distraction up to two inches.[34] However, the spinal cord can stretch only a quarter of an inch. A longitudinal traction force caused by the difference between the inherent elasticity of the spinal column and the lessor elasticity of the dura and its contents may cause disruption over several cord segments. About 70 per cent of spinal injuries at birth occur with breech deliveries, and 30 per cent with cephalic presentations.[20, 31, 32, 35, 43–45] In breech delivery, traction force is applied to the torso while uterine contractions grip the after-coming head. This is worse in the extended position. The spinal cord is fixed by the lumbar and cervical roots, and the delicate thoracocervical junction or the upper cervical spinal cord bears the brunt of the traction injuries. Multisegment stretching can cause injury to the ligaments, producing prevertebral soft tissue injury and cord damage without fracture. This was seen in 12 autopsies reported by Aufdermaur.[29]

The unique structural characteristics of the infant vertebral column allow traction and elongation of the spinal column to occur.[34, 46–48] In a study on occipitoatlantal mobility in 17 newborn cadavers, hyperextension in ten allowed the posterior atlantal arch to invaginate into the foramen magnum, causing dorsal cervicomedullary compression.[49] In four of the 17 infants, a vertical translation of the odontoid occurred in hyperflexion with ventral compression on the lower medulla oblongata. Momentary distortion or compression of the spinal cord may occur with displacement of the vertebrae or stretching of the spinal column by cervical hyperflexion. This can also lead to selective compromise of the segmental cord blood supply. Cadaveric studies have shown that forceful traction applied to the infant tends to produce injuries at the brainstem, with the medulla oblongata being drawn into the foramen magnum.[35, 50, 51] The cerebellum and the medulla oblongata are both at risk to be impaled by bony structures, as previously described, as well as subject to pressure and laceration by the edges of the foramen magnum. The findings of Yates[52] that distortional trauma to the cervical spine can occur at birth and can result in damage to the cervical portions of the vertebral arteries was further investigated by Jones.[32] Of 320 necropsies performed at the Birmingham Children's Hospital during 1967, 78 were stillbirths and 114 neonatal deaths. A random selection of 30 fetuses was made, and the spinal cord and vertebral arteries were carefully examined. In 19 patients there was evidence of hemorrhage around one or both vertebral arteries or crescentic adventitial hematoma.[32] These stretch injuries affect the dura and the spinal cord, as well as the vertebral arteries, and may account for the perinatal mortality and morbidity rates reported.

There is a preponderance of atlas and axis injuries in infants and young children that is related to the developmental anatomy of the high cervical region.[4, 5, 20, 53–56] A large infantile head on a small body results in high torque being applied to the neck with acceleration and deceleration stresses.[57] The cervical musculature only becomes supportive at puberty. The ligaments and joint capsules are lax in small children, allowing for mobility at the cost of stability.[9, 20, 56, 58] The facets in the upper three cervical vertebrae have a horizontal orientation to the articular surfaces, and this permits increased translation motion.[53, 56, 59] These facets never become as oblique as in the lower cervical spine. There is an incomplete development and flattening of the uncinate processes in children younger than 10 years of age. This makes them unable to withstand flexion and rotation forces.[2, 60, 61] Finally, the fulcrum of cervical movement may be located higher in young children than in adolescents and adults.[1] Because the immature spine is progressively ossifying, the injuries in patients under 8 years of age tend to be avulsions, epiphyseal separations, or fractures of the growth plate rather than true fractures. This mechanism pertains to all spinal injuries in this age group, but is most commonly seen in the odontoid fractures. Here the line of separation is through the basal synchondrosis, which is below the level of the superior facets.[9, 56, 62, 63] Minor trauma has precipitated instability in children who already have a structural defect in their bony elements (e.g., assimilation of the atlas, os odontoideum) or ligamentous complex (e.g., inflammatory states, Down's syndrome).[60, 61] Absence of the posterior elements of the upper cervical spine may lead to soft tissue wedging into the upper cervical canal during neck extension. This may indent the unprotected spinal cord. Hangman's fracture may also occur with violent forces.[42, 50, 64]

Cattell and Filtzer studied the normal cervical spines in 160 children between the ages of 1 and 16.[59] Ten children were grouped at each year. Flexion-extension lateral cervical spine x-ray films were done in a standardized manner. Twenty per cent of the children in all age groups had a predental space (space between the anterior arch of the atlas and the odontoid process) of 3 to 5 mm (Fig. 23–1A and B). An overriding of the atlas anterior arch on the odontoid process occurred in 20 per cent during extension. A pseudosubluxation be-

tween the second and third cervical vertebrae was visualized in 45 per cent of normal children. There was an absence of uniform angulation between the adjacent vertebrae in 16 per cent during neck flexion. The neurocentral synchondrosis of the axis was present in 100 per cent of individuals under 3 years of age, in 50 per cent of those 3 to 6 years of age, and in an extreme few older than 8 years of age. The pseudosubluxations that occurred in the cervical spine in infants and young children are due to the anterior wedging of the vertebral bodies, poorly developed joints of Luschka, ligamentous laxity, and the relative horizontal plane of the articular processes.[53, 59, 61, 63, 65]

PATHOLOGY AND PATHOPHYSIOLOGY OF SPINE AND SPINAL CORD INJURY

SPINAL COLUMN TRAUMA

The special anatomic features of the immature spine that predispose to certain types of injury have already been mentioned. The pathologic findings share some characteristics with those in adults, but others are unique to the pediatric population. Aufdermaur, in 1974, reviewed a series of 100 spinal autopsies, 12 of which were in children.[29] A cervical epidural hematoma was the most common finding, along with ligamentous disruption. The injuries consisted of severance of the cartilaginous end plate with fracture of the growth plate. Seven spinal cord injuries were located in the cervical spine, four in the thoracic region, and one in the lumbar spine. Birth injuries accounted for two cord injuries and motor vehicles for the remaining ten.

Spinal cord injury in the neonate accounts for 10 per cent of all neonatal deaths.[32, 43] The injuries occur with

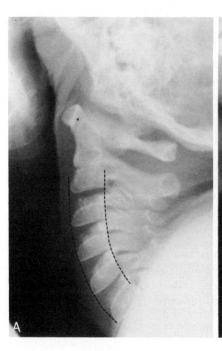
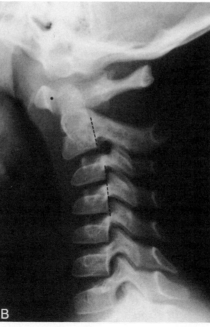

FIGURE 23–1. Normal laxity of the cervical spine in a 4-year-old child seen on lateral radiographs. *A,* Extension position. Lines drawn tangent to the anterior and posterior margins of the vertebral bodies are smooth *(dotted lines). B,* Flexion position. There is anterior "subluxation" of C2 on C3 with interruption of the tangent lines *(dotted lines).* The predental space has widened to 5 mm *(dot).*

breech presentation, transverse lie, and internal podalic version. In the "star gazing position" of breech presentation[28, 45, 66] or the "flying fetus" position[67] of transverse lie, the hyperextended head is particularly prone to injury with vaginal delivery. No case of cesarean birth has had permanent spinal cord injury. The lower cervical and upper thoracic spine are particularly vulnerable to longitudinal stress leading to epidural hemorrhage, cord injury, and hematomyelia. LeBlanc and Nadell reported on three children under 3 years of age who had disruptions of the lower cervical and upper thoracic dural sacs with severe cord injury and disruption.[48] Fractures were seen in this situation. A similar example is seen in Figure 23–2A through D.

Trauma to the upper cervical spine has resulted in occipitoatlantal and atlantoaxial dislocations, rotary luxations, and, in some instances, a delayed development of an os odontoideum.[64, 65, 68–72] A total of 15 to 70 per cent of spinal cord injuries in the pediatric population have no demonstrable fracture or dislocation. Present investigations into the syndrome of spinal cord injury without radiographic abnormalities in children have been undertaken utilizing magnetic resonance imaging and positron emission tomography.[64, 73–75] These modalities have revealed abnormalities within the spinal cord as well as in the ligamentous structures.

The mechanics of spinal trauma can be classified into five categories:[15, 20, 76–80] (1) flexion dislocation, (2) flexion compression, (3) compression burst, (4) extension, and (5) gunshot and penetrating injuries. In addition, a rare distraction injury may occur that is coupled with a rotational phenomenon. Flexion dislocations are associated with maximal ligamentous damage with minimum bone pathology, unilateral or bilateral locked facets, and severe neurologic deficits. In flexion-compression injuries, the most anterior aspect of the vertebral body is reduced in height with associated posterior ligamentous disruptions (Fig. 23–3A through C). During compression burst fractures resulting from axial loading, the vertebral bodies may be shattered, but the ligaments are commonly preserved. In severe extension injuries, there may be fractures of the spinous processes, laminae, and interarticular facets and avulsion fractures of the anterior portions of the vertebral bodies. With the penetrating injuries, the damage to the nervous system constitutes the most serious problem, and the spinal column is usually stable. The penetrating object and the resultant shock wave combine to result in various degrees of neurologic deficit. Distraction injuries are especially prominent at the occipitoatlantal and atlantoaxial joints. The easiest form of classification of vertebral column fractures is that by Holdsworth, wherein they have been categorized as a stable and an unstable variety.[78] Fracture-dislocations, accompanied by rupture of the ligamentous complex and facet interlock, are unstable. Rotational fracture-dislocations are the most unstable of all vertebral fractures and are the result of rotational flexion forces, disruption of the posterior ligament complex, and lateral displacement of the upper vertebral body on the lower. Burst fractures associated with fractures of the neural arch, referred to

as "shear" fractures, are limited to the lower thoracic and lumbar regions and frequently occur as the result of seat-belt injuries. Such fractures are unstable. The stable fractures are simple wedge fractures of flexion, with impaction of fracture fragments, and extension fractures localized to the cervical spine. In these cases, the posterior ligaments are intact, maintaining stability in neutral and flexed positions. Burst fractures have to be considered unstable unless there is impaction of the fracture fragments, as in the lumbar spine. However, in the cervical spine, they may be frequently associated with severe neurologic deficit and instability.

In the upper thoracic spine (second to tenth thoracic vertebrae), considerable violence is necessary to produce a fracture or dislocation. The narrow spinal canal makes it almost inevitable that these children should sustain neurologic injury. These fractures are stable as a result of the support of the rib cage, but the major consideration is the degree of spinal cord compromise. The axial loading of wedge compression fractures, as well as anterior subluxations, are stable.[76, 77] Because there is very little rotary motion of the upper part of the thoracic spine, most of the injuries occur in flexion, with axial loading. The "sagittal slice fracture" occurs when the vertebra above slices in the sagittal plane through the vertebra below, displacing half of the lower vertebra to a lateral position. Spinal dislocation in this instance results from total disruption of the posterior and anterior ligaments as well as the disc. The resultant instability may be further compounded by an inappropriate laminectomy during which the posterior supporting elements are removed when an anterior compression fracture is present. In this situation, surgical intervention with decompression and internal fixation and arthrodesis is essential for neurologic recovery and prevention of kyphosis.

The majority of fractures of the thoracic and lumbar spine occur at the fulcrum of motion where the thoracic and lumbar portions of the spine meet (Fig. 23–4A and B). Neurologic injury in this area may affect the conus medullaris or the cauda equina. The five types of fractures previously described can occur here. Acute fractures of the thoracolumbar spine should be considered initially unstable and must be immobilized. Vertebral compression fractures with reduction of more than 40 per cent of the normal height require stabilization. The most unstable fracture in this region is the rotary fracture-dislocation, for which early reduction with internal fixation and arthrodesis is the preferred treatment.

Multiple levels of injury may occur. Fifteen of 53 patients reported by Kewalramani showed multiple segments involved in the spinal canal.[1] Multiple-level injuries are most common to the thoracic spine, as reported by McPhee.[18]

The cervical spine is the most commonly affected in the pediatric population, especially among those below the age of 8 years. Hadley et al., in a review of the Barrows Neurological Institute series, found 72 per cent of injuries to be located in the cervical spine.[4] Fifty per cent of these were between the occiput and C2. In 16

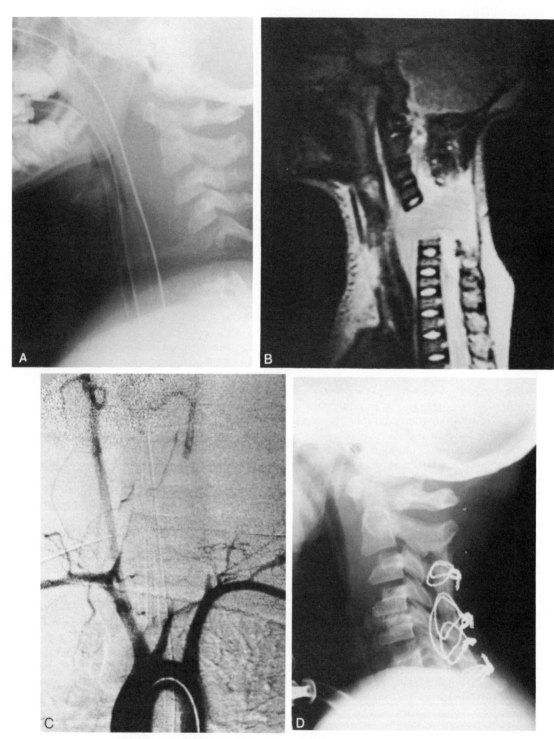

FIGURE 23–2. Severe spinal column and cord disruption in a 4-year-old boy involved in a motorcycle mishap. *A,* Lateral cervical radiograph shows an avulsion fracture of the C5 vertebral body with distraction of the proximal and distal spinal segments. Note the huge prevertebral swelling. *B,* Midsagittal T2-weighted MRI of cervical spine reveals the growth plate avulsion of the C5 vertebral body and pseudo-meningoceles. *C,* Arch aortogram reveals occlusion of both vertebral and left carotid arteries. *D,* Postoperative lateral cervical roentgenogram demonstrates normal cervical alignment after dorsal interlaminar C3–C7 rib graft fusion.

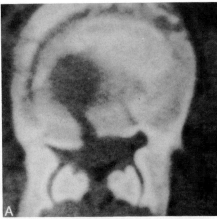

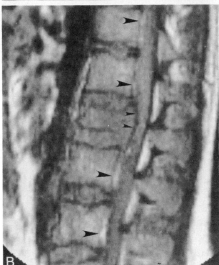

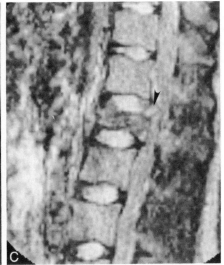

FIGURE 23–3. *A,* Axial CT scan reveals a burst fracture of T12 with posterior displacement of the fracture fragments, compromising the sagittal diameter of the spinal canal. *B,* Midsagittal T1-weighted MRI of the thoracolumbar spine (T-L) reveals cord compression at T12 *(small arrowheads).* The bright signal intensity of normal epidural fat, well seen above and below *(large arrowheads),* is obliterated at T12. *C,* Midsagittal T2-weighted MRI of T-L region better demonstrates the T12 vertebral body collapse. A small fragment of bone is displaced posteriorly *(arrowhead)* into the spinal canal.

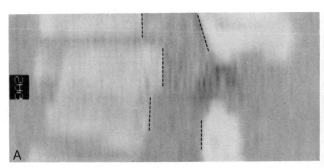

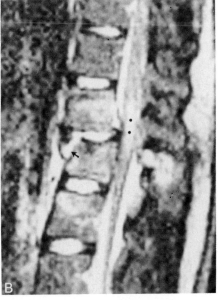

FIGURE 23–4. L1 compression fracture with conus medullaris compression in a 15-year-old. *A,* Midsagittal reformatted CT demonstrates a compression fracture of the L1 vertebral body with posterior displacement into the spinal canal. (The spinal canal is indicated by the dotted lines.) *B,* Midsagittal T2-weighted MRI reveals obliteration of the high signal intensity CSF at the L1 level. There is hemorrhage under the anterior longitudinal ligament *(arrow)* and hemorrhage in the conus medullaris *(dots).*

patients, multiple levels of injury occurred. The University of Iowa Hospitals and Clinics series on pediatric spinal column trauma showed that the cervical spine was affected in 79 per cent of cases.[20] The thoracolumbar junction and the upper lumbar regions were affected in the adolescent. Seventy-three per cent of patients had neurologic deficit when the lower cervical spine was involved, as opposed to 36 per cent who had a deficit when the upper cervical spine was involved. Peculiarly, the involvement of the upper cervical spine in orthopaedic series is low and may reflect the patient population treated by individual services.[9, 14, 18]

SPINAL CORD INJURY

The majority of spinal cord injuries resulting in permanent loss of sensory and motor function do not involve initial physical transection, but rather compression and contusion.[77, 81] As a result, during the initial few hours after injury, impulse generation and conduction cease, blood flow to the injured segment decreases, and consequent ischemia or hypoxia triggers extensive tissue destruction.[82–95] Experimental studies have demonstrated the presence of central hemorrhages and edema in the spinal cord during the first few hours after injury. It is believed that ischemia plays a significant role in the continuum of pathologic processes leading to spinal cord dysfunction. The greatest neurologic dysfunction occurs at impact, and the deficit may improve with time. However, the pathologic picture is the reverse. Even in the face of improved neurologic function, the gross pathologic picture evolves, over 5 to 7 days, from a small central necrotic area to extensive central and peripheral necrosis, depending on the severity of the trauma. Studies of early alterations in the traumatized spinal cord have included pial circulation, histopathology, electric conduction, biochemical changes, and circulatory changes within the intrinsic vasculature.[2, 44, 84, 89, 91–98]

Within seconds of traumatic impact on the spinal cord, small flame-shaped hemorrhages appear in the gray matter and beneath the pia-arachnoid membrane. Within 10 minutes, the hemorrhage spreads to the white matter. As this develops, it affects the general cord microcirculation, as evidenced by capillary wall thickening, extravasation of blood and fluid from the vessel lumen, and morphologic alterations of the myelin sheath and the periaxonal space. The predominant pattern is a central to peripheral spread of the pathologic condition. The central gray matter is involved before the peripheral gray matter. The more central white matter changes before the peripheral white matter. Significant formation of edema is noted by the end of the second day following a moderately severe concussion injury (Fig. 23–5). The appearance of edema is related to the time elapsed following trauma and the severity of the injury. In severe compression injuries, edema may be seen as early as 4 hours followed by tissue necrosis. This is characterized by the shrinkage of neurons, cytolysis, and glial scar formation at the injury

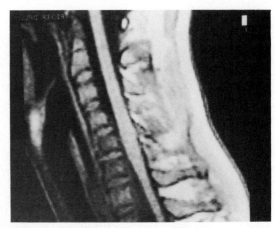

FIGURE 23–5. Midsagittal T1-weighted MRI of cervical spine of a 13-year-old male made 28 hours after cervical spinal cord injury following a diving incident. There is focal cord swelling at the C5–C6 level. No disc hernia or epidural clot was seen.

site. The initial hemorrhagic infarction is followed by removal of necrotic parenchyma and the development of adhesive arachnoiditis and intramedullary cavitation (Fig. 23–6A through D).

The ultrastructural changes following moderately acute impact lesions in monkeys correlates with the light microscopic changes. Within several hours, varying degrees of damage are seen, ending in shrunken axons and excessive tissue necrosis. Electron microscopic examinations have shown that microcysts develop from the myelin, forming sacks filled with fluid under tension and containing a swollen axon. These rupture into the extracellular space, creating larger cavities in the spinal tissue, presumably by release of lytic enzymes. There is platelet and red cell infiltration into the perivascular spaces, adding to the cellular necrosis. Damage to the vascular endothelium reduces the synthesis and release of prostacyclin and promotes additional platelet aggregation, resulting in a decrease in blood flow to that region of the tissue. Changes in the spinal cord blood flow (SCBF) begin shortly after impact. This decrease in the SCBF is due to vasospasm, stasis, and thrombosis of vessels of the gray matter. There is a rapid decrease in the spinal cord oxygen partial pressure (SCP_{O_2}) and a persistent state of hypoxia for several hours thereafter. A significant and common finding in traumatized spinal cord tissue is accumulation of lactate distal and proximal to the area of the lesion. Lactic acidosis negatively affects the glucose and oxygen consumption in aerobic metabolism, as well as the ionic sodium–potassium triphosphate-dependent (ATP-dependent) cell pump. The decrease in cellular oxidative phosphorylation sets in motion chemical transformations, involving membrane phospholipids and production of circulating prostaglandins, along with stimulation of adenosine diphosphate (ADP). Prostaglandins of the F series (which have vasoconstrictive properties) are increased in the acutely contused spinal cord of the cat.[99] Of greater significance is the injury-induced released of prostaglandin precur-

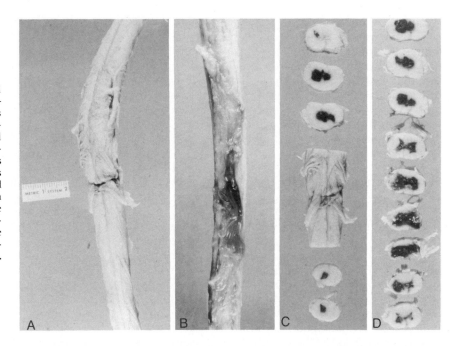

FIGURE 23–6. Autopsy specimen of cervical spinal cord from a 16-year-old male with C6–C7 fracture-dislocation occurring 5 weeks previously. *A,* The impact to the external ventral aspect of the spinal cord is seen. *B,* Dorsal external surface of spinal cord shows diminished caliber of the cord with arachnoiditis and resolving surface hemorrhage. *C,* Cross sections above and below the unsectioned (impact) spinal cord. Hematomyelia is seen in the central gray matter above and below the injury site. *D,* Cross sections through the injured spinal cord. Early cavitation and white matter disruption are seen. Note the ascending and descending central cord hemorrhages.

sor arachidonic acid, which increases the formation of thromboxanes. Thromboxane A$_2$ is an important vasoconstrictor and promoter of platelet aggregation. Under normal circumstances its actions are counteracted by the production of prostacyclin in the vascular endothelium. However, in injured spinal cords, endothelial lipid peroxidation leads to a selective decrease in prostacyclin production, and the primary action of thromboxane A$_2$ goes unopposed.

Free radicals generated as a result of the injury-induced tissue hypoxia initiate peroxidative reactions within the lipid bilayer of cell and organelle membranes. These lipid peroxidation reactions are catalyzed by the blood or hemoglobin and the contents of disrupted organelles. The free radicals attack unsaturated lipids in the membranes, leading to the inhibition of key neuronal enzymes and ultimately to the disruption of membrane function to the point that impulse generation cannot take place. Free radicals may rise in the injured spinal cord secondary to synthesis of prostaglandins or thromboxanes. Interestingly, calcium ions accumulate rapidly in the injured spinal cord, favoring prostaglandin production. The lipid peroxides inhibit production of prostacyclin and indirectly enhance platelet and granulocyte adhesiveness and free radical production. The end result is a self-perpetuating process resulting in tissue death.

Spinal cord injuries are classified as:

1. Complete lesions with loss of motor, sensory, and autonomic function distal to the injury.

2. Anterior cord syndrome, akin to the syndrome of the anterior spinal artery. Here touch and proprioception are preserved, although there is a loss of all other cord functions. This is an indication for visualizing the spinal cord and subarachnoid sac to exclude the presence of disc or bone fragments compressing the spinal cord. Magnetic resonance imaging is invaluable.

3. Posterior cord syndrome, in which only crude touch sensation is present.

4. Central cord syndrome. Children with this problem may go on to significant recovery.

5. Partial spinal cord syndrome of Brown-Séquard.

6. Root syndrome. Pain in a radicular distribution may indicate reversible injury to the root at that level, even when associated with sensory motor or reflex loss. One cannot overemphasize the value of functional recovery of even a single nerve root at the level of the brachial plexus or the thoracolumbar junction.

CURRENT APPLIED RESEARCH IN SPINAL CORD INJURY

There are six steps in the care of a child with spinal cord injury and neurologic deficit. Each phase of treatment may influence the final neurologic outcome. The steps are as follows:

1. Splinting and immobilization.
2. Medical stabilization.
3. Alignment of the spine.
4. Diagnostic procedures.
5. Decompression of the compressed neural elements.
6. Stabilization of the spine.

Once medical stabilization is accomplished, realignment of the spinal column is of paramount importance. The initial anatomic integrity of the spinal cord observed following some types of injury suggests that recovery could be facilitated if appropriate therapy were aimed at (1) preventing ischemia-related tissue degeneration, (2) supporting excitability of surviving spinal neurons, and (3) enhancing blood flow within the injured spinal segment. To this end various surgical and pharmacologic therapies have been tried with varying success.

Laminectomy to "decompress the swollen spinal cord" has proved ineffectual and detrimental to the patient. Midline myelotomy to relieve the "tension and pressure" within the spinal cord and prevent progression of the ischemic hemorrhagic tissue destruction has not proved efficacious. Dorsal rhizotomy above the level of the injury and myelotomy as proposed by Osterholm in the early 1970s have not changed the final outcome in these patients.

PHARMACOLOGIC INTERVENTION

The efficacy of corticosteroids in patients with spinal cord injury has been controversial. The rationale for the use of corticosteroids is based on the ability to maintain cellular and vascular membrane integrity, stabilize lysosomal membranes, and improve regional spinal cord blood flow. Earlier studies failed to demonstrate any beneficial effects of methylprednisolone in observed neurologic recovery.[100, 101] Recently, results of the second National Spinal Cord Injury Study (NASCIS II) were published.[102, 103] Overall, 487 patients were randomized to receive treatment with either methylprednisolone (30 mg/kg bolus followed by 5.4 mg/kg/hour for 23 hours—162 patients) or naloxone (5.4 mg/kg bolus and 4.0 mg/kg/hour—154 patients) or placebo (171 patients). All eligible patients were randomized within 12 hours of injury. Neurologic function was assessed 6 weeks and 6 months following injury. Analysis of the data revealed that after 6 months, patients who received methylprednisolone within 8 hours of injury had a statistically better recovery of motor and sensory function than occurred in those who received placebo. None of the differences in recovery in patients who received naloxone reached statistical significance, nor did the differences in patients initially treated outside the 8-hour window following injury. Benefit from methylprednisolone was noted in patients initially classified as having complete neurologic lesions as well as those with incomplete lesions. Following publication of this study, methylprednisolone was implemented as part of the standard treatment protocol in all patients with spinal cord injury. Recently, the 1-year follow-up of the same study was published and revealed that the increased recovery of neurologic function seen at 6 weeks and 6 months continued to be observed at 1 year.[103] This improvement in recovery was significant for motor function and was observed in patients with both complete and incomplete spinal cord injuries. Furthermore, the authors believed that continued treatment of patients with the study dose of methylprednisolone was justified owing to the low morbidity associated with treatment. Interestingly, it was noted that patients who were administered methylprednisolone more than 8 hours following injury had worse results than did the group receiving placebo, although the differences were not significant. Because there is some evidence suggesting that steroids may interfere with the ability of neurons to regenerate, it has been speculated that delayed administration of methylpred-

nisolone offers little of the benefits of inhibition of lipid peroxidation while interfering with the regenerative processes that may occur following injury.

Despite the encouraging results of NASCIS II, there remain several unresolved key issues regarding neural protection in acute spinal cord injury. First, it is possible that the efficacy of methylprednisolone could be augmented if treatment could be initiated even earlier, possibly at the scene of the accident. A second issue involves the optimal duration of therapy with methylprednisolone. Based upon the pathophysiology of spinal cord injury and lipid peroxidation, there is reason to believe that doses in excess of 24 hours may be beneficial in attenuating the tissue damage and improving recovery. Hall has suggested that the optimal duration of steroid administration will encompass the time required for hemorrhage within the spinal cord to be resorbed. The rationale for this is that as blood within the spinal canal is broken down and absorbed, hemoglobin is liberated which can drive the process of lipid peroxidation. However, prolonged administration of methylprednisolone would increase the risk of serious glucocorticoid side effects. It is possible that the anti-inflammatory effect of methylprednisolone could potentially prolong the presence of hematomyelia. These limitations have caused investigators to search for a drug with potent antioxidant but minimal steroidal side effects. Hall has speculated that the protective effect of methylprednisolone is not actually by glucocorticoid receptors.[99] This has led to the development of a series of methylprednisolone analogues that lack the 11-beta hydroxyl group, which is essential for glucocorticoid receptor binding, yet retain their antioxidant property. A recent discovery, substituting the complex amine for the 21-hydroxyl group, resulted in a dramatic augmentation of lipid antioxidant effects.[81] These have proved effective in preventing iron-catalyzed lipid peroxidation in rat brain homogenates. Tirilazad mesylate (U-74006F) has demonstrated excellent activity in experimental models of brain and spinal cord injury.

In an effort to answer some of the questions posed by the NASCIS II and current research regarding the 21-aminosteroids, the third NASCIS study has been designed and initiated. This protocol is meant to compare the efficacy of Tirilazad mesylate (2.5 mg/kg every 6 hours for 48 hours) with methylprednisolone administered for 24 hours or 48 hours. It is hoped that this study will provide answers to some of these unsolved issues.

Although methylprednisolone has received most of the attention, other pharmacologic agents have also been studied concerning their efficacy in spinal cord injury. Naloxone, a narcotic antagonist, was used with success in animals subjected to spinal cord injury.[85] Motor function returned earlier in those treated with naloxone than in control subjects. Faden and colleagues demonstrated that naloxone reversed the hypotension caused by transection of the cervical spinal cord, implicating endorphins in the pathophysiology of spinal shock. It was believed that restoration of blood pressure augmented the spinal cord blood flow and reduced subsequent ischemia.[85, 86, 104] The phase I trial of naloxone treatment in acute spinal cord injury in a clinical setting has shown that patients treated with naloxone showed a greater trend to recovery of evoked potentials over a period of 6 weeks to 6 months after injury. However, in NASCIS II, naloxone was shown to have no significant statistical effect on recovery of spinal cord function at 6 months to 1 year.

Faden et al. have shown that treatment with thyroxine-releasing hormone resulted in significant improvement in function in experimental spinal cord injury. It is believed that thyrotropin-releasing hormone functions as a physiologic opiate antagonist.[84, 85] Despite all these efforts, the mortality rates in spinal cord-injured patients ranges from 11 to 14 per cent.

CLINICAL DIAGNOSIS: PRESENTATION AND NEUROLOGIC DEFICITS

The diagnosis of spinal cord injury in the general population is usually made on the basis of recognized trauma, followed by immediate rapid development of the classic clinical syndrome of paralysis and spinal cord shock. This is not the case in children. The peculiar features of the pediatric spine allow for longitudinal distraction and rotational forces to cause injuries in the spinal cord at various levels without fracture or dislocation. A significant number may have a delayed onset of neurologic deficits. The time interval between injury and the appearance of objective sensori-motor dysfunction, termed the "latent period," can range from a few minutes to 3 or 4 days.[23, 24, 105]

The leading cause of neonatal spinal cord injury is delivery of the fetus with a hyperextended head from either a transverse lie or a breech presentation. The infant is often hypotonic, and there is difficulty in establishing respiration. These infants are noted to have abdominal breathing and to move the arms and legs infrequently. In the immediate newborn, a weak cry, poor feeding, and floppy lower extremities are clues to the presence of spinal cord injury. Repeated bouts of pneumonia, urinary tract infection, the development of spasticity in the lower extremities, and Horner's syndrome point to a cervicothoracic junction spinal cord lesion. Allen found that on re-examination of 31 infants initially diagnosed as having Werdnig-Hoffmann disease, 19 were suffering from spinal cord injuries.[43] Transverse myelitis and spinal cord tumors should be considered in children who had a normal neonatal period followed by paralysis. A diagnostic dilemma occurs in infants with bilateral brachial plexus palsy, who may also have sensory or motor loss or Horner's syndrome and fit into the category for central cord injury. Spinal radiographs are usually normal in this group, although the chest radiograph is abnormal with a bell-shaped chest appearance indicative of loss of the external muscles of respiration. Visualization of the spinal cord with magnetic resonance imaging is important because it usually demonstrates a block in the subarachnoid space. In the past, myelography and computed tomography were utilized.[44–46, 73, 74, 106] Infrequently, localized spinal cord atrophy may be identified.

A high index of suspicion is required for the diagnosis of spinal cord injury in the acutely injured, unconscious child. Vertebral column or spinal cord injury should be suspected in the conscious individual with symptoms of neck or back pain or localized tenderness, and in a child in whom an asymmetric response to stimulation is obtained. Frontal or occipital head trauma and limitation of neck movement must alert the clinician to possible hyperextension or hyperflexion injuries to the cervical spine.[107] Bruising over the cervical, thoracic, or lumbar spine usually indicates underlying osseous injury. Abdominal distention with hypotonia in the lower extremities is a clue to spinal cord injury in the young child. An underlying preexisting pathologic condition, such as inflammatory disease of the upper respiratory system, may make the cervical spine prone to atlantoaxial instability with minor trauma.[107]

An additional complication in the evaluation of the child with spinal injury is that 15 to 70 per cent of patients with major neurologic involvement have normal radiographs. Therefore, accurate diagnosis may depend upon several observations and examinations. This cannot be repeated often enough. In the awake, cooperative child, sensory, motor, and reflex examination allows one to assess reliably the level of cord injury. In spinal shock, there is flaccid paralysis below the level of the lesion, and the deep tendon reflexes are lost. There is urinary retention and autonomic imbalance resulting in hypotension. If the injury is not too severe, voluntary control is reestablished and recovery begins within a few hours of injury. However, if the injury is severe, the spinal cord distal to the injury is isolated, and mass reflexes set in unaccompanied by any evidence of improvement in voluntary motor activity or sensory perception. Assessment of reflexes is helpful in determining the level of lesions in infants and children with cervical spinal cord and cauda equina injuries. The reflex loss is generally appropriate to the degree of motor involvement. Thus, spinal cord injury may result in a complete loss of function, a partial loss of function with or without cauda equina sparing, or root dysfunction. Neural trauma motor index scoring is useful in comparing patients and results from various treatment regimens.[83] We have found it extremely useful in the day-to-day treatment of a patient and helpful in assessing efficacy of treatment.

In the series published from the University of Iowa Hospitals and Clinics, Osenbach and Menezes reviewed 179 children with spinal column and cord injuries.[20] Fifty-two per cent sustained neurologic injury. The neurologic outcome was dependent on the severity of initial injury. Only one patient with complete injury became ambulatory. The majority of children with mild to moderate injury regained complete function. There was no difference between patients managed operatively or conservatively. Hadley et al. reported a series in which 50 per cent of patients had neurologic deficit.[4] In 33 per cent the injury was incomplete, and in 17 per cent it was complete. There was a high incidence of neurologic injury in the younger age group. In 13 of 20 patients with complete injury, the injury remained complete. Three of 20 patients improved to a Frankel D, one of the 20 improved to Frankel C, and three died. Eighty-nine per cent of incomplete injuries improved. Improvement was even experienced relatively late in the course of the disease and was believed to be due to the plasticity of the nervous system. In the series by Kewalramani et al., 50 of 62 patients with cervical injuries (81 per cent) remained quadriplegic.[1] Twenty-nine of 35 patients with thoracolumbar injuries (83 per cent) remained paraplegic. The complete lesions did not improve regardless of surgery, and surgery made no difference in the recovery in incomplete neurologic deficits in children.

Thus, in regard to prognosis for children with traumatic quadriplegia, 85 per cent of all patients who were initially "complete" remained complete, and a small percentage regained some motor function in their legs. The few patients who improve may do so because of aggressive therapy or because initial examination reflected a shock or concussive wave. In severe partial lesions, 8 to 25 per cent may recover. In central cord lesions with relatively preserved function in the legs, recovery of lost motor power occurs between 75 and 80 per cent of the time. Paraplegia has been similarly analyzed. Data pertaining to thoracic lesions are practically identical to data pertaining to cervical lesions. However, in the thoracolumbar junction, it appears that as many as 30 per cent of those with initially complete lesions will regain motor function.

RADIOGRAPHIC EVALUATION

Integrity of the posterior osseoligamentous complex of the spinal canal is essential for spinal column stability, together with the middle column.[108, 109] Consequently, anterior vertebral injuries involving the vertebral bodies, ligaments, and disc are relatively more stable than those that involve the posterior and lateral complex. Imaging of the child with presumed spinal trauma should aim to diagnose the entire extent of the injury. In doing so, one has to consider the likelihood of worsening the patient's condition in attempting to fully define the extent of trauma. A number of spinal imaging techniques are currently available. It is essential that the treating physician keep in mind the different modalities of imaging, as well as the order in which these should be implemented. The diagnostic studies should complement one another and provide maximal information in a relatively short time. Thus, each component of the diagnostic process should be undertaken with an appreciation for its limitations and timeliness.[64] The imaging modalities currently available are plain radiographs, flexion-extension films, fluoroscopy, dynamic motion studies, computerized tomography with or without myelography, and magnetic resonance imaging.

Conventional radiography encompasses spine films in the frontal, lateral, and oblique positions, especially in the cervical spine.[107] An open-mouth odontoid view is difficult to obtain in a young child or infant. Pleuridirectional tomography and computerized axial tomography are important diagnostic tools to assess the degree of bony and soft tissue disruption and the maintenance of midline and lateral column alignment. Suspicion of spinal cord injury in the absence of fracture or dislocation on plain radiographs requires the visualization of the spinal cord and spinal column by the use magnetic resonance imaging in the T1 and T2 modes (Fig. 23–7A and B).[63, 64, 73, 74, 106, 110, 111]

Plain radiographs are the mainstay of cervical and thoracolumbar spine imaging. In the cervical spine, imaging consists of the anterior-posterior view, the lateral cervical radiograph, oblique views with 30-degree angulation of the filming x-ray unit to the right and left, and open-mouth views to visualize the atlas and axis vertebrae. These films can demonstrate the presence, the extent, and the severity of an injury. Lateral radiographs must clear the C7–T1 interspace, and this frequently requires that the patient's shoulders be depressed for a swimmer's view in a lateral projection. An inadequate examination can lead to missed fractures. A high suspicion of spinal trauma must be entertained in children who are not awake or who have multiple injuries. In addition, a painful injury may mask evidence of cervical spine instability due to muscle spasm. The retropharyngeal soft tissue space must be appraised, and the cervical alignment checked. Immobilization may be required until the spasm resolves and radiographs are repeated.

The following criteria have been used to detect instability at the craniocervical junction in children:[64]

1. Predental space of more than 5 mm in those below the age of 8 years and more than 3 mm in those over 8 to 10 years of age.
2. Separation of atlas lateral masses of more than 7 mm in the open-mouth view suggests a Jefferson (C1) burst fracture and the possibility of disruption of the transverse portion of the cruciate ligament.
3. Vertical clivus odontoid translation of more than 2 mm.
4. The gap between the occipital condyles and the atlas facets should be minimal, so that the occipital condyles are never visible on their own. "Bare" occipital condyles indicate an occipitocervical dislocation.
5. Any abnormal relationship between the spinal canal and foramen magnum is pathologic, except for widening of the interspace between the occiput and C1 and between C1 and C2 posteriorly.
6. Abnormal cervicocranial motion dynamics.

With cervical spine injuries, the absence of neurologic deficit and the presence of a stable cervical spine necessitates dynamic views in the flexed and extended position to assess stability. In a patient with an unstable fracture of the cervical spine, skeletal traction with increasing weight may be required to reduce the defor-

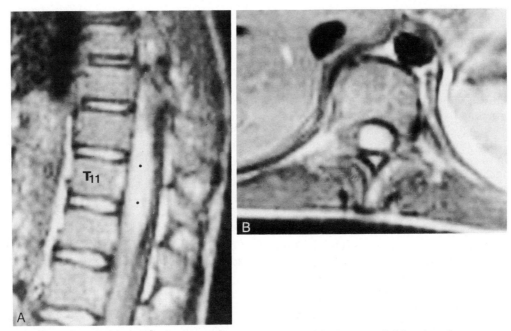

FIGURE 23–7. MR imaging in a 13-year-old gymnast with acute back pain and delayed (54 hours) onset of paraparesis. Plain radiographs and CT scan of the thoracolumbar region (T-L) were unremarkable. *A,* Midsagittal T1-weighted MRI of the T-L region demonstrates high signal intensity within the spinal cord *(dots),* consistent with hemorrhage. *B,* Axial T1-weighted MRI at the T11 vertebral level. Note the hemorrhage in the spinal cord.

mity. The effects of traction are documented with appropriate radiographs. In 5 per cent of children, a symptomatic disc herniation may be present, and this must be identified so that appropriate treatment measures can be followed.[53, 59, 83]

Acute-injury extension lateral radiographs are commonly used to assess the integrity of the ligamentous structures in patients with suspected injury. The patient is instructed to voluntarily flex and extend the spine as far as possible. No attempt is made to increase the patient's range of motion. The extent of subluxation can easily be measured on the radiographs. These motion studies employing plain radiographs can be substituted with CINE or fluoroscopic technique. The disadvantage is the impermanency of the image.

Pleuridirectional tomography and CT have greatly enhanced our understanding of the bony pathology. The latter has become the mainstay of imaging of spinal cord and spinal column injuries. The bony detail is exquisite with demonstration of even small cortical disruptions. The extent of bony encroachment on the spinal canal becomes obvious, and the configuration of the spinal column can only be evaluated with contiguous 2-mm thin section axial views to permit reconstruction, and at times 3D imaging. This is extremely important in the thoracic and lumbar spine when consideration is to be given for stabilization and instrumentation. It is important to be able to assess the integrity of the anterior, middle, and posterior columns of the spine at least 3 to 4 motion segments above and below the injury site. However, there are pitfalls in CT examination of the spine. This is particularly so when fractures parallel the plane of the scan and involve the facets or when fractures through the pedicles are missed on the axial sections. Unfortunately, the intraspinal contents require contrast enhancement. Most of the time anatomic arrangement of the spine can be better appreciated with 3-dimensional reformatted images. We believe that CT myelography is not useful in the determination of spinal instability or the extent of the spinal cord injury. Magnetic resonance imaging has superseded this.

MRI has the advantage of imaging long vertebral segments, identifying spinal and spinal cord pathology, as well as ligamentous disruptions or disc herniations in the presence or absence of hematoma. The role of magnetic resonance imaging has evolved significantly within the past decade. The ability to evaluate soft tissue, including detailed assessment of the intervertebral discs and ligaments, has been of great advantage in planning surgical therapy. It has to be used in conjunction with CT when osseous anatomy needs to be depicted in fine detail. MRI-compatible cervical traction devices are routinely available in emergency facilities. The tissue parameters in the T1- and T2-weighted modes must be obtained with sagittal as well as coronal and axial imaging.

We recommend immediate identification of bony pathology with plain radiographs to be followed by magnetic resonance imaging as soon as possible in all cases of spinal cord injury and involvement of the spine. CT complements the MRI.

AGE-RELATED PROBLEMS

SPINAL CORD INJURIES DURING BIRTH

Certain factors stand out as being important apart from injuries to the fetal spinal cord. These are longitudinal stretching of the vertebral column in breech presentation, torsional forces applied in rotating the head in cephalic deliveries, distortion of the shoulder with traction being transmitted to the spinal cord, and hyperextension of the head in breech delivery.

A state of shock and difficulty in initiating respiration are common with these lesions. The motor manifestations vary with the site of the injury. Those injuries that occur above the C3–C4 cervical spinal level are promptly fatal, unless the infant is given constant respiratory support. Damage to the lower cervical and upper thoracic spinal cord, often associated with brachial plexus injury, produces flaccidity of the arms and hands, respiratory embarrassment with paradoxical respiration, and occasionally Horner's syndrome (Fig. 23–8A and B). There are varying degrees of flaccidity of the legs following injury to the lumbosacral segments. Bladder paralysis is common, but a newborn's problem can usually be managed without catheterization. Radiographs of the spine are usually normal; however, they are useful in excluding congenital anomalies, especially spina bifida, and may occasionally demonstrate vertebral dislocation. At the present time, we believe that magnetic resonance imaging should be performed as soon as possible to permit visualization of the posterior fossa and its contents as well as the spinal canal.

The state of "spinal shock" subsides within a few weeks, and then it becomes possible to establish a reasonably accurate and durable assessment of the infant's neurologic status. Thus it is important that repeated examinations be performed. The infant is alert with few, if any, cranial nerve abnormalities, unless the brainstem was injured with traction or by damage to its blood supply. Reflex movements develop in response to noxious stimuli over a wide receptive area in the arms and legs. Spasticity leads to contractures and this is unusual. It is seen in the hips and femoral muscles. Koch reviewed the long-term prognosis of 14 infants with neonatal spinal cord injuries.[111] Eight of the 14 died: four patients at less than 3 months of age, three patients between 3 months and 1 year of age, and one patient at 3 1/2 years. Six children survived for more than 2 years for a follow-up examination. The quality of survival for those with functional levels of C8–T1 and below depends on the presence and severity of medical complications. Supportive measures for such patients include bracing of the thoracolumbar spine as the infant grows.

TRAUMA OCCURRING TO PATIENTS UNDER 8 YEARS OF AGE

A significant proportion of spinal canal and spinal cord trauma occurs in the cervical spine. In most children below the age of 6 years, this is referable to the level above C3. The odontoid process is the most affected at the neurocentral synchondrosis. The superior segment angulates forward along with the atlas vertebra (Fig. 23–9A and B). In the youngest infant in our series in whom this occurred, the injury was the result of birth trauma, and this infant had an associated epidural intracranial hematoma.[107] Radiographs may also reveal fractures of the pedicles with anterior subluxation of the atlas and the body of C2 on C3, typical hangman's fractures. These are unstable.[64] Reduction is best achieved with the head and neck placed in a hyperextended position over the edge of a mattress. Should positioning not succeed in accomplishing reduction, halo ring immobilization should then be utilized. Once adequate reduction of the spinal deformity has been achieved, rigid external immobilization can be obtained by the use of the halo vest. This offers the ad-

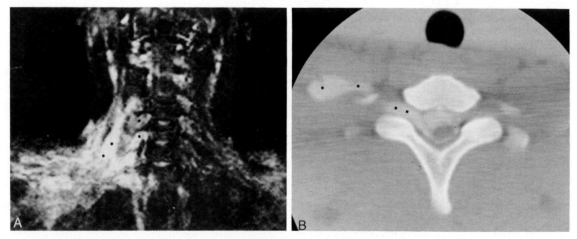

FIGURE 23–8. Brachial plexus root avulsion. *A,* Coronal T2-weighted MRI of cervical and upper thoracic spine to visualize the brachial plexus. Note the CSF extravasation at C7 and C8 into the soft tissues of the neck *(dots). B,* CT metrizamide-enhanced myelogram at C7. There is contrast extravasation outside the spinal canal along the tract of the C8 nerve root *(dots).*

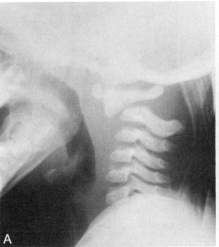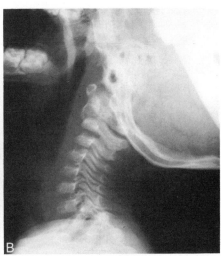

FIGURE 23–9. *A,* Lateral cervical radiograph in a 14-month-old child with odontoid fracture dislocation. There is avulsion at the neurocentral synchondrosis. *B,* Radiograph done 10 weeks after halo traction and immobilization. There is healing at the axis odontoid fracture site with good alignment.

vantage of prolonged immobilization and active early rehabilitation.

Skeletal traction in the toddler or young child can be safely applied provided attention is given to such factors as skull thickness, age, and anatomic and biomechanical properties of the pediatric spine. In older children, whose skull is of adequate thickness, traction can be applied by means of a standard halo ring or a crown halo. At our institution, magnetic resonance imaging is obtained acutely in all children with spinal cord injury to exclude a surgical lesion; therefore, MRI-compatible skeletal tongs or MRI-compatible halo is preferred. In young children, a halo ring can be used with eight pins for fixation to evenly distribute the forces at 2 pounds per square inch pressure in those under 4 years of age. In those under 2 years of age, finger tightening between the index finger and thumb allows for pressures between 1 and 2 pounds. The amount of weight required to achieve reduction of a cervical spine subluxation is considerably less than that needed in teenagers or adults. It is imperative that frequent films be obtained to ensure that overdistraction does not occur at the site of injury as this can result in a worsening of neurologic deficit or, in some instances, promote the formation of an os odontoideum.[60, 107] Once reduction is achieved, alignment must be maintained. Careful attention should be paid to cleanliness of the pins and the tong sites. Symptoms of local pain and headache may indicate penetration of the skull, leading to osteomyelitis or even cerebritis.

Cervical spine fractures in the older child are managed with reduction and immobilization. The presence of disc herniation, bone fragments, or hematoma impinging on the spinal cord requires decompression and fusion. This may be accomplished via the anterior or posterior routes. It is then followed by external immobilization and early rehabilitation.

We have performed anterior cervical discectomy at the C3–C4 level in nine patients 6 to 8 years of age with good results. Thus, surgery is indicated for stabilization of an unstable fracture, reduction of locked facets that are irreducible, debridement of compound wounds, and removal of bone fragments and disc material from the spinal canal.[80, 107, 112–114]

When posterior fusion is necessary in the cervical spine, wire fixation alone does not serve the purpose. This is because the ultimate fusion construct should be osseous. The wire may cut through the thin, poorly ossified lamina or spinous process. As a child grows, a position of hyperextension may occur or subsequent disruption of the wire with impingement of the spinal cord may result.[17, 20, 60] The treatment of choice is wiring of bone to each individual lamina or facet, so that once incorporation of the bone has taken place, the bone will grow with the child. Our experience with over 200 such cervical fusions in children over the past 15 years has shown no decrease in the growth potential or exaggerated lordosis. From a neurosurgical perspective, the bone may be harvested from rib or the posterior iliac crest, or the tibia. We prefer to use rib for posterior cervical fusions.

SPINAL CORD TRAUMA IN PATIENTS 8 TO 16 YEARS OF AGE

Cervical injuries predominate in this age group and account for 60 to 70 per cent of injuries. Thoracic and thoracolumbar junction injuries are related to violent forces that occur with football injuries, crush injury, falls from a height, and automobile accidents.[107, 115, 116] The principles of management of unstable cervical spine injuries are the same as previously described. Unstable thoracic or thoracolumbar spine fractures, whether complete or incomplete, require stabilization (Fig. 23–10*A* through *C*). This should be accomplished via the anterior route.[76, 79, 107, 117] The transthoracic anterior approach to resect the involved vertebral body and disc allows visualization of the ventral dural sac and confirmation of decompression. A rib graft with attached vascular pedicle is then rotated into position and wedged between the vertebra above and the vertebra below the level of injury. This allows for removal of the compressed, disrupted bony segment that is in-

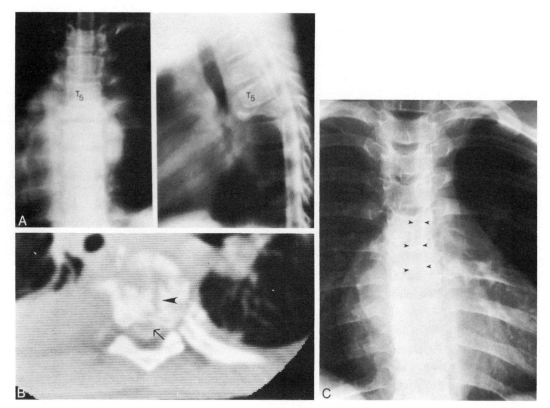

FIGURE 23–10. Twelve-year-old male with T6 vertebral body compression fracture and incomplete spinal cord injury. *A,* Composite of frontal and lateral thoracic metrizamide-enhanced myelotomogram. There is a burst fracture of T6 with ventral cord angulation. *B,* Axial CT myelogram with metrizamide at the T6 level. The spinal cord *(arrow)* is ventrally located. There is comminution of the vertebral body *(arrowhead).* *C,* Anterior-posterior view of thoracic spine done 3 months after transthoracic anterior vertebral decompression of the spinal cord at T6. A vascularized T6 rib graft bridged T5–T7 for fusion *(arrowheads).*

volved. Removal of the segment prevents kyphosis, and the vascularized rib graft shows incorporation into the recipient site within 6 to 8 weeks (Fig. 23–10*C*). It is our view that thoracic fractures can also be handled via the transpedicular or costotransversectomy posterolateral routes. This can allow for satisfactory ventral decompression with posterior column instrumentation done simultaneously.

We believe that thoracolumbar junction fractures are best approached by a posterolateral decompressive route, which allows for visualization of the dura mater and the spinal cord.[20, 107] A concomitant transpedicular approach to the ventral spinal canal permits the anterolateral bony decompression to be performed. Segmental stabilization is preferable to the long Harrington rod or Luque fixation. Bony fusion is mandatory. Surgical intervention in this fashion has allowed immediate stabilization and rehabilitative measures to be instituted.

In summary, the care of the child or the young adult with spinal injury and neurologic deficit is divided into six phases. These comprise immobilization, medical stabilization, restitution of alignment of the spine, diagnostic procedures, surgical decompression if there is compression of the neural elements, and stabilization of the spine. Rehabilitation must be instituted from the time of admission following the acute spinal cord insult.

SPECIAL CONSIDERATIONS

LESIONS OF THE CRANIOVERTEBRAL JUNCTION

This is a transition zone between the skull and the vertebral joints and is unique in that it allows extensive movement, and yet its vertebrae are interlocked in an amazingly stable three-dimensional structure.[118] The complex interaction between the occipital bone, the atlas and the axis vertebrae, and their associated ligaments strongly suggests that this complex acts as a unit. The atlas serves as a washer or bearing between the occipital condyles and the axis vertebra. The diagnosis and treatment of trauma to this region require a thorough understanding of the osseous anatomy, ligamentous structures and their functional properties, together with the joint kinematics. Injuries to the occipitoatlantoaxial complex are divided into the following:[56, 64]

1. *Osseous injuries*
   a. Occipital condyle fracture
   b. The Jefferson fracture (C1)
   c. Odontoid fractures (C2)
2. *Ligamentous injuries*
   a. Occipitoatlantal dislocation
   b. Atlantoaxial dislocation

3. *Complex injuries*
   a. Transaxial cervicomedullary junction injury
   b. Traumatic spondylolisthesis of C2 (Hangman fracture)
   c. Combined osseoligamentous disruptions.

JEFFERSON FRACTURE

The Jefferson fracture is caused by excessive axial loading, which results in divergent lines of force passing through the lateral masses of the atlas vertebra. The lateral atlantal masses are wedge shaped and thus can be easily displaced in an outward manner, with bursting of the C1 ring at the vertebral artery groove, which is its weakest point. It has been said that atlas fractures are uncommon in children, but this is not the case.[56, 64, 107] Posterior arch fractures are the most common. However, the anterior C1 arch fracture may occur with axial loading in extreme flexion. These were described as a four-part burst fracture by Jefferson. In most instances, the Jefferson fracture is considered to be a stable injury that responds well to conservative management with Philadelphia collar immobilization, or in rare instances with combination fractures, a halo immobilization may be required.

FRACTURES OF THE ODONTOID PROCESS

Injuries in children present problems that are different from those in the adult. Odontoid fractures in children are avulsion injuries at the neurocentral synchondrosis, particularly in children under the age of 8 to 10 years. In addition, ligamentous laxity and incomplete ossification in young children make them more prone to this sort of injury. The treatment comprises realignment and complete immobilization for 8 to 10 weeks in a halo vest or a Minerva cast.[4, 20] In those above the age of 8 to 10 years, fractures that occur can be divided into the adult forms of type I, type II, and type III fracture. Type I fracture has an oblique line that goes through the upper one third of the odontoid process. This represents an avulsion fracture where the alar ligament attaches. Type II fracture occurs at the lower third of the odontoid at the junction of the odontoid process and the body of C2. The type III fracture extends down into the cancellous portion of the body of the axis, and the fracture line usually extends to the superior articular facets of C2.

OCCIPITOATLANTAL DISLOCATION

The literature concerning traumatic occipitoatlantal dislocation is limited, and the majority of reports have appeared in the past decade.[118–121] The condition is not uncommon and appears to be associated with an extremely high mortality at the scene of the accident. Hence, this had been presumed to be a rare occurrence. The actual incidence is obscured by the devastating na-

ture of the injury itself. In a review of 112 victims of trauma who died at the scene of the injury, Bucholz and Burkhead discovered that 26 had cervical spine injury.[119] Of the 26, nine had a traumatic atlantooccipital dislocation and five had an odontoid fracture. Alker and co-workers, in a similar experience, found that 19 per cent had occipitoatlantal dislocation. The number of survivors with this injury has increased dramatically owing to improved on-site resuscitation and transportation by emergency units. Our own neurosurgical experience encompasses 18 patients with traumatic occipitoatlantal dislocation and four with lesser forms of ligamentous occipitoatlantal injury.[118] Six patients succumbed to their injury.

Several mechanisms have been implicated as the cause of occipitoatlantal dislocation. We believe that the most frequent mechanism of injury is hyperflexion of the skull in relation to the upper cervical spine, with distraction. The resulting separation of the posterior elements of the atlas and the axis is well visualized with MRI. Several authors have implicated lateral flexion as a major etiology, while others have invoked extreme hyperextension leading to disruption of the tectorial membrane.[60, 64, 68, 120, 121] Ligamentous disruption of the anterior occipitoatlantal ligament, the tectorial membrane, the alar ligaments, and the posterior element of the occipitoatlantoaxial complex produces forward displacement of the cranium on the atlas. Although anterior occipitoatlantal injury is the most common, lateral occipitoatlantal dislocation as well as posterior cranial displacement have been reported.

Based upon a review of the literature and our own series of patients, occipitoatlantal dislocation is classified as follows:

1. Anterior displacement of the cranium with respect to the atlas.

2. Posterior displacement of the cranium on the atlas.

3. Longitudinal distraction with separation of the skull from the spine.

Avulsion of the cranial nerves, as well as transection of the medulla oblongata and the upper cervical cord, have been reported in postmortem studies. Infants and young children who survive are usually comatose with a hemiparesis, quadriparesis, or diaphragmatic breathing. In other instances, the patients may have altered levels of consciousness with abnormal lower cranial nerve function and a combination of spinal cord abnormalities.

Several radiographic criteria of the diagnosis of occipitoatlantal dislocation have been proposed to aid in the early diagnosis with lateral cervical radiographs. However, an obvious dislocation is easily seen by checking with the normal reference points at the craniovertebral junction. Magnetic resonance imaging best identifies the ligamentous disruption, as well as the spinal cord and brainstem hemorrhagic contusion and the possible presence of epidural hematoma external to the tectorial membrane (Fig. 23–11*A* through *C*). We recommend

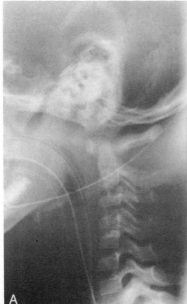

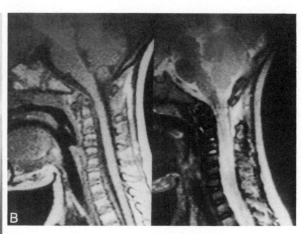

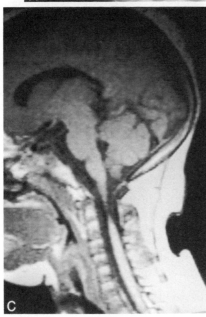

FIGURE 23–11. Occipitoatlantal injury with cervicomedullary junction dysfunction in a 6-year-old female. *A*, Lateral craniocervical radiograph reveals swelling in front of the craniovertebral junction; "bared occipital condyles" and widening of the interspinous space at C1–C2. *B*, Composite of midsagittal T1-weighted *(left)* and T2-weighted *(right)* MRI of craniovertebral junction (CVJ) 4 days after injury. Note the dorsal odontoid position *(left)*, the hemorrhage in the spinal cord at the C1 level *(right)*, and the soft tissue injury in the interspinous C1–C2 space. *C*, Midsagittal T1-weighted MRI of CVJ made 7 months after injury. The spinal cord at C1–C2 level is atrophic.

CT scanning using 3-mm slice thickness in routine multiplane sagittal and coronal reconstructions to evaluate all patients with suspicious upper cervical spine radiographs. This is particularly recommended for those who have signs of brainstem injury or unexplained quadriparesis or cranial nerve palsies. Cervical traction should never be used in patients with suspected occipitocervical instability. Angiography may reveal stenosis or occlusion of the vertebral arteries.

Occipitocervical dislocation requires immediate fixation in a halo vest and immobilization. A contoured-loop occipitocervical fixation would be ideal and should be implemented as soon as the patient's condition is stable and allows it. Osseous integration can be achieved by utilizing bone grafts at the same time.

ATLANTOAXIAL INSTABILITY AND LUXATION

Luxation refers to a complete and lasting disruption of the articular facets of the synovial joints. Examples of this are the interlocking of the articular facets or the marked diastasis that occurs with hyperflexion fracture luxation. Atlantoaxial luxations (C1–C2) can be divided into the anterior, posterior, and rotational types. Fielding and Hawkins, in a biomechanical study of the strength of the atlantoaxial ligament complex, showed that the force required to fracture the odontoid process was much less than the force required to cause failure of all the ligaments in the same specimen.[69, 70] In the clinical setting the frequency of fracture of the odontoid process in children is much greater than atlantoaxial luxation secondary to trauma. The anterior and the rare posterior atlantoaxial luxation are a finding in acute, as well as chronic, nonunited fractures of the odontoid process. The rotary luxations require more attention and will be discussed in greater detail.

The rotary atlantoaxial luxation is not an uncommon finding in children with infections of the upper respiratory system or other inflammatory conditions.[12, 60, 69, 70, 122] In normal patients, rotation of the atlas and the axis is within the range of 35 degrees.[123] This may also occur in a traumatic situation, but if the rotation exceeds 40 degrees, facet interlock occurs.[60, 69, 123] In our series of 36 patients with atlantoaxial rotary luxations, trauma was a causative factor in each and every one.[118] Football spearing injury occurred in a significant number, followed by motor vehicle accidents and wrestling injuries. An associated occipitoatlantal rotary luxation is not uncommon. This series does not include the patients with Down's syndrome. An associated occipitoatlantal rotary luxation leads to a characteristic "cock robin" appearance.[56] This abnormality has been reported following surgical repair of cleft lip and cleft palate and removal of orthodontic devices and a body cast. It may go unrecognized if the symptoms are minor, or it may be diagnosed when associated with brainstem dysfunction or cervical myelopathy.

Children with rotatory atlantoaxial luxation have been erroneously diagnosed as having brainstem vascular insult, cerebellar tumor, Chiari malformation, cervical migraine, syringo-hydromyelia and ocular palsies.[60] All patients present with a torticollis and diminished range of motion of the neck. Facial flattening is prominent and symptoms of neural compression occur when the atlas is separated from the odontoid process by more than 5 mm, allowing a rotation of the atlas and the axis, and thus compromise of the spinal canal. The diagnostic procedures utilized are lateral cervical radiographs, pleuridirectional tomography, CINE radiographs, CT scans, and magnetic resonance imaging. The entity may be difficult to diagnose owing to radiographic problems in visualizing the complex anatomic structures in the area.

Overriding of the atlas in relationship to the axis on the AP view is abnormal and a clue to the diagnosis. On the lateral radiographs of the skull and cervical spine, there should be normal alignment of the facet joints of the upper cervical spine. Rotation of the atlas is usually seen in relation to the axis with a forward projection of the atlantal lateral masses anterior to the odontoid process (Fig. 23–12A through C). This represents a large bulk of bone in front of the odontoid process, which should be a clue to the diagnosis. If the skull and the atlas are in a true lateral position, the cervical spine then shows a prominence of the facet joints rather than a true lateral picture in the subaxial location. There is persistent asymmetry in the atlantoaxial relationship that is not corrected by rotation unless it is reduced (Fig. 23–12D). This is easily seen on the CINE CT or CINE radiographs, which show that the subluxed axis and the atlas move as a unit during neck rotation.

The best conceptualization of the abnormality and definition of a possible interlock of the facets are provided by illustrating the pathologic state in a third dimension such as CT scanning and magnetic resonance imaging (Fig. 23–13A and B). A functional or dynamic study using CT or MRI can be obtained through the craniovertebral complex.[64, 118] No motion is seen at the C1–C2 articulation in a fixed luxation, be it unilateral or bilateral. This is visualized on CT scanning with the head turned to the extreme right and turned to the extreme left. Magnetic resonance imaging provides indirect information regarding the patency of the vascular structures as well as possible neural compromise.

Fielding and Hawkins classified the atlantoaxial rotary fixed luxation.[69, 70] This is dependent upon the integrity of the transverse ligament and the secondary support ligament complex. If the transverse ligament ruptures during such an accident, the atlas arch is displaced forward, causing compromise of the spinal canal diameter. This requires reduction and surgical immobilization.

SPINAL CORD INJURY WITHOUT RADIOGRAPHIC ABNORMALITY (SCIWORA)

Spinal cord injury without radiographic abnormality (SCIWORA) is a syndrome that describes injuries in which traumatic myelopathy occurs in the absence of demonstrable contiguous osseous or ligamentous injury. The concept initially was theorized that transient subluxation of the spine could occur without bony fracture or overt ligamentous instability and then elastic recoil would return the spinal column to its normal alignment. Thus, spinal cord injury could occur in the absence of radiographic abnormality. This concept dates back to the early twentieth century. Pang and Weilberger reported a large group of children who sustained traumatic spinal cord injury despite normal radiographic studies and subsequently coined the term SCIWORA.[24] Other authors had previously reported similar cases of spinal cord injury which would fall into this category.[13, 16, 24, 107, 124, 125]

This lesion has been compared with the acute central cord syndrome in adults. The incidence of SCIWORA varies considerably, ranging between 5 and 70 per cent of all pediatric spinal cord injuries. SCIWORA occurs almost exclusively in the pediatric population, with the majority of cases occurring in children less than 8 years of age. The mechanisms of neural damage include flexion, hyperextension, longitudinal distraction, and ischemia. There is reason to believe that flexion recoil can occur in young children but not in adolescents and young adults. In hyperextension, the cervical spine may have buckling of the ligamentum flavum resulting in a decreased sagittal diameter of the spinal canal. Hyperextension, in addition, can lead to spasm and compression of the vertebral arteries, which might lead to spinal cord ischemia and infarction. Flexion injuries tend to occur more commonly in the very young. Excessive distraction has been implicated as an important

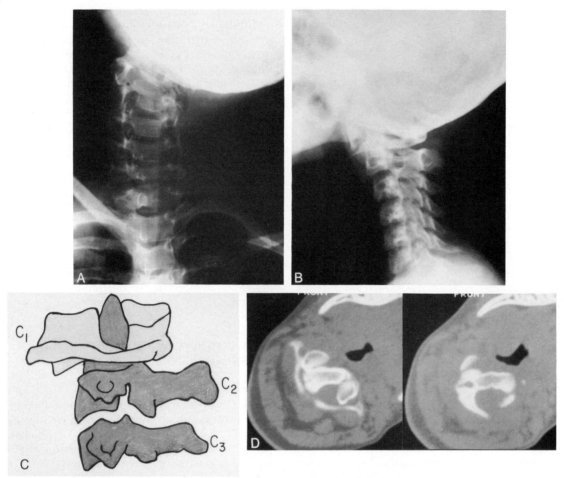

FIGURE 23–12. Rotatory atlantoaxial (C1–C2) luxation with bilateral facet interlock. This 10-year-old male was unable to "straighten" his neck and head after a motor vehicle accident. *A,* Anterior posterior view of neck showing acute head rotation and dislocation above the C2 vertebra. *B,* Lateral cervical spine x-ray. This reveals rotation of the head and C1 so as not to present a lateral view. The lateral mass of C1 is in the midline. *C,* Illustration of rotatory C1–C2 luxation with bilateral facet interlock. *D,* Composite of axial CT through C1 *(left)* and C2 *(right).* Note the facet interlock at C1 bilaterally. This was unchanged with the head turned to the right or left.

mechanism in regard to injuries at birth and in the young child. Leventhal described the pathologic anatomy of birth injuries and correlated these findings with the mechanism of injury.[34] He showed that the neonatal spine has sufficient elasticity to be stretched as much as 2 inches without being disrupted. However, the spinal cord and meninges can be stretched only one quarter of an inch before anatomic disruption occurs. Thus, problems are seen at the area where the dentate ligament first arises in the uppermost portion of the

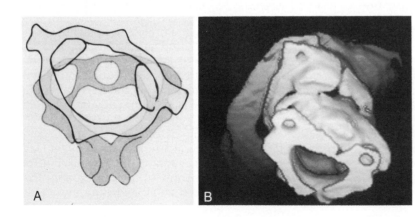

FIGURE 23–13. *A,* Illustration of unilateral interlock with C1–C2 rotational luxation. *B,* 3D CT scan of occiput–C1–C2–C3 in a 3-year-old child with C1–C2 rotatory luxation. There is a bifid anterior atlas arch with malalignment of the vertebral artery canal at C1–C2. The right lateral C1 mass is anterior to the right C2 facet.

cervical spine and the cervicothoracic junction relating to the tethering effect of the nerve roots.

Dickman et al. reviewed the literature on SCIWORA and were able to find reports of 201 cases, of which 104 had adequate data from which conclusions could be drawn.[105] They showed that cervical and thoracic injuries occurred with about equal frequency (44 per cent and 48 per cent, respectively). When one considers the length and the number of vertebrae in the cervical spine, it is injured disproportionately. Osenbach and Menezes (1991) reported on 31 children with SCIWORA, of which 26 (84 per cent) were affected in the cervical spine.[23] All upper cervical injuries occurred in children less than 8 years of age.

The neurologic injuries in young children with SCIWORA tend to be particularly severe, in contrast to teenagers and the occasional adult with SCIWORA, who tend to suffer milder central cord injuries. In 52 per cent of children with this form of injury, the onset of paralysis is delayed for as long as 4 days after injury, and most of these children recall transient paresthesias, numbness, and subjective motor loss. The neurologic examination at the time of initial evaluation reveals four individual syndromes: complete physiologic transection, central cord syndrome, Brown-Séquard syndrome, and a partial dysfunction of the spinal cord. In retrospect, a history of premonitory neurologic symptoms such as paresthesias or subjective feelings of weakness can be elicited. Indeed, any neurologic symptom, no matter how trivial, in a child with spinal injury must be taken seriously so as to avoid a potentially preventable disaster. In a significant number of football and gymnastic injuries, a burning sensation has been described by patients prior to the onset of neurologic devastation.

Magnetic resonance imaging has made the term SCIWORA inaccurate, although we believe the term is still useful in describing this type of injury (see Fig. 23–7). Fracture or instability has been excluded. Plain radiographs, including flexion-extension dynamic views, should be obtained. Multiplane or polytomography and thin-section CT scanning are essential to identify bony pathology as well as spinal alignment. Surgical lesions such as a herniated disc and epidural hematoma are excluded with magnetic resonance imaging.

It is not uncommon for children who are partially affected with neurologic dysfunction to have a recurrent episode a few weeks following the initial insult. For this reason, these children should be braced after the initial neurologic injury and kept so for 3 months so as to regain ligamentous stability. This particularly refers to the injuries affecting the cervical spinal cord.

COMPLICATIONS OF PEDIATRIC SPINAL CORD INJURY

Improvements in the acute and chronic care of children with paraplegia and quadriplegia have resulted in a significant increase in the number of those who survive to adulthood. Because of the increased life expectancy, attention has been directed to the complications of spinal cord injury. A large number of these problems are similar to those encountered in the adult. These include decubitus ulcers, genitourinary infections, pulmonary infections, myositis ossificans, and a variety of psychological problems. However, there are two complications that require mention and attention: post-traumatic spinal deformity and post-traumatic syringomyelia.

POST-TRAUMATIC SPINAL DEFORMITY

This problem is unique to the growing child. It is relatively uncommon in patients who are near the end of the growth period. The deformities encountered include scoliosis, kyphosis, and lordosis, each with a different etiology. The major factors that contribute to progressive spinal curvature are paralysis of the postural muscles of the spine below the level of the injury and epiphyseal damage to the growth plates, which interfere with the normal growth of the spine and lead to the development of scoliosis. Lesions caudal to T12–L1 are less likely to result in scoliosis because most of the postural muscles remain innervated. As the scoliotic curve develops, additional changes occur in the vertebral bodies. On the concave side of the curve, there is deficient growth of the lamina and the articular processes with excessive growth of the vertebral body and discs on the convex side.[126]

The incidence of progressive spinal deformity in series with pediatric spinal injury with long-term follow-up is high, exceeding 90 per cent in some cases.[127–132] Spinal curves may progress rapidly during the periods of growth. The development of a significant spinal deformity leads to pelvic obliquity and ischial weight bearing, which predisposes to decubitus ulcers. Curves that exceed 60 per cent may compromise cardiopulmonary function and result in intestinal and bladder dysfunction.

Age at the time of the injury seems to be the most important risk factor for the development of scoliosis. It is believed by most authors that in children with unstable thoracolumbar fractures and spinal cord injury, early instrumentation and fusion are indicated. In young children with complete spinal cord injury, one should consider extending the fusion several segments more than normally would be required for stability alone. External orthosis as a temporary means for delaying spinal fusion is acceptable, but is inadequate as a definitive treatment. Surgical fusion is required in the majority of children and will result in improved sitting balance in all cases.

POST-TRAUMATIC SYRINGOMYELIA

The development of a cyst or syrinx within the spinal cord following traumatic injury is a well-documented occurrence. Barnett et al.[133] reviewed 319 patients with post-traumatic paraplegia and documented clinical features suggestive of a syrinx in 1.8 per cent. This was in the pre-CT and pre-MRI era. Experimental studies in animals have documented the presence of myelin microcysts within the vicinity of the spinal cord transection. Kao et al. suggested that these microcysts rupture and coalesce to form the syrinx cavity.[134] They further postulated that syrinx formation appears to be associated with ineffective attempts at regeneration by the spinal cord. It is felt that tethering of the spinal cord at the site of injury, together with elevation of central venous pressure, will ultimately result in transmission of this elevation and pressure to the epidural veins. Subsequently, this alters the tension within the syrinx and leads to dilatation and extension of the cyst.[135–137]

Post-traumatic spinal cord cavitation may become clinically symptomatic relatively early following spinal cord injury. Alternatively, symptoms may be delayed in their onset for several years. The clinical onset is usually heralded by pain in the most rostral area of dysfunction. In many instances, pain may originate in the neck and radiate into the upper extremities. The pain is commonly exacerbated by sneezing or coughing. There is often an upward migration of the lowest area of hypesthesia. With progressive involvement of the cervical cord, weakness and atrophy involving the arm muscles develop and deep tendon reflexes become hypoactive. In patients with incomplete spinal cord lesions, the symptoms consist of increased weakness and spasticity, along with progressive loss of bowel, bladder, and sexual function. The cavity can extend into the rostral brainstem and lead to cranial nerve dysfunction or paroxysmal episodes of unconsciousness. Diagnosis is best made by means of magnetic resonance imaging, which accurately demonstrates the extent of the syrinx and effectively excludes other pathologic processes (Fig. 23–14).

Mere documentation of an asymptomatic post-traumatic syrinx is not an indication for surgery. The clinical symptoms are what should guide the physician in deciding whether or not an operative procedure is indicated. We prefer to perform a syringosubarachnoid shunt as the primary procedure for a post-traumatic syrinx. Intraoperative ultrasonography locates the syrinx cavity and the region of maximum dilatation. Placement of a syringosubarachnoid shunt requires meticulous attention to preservation of the arachnoid membrane during dural opening. The operating microscope facilitates the procedure and is imperative for the dissection. Median myelotomy is performed and a fine silicone catheter inserted cephalad for 2 to 3 cm into the cavity. The catheter is then anchored to the arachnoid at the myelotomy site and passed caudally into the subarachnoid space for several centimeters. The long-term follow-up in 14 patients with post-traumatic syringomyelia has shown improvement in 12.[138] In cases where there is significant arachnoiditis, a syringoperi-

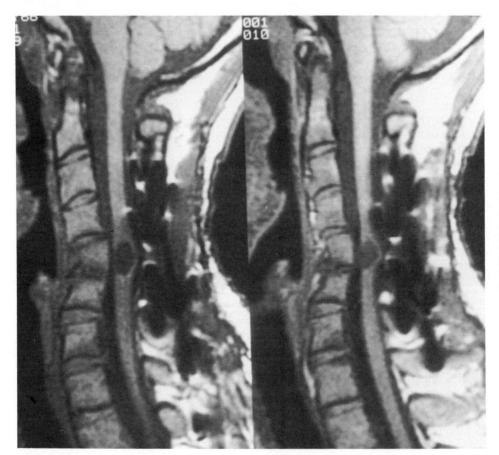

FIGURE 23–14. Midsagittal and parasagittal T1-weighted MRI of the cervical spine. This 21-year-old male presented with neck pain and hand paresthesias. He had sustained a C5 burst fracture at age 13 years and was treated with decompressive laminectomies and C3–C7 dorsolateral fusion. Note the intramedullary cavity at the C5 level.

toneal shunt is preferred. If pain persists despite the demonstration of compression of the syrinx on magnetic resonance imaging, a dorsal root entry zone lesion may be considered for pain control.[138]

SUMMARY

The pediatric spine and its supporting structures are in a process of progressive development and ossification. Specific pathologic states occur at different ages, and it is essential that one be familiar with this when treating a young individual with spine or spinal cord injury. The long-term management of paraplegic and quadriplegic children shares many of the problems seen in the adults so affected. Early recognition and treatment are imperative to prevent functional deformity.

REFERENCES

1. Kewalramani LS, Kraus JF, Sterling HIN: Acute spinal cord lesions in a pediatric population: Epidemiological and clinical features. Paraplegia 18:206, 1980.
2. Bracken MB, Freeman DH, Jr, Hellendrand KA: Incidence of acute traumatic hospitalized spinal cord injury in the United States, 1970–1977. Am J Epidemiol 113:615, 1981.
3. Bruce DA, Schut L, Sutton L: Brain and cervical spine injuries occurring during organized sports activities in children and adolescents. Primary Care 11:175, 1984.
4. Hadley MN, Zabramski JM, Browner CM, et al.: Pediatric spinal trauma. Review of 122 cases of spinal cord and vertebral column injuries. J Neurosurg 68:18, 1988.
5. Ruge JR, Sinson GP, McLone DG, et al.: Pediatric spinal injury: The very young. J Neurosurg 68:25, 1988.
6. Gelehrter G: Fracture of the vertebrae in children and adolescents. Arch Orthop Unfallchir 49:253, 1957.
7. Hubbard DD: Injuries of the spine in children and adolescents. Clin Orthop 100:56, 1974.
8. Papavasiliou V: Traumatic subluxation of the cervical spine during childhood. Orthop Clin North Am 9:945, 1978.
9. Sherk HH: Fractures of the odontoid process in young children. J Bone Joint Surg (Am) 60:921, 1978.
10. Hachen HJ: Spinal cord injury in children and adolescents. Diagnostic pitfalls in therapeutic considerations in the acute state. Paraplegia 15:55, 1977–1978.
11. Andrews LA, Jung SK: Spinal injury in children in British Columbia. Paraplegia 17:442, 1979.
12. Gehweiler JA, Osborne RL, Becker RF: Atlantoaxial rotatory fixation. In Gehweiler JA, et al.: The Radiology of Vertebral Trauma. Philadelphia, WB Saunders Co, 1980, pp 145–147.
13. Hill SA, Miller CA, Kosnik EJ, et al.: Pediatric neck injuries: A clinical study. J Neurosurg 60:700, 1984.
14. Anderson JM, Schutt AH: Spinal injury in children. A review of 156 cases seen from 1950 through 1980. Mayo Clin Proc 55:499, 1980.
15. Babcock JL: Cervical spine injuries. Diagnosis and classification. Arch Surg 111:646, 1976.
16. Burke DC: Traumatic spinal paralysis in children. Paraplegia 11:268, 1974.
17. Hause M, Hoshino R, Omata S, et al.: Cervical spine injuries in children. Fukushima J Med Sci 20:114, 1974.
18. McPhee IB: Spinal fractures and dislocations in children and adolescents. Spine 6:533, 1981.
19. Micheli LJ: Back injuries in gymnastics. Clin Sports Med 4:85, 1985.
20. Osenbach RK, Menezes AH: Pediatric spinal cord and vertebral column injury. Neurosurgery 30:385, 1992.
21. Lesoin F, Kabbaj K, Dhellemmes P, et al.: Fractures du rachis chez l'enfant. Problemes diagnostiques et therapeutiques. A propos de 67 observations. Neurochirurgie 30:289, 1984.
22. Kewalramani LS, Tori JA: Spinal cord trauma in children. Neurologic patterns, radiologic features, and pathomechanics of injury. Spine 5:11, 1980.
23. Osenbach RK, Menezes AH: Spinal cord injury without radiographic abnormality (SCIWORA) in children. Pediatr Neurosci 15:168, 1989.
24. Pang D, Wilberger JE, Jr.: Spinal cord injury without radiographic abnormalities in children. J Neurosurg 57:114, 1982.
25. Walsh JW, Stevens DB, Young BA: Traumatic paraplegia in children without contiguous spinal fracture or dislocation. Neurosurgery 12:439, 1983.
26. Melzak J. Paraplegia among children. Lancet ii:45, 1969.
27. Choi JU, Hoffman HJ, Hendrick EB, et al.: Traumatic infarction of the spinal cord in children. J Neurosurg 65:608, 1986.
28. Abroms IF, Bresnan MJ, Zukerman JE, et al.: Cervical cord injuries secondary to hyperextension of the head in breech presentation. Obstet Gynecol 41:369, 1973.
29. Aufdermaur M: Spinal injuries in juveniles. J Bone Joint Surg (Br) 3:513, 1974.
30. Byers RK: Spinal cord injuries during birth. Dev Med Child Neurol 17:103, 1975.
31. Franken EA: Spinal cord injury in the newborn infant. Pediatr Radiol 3:101, 1975.
32. Jones EL: Birth trauma and the cervical spine. Arch Dis Child 45:147, 1970.
33. Jones ET, Hensinger RN: C2-C3 dislocation in a child. J Pediatr Orthop 1:419, 1981.
34. Leventhal HR: Birth injuries of the spinal cord. J Pediatr 56:447, 1960.
35. Towbin A: Latent spinal cord and brain stem injury in newborn infants. Dev Med Child Neurol 11:54, 1969.
36. Campbell J, Bonnett C: Spinal cord injury in children. Clin Orthop 112:114, 1975.
37. Campbell JB, DeCrescito V, Tomasula JJ, et al: Effects of antifibrinolytic and steroid therapy on the contused spinal cord of cats. J Neurosurg 40:726, 1974.
38. Dunlap JP, Morris M, Thompson RG: Cervical spine injuries in children. J Bone Joint Surg (Am) 40:681, 1958.
39. Ewald FC: Fracture of the odontoid process in a seventeen month infant treated with a halo. J Bone Joint Surg (Am) 53:1636, 1971.
40. Gaufin LM, Goodman SJ: Cervical spine injuries in infants. Problems in management. J Neurosurg 42:179, 1975.
41. Marlin AE, Williams GR, Lee JF: Jefferson fractures in children. Case report. J Neurosurg 58:277, 1983.
42. Weiss MH, Kaufman B: Hangman's fracture in an infant. Am J Dis Child 126:268, 1973.
43. Allen JP: Birth injury to spinal cord. Northwest Med 69:323, 1970.
44. Bell HJ, Dykstra DO: Somatosensory evoked potentials as an adjunct to diagnosis of neonatal spinal cord injury. J Pediatr 106:298, 1985.
45. Stern WE, Rand RW: Birth injuries to the spinal cord. A report of 2 cases and review of the literature. Am J Obstet Gynecol 78:498, 1959.
46. Glasauer FE, Cares HL: Traumatic paraplegia in infancy. JAMA 219:38, 1972.
47. Glasauer FE, Cares HL: Biomechanical features of traumatic paraplegia in infancy. J Trauma 13:166, 1973.
48. LeBlanc JH, Nadell J: Spinal cord injuries in children. Surg Neurol 2:411, 1974.
49. Gilles FH, Bina M, Sotrel A: Infantile atlantooccipital instability. Am J Dis Child 133:30, 1979.
50. Schneider RC, Crosby EC: Vascular insufficiency of brain stem and spinal cord in spinal trauma. Neurology (Minneap) 9:63, 1959.
51. Turnbull LM: Microvasculature of the human spinal cord. J Neurosurg 35:141, 1971.
52. Yates DO: Birth trauma to the vertebral arteries. Arch Dis Child 311:436, 1959.
53. Bailey DK: The normal cervical spine in infants and children. Radiology 59:712, 1952.

54. Bailey RW, Badgeby CE: Stabilization of the cervical spine by anterior fusion. J Bone Joint Surg 42:565, 1960.

55. Vigouroux RP, Baurand C, Choux M, et al.: Les traumatismes du rachis cervical chez l'enfant. Neurochirurgie 14:689, 1968.

56. Von Torklus D, Gehle W: The upper cervical spine. Regional anatomy, pathology and traumatology. In Verlag GT (ed): A Systemic Radiological Atlas and Textbook. New York, Grune & Stratton, 1972, pp 2–91.

57. Silverman FN, Kaltan KR: Trauma and non-trauma of the cervical spine in pediatric patients. In Kattan KR (ed): Trauma and No Trauma of the Cervical Spine. Springfield, Ill, Charles C Thomas, 1975, pp 206–241.

58. Caffey J: The whiplash-shaken infant syndrome. Manual shaking by the extremities with whiplash-induced intracranial and intraocular bleedings, linked with residual premanent brain damage and mental retardation. Pediatrics 54:396, 1974.

59. Cattell HS, Filtzer DL: Pseudosubluxation and other normal variations in the cervical spine in children. J Bone Joint Surg 47:1295, 1965.

60. Menezes AH: Traumatic lesions of the craniovertebral junction. In VanGilder JC, Menezes AH, Dolan K (eds): Textbook of Craniovertebral Junction Abnormalities. Mount Kisco, Futura Publishing Company, 1987, pp 1–255.

61. White AA, III, Panjabi MM: The clinical biomechanics of the occipito-atlantoaxial complex. Orthop Clin North Am 9:867, 1978.

62. Griffiths SC: Fracture of the odontoid process in children. J Pediatr Surg 7:680, 1972.

63. Holmes JC, Hall JE: Fusion for instability and potential instability of the cervical spine in children and adolescents. Orthop Clin North Am 9:923, 1978.

64. Menezes AH, Piper JG: Anatomy and radiographic pathology of injury to the occipito-atlanto-axial complex. In Wilkins RH (ed): AANS Publication. Baltimore, Williams & Wilkins, 1992.

65. Fielding JW, Stillwell WT, Chynn KY, et al.: Use of computed tomography for the diagnosis of atlanto-axial rotatory fixation. A case report. J Bone Joint Surg (Am) 60:1102, 1978.

66. Barnett E, Nairn A: A study of fetal attitude. Br J Radiol 38:338, 1965.

67. Knowlton RW: A flying faetus. J Obstet Gynaecol Br Emp 45:834, 1938.

68. Evarts CM: Traumatic occipito-atlantal dislocation. Report of a case with survival. J Bone Joint Surg (Am) 52:1653, 1970.

69. Fielding JW, Hawkins RJ: Atlanto-axial rotatory fixation. J Bone Joint Surg (Am) 59:37, 1977.

70. Hawkins RJ, Fielding JW, Thompson WJ: Os Odontoideum: Congenital or acquired. J Bone Joint Surg (Am) 58:413, 1976.

71. Kalsbeck WD, McLaurin RL, Harris BS, III, et al.: The national spinal cord injury survey: Major findings. J Neurosurg 53:19, 1980.

72. Riccardi JE, Kaufer H, Louis DS: Acquired os odontoideum following acute ligament injury. J Bone Joint Surg (Am) 58:410, 1976.

73. Bates D, Ruggierri P: Imaging modalities for evaluation of the spine. Radiol Clinic North Am 29:675, 1991.

74. Beers GJ, Ragne GH, Wagner GG: MR imaging in acute cervical spine trauma. J Comput Assist Tomogr 12:755, 1988.

75. Schaeffer DM, Flanders AE, Osterholm JL, et al.: Prognostic significance of magnetic resonance imaging in the acute phase of cervical spine injury. J Neurosurg 76:218, 1992.

76. Bohlman H: Treatment of fractures and dislocations of the thoracic and lumbar spine. J Bone Joint Surg (Am) 57:165, 1985.

77. Ducker TB, Kindt GW, Kempe LG: Pathological findings in acute experimental spinal cord trauma. J Neurosurg 35:700, 1971.

78. Holdsworth F: Fractures, dislocations and fracture-dislocations of the spine. J Bone Joint Surg (Am) 52:1534, 1971.

79. Seljeskog EL: Thoracolumbar injuries. Clin Neurosurg 30:626, 1983.

80. Venes JL: Spinal cord injury. In McLaurin RL (ed): Pediatric Neurosurgery. New York, Grune & Stratton, 1982, pp 333–343.

81. Tator CH, Fehlings MG: Review of the secondary injury theory of acute spinal cord trauma with emphasis on vascular mechanisms. J Neurosurg 75:15, 1991.

82. de La Torre JC: Spinal cord injury: Review of basic and applied research. Spine 6:315, 1981.

83. Ducker TB, Lucas J, Wallace CA: Recovery from spinal cord injury. Clin Neurosurg 30:495, 1983.

84. Faden AI, Jacobs TP, Mougey E, et al.: Endorphins in experimental spinal injury: Therapeutic effect of naloxone. Ann Neurol 10:326, 1981.

85. Faden AI, Jacobs TP, Mougey E, et al.: Opiate antagonist improves neurological recovery after spinal injury. Science 211:493, 1981.

86. Flamm ES, Young W, Collins WF, et al.: A phase I trial of naloxone treatment in acute spinal cord injury. J Neurosurg 63:390, 1985.

87. Gerber AM, Olson WL, Harris JH: Effect of phenytoin on functional recovery after experimental spinal cord injury in dogs. Neurosurgery 7:472, 1980.

88. Means ED, Anderson DK, Waters TR, et al.: Effect of methylprednisolone in compression trauma to the feline spinal cord. J Neurosurg 55:200, 1981.

89. Senter JH, Venes JL: Loss of autoregulation and post-traumatic ischemia following experimental spinal cord trauma. J Neurosurg 50:198, 1979.

90. Taylor S, Ashby P, Verrier M: Neurophysiological changes following traumatic spinal lesions in man. J Neurol Neurosurg Psychiatry 47:1102, 1984.

91. Tator CH: Spine-spinal cord relationships in spinal cord trauma. Clin Neurosurg 30:479, 1983.

92. Wagner FC, VanGilder JC, Dohrmann GJ: Pathological changes from acute to chronic in experimental spinal cord trauma. J Neurosurg 48:92, 1978.

93. Wallace MC, Tator CH, Frazee P: Relationship between post-traumatic ischemia and hemorrhage in the injured rat spinal cord as shown by colloidal carbon angiography. Neurosurgery 18:43, 1986.

94. Guha A, Tator CH, Piper I: Effect of a calcium channel blocker on post-traumatic spinal cord blood flow. J Neurosurg 66:423, 1987.

95. Panjabi MM, Thibodeau LL, Crisco JJ: What constitutes spinal instability. Clin Neurosurg 34:314, 1988.

96. Dohrmann GJ, Wick KM, Bucy PC: Spinal cord blood flow patterns in experimental traumatic paraplegia. J Neurosurg 38:52, 1973.

97. Osterholm JL: The pathophysiological response to spinal cord injury. J Neurosurg 40:5, 1974.

98. Pincus JH, Lee S: Diphenylhydantoin and calcium: Relation to norepinephrine release from brain slices. Arch Neurol 29:239, 1973.

99. Hall ED, Braughler JM: Glucocorticoid mechanism in acute spinal cord injury. A review and therapeutic rationale. Surg Neurol 18:320, 1982.

100. Bracken MB, Collins WF, Freeman DF, et al.: Efficacy of methylprednisolone in acute spinal cord injury. JAMA 251:45, 1984.

101. Bracken MB, Shepard MJ, Hellendrand KA, et al: Methylprednisolone and neurological function 1 year after spinal cord injury. Results of the National Acute Spinal Cord Injury Study. J Neurosurg 63:704, 1985.

102. Bracken MB, Shepard MJ, Collins WF, et al.: A randomized, controlled trial of methylprednisolone or naloxone in the treatment of acute spinal cord injury. Results of the Second National Acute Spinal Cord Injury Study. New Engl J Med 322:1405, 1990.

103. Bracken MB, Shepard MJ, Collins WF, et al.: Methylprednisolone or naloxone treatment after acute spinal cord injury: 1-year follow-up data. J Neurosurg 76:23, 1992.

104. Hamilton AJ, McBlack P, Carr DB: Contrasting actions of naloxone in experimental spinal cord trauma and cerebral ischemia: A review. Neurosurgery 17:845, 1985.

105. Dickman CA, Rekate HL, Sonntag VKH, et al.: Pediatric spinal trauma: Vertebral column and spinal cord injuries in children. Pediatr Neurosci 15:237, 1989.

106. Karnaze MG, Gado MH, Sartor KJ: Comparison of MR and CT myelography in imaging the cervical and thoracic spine. AJR 150:397, 1988.

107. Menezes AH, Godersky JC, Smoker WRK: Spinal cord injury. *In* McLaurin RL, Schut L, Venes JL, Epstein F (eds): Pediatric Neurosurgery: Surgery of the Developing Nervous System, 2nd ed. Philadelphia, WB Saunders, 1989, pp 198–317.

108. Atlas SW, Regenbogen V, Rogers LF, et al.: The radiographic characterization of burst fractures of the spine. AJR 7:675, 1986.

109. Babcock JL: Spinal injuries in children. Pediatr Clin North Am 22:487, 1975.

110. Berquist TH: Imaging of adult cervical spine trauma. Radiographics 8:667, 1988.

111. Koch BM, Eng GM: Neonatal spinal cord injury. Arch Phys Med Rehabil 60:378, 1979.

112. Cloward RB: Treatment of acute fractures and fracture-dislocations of the cervical spine by vertebral bony fusion. J Neurosurg 18:201, 1961.

113. Roy L, Gibson A: Cervical spine fusions in children. Clin Orthop 73:146, 1970.

114. Wickboldt J, Sorensen N: Anterior cervical fusion after traumatic dislocation of the cervical spine in childhood and adolescence. Childs Brain 4:120, 1978.

115. Dzilba RB, Gervin AI: Irreversible spinal deformity in Olympic gymnasts. Annual meeting, American Orthopaedic Society for Sports Medicine, Anaheim, California, March, 1983.

116. Garrick JA, Requa RK: Injuries in high school sports. Pediatrics 61:465, 1978.

117. Paul RL, Michael RH, Dunn JE, et al.: Anterior transthoracic surgical decompression of acute spinal cord injuries. J Neurosurg 43:299, 1975.

118. Menezes AH, Muhonen M: Management of occipito-cervical instability. *In* Cooper PR (ed): Neurosurgical Topics, vol. 1. Baltimore, Williams & Wilkins, 1990, pp 65–76.

119. Bucholz RW, Burkhead WF: The pathological anatomy of fatal atlanto-occipital dislocations. J Bone Joint Surg (Am) 61:248, 1979.

120. Pang D, Wilberger JE: Traumatic atlanto-occipital dislocation with survival: Case report and review. Neurosurgery 7:503, 1980.

121. Powers B, Miller MD, Kramer RS, et al.: Traumatic anterior atlanto-occipital dislocation. Neurosurgery 4:12, 1979.

122. Sullivan CR, Bruwer AJ, Harris LE: Hypermobility of the cervical spine in children. A pitfall in the diagnosis of cervical dislocation. Am J Surg 95:636, 1958.

123. Selecki BR: The effects of rotation of the atlas on the axis. Experimental work. Med J Aust 1:1012, 1969.

124. Ahmann PA, Smith SA, Schwartz JF, et al.: Spinal cord infarction due to minor trauma in children. Neurology 25:301, 1975.

125. Kraus JF: Epidemiological aspects of acute spinal cord injury: A review of incidence, prevalence, causes, and outcome. *In* Becker DP, Povlishock JT (eds): Central Nervous System Trauma Status Report. Bethesda, National Institute of Neurological and Communicative Disorders and Stroke, National Institutes of Health, 1985, pp 313–322.

126. Roaf R: Scoliosis secondary to paraplegia. Paraplegia 8:42, 1970.

127. Banniza VB, Paeslack UK: Scoliotic growth in children with acquired paraplegia. Paraplegia 11:277, 1974.

128. Bedbrook GM: Correction of scoliosis due to paraplegia sustained in paediatric age group. Paraplegia 14:90, 1977–1978.

129. Bradford DS: Deformities of the thoracic and lumbar spine secondary to spinal injury. *In* Bradford DS, Lonstein JE, Moe JH, Oglivie JW, Winter RB (eds): Moe's Textbook of Scoliosis and Other Spinal Deformities, 2nd ed. Philadelphia, WB Saunders, 1987, pp 435–463.

130. Kilfoyle RM, Foley JJ, Norton PL: Spine and pelvic deformity in childhood and adolescent paraplegia. A study of 104 cases. J Bone Joint Surg (Am) 47:659, 1965.

131. Lancourt JE, Dickson JH, Carter RE: Paralytic spinal deformity following traumatic spinal cord injury in children and adolescents. J Bone Joint Surg (Am) 63:47, 1981.

132. Mayfield JK, Erkkila JC, Winter RB: Spine deformity subsequent to acquired childhood spinal cord injury. Am Acad Orthop Surgeons 3:281, 1979.

133. Barnett HJM, Bottrell EH, Jouse AT, et al.: Progressive myelopathy as a sequel to traumatic paraplegia. Brain 89:159, 1966.

134. Kao CC, Chang LW, Bloodworth JR: The mechanism of spinal cord cavitation following spinal cord transection. J Neurosurg 46:745, 1977.

135. Gabriel KR, Crawford AH: Identification of acute post-traumatic spinal cord cyst by magnetic resonance imaging: A case report and review of the literature. J Pediatr Orthop 8:710, 1988.

136. McComas DF, Frost JL, Schochet SS: Post-traumatic syringomyelia with paroxysmal episodes of unconsciousness. Arch Neurol 40:322, 1983.

137. Shannon N, Symon L, Logue A, et al.: Clinical features, investigation and treatment of post-traumatic syringomyelia. J Neurol Neurosurg Psychiatry 44:35, 1981.

138. Menezes AH, Smoker WRK, Dyste GN: Syringomyelia, Chiari malformations and hydromyelia. *In* Youmans J (ed): Textbook of Neurological Surgery, 3rd ed. Philadelphia, WB Saunders Co, 1990, pp 1421–1459.

Chapter 24

PERIPHERAL NERVE INJURIES

JOHN P. LAURENT, M.D.

Although many peripheral nerve lesions seen in adults are also seen in children, this chapter will deal only with common pediatric peripheral nerve injuries. Injection and traction injuries occur more frequently in children than in adults.

PATHOPHYSIOLOGY

Seddon's classification of traumatic nerve injuries is universally accepted.[1] *Neurapraxia* is a temporary block in nerve conduction without transection; full recovery is expected. *Axonotmesis* is a nerve lesion in which axons are interrupted while the nerve sheath remains intact; recovery is possible with axon regeneration. *Neurotmesis* (rupture) is the interruption of both the neuron sheath and the axons; recovery is likely to be incomplete because proximal axon sprouting may not reach the distal stump. *Avulsion* occurs when nerve rootlets are traumatically detached from the spinal cord; no recovery may be expected. Various combinations of these lesions are typically present following traumatic nerve injuries.

Regeneration of a nerve is usually more successful the less distance there is between the regeneration site and the organ. In neurotmesis, antegrade (wallerian) degeneration occurs at the distal stump. The lag time between rupture and the onset of distal degeneration varies with fiber type; the thin fibers begin to degenerate in 24 hours, whereas deterioration of the thick fibers begins 48 hours after injury.[2] The rate of distal wallerian degeneration of thin fibers is approximately 250 mm/day, and of thick fibers, 45 mm/day. Dissolution of the myelin sheath follows degeneration.

Concurrent with distal degeneration of axons and myelin sheaths, Schwann cells increase in number, arranging themselves in longitudinal columns and eventually demarcating the distal nerve stump. If no axonal regeneration from the proximal stump occurs through these columns of Schwann cells, they will reduce in size by 50 per cent during the first year and continue to decrease thereafter. In the absence of Schwann cell columns, regeneration of neuronal sprouts into the distal nerve sheath will be incomplete.

As antegrade (wallerian) degeneration continues, retrograde degeneration to the first nodal site occurs, demarcating the proximal nerve stump. Regeneration of the proximal stump begins at 10 to 21 days; this is called the growth bulb and is composed of axonal sprouts. For regeneration to be successful, it is critical that the axonal sprouts from the growth bulb reach the distal stump and be guided by the longitudinal Schwann cell columns to the end organ. The rate of axonal regeneration fluctuates between 1 and 5 mm/day, depending on several factors.[3] Regeneration is most rapid proximally, closest to the neuronal cell body, and slows as distance from the cell body increases. Neuronal function reestablishes rapidly in children, and regeneration, particularly in the very young child, is thought to occur at a rate of as much as 5 mm/day.

Structural changes to end organs denervated for 12 months or more preclude successful functional reinnervation.[4] This depends to some extent on the volume of nerve fibers reaching a functional distal organ. A neuroma forms when the axonal sprouts from the growth bulb fail to properly reach the distal stump. Neuroma incontinuity occurs when axonal sprouts partially exit the damaged nerve sheath and fail to re-enter the distal stump. Grafting can provide a Schwann cell tube for the proximal sprouting of axons to grow to the Schwann cell columns of the distal nerve.

INVESTIGATION

Radiologic studies should routinely be done on children with suspected peripheral nerve injuries. Dia-

344

phragm function studies and spinal and pelvic roentgenograms will show fractures or dislocations and help to determine the etiology of a particular peripheral nerve injury or palsy. Magnetic resonance imaging (MRI) of the spine and peripheral nerves has not been especially helpful in delineating peripheral nerve lesions. In a cohort of 20 infants (<5 months) undergoing surgery for brachial plexus lesions at Texas Children's Hospital, MRIs of the cervical spine were compared with computerized tomography (CT) myelograms. The CT myelograms consistently defined nerve root lesions better than the MRIs. A comparison between operative evoked potentials for individual nerve roots and CT myelogram findings demonstrated a correlation coefficient for pseudomeningocele (0.8) and avulsed nerve rootlets (0.9). CT myelograms serve to confirm clinical suspicions (Fig. 24–1).

Electrophysiologic studies (EMG, nerve conduction studies, H-reflexes, and evoked responses), which confirm a preoperative impression, do not alter the preoperative management. Clinical functional improvement may not correspond to electrical improvement. Electrophysiologic studies, on the other hand, are extremely useful intraoperatively in delineating and clarifying the anatomic dissection.

It is important that anesthesia personnel be experienced with intraoperative analgesia and anesthetic medications that will not interfere with the ability to perform EMGs, nerve conduction studies, and evoked responses on the operating table. Intravenous access may be limited to one limb if the other limbs are used for harvesting nerve grafts. A neuroma incontinuity is the most difficult lesion to assess without electrophysiologic studies. A decrease in amplitude of 50 per cent of the stimulated EMG of a particular muscle across the neuroma suggests that conduction through the nerve is inadequate and that the neuroma incontinuity should be excised. Intraoperative evoked responses to the biparietal areas and C1–C2 are necessary to diagnose nerve rootlet avulsions. The C1–C2 response is important in neonates, since myelination may not have progressed sufficiently for a parietal response. Evoked responses should be correlated with CT myelograms.

INTERVENTION

Timing for operative intervention is determined by injury type. *Immediate exploration* is indicated for a sharp laceration with no other injury. *Delayed exploration* (<4 months) is indicated when other injuries take precedence over the nerve injury. *Late exploration* (>4 months) is indicated in those patients for whom recovery is a possibility; such lesions are usually caused by fractures, blunt trauma, traction injuries, or injection injuries. Late exploration is also recommended when recovery is partial. Partial recovery of function may lead to misplaced confidence on the part of parents and physician; one element of the nerve lesion may have recovered while others remain injured. Functionality of the end organ should be the primary consideration.

CLINICAL EVALUATION

The neurologic evaluation is of primary importance in diagnosing a pediatric peripheral nerve injury. In a child older than 6 years of age, this examination is similar to that performed in adults. Evaluation of a younger child, however, may well require lengthy observation and reward-based induced movements.

TREATMENT

The surgical techniques available include internal and external neurolysis, nerve grafting, primary anastomosis, and excision or reduction of neuroma incontinuity. Each of these methods has been extensively

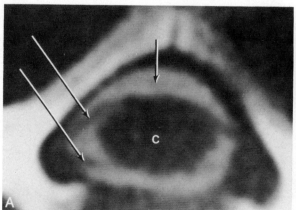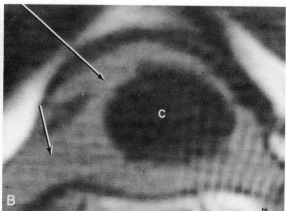

FIGURE 24–1. CT-metrizamide-myelograms. *A,* Normal C–5 level. Subarachnoid space *(short arrow),* nerve rootlets *(long arrow),* spinal cord (c). *B,* Abnormal C–7 level. Pseudomeningocele *(short arrow),* nerve rootlet avulsion *(long arrow),* spinal cord (c).

discussed in the literature and will not be reviewed in this chapter.[5]

Although physiotherapy does not aid in nerve regeneration, it is strongly recommended as a means of preventing contractures. Neonates who have sustained nerve injuries should begin physiotherapy 10 to 14 days following the injury or surgery.

Reconstructive surgery involving tendon and muscle transfers is in the armamentarium of both orthopedic and plastic surgeons; such procedures may be used to treat old injuries or instances of failed regeneration. A review of the plastic surgery and orthopedic literature reveals many accounts of successful muscle and tendon transfers.[5]

LESIONS OF THE CERVICAL NERVES

PHRENIC NERVE

Phrenic nerve paralysis at birth from bilateral brachial plexus injury has been observed in three of the 70 brachial plexus explorations completed at Texas Children's Hospital. These three infants and those with phrenic nerve damage secondary to cardiac surgery have undergone direct intercostal-phrenic nerve grafts, which have been remarkably successful. Normal diaphragmatic movement has been recovered unilaterally, allowing these children to be weaned from respirators (Fig. 24–2).

SPINAL ACCESSORY NERVE

Although the spinal accessory nerve is not a true peripheral nerve but a cranial nerve, it is considered in the context of pediatric peripheral nerve injuries because of the frequency of lymph node biopsies in children. The lateral triangle of the neck, where the lymph nodes are located, is the distal site of the spinal accessory nerve. Injury to this nerve may paralyze the trapezius and sternocleidomastoid muscles, causing a disfiguring shoulder drop. The anatomy of the spinal accessory nerve has been well described in anatomy texts.[6] Aside from injuries occurring in the course of lymph node biopsies, spinal accessory nerve lesions are seldom seen in children. Because the prognosis for these lesions is poor, intervention is indicated. Retraction of the proximal and distal nerve portions following injury makes primary anastomosis difficult. Electrical stimulation aids in locating the nerve ends so that nerve grafts can be inserted.

BRACHIAL PLEXUS

Brachial plexus injuries represent the peripheral nerve injury most frequently seen by the pediatric neurosurgeon; the incidence of birth-related brachial plexus injury is 1/1000 live births (Fig. 24–3). The incidence of these injuries is higher in the delivery room than at discharge from the hospital because many children are "cured" prior to being seen by a consultant. We at Texas Children's Hospital have followed more than 300 birth-related brachial plexus injuries. Of these infants, 70 required surgical intervention for such lesions as nerve root avulsion, neuroma, neuroma incontinuity, and neurotmesis (rupture). Those children with axonotmesis and neuropraxic lesions usually recover within 4 to 6 months and do not require surgery. Kline et al. have described the treatment and prognosis for older individuals with brachial plexus injuries.[7]

A dominant lesion (upper, lower, or combined) will be established in an infant with birth-related brachial plexus injury by 8 weeks after delivery. Upper and combined lesions are more common than lower plexus injuries. Neurologic improvement occurs in 2 to 3 months in 90 per cent of infants with birth-related brachial plexus injuries and in 4 to 5 months in 98 per

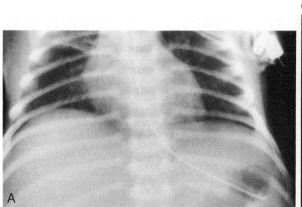
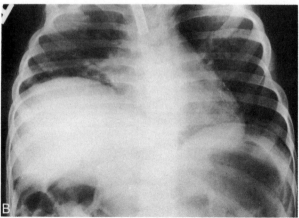

FIGURE 24–2. Types of birth injury lesions to the brachial plexus. *A,* Chest roentgenogram of bilateral combined brachial plexus birth injury with bilateral diaphragmatic palsy (inspiration). *B,* Nine months postoperative chest roentgenogram in same child following intercostal sural graft phrenic repair on left side with functional diaphragm (inspiration).

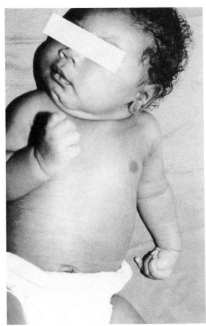

FIGURE 24–3. Upper brachial plexus birth injury (C5–C6–C7). Classic appearance of "Erb's palsy" "waiter's tip" position.

cent of these infants. The neurologic examination is the primary means of determining whether surgery should be considered. Although CT myelograms and electromyography usually confirm the neurologic examination, they are not regarded as indicators for surgical intervention. The operative window for birth-related brachial plexus injuries is similar to that for traumatic brachial plexus injuries occurring later in life, i.e., 4 to 6 months after injury if no functional recovery is observed.

The 75 infants in our study with upper plexus injuries who demonstrated no neurologic improvement by 4 to 6 months of age showed 90 per cent improvement 9 months after surgery ($p < .05$). The operative procedures in order of frequency included nerve grafting, excision of neuroma incontinuity, and neurolysis.

RADIAL NERVE

The radial nerve is the largest branch of the brachial plexus and innervates the dorsal extensors of the arms and hands. Its circular course along the dorsal aspect of the humerus renders it vulnerable to injury during mid and upper humeral fractures. Anatomic descriptions abound in the literature.[6]

Proximal radial nerve injury causes tricep weakness; the injury is neuropraxic and recovery is expected. Proximal lesions of the radial nerve in children can be caused by the use of crutches. Radial nerve palsy secondary to fracture of the shaft of the humerus is usually neuropraxic and begins at the time of fracture. Recovery is often complete by 2 to 3 months after injury. If there is slow or continued paralysis 3 to 4 months after

injury, the lesion should be explored for scarring or bony callous formation around the nerve. Nerve grafting is seldom required.

LESIONS OF THE LUMBOSACRAL NERVES

SCIATIC NERVE

The sciatic nerve, formed by the L4 through S3 nerve roots, leaves the pelvis through the intrapiriform foramen and is the longest peripheral nerve in the body. Two distinct nerve bundles (the tibial and peroneal) can be discerned along the initial course of the nerve, which is covered by the gluteus maximus muscle. Loose adipose tissue around the nerve contains an abundance of arteries and veins; this subgluteal segment may contain loculi of hematomas and infections. Inappropriately placed injection solutions in this area endanger the sciatic nerve, which continues on to the popliteal fossa and its divisions. The vascular supply of the proximal portion of the sciatic nerve is through the branches of the inferior gluteal artery, which anastomoses distally with the circumflex artery of the femur. Umbilical artery catheters in neonates may extend into the inferior gluteal artery.

The sciatic nerve provides motor innervation for the hamstring muscles of the thigh and all the muscles of the lower leg and foot. The peroneal portion of the sciatic nerve is affected more frequently than the tibial portion. The greater susceptibility of the peroneal segment is related to its fewer nerve bundles and lesser vascularity. Poor vascular supply to the peroneal portion of the sciatic nerve has been demonstrated in animal experiments in which the lower aorta is compressed, producing peroneal palsy.[8]

Sciatic nerve injuries in children have been seen following gunshot injuries and orthopedic procedures for fractures of the femoral neck and hip dislocations. The most likely pathogenesis is neuropraxic injury to the nerve, and the prognosis is good without surgical intervention. If recovery is not apparent in 4 to 6 months after injury, exploration is indicated.

Hemorrhage into the ischial musculature near the sciatic nerve, sometimes caused by anticoagulation problems in chemotherapy for tumors and by trauma to the gluteal muscle, can be responsible for sciatic nerve paresis. Most such hemorrhages will be demonstrated on computerized tomography. Interventional therapy depends upon the patient's general medical condition.

Tumors arising from the sciatic nerve outside the intrapiriform foramen have been described; these tumors occur more commonly in the thigh than in the gluteal area. Approximately 20 per cent of these are neurofibromas, 20 per cent are schwannomas, and the remaining 60 per cent are highly malignant neurofibrosarcomas.[9] CT scan and MRI are helpful in diagnosis. Surgical intervention is not likely to aid the child.

Pressure palsies of the sciatic nerve have been described in children and more commonly involve the peroneal portion of the nerve than the tibial. One account deals with a 10-year-old who sat for a long period of time on a stone step; the resulting pressure palsy was treated conservatively, and the child had functional recovery 9 months after the injury.[10]

Damage to the sciatic nerve may be caused by direct parenteral injection into the gluteal area or through the umbilical artery. If the injection reaches the subgluteal adipose space, gluteal skin necrosis may result. Damage usually involves the proximal portion of the sciatic nerve. If function fails to return in 4 to 6 months, exploration to assess the degree of damage should be carried out. A typical presentation of this type of nerve injury involved a premature neonate with an umbilical artery catheter who had had an intra-arterial injection that resulted in complete gluteal skin necrosis and sciatic nerve damage. Exploration of the gluteal segment of the nerve when the infant was 5 months old revealed normal distal conduction to all muscles supplied by the sciatic nerve. Evoked response showed a proximal lesion. Exploration of the pelvic fossa demonstrated damage at the sciatic nerve rootlets, and an intercostal graft to the gluteal portion of the nerve was performed.

TERMINAL BRANCHES OF THE SCIATIC NERVE

The sciatic nerve has two major divisions, the common peroneal nerve and the tibial nerve, which appear to be individual bundles as far proximal as the original tract of the sciatic nerve. The common peroneal nerve is more frequently injured than the tibial nerve. It exits the popliteal fossa and divides at the head of the fibula into the superficial and deep peroneal nerves. A more detailed description can be found in most anatomy texts.[6]

Tibial Nerve

The tibial nerve supplies the posterior tibialis and gastrocnemius muscles for plantar flexion of the foot. Tibial nerve injuries, other than those associated with proximal traumatic nerve injuries, are uncommon in children and will not be discussed.

Common Peroneal Nerve

Pressure on the lateral head of the fibula as the nerve crosses and divides into the deep and superficial peroneal nerves is the most usual cause of common peroneal nerve palsy. This injury is seen in children playing on a gym set or performing cartwheels. The lesion is probably neuropraxic with a good prognosis; surgical exploration is not helpful.

Arthroscopy of the knee can cause damage to the common peroneal nerve at the incision site. Exploration is indicated if neurologic function does not return

4 to 6 months post-arthroscopy. Primary nerve anastomosis, neurolysis, or grafting procedure is the treatment of choice. Prognosis for this type of common peroneal nerve injury is guarded; only 30 per cent of patients will experience some return of function following surgical exploration.[11]

DEEP AND SUPERFICIAL PERONEAL NERVES

Injury to the deep and/or superficial peroneal nerves commonly manifests as anterior compartment syndrome. The muscles in the anterior tibial compartment (e.g., tibialis anterior, extensor hallucis longus, extensorum digitorum longus) are tightly surrounded by connective and osseous tissue. Edema may develop within these compartments as a result of overexertion. This is particularly common in children who have increased their school sports activity level (e.g., soccer). A cycle consisting of edema followed by compression followed by more edema may be established and result in damage to these two nerves. Treatment is surgical splitting of the anterior fascia. The prognosis for recovery is less than 30 per cent.

SUMMARY

The pediatric neurosurgeon needs to take a more active role in the surgical exploration of peripheral nerve and brachial plexus injuries. Encouraged by a better understanding of the published data from both prospective and retrospective studies, non-neurologically trained surgeons have become involved in the treatment of these conditions. It is important that pediatric neurosurgery maintain a dominant role in treating such neurologic disorders.

REFERENCES

1. Seddon HJ: Surgical Disorders of Peripheral Nerves. 2nd ed. London, Churchill, 1975.
2. Gutmann E, Holubar J: The degeneration of peripheral nerve fibers. J Neurol Neurosurg Psychiatry 13:89, 1950.
3. Lubinska L: Early course of wallerian degeneration in myelinated fibers of the rat phrenic nerve. Brain Res 130:47, 1977.
4. Sunderland SRD: Nerve and Nerve Injuries. 2nd ed. Edinburgh, Livingstone, 1978.
5. Terzis JK: Microreconstruction of Nerve Injuries. Philadelphia, WB Saunders Company, 1987.
6. Carpenter MB: Human Neuroanatomy. 7th ed. Baltimore, Williams & Wilkins, 1976.
7. Kline DG, Judice DJ: Operative management of selected brachial plexus lesions. J Neurosurg 58:631, 1983.
8. Mumenthaler M, Schliack H: Peripheral Nerve Lesions. New York, Thieme Medical Publishers, Inc., 1991.
9. Thomas JE, Piepgras DG, Scheithauer B, et al.: Neurogenic tumors of the sciatic nerve. Mayo Clin Proc 58:640, 1983.
10. Deverell MW, Ferguson JH: An unusual case of sciatic nerve paralysis. JAMA 205:699, 1968.
11. Wood MB: Peroneal nerve repair. Clini Orthoped 267:206, 1991.

PART

IV

NEOPLASMS

Chapter 25

INTRODUCTORY SURVEY OF BRAIN TUMORS

LUCY BALIAN RORKE, M.D.

Primary tumors of the central nervous system (CNS) are the most common type of solid neoplasm in children.[1] Although the prospect of survival has improved because of advances in diagnosis, surgical techniques, anesthesia and critical care, new chemotherapeutic agents, and new treatment protocols, major problems nevertheless remain. These are not necessarily related solely to the histologic malignancy of many of these neoplasms and lack of response to therapy but, as with CNS tumors in individuals at all ages, are often a function of their location either because of their effect on the function of the tissue in which they are growing or because of their effect on adjacent structures. For example, the craniopharyngioma, a common childhood tumor, is always histologically benign, but its location in the parasellar region in proximity to the optic nerves and chiasm, infundibulum, and diencephalon accounts for the disturbingly frequent and often unavoidable permanent visual and endocrine disturbances that follow surgery.

Some tumors can be only biopsied because they grow in vital structures, such as the optic nerves, diencephalon or brainstem. Although the majority of these neoplasms are histologically benign, at least when initially diagnosed, they produce serious deficits and, all too often, death of the child.

At the same time, one of the most histologically malignant tumors, the primitive neuroectodermal tumor/medulloblastoma (PNET/MB), carried a dismal prognosis in the past, but now often responds well to treatment.[2] However, prolonged survival after successful treatment has introduced two new problems: fixed neuropsychological deficit and an increased risk of developing a second tumor, both often a consequence of the therapy.[3–5] Thus, the clinician walks a narrow line in efforts to destroy the tumor while leaving intact the developmental integrity of the child.

The incidence of two to five new cases per 100,000 per year remains relatively stable throughout the world.[6–9] Some have claimed a greater frequency of CNS tumors in males,[8–10] whereas others suggest that the ratio of 1.2:1 generally cited in favor of males merely reflects the normal sex ratio in the population at any point in time.[11] The male to female ratio among 744 children 18 years of age or younger who were diagnosed and/or treated at The Children's Hospital of Philadelphia (CHOP) during the period from July, 1979 to January, 1992 is 1.4:1. However, if the M:F ratio is calculated for specific tumor types, more striking differences are observed (Tables 25–1 and 25–2). Twenty subtypes of tumors occur with a ratio of 1.4:1 or greater in males than females, five of which are relatively common childhood neoplasms, namely, PNET, craniopha-

TABLE 25–1. RATIO OF SPECIFIC BRAIN TUMOR TYPES IN MALES AND FEMALES

M:F RATIO 1.4 TO 1.9:1	M:F RATIO 2 TO 4:1
PNET	Malignant cerebral astrocytoma
Malignant cerebellar astrocytoma	Cerebellar ganglioglioma
Cerebral pilocytic astrocytoma	Germ cell tumor—pineal
Subependymal giant cell tumor	Oligodendroglioma
Gliomatosis cerebri	Lymphoma
Mixed glioma—cerebral	Metastases
Craniopharyngioma	Choroid plexus tumors
Epidermal/dermoid cyst	Meningioma—infratentorial and spinal
Brainstem glioma	Neurofibroma
	ATT/rhabdoid*
	Ependymoma

M:F RATIO > 4:1	F:M RATIO 1.4–1.9:1
Pituitary adenoma	Cerebral astrocytoma ("benign")
	Mixed glioma—cerebellar
	Meningioma—supratentorial
	Hamartoma—neuronal/glial

*Atypical teratoid tumor/rhabdoid.

TABLE 25–2. CNS TUMORS OCCURRING WITH EQUAL FREQUENCY IN MALES AND FEMALES

M:F 1:1–1.3:1
Cerebellar pilocytic astrocytoma
Optic nerve glioma
Ganglioglioma—cerebral
Germ cell tumors—nonpineal
Pineocytoma
Rathke's cleft cyst
Medulloepithelioma
Mesenchymal chondrosarcoma
Schwannoma
Chordoma

ryngioma, brainstem glioma, ependymoma, and germ cell tumors arising in the pineal. The most striking disparity between the sexes is the 7:1 ratio of pituitary adenoma in favor of males.

A female preponderance is found for only three tumor types, the cerebellar mixed glioma being the most important of these. Previous evaluation of the M:F distribution of 382 CNS tumors in children (all of whom are included in this larger group) had indicated a female predominance for ependymomas and optic nerve gliomas.[12] Thus there has been a shift toward male predominance for the ependymomas in the past 5 years, and there is now no apparent gender predisposition in the distribution of optic nerve gliomas.

Over 90 per cent of primary CNS tumors in children are located within the intracranial cavity and involve the brain, meninges, pineal gland, optic nerves, or parasellar regions. Tumors of the cranial nerve roots are rare. The majority of older statistical studies analyzing distribution of CNS tumors in children have emphasized their predilection for posterior fossa structures.[13] However, more recent analyses demonstrated a reversal of these percentages. In fact, 54 per cent of the 744 tumors diagnosed or operated upon at CHOP were located in the supratentorial space, whereas only 41 per cent were found in the posterior fossa; the remaining 5.1 per cent grew in the spinal canal (Table 25–3). Aside from the general distribution of primary CNS tumors, these growths during the childhood years tend to favor certain sites that are different from site predilection in adults. These include the cerebellum, brainstem, optic nerve, parasellar region, and pineal gland. The cerebrum, meninges, and nerve roots, in contrast, are most commonly involved among older individuals.

Figures based upon biopsy specimens are not necessarily accurate indications of the true distribution of CNS tumors in children. For example, such figures underestimate the incidence of optic nerve and brainstem gliomas, as tumors in these locations are often treated without benefit of a tissue diagnosis. Moreover, in Japan, a tumor clinically and radiologically identified in the pineal region is presumptively diagnosed as a germ cell neoplasm and is treated as such without biopsy confirmation.

A major factor in the shift in the supra- versus infratentorial distribution probably reflects advances in neu-

rosurgical technique and widespread use of the operating microscope, combined with progress in pediatric anesthesia and critical care. This combination has reduced both morbidity and mortality in children with CNS tumors in regions previously regarded as inaccessible (e.g., the pineal gland).

There has also been remarkable progress in radiologic techniques, namely, widespread use of the CT scanner, magnetic resonance imaging (MRI), and use of gadolinium for enhancement. These have allowed earlier diagnosis when symptoms are subtle or the lesions are small or poorly defined, as is often the case, for example, with gangliogliomas or gliomatosis cerebri. Perhaps the most accurate figures on the site of origin of CNS tumors could be obtained from the diagnostic neuroradiologist.

It has long been known that almost all types of primary CNS neoplasms may be found at any age but that certain tumors are more common among infants and children than among older individuals. Moreover, several rare types have, to date, been identified only in the first years of life. These include medulloepithelioma,[14] atypical teratoid/rhabdoid tumors,[15] and a small group consisting of a mixture of astrocytes and fibrocollagenous tissue with or without primitive neuroepithelial cells or mature neurons.[16, 17]

Among the most common childhood tumor types are the primitive neuroectodermal tumors, most frequently located in the cerebellum (medulloblastoma); cerebellar, diencephalic, optic nerve and brainstem astrocytoma (most frequently histologically benign); ganglioglioma; craniopharyngioma; ependymoma; mixed glioma; germ cell tumor; and solid and cystic hamartomas (Table 25–4). In contrast, the four most common tumor types afflicting adults are astrocytomas (primar-

TABLE 25–3. DISTRIBUTION OF 744 CNS TUMORS AND HAMARTOMAS IN CHILDREN 0–18 YEARS OF AGE DIAGNOSED AT CHOP DURING THE PERIOD JULY, 1979 TO JANUARY, 1992

LOCATION	NUMBER	PERCENTAGE
Supratentorial		400	54
Cerebral (incl intraventricular)	264	
Optic nerve	14	
Meningeal	16	
Parasellar	63	
Pineal	42	
Cranial nerve roots	1	
Infratentorial		304	41
Cerebellar (incl intraventricular)	262	
Brainstem	38	
Meningeal	2	
Cranial nerve root and bone	2	
Spinal		38	5.1
Spinal cord	31	
Spinal roots	5	
Meningeal	2	
Unknown	2		0.3

TABLE 25–4.   COMPARATIVE FREQUENCY OF SPECIFIC TUMOR TYPES IN BRAINS OF CHILDREN AND ADULTS IN SURGICAL SERIES

DIAGNOSIS	CHILDREN (%)* N = 744	ADULTS (%)† N = 358
Astrocytoma (all types)	32.7	46.9
PNET	17.6	3.3
Ganglioglioma	7.9	—
Craniopharyngioma	5.8	1.1
Ependymoma	5.7	2.5
Germ cell tumor	4.2	1.4
Mixed glioma	3.6	—
ATT/rhabdoid‡	1.2	—
Choroid plexus tumors	2.6	1.4
Meningioma	2.7	13.4
Oligodendroglioma	1.9	1.9
Pituitary adenomas	1.1	8.7
Pineocytoma	0.5	0.8
Metastatic tumors	1.0	10.6

*Data from CHOP series.
†Data from Salcman M: The morbidity and mortality of brain tumors. Neurol Clin 3:229, 1985.
‡Atypical teratoid tumor/rhabdoid.

ily cerebral and histologically malignant); meningiomas; metastatic tumors; and pituitary adenomas.[18, 19]

An interesting and perhaps ominous change has occurred in the 5½-year interval between analysis of a group of 362 childhood brain tumors diagnosed and/or treated at CHOP and the larger group of 744 cases (which includes the previous 362). That is, astrocytomas have not only increased in frequency, but there has been a dramatic jump in the percentage of these tumors that are histologically malignant at the time of initial biopsy.[12] Among the smaller group of children, only 6.1 per cent were in that category, but the current figure now stands at 21 per cent.

Gangliogliomas, more common in children than in adults, are most often located in the cerebral hemispheres (86 per cent), whereas the mixed gliomas tend to occur more often in the cerebellum (60 per cent). With one exception, all gangliogliomas that we studied were histologically and biologically benign. The mixed gliomas were also histologically benign. The most common combination of neoplastic cells in these mixed tumors consisted of astrocytes and oligodendrocytes (58 per cent). The other combinations consisted of astrocytes and ependymal cells (29 per cent) and ependymal cells and oligodendroglia (13 per cent). Several complex combinations that also contained ganglion cells were placed in the ganglioglioma category.

An inescapable problem in comparing statistics from one institution to another of various brain tumor types consists of lack of uniformity of classification systems utilized by pathologists throughout the world. Most commonly used in English-speaking nations are the classification and modifications thereof proposed by Bailey and Cushing in 1926.[20] A variation of the Bailey and Cushing scheme prepared by Zülch[21] was popular in Germany and other European countries, whereas Spanish pathologists followed the classification set forth

by del Rio Hortega.[22] The World Health Organization made an effort in the 1970s to bring these disparate schemes into a classification system that would be acceptable world-wide. To this end, a group of internationally renowned neuropathologists convened in Geneva and, after considerable deliberation, published their consensus document in 1979.[23] This did not enjoy universal acceptance, and a revision of the classification scheme, produced by a second international group of neuropathologists, is scheduled for publication in 1993. The special aspects of nomenclature for childhood tumors have, to date, been addressed by only two groups: the Japanese Society of Neuropathologists in 1983 and a small group of North American pediatric neuropathologists, who proposed a modification of the 1979 WHO classification and published this in 1985.[24] It has been argued by some that a separate classification system for CNS tumors occurring in childhood is not necessary.

Like many other things in the world, no classification system currently in use is ideal, and in fact, all have been changed in the past and are subject to change in the future. This is a consequence partly of fundamental differences among pathologists, the biology of neoplasia, and continuing expansion of our knowledge of the cellular characteristics of the tumors.

Tumors are generally classified on the basis of their resemblance to normal cells of the organ in which they arise. Thus, a brain tumor composed of cells resembling astrocytes is called an astrocytoma, or one formed by ependymal-appearing cells is an ependymoma. This system works fairly well if the tumor cells are sufficiently differentiated to allow such easy recognition. However, about one fifth of the childhood CNS tumors are formed by primitive or poorly differentiated cells whose identity is not obvious on examination with routine cell stains such as hematoxylin and eosin. Past generations of pathologists achieved some measure of success in more precise identification of the cells by developing specialized histochemical techniques such as the PTAH stain for astrocytes or the Bielschowsky method for identification of neurons and their processes.

Introduction of immunohistochemical techniques in 1970[25] has led to a revolution in our concepts of tumor biology, the unique cytologic characteristics of neoplastic cells, and classification of tumors on the basis of their specific features.[26] The immunocytochemical techniques have been of particular value in identification of specific types of intermediate filament cytoskeletal proteins such as vimentin, glial fibrillary acidic protein (GFAP), neurofilament proteins (NFP), keratin, desmin, and most recently nestin.[27] Utilization of monoclonal antibodies recognizing these proteins along with a large number of other cellular antigens has expanded our knowledge of the primitive neuroectodermal tumors, the specific nature of which has stimulated considerable, sometimes acrimonious, debate since the prototype tumor in this category, the medulloblastoma, was first described by Bailey and Cushing in 1925.[28–31] Although the majority of these tumors arise in the cerebellar vermis, histologically and biologically identical neoplasms may be primary in the pineal, cerebrum, brainstem, or spinal cord. Studies by several groups of investigators have established similar cytoskeletal profiles of these tumors regardless of their location in the CNS, as well as a remarkable complexity of the cells comprising the tumors.[32–34] The PNETs may be subdivided into categories depending upon expression of specific intermediate filament proteins. Some tumors express none, whereas others contain clones of NFP-positive cells and/or GFAP-positive cells. A small percentage of cells express desmin and there is considerable co-expression of intermediate filament proteins such as vimentin-NFP, vimentin-GFAP, NFP-GFAP, and others, features that have not been identified in normal CNS cells. Both smooth and striated muscle, as well as melanin-bearing cells, have been observed in these tumors by routine light microscopy. All PNETs express synaptophysin, and some contain retinal antigens as well.

Utilization of panels of monoclonal antibodies in the study of CNS tumors in children has also assisted in identification of tumor types hitherto unknown or misclassified. In this category is the superficial astrocytoma of infancy, a supratentorial tumor typically adherent to the dura and originally thought to be a low-grade fibrosarcoma because of abundant fibrocollagen.[35] Taratuto et al,[16] however, established the astrocytic component by use of GFAP and redefined the true nature of the tumor.

Similarly, another tumor that, to date, appears to be restricted to infants and children, namely, the atypical teratoid/rhabdoid tumor,[15] has been separated from the group of PNETs with which it was classified before the unique histologic and immunocytochemical features were identified.

Cytogenetic studies provide yet another dimension in expanding our understanding of childhood brain tumors, although considerably more is known of chromosomal aberrations in adult tumors, specifically malignant gliomas and meningiomas.[36, 37] Recent systematic studies of the childhood tumors have yielded intriguing findings, such as identification of an iso 17q abnormality in about one third of PNETs and deletion of chromosome 22 in the atypical teratoid/rhabdoid tumors.[38–40] Curiously, histologically benign CNS tumors rarely exhibit chromosomal abnormalities.

Contribution of the neurosurgeons to this expansion of knowledge of CNS tumors in children should not be underestimated. In past years, there was a tendency to submit a tiny specimen for pathologic examination and to suction away or otherwise discard the rest of the tumor. The pathologist was therefore forced to make a diagnosis on a minute scrap of tissue, and little or none was available for tissue culture or for cytogenetic or other research studies. Unfortunately, diagnosis made on this inadequate sample was used as a guide for both prognosis and selection of a treatment regimen. Since CNS tumors frequently display cellular heterogeneity, it is not surprising that such a limited view of the histologic features led to inappropriate therapy and, sometimes, incorrect prognostic expectations.

Current neurosurgical practice of subtotal or total extirpation of tumor, when feasible, has had several effects. First, it provides the pathologist the opportunity to gain a broader picture of the histologic character and variations of tumors within general diagnostic categories. Second, tissue has become available for cytogenetic studies, development of genetic probes, and growth of tumor in tissue cultures for, among other things, testing of the efficacy of chemotherapeutic agents. Only through intensive study of the histology and biology of these neoplasms that threaten the lives of children can we hope to treat and ultimately cure them.

REFERENCES

1. Silverberg BS, Lubera JA: Cancer statistics, 1988. Ca—A Cancer Journal for Clinicians 38:5, 1988.
2. Packer RJ, Sutton LN, Goldwein JW, et al.: Improved survival with the use of adjuvant chemotherapy in the treatment of medulloblastoma. J Neurosurg 74:433, 1991.
3. Duffner PK, Cohen ME, Thomas P: Late effects of treatment on the intelligence of children with posterior fossa tumors. Cancer 51:233, 1983.
4. Hawkins MM, Draper GJ, Kingston JE: Incidence of second primary tumours among childhood cancer survivors. Br J Cancer 56:339, 1987.
5. Ron E, Modan B, Boice JD, et al.: Tumors of the brain and nervous system after radiotherapy in childhood. N Engl J Med 319:1033, 1988.
6. Dahnmann GJ, Farwell JR: Intracranial neoplasms in children: A comparison of North America, Europe, Africa and Asia. Dis Nerv Syst 37:696, 1976.
7. Gjerris F, Harmsen A, Klinken L, et al.: Incidence and longterm survival of children with intracranial tumors treated in Denmark, 1935–1959. Br J Cancer 38:442, 1978.
8. Madon E, Besenzon L, Broch del Prever A, et al.: Results of a multicenter retrospective study on pediatric brain tumors in Italy. Tumori 72:285, 1986.
9. Schoenberg BS, Schoenberg DG, Christine BW, et al.: The epidemiology of primary intracranial neoplasms of childhood. Mayo Clin Proc 51:51, 1976.
10. Oi S, Kokunai T, Matsumoto S: Congenital brain tumors in Japan (ISPN Cooperative Study): Specific clinical features in neonates. Child's Nerv Syst 6:86, 1990.
11. Farwell JR, Dahnmann GJ, Flannery JT: Central nervous system tumors in children. Cancer 40:3123, 1977.
12. Rorke LB, Schut L: Introductory survey of pediatric brain tumors. In McLaurin RL, Schut L, Venes JL, et al. (eds): Pediatric Neurosurgery. 2nd ed. Philadelphia, WB Saunders, 1989.
13. Leetsma JE: Brain tumors—teaching monograph. Am J Path 100:243, 1980.
14. Karch SB, Urich H: Medulloepithelioma: Definition of an entity. J Neuropath Exp Neurol 31:27, 1972.
15. Lefkowitz IB, Rorke LB, Packer RJ, et al.: Atypical teratoid tumor of infancy: Definition of an entity. Ann Neurol 28:448, 1987.
16. Taratuto AL, Monges J, Lylyk P, et al.: Superficial cerebral astrocytoma attached to dura. Report of six cases in infants. Cancer 54:2505, 1984.
17. VandenBerg SR, May EE, Rubinstein LJ, et al.: Desmoplastic supratentorial neuroepithelial tumors of infancy with divergent differentiation potential (desmoplastic infantile gangliogliomas). Report on 11 cases of a distinctive embryonal tumor with favorable prognosis. J Neurosurg 66:58, 1987.
18. Helseth A, Langmark F, Mork SJ: Neoplasms of the central nervous system in Norway. II. Descriptive epidemiology of intracranial neoplasms 1955–1984. Acta Path Microbiol Immunol Scand 96:1066, 1988.
19. Salcman M: The morbidity and mortality of brain tumors. Neurol Clin 3:229, 1985.

20. Bailey P, Cushing H: A Classification of Tumors of the Glioma Group of a Histologic Basis with a Correlated Study of Prognosis. Philadelphia, JB Lippincott, 1926.
21. Zülch KJ: Biologie und Pathologie der Hirngeschwülste Handbuch der Neurochirugie, vol III. Springer, Berlin, 1956.
22. del Rio Hortega P: Nomenclatura y classificacion de los tumores del sistemo nervisso. Lopez and Etchefazen, Buenos Aires. Arch Histol 3:5, 1945.
23. Zülch KG: Histological Typing of Tumors of the Central Nervous System. Geneva, World Health Organization, 1979.
24. Rorke LB, Gilles FH, Davis RL, et al.: Revision of the World Health Organization classification of brain tumors for childhood brain tumors. Cancer 56:1869, 1985.
25. Sternberger LA, Hardy PH Jr, Cuculis JJ, et al.: The unlabelled antibody enzyme method of immunohistochemistry. Preparation and properties of soluble antigen-antibody complex (horseradish-antihorseradish peroxidase) and its use in identification of spirochetes. J Histochem Cytochem 18:315, 1970.
26. Gould VE: Histogenesis and differentiation: A re-evaluation of these concepts as criteria for the classification of tumors. Human Pathol 17:212, 1986.
27. Tohyama T, Lee VM-Y, Rorke LB, et al.: (LI-9614) Nestin expression in embryonic human neuroepithelium and in human tumor neuroepithelial cells. Lab Invest 66:303, 1992.
28. Bailey P, Cushing H: Medulloblastoma cerebelli: a common type of midcerebellar glioma of childhood. Acta Neurol 14:192, 1925.
29. Rorke LB: The cerebellar medulloblastoma and its relationship to primitive neuroectodermal tumors. J Neuropathol Exp Neurol 42:1, 1983.
30. Rorke LB: Primitive neuroectodermal tumor—a concept requiring an apologia? In Fields WS (ed): Primary Brain Tumors: A Review of Histological Classification. New York, Springer-Verlag, 1989.
31. Rubinstein LJ: Embryonal central neuroepithelial tumors and their differentiating potential. J Neurosurg 62:759, 1985.
32. Gould VE, Jansson DS, Molenaar WM, et al.: Primitive neuroectodermal tumors of the central nervous system—patterns of expression of neuroendocrine markers, and all classes of intermediate filament proteins. Lab Invest 62:498, 1990.
33. Gould VE, Rorke LB, Jansson DS, et al.: Primitive neuroectodermal tumors of the central nervous system express neuroendocrine markers and may express all classes of intermediate filaments. Human Pathol 21:245, 1990.
34. Molenaar WM, Jansson DS, Gould VE, et al.: Molecular markers of primitive neuroectodermal tumors and other pediatric central nervous system tumors. Lab Invest 61:635, 1989.
35. Bailey OT, Ingraham FD: Intracranial fibrosarcoma of the dura mater in childhood. J Neurosurg 2:1, 1945.
36. Bigner SW, Mark J, Burger PC, et al.: Specific chromosomal abnormalities in malignant human gliomas. Cancer Res 48:405, 1988.
37. Collins VP, Nordenskjöld JP, Dumanski JP: Molecular aspects of meningiomas. Brain Pathol 1:19, 1990.
38. Biegel JA, Rorke LB, Packer RJ, et al.: Isochromosome 17q in primitive neuroectodermal tumors of the central nervous system. Genes Chromosome Cancer 1:139, 1989.
39. Biegel JA, Rorke LB, Packer RJ, et al.: Monosomy 22 in rhabdoid or atypical teratoid tumors of the brain. J Neurosurg 73:710, 1990.
40. Griffin CA, Hawkins AL, Packer RJ, et al.: Chromosome abnormalities in pediatric brain tumors. Cancer Res 48:175, 1988.

Chapter 26

CEREBELLAR ASTROCYTOMAS

MARK S. O'BRIEN, M.D., and ALI KRISHT, M.D.

Cerebellar astrocytomas are the most benign of the neuroectodermal tumors of childhood, both by location and by postoperative prognosis. Although recurrences after 20 to 30 years have been documented, the 25-year tumor-free survival rate is near 90 per cent for those children with histologically benign tumors not invading the brainstem.

CLINICAL PRESENTATION

Unlike the other, more malignant, posterior fossa tumors such as medulloblastomas, the clinical symptomatology in cerebellar astrocytomas is more insidious. The most common presentation is headache associated with nausea and vomiting. The headache is usually frontal in location. If occipital, it is then associated with neck stiffness and opisthotonus; this suggests the occurrence of tonsilar herniation. Nausea usually occurs in the morning and subsides later during the day. The child may present with a long history of intermittent vomiting that gradually becomes persistent and projectile. It is not unusual for a child with cerebellar astrocytoma to be treated for gastrointestinal disease initially and for a long period of time before the diagnosis of a brain tumor is made.

Papilledema occurs in up to 90 per cent of the cases.[1] Prolonged papilledema may lead to optic atrophy and decrease in visual acuity. This is usually seen as optic pallor on funduscopy.

Up to 95 per cent of the children have ataxia at the time of presentation.[1] The ataxia may be truncal or peripheral. It is usually noticed as an unsteady gait in younger children and as "clumsiness" in older children. Dysmetria and nystagmus are present in the majority of patients. These are usually easier to detect in older children, who are more cooperative during the physical examination. When nystagmus is present, it is worse on lateral gaze to the side of the lesion.

An increase in head circumference may be seen in children with cerebellar astrocytomas who are less than 2 years of age. However, this is more common in patients with medulloblastomas who have an earlier presentation when the cranial sutures are still open. A small number of patients present with diplopia due to a cranial neuropathy. This most commonly involves the sixth cranial nerve, and it is secondary to hydrocephalus. The facial nerve may be involved in up to 26 per cent of these cases.[1]

The advent of computerized tomography (CT) has allowed an earlier diagnosis of posterior fossa tumors, thereby decreasing the number of patients presenting late in the course of their disease with deterioration in the level of consciousness. Decreased consciousness may still occur in some patients, and it is usually due to severe, noncommunicating hydrocephalus. The hydrocephalus results from deformation or obstruction of either the fourth ventricle or the sylvian aqueduct. This should be considered a medical emergency and should be treated by immediate insertion of a ventriculostomy or a ventriculoperitoneal shunt.

DIAGNOSTIC STUDIES

An increase in head circumference secondary to hydrocephalus may lead to suture separation, which can be readily seen on skull radiographs of children with posterior fossa tumors. This is not so common in astrocytomas as it is in medulloblastomas because they usually present in older children after closure of the cranial sutures.

The CT scan is diagnostic in the majority of cases.[2–4] It may show either a midline (vermian) solid mass or a lateral (hemispheric) cystic tumor. The tumor is iso- or hypodense on noncontrasted scans. It does not enhance in the majority of cases, although it may occasionally show areas of enhancement. Areas of calcification may be apparent. There may be deformation of the fourth ventricle with secondary hydrocephalus (Fig. 26–1). Solid tumors may be difficult to differentiate from other childhood posterior fossa tumors such as ependymomas and medulloblastomas. The cystic astrocytomas may look similar to the cystic hemangioblastomas that have a large cyst and a contrast-enhancing mural nodule (Fig. 26–2). In children, it is more often diagnostic of astrocytoma, since hemangioblastomas are extremely rare in the pediatric age group.

In addition to CT, we routinely obtain a magnetic resonance imaging (MRI) study of the head unless the condition of the patient contraindicates it. The high resolution and multiplanar capabilities of MRI help to delineate the margins of the tumor and its relationship to the floor of the fourth ventricle. We find these details helpful in planning surgery. Cerebellar astrocytomas are usually iso- or hypointense on T1-weighted images and hyperintense on T2-weighted images (Fig. 26–3).[3–5] Contrast enhancement is seen in the mural nodule of the cystic variety and in some areas of the solid variety.

EPIDEMIOLOGY

Seventy to 80 per cent of cerebellar astrocytomas are found in children.[1] They account for up to 28 per cent of tumors in the pediatric age group.[5] They also constitute one third of the childhood posterior fossa tumors.[6]

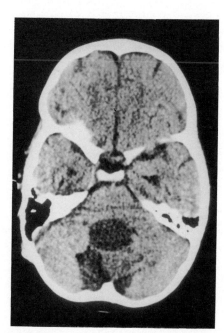

FIGURE 26–1. A noncontrasted CT scan shows a cystic midline cerebellar astrocytoma that had obliterated the fourth ventricle and resulted in secondary noncommunicating hydrocephalus documented with the dilated temporal horns.

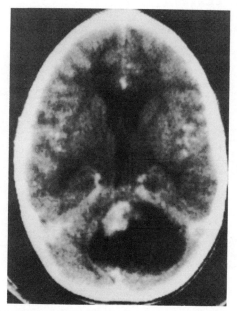

FIGURE 26–2. A contrast-enhanced CT scan shows a cystic cerebellar astrocytoma with a contrast-enhancing mural nodule. This is similar to a cerebellar hemangioblastoma.

Even though some studies found a higher incidence of cerebellar astrocytomas in males,[6] these tumors are considered to have no sex predilection.[1, 7] These lesions are considered a disease of children and young adults, but may rarely occur at the two extremes of age.[6] The typical patient is an otherwise healthy child between 5 and 15 years of age, presenting with intermittent symptoms of headaches associated with nausea and occasional vomiting.

MANAGEMENT

Cerebellar astrocytomas are benign brain tumors that are potentially curable. The potential for cure increases proportionately with the extent of radical excision.[1, 3, 4, 8–11]

Preoperative Management

Preoperative management varies with the patient's neurologic status. Children with signs and symptoms of increased intracranial pressure and with no hydrocephalus on the CT scan benefit from high-dose steroids to decrease the peritumoral swelling. Decadron is started at 0.1 mg/kg/dose every 6 hours. The decrease in peritumoral swelling may restore the patency of the cerebrospinal fluid (CSF) pathways and result in partial relief of hydrocephalus. Steroids are continued through the postoperative period and then gradually discontinued.

The insertion of a CSF shunt remains a controversial issue. It has been reported that only 30 per cent of

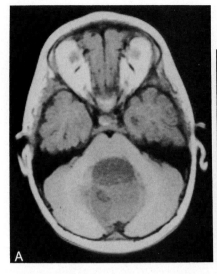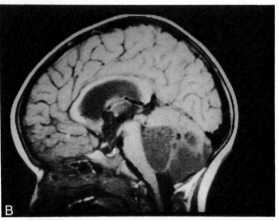

FIGURE 26–3. Axial (A) and sagittal (B) T1-weighted MRIs of the same patient shown in Figure 26–1, which show a hypointense, multicystic, midline posterior fossa mass that is obliterating the fourth ventricle and compressing the brainstem.

patients with cerebellar astrocytoma will need a permanent ventriculoperitoneal shunt.[5] For this reason, some neurosurgeons advocate a CSF drainage procedure only if corticosteroids fail to improve the neurologic status and the child continues to deteriorate.[12] Other neurosurgeons advocate the use of external ventricular drainage as a temporary measure until the tumor is excised and patency of the CSF pathway is established. The rationale for this attitude is to avoid the potential complications related to shunt procedures that include tumor hemorrhage,[3, 4] upward cerebellar herniation, and dissemination of malignant cells to the peritoneum and systemic circulation.[13]

Others believe that the benefits obtained from inserting a ventriculoperitoneal shunt outweigh the above-mentioned risks, which are not proved beyond doubt. Albright and Reigel found that preoperative CSF drainage leads to lower postoperative mortality and morbidity.[12] The neurologic improvement achieved provides ample time to plan operation on an elective basis and to obtain an MRI of the head with gadolinium before tumor excision. It will also provide the surgeon with a relaxed posterior fossa during surgery. The family is also provided with an additional period of adjustment.

Intraoperative Management

In the operating theater, we recommend that the patient be positioned in the way that best suits the preference and experience of the neurosurgeon. We usually place the child prone with the head rested on either a horseshoe or a three-point head holder for older children (Fig. 26–4). Younger children less than 5 years of age are usually put in the lateral decubitus position with the side of maximum tumor involvement superior (Fig. 26–5). We usually avoid placing the child in the sitting position owing to the known risks of air embolism and possible pneumocephalus.

A midline skin incision is made, extending from the

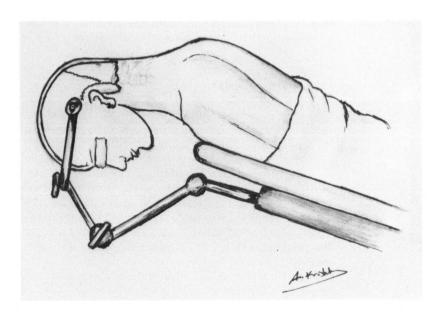

FIGURE 26–4. Operative positioning used for older children shows the child placed prone with the head in a three-point head holder.

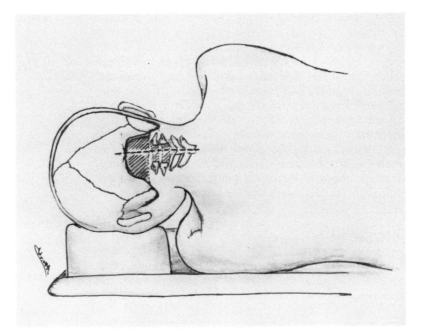

FIGURE 26–5. Operative positioning used for younger children under 5 years of age shows the child placed in the lateral decubitus position with the side of maximum tumor involvement superior. The midline skin incision extends from the external occipital protuberance to the midvertebral region to facilitate removal of the lamina of C1 and C2 vertebrae, if necessary.

external occipital protuberance to the midcervical region. The exposure is made to permit removal of the laminae of C1 and C2 vertebrae, if needed (Fig. 26–5). We prefer a craniectomy over a craniotomy for opening the posterior fossa, although craniotomy is a valid option used by many neurosurgeons.

When a cyst is present, needle aspiration is done to decompress the posterior fossa. A Y-shaped durotomy is used for opening the dura, and ultrasonography is used to better define the tumor margins. Since it is a potentially curable tumor, total surgical excision of the astrocytoma should be the goal. This is fortunately achievable in the majority of cases unless the tumor invades the brainstem or envelops the surrounding blood vessels and/or cranial nerves. At the end of the procedure, watertight dural closure is done primarily or by use of a dural graft.

Postoperative Management

In the postoperative period, the patient is kept in the intensive care unit for a day or two. In the presence of lower cranial neuropathies, it is advisable to keep the endotracheal tube in place until the patient is fully awake and able to clear the airway of secretions. High-dose steroids are used for 48 to 72 hours and are tapered over 5 to 7 days.

COMPLICATIONS

In the event of a neurologic deterioration or if the patient does not wake up in the immediate postoperative period, a CT scan should be performed to rule out a postoperative hematoma or persistent hydrocephalus.

The latter may be due to incomplete decompression of the CSF pathways or blockage of the CSF drainage system.

Postoperative aseptic meningitis may occur after excision of cerebellar astrocytomas. It usually takes 4 to 7 days postoperatively to manifest itself. The child may complain of headache that is associated with fever, neck stiffness, and pleocytosis in the CSF. This is usually due to spillage of either tumor-cyst fluid or blood in the subarachnoid spaces. These patients improve on their own, and the symptoms are alleviated by the use of steroids.

If the postoperative course is uneventful, the patient is transferred to "floor care" and started on a regular diet, while gradually increasing his or her activities. Either a CT scan or an MRI of the head is obtained as a baseline study for future follow-up before the patient is discharged.

PATHOLOGY

Cerebellar astrocytomas have a benign biologic behavior. Unlike other intra-axial brain tumors, a cure is possible when total surgical excision is achieved. Grossly, the tumors are well-circumscribed lesions that occupy the cerebellar hemisphere. They are formed of either a large cyst with a mural nodule or a solid mass with multiple cystic areas. They are entirely solid in 22 per cent of cases, with the remaining cases tending to be cystic.[14] The cysts contain a yellowish proteinaceous fluid. These lesions compress the fourth ventricle and lead to secondary hydrocephalus. Occasionally, they invade the brainstem, usually through the cerebellar peduncles. Ilgren et al. reported brainstem invasion in 8 per cent of their cases.[14]

The microscopic features of cerebellar astrocytomas are characteristic. A biphasic pattern is seen that is formed of dense and compact areas with elongated (pilocytic) cells that alternate with loose areas containing stellate astrocytes and microcysts.[14, 15] The nuclei are uniform, regular, and nonpleomorphic. The cells may contain intracytoplasmic eosinophilic inclusions, termed *Rosenthal bodies*.[15] On electron microscopy, the Rosenthal bodies consist of cytoplasmic aggregates of glial filaments. Vascular proliferation may be seen in cerebellar astrocytomas. Unlike other gliomas, this proliferation does not indicate a more aggressive behavior of the tumor. Calcifications may be seen.

OUTCOME

Pediatric cerebellar astrocytomas have a good prognosis. A 20-year survival rate of up to 80 per cent has been documented.[5] Garcia et al. reviewed the outcome in 84 children (aged 19 years or less) with cerebellar astrocytomas.[8] The 5-, 10-, and 25-year disease-free survival rates for the entire group were 92, 88, and 88 per cent, respectively. Extent of surgical excision was a prognostic factor, but postoperative radiation did not affect the outcome. Seventy-five per cent of the patients were employed or attended school at the time of the study.

There is enough evidence in the literature to indicate that if total surgical excision of a benign cerebellar astrocytoma is achieved, no further adjuvant therapy, specifically radiation, is needed.[16] This is supported by data that indicate a low recurrence rate after total excision. Garcia et al. reviewed 80 children with cerebellar astrocytomas.[16] Recurrence was noted in 2.5 per cent of patients who had total removal of their tumors and in 35 per cent of patients who had subtotal removal. Radiation did not affect the outcome of patients who had subtotal excision.

Subtotal resection is compatible with long-term survival.[8, 9, 11, 16, 17] In a study by Ilgren and Stiller,[9] two thirds of the patients who had subtotal resection of their tumors were alive 10 years or more after surgery. Recurrence of cerebellar astrocytomas may not be as predictable in some children. Although a 25-year disease-free survival is equivalent to a cure, recurrence was reported 36 years after radical removal.[18] In another case reported by Budka, a malignant recurrence occurred 28 years after original excision.[19] Although cerebellar astrocytomas have a benign course in the majority of cases, they may lead to a less favorable outcome when invading the brainstem[19, 20] or if the histologic features of the tumor indicate a more aggressive potential.[14, 17, 21]

Based on our present knowledge of cerebellar astrocytomas, radiation is recommended when there is a recurrence and further surgical excision is not feasible, and if the recurrent tumor has malignant histology (Table 26–1). Chemotherapy is indicated in the malignant recurrences that do not respond to radiation.

TABLE 26–1. TREATMENT FOR PEDIATRIC CEREBELLAR ASTROCYTOMAS

EXTENT OF SURGICAL RESECTION	RECURRENCE	TREATMENT
Total	−	No radiation therapy
	+ (resectable)	Surgery
	+ (nonresectable)	Radiation therapy
Subtotal	−	No radiation therapy
	+	Radiation therapy ± surgery
	Malignant recurrence	Radiation therapy ± surgery and ± chemotherapy

SUMMARY

Pediatric cerebellar astrocytomas are the most common posterior fossa tumors in children. Clinically, they present with signs and symptoms related to raised intracranial pressure and cerebellar dysfunction. They have characteristic CT and MRI findings. Fortunately, they have a benign biologic behavior. They are best treated with surgical excision, and after total surgical excision, they carry an excellent prognosis with an average 25-year disease-free survival.

REFERENCES

1. Davis CH, Joglekar VM: Cerebellar astrocytomas in children and young adults. J Neurol Neurosurg Psychiatry 44:820, 1981.
2. Zimmerman RA, Bilanink LT, Pahlajani H: Spectrum of cerebellar astrocytoma. Am J Roentgenol 130:929, 1978.
3. Epstein F: Pediatric posterior fossa tumors. Part I. Contemp Neurosurg 8:17, 1986.
4. Epstein F: Pediatric posterior fossa tumors. Part II. Contemp Neurosurg 8:18, 1986.
5. Sutton LN, Schut L: Cerebellar astrocytomas. *In* McLaurin RL et al. (eds): Pediatric Neurosurgery: Surgery of the Developing Nervous System. 2nd ed. Philadelphia, WB Saunders Company, 1989, pp 338–346.
6. Rorke LB, Schut L: Introductory survey of pediatric brain tumors. *In* McLaurin RL et al. (eds): Pediatric Neurosurgery: Surgery of the Developing Nervous System. 2nd ed. Philadelphia, WB Saunders Company, 1989, pp 335–337.
7. Gjerris F, Klinken L: Long-term prognosis in children with benign cerebellar astrocytoma. J Neurosurg 49:179, 1978.
8. Garcia DM, Latifi HR, Simpson JR, Pickens S: Astrocytoma of the cerebellum in children. J Neurosurg 71:661, 1989.
9. Ilgren EB, Stiller CA: Cerebellar astrocytomas: therapeutic management. Acta Neurochir (Wien) 81:11, 1986.
10. Klein DM, McCullough DC: Surgical staging of cerebellar astrocytomas in childhood. Cancer 56:1810, 1985.
11. Undjian S, Marinov M, Georgieve K: Long-term follow-up after surgical treatment of cerebellar astrocytomas in 100 children. Childs Nerv Syst 5:99, 1989.
12. Albright L, Reigel DH: Management of hydrocephalus secondary to posterior fossa tumors. J Neurosurg 46:52, 1977.
13. Kessler LA, Dugan P, Coucannon JP: Systemic metastases of medulloblastoma promoted by shunting. Surg Neurol 3:147, 1975.

14. Ilgren EB, Stiller CA: Cerebellar astrocytomas. Part I. Macroscopic and microscopic features. Clin Neuropathol 6:185, 1987.
15. Russell DS, Rubinstein LJ: Pathology of Tumors of the Nervous System. 4th ed. Baltimore, Williams & Wilkins, 1977, pp 183–190.
16. Garcia DM, Marks JE, Latifi HR, Kliefoth AB: Childhood cerebellar astrocytomas: is there a role for postoperative irradiation? Int J Radiat Oncol Biol Phys 18:815, 1990.
17. Cushing H: Experiences with cerebellar astrocytomas: a critical review of 76 cases. Surg Gynecol Obstet 52:129, 1931.
18. Pagni CA, Giordama MT, Canarero S: Benign recurrence of a pilocytic cerebellar astrocytoma 36 years after radical removal: case report. Neurosurgery 28:606, 1991.
19. Budka H: Partially resected and irradiated cerebellar astrocytoma of childhood: malignant evolution after 28 years. Acta Neurochir 32:139, 1975.
20. Ilgren EB, Stiller CA: Cerebellar astrocytomas: clinical characteristics and prognostic indices. J Neurooncol 4:293, 1987.
21. Casadei GP, Arrigoni GL, Dangelo V, Bizzozero L: Late malignant recurrence of childhood cerebellar astrocytoma. Clin Neuropathol 9:295, 1990.

Chapter 27

MEDULLOBLASTOMAS

LESLIE N. SUTTON, M.D., and ROGER J. PACKER, M.D.

The clever man takes advantage of everything, neglects nothing that may give him some added opportunity.

BONAPARTE TO TALLYRAND
September, 1797

Medulloblastomas were first described in 1925 by Bailey and Cushing, who reported a group of patients with tumors presenting for the most part in the region of the fourth ventricle that had clinical and histologic features distinctive from previously reported neoplasms. They concluded that "this was a very cellular tumor of a peculiar kind."[1] These authors coined the term *medulloblastoma*, suggesting that these tumors arose from a primitive pleuripotential cell, the *medulloblast*. This putative cell has never been found, making the term medulloblastoma confusing. Furthermore, tumors that occur in the cerebral hemispheres and in the pineal region may have a histologic appearance identical to that of the classic fourth ventricular medulloblastoma, yet have been called by other names, such as *central neuroblastoma* or *pineoblastoma*. Recently, Rorke suggested that all such malignant small cell tumors be designated *primitive neuroectodermal tumors* (or *PNETs*), independent of their site within the central nervous system.[2] This terminology has not yet gained universal acceptance,[3] and the term medulloblastoma has become so entrenched in the literature that for purposes of this chapter the older term will be used.

The early surgical experience suggested that medulloblastomas were never removable, and that attempts at radical excision conferred little benefit and carried significant operative mortality.[4] By 1934, the standard treatment of medulloblastoma was palliative decompression, followed by roentgen therapy,[5] and by 1953 a 3-year survival rate of 53 per cent was reported utilizing prophylactic whole-neuraxis irradiation.[6] The treatment of medulloblastoma changed little until the past decade, during which time the morbidity associated with craniospinal irradiation therapy in the young child became apparent.[7] Concurrently, the value of chemotherapy for certain patients with medulloblastoma became established.[8, 9] Using adjuvant craniospinal axis irradiation and chemotherapy in a fashion determined by staging criteria, recent series of children with newly diagnosed medulloblastoma are reporting 5-year survival rates in the range of 60 to 70 per cent.[10, 11] The treatment of childhood medulloblastoma has become truly multidisciplinary, requiring close cooperation between the neurosurgeon, radiation therapist, neuroradiologist, and neuro-oncologist.

EPIDEMIOLOGY AND ETIOLOGY

Medulloblastoma is the most common malignant central nervous system tumor of childhood, comprising 15 to 20 per cent of childhood brain tumors.[12, 13] Medulloblastomas account for about one third of all childhood posterior fossa neoplasms.[14] There is a peak in incidence between 3 and 8 years of age, and these tumors tend to cluster at the older portion of this age range. They may occur, however, at any age, including the newborn period. They less commonly present in adults,[15] and have been reported in patients in the seventh decade of life. There is a slight predominance in males.[16]

The cause of medulloblastoma is unknown. Rare instances of familial medulloblastomas have been reported, and there are anecdotal reports of siblings with the disease. There is no clear environmental factor that appears to predispose children to medulloblastoma, and recent research on etiology has focused on genetic factors. Chromosomal studies carried out on tissue obtained at surgery have revealed numerous cytogenetic abnormalities, involving chromosomes 5, 6, 11, 16, and 17. The most consistent abnormality has been an isochromosome 17q, which is present in about one third of cases.[17] This abnormality is not specific for medulloblastomas, however, and it is not clear what relationship this may have to tumor development or progression.

362

PATHOLOGY

Medulloblastomas are most commonly found in the region of the fourth ventricle, arising within the vermis. They may also arise in the cerebellar hemisphere or in the cerebellopontine angle. Rarely, they may be found initially in the spinal subarachnoid space or spinal cord, but these cases generally represent "drop metastases" from a primary tumor within the posterior fossa. The tumors grossly are reddish in color, friable, and in most cases highly vascular. In about 15 per cent of cases they are grossly hemorrhagic.[16, 18] A "desmoplastic" variant has been described, characterized by a firm, well-demarcated mass, which tends to occur more frequently in older children and adults.

A characteristic of these tumors is their ability to spread via the cerebrospinal pathways into the spinal or cerebral subarachnoid spaces of the ventricles. Such dissemination may take the form of nodular tumor deposits or a diffuse coating known as "sugar coating." Dissemination may already be present at the time of initial diagnosis or may occur later in the course of the disease.

Histologically, the classic medulloblastoma is composed of densely packed cells with hyperchromatic nuclei and very little cytoplasm (Fig. 27–1). This gives histologic slides stained with hematoxylin and eosin the gross appearance of "blue tumors," distinguishing them from juvenile astrocytomas, which are pink. Under the microscope, mitoses may be abundant. Rosettes of the Homer Wright type (Fig. 27–1) are seen in about 20 per cent, although perivascular "pseudorosettes," as initially described by Bailey and Cushing,[1] and Flexner-Wintersteiner rosettes may also be found. Histologic features vary and are unpredictable from one tumor to the next. The tumor may be composed entirely of a population of apparently undifferentiated neuroepithelial cells or contain neuronal or glial cells exhibiting varying degrees of maturity. Rarely, melaninin-containing cells and smooth or striated muscle are also components of these tumors. Nests or fields of neoplastic astrocytes are seen more frequently than are mature ganglion cells, although a recognizable pattern of somewhat lobular and linear growth of cells resembling primitive brain development is characteristic of a subtype of medulloblastoma, which has been designated "neuroblastic medulloblastoma."

Increasing utilization of a panel of monoclonal antibodies for immunohistochemical identification of specific cytoskeletal proteins has greatly expanded knowledge of the nature and differentiating potential of the neuroepithelial cells forming these tumors.[19, 20] By use of such techniques, medulloblastomas may be divided into several subgroups: (1) tumors entirely composed of undifferentiated neuroepithelial cells; (2) tumors composed of undifferentiated cells and a population manifesting neuronal differentiation; (3) tumors composed of undifferentiated cells and a population manifesting glial (basically astrocytic) differentiation; (4) tumors composed of all three cell types; and (5) tumors composed of undifferentiated cells, possibly neurons and/or glia, and melanin-bearing cells or muscle. More often than not, the neoplastic cells that stain positively for the presence of specific intermediate filament proteins (IFP), such as neurofilament protein (NFP), glial filament protein (GFP), and desmin cannot be distinguished by light microscopy from cells without such IFPs. Moreover, studies utilizing immunoflourescence techniques have also disclosed that many tumor cells may co-express two or even three different cytoskeletal proteins, for example, NFP-GFP, NFP-desmin, or NFP-vimentin. Normal cells of the central nervous system do not demonstrate such features. The importance of expression of specific neurofilament proteins in determining prognosis is not yet clear.

CLINICAL FEATURES

Children with medulloblastoma typically present with the "midline syndrome" of headache, lethargy, and vomiting. These symptoms are nonspecific manifestations of increased intracranial pressure, and a similar picture is seen with cerebellar astrocytomas and ependymomas. Because all of these tumors arise in the

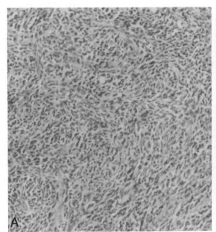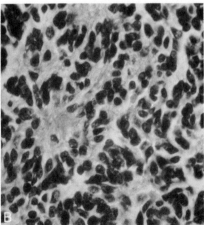

FIGURE 27–1. Pathology of a typical medulloblastoma. *A*, On light microscopy (hematoxylin & eosin), medulloblastomas appear as a field of densely packed small round cells which stain blue. *B*, On higher magnification, Homer Wright rosettes can be seen in 20 per cent of cases.

region of the fourth ventricle, obstructive hydrocephalus occurs early, and is usually the cause of the early symptomatology. The midline syndrome typically begins insidiously, with occasional morning headache and vomiting that improve throughout the rest of the day and may be initially attributed to a viral illness. Later in the course of the disease, symptoms become more persistent, and if the diagnosis is not made at this stage, signs of truncal ataxia, nystagmus, and sixth nerve palsies due to hydrocephalus may develop. Some patients may develop head tilt from tonsillar impaction into the cervical spinal canal. If the tumor is permitted to progress at this point, pressure waves, opisthotonus, bradycardia, apnea, and death ensue. The median duration of symptoms prior to radiologic diagnosis is 6 to 7 weeks, which is considerably shorter than that seen in cerebellar astrocytomas and reflects the more rapid growth rate of medulloblastomas.[16, 21]

Atypical presentations are not uncommon. Infants with open sutures may escape other signs of intracranial hypertension and present with asymptomatic head enlargement. Patients with diffuse subarachnoid spread of tumor at the time of diagnosis may present with meningeal signs, such as neck stiffness and photophobia. Medulloblastoma cells may be confused with lymphocytes on cerebrospinal fluid analysis, and disseminated medulloblastoma must be considered in the differential diagnosis of a child or infant with subacute meningitis. Some children may present with signs and symptoms of cauda equina or spinal cord compression as the first manifestations of their disease, and imaging studies directed at the posterior fossa may be indicated prior to undertaking laminectomy in a child with multiple intradural spinal mass lesions. Tumors arising in the cerebellopontine angle may present with multiple cranial nerve palsies. Occasionally, a medulloblastoma will present as a catastrophic intratumoral hemorrhage leading rapidly to coma, suggestive of a ruptured arteriovenous malformation.[16, 22] It is thus important to obtain biopsy material when exploration is undertaken for an unexplained hematoma in a child with a spontaneous intracerebral or intracerebellar hemorrhage.

IMAGING FEATURES

Modern imaging techniques have revolutionized the diagnosis of posterior fossa tumors of childhood, and older modalities such as pneumoencephalography and conventional angiography are now only of historical importance in this context. The features of medulloblastoma on computerized tomography (CT) and magnetic resonance imaging (MRI) are sufficiently characteristic that the diagnosis is suspected prior to surgery in a high percentage of cases.

On CT, the tumor appears as a well-marginated homogeneously hyperdense mass that arises from the vermis and fills the fourth ventricle. The mass typically enhanced brilliantly and uniformly with the administration of contrast material (Fig. 27–2).[18] Less fre-

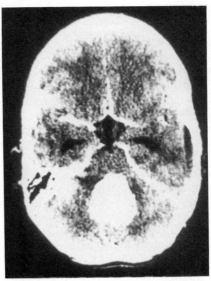

FIGURE 27–2. Contrast-enhanced CT scan of a typical medulloblastoma. The tumors typically enhance brilliantly and homogeneously.

quently, the tumor is isodense on precontrast images and/or demonstrates patchy enhancement. Calcification is uncommon and occurs in only about 15 per cent of cases. Although cystic and necrotic areas are usually considered uncommon in medulloblastomas, some series reported these findings in 47 per cent of cases.[23, 24] Mild to moderate edema surrounds the tumor in most cases,[25] and hydrocephalus is associated in 95 per cent of patients. Intratumoral hemorrhage is unusual.

In some instances, the tumor extends beyond the boundaries of the fourth ventricle. Tumor may fill the cisterna magna or even extend to the cervical subarachnoid space. Superiorly, medulloblastomas may grow to the level of the third ventricle. The presence of such extensions and the size of the tumor appear to be important in prognosis.[26]

Recently, MRI has replaced or supplemented CT for the imaging of brain tumors in many centers.[27] This is due to its greater resolution, its ability to provide multiplanar images, its lack of artifact in the posterior fossa due to lack of bone artifact, and its ability to distinguish aneurysms or other vascular malformations, which may be confused with tumors in rare cases. On MRI, the appearance of medulloblastoma is less specific than on CT.[25] The tumor may be seen to arise from the vermis and is usually relatively hypodense on short TR/TE (T1-weighted) images (Fig. 27–3), becoming brighter on proton density (intermediate-weighted) images.

Medulloblastomas may demonstrate relative hypointensity on long TR/TE (T2-weighted) images, presumably owing to dense cellularity with a relatively low free water content. This pattern is by no means specific, however, and the signal may be hyperintense on T2-weighted images. The pattern of enhancement after injection of gadolinium-DTPA is similar to that after injection of iodinated contrast with CT. The presence of

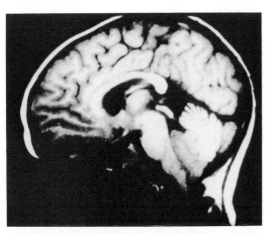

FIGURE 27–3. T1-weighted MRI of a posterior fossa medulloblastoma. The mass fills the fourth ventricle, obstructing the flow of cerebrospinal fluid. The tumor is plastered against the dorsal surface of the brainstem.

subarachnoid seeding or cerebral metastases would favor the diagnosis. Newer diagnostic techniques, such as magnetic resonance spectroscopy, may soon supplement MRI and render it more specific.[28, 29]

OPERATIVE MANAGEMENT

With current surgical techniques, the vast majority of patients with medulloblastoma can be operated on safely, and the perioperative mortality approaches zero in experienced hands. Safe surgery depends on a thorough understanding of the anatomy of the structures surrounding the tumor.

The fourth ventricle is roughly a pyramid, its floor formed by the dorsal pons and medulla, and its roof by the superior medullary velum and the inferior medullary velum. The lateral boundaries are composed of the superior, middle, and inferior cerebellar peduncles. The inferior apex opens into the cisterna magna by way of the midline foramen of Magendie. If the cisterna magna is exposed and the tonsils are retracted laterally, the inferior portion of the fourth ventricle may be visualized.

If the vermis is divided and the ventricle is entered, the structures forming the ventricular floor are visible. Inferiorly, the obex, hypoglossal trigone, and area postrema are seen. The stria medullaris forms a transverse band at the midportion of the ventricle and dips into the median sulcus. More rostrally, the median sulcus is flanked by the facial colliculi. At the rostral apex, the cavity of the fourth ventricle curves gently downward (anteriorly), and the cerebral aqueduct leads to the third ventricle. The lateral apices of the ventricle form the lateral recesses, from which the choroid plexus originates. The choroid plexus protrudes from the lateral foramen and is immediately over the ninth cranial nerve and slightly posterior to the facial and vestibulocochlear nerves. The blood supply to the structures of the inferior fourth ventricle derives from the tonsilar hemispheric branch of the posterior inferior cerebellar artery, which originates at the choroidal area and follows the inferior and medial surface of the tonsil.

Medulloblastomas typically arise from the medullary velum and fill the cavity of the fourth ventricle. They often attach laterally to the cerebellar peduncles and derive blood supply inferolaterally from the tonsilar hemispheric arteries. In about a third of cases, there is infiltration of the dorsal brainstem.[16]

Preoperative planning begins with careful review of the radiologic studies. In most cases, this will include computed tomography (CT) scans, magnetic resonance imaging (MRI) scans with contrast enhancement, or both. The presence of hydrocephalus is noted. The midsagittal MRI scan (see Fig. 27–3) is helpful in determining the superior and inferior extent of the exposure needed for the resection. In addition, areas of possible brainstem infiltration may be determined.

Children with medulloblastomas are often acutely ill at the time of presentation. They are often vomiting, lethargic, and complaining of severe headache. These symptoms are usually the result of acute obstructive hydrocephalus rather than the mass itself, and considerable controversy has centered on the management of this hydrocephalus. Options include preoperative steroids followed by tumor excision,[30, 31] external ventricular drainage,[32] and placement of a cerebrospinal fluid (CSF) shunt before tumor removal.[33–38] Those who favor the use of preoperative shunting point out that (1) time is afforded to prepare the patient and the family for surgery, perform diagnostic tests, and schedule major surgery electively; and (2) a safer surgical procedure is potentially permitted in the posterior fossa after the intracranial pressure is decreased. In one series, the operative mortality rate was decreased with preoperative shunting.[34] Others point out, however, that there are disadvantages with this strategy: (1) not all patients will require shunts after the tumor has been excised, and preoperative shunting condemns the entire group to the possibility of shunt-related complications; (2) a preoperative shunt delays definitive treatment of the tumor; and (3) shunts serve as a source of dissemination of the medulloblastoma, which may spread by the CSF pathways.[32, 39] The use of millipore filters has been described to prevent this problem,[16] but these frequently obstruct, resulting in shunt failure.[4] Upward herniation[40] and tumor hemorrhage[41, 42] have been reported after acute decompression of the supratentorial compartment when the posterior fossa mass is left behind.

McLaurin has concluded that these risks and benefits probably balance each other, and therefore either approach is acceptable.[40] It is our policy to begin dexamethasone (1 mg per kg per day) on admission, avoid preoperative shunting, and perform surgery on the next elective operative day. If the child's condition deteriorates suddenly, the tumor is removed on an emergency basis.

Proper anesthetic management is crucial to the safe conduct of posterior fossa surgery. Patients with posterior fossa tumors are presumed to have a "full stomach and tight head,"[43] meaning that precautions should be taken to fit the conditions of a full stomach and reduced intracranial compliance. The patient is lightly premedicated or is not premedicated at all, and narcotics are avoided. Atropine is given to dry oral secretions. Induction of anesthesia is accomplished once a secure intravenous line is inserted. The patient is preoxygenated using a bag and mask, then pancuronium is given, followed by thiopental. As the patient loses consciousness, cricoid pressure is applied to occlude the esophagus and prevent regurgitation, and hyperventilation is instituted. When paralysis ensues, the endotracheal tube is inserted, and the stomach is emptied via a nasogastric tube. Monitoring consists of electrocardiography, end-tidal carbon dioxide analysis and analysis of other exhaled gases using mass spectrometry, arterial blood pressure by cuff and arterial line, stethoscope, and frequent blood gas analysis. Maintenance anesthesia employs the technique of nitrous-narcotic-relaxant-barbiturate.

For surgery on posterior fossa tumors, the patient may be placed in the prone position. The risk of air embolism, frontal pneumocephalus, and systemic hypotension associated with the sitting position are minimized with this position. Children 3 years of age or older are flexed and held in position with three-point pin fixation. In younger children in whom pins might perforate the skull, the head is supported with a padded horseshoe-shaped rest. By standing at the side of the patient facing cephalad, the operating surgeon obtains an excellent view, and exposure is excellent as far upward as the upper vermis and tentorial notch.

Surgery is begun by placing an occipital burr hole to provide access to the ventricle. In patients with hydrocephalus, a catheter may be inserted into the ventricle and tunneled subcutaneously. Cerebrospinal fluid may then be vented as the dura is opened and during the postoperative period if necessary.

A midline vertical incision is made from the inion to the mid-cervical region, and a wide craniectomy is performed from the transverse sinuses to the foramen magnum. Free craniectomy flaps for posterior fossa procedures have been described,[44] but the presence of large dural sinuses and midline keels of bone have made craniectomy the procedure preferred by many pediatric neurosurgeons. The arch of C1 is usually removed when the tumor is large, since the tumor may extend into the cisterna magna and the tonsils are often impacted.

The dura is opened with a Y-shaped incision extending to the level of C1. Large dural venous sinuses are frequent at the level of the foramen magnum in children; they are occluded with MRI-compatible dural clips or oversewn. Cerebrospinal fluid is vented through the ventriculostomy at this point to reduce the tension in the posterior fossa; if the ventricles are small, mannitol is used for this purpose. The cisterna magna is opened, and the cerebellar tonsils separated with self-retaining retractors. The tumor may be visible as a red, semicircumscribed mass presenting in the vallecula

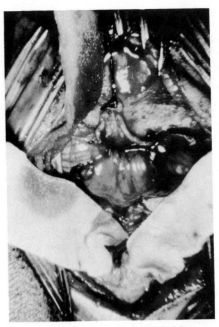

FIGURE 27–4. Gross appearance of a medulloblastoma at surgery. The mass is red and friable, and it is readily distinguished from normal brain.

(Fig. 27–4). The vermis is then opened in the midline using bipolar cautery and gentle suction, until the dorsal surface of the tumor is totally exposed. Tomita and McLone have shown that CSF or arachnoid from the cisterna magna almost always demonstrates evidence of seeding of medulloblastoma cells.[44] The significance of this finding is unknown, but it is not a contraindication for radical resection of the tumor.

Medulloblastomas are not truly encapsulated, but a clear interface can often be developed between the tumor and surrounding brain. A gross total excision can be accomplished if effort is spent to define this plane circumferentially around the tumor, as the inside of the tumor is gutted using suction or the Cavitron ultrasonic surgical aspirator (CUSA). The dissection is accomplished using bipolar cautery, suction, and cottonoid sponges as the retraction is gradually deepened. Retraction must be done gently, under direct vision. Shoving cottonoid sponges blindly into the depths of the dissection may injure the brainstem, resulting in prolonged coma, respiratory disturbances, or extraocular muscle palsies. The tumor usually is not removed as a single specimen, but internally decompressed as the margins are defined. The midsagittal MRI scan is useful to delineate where CSF of the fourth ventricle separates tumor from brainstem, and these portions of the tumor are removed first. Removal of areas where the brainstem may be attached is deferred until there is less tumor bulk to obscure the anatomy. Medulloblastomas are frequently highly vascular, and often the best way to control blood loss is to work quickly. Bleeding will stop once the major part of the tumor has been removed. At the superior depth of the tumor, a tongue of tumor will often occlude or fill the aqueduct, and this is removed with suction. If the tumor is attached to the brainstem or peduncles, this is carefully shaved down, but no attempt is made to enter the substance of the brainstem itself. Unlike some focal brainstem gliomas, in which the tumor is separate from functional brainstem neural tissue, medulloblastomas tend to infiltrate, and attempts to remove this tissue will result in permanent neurologic damage to the child. Furthermore, removal of small bits of tumor has not been shown to improve survival in patients who require postoperative radiation therapy or chemotherapy anyway.[45] The goal of surgery is total resection of gross visible tumor except that located within the brainstem or cerebellar peduncles.

Meticulous hemostasis is achieved, and the wound is irrigated to remove as much blood as possible. Absorbable hemostatic agents may be used in troublesome areas of the tumor bed, but may float free and occlude the CSF pathways. Dural closure is difficult at best. The posterior fossa dura shrinks during the procedure, and a watertight closure is often impossible without a graft. Pericranium or freeze-dried dura may be used.

During the first 24 to 48 hours, the ventriculostomy is drained at 100 mm H_2O by elevating the drainage bag or by attaching the system to a pressure transducer and intermittently opening the system to drainage when needed. During the next 24 hours, the drain is clamped, and if this is well tolerated, the ventriculostomy is removed. Some surgeons believe that intermittent spinal taps are useful for a few days to promote CSF drainage and to clear blood. This requires that the CSF pathways be open and may be hazardous if there is tumor or blood clot within the aqueduct or fourth ventricle. If a large subcutaneous CSF collection develops at the operative site or if symptoms of hydrocephalus occur with cessation of CSF drainage, a shunt will be required.

It is common in the immediate postoperative period for patients to be extremely irritable, photophobic, and nauseous. Splitting the vermis results in transient truncal ataxia and disconjugate gaze, which usually resolve over a couple of weeks. Persistent ipsilateral dysmetria is the rule in patients whose tumors arise from the peduncle, but it is usually well tolerated. Patients with tumors that involve the brainstem may have more serious postoperative sequelae, including apnea, chronic aspiration, and facial or extraocular palsies. Rarely, patients will have an expressive aphasia postoperatively, the etiology of which is obscure. This usually clears over several weeks.

POSTOPERATIVE STAGING

It has been known for over 30 years that surgical excision alone is inadequate treatment for medulloblastoma. The addition of prophylactic whole-brain and spinal axis irradiation has markedly improved survival, and many series now report 5-year disease-free survival rates in the range of 50 to 70 per cent,[10, 16, 46–49]

and for some long-term survivors, one is even tempted to speak of "cure."[50] It has been suggested, for example, that patients with survival periods greater than the patient's age at diagnosis plus 9 months are no longer at risk of recurrence (Collins' law),[51, 52] although numerous cases of relapse beyond the Collins period of risk have been reported.[50] As the outlook for survival has improved, however, so has concern that whole-brain irradiation (WBI) in the child results in significant neuropsychological and cognitive dysfunction. Numerous attempts have been made to develop staging criteria to maximize tumor-free survival and at the same time to minimize the adverse effects of whole-brain irradiation. In patients assigned to "good risk" groups, the radiation dose is reduced, whereas in patients in "poor risk" groups, adjuvant chemotherapy is added to improve survival. This concept has recently been questioned, since adjuvant chemotherapy appears to confer greater benefit to poor-risk patients than that obtained in so-called "good-risk" patients treated with radiation alone.[10] Even if future protocols call for chemotherapy in all patients with medulloblastoma, however, some form of postoperative evaluation for extent of disease will be necessary to guide radiation boosts for lump disease in the spine, and to allow comparison of outcome in series treated with different regimens.

Extent of Surgical Resection. Although it seems intuitive that a patient who undergoes a "total" resection will fare better than a patient with a subtotally resected tumor, this has yet to be proved. In part, this relates to lack of agreement among clinicians as to what constitutes a total resection. It has become clear that postoperative imaging studies are superior to the subjective impression of the surgeon in gauging extent of resection with posterior fossa tumors. An exception might be very small amounts of residual tumor in the brainstem, which may be below the limit of resolution of current scanners but are visible to the operating surgeon. "Total resection" in the strictest sense would then be no visible tumor in the operative bed *as well as* no visible tumor seen on the postoperative enhanced MRI scan. A resection is deemed "subtotal" if the surgeon thought that a small amount of tumor had been left, or if the postoperative scan shows lumps of enhancing tissue in the operative bed. In most cases, this will mean a small nodule within the substance of the brainstem or cerebellar peduncle. Using these strict criteria, there does not appear to be a significant difference in outcome between the two groups.[45] This result does not justify conservative surgery, since partial excision and biopsy are associated with poorer outcome than more aggressively resected tumors.[45] Radical surgery is generally safe and appropriate, but there is no benefit to be gained by surgical attempts to remove tumor from within the brainstem, or by reoperating on patients with very small amounts of postoperative residual disease prior to radiotherapy or chemotherapy.

Tumor Size. For years, the Chang staging system has been widely employed to quantitate tumor size at the time of diagnosis[26] (Table 27–1). In this system, the surgeon's intraoperative impressions are used to cate-

TABLE 27–1.   CHANG STAGING SYSTEM FOR MEDULLOBLASTOMA

TUMOR STAGE	DEFINITION
T1	Tumor less than 3 cm in diameter and limited to the midline position in the vermis, roof of the fourth ventricle, and less frequently to the cerebellar hemispheres
T2	Tumor more than 3 cm in diameter, further invading one adjacent structure or partially filling the fourth ventricle
T3a	Tumor invading 2 adjacent structures or completely filling the fourth ventricle with extension into the aqueduct of Sylvius, foramen of Magendie, or foramen of Luschka, thus producing marked obstructive hydrocephalus
T3b	Tumor arising from the floor of the fourth ventricle or brainstem and filling the fourth ventricle
T4	Tumor further spreading through the aqueduct of Sylvius to involve the third ventricle or midbrain or tumor extending to the upper cervical cord
METASTASIS STAGE	
M0	No evidence of gross subarachnoid or hematogenous metastasis
M1	Microscopic tumor cells found in CSF
M2	Gross nodule seedings demonstrated in the cerebellum, cerebral subarachnoid space, or in the third or lateral ventricles
M3	Gross nodule seedings in the spinal subarachnoid space
M4	Extraneuroaxial metastasis

gorize the tumor into stages, although more recently preoperative imaging studies have been used as well. Chang stage T1 and T2 lesions are small tumors and are seen relatively infrequently. Chang stage T3 and T4 lesions fill the fourth ventricle and cause hydrocephalus, invade the brainstem, or coat the upper cervical cord. In several older series, patients with these larger tumors were found to fare more poorly; however, it is unclear whether the effect of the size of the tumor at diagnosis can be negated by the extent of resection. In fact, more recent studies have shown T stage to be of no predictive value. Laurent et al.[53] have suggested that a postoperative CT scan (or, alternatively, MRI scan) could replace the Chang system.

Dissemination. The presence or absence of dissemination of tumor through the neuraxis at diagnosis is the most significant factor in predicting survival in patients with medulloblastoma, and the Chang system also provides for an "M stage" to account for this factor (Table 27–1). Dissemination is detected in approximately 20 to 30 per cent of children at the time of diagnosis and may be present in as many as 50 per cent of infants.[54]

To some extent, successful identification depends on the diagnostic method used. Until recently, postoperative patients usually underwent a staging myelogram for the evaluation of spinal dissemination prior to therapy.[55] Many centers are now using spinal MRI with and without contrast for this purpose, but the relative sensitivity and specificity of this modality compared with

myelography remains a matter of dispute. Recent evidence suggests that MRI is superior to myelography in delineating cord nodules and "sugar coating," but myelography with postcontrast CT may better define subtle root lesions (Fig. 27–5).[56] A problem with both techniques is the distinguishing of tumor from blood clots on immediate postoperative studies. In typical cases in which the initial imaging studies suggest a medulloblastoma, it is preferable to perform the spine MRI study preoperatively to avoid this source of error.

As with postoperative imaging studies, CSF cytologies obtained immediately after surgery may be difficult to interpret. Malignant cells may be dislodged by the surgical procedure, giving false-positive results. In some institutions, protocols call for repeat CSF cytologic examination 10 to 14 days after surgery if the only positive study is a positive cytology in the immediate postoperative period. Some centers are also measuring CSF polyamines (putrescine and spermidine) as evidence of dissemination.[57]

Age. For unknown reasons, younger children, especially infants, do not fare as well as older children with medulloblastoma. The factor of age is a complex one, since younger children are more likely to have disseminated disease at the time of diagnosis, and since the immature brain is more susceptible to the adverse effects of radiation, younger patients usually receive less aggressive treatment.[58]

Histology. The presence of a desmoplastic component within a medulloblastoma has been related by some authors to a somewhat improved survival.[59–61] Others, however, have associated this histologic variant with a worse prognosis,[21, 62] and its significance remains uncertain.

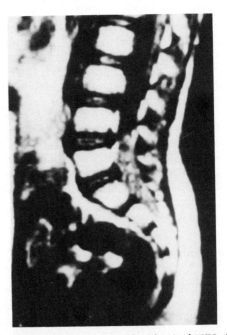

FIGURE 27–5. Gadolinium-enhanced midsagittal MRI of the lumbosacral spine in a patient with drop metastases from a medulloblastoma, filling the caudal thecal sac.

TABLE 27-2.   RISK FACTORS FOR CHILDREN WITH MEDULLOBLASTOMA

FACTOR	GOOD RISK	POOR RISK (1 OR MORE)
Extent of disease	Nondisseminated	Disseminated
Size of primary tumor	Chang T1-T2	Chang T3-T4
Resection	?Total	? Subtotal
Age	4 years or older	Younger than 4 years

More recently, the presence within the tumor of differentiation along identifiable cell lines (glial, neuronal, ependymal) by light microscopy has been linked with an unfavorable prognosis.[45] Others have not been able to document such a correlation, however.[47] The introduction of immunohistochemical stains for precise identification of intermediate filaments has greatly added to the understanding of the nature of these poorly differentiated tumors,[19] but the issue of differentiation utilizing these techniques as a prognostic factor is unsettled.

Based on all of the above factors, it is possible to stratify patients into "good-risk" and "poor-risk" groups (Table 27–2). From Children's Cancer Study Group (CCSG) data, it can be estimated that for the poor-risk group, overall survival is approximately 36 per cent at 5 years with standard postoperative craniospinal axis irradiation versus 60 to 70 per cent for children without adverse risk factors. These staging criteria have been used at a number of centers to place poor-risk patients into chemotherapy protocols and to attempt reduction in the dose of cranial irradiation in "good-risk" patients in an attempt to diminish late sequelae.

RADIATION THERAPY AND NEUROPSYCHOLOGICAL SEQUELAE

The optimal dose of radiation therapy required for medulloblastoma remains controversial. Most series have employed a local tumor dose of 5000 to 5500 cGy, with a dose of 3600 to 4000 cGy to the neuraxis.[7, 8, 45, 46, 54] It has been suggested, but not proved, that patients who are carefully staged and found to have only localized disease can be equally well treated with reduced-dose whole-brain and spinal therapy.[44] Such studies are important, because it has become clear that children surviving medulloblastoma and its therapy are at risk for adverse late effects.[7, 63–66] A 4-year-old child receiving a standard dose of whole-brain irradiation might expect a decrease of 40 IQ points 2 years after treatment, whereas children older than 10 appear to suffer no measurable decline in IQ (Fig. 27–6). Neurocognitive sequelae are dependent on age at diagnosis and almost certainly on whole-brain radiation dose as well (Fig. 27–7). Significant endocrinologic problems may also occur in long-term survivors of medulloblastoma,

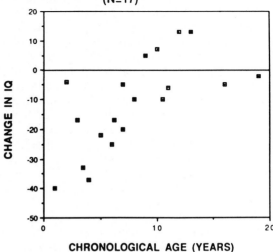

CHANGE IN IQ AT 3 & 4 YEAR FOLLOWUP (N=17)

FIGURE 27–6. Drop in IQ at 3 and 4 years of follow-up for patients with medulloblastoma treated with whole-brain radiation. Neurocognitive impairment is age-dependent, with younger children suffering the greatest degree of damage.

notably hypothyroidism and growth failure due to growth hormone deficiency.[63] Endocrine hormone replacement may be instituted as necessary.

In order to reduce these late effects, some institutions have attempted to reduce the dose of whole-brain irradiation, and recent reports from two separate institutions suggest that whole-brain doses in the range of 2400 to 2500 cGy may be as effective as the higher dose.[60, 67] However, a recent randomized prospective trial demonstrated an increased frequency of exo-primary site (primarily spinal) recurrence in patients treated with 2340 cGy of craniospinal radiation as com-

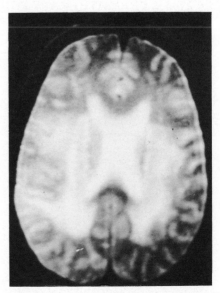

FIGURE 27–7. T2-weighted MRI of a patient 3 years after craniospinal axis irradiation for medulloblastoma. Extensive periventricular white matter abnormalities are seen.

pared to patients treated with the more conventional (3600 cGy) dose.[68] This has led to general abandonment of attempts to reduce the amount of craniospinal radiotherapy alone, but there is hope that the use of adjuvant chemotherapy could substitute for some of the radiation and that the use of chemotherapy might allow employment of lower radiation doses. At our institution between 1988 and 1989, patients in the 18-month to 5-year age group without dissemination were placed on a protocol in which the neuraxis dose was reduced to 1800 cGy, while maintaining the local tumor dose at 5040 to 5580 cGy. Adjuvant chemotherapy with vincristine, CCNU, and cisplatin was used in an attempt to prevent relapse. At a mean of 2 years of follow-up, 3 of 10 patients have relapsed, and in all cases the relapse involved sites outside the tumor bed. There was no measurable drop in IQ, however, suggesting that this dose of whole-brain radiation is well tolerated in this age group.[69] In view of these results, efforts are now under way utilizing 2340 cGy of craniospinal radiotherapy with chemotherapy to control disease with fewer sequelae. For entry into the study, patients must be carefully staged and free of disseminated disease. Another approach is the use of hyperfractionated radiation, which delivers doses that are "reduced" with respect to late sequelae, but are "standard" with respect to tumor control.[70]

CHEMOTHERAPY

Medulloblastomas are theoretically excellent tumors for chemotherapeutic intervention.[71] They are well vascularized and have a high growth fraction. In vivo and in vitro studies of human medulloblastomas have demonstrated responsiveness of the tumor to a variety of chemotherapeutic agents. Clinical evidence for the benefit of chemotherapy has been substantiated by analysis of patients at the time of disease recurrence and by pre-irradiation therapy trials during which therapy is given after surgery and before radiation therapy.[71]

Efficacy of Chemotherapy at the Time of Disease Recurrence. A variety of different drugs, or drug combinations, have been shown to be effective at the time of disease recurrence (Table 27–3).[71–82] Active drugs include cyclophosphamide, cisplatin, vincristine, and methotrexate. The utility of these drugs is somewhat limited by associated toxicities. For example, methotrexate, although clearly an active agent, may cause significant leukoencephalopathy, especially when used after radiotherapy. Overall response rates to single agents are relatively high, but most children with recurrent disease will ultimately relapse and die of their illness.

In an attempt to improve the efficacy of chemotherapy for children with medulloblastoma, multi-agent drug combinations are now more frequently employed.[71] This is primarily based on the concept that a tumor is less likely to be resistant to multiple agents administered simultaneously than it is to be resistant to individual agents; and if drugs are given over a relatively short period of time, myelosuppression should be less because damage to hematopoietic precursor cells is partially dependent on duration of exposure. The most aggressive application of rapid-sequence, multi-agent chemotherapy has been the 8-drug-in-one-day treatment approach: eight agents (vincristine, CCNU, cisplatin, hydroxyurea, prednisone, cyclophosphamide, arabinosyl cytosine, procarbazine hydrochloride) are given over a 24-hour period.[79] Long-term therapeutic advantage in medulloblastoma for this combination as com-

TABLE 27–3.   CHEMOTHERAPY FOR RELAPSED MEDULLOBLASTOMA: SELECTED TRIALS

AUTHOR	NUMBER OF PATIENTS	THERAPY	NUMBER OF PATIENTS RESPONDING (%)	MEDIAN LENGTH OF RESPONSE (MONTHS)
Crafts	16	Procarbazine CCNU VCR	14(87.5)	11
Walker and Allen	12	Cisplatin	9(75)	8
Sexauer	10	Cisplatin	5(50)	3.5
Allen and Helson	8	Cyclophosphamide	8(100)	6
Allen and Walker	14	Carboplatin	6(42.8)	10+
Freidman	15	Carboplatin	1(7)	NA
Rosen	7	HDMTX BCNU VCR	5(71.4)	9
Bertolone	12	Cisplatin	3(25)	NG
Pendergrass	11	"8-in-1"	8(72.7)	16
Duffner	8	IV MTX IV MTX BCNU VCR Prednisone	8(100)	18.8
Lefkowitz	6	CCNU/VCR/ Cisplatin	6(100)	18.5

HDMTX = high dose methotrexate; VCR = vincristine; NG = not given; NA = not available; IV MTX = intravenous methotrexate; "8-in-1" = prednisone, vincristine, CCNU, procarbazine, hydroxyurea, cisplatin, arabinosyl cytosine, and cyclophosphamide.

pared to less complicated drug regimens has never been demonstrated.

Efficacy of Chemotherapy for Patients with Newly Diagnosed Disease. Two independent multi-institutional randomized trials undertaken in the mid-1970s demonstrated a benefit for the addition of chemotherapy when used after radiation therapy for some patients with medulloblastoma.[83, 84] The addition of vincristine during radiation therapy and postradiation cycles of CCNU and vincristine were shown to improve the duration and frequency of survival for children with more extensive disease. Although studies performed in the 1970s are difficult to directly apply to current management, since neuro-imaging techniques have improved over this period of time and postoperative surveillance studies are now more routinely obtained, the information obtained from the Children's Cancer Study Group trial and the trial undertaken by the International Society for Pediatric Oncology suggests that patients with larger tumors, especially those which had disseminated within the neuroaxis prior to diagnosis, were most likely to benefit from chemotherapy. In 30 patients with the most extensive tumors, both large primary site disease and metastatic disease, event-free survival was markedly better in the group receiving chemotherapy (48 per cent versus 0 per cent, $p = 0.006$).[83] Smaller, nonrandomized trials have also suggested a benefit of adjuvant chemotherapy.

Even more recently, information from the Children's Hospital of Philadelphia has also substantiated the role of adjuvant chemotherapy.[10] In this single-arm trial, weekly vincristine was given during radiotherapy, and cisplatin, CCNU, and vincristine were delivered after radiotherapy in children with high-risk disease. To date, over 55 children with either metastatic disease or partially resected primary site disease have been treated in this manner, and actuarial 5-year, disease-free survival is nearly 90 per cent (Fig. 27–8). Other trials are currently under way, some utilizing chemotherapy during and following radiotherapy and others administering drugs prior to radiotherapy. Only randomized trials pitting one drug regimen against another will determine which is most efficacious.

Results of these adjuvant trials raises significant questions concerning the use of chemotherapy in children with newly diagnosed medulloblastoma. The first is whether chemotherapy is indicated in all patients, regardless of risk factors. This question is unanswerable at present; however, it does seem that children with high-risk disease now treated with adjuvant chemotherapy are faring as well as, or possibly even better than, patients with so-called "good-risk" disease receiving radiotherapy alone.[10] A second important issue is whether chemotherapy can be used to reduce the amount of radiotherapy required for patients with newly diagnosed disease. It has been well established that children surviving medulloblastoma often have significant, long-term sequelae. Craniospinal radiation therapy has been incriminated as the major cause for intellectual and endocrinologic long-term dysfunction. As stated previously, attempts to reduce the amount of craniospinal radiotherapy, even in patients with non-metastatic disease at the time of diagnosis, have failed; children receiving reduced-dose radiotherapy have a higher rate of both local and disseminated relapse.[68] Trials are currently under way to evaluate the ability of reduced-dose radiotherapy (in the 2400 cGY range) to control disease when adjuvant chemotherapy is added.

A third issue concerning the use of chemotherapy is whether a more aggressive or rational use of chemotherapy could improve survival for children at highest risk for disease relapse after radiotherapy alone, namely those with diffuse metastatic disease at the time of diagnosis. Given the difficulty in utilizing high-dose chemotherapy following craniospinal radiation, there are, at present, attempts to utilize chemotherapy prior to radiation. It is believed that pre-radiation chemotherapy will allow more treatment to be given and better drug delivery to the tumor site. However, to date, there is no evidence for long-term benefit from this approach.

Chemotherapy Alone for Very Young Children with Medulloblastoma. Possibly the most important ultimate use of chemotherapy for children with medulloblastoma will be in very young children who are likely to be severely damaged by therapeutic doses of

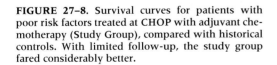

FIGURE 27–8. Survival curves for patients with poor risk factors treated at CHOP with adjuvant chemotherapy (Study Group), compared with historical controls. With limited follow-up, the study group fared considerably better.

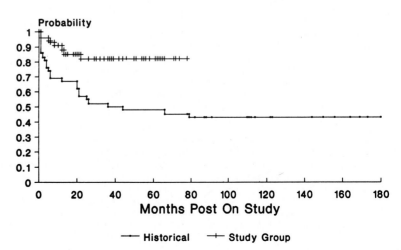

craniospinal radiation therapy. MOPP chemotherapy (mechlorethamine hydrochloride, vincristine, procarbazine, and prednisone) has been used for many years for infants with malignant tumors, including medulloblastoma.[85] Eight of 18 children with medulloblastoma treated with MOPP in one study are in complete remission without radiotherapy for follow-up periods ranging from 6 to 150 months (mean 73 months).[85] The Pediatric Oncology Group has used cisplatinum, high-dose cyclophosphamide, etoposide, and vincristine for children younger than 3 years of age with a variety of malignant tumors, including medulloblastoma.[86] In the majority of patients, craniospinal and local radiotherapy could be delayed until children were 24 to 36 months of age. Since radiotherapy was mandated in this study for all children at the completion of treatment, or at 3 years of age, it is unclear whether children actually needed radiotherapy. Studies are under way at present to determine whether radiotherapy can safely be omitted in those patients without evidence of residual disease after treatment with surgery and chemotherapy.

REFERENCES

1. Baily P, Cushing H: Medulloblastoma cerebelli: A common type of midcerebellar glioma of childhood. Arch Neurol Psych 14:192, 1925.
2. Rorke L: The cerebellar medulloblastoma and its relationship to primitive neuroectodermal tumors. J Neuropathol Exp Neurol 42:1, 1983.
3. Russell D, Rubenstein L: Pathology of Tumors of the Nervous System. 5th ed. Baltimore, Williams & Wilkins, 1989, pp 251–279.
4. Elsberg C, Gotten N: Results of conservative compared with radical operations in cerebellar medulloblastoma. Bull Neurol Inst 3:33, 1933.
5. Wanke R: Sur anatomie und chirurgie der kleinhirngechwulste. Arch Klin Chir 180:428, 1934.
6. Patterson E, Farr R: Cerebellar medulloblastoma treated by irradiation of the whole CNS. Acta Radiol 39:323, 1953.
7. Hirsch J, Renier D, Czernichow P, et al.: Medulloblastoma in childhood. Survival and functional results. Acta Neurochir 48:1, 1979.
8. Gerosa M, DiStefano E, Oliva A, et al.: Multidisciplinary treatment of medulloblastoma. A 5-year experience with the SIOP trial. Childs Brain 8:107, 1981.
9. Allen J, Bloom J, Ertel I, et al.: Brain tumors in children. Current cooperative and institutional chemotherapy trials in newly diagnosed and recurrent disease. Semin Oncol 13:110, 1986.
10. Packer R, Sutton L, Goldwein J, et al.: Improved survival with the use of adjuvant chemotherapy in the treatment of medulloblastoma. J Neurosurg 74:433, 1991.
11. Levin V, Rodriguez L, Edwards M, et al.: Treatment of medulloblastoma with procarbazine, hydroxyurea, and reduced radiation doses to whole brain and spine. J Neurosurg 68:383, 1988.
12. Koos W, Miller M: Intracranial Tumors of Infants and Children. Stuttgart, George Thieme, 205, 1971.
13. Matson D: Neurosurgery of Infancy and Childhood. Springfield, Ill, Charles C Thomas, 1969, pp 448–456.
14. Humphreys R: Posterior cranial fossa brain tumors in children. In Youmans J (ed): Neurological Surgery. 2nd ed. Philadelphia, WB Saunders, 1982, pp 2730–2752.
15. Hubbard J, Scheithauer B, Kispert D, Carperter S, Wick M, Laws E: Adult cerebellar medulloblastomas: the pathological, radiographic, and clinical disease spectrum. J Neurosurg 70:536, 1989.
16. Park T, Hoffman H, Hendrick E, Humphreys R, Becker L: Medulloblastoma, clinical presentation and management. Experience at the Hospital for Sick Children, Toronto, 1950–1980. J Neurosurg 58:543, 1983.
17. Biegel J, Rorke L, Packer R, et al.: Isochromosome 17q in primitive neuroectodermal tumors of the central nervous system. Genes Chromosomes Cancer 1:139, 1989.
18. Zimmerman R, Bilaniuk L, Pahlajani H: Spectrum of medulloblastoma demonstrated by computed tomography. Radiology 126:137, 1978.
19. Gould V, Jansson D, Milenaar W, et al.: Primitive neuroectodermal tumors of the central nervous system. Patterns of expression of neuroendocrine markers, and all classes of intermediate filament proteins. Lab Invest 62:498, 1990.
20. Katsetos C, Liu H, Zacks S: Immunohistochemical and ultrastructural observations on Homer-Wright rosettes and the "pale islands" of human cerebellar medulloblastoma. Hum Pathol 19:1219, 1988.
21. Choux M, Lena G: Medulloblastoma. Neurochirurgie 28:13, 1982.
22. Laurent J, Bruce D, Schut L: Hemorrhagic brain tumors in pediatric patients. Childs Brain 8:263, 1981.
23. Zee C-S, Segall H, Miller C, et al.: Less common CT features of medulloblastoma. Radiology 144:97, 1982.
24. Sandhu A, Kendall B: Computed tomography in management of medulloblastomas. Neuroradiology 29:444, 1987.
25. Gusnard D: Cerebellar neoplasms in children. Semin Roentgenol XXV:263, 1990.
26. Chang C, Housepian E, Herbert C Jr.: An operative staging system and a megavoltage radiotherapeutic technique for cerebellar medulloblastomas. Radiology 93:1351, 1969.
27. Heafner M, Schut L, Packer R, Bruce D, Bilaniuk L, Sutton L: Discrepancy between computed tomography and magnetic resonance imaging in a case of medulloblastoma. Neurosurgery 17:487, 1985.
28. Sutton L, Wang Z, Gusnard D, et al.: Proton magnetic resonance spectroscopy of pediatric brain tumors. Neurosurgery 31:195, 1992.
29. Sutton L, RE L, BH C, Packer R, Zimmerman R: Localized 31P magnetic resonance spectroscopy of large pediatric brain tumors. J Neurosurg 72:65, 1990.
30. Lapras C, Palet J, Lapras C, et al.: Cerebellar astrocytomas in childhood. Childs Nerv Syst 2:55, 1986.
31. Wilson C: Diagnosis and surgical treatment of childhood brain tumors. Cancer 35:950, 1975.
32. Kessler L, Dugan P, Concannon J: Systemic metastases of medulloblastoma promoted by shunting. Surg Neurol 3:147, 1975.
33. Abraham J, Chandy J: Ventriculo-atrial shunt in the management of posterior fossa tumor—preliminary report. J Neurosurg 20:252, 1963.
34. Albright L, Reigel D: Management of hydrocephalus secondary to posterior fossa tumors. J Neurosurg 46:52, 1977.
35. Elkins C, Fonesca J: Ventriculo-venous anastamosis in obstructive and acquired hydrocephalus. J Neurosurg 18:134, 1961.
36. Hekmatpanah J, Mullan S: Ventriculo-caval shunt in the management of posterior fossa tumors. J Neurosurg 26:609, 1967.
37. Jane J, Kaufman B, Nulsen F, et al.: The role of angiography and ventriculovenous shunting in the treatment of posterior fossa tumors. Acta Neurochir 28:13, 1973.
38. Raimondi A, Yashon D, Matsumoto S, et al.: Increased intracranial pressure without lateralizing signs: the midline syndrome. Neurochirurgia 10:197, 1967.
39. Hoffman H, Hendrick E, Humphreys R: Metastasis via ventriculoperitoneal shunt in patients with medulloblastoma. J Neurosurg 32:83, 1970.
40. McLaurin R: On the use of precraniotomy shunting in the management of posterior fossa tumors in children. A cooperative study. In Chapman P (ed): Concepts in Pediatric Neurosurgery. Vol 6. Basil, Karger, 1985, pp 1–5.
41. Waga S, Shimizo T, Shimosaka S, et al.: Intratumoral hemorrhage after a ventriculo-peritoneal shunting procedure. Neurosurgery 9:249, 1981.
42. Vaquero J, Cabezudo J, DeSola R: Intratumoral hemorrhage in posterior fossa tumors after ventricular drainage. J Neurosurg 54:406, 1981.

43. Swedlow D: Anesthesia for neurosurgical procedures. *In* Gregory G (ed): Pediatric Anesthesia. New York, Churchill Livingstone, 1983, pp 679–705.

44. Tomita T, McLone D: Medulloblastoma in childhood: results of radical resection and low-dose neuroaxis radiation therapy. J Neurosurg 64:602, 1987.

45. Packer R, Sutton L, Rorke L, et al.: Prognostic significance of cellular differentiation in medulloblastoma of childhood. J Neurosurg 61:296, 1984.

46. Berry M, Jenkin P, Keen C, et al.: Radiation treatment for medulloblastoma—a 21-year review. J Neurosurg 55:43, 1981.

47. Caputy A, McCullogh D, Manz H, et al.: A review of the factors influencing the prognosis of medulloblastoma. The importance of cellular differentiation. J Neurosurg 66:80, 1987.

48. Inoya M, Takakura K, Shatara N, et al.: Treatment of medulloblastoma. Prog Exp Tumor Res 30:91, 1987.

49. Norris D, Bruce D, Byrd R, et al.: Improved relapse-free survival in medulloblastoma using modern techniques. Neurosurgery 9:661, 1981.

50. Belza M, Donaldson S, Steinberg G, Cox R, Cogan P: Medulloblastoma: freedom from relapse longer than 8 years—a therapeutic cure? J Neurosurg 75:575, 1991.

51. Collins V. The treatment of Wilms' tumor. Cancer 11:89, 1958.

52. Silverman C, Simpson J: Cerebellar medulloblastoma: the importance of posterior fossa dose to survival and patterns of failure. Int J Radiat Oncol Biol Phys 8:1869, 1982.

53. Laurent J, Chang C, Cohen M: A classification system for primitive neuroectodermal tumors (medulloblastoma) of the posterior fossa. Cancer 56:1806, 1985.

54. Allen J, Epstein F: Medulloblastoma and other primary malignant neuroectodermal tumors of the CNS. The effect of patient's age and extent of disease on prognosis. J Neurosurg 57:446, 1982.

55. Deutch M, Laurent J, Cohen M: Myelography for staging medulloblastoma. Cancer 56:1763, 1985.

56. Kramer E, Rafto S, Packer R, Zimmerman R: Comparison of myelography with computed tomography follow-up vs. gadolinium magnetic resonance imaging for subarachnoid metastatic disease in children. Neurology 41:46, 1991.

57. Marton L, Edwards M, Levin V, et al.: CSF polyamines: a new and important means of monitoring patients with medulloblastoma. Cancer 47:757, 1984.

58. Packer R, Sutton L, Rorke L, et al.: Management of children with primitive neuroectodermal tumors of the posterior fossa/medulloblastoma. Pediatr Neurosci 12:272, 1986.

59. Chatty E, Earle K: Medulloblastoma: a report of 201 cases with emphasis on the relationship of histologic variants to survival. Cancer 28:977, 1971.

60. Hughes E, Shillito J, Sallan S, Loeffler J, Cassady J, Tarbell N: Medulloblastoma at the Joint Center for Radiation Therapy between 1968 and 1984. The influence of radiation dose on the patterns of failure and survival. Cancer 61:1992, 1988.

61. Hughes P: Cerebellar medulloblastoma in adults. J Neurosurg 60:994, 1984.

62. Hoffman H, Hendricks E, Humphreys R: Management of medulloblastoma in childhood. Clin Neurosurg 30:226, 1982.

63. Duffner P, Cohen M, Anderson S, et al.: Long-term effects of treatment on endocrine function in children with brain tumors. Ann Neurol 14:528, 1983.

64. Duffner P, Cohen M, Thomas P: Late effects of treatment on the intelligence of children with posterior fossa tumors. Cancer 51:233, 1983.

65. Duffner P, Cohen M, Thomas P: The long-term effects of treatment on the intelligence of children with posterior fossa tumors. Cancer 56:1841, 1985.

66. Packer R, Sutton L, Atkins T, et al.: A prospective study of cognitive function in children receiving whole-brain radiotherapy and chemotherapy: 2-year results. J Neurosurg 70:707, 1989.

67. Brand W, Schneider P, Tokars R: Long-term results of a pilot study of low dose craniospinal irradiation for cerebellar medulloblastoma. Int J Radiat Oncol Biol Phys 13:1641, 1987.

68. Deutsch M, Thomas P, Boyett J, et al.: Low-stage medulloblastoma: A Children's Cancer Study Group (CCSG) and Pediatric Oncology Group (POG) randomized study of standard versus reduced neuraxis irradiation. Proc ASCO 10:124, 1991.

69. Goldwein J, Radcliffe J, Packer R, Sutton L: Results of a pilot study of low-dose craniospinal radiation therapy plus chemotherapy for children younger than 5 years with primitive neuroectodermal tumors. Cancer 71:2647, 1993.

70. Withers J: Cell cycle redistribution as a factor in multifraction irradiation. Radiology 114:199, 1975.

71. Packer R: Chemotherapy for medulloblastoma/primitive neuroectodermal tumors of the posterior fossa. Ann Neurol 28:823, 1990.

72. Crafts D, Levin VA, Edwards M, et al.: Chemotherapy of recurrent medulloblastoma with combined procarbazine, CCNU, and vincristine. J Neurosurg 49:589, 1978.

73. Walker R, Allen JC: Cisplatin in the treatment of recurrent childhood primary brain tumors. J Clin Oncol 6:62, 1988.

74. Sexauer C, Khan A, Burger P, et al.: Cisplatin in recurrent pediatric brain tumors; a POG phase II study. Cancer 56:1497, 1985.

75. Allen J, Walker R, Luks E, et al.: Carboplatin and recurrent brain tumors. Clin Oncol 5:459, 1987.

76. Allen J, Helson L: High-dose cyclophosphamide chemotherapy for recurrent CNS tumors in children. J Neurosurg 55:749, 1981.

77. Bertolone S, Baum E, Krivit W, Hammond D: Phase II trial of cisplatinum diamino-dichloride (CPDD) in recurrent childhood brain tumors; a CCSG trial. Proc Am Soc Clin Oncol 2:72, 1983.

78. Rosen G, Ghavimi F, Nirenberg A, et al.: High-dose methotrexate with citrovorum factor rescue for the treatment of central nervous system tumors in children. Cancer Treat Rep 61:681, 1977.

79. Pendergrass T, Milstein JM, Geyer J, et al.: Eight-drugs-in-one-day chemotherapy for brain tumors; experience in 107 children and rationale for preradiation chemotherapy. J Clin Oncol 5:1221, 1987.

80. Lefkowitz I, Packer R, Siegel KR, et al.: Results of treatment of children with recurrent primitive neuroectodermal tumors/medulloblastoma (PNET/MB) with CCNU, cisplatin (CPDD), and vincristine (VCR). Proc Am Soc Clin Oncol 6:771, 1987.

81. Duffner P, Cohen M, Thomas P, et al.: Combination chemotherapy in recurrent medulloblastoma. Cancer 43:41, 1979.

82. Friedman M: Treatment of children with progressive or recurrent brain tumors with carboplatin or iproplatin; a Pediatric Oncology Group randomized phase II study. J Clin Oncol 10:249, 1992.

83. Evans A, Jenkin R, Sposto R, et al.: The treatment of medulloblastoma; the results of a prospective randomized trial of radiation therapy with and without chloroethylcyclohexyl nitrosourea, vincristine, and prednisone. J Neurosurg 72:572, 1990.

84. Tait D, Thornton-Jones M, Bloom H, et al.: Adjuvant chemotherapy for medulloblastoma; the first multi-centre control trial of the International Society of Pediatric Oncology. Eur J Cancer 26:464, 1990.

85. Alter J, Woo S, Van Eyes J: Update on MOPP chemotherapy as primary therapy for infant brain tumors. Pediatr Neurosci 14:153, 1988.

86. Duffner P, Cohen M: Treatment of brain tumors in babies and very young children. Pediatr Neurosci 12:304, 1985–1986.

Chapter 28

BRAINSTEM TUMORS:
Surgical Indications

RICK ABBOTT, M.D., JOHN RAGHEB, M.D.,
and FRED J. EPSTEIN, M.D.

Intrinsic tumors of the brainstem are relatively common in children, representing 10 to 20 per cent of the tumors that arise within the central nervous system (CNS).[1-3] Their treatment has evolved over the last several decades, reflecting the evolution in imaging technology and microsurgical technique. In the early part of the century, surgeons viewed these neoplasms with a sense of hopelessness. Bailey, Bucy, and Buchanan stated that "Until some effective treatment other than surgery is devised, gliomas of the brainstem will be hopeless problems for treatment.[4] Surgery was only employed to establish the diagnosis when it was in doubt. With the introduction of pneumoencephalography and ventriculography, physicians could differentiate these tumors from other types within the posterior fossa without the need for exploratory surgery. Criteria were established, which included the patient's age, clinical symptoms, cerebrospinal fluid (CSF) characteristics, and appearance of the aqueduct and fourth ventricle on contrasted radiographic studies.[1] Matson stated that "Exploration for confirmation of the diagnosis should be avoided if possible, since such surgery is useless, but care must be taken not to miss another more favorable lesion."[1] These tumors came to be viewed as a homogeneous group because of the lack of sensitivity in the imaging technology. Treatment recommendations consisted mainly of radiation, with only palliative benefit being expected. However, hints as to the true heterogeneity of these neoplasms did appear in the literature. In 1968 Pool reported on three patients who were successfully operated on and survived, apparently cured of their disease (survival of 11 to 23 years without clinical progression).[5] The histology varied (astroblastoma, fibrillary astrocytoma, and astrocytoma). Articles also appeared describing two subgroups for these tumors, those that respond to radiation and those that did not. Bray stated that patients with brainstem tumors tended to respond to radiation if they did not exhibit involvement of multiple cranial nerves (a current-day descriptor of malignant brainstem gliomas).[6] Panitch found that children with high-grade gliomas of the brainstem could expect to survive only 6.4 months after diagnosis and radiation, whereas children with low-grade gliomas experienced an average survival of 32.4 months.[7] The introduction of the computerized tomographic (CT) scanner improved considerably the evaluation of children with this neoplasm and resulted in changes in treatment recommendations. First came a report by Hoffman et al. describing a distinct subgroup of brainstem gliomas, which had exophytic components that could be surgically resected and behaved in a clinically benign fashion.[8] In 1986 two groups, Epstein et al. and Stroink et al., reported classification schemes based upon CT appearance of the tumors which described surgically treatable subgroups of brainstem gliomas.[9, 10] Since that time, magnetic resonance imaging (MRI) has been added to our armamentarium. It has allowed us to further appreciate the true heterogeneity of these tumors and to even describe new subcategories of tumors not previously appreciated. Now, after having applied these new classification schemes and their treatment recommendations, an understanding of the pathologic spectrum of brainstem tumors, their clinical presentation, and anatomic location has emerged. This has led to a better understanding of which children may benefit from surgery and which should be spared a senseless procedure.

Since 1981 we have had the opportunity to participate in the management of over 200 patients with brainstem tumors at New York University Medical Center (NYUMC) and have current follow-up on 75. From this experience, we present a classification system and management scheme with recommendations for which patients should or should not undergo operation.

PRESENTATION

Brainstem tumors may be divided broadly into four categories: diffuse, focal, exophytic, and cervicomedullary. The last category is used primarily to emphasize that this type of tumor frequently does not involve the brainstem. Each category has a typically unique presentation.

DIFFUSE TUMORS

This is the historical stereotype of a brainstem neoplasm. The majority of brainstem tumors probably reside in this group. While earlier reports based upon CT scans showed these tumors to comprise only 14 to 36 per cent of brainstem gliomas, studies based upon MR imaging show that tumors which appear focal on CT scan can, in truth, extensively involve the brainstem and cerebellum.[11] It is our sense that 60 to 70 per cent of brainstem tumors probably belong in this group.

The clinical evolution of this tumor is rapid: symptoms are gait instability and multiple dysfunctional cranial nerves. Examination demonstrates involvement of multiple cranial nerve nuclei as well as pyramidal tracts and the cerebellum. The most frequently involved cranial nerves are V, VI, VII, IX, and X. Typically there is mild motor weakness, hyperreflexia, and ataxia.

The MRI scan shows an expanded pons or medulla which is hypointense on T1 images. Fig. 28–1. The extent of tumor involvement is best appreciated on T2 imaging, with the tumor having a hyperintense signal. The MRI scan characteristically reveals a neoplasm more extensive than the CT scan would suggest and is much more supportive of the clinical examination. There are variable patterns of enhancement, and frequently there is evidence of growth from the epicenter to involve adjacent segments of the brainstem and, occasionally, the thalamus and upper cervical cord.

FOCAL TUMORS

These tumors can arise anywhere within the brainstem.[9, 10, 12] There are two types of focal tumors: solid and cystic. The solid tumors are less than 2.5 cm in diameter and have an intrinsic epicenter. Occasionally they can erupt to present an exophytic component either dorsally, laterally, or anteriorly. It is the extent of intrinsic tumor that differentiates these from the classic exophytic tumors, which arise in the subependyma with over 90 per cent of their mass being outside the stem.[8] An interesting subgroup of the focal solid tumors is that of the tectal gliomas. Many of these tumors were missed in the CT scan era, and children having them carried the diagnosis of late-onset aqueductal stenosis.[13] The cystic tumors may have a mural nodule similar to that seen with pilocystic astrocytomas of the cerebellum or tumor may line the wall of the cyst.

Typically, these tumors have a history that spans many months to years. Not infrequently these children

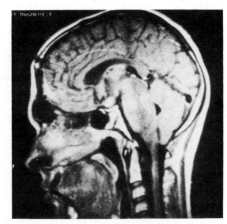

FIGURE 28–1. A diffuse brainstem glioma involving the pons and midbrain.

have had extensive gastrointestinal, ophthalmologic or otolaryngologic evaluations for persisting complaints of nausea or vomiting, poor weight gain, visual difficulties, or hoarseness. The symptoms speak of a focal area of involvement of the stem which is, at worst, slowly progressive. Rarely, there may be signs of increased intracranial pressure if the tumor has a large exophytic component blocking the outlets of the fourth ventricle or the aqueduct. The clinical examination supports the clinical focality, with only unilateral focal cranial nerve dysfunction being demonstrated. Children with tectal gliomas typically present with long histories of headache and may have macrocephaly. Scans show hydrocephalus. Infrequently, Parinaud's syndrome may be present.

The solid portion of these focal solid and cystic tumors typically enhances with gadolinium except in the case of the tectal gliomas, which are frequently nonenhancing (Fig. 28–2). In the past, when CT scanning of these children was more common, we would be presented with children whose scans showed focal tumors, but whose clinical examination showed more extensive involvement of the stem. The MRI scan invariably clarified the situation, for it would disclose much more extensive involvement of the stem. The tectal gliomas will frequently demonstrate calcification on CT scans (4/6 patients of May et al.).[13] Usually the focal tumors of the brainstem do not have a surrounding halo of hypointensity (edema). Konovalov has described a classification scheme that focuses on this point: tumors exhibiting tumors with surrounding zones of "edema" are infiltrative and therefore of a higher grade than tumors not showing this zone on imaging.[14] While this may be a useful concept, we do not have the clinical experience to comment on this.

EXOPHYTIC TUMORS

These tumors arise from subependymal glial tissue and fungate into the fourth ventricle. The majority of the stem is spared involvement, with >90 per cent of the tumor residing within the ventricle. As with the

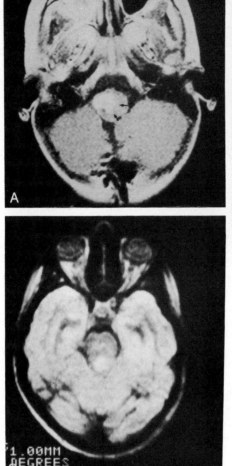

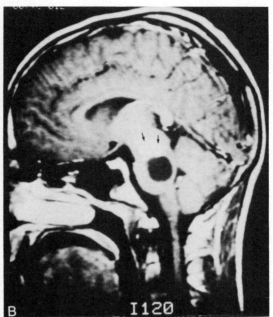

FIGURE 28–2. *A,* A solid, focal ganglioglioma of the medulla that homogeneously enhances with gadolinium. *B,* A cystic, focal astrocytoma of the medulla with homogeneously enhancing tumor lining its walls. *C,* A focal tumor of the midbrain's tectum that has obliterated the aqueduct. Note the relative preservation of the surrounding structures.

focal tumors, the clinical history is long. Because of its potential for obstructing CSF pathways, symptoms of increased intracranial pressure are present and ventriculomegaly is seen on scanning. Infants with this tumor frequently have a history of ". . . intractable vomiting and failure to thrive."[8] Ataxia and nystagmus are commonly seen on examination.

This tumor can be difficult to differentiate from PNETs and astrocytomas of the vermis. On several occasions we have been surprised to find that a tumor diagnosed preoperatively as a PNET was in truth an exophytic glioma with a relatively small pedicle of attachment to the subependymal tissue from which it arose. These tumors are isointense to surrounding tissue and tend to enhance with gadolinium in a homogeneous fashion. (Fig. 28–3).

CERVICOMEDULLARY TUMORS

Cervicomedullary gliomas are tumors that involve the cervical cord and the medulla. They either arise within the upper cervical cord and grow rostral or within the cervicomedullary junction with intrinsic growth occurring both within the cervical cord and the medulla. The majority of these tumors appear to represent cervical spinal cord tumors in which the rostral growth has been blocked at the level of the decussating white matter tracts of the medulla.[15] Because of this blockage, the tumor turns dorsally to erupt into the cisterna magna and outlet of the fourth ventricle. Patients presenting with this tumor complain of long-standing neck pain, Lhermitte's sign, and slowly evolving weakness in the arms and legs with sensory dysesthesias. Cranial nerve dysfunction is unusual and, when present, is an indication of a tumor that arose within the caudal medulla and not within the spinal cord. There can be symptoms of increased intracranial hypertension if the outlets of the fourth ventricle have been blocked by the rostral pole of the tumor. On examination a torticollis may be noted, as well as arm and leg weakness, hyperreflexia, and sensory anomalies.

CT scanning is of little value in imaging these tumors because of the bone artifact at the foramen magnum. MRI scan of a tumor arising within the upper cervical cord will show an enlarged upper cervical cord with

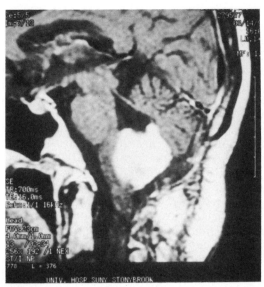

FIGURE 28–3. A classic dorsally exophytic brainstem glioma that is filling the fourth ventricle. Note the lack of infiltration into the pons.

distortion of the medulla (Fig. 28–4A). There is usually an exophytic component growing into the cisterna magna. The tumor can homogenously or inhomogeneously enhance with gadolinium. These low-grade tumors push neural structures out of their way as they grow rostrally. Tumors arising at the cervicomedullary junction show enlargement of the lower medulla as well as tumor infiltrating the upper cervical cord (Fig. 28–4B). Rarely, malignant tumors arising within the upper cervical cord can grow rostrally through the decussating fibers of the lower medulla to diffusely infiltrate the medulla. Symptoms will reflect this with rapidly evolving, bilateral lower cranial nerve deficits in addition to symptoms referable to the upper cervical cord involvement.

TREATMENT

Treatment options are dictated by the tumor's category. Retrospective analysis has made it obvious that

surgery is only potentially beneficial for low-grade gliomas, and therefore it is essential to utilize clinical and neurodiagnostic studies to help identify these patients in advance.

The most common brainstem neoplasm is the diffuse glioma, and this is invariably a malignant astrocytoma. The characteristic hypodense appearance on T1 images and hyperintense signal on T2 images is not edema but infiltrating malignant tumor.[16] Regardless of treatment, these children are destined to die within 12 months, and as a consequence treatment is palliative.[17] Just as it is important to identify tumors that will not respond to treatment, it is also important to identify those that do not require it. Indolent tumors of the midbrain causing an obstructive hydrocephalus require shunting of the hydrocephalus and only observation of the tumor.[13]

GENERAL PRINCIPLES

Surgery is only potentially beneficial for patients with focal, exophytic, or cervicomedullary tumors. Before these groups are discussed individually, it is important to recognize some general principles of brainstem tumor surgery. The first, and perhaps most important, is that the surgeon must recognize that it is impossible to excise a glioma completely and to attempt to do so in the brainstem is potentially catastrophic. Rather, the goal of the surgery should be to reduce the tumor burden and to obtain adequate tissue for a histologic diagnosis. Although it is not uncommon for us to leave the operating room heartened by an impression that we have obtained a near-total resection, we typically accomplish a 50 to 80 per cent reduction in the mass of the tumor as shown on postoperative MRI scan. This speaks to the infiltrative nature of these tumors and why the outcome of the surgery is so dependent on the biological nature of the tumor, that is, subtotally excised malignant tumors will rapidly grow back, overcoming any palliative effect of the surgical debulking. The second surgical principle is that there is never a cleavage plain between these gliomas and the surrounding brainstem. For this reason, the surgeon must

FIGURE 28–4. A, A cervicomedullary tumor that arose in the upper cervical cord and whose rostral growth has respected the cervicomedullary junction *(arrows)*. Note how the tumor has turned dorsal to erupt into the cisterna magna instead of invading the medulla. B, A cervicomedullary tumor that arose in the medulla and subsequently grew down into the cervical cord.

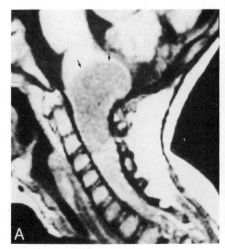
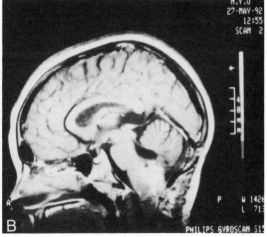

not attempt to define a tumor-brain interface. We have found this interface to be exceedingly vulnerable to injury, and approaching it aggressively results in protracted cranial nerve deficits. These tumors may be removed with relative safety only if the resection proceeds from the central core of the tumor outward. The resection proceeds until normal white matter begins to peek through the tumor circumferentially. At this point, the resection is suspended and its extent is evaluated with ultrasonography. The resection is stopped when no significant lumps of tumor are seen on ultrasonography. This technique will avoid permanent injury to neural tissue, since low-grade tumors tend to displace functioning neural elements and are minimally infiltrative by nature.

There have been several reports on the utility of intraoperative monitoring of evoked potentials in avoiding injury to the brainstem.[18, 19] As our experience with this technology has increased, we have grown to recognize its limitations.[20] First, if a large number of signals must be averaged to obtain reliable reproducibility, the neurophysiologist will not recognize the injury until long after it has occurred. Consequently, we now use a special electrode that lies on the floor of the fourth ventricle or within the aqueduct. Since the potentials recorded with this electrode are so robust, a much smaller number are needed to generate a reproducible averaged signal. Typically, our averaged signal is updated every 7 to 15 seconds, allowing greater opportunity to stop activity that is injurious before permanent injury is inflicted. Second, and the most important limitation, is that the functions monitored by this modality are not those that seem most vulnerable and whose loss would account for the greatest morbidity seen with this surgery. At this time, there is no way to monitor the visceral motor function of the lower cranial nerves, and it is the loss of this function, with the resultant need for feeding gastrostomy and tracheostomy, that we most dread.

Diffuse Tumors

These are malignant tumors with a dismal outlook. No treatment has been shown to be effective in causing a significant survival in children with this type of tumor. Early in our experience, several children with this type of tumor were operated upon with no impact on the duration of their survival. Radiation has been shown to have a palliative effect and to increase survival.[6, 21, 22] Earlier chemotherapy trials failed to demonstrate efficacy, but more aggressive regimens are currently under evaluation.[23]

Focal Tumors

These slow-growing benign tumors cause slowly progressive, clinically focal symptoms. The MRI scan confirms this. If there is conflict between the clinical history and examination and the MR image with regard to the biological nature of the tumor, the wisdom of surgery should be questioned. That is not to say that surgery should be avoided if there is the possibility that the tumor is benign (slowly evolving history with focal deficits or MRI scan showing a focal lesion). Rather, the surgeon should maintain a high degree of suspicion at the time of surgery, obtaining frozen sections before embarking on a radical resection. There are three surgical subtypes in the category: the solid intrinsic tumor, the cystic tumor with a mural nodule, and the exophytic tumor. The risks of surgery vary with each, and each is approached in a different manner.

The solid, intrinsic tumor, while potentially very responsive to radical resection, is a tumor whose resection is associated with the risk of some of the greatest morbidity seen with neurosurgical procedures, particularity when it resides within the medulla. In operating on these tumors the surgeon must be prepared to accept the morbidity of complete loss of swallowing and airway protection, resulting in the need for feeding gastrostomy and tracheostomy. Diplopia due to internuclear ophthalmoplegia, sixth nerve and seventh nerve weakness, is a given when resecting focal solid tumors of the pons. Although the patients usually recover these functions over a period of several months, this recovery is by no means guaranteed. The pyramidal tracts or dorsal columns seem to be fairly resilient to the surgery. These risks need to be paramount in the mind of the surgeon when he or she is discussing the surgical option with the family and when he or she is performing the operation. At surgery, time is spent on obtaining an adequate exposure to visualize not only the anticipated point of entry, but also surrounding landmarks that will be used during the resection for orientation and protection of important structures. This is especially important in cases of eccentric tumors, which extend well laterally. We have observed a tendency to lose heart when, on extending the resection laterally, we lose our sense of location of the lateral wall of the stem with the large branches of the basilar and vertebral arteries coarsing over it. Consequently, time is spent unroofing the fourth ventricle so that the margins of the tumor bulge are seen well. Similarly, the CP angle is exposed for operations on eccentric tumors in the caudal brainstem. With this visual orientation, we are much more aggressive with the rostral pole of the tumor. Care is taken with eccentric tumors of the lower brainstem to shave the ring of the foramen magnum down laterally so that it is not jutting out over the dorsolateral surface of the stem.

Generally, the solid, intrinsic tumor is approached along the shortest path. Typically the point of entry into the brainstem will be marked by a small area of discoloration seen through the ependyma or pia arachnoid. After ultrasonography of the tumor, the ependyma or pia is incised sharply or with a laser, and the fibers of the white matter are spread bluntly until the discolored tumor tissue is encountered. As soon as tumor is encountered, biopsy should be obtained *immediately* to ensure that an adequate biopsy is obtained, since these small tumors can quickly be aspirated by suctioning or an ultrasonic aspirator. If there is conflict between the clinical history and MRI (e.g., one suggested a benign tumor while the other suggests a malignant one), a frozen section is obtained. An aggressive resection is not indicated if a malignant tumor is found. Initially, the central portion of the tumor is resected using aspiration or ultrasonic aspiration. To minimize the extent of the incision through the normal white matter, the assistant exposes the lateral aspects of the tumor by retracting first in one direction then another as the surgeon works on the lateral aspects of the tumor. Either the laser or gentle aspiration is used at the periphery of the lesion for better control. The resection is halted when the consistency of the tissue begins to change toward normal. Bleeding vessels should not be chased into the parenchyma, and any bleeding is controlled with packing and hemostatic agents. Time is spent at the end of the procedure irrigating out the blood and hemostatic debris prior to closure.

Focal cystic tumors are clinically analogous to cystic cerebellar astrocytomas and are handled in a similar manner surgically. Others have advocated aspiration as a treatment for these neoplasms, but we believe that this will result in only temporary benefit, with the cyst reforming over a short period of time.[24] Not as much effort is needed in exposing the margins of these tumors since the anatomy will be clearly laid out once the cyst has been entered. The cysts are approached via the most direct route. Once the cyst is entered, the solid portion of the tumor is resected. Mural nodules lend themselves to a more radical resection than en plaque tumors since by their nature they are much less infiltrative. Hemostasis is obtained with hemostatic agents and gentle packing.

The use of adjuvant therapies (radiation and chemotherapy) for focal tumors generally is not indicated when the histology is benign. Rather, the child is simply observed by follow-up with serial MRI scans. Should there be recurrent growth, consideration is given to reoperation as well as radiotherapy. Occasionally, radiotherapy may be indicated for a low-grade tumor that is causing debilitating symptoms which were not ameliorated by surgery. This is exceedingly rare and should only be chosen after careful consideration. Children with focal anaplastic gangliogliomas and high-grade astrocytomas require radiotherapy. Chemotherapy has been employed in a protocol setting, with earlier trials being disappointing. More aggressive regimens are currently under investigation.[23]

The intrinsic tumor with an exophytic component is approached via the exophytic component. Tumors with a dorsally exophytic component provide a broad path of entry into the heart of the tumor. This results in better visualization and less need for retraction. A discolored tumor mass defines the margins of incision through the ependyma and pia. Once the tumor has been uncapped, a central resection proceeds with minimal retraction. The broad exposure allows for the use of the ultrasonic aspirator, whose aspiration force can be used to advantage, pulling the lateral tumor into the center of the resection cavity. More gentle technique can be used at the tumor's periphery. It is our impression that patients with this type of tumor seem to be at less risk for lower cranial nerve dysfunction postoperatively, although we have seen these complications in this subgroup. Laterally exophytic tumors are approached either via the cerebellopontine (CP) angle or a subtemporal-transtentorial route. These tumors occasionally may be erroneously diagnosed on MRI. In several of our cases, tumors appearing to have exophytic components on MRI scan have been found at surgery to be intrinsic. When confronted with this, the surgeon must decide whether to reorient his approach to a dorsal one or continue with the approach through the lateral wall of the stem. In our experience, a radical resection has been more difficult with the lateral approach because cranial nerves obscure the view of the resection, and it is difficult to maneuver instruments between the cranial nerves. Extensive normal-appearing tissue dorsal to the tumor may prohibit a dorsal approach, however.

Neoplasms of the cerebral peduncle are approached subtemporally, and incision of the tentorium frequently is required for adequate exposure. Following incision of the arachnoid covering the upper midbrain cisterns, a bulging peduncle is usually obvious. The pia is incised at the point of maximal bulging, and blunt dissection is used until the tumor is encountered. The pial incision is then lengthened parallel to the fiber tracts to expose the length of the tumor. An internal debulking of the tumor then is done until the borders of the tumor start to blend with normal-appearing white matter. Ultrasonography is used to confirm that resection of the solid portion of the tumor is adequate and that all cysts have been drained.

DORSALLY EXOPHYTIC TUMORS

Tumors in this location are approached as midline cerebellar neoplasms. Not infrequently, the provisional diagnosis preoperatively is PNET or vermian astrocytoma. As the tumor is debulked, its origins become apparent. It is because of this that all large midline tumors filling the fourth ventricle must be approached with caution. The floor of the fourth ventricle must be identified prior to debulking the more ventral portions of the tumor. We use Lapras's technique of horizontally splitting the vermis, carrying this incision into the hemispheres bilaterally for 1 cm to approach the rostral surface of the tumor. This incision is carried dorsally just skirting the rostral surface of the tumor until the aqueduct is encountered. The tumor is then gently rolled caudally, and the rostral floor of the fourth ventricle is protected with a cottonoid. The vermis can then be split longitudinally from the rostral pole of the tumor caudally to the foramen of Magendie. In this fashion the position of the floor is appreciated caudally. A debulking of the tumor is then done; during the debulking the location of the floor of the ventricle is checked frequently. The goal is to shave the tumor flush with the surrounding floor of the ventricle and not to go ventral to this plane. It is important to emphasize that there is no effort to excise that part of the tumor within the stem since this represents the absolute margin of the tumor with normal brainstem structures being just anterior to it, which are easily damaged.

These tumors are benign by nature and require only routine follow-up with repeated MRI. Tumor recurrence is probably best addressed with repeat surgery.

CERVICOMEDULLARY TUMORS

Tumors arising within the cervical cord and respecting the decussating fibers of the medulla are more appropriately thought of as spinal cord tumors. Their growth pattern, once in the medulla, speaks to their histologic nature as mentioned earlier. Benign tumors are not infiltrative and thus do not penetrate fiber pathways easily. Consequently, when one of these tumors encounters the decussating fibers of the pyramidal tract and dorsal columns, the growth of the tumor is curved dorsally and it grows exophytically into the cisterna magna and caudal fourth ventricle. If this is not the pattern of growth observed, the overwhelming probability is that the tumor is a high-grade infiltrating glioma or a tumor that has arisen within the medulla. The surgical approach to this tumor is similar to that for a spinal cord tumor. In this case, unlike the case of tumor confined to the medulla, intraoperative physiologic monitoring can be useful. Typically we monitor both sensory evoked potentials and motor evoked potentials. The evoked potentials in response to sensory nerve stimulation are recorded by means of an electrode resting on the rostral floor of the fourth ventricle. This allows for much more rapid updating of the averaged signal and, as a result, approaches a real-time monitoring situation. Similarly, epidural electrodes are placed caudal to the tumor to pick up potentials evoked by transcranial stimulation of the motor cortex. Use of these electrodes allows muscle paralysis and thus prevents patient movement during the surgery. Typically, the cord portion of the tumor is intraparenchymal. Consequently, a midline myelotomy is made and the fiber pathways of the dorsal columns bluntly separated to expose the dorsum of the tumor. A central debulking of the tumor is then done with the ultrasonic aspirator followed by the removal of the tumor at its periphery using gentle suction or the laser. This resection is carried rostrally to the level of the medulla, where the resection becomes more conservative. The exophytic component of the tumor is then removed carefully to avoid injury to the posterior inferior cerebellar artery (PICA), which typically lies wedged between the tumor, inferior cerebellar hemisphere, and medulla where the three meet. Some idea of the location of this vessel can be gained by looking at the lateral aspect of the lower medulla, where PICA passes from the vertebral artery dorsally toward the cerebellum. The intraparenchymal medullary component of the tumor is then addressed by first centrally debulking it with the ultrasonic aspirator and removing the tumor at its periphery with gentle aspiration or the laser.

The dura is closed in all cases. We typically use a high-speed craniotome to perform a craniotomy and so the bone window is replaced during the closure. This improves the cosmetic result and, should reoperation be required, the replacement of the bone makes the reopening much easier by eliminating the risk of incising the dura during the muscle dissection.

POSTOPERATIVE CARE

Surgery for intrinsic tumors of the medulla is associated with a risk for progressive CO_2 retention followed by respiratory collapse. We have seen this occur in four of seven patients we operated upon for focal tumors of the medulla.[20] None of these patients exhibited signs of injury to their lower cranial nerves after their surgery. They all experienced respiratory collapse within 48 hours of their surgery, and all exhibited changes consistent with injury to a portion of their medulla. They had severe compromise in their ability to protect their airways and to eat, resulting in the need for tracheostomies and feeding gastrostomies. Since noting this, we have kept all patients undergoing surgery for intrinsic solid tumors of the medulla and cervicomedullary junction intubated postoperatively, regardless of their physical status, for a minimum of 24 hours until they show no evidence of CO_2 retention. Children with tumors of the pons and midbrain or dorsally exophytic tumors are not as vulnerable and therefore usually do not require this level of ventilatory support.

DISCUSSION

Perhaps the most important contribution to the management of brainstem neoplasms is the recognition that they are not a single entity but, in fact, consist of different tumors that may be classified according to location and biologic activity. Although diffuse tumors are the most common, the other categories are not rare, and surgical options can be considered for most of them.

In our experience, surgery is beneficial only for ganglliogliomas, benign astrocytomas, and intrinsic cervicomedullary ependymomas. No patient with a malignant astrocytoma or glioblastoma has lived longer than 12 months after surgery. Therefore, if the surgical option is to be considered, it is essential that there be some relatively reliable preoperative assessment of the tumor's biologic activity. The relationship of this to the patient's clinical course and to the extent and appearance of the tumor on neurodiagnostic imaging then becomes important in determining who should undergo these relatively risky operations.

DIFFUSE TUMORS

All diffuse brainstem tumors are malignant. At present, there is no justification for attempts at surgical excision or biopsy of these tumors when the clinical course and MRI support the diagnosis. The only therapeutic option consists of radiation and, possibly, adjuvant chemotherapy.

Focal Tumors

These typically low-grade tumors are amenable to surgical resection. The surgeon must take care that the MRI is complete (including T2-weighted images) to ensure that the tumor is truly focal. In addition, the surgeon's suspicions should be raised when the clinical history reveals a rapid development of symptoms. We have seen several children with focal glioblastomas who presented with rapidly evolving focal tumors on MRI scans and underwent radical resections of their tumors. All died within 12 months despite aggressive surgical and adjuvant therapies.

Tumors of the tectum of the midbrain, which cause an obstructive hydrocephalus, appear to be a unique subset of the focal tumors of the brainstem. These tumors do not require surgical intervention at the time of their diagnosis. Since there have been several reports as to the indolent nature of many of these tumors, the hydrocephalus is treated and the tumors observed with serial MRI scans.[13, 25] Only those tumors that show progressive growth require further treatment. Although several reports have attested to the malignant nature of these tumors when they grow, we believe that as time passes and more cases appear in the literature, the same heterogeneity that exists in the rest of the stem will also exist here.

Dorsally Exophytic Tumors

These minimally invasive tumors have long been recognized as being amenable to radical resection. They are usually low-grade astrocytomas, and with radical resection, long-term survival is to be expected.

Cervicomedullary Tumors

Cervicomedullary tumors arising in the upper cervical cord are typically low-grade astrocytomas, gangliogliomas, and, rarely, ependymomas. These tumors are often favorably affected by radical resection. The cervicomedullary junction is respected with regard to the clinical history and the growth of the tumor. Cervicomedullary tumors arising within the lower medulla and growing caudally into the brainstem have clinical histories mimicking the focal tumors of the medulla, except for the added symptoms of cervical cord involvement. These tumors may be viewed as intermediate between the tumors of the cervical cord and tumors of the brainstem. Primary surgical extirpation may be most appropriate for these tumors unless the clinical history and MRI scan suggest a malignant tumor.

SUMMARY

Brainstem tumors in children are a heterogeneous group of neoplasms that may be classified according to clinical and neurodiagnostic criteria. We have described a simple anatomic classification that has significance pathologically, surgically, and prognostically. Although there is no surgical option for the most common diffuse brainstem neoplasms, the other subtypes may be operated upon if the clinical and radiographic information warrants. Surgical resection of the focal and exophytic brainstem tumors has been well tolerated and often beneficial. We expect data to be forthcoming to support the surgical management of benign brainstem neoplasms.

REFERENCES

1. Matson DD: Neurosurgery of Infancy and Childhood. 2nd ed. Springfield, Charles C Thomas, 1969, pp 469–477.
2. Schoenberg BS, Schoenberg DG, Christine BW, et al.: The epidemiology of primary intracranial neoplasms of childhood: A population study. Mayo Clin Proc 51:51, 1976.
3. Yates AJ, Becker LE, Sachs LA: Brain tumors in childhood. Childs Brain 5:31, 1979.
4. Bailey P, Buchanan DN, Bucy P: Intracranial Tumors of Infancy and Childhood. Chicago, University of Chicago Press, 1939, p 188.
5. Pool JL: Gliomas in the region of the brainstem. J Neurosurg 29:164, 1968.
6. Bray PF, Carter S, Taveras JM: Brainstem tumors in children. Neurology 8:1, 1958.
7. Panitch HS, Berg BO: Brainstem tumors of childhood and adolescence. Am J Dis Child 119:465, 1970.
8. Hoffman HJ, Becker L, Craven MA: A clinically and pathologically distinct group of benign brainstem gliomas. Neurosurgery 7:243, 1980.
9. Epstein F, McCleary EL: Intrinsic brainstem tumors of childhood: Surgical implications. J Neurosurg 64:11, 1986.
10. Stroink AR, Hoffman HJ, Hendrick EB, et al.: Diagnosis and management of pediatric brainstem gliomas. J Neurosurg 65:745, 1986.
11. Smith RR, Zimmerman RA, Packer RJ, et al.: Pediatric brainstem glioma: Post-radiation clinical and MR follow-up. Neuroradiology 32:265, 1990.
12. Vandertop WP, Hoffman HJ, Drake JM, et al.: Focal midbrain tumors in children. Neurosurgery 31:186, 1992.
13. May PL, Blaser SI, Hoffman HJ, et al.: Benign intrinsic tectal "tumors" in children. J Neurosurg 74:867, 1991.
14. Konovalov A, Atieh J: The surgical treatment of primary brain stem tumors. In Schmidek HH, Sweet WH (eds): Operative Neurosurgical Techniques. Indications, Methods and Results. Orlando, Grune & Stratton, 1988, pp 709–720.
15. Epstein FJ, Farmer JP: Brainstem glioma growth patterns. J Neurosurg 78:408, 1993.
16. Albright AL, Guthkelch AN, Packer RJ, et al.: Prognostic factors in pediatric brain-stem gliomas. J Neurosurg 65:751, 1986.
17. Golden GS, Ghatak NR, Hirano A, et al.: Malignant glioma of the brainstem: A clinicopathological analysis of 13 cases. J Neurol Neurosurg Psychiatry 35:732, 1972.
18. Albright AL, Sclabassi RJ: Use of the ultrasonic surgical aspirator and evoked potentials for the treatment of thalamic and brainstem tumors in children. Neurosurgery 17:564, 1985.
19. Epstein F, Wisoff JH: Surgical management of brain stem tumors of childhood and adolescence. Neurosurg Clin North Am 1:111, 1990.

20. Abbott R, Shiminske-Maher T, Wisoff JH, Epstein FJ: Intrinsic tumors of the medulla: Surgical complications. Pediatr Neurosurg 17:239, 1991–92.
21. Edwards MSB, Wara WM, Urtasun RC, et al.: Hyperfractionated radiation therapy for brainstem glioma: A phase I-II trial. J Neurosurg 70:691, 1989.
22. Packer RJ, Allen JC, Goldwein JL, et al.: Hyperfractionated radio-therapy for children with brainstem gliomas: A pilot study using 7,200 cGy. Ann Neurol 27:167, 1990.
23. Finlay JL, August C, Packer RJ, et al.: High-dose chemotherapy followed by bone-marrow rescue for malignant astrocytomas of childhood and adolescence. J Neurooncol 9:239, 1990.
24. Hood TW, Gebarski SS, McKeever PE, et al.: Stereotaxic biopsy of intrinsic lesions of the brain stem. J Neurosurg 65:172, 1986.

MISCELLANEOUS POSTERIOR FOSSA TUMORS

The posterior fossa is a common site for various tumors to occur during childhood. Table 29–1 shows the histologic distribution of 279 posterior fossa tumors in childhood diagnosed by computed tomography from 1978 to 1990 at the Children's Memorial Hospital. The most common histologic types were astrocytomas and medulloblastomas (approximately 80 per cent). Mesenchymal tumors such as acoustic neurinomas, meningiomas, and hemangioblastomas rarely occur in childhood; they are more prevalent in adults. Ependymomas, on the other hand, are not uncommon in the posterior fossa of children, and their incidence is significant in the differential diagosis of pediatric posterior fossa tumors. Choroid plexus papillomas may occur in the fourth ventricle or cerebellopontine angle, but they are more often located in the supratentorial location in children. Embryonal tumors, such as teratomas and dermoid cyst, can also occur in the posterior fossa.

This chapter will focus on neuroepithelial tumors (ependymomas, choroid plexus papillomas), embryonal tumors (dermoid cysts, epidermoid cysts, teratomas) and mesenchymal tumors (meningiomas, acoustic neuromas) occurring in the posterior fossa in childhood.

EPENDYMOMAS

Ependymomas occur in various locations of the central nervous system in children. Of these, the most common location (70 per cent) is the posterior fossa; less common are the supratentorial location and the spinal cord.[1] They occur most commonly in young and frequently preschool children. Presenting symptoms are similar to those of other common pediatric cerebellar—fourth ventricular tumors such as medulloblastomas and cerebellar astrocytomas. Headaches, vomiting, double vision, and gait ataxia are common symptoms. Papilledema and cerebellar ataxia are prominent neu-

rologic signs. These symptoms and signs are more or less directly related to hydrocephalus rather than to the mass in the posterior fossa.[2]

A great majority of ependymomas in the posterior fossa occupy the fourth ventricle and often extend to the subarachnoid space through the foramina. These tumors frequently adhere to or invade the floor or the wall of the fourth ventricle. Hydrocephalus is almost invariably present in association with posterior fossa ependymomas.

TABLE 29–1. HISTOLOGIC DISTRIBUTION OF 279 POSTERIOR FOSSA TUMORS. CHILDREN'S MEMORIAL HOSPITAL (1978–1990)

Cerebellum–fourth ventricle	197
Medulloblastomas	81
Benign astrocytomas	75
Ependymomas	23
Dermoids	6
Malignant ependymomas	4
Malignant astrocytomas	3
Teratomas	2
Hemangioblastoma	1
Choroid plexus papilloma	1
Meningioma	1
Brainstem	75
Pons	
Malignant astrocytomas	19
PNET	3
Benign astrocytomas	2
Unknown	24
Medulla oblongata	
Benign astrocytomas	9
Malignant astrocytomas	3
Midbrain	
Benign astrocytomas	5
Malignant astrocytoma	1
Cerebellopontine angle	9
Ependymomas	2
Meningiomas	2
Others	5*

*Chondrosarcoma, chordoma, epidermoid, neurinoma, melanoma.

Histologically, ependymoma is composed of well-differentiated cells that are often arranged around blood vessels, forming perivascular rosettes. Some may form a true rosette with cells arranged around a lumen, resembling the central canal of the spinal cord. Under high-power magnification blepharoplasts, basal bodies of cilia, may be observed in these cells, and are diagnostic of ependymomas. Malignant ependymomas have nuclear pleomorphysm, mitosis, necrosis, or other features of anaplasia,[3, 4] but are relatively uncommon.

Computerized tomography (CT), with and without intravenous contrast agents, is often diagnostic for posterior fossa ependymomas. Prior to contrast infusion, ependymomas appear either iso- or hyperdense, with mixed density in the tumor. Some areas of tumor are hyperdense (calcification), while others are hypodense (cyst formation or necrotic center). Enhancement after contrast infusion varies from marked enhancement to little or no enhancement. Magnetic resonance imaging (MRI), in the past several years, has provided better information regarding location and extension of the posterior fossa tumors. Even a nonenhancing or ill-defined tumor on CT can be clearly demonstrated on T1- and T2-weighted images. Multidimensional MRI images, in particular, distinctly demonstrate ependymoma extension to the basal cisterns and cervical canal from the fourth ventricle. The great majority of posterior fossa ependymomas are located in the fourth ventricle. They may also be located, though rarely, in the cerebellar hemisphere or in the cerebellopontine angle. The most characteristic appearance on neuro-imaging studies is the various extension into the subarachnoid space from the fourth ventricle. They may extend into the cerebellopontine/medullary cistern through the lateral recess (Fig. 29–1), and a caudal extension into the cervical spinal canal is not uncommon. The ventrolateral subarachnoid extension is the hallmark of ependymomas, as medulloblastomas and cerebellar astrocytomas seldom show this characteristic. With CT and MRI techniques, further diagnostic measures such as angiography are rarely necessary.

Surgery aims to establish histologic diagnosis, restore the CSF circulation, and effect maximum cytoreduction. For coexisting hydrocephalus, precraniotomy CSF diversion has been practiced in the past.[2] Although patients improve and often become asymptomatic after a precraniotomy shunt, the loss of CSF space in the rostal fourth ventricle and the upward shift of the fourth ventricle tumor toward or into the aqueduct of Sylvius after the shunting procedure make surgical resection of the fourth ventricle tumor difficult.[1] The most serious side effects of a precraniotomy shunt are upward herniation and intratumoral hemorrhage, which are uncommon but often fatal.[1] Thus, although precraniotomy shunt is not necessary in a great majority of cases, if needed, an urgent posterior fossa craniotomy with resection of the posterior fossa tumor is warranted.

Posterior fossa craniotomy is done under general anesthesia with the patient in a prone position. A burr hole is made in the parieto-occipital junction for ventricular cannulation. Initially, ventricular CSF is allowed to drain minimally to obtain a sample for cytologic studies. The ventricular cannula is left in place for postoperative external ventricular drainage (EVD). For midline tumors, a midline skin incision is made from the inion to the level of the C3 spinous process. If the preoperative neuro-imaging study indicates that the tumor extends to a unilateral cerebellopontine/medullary cistern, a hockey-stick incision (a midline incision with upper limb extending toward the ipsilateral mastoid process) is made. This permits a wider craniotomy toward the ipsilateral occipital bone. After stripping the pericranium from the squamous portion of the occipital bone and exposing the rim of the foramen magnum, two burr holes are made just below the lateral sinus, 2.5 to 3 cm from the midline bilaterally. A sagittal MRI is helpful to measure the distance from the foramen magnum to the torcular Herophili (usually 3.5 to 5 cm, depending on the patient's age). In older patients with a prominent internal protuberance, a third burr hole is made in the midline below the torcular, which facilitates verification of the dura mater. Subsequently, the foramen magnum is freed from the periosteum by a

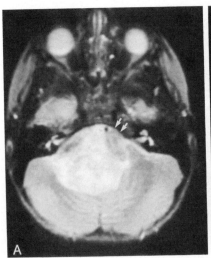
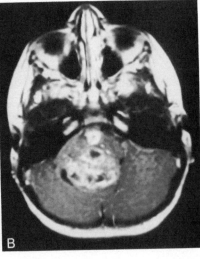

FIGURE 29–1. *A*, Axial T2-weighted MRI showing extension of fourth ventricle ependymoma into the cerebellomedullary cistern. Note a contralateral displacement of the medulla oblongata (*arrows*). *B*, Axial gadolinium-enhanced MRI showing inhomogeneous enhancement of posterior fossa ependymoma.

sharp dissector, and then the posterior fossa dura is separated from the inner table of skull by means of a Penfield dissector. The pediatric posterior fossa dura is rarely adherent to the skull. With a pneumatic craniotome, a posterior fossa craniotomy is done with the caudal end crossing the foramen magnum. Craniotomy is preferable to craniectomy because of the thin suboccipital musculature and the growing skull structures in young children, and for prevention of a pseudomeningocele, which often occurs after posterior fossa craniectomy. A resection of the posterior arch of C1 is rarely necessary. Even if the tumor extends to C1 or C2, this portion of tumor is readily pulled out because it does not adhere to the spinal cord.

The dura is incised in a Y configuration. Upon opening the dura, one can drain ventricular CSF through the ventriculostomy catheter, depending on the tension of the cerebellum. Specimens of the CSF and arachnoid membrane from the cisterna magnum are routinely obtained for pathologic evaluation of tumor dissemination.[5] If the tumor is not protruding into the cisterna magnum, it is exposed by exploration of the cerebellar vallecula by displacing the cerebellar tonsils laterally. The posterior inferior cerebellar artery is often shifted laterally, or it may be wrapped in the tumor mass.

An initial procedure for fourth ventricle tumors is to identify the upper cervical cord, the obex, and the calamus scriptorius. Once the floor of the fourth ventricle is identified, the tumor mass is gently elevated, and the floor of the fourth ventricle is further explored rostrally. If the tumor does not involve the ventricular floor, one can safely place a cottonoid covering to protect the floor. If the tumor is invading the floor, tumor resection is directed from the dorsal aspect of the tumor. Approximately 10 to 25 per cent of posterior fossa ependymomas are invasive of the fourth ventricular floor.[1, 6] Usually, the inferior vermis is sectioned between the inferior vermian veins to reach the dorsal dome of the tumor. Involvement of the cerebellar peduncle is common, occurring in about 80 per cent of cases.[1] Preoperative neuro-imaging studies show the invasiveness of ependymoma to the lateral wall of the fourth ventricle by an ill-defined border. The lateral tumor dissection should be carried out from the non-invasive side. Resection of a tumor that extends to the cerebellopontine/medullary cistern should be started from the wall of the contralateral side. Once the lateral and dorsal margins of the tumor are separated and internal decompression is performed, the most rostral portion of tumor is reached. Subsequently, that portion of tumor is lifted, and the aqueduct of Sylvius is identified. Once the aqueduct and the rostral floor of the fourth ventricle are secured and protected by another cottonoid, further tumor resection is done. Usually, the superior cerebellar peduncles are not invaded by ependymomas; thus the superior cerebellar peduncle of the other side is freed from the tumor up to the point where the tumor invades the inferior cerebellar peduncle. One should be extremely careful to resect the tumor from the floor of the fourth ventricle using microscopic magnification, although total resection is not

recommended. A carbon dioxide laser is helpful in resecting the tumor from these critical regions with minimal mechanical manipulations.

Ependymomas often invade, or perhaps originate in, the lateral recess, particularly in cases with inferior cerebellar peduncle involvement.[1, 7] The portion of the tumor invading the inferior cerebellar peduncle can be resected radically under the surgical microscope although patients often experience a transient cerebellar ataxia postoperatively.[8] Even after the fourth ventricular ependymoma is removed, it is advisable to explore the lateral recess and the cerebellomedullary fissure by merely lifting the tonsil and hemisphere of the ipsilateral side to ensure completeness of tumor resection.[1, 9] This technique is also used to remove ependymomas that are extending in a dumbbell fashion from the fourth ventricle to the cerebellopontine/medullary fissure through the lateral recess or the cerebellomedullary fissure. In the cistern, the regional arteries and cranial nerve roots are compressed or wrapped by the ependymoma. However, it is possible to remove these tumors with minimum damage to cranial nerves and arteries by means of microscopic magnification and meticulous dissection. The cerebellopontine/medullary angle is approached through the wider craniotomy of the ipsilateral side. The tumor often extends through the spaces between the nerve roots, rootlets, and arteries. Some may extend into the jugular foramen or the internal auditory canal, and these can be removed. If the continuity of cranial nerves is preserved, complete or nearly complete recovery is the rule despite possible transient dysfunctions.

Once maximum cytoreduction is completed, the dura mater is closed in a watertight fashion. If a dural graft is needed, a piece of autologous pericranium or commercially available cadaver dura is used. The free bone flap is replaced and secured to the craniotomy edge. A multilayer closure is undertaken for the suboccipital musculature.

Postoperatively, the ventricular CSF is drained through the EVD at the level of 10 cm H_2O for 3 days, followed by closed ICP monitoring for 2 days. About 80 per cent of the children become shunt-free after successful surgical resection of the cerebellar—fourth ventricle tumor.[10]

Postoperative tumor staging is important for the selection of further therapy. Myelography and CSF cytology have been done to rule out intraspinal seedings. More recently, the combination of gadolinium-enhanced spine MRI and CSF cytology by lumbar puncture may be sufficient for the evaluation of spinal dissemination. The incidence of subarachnoid dissemination of benign ependymomas varies in the literature, but is generally regarded to be as low as 3 per cent.[11, 12]

Ependymomas of the posterior fossa need adjuvant therapy, although Nazar et al. have reported that radiation therapy (RT) is not required after total resection.[13] RT is indicated if patients are old enough to receive it. Although there has been controversy regarding the field of RT,[1, 11, 12] current methods irradiate only the posterior fossa provided tumor staging tests show no evidence of subarachnoid dissemination. The Pediatric Oncology Group currently treats posterior fossa ependymomas with a hyperfractionated RT technique.

To date, the efficacy of single-agent chemotherapy is doubtful. Also clinical experience with multi-agent chemotherapy shows little or no favorable response, particularly in patients with recurrent tumors. On the other hand, baby POG protocol (POG #8633/34) including cisplatin, cyclophosphamide, etoposide, and vincristine for ependymomas in children younger than 3 years of age demonstrated some clinical response. The disease control interval was 60 per cent at 12 months and 48 per cent at 24 months.[14]

Ependymomas usually recur within 2 years after incomplete resection and RT, and they may recur in 2 to 3 years even after visible total resection and RT.[1] These recurrent tumors probably need further surgical resection, should the location of recurrence permit. The prognosis for patients with posterior fossa ependymomas appears to be related to the extent of surgical resection.[3, 12, 13, 15] Radical resection usually leads to prolonged remission. Patients of younger age at diagnosis, with brainstem involvement and incomplete resection, have the bleakest prognosis.[3, 11, 13] Pathologic features such as high mitotic index and dense cellularity may also indicate poor prognosis.[4, 13]

CHOROID PLEXUS PAPILLOMAS

Choroid plexus papillomas are unique because of their CSF secretory function. These tumors of childhood occur primarily in the very young, about 80 per cent in the first 24 months of life.[16] The most common location is the lateral ventricle; the fourth ventricle location is uncommon, constituting 6 to 17 per cent of childhood choroid plexus papillomas.[16, 17] This incidence is contrary to that in adults, in whom the posterior fossa is the most common location for choroid plexus papillomas.[18, 19] Because of their obstructive nature compounded with CSF overproduction, fourth ventricle papillomas almost invariably present with hydrocephalus.[16]

Choroid plexus papillomas are histologically similar to the normal choroid plexus, composed of cuboidal cells arranged in fronds. Malignant papillomas are unusual, although some authors have reported as many as 26 per cent of childhood choroid plexus papillomas to be malignant.[17] Malignant choroid plexus papillomas (carcinomas) in the posterior fossa are extremely unusual, and only a few have been reported.[19, 21]

CT shows a solid, lobulated mass (Fig. 29–2). Occasional calcifications occur in older patients. Solid portions of the tumor invariably enhance after intravenous infusion of contrast material. MRI demonstrates the vascular nature of the papillomas within the tumor mass. Fourth ventricle papillomas may extend through the apertures of the ventricle. These neuro-imaging findings, however, are not specific for choroid plexus papillomas, and histologic diagnosis cannot be made on the basis of these imaging studies. Vertebral angiography can show large posterior inferior cerebellar arteries (PICAs) with neovascularization and large inferior vermian or, sometimes, precentral veins.

Placement of precraniotomy shunt is not recommended because of the aforementioned reasons. Additionally, owing to oversecretion of the CSF and the small peritoneal space of newborns and infants, a ventriculoperitoneal shunt tends to be complicated by severe abdominal distention due to CSF ascites.[16] Two deaths have been reported after shunting for hydrocephalus secondary to fourth ventricle choroid plexus papillomas.[21]

The initial steps in the surgical approach are the same

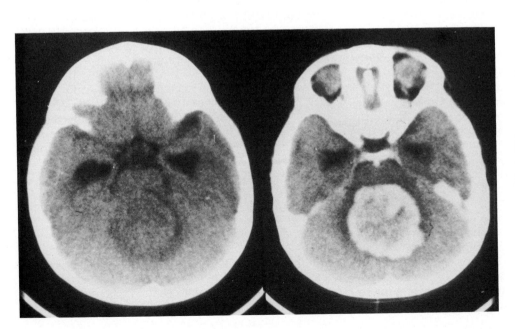

FIGURE 29–2. Axial CT scans before *(left)* and after *(right)* contrast infusion showing a choroid plexus papilloma of the fourth ventricle.

as those described for ependymomas. After the dura is opened, the tumor mass is often noticed protruding through the vallecula to the cisterna magnum. The inferior vermian vein may be hypertrophic and, sometimes, arterialized owing to rapid arteriovenous shunting in the papilloma. The identification of the posterior inferior cerebellar arteries (PICA) is important as the blood supply to the tumor is through them. In order to identify the PICAs, the cerebellar tonsil is laterally retracted, and the tonsillomedullary fissure is entered where the PICA is located. If the cerebellar vallecula is occupied by the papilloma, the tumor size is first reduced by bipolar cautery. Papillary portions of the choroid plexus papilloma are easily reduced in size by bipolar cautery and suction. Once choroidal points are identified and supplying blood vessels are secured and transected, tumor vascularity is markedly reduced. As choroid plexus papillomas rarely invade the fourth ventricular wall and the floor of the fourth ventricle, the remaining tumor resection is relatively straightforward. The fourth ventricle is entered through the split inferior vermis, and the tumor is dissected away from the cavity. The ependymal wall of the ventricle often shows xanthochromic discoloration, which is not a sign of tumor invasion but is due to previous hemorrhage. The portion extending into the aqueduct of Sylvius and lateral recess is removed with relative ease.

Once a total resection is achieved, the patient's prognosis is excellent. Malignant transformation or recurrence of choroid plexus papillomas is almost nonexistent. Despite a total resection, hydrocephalus may recur or persist and needs special attentive long-term care. Choroid plexus carcinomas, however, tend to recur or disseminate through the CSF pathway. Multi-agent chemotherapy has been used for carcinomas instead of radiotherapy due to the young age of patients.[22, 23] If the patients are older, radiation therapy is the treatment of choice for malignant choroid plexus papillomas, and radiation fields should include the craniospinal axis.

DERMOID CYSTS

Intracranial dermoids commonly occur in either the posterior fossa or the frontonasal location. These tumors are associated with a cutaneous dermal sinus in these locations. These dermal sinuses are defects in the closure of the ectoderm and may be produced by a failure of the anterior neuropore to close at the end of the fourth week of gestation. Posterior fossa dermoids have dermal sinus tracts near the inion, which extend through the bony defect into the intracranial space. Transdural extensions are located, almost always, just under the torcular Herophili. Posterior fossa dermoids are rarely associated with dermal sinus tracts of a supratentorial location.[24] The end of a dermal sinus forms a dermoid cyst, which may be located between the two leaves of the dura, in the subdural space, in the cerebellar parenchyma, or in the fourth ventricle. The dermoid forms a well-encapsulated mass, with the cyst wall composed of epidermis and dermis including hair follicles and sebaceous and sweat glands. The dermoid cyst contains desquamated epithelium, sweat, hair, and sebaceous materials, and shows slow but continuous growth.

Presenting symptoms are associated with infectious complications, mass effects, or a draining dermal sinus. One well-known presentation is repetitive bouts of bacterial meningitis.[24, 25] The common offending organism is *Staphylococcus epidermidis* or *aureus*, unlike meningitis secondary to spinal dermal sinus, which is usually associated with *Escherichia coli* or other gram-negative organisms. In some instances, dermoids can form a bacterial abscess. Purulent or sebaceous discharges from the cutaneous dermal sinus may be overlooked because of the presence of hair. If one suspects dermal sinus, a careful examination is needed to identify the cutaneous lesion, which is often surrounded by a hemangioma. On other occasions, a dermal tumor is detected incidentally during the evaluation of posterior fossa cysts or occipital meningoencephaloceles.

CT scans usually show a hypodense mass with subtle enhancement of the cyst wall after contrast infusion (Fig. 29–3). CT with bone window can disclose an occipital bone defect. Sagittal MRI is particularly useful to evaluate the relationship between the dermal sinus tract and torcular Herophili (Fig. 29–4).

Surgical resection should include both dermal sinus and cyst. The patient is placed in a prone position. After the occipital region is shaved, further inspection is made to identify the dermal sinus, which is located near the inion. If there is an associated posterior fossa cyst, the position of the inion is higher than usual. The skin incision is made in the midline and its upper end should include the dermal sinus. The dermal sinus is dissected and the bone defect widened by curettage. As the torcular Herophili is located just rostral to the dermal sinus, one should be careful not to traumatize the venous sinus. Further posterior fossa craniotomy is done in a size appropriate to the location of the dermoid cyst and the bony defect. The dural incision starts from the dermal sinus tract caudally toward the foramen magnum. The intradural dermal sinus tract is traced and the dermoid tumor identified. As the cyst capsule is well demarcated and there is little or no adhesion to the surrounding cerebellum, the resection of the dermoid tumor is relatively straightforward. An en bloc resection is possible. Once total resection of the dermoid and dermal sinus is achieved, these conditions do not recur.

EPIDERMOID CYSTS

In contrast to the dermoid, the epidermoid can occur without association with a dermal sinus in the posterior fossa. The most common site for a posterior fossa epidermoid is the cerebellopontine angle, but it may occur in the brainstem.[26] In most of the reported cases, the

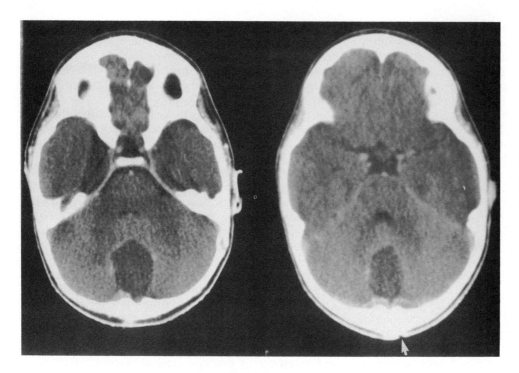

FIGURE 29–3. Axial CT scans after contrast infusion showing a posterior fossa dermoid cyst. Note a faint enhancement in the cyst wall and the presence of a dermal sinus tract (arrow).

patients are adults, despite the fact that the epidermoid originates in displaced epithelial tissues during an early embryonal stage. The lateral location of epidermoid cyst is explained by the theory that epithelial rests may be carried into the region of the cerebellopontine angle with the developing otic vesicles.[27]

An epidermoid cyst in the posterior fossa can cause aseptic meningitis due to leakage of the desquamated materials.[26] Bouts of meningitis due to a dermoid are usually bacterial. Other presentations of a posterior fossa epidermoid are those related to local mass effects.

The epidermoid cyst contains desquamated epidermal cell debris from the inner epithelial lining of the tumor capsule. The cyst contents are rich in cholesterol and usually solid in nature, consisting of flaky milky white material. Liquid cyst contents may range from creamy in nature to a lighter greenish to yellowish fluid.

CT appearance of these tumors is almost invariably a hypodense mass with occasional calcifications in the cyst wall. On MRI, epidermoid cysts may be hyperintense or may resemble CSF intensity. Neighboring bone may show erosion due to chronic local compression.

For cerebellopontine angle lesions, the patient is placed in a supine position with the ipsilateral shoulder elevated 45 degrees and with the head turned 45 degrees further so that the sagittal plane of the head is parallel to the operating room floor. In younger children, this position provides sufficient surgical exposure. In older patients, a lateral recumbent position or a park-bench position is used.

A paramedian, retromastoid skin incision is made. Craniotomy is again preferable to craniectomy so as to avoid postoperative pseudomeningocele. Craniotomy is made ipsilaterally through burr holes with one in the superolateral corner subjacent to the venous sinus and another in the midline caudal to the torcular Herophili. Craniotomy is done unilaterally with further bone removal from the ipsilateral foramen magnum caudally, and up to the sigmoid sinus laterally. The dura is opened parallel to the sigmoid sinus. The cerebellar hemisphere is gently retracted medially and superiorly. After drainage of the CSF from the basal cistern, further retraction of the cerebellum is easier because of gravity. Once the arachnoid membrane is opened, the lower cranial nerves should be identified. These are usually caudally displaced by the tumor mass. Under microscopic magnification, these nerves are separated from the tumor and protected by a cottonoid. The tumor capsule is opened and the contents removed. After this internal decompression, the cyst is easily mobilized in the cerebellopontine angle. Epidermoid capsules in

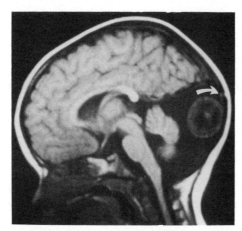

FIGURE 29–4. Sagittal T1-weighted MRI showing a dermoid cyst in enlarged cisterna magnum. Note a dermal sinus tract (arrow).

adults invariably adhere to the brainstem and sub-arachnoid neurovascular structures and show finger-like protrusions between the cranial nerves; whereas epidermoids in children show a less invasive nature and a visible total resection is possible. However, one should not forcibly remove the epidermoid capsule if there are severe adhesions to the vital structures. Residual capsule may lead to a cystic recurrence in a number of years. It can be acceptable in adults not to perform radical resection as the growth rate is slow.[27] Resecting the recurrent epidermoid from the cerebellopontine angle is often difficult due to adhesions of the capsule to the brainstem. An internal decompression alone may be justified, but further recurrence is inevitable. Perhaps internal irradiation with radioisotopes, as used for cystic craniopharyngiomas, may be considered.[28] The value of external beam radiation therapy for intracranial epidermoids has yet to be established.

TERATOMAS

Teratomas are rare tumors and usually occur in infancy and childhood. Their histologic type is one of the most common among neonatal brain tumors.[29] They are often located in the skull midline, with the para-third ventricular region being the common site of occurrence.

Histologically, teratomas are composed of several types of tissue representing more than one germ layer. The tissues in a teratoma are either well differentiated or immature. The latter contains varying amounts and proportions of embryonal and fetal tissues. In the posterior fossa, teratomas are usually located in the fourth ventricle,[30] but may be located in the cerebellopontine angle.[31] Some neonatal teratomas are so massive that the normal posterior fossa architecture may be obscured (Fig. 29–5), or the brainstem may be replaced by teratoma.[32] Although they are well demarcated and encapsulated, teratomas in young patients are often large and located in the midline, making surgical resection hazardous. Posterior fossa teratomas invariably present with hydrocephalus owing to their obstructive nature.

Teratomas are noted to have varying degrees of calcification and cyst formation within the tumor mass, and some may show the presence of fat or of cartilage formations. Teratomas with cyst formations or calcification are more benign in nature; malignant teratomas are usually solid and show a lower incidence of calcification and more enhancement after intravenous contrast infusion.[30, 33]

Surgical resection is the treatment of choice for benign teratomas. However, neonatal teratomas need special surgical care owing to their magnitude, their vascular nature, and the newborn's limited blood volume. These tumors carry a particularly high mortality rate.[32, 34] Cyst contents vary in nature, ranging from light liquid to thick mucoid material, depending on the varying secretory glandular components.

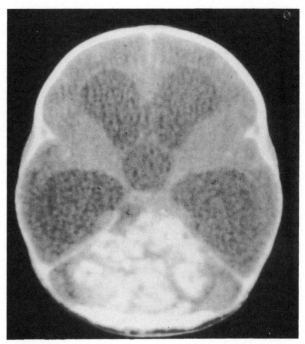

FIGURE 29–5. Axial CT after contrast infusion showing a massive teratoma of the posterior fossa in a newborn.

Successful resection of benign teratomas provides an excellent prognosis. However, immature teratomas are unpredictable in outcome; some may mature histologically and lose their malignant potential,[30] whereas others may develop into teratocarcinomas, which tend to recur and disseminate. Because of their occurrence in young children, radiation therapy is not recommended for these malignant tumors, though they may be radiosensitive. Chemotherapy may be useful in tumor control.[35]

MENINGIOMAS

Meningiomas, which are common in adults, are rare in infancy and childhood. Only 1 per cent of meningiomas occur in childhood.[36] Posterior fossa meningiomas are even more unusual, although an unusually high incidence at this site was noted among pediatric meningiomas (19 percent).[37] They may be associated with neurofibromatosis or previous exposure to cranial irradiation. In the posterior fossa of children, meningiomas occur usually in the petrous ridge or cerebellopontine angle, but they may occur in the fourth ventricle or cerebellar convexity. There are contradicting reports regarding the incidence of malignant transformation of meningiomas; some claim it is infrequent,[37] while others report it to be as high as 30 per cent.[38]

CT shows the meningioma to be a well-circumscribed, slightly hyperdense mass and to exhibit bright enhancement after intravenous infusion of contrast. Neighboring bony changes may be present. Petrous ridge meningiomas tend to extend to the middle cranial fossa. MRI provides clear information regarding the relationship of meningioma with vital structures such as the brainstem, venous sinuses, and basilar artery. Angiography may be indicated if the origin appears to be the ventral dura or the tentorium, or if MRI indicates a vascular tumor.

Meningioma is a surgical disease; thus an effort must be made to surgically resect this histologically benign tumor. Petrous ridge meningiomas are best removed through a subtemporal approach, a lateral posterior fossa craniotomy, or a combination of both. A wide resection of adjacent dura is needed in order to ensure complete meningioma resection.

Meningiomas rarely recur after total resection. However, they do recur after incomplete resection or insufficient resection of the dura surrounding the meningioma. Recurrent or residual tumor can be treated with radiation therapy. Local high-intensified radiation therapy using a gamma knife or Linac system may be considered for that purpose. Hormonal therapy with antiestrogen or antiprogestin agents has been considered for meningiomas. However, our experience with five pediatric meningiomas showed little or no estrogen and progestin binding capacity; hence hormonal manipulation therapy was not warranted for these pediatric meningiomas. The value of chemotherapy for meningiomas has yet to be determined.

NEURINOMAS

Neurinomas in childhood are rare, and only a limited number of patients are reported in the literature. In the posterior fossa they occur in the cerebellopontine angle, and their origin is usually the acoustic nerve. They may be also localized in the foramen magnum, developing from the lower cranial nerves.[39] These usually occur without the cutaneous manifestation of neurofibromatosis, whereas acoustic neurofibromas are associated with neurofibromatosis and tend to occur bilaterally. At the time of diagnosis, most pediatric acoustic neurinomas are large, because unilateral auditory dysfunction may go unnoticed by children for a prolonged period.[40] Although hearing loss is the major symptom, various symptoms such as cerebellar compression, other cranial nerve signs, and hydrocephalus are present by the time of their diagnosis.

Neurinomas on neuro-imaging studies show an extrinsic cerebellopontine angle mass with contrast enhancement. In the case of acoustic neurinoma, the internal auditory meatus is enlarged. The clear extrinsic character is distinct on MRI, as tumor density is distinguished from compressed brainstem density. MRI is particularly useful in differentiating acoustic neurinoma or other extrinsic tumors from ventrally exophytic brainstem tumors, which are more commonly located in the cerebellopontine angle in childhood. Some acoustic neurinomas are vascular, supplied by the external carotid system.[41]

Surgical resection is the treatment of choice for acoustic neurinomas. Although their growth rate is slow, they recur if resection is not complete. Acoustic neurinomas or foramen magnum neurinomas are best approached via a lateral posterior fossa craniotomy. If tumor vascularity is significant, a preoperative embolization is recommended and may substantially reduce tumor vascularity.[41] Protection of the lower cranial nerves and sparing of the facial nerve are usually achieved by a microsurgical technique, although childhood neurinomas pose a significantly high risk because of the magnitude of these tumors.

Totally resected neurinomas carry a good prognosis, provided vital neurologic functions are preserved. Recurrent or small residual tumors may be treated by a local high-intensified irradiation technique, but its long-term effect in childhood needs further investigation.

SUMMARY

The posterior fossa is a common site for tumor occurrence in childhood. Other than common pediatric tumors such as medulloblastomas, cerebellar astrocytomas, ependymomas, and brainstem tumors, one should keep in mind that tumors of various pathology, though rare, occur in the posterior fossa. Advanced neuro-imaging (CT and MRI) is helpful in identifying the location, extension, and nature of the lesion. The histologic nature of these tumors may be predicted based on this information. Hydrocephalus is often the cause of presenting symptoms and, in a great majority of cases, is resolved after successful tumor resection. Tumors occurring in the cerebellopontine angle usually present with localized mass effects. Significant improvements in diagnostic neuro-imaging technology, surgical instrumentation, and pediatric subspecialization over the past few decades enable surgeons to resect posterior fossa tumors in childhood with an acceptable morbidity while striving toward maximum cytoreduction. One should make every effort to effect this surgical purpose with safety. Careful surgical planning and a knowledge of the strategic relationship between tumor and vital structures such as the brainstem, cerebellar peduncle, cranial nerves, and vertebrobasilar system are critical for successful tumor resection. Unresectable and malignant tumors need further adjuvant therapy. External beam irradiation remains problematic in young children because of its late toxicity to the developing central nervous system. Currently available "radiosurgery" techniques deliver a localized intensified radiation dose to a limited target, but radionecrosis in the brainstem should be a concern. The role of adjuvant chemotherapy in the management of malignant brain tumors in infants and young children has gained significant recognition, but improved chemotherapeutic agents and protocols need exploration.

REFERENCES

1. Tomita T, McLone DG, Das L, et al.: Benign ependymomas of the posterior fossa in childhood. Pediatr Neurosci 14:277, 1988.

2. Raimondi AJ, Tomita T: Hydrocephalus and infratentorial tumors: Incidence, clinical picture and treatment. J Neurosurg 55:174, 1981.
3. Healey EA, Barnes PD, Kupsky WJ, et al.: The prognostic significance of postoperative residual tumor in ependymoma. Neurosurgery 28:666, 1991.
4. Schiffer D, Chio A, Cravioto H, et al.: Ependymoma: internal correlation among pathological signs: The anaplastic variant. Neurosurgery 29:206, 1991.
5. Tomita T, Mclone DG: Spontaneous seeding of medulloblastoma: results of CSF cytology and arachnoid biopsy from the cisterna magnum. Neurosurgery 12:265, 1983.
6. Krichef II, Becker M, Schneck A, et al.: Intracranial ependymomas; factors influencing prognosis. J Neurosurg 21:7, 1964.
7. Courville CB, Broussalian SL: Plastic ependymomas of the lateral recess. Report of eight verified cases. J Neurosurg 18:792, 1961.
8. Tomita T: Surgical management of cerebellar peduncle lesions in childhood. Neurosurgery 18:568, 1986.
9. Matsushima T, Fukui M, Inoue T, et al.: Microsurgical and magnetic resonance imaging anatomy of the cerebellomedullary fissure and its application during fourth ventricle surgery. Neurosurgery 30:325, 1992.
10. Tomita T, Rosenblatt SS: Management of hydrocephalus secondary to posterior fossa tumor in childhood. In Matsumoto S, Tamaki N (eds): Hydrocephalus—Pathogenesis and Treatment. New York, Springer-Verlag, 1991, pp 306–310.
11. Lyons MK, Kelly PJ: Posterior fossa ependymomas: report of 30 cases and review of the literature. Neurosurgery 28:659, 1991.
12. Shaw EG, Evans RG, Scheithauser BW, et al.: Postoperative radiotherapy of intracranial ependymoma in pediatric and adult patients. Int J Radiat Oncol Biol Phys 13:1457, 1987.
13. Nazar GB, Hoffman HJ, Becker LE, et al.: Infratentorial ependymomas in childhood: Prognostic factors and treatment. J Neurosurg 72:408, 1990.
14. Duffner P, Cohen M, Horowitz M, et al.: Postoperative chemotherapy and delayed radiation therapy in infants with intracranial ependymomas: A POG group-wide protocol. Ann Neurol 28:442, 1990.
15. Hendrick EB, Raffel C: Tumors of the fourth ventricle: ependymomas, choroid plexus papillomas and dermoid cysts. In McLaurin RL, Schut L, Venes JL, Epstein F (eds): Pediatric Neurosurgery. 2nd ed. Philadelphia, WB Saunders, 1989, pp 366–372.
16. Tomita T, McLone DG, Flannery AM: Choroid plexus papillomas of neonates, infants and children. Pediatr Neurosci 14:23, 1988.
17. Humphreys RP, Nemoto S, Hendrick EB, et al.: Childhood choroid plexus tumors. Concepts Pediatr Neurosurg 7:1, 1987.
18. Laurence KM: The biology of choroid plexus papilloma in infancy and childhood. Acta Neurochir (Wien) 50:79, 1979.
19. McGirr SJ, Ebersold MJ, Scheithauer BW, et al.: Choroid plexus papillomas: Long-term follow-up results in a surgically treated series. J Neurosurg 69:843, 1988.
20. Vazquez E, Ball WS, Prenger EC, et al.: Magnetic resonance imaging of fourth ventricular choroid plexus neoplasms in childhood. A report of two cases. Pediatr Neurosurg 17:48, 1991–1992.
21. Pascual-Castroviejo I, Roche MC, Villarejo F, et al.: Choroid plexus papillomas of the fourth ventricle: Report of three cases. Childs Brain 9:373, 1982.
22. Allen J, Wissof J, Helson L, et al.: Choroid plexus carcinoma: Responses to chemotherapy alone in newly diagnosed young children. J Neurooncol 12:69, 1992.
23. Griffin BR, Stewart GR, Berger MS, et al.: Choroid plexus carcinoma of the fourth ventricle: Report of a case in an infant. Pediatr Neurosci 14:134, 1988.
24. Schijman E, Monges J, Cragnaz R, et al.: Congenital dermal sinuses, dermoid and epidermoid cysts of the posterior fossa. Childs Nerv Syst 2:83, 1986.
25. Altman RS: Dermoid tumours of the posterior fossa associated with congenital dermoid sinus: Report of a case and review of the literature. J Pediatr 62:565, 1963.
26. Leal O, Miles J: Epidermoid cyst in the brain stem. Case report. J Neurosurg 48:811, 1978.
27. Berger MS, Wilson CB: Epidermoid cysts of the posterior fossa. J Neurosurg 62:214, 1985.
28. Kobayashi T, Kageyama N, Ohara K: Internal irradiation for cystic craniopharyngioma. J Neurosurg 55:898, 1981.
29. Wakai S, Arai T, Nagai M: Congenital brain tumors. Surg Neurol 21:597, 1984.
30. Drapkin AJ, Rose WS, Pellmer MB: Mature teratoma in the fourth ventricle of an adult: Case report and review of the literature. Neurosurgery 21:404, 1987.
31. Waters DC, Venes JL, Zis K: Case report: Childhood cerebellopontine angle teratoma associated with congenital hydrocephalus. Neurosurgery 18:784, 1986.
32. Radkowski MA, Naidich TP, Tomita T, et al.: Neonatal brain tumors: CT and MRI findings. J Comput Assist Tomogr 12:10, 1988.
33. Iplikcioglu AC, Ozer F, Benli K, et al.: Malignant teratoma of the cerebellopontine angle: Case report. Neurosurgery 27:137, 1990.
34. Ventreyra ECG, Herder S: Neonatal intracranial teratoma: Case report. J Neurosurg 59:879, 1983.
35. Allen JC: Management of primary intracranial germ cell tumors of childhood. Pediatr Neurosci 13:152, 1987.
36. Chan RC, Thompson GB: Intracranial meningiomas in childhood. Surg Neurol 21:319, 1984.
37. Merten DF, Godding CA, Newton TH, et al.: Meningiomas of childhood and adolescence. J Pediatr 84:696, 1974.
38. Cooper M, Dohn DF: Intracranial meningiomas in childhood. Cleve Clin Q 41:197, 1974.
39. Martinez R, Vaquero J, Cabezudo J, et al.: Neurinomas of the jugular foramen in children. J Neurosurg 54:693, 1981.
40. Vassilouthis J, Richardson AE: Acoustic neurinoma in a child. Surg Neurol 12:37, 1979.
41. Rushworth RG, Sorby WA, Smith SF: Acoustic neuroma in a child treated with the aid of preoperative arterial embolization. Case report. J Neurosurg 61:386, 1984.

Chapter 30

TUMORS OF THE CEREBRAL HEMISPHERES

JEFFREY H. WISOFF, M.D.

Central nervous system tumors are the second most common form of neoplasia to affect the pediatric population and the third leading cause of death in children under 16 years old.[1-3] Brain and spinal cord tumors account for 20 per cent of all pediatric cancers compared to 1 to 2 per cent of all adult malignancies.[2] Their incidence appears to be increasing in frequency; from 2.4 new cases/100,000 children/year in 1973 to 3.3 cases/100,000 children/year in 1986.[1, 4-8] There are approximately 1500 new central nervous system tumors annually.[3, 5, 7]

Supratentorial tumors are a heterogeneous assortment of predominantly neuroectodermal tumors that account for 30 to 55 per cent of pediatric brain tumors.[9-11] Approximately one third of these neoplasms involve the cerebral hemispheres.[9, 12] The most common tumor is the low-grade astrocytoma (grades 1 and 2 of Kernohan[13] or grade 2 WHO[14]) composed of fibrillary or protoplasmic neoplastic astrocytes. Other low-grade tumors include the juvenile pilocytic astrocytoma, oligodendroglioma, ependymoma, mixed glioma, and ganglioglioma.[2, 15] Approximately 20 per cent of supratentorial tumors will be malignant neoplasms: anaplastic gliomas and glioblastomas.[2, 15] During the first 2 years of life, supratentorial tumors predominate; most are malignant neoplasms with a relatively high incidence of teratomas, choroid plexus tumors, and primitive neuroectodermal tumors (PNET).[10, 15, 16]

The pathogenesis of pediatric brain tumors remains obscure. Recent advances in molecular biology and cytogenetics have begun to identify possible sites of oncogenesis. Chromosomal abnormalities associated with brain tumors include deletions of chromosome 22 (meningiomas, acoustic neuromas), alterations of chromosome 17 (medulloblastoma, astrocytoma), and loss on chromosome 10 (glioblastoma).[17-21]

Central nervous system tumors can be part of the clinical manifestation of one of the phakomatoses (Fig. 30-1). Tuberous sclerosis is associated with subependymal giant cell astrocytomas. Optic pathway gliomas, hemispheric astrocytomas and hamartomas, nerve sheath tumors, and meningiomas may be seen in children with neurofibromatosis. Cerebellar hemangioblastoma presenting in childhood is pathognomonic of von Hippel–Lindau disease.

The initial treatment of all hemispheric tumors is surgical resection with the intent of obtaining a gross total removal. Intraoperative real-time ultrasonography accurately delineates subcortical pathology, facilitating the surgical approach and minimizing damage to adjacent normal structures. Neurophysiologic monitoring and intraoperative electroencephalographic (EEG) corticography precisely identify eloquent cortical areas serving such functions as speech and primary motor control. Use of advanced surgical technology including the operating microscope, ultrasonic surgical aspirator, and the CO_2 laser allows radical resection with minimal risk throughout the supratentorial compartment. Even deep tumors previously considered forbidden territory may be resected with minimal morbidity. The operative mortality in pediatric neurosurgical centers approaches zero.

This chapter will discuss the childhood tumors of the cerebral hemispheres, their current treatment, long-term prognosis, late sequelae of therapy, and future directions in pediatric neuro-oncology.

ASTROCYTOMAS

Supratentorial astrocytomas comprise one third of cerebral hemisphere neoplasms.[9, 12] There is equal distribution between the sexes with a peak incidence between the ages of 8 and 12 years.[22-25] The most common tumor is the low-grade astrocytoma (grade 1

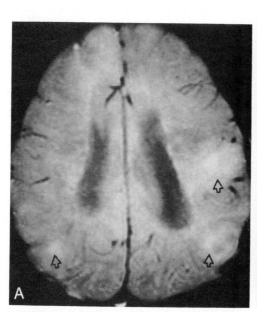
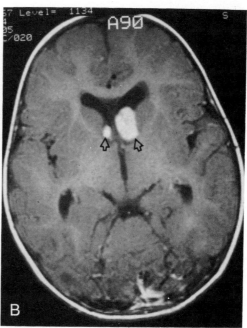

FIGURE 30–1. Tuberous Sclerosis. *A*, T2-weighted MRI shows multiple cortical hamartomas (tubers) *(arrows)*. *B*, T1-weighted gadolinium-enhanced MRI. Note subependymal giant cell astrocytomas *(arrows)*.

WHO[14]) composed of fibrillary or protoplasmic neoplastic astrocytes. Ten to 20 per cent may be juvenile pilocytic astrocytomas, which have a distinct pathologic pattern consisting of alternating areas of high and low cellularity, abundant Rosenthal fibers, and microcysts.[2, 15] Malignant histology (anaplastic astrocytomas and glioblastomas) is seen in approximately 20 to 30 per cent of the cases.[2, 15, 22] Tumor cysts are seen in 36 to 54 per cent of the children[23, 26] (Fig. 30–2). The cyst wall is lined with neoplastic cells 70 per cent of the time and with a mural tumor nodule and an associated non-neoplastic reactive cyst in the remainder.[11, 23–25]

Within each of these pathologic entities, the biological behavior may be variable. Studies of cell cycle ki-

netics, cytogenics, and cytometrics have shown slow growth rates in the majority of histologically well-differentiated astrocytomas.[27–30] Clinical experience supports the indolent nature of many of these low-grade tumors, with prolonged survival occurring commonly.[1, 31, 32]

In spite of benign histology, only 60 to 70 per cent of children with low-grade gliomas will be long-term survivors.[5, 7, 12, 31–33] The heterogeneity in location, treatment regimens, neurodiagnostic evaluation, and the unclear natural history have resulted in extensive controversy and debate in the literature, with 10-year survivals ranging from 10 to 94 per cent.[1, 5, 7, 9, 26, 32, 34, 35]

In contrast to the low-grade tumors, malignant astro-

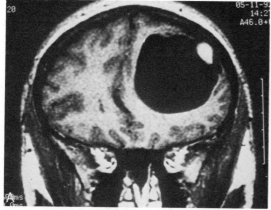
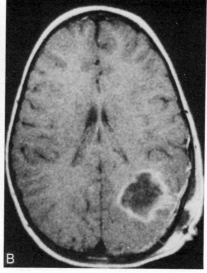

FIGURE 30–2. Cystic astrocytomas. *A*, T1-weighted gadolinium-enhanced MRI with mural nodule and reactive cyst. *B*, T1-weighted gadolinium-enhanced MRI with neoplastic cyst walls.

cytomas carry a poor prognosis similar to that for adult tumors. Children with glioblastomas have a dismal outcome, with 5-year survival ranging from 5 to 15 per cent.[36-38] Anaplastic astrocytomas fare better with 20 to 40 per cent long-term survival.[37] Leptomeningeal dissemination may occur in approximately 10 per cent of children with malignant astrocytomas, especially tumors located adjacent to the ventricles.[39] Routine postoperative neuraxis staging is recommended for these patients.

PRESENTATION

The signs and symptoms of supratentorial gliomas are dependent on anatomic localization and histologic grade. Brief prodromes are more characteristic of malignant gliomas. Symptoms of increased intracranial pressure occur in most patients, with a fulminant course typical of malignant tumors. Obstructive hydrocephalus is common with deep tumors of the basal ganglia and thalamus that impinge on the ventricles, whereas superficial hemispheric gliomas rarely present with hydrocephalus. Macrocrania may be the only sign of large cerebral tumors in infants. Among the older children, over one half with hemispheric tumors complain of headache, usually worse in the morning and associated with emesis. In rare instances, patients with chronic increased intracranial pressure and papilledema may present with intermittent visual obscurations, visual loss, or even blindness.

Focal signs and symptoms are related to the location of the neoplasm. Most children with hemispheric astrocytomas will have some involvement of the posterior frontal lobe (motor cortex) or basal ganglia, resulting in monoparesis or hemiparesis. Occipital lobe tumors will often result in visual field abnormalities. Other neurologic deficits may be more subtle and insidious (e.g., sensory loss, personality changes, and deteriorating school performance). Seizures occur in approximately 40 to 60 per cent of children with hemispheric gliomas.[9, 40] Like the focal neurologic deficits, the seizure pattern will reflect the location of the tumor (e.g.,

complex seizures with temporal lobe tumors and focal motor seizures with frontoparietal neoplasms). Since the advent of computerized tomography (CT) and magnetic resonance imaging (MRI), unsuspected low-grade tumors frequently have been identified as the etiology of chronic epilepsy.[26, 32]

TREATMENT

Surgery

Surgical intervention has been the primary therapy for the vast majority of low-grade gliomas of childhood. Most pediatric neurosurgeons believe that gross total excision of low-grade tumors offers the potential for long-term event-free survival or possible cure. Approximately 18 per cent of supratentorial low-grade gliomas are superficial in location and amenable to gross total surgical excision.[9, 23-25, 31] Long-term disease-free survival (>10 years) and probable cure following gross total resection ranges from 50 to 82 per cent in recent retrospective series (Fig. 30–3).[24, 26, 31, 34, 41]

Unfortunately, the many low-grade gliomas of childhood extend into vital areas or arise in deep midline structures (e.g., chiasmatic-hypothalamic, thalamic, basal ganglia), rendering complete surgical excision impossible (Fig. 30–4). The role of radical subtotal resection of these tumors is less clear. Laws et al. found the rate of survival beyond 5 years to be similar for total resections and radical subtotal resections, but not for biopsy or partial resection.[31] Radical subtotal resection as the sole treatment modality has been promulgated for hemispheric tumors extending deep into midline structures. Support for this management strategy is based on encouraging preliminary reports of prolonged progression-free survival following radical subtotal resection for thalamic,[42] septal,[43] hypothalamic,[44, 45] and dorsal exophytic brainstem tumors.[46, 47]

Radical resection of malignant gliomas of childhood has been correlated with improved disease-free survival and overall survival in two prospective Children's Cancer Study Group (CCSG) (65, CCSG-945 personal communication, Wisoff JH and Boyett J, 1992). This sur-

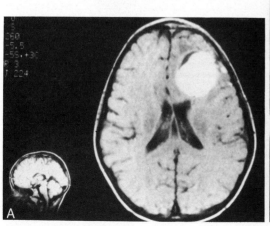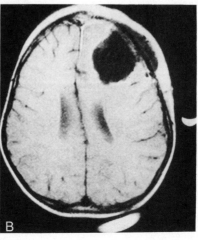

FIGURE 30–3. Gross total resection of hemispheric anaplastic astrocytoma. *A*, T1-weighted gadolinium-enhanced MRI (preoperative). *B*, T1-weighted gadolinium-enhanced MRI (postoperative).

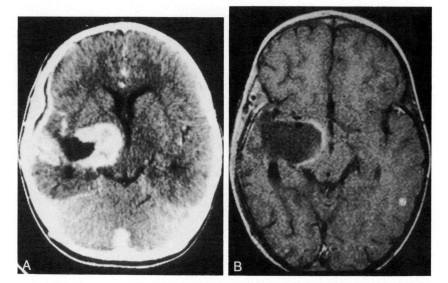

FIGURE 30–4. Radical subtotal resection of deep low-grade astrocytoma. *A*, T1-weighted gadolinium-enhanced MRI (preoperative). *B*, T1-weighted gadolinium-enhanced MRI (postoperative).

vival advantage is independent of adjuvant radiation, chemotherapy, and tumor location. The recent CCSG-945 study showed the greatest benefit with >90 per cent tumor resection.

Irradiation

Although there is no consensus about the optimal treatment of subtotally resected low-grade tumors, therapeutic irradiation has been the traditional adjuvant treatment in these patients in spite of conflicting reports concerning efficacy.[5, 31, 34, 35, 42, 48–50] The use of irradiation is limited by a relatively narrow therapeutic window. Doses in excess of 4000 cGy are required to delay tumor progression.[48–50] There is no prospective or randomized study examining long-term efficacy, late effect, or quality of survival following irradiation for low-grade gliomas. The question of efficacy is especially important, since tumors are being diagnosed at an earlier stage and age as a result of routine screening of minimally symptomatic children with MRI and CT scans.

There is clear benefit of adjuvant irradiation for children with malignant gliomas.[36, 37] Doses of 5400 cGy to 6000 cGy appear to offer longer survival time than doses under 5000 cGy.[37] Although whole-brain irradiation was frequently recommended in the past, most centers have adopted a focal field with generous margins around the tumor.[37, 40] As in medulloblastoma, irradiation has been associated with intellectual deterioration, developmental delay, endocrine dysfunction, and the development of irradiation-induced tumors.[51–59]

Chemotherapy

Postirradiation adjuvant chemotherapy has been shown to significantly increase survival in children with malignant astrocytomas.[38] A randomized CCSG trial of a nitrosourea-based regimen increased 5-year

survival to 43 per cent compared to 13 per cent of children receiving only irradiation.[38] This effect on survival was most significant for children with glioblastoma. Preirradiation chemotherapy has been proposed to facilitate the efficacy of radiotherapy by providing further tumor "debulking." Several antineoplastic agents such as cisplatin have also demonstrated radiosensitizing properties that could potentially augment the efficacy of irradiation. Currently there are several institutional and cooperative group trials of neo-adjuvant intensive chemotherapy for children under 3 years of age that are intended to delay the initiation of irradiation and thus protect the immature brain.

EPENDYMOMA

Ependymomas constitute 8 to 10 per cent of all central nervous system tumors of childhood.[2] They have a predilection for younger children, with over half occurring before the age of 2 years. Approximately 30 to 50 per cent originate supratentorially. Unlike the posterior fossa ependymomas, which are located almost exclusively in the fourth ventricle, these supratentorial tumors arise within the parenchyma of the cerebral hemispheres from ectopic rests of ependymal cells adjacent to the ventricles[2, 60, 61] (Fig. 30–5). Macrocysts occur in 50 per cent of supratentorial ependymomas but do not connote benign histology.[60]

Pathologically, the grading of these tumors is analogous to the grading of astrocytomas. The low-grade tumors have features that recapitulate normal ependymal cell morphology, whereas the anaplastic tumors have varying degrees of pleomorphism, increased cellularity, mitotic activity, necrosis, and endothelial hyperplasia. The significance of histologic grading is controversial, with most studies demonstrating a tendency toward a worse prognosis with increasing anaplasia. A primitive, extremely malignant neoplasm, the ependy-

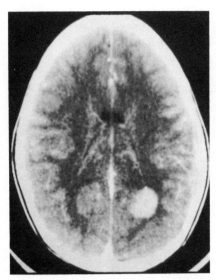

FIGURE 30–5. Ependymoma. Note extraventricular location on T1-weighted gadolinium-enhanced MRI.

moblastoma is now considered to be a variant of PNET.[14]

The duration of symptoms and clinical presentation are related to the anatomic location; headache, vomiting, macrocrania, and seizures constitute the most common presentation. Radical surgical excision should be attempted in all patients. Supratentorial tumors can be totally resected in the majority of cases; involvement of the thalamus, hypothalamus, and basal ganglia may preclude complete removal. Postoperative staging includes assessment of residual tumor, CSF cytology, and gadolinium-enhanced MRI of the spine.

Risk of tumor recurrence has been related to several prognostic factors: leptomeningeal dissemination, young age (<2 to 3 years), and subtotal surgical resection.[61–65] As discussed above, histologic grading of anaplasia has an uncertain impact on prognosis. Overall 5-year disease-free survival is between 40 and 60 per cent.[61, 63, 64] Children with gross total resection of their tumor, including no identifiable tumor on postoperative scans, have the best survival, approaching 85 per cent in recent series.[63]

Adjuvant irradiation is clearly of benefit in patients with residual tumor, disseminated tumor, and anaplastic histology.[33, 61, 63, 65, 66] Between 5000 and 6000 cGy are required for tumor control. The incidence of dissemination is extremely low for supratentorial ependymoma, and involved field irradiation is adequate.[61] Most centers recommend neuraxis irradiation for anaplastic ependymomas because 80 per cent of the patients who ultimately develop metastasis have high-grade pathology.[61, 65, 66] However, dissemination is almost never seen without recurrence at the primary site, suggesting that tumor spread is secondary to failure of local control of the ependymoma.[62] A recent trial of local irradiation by the Pediatric Oncology Group (POG) identified no secondary dissemination.[40] The issue of craniospinal irradiation is of particular impor-

tance, since the majority of children with ependymoma are young and are thus the most prone to develop long-term sequelae.

Although recurrent ependymomas have been shown to be chemosensitive tumors, responding to the same agents as medulloblastomas, prospective therapeutic trials of newly diagnosed ependymomas, combining craniospinal irradiation and chemotherapy by CCSG and International Society of Pediatric Oncology (SIOP), have failed to demonstrate an increase in disease-free survival or overall survival.[67] Future innovations in treatment may include deferred irradiation for older children with totally resected tumors, increased tumor resectability utilizing intraoperative neurophysiologic monitoring to pursue tumors into deep structures, and adjuvant chemotherapy in combination with either local irradiation, hyperfractionated irradiation, or reduced-dose neuraxis irradiation.

OLIGODENDROGLIOMAS

Oligodendrogliomas are rare tumors in the pediatric age group. Only 2 to 3 per cent of hemispheric neoplasms are pure oligodendrogliomas, although up to 30 per cent of supratentorial gliomas may have a mixed population of astrocytes and oligodendrocytes (mixed glioma, oligoastrocytoma).[22, 68] The peak incidence during childhood is between the ages of 6 and 12 years with a strong male predominance.[68, 69]

These tumors are most frequently located in the frontal lobes (Fig. 30–6). Pathologically the cells are arranged in uniform, monotonous sheets with perinuclear clear zones or halos producing a "fried egg" appearance. Calcification, thin-walled capillaries, and microscopic hemorrhages are common.[2, 14] Although an admixture of astrocytes is frequently present, the term "mixed glioma" is reserved for tumors that have more than 25 per cent astrocytes. The histologic grading system is similar to that for astrocytomas. Microscopic involvement of leptomeninges may be seen in one third of the patients but does not have any prognostic significance.[2] Neuraxis dissemination is rare.

A history of seizures for several years is present in almost all children. Symptoms of increased intracranial pressure, behavioral changes, and focal neurologic deficits may be present, usually for less than 1 year. A short prodrome may suggest an anaplastic tumor.

There is no pathognomonic radiographic picture for oligodendrogliomas. CT scans and plain skull radiographs show the calcifications. Patchy contrast enhancement is seen on CT and MRI. Tumor cysts are common.

Radical surgical resection is the most effective therapy. Extent of resection may be limited by dense calcifications and the infiltrative growth pattern of these tumors. The role of adjuvant irradiation of these tumors is controversial but may improve survival in subtotally resected and anaplastic tumors. Five-year survival for pure oligodendrogliomas ranges from 75 to 85 per

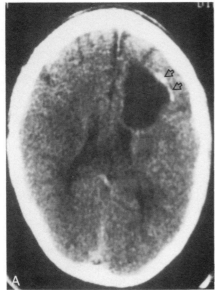

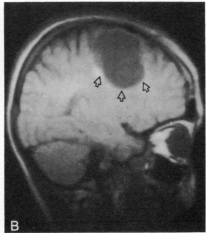

FIGURE 30–6. Oligodendroglioma. *A*, CT showing cyst with calcifications *(arrows)*. *B*, MRI shows diffuse cyst wall enhancement *(arrows)*.

cent.[40, 68, 69] Children with anaplastic tumors fare poorly, with few long-term survivors. Recent experience with chemotherapy (procarbazine, CCNU, and vincristine—PCV) showed significant responses in recurrent anaplastic oligodendrogliomas.[40] Current multi-institutional and cooperative group trials are addressing the role of chemotherapy for newly diagnosed anaplastic tumors.

GANGLIOGLIOMA

Ganglioglioma, a mixed tumor composed of neoplastic ganglion cells and astrocytes,[2, 70] accounts for 4 to 8 per cent of pediatric brain tumors. The histologic grading is analogous to that of astrocytomas;[15] only the astrocytic component of the tumor is evaluated for features of anaplasia. Although gangliogliomas may arise at any site throughout the central nervous system, they appear to have a predilection for the medial temporal lobe[2, 70] (Fig. 30–7). They may occur throughout childhood, most often in males.

For most affected children, the presenting complaint is a poorly controlled seizure disorder, often with associated behavioral abnormalities. Focal neurologic deficits are less common. An MRI demonstrating a well-demarcated, cystic temporal lobe mass without edema in a child is almost pathognomonic of a ganglioglioma. The slow growth of these tumors is occasionally shown by erosion and remodeling of the adjacent inner table of the calvarium on CT scan.

The indolent nature of these tumors, frequent superficial location, and demarcation from surrounding white matter mandates surgery with the intent to perform a curative gross total resection. In patients with

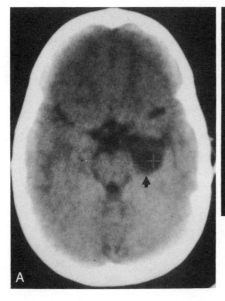

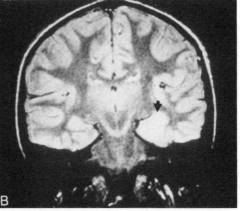

FIGURE 30–7. Ganglioglioma of temporal lobe. *A*, CT scan. Note hypodense medial temporal lesion *(arrow)*. *B*, T2-weighted MRI coronal demonstrates tumor *(arrow)*.

refractory epilepsy, intraoperative electrocorticorgraphy may be of benefit in delineating the epileptogenic foci and guiding resection of adjacent non-neoplastic cortex.[71] Long-term disease-free survival is 75 to 90 per cent following radical surgery.[40, 70] Adjuvant irradiation does not appear to have any value in totally resected tumors. The role of irradiation in treating subtotally resected tumors and those with anaplastic features is controversial.

PRIMITIVE NEUROECTODERMAL TUMORS (PNET)

PNET of the cerebral hemispheres is a rare tumor that is histologically and biologically similar to medulloblastoma. World Health Organization (WHO) classification of pediatric CNS tumors considers all undifferentiated neoplasms, regardless of location, as derived from a common primitive neuroepithelial cell and categorizes them as primitive neuroectodermal tumors (PNET).[14]

Children usually present with a short prodrome of symptoms of increased intracranial pressure typical of a rapidly growing neoplasm. As with other hemispheric tumors, focal signs are referable to the tumor's anatomic location. Neuroradiographic studies demonstrate a large, relatively well-demarcated lesion with a more heterogenous enhancement pattern than that of medulloblastomas. Cysts, areas of calcification, and hemorrhage are frequently present.

The initial treatment is radical surgical resection. The recent CCSG-921 study demonstrated a significant disease-free survival advantage for gross total resection of cerebral PNET. The gadolinium-enhanced MRI determines the extent of surgical resection and the presence of residual disease. The propensity for leptomeningeal dissemination mandates postoperative staging, both for treatment planning and prognosis. Gadolinium-enhanced MRI of the spine or a CT myelogram and CSF cytology complete the CNS evaluation.

Adjuvant treatment is identical to that for "poor risk" medulloblastoma: craniospinal irradiation and chemotherapy. In children under 2 years of age, multi-agent chemotherapy alone has been utilized to delay the time to irradiation in the hope of avoiding severe late neuropsychological impairment. The overall prognosis for cerebral PNET is poor, with less than 30 per cent surviving for 5 years.[2]

MENINGIOMAS

Meningiomas are rare, representing between 1 and 3 per cent of all brain tumors in children.[72, 73] They are found predominantly in females and, in adolescents, may be associated with neurofibromatosis. At diagnosis they are often relatively large and may have no evidence of a dural attachment (Fig. 30–8). One quarter of pediatric meningiomas are intraventricular.

Although the pathologic features of pediatric menin-

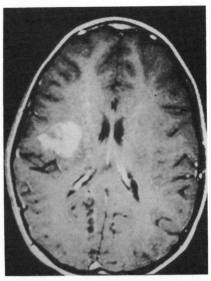

FIGURE 30–8. Meningioma. T1-weighted gadolinium-enhanced MRI. Note lack of dural attachment.

giomas often suggest aggressive biological behavior, the outcome following resection is identical to that in the adult population. An arachnoidal plane separating the tumor from parenchyma is usually present. En bloc resection with removal of adjacent dura and involved bone is curative in 70 to 90 per cent of cases of pediatric meningioma.[33, 72] Recurrence is common following subtotal resection.

TERATOMAS

Teratomas are the most common supratentorial congenital tumor.[10, 74] Over 50 per cent occur in the pineal region; location of the remainder is suprasellar or intraventricular. In infants, the tumors—often of massive size—present with macrocrania and signs of intracranial hypertension.

Complete resection of benign teratomas is usually curative. Malignant teratomas have a poor prognosis following surgical resection. Infants with malignant teratomas have only a 7 per cent one-year survival rate.[74] Neo-adjuvant chemotherapy and subsequent irradiation have shown encouraging early results in limited institution trials (Allen J, personal communication, 1992).

Dermoid and epidermoid tumors most commonly occur in the cerebellopontine angle or parasellar region. They occasionally occur in the cerebral hemisphere (Fig. 30–9). Operative resection is the only therapeutic option.

CEREBRAL METASTASES

Compared with the adult population, metastatic tumors are uncommon in children, accounting for only 2

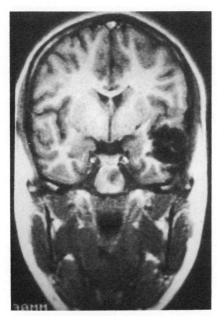

FIGURE 30–9. Epidermoid of temporal lobe.

to 8 per cent of brain tumors[10, 75] (Fig. 30–10). Approximately 6 per cent of pediatric solid tumors will have a cerebral hemispheric metastasis; neuroblastoma, rhabdomyosarcoma, and Wilms' tumor are the most frequent primary neoplasms.[10, 75] Over half the patients will have multiple tumor nodules. Systemic dissemination with pulmonary metastasis is invariably present at the time of central nervous system involvement.[75] The prognosis is poor, with survival ranging from 2 to 20 months, depending on primary tumor histology, location and multiplicity of cerebral lesions, and extent of systemic disease.

LATE EFFECTS

Although much has been published concerning these survival rates, until recently relatively little has been published to evaluate and compare the quality of survival of children with specific types of tumors. As aggressive multimodality therapy has improved the survival of children with brain tumors, increasing numbers of these patients are presenting with the late sequelae of treatment: endocrine dysfunction, neuropsychological deficits, and secondary oncogenesis. Most of these problems are related to the long-term effects of irradiation.

Most of the children receiving radiation therapy will experience endocrine or growth disturbances. Irradiation of the spinal column before puberty retards axial growth, whereas involvement of the hypothalamic-pituitary axis in the radiation portals will usually result in growth hormone deficiency. Hypothyroidism occurs in at least 25 per cent of children either from radiation injury to the pituitary or, when the cervical spine is irradiated, the thyroid.

Although most patients can compensate for neurologic deficits and endocrinologic deficiencies, cognitive and psychosocial sequelae of treatment may be functionally devastating, interfering with education, limiting independence, and adversely affecting the quality of life as these children approach adulthood. In a careful review of the literature on neuropsychological sequelae of pediatric brain tumors,[55] several observations were presented: (1) overall, children with brain tumors display a high incidence of intellectual impairment and emotional/behavioral problems; (2) hydrocephalus preoperatively does not significantly affect postoperative functional outcome; (3) CNS irradiation, especially whole-brain radiation, is associated with decreased neuropsychological functioning; (4) younger children do not do as well neuropsychologically as their older counterparts; and (5) children with supratentorial tumors do not do as well as those with infratentorial tumors.

Kun, Mulhern, et al. have serially followed a group of 26 pediatric patients with primary brain tumors of mixed etiology and localization.[55, 56] Of 15 children studied after cranial irradiation, 8 had subnormal IQ scores. Serial postirradiation testing in 10 patients showed improvement in two, stability in five, and further deterioration in three. The only neuropsychological study involving irradiated astrocytoma patients, by Hochberg and Slotnick,[54] demonstrated diffuse cortical dysfunction involving deficient problem-solving and an inability to cope with novel situations, while psychometric intelligence as a whole remained consistent with premorbid levels. Location of lesion and presence of hydrocephalus did not appear to be determining factors.

Neuropsychological testing, together with periodic systems review and endocrine evaluation, can provide interim assessments of change in the patient's clinical

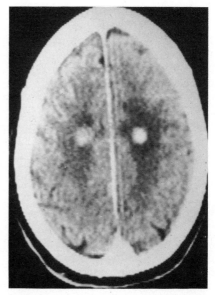

FIGURE 30–10. Bilateral parasagittal metastatic tumors presenting as paraparesis.

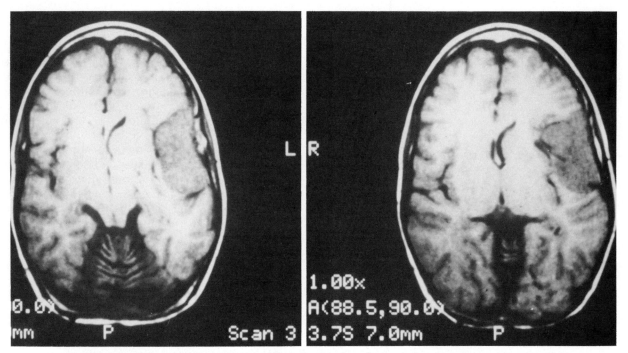

FIGURE 30–11. T1-weighted gadolinium-enhanced MRI of a radiation-induced meningioma 7 years after craniospinal irradiation for medulloblastoma.

status and monitor the development of damage to CNS functioning prior to disease recurrence or death. This allows appropriate intervention or remedial strategies to be instituted earlier, thus directly affecting the patient's "quality of survival." As long-term survival and possible cure become a reality for the majority of children with brain tumors, the quality of life will gain in importance.

Although relatively uncommon at this time, rising numbers of second tumors are occurring in long-term survivors. Both irradiation and certain chemotherapeutic agents (e.g., alkylators) may be carcinogenic. Secondary neoplasms may be induced within the radiation portals following high-dose irradiation for primary brain tumors. Meningiomas, sarcomas, and anaplastic gliomas are the most frequent secondary lesions (Fig. 30–11). These tumors tend to be biologically aggressive and, with meningiomas in particular, often multiple and prone to recurrence after excision. Thyroid carcinoma may occur following spinal irradiation, and leukemias may result from alkylator chemotherapy. Treatment options are limited in view of previous high-dose irradiation or intensive chemotherapy.

SUMMARY

Brain tumors are the most common solid neoplasm of childhood and are second only to leukemia in overall incidence. Supratentorial tumors account for 30 to 55 per cent of pediatric brain tumors, with hemispheric neoplasms comprising approximately one third. Clinical presentation includes seizures, headache, symptoms of increased intracranial pressure, and, depending on location, focal neurologic deficits. The most common tumors are astrocytomas.

Over the past decade, advances in neuroradiographic evaluation, neurosurgical technique, physiological monitoring, and anesthetic management have permitted aggressive surgical resection with decreased morbidity and minimal mortality. Gross total surgical resection of benign tumors results in prolonged disease-free survival and possible cure. Radical surgical resection combined with irradiation and multi-agent chemotherapy has led to improved survival in children with malignant neoplasms. Future innovations in therapy will seek to further improve cure rates while diminishing the long-term sequelae of treatment.

REFERENCES

1. Cohandon F, Aouad N, Rougier A, et al.: Histologic and non-histologic factors correlated with survival time in supratentorial astrocytic tumors. J Neurooncol 3:105, 1985.
2. Russell DS, Rubinstein LJ: Pathology of Tumors of the Nervous System. 4th ed. Baltimore, Williams & Wilkins, 1977.
3. Silverberg E, Lubera J: Cancer statistics, 1986. CA 36:9, 1986.
4. Carrea R, Zingale D: Epidemiology of neoplasms of the central nervous system in infancy and childhood. In Amador LV (ed): Brain Tumors in the Young. Springfield, IL, Charles C Thomas, 1983.
5. Farwell JR, Dohrmann GJ, Flannery JT: Central nervous system tumors in children. Cancer 40:3123, 1977.
6. Horm JW, Asire AJ, Young IL, et al.: SEER Program: Cancer Incidence and Mortality in the United States 1973–1981. Bethesda, National Institutes of Health Publication No. 85–1837, 1984.

7. Young JL, Miller RW: Incidence of malignant tumors in U.S. children. J Pediatr 86:254, 1975.
8. Young JL, Ries LG, Silverberg E, et al.: Cancer incidence, survival, and mortality for children younger than age 15 years. Cancer 58:598, 1986.
9. Hoffman, HJ: Supratentorial brain tumors in children. In Youman JR (ed): Neurological Surgery. Philadelphia, WB Saunders, 1982.
10. Jooma R, Hayward RD, Grant DN: Intracranial neoplasms during the first year of life: Analysis of one hundred consecutive cases. Neurosurgery 14:31, 1984.
11. Mason DD: Gliomas of the cerebral hemispheres. In Matson DD, Ingraham FD (eds): Neurosurgery of Infancy and Childhood. 2nd ed. Springfield, Il, Charles C Thomas, 1969, pp 480–522.
12. Dohrman GJ, Farwell JR, Flannery JT: Astrocytomas in childhood: A population based study. Surg Neurol 23:64, 1985.
13. Kernohan JW, Mabon RF, Svien HJ, et al.: Symposium on new and simplified concept of gliomas: A simplified classification of the gliomas. Proc Mayo Clin Staff Meet 24:71, 1949.
14. Rorke LB, Gilles FH, Davis RL: Revision of the World Health Organization Classification of Brain Tumors for Childhood Brain Tumors. Cancer 56:1869, 1985.
15. Burger PC, Vogel FS: Surgical Pathology of the Nervous System and Its Coverings. 2nd ed. New York, John Wiley & Sons, 1982.
16. Farwell JR, Dohrman GJ: Intracranial neoplasms in infants. Arch Neurol 35:533, 1978.
17. Cogen PH, Daneshvar L, Metzger AK, et al.: Deletion mapping of the medulloblastoma locus on chromosome 17p. Genomics 8:279, 1990.
18. James CD, Carlbo E, Dumanski JP, et al.: Clonal genomic alterations in glioma malignancy stages. Cancer Res 48:5546, 1988.
19. James CD, Carlbom E, Nordenskold M, et al.: Mitotic recombination of chromosome 17 in astrocytomas. Proc Natl Acad Sci USA 86:2858, 1989.
20. Seizinger BR, Martuza RL, Gusella JF: Loss of genes on chromosome 22 in tumorigenesis of human acoustic neuroma. Nature 322:644, 1986.
21. Seizinger BR, De La Monte S, Atkins L, et al.: Molecular genetic approach to human meningioma: Loss of genes on chromosome 22. Proc Natl Acad Sci 84:5419, 1987.
22. Duffner PK, Cohen MD, Myers MH, et al.: Survival of children with brain tumors: SEER Program 1973–1980. Neurology 36:597, 1986.
23. Mercuri S, Russo A, Palma L: Hemispheric supratentorial astrocytomas in children. J Neurosurg 55:170, 1981.
24. Palma L, Russo A, Mercuri S: Cystic cerebral astrocytomas in infancy and childhood: Long-term results: Childs Brain 10:79, 1983.
25. Palma L, Guidetti B: Cystic pilocytic astrocytomas of the cerebral hemispheres. Surgical experience with 51 cases and long-term results. J Neurosurg 62:811, 1985.
26. Hirsch JF, Sainte Rose C, Pierre-Kahn A, et al.: Benign astrocytic and oligodendrocytic tumors of the cerebral hemispheres in children. J Neurosurg 70:568, 1989.
27. Hoshino T: A commentary on the biology and growth kinetics of low-grade and high-grade gliomas. J Neurosurg 61:895, 1984.
28. Hoshino T, Nagashima T, Murovic J, et al.: In situ cell kinetics studies on human neuroectodermal tumors with bromodeoxyuridine labeling. J Neurosurg 64:453, 1986.
29. Hoshino T, Wilson CB: Cell kinetic analyses of human malignant brain tumors (gliomas). Cancer 44:956, 1979.
30. Shitara N, McKeever PE, Whang-Peng J, et al.: Flow-cytometric and cytogenetic analysis of human cultured cell lines derived from high- and low-grade astrocytomas. Acta Neuropathol 60:40, 1983.
31. Laws ER, Taylor WF, Clifton MB, et al.: Neurosurgical management of low-grade astrocytoma of the cerebral hemispheres. J Neurosurg 61:665, 1984.
32. Spencer DD, Spencer SS, Mattson RH, et al.: Intracerebral masses in patients with intractable partial epilepsy. Neurology 34:432, 1984.
33. Leibel SA, Sheline GE: Radiation therapy for neoplasms of the brain. J Neurosurg 66:1, 1987.
34. Cohen ME, Duffner PK: Brain Tumors in Children: Principles of Diagnosis and Treatment. New York, Raven Press, 1984.
35. Sheline GE: Radiation therapy of brain tumors. Cancer 39:873, 1977.
36. Dohrman GJ, Farwell JR, Flannery JT: Glioblastoma multiforme in children. J Neurosurg 44:442, 1976.
37. Marchese MJ, Chang CH: Malignant astrocytic gliomas in children. Cancer 65:2771, 1990.
38. Sposto R, Ertel IJ, Jenkin RDT, et al.: The effectiveness of chemotherapy for the treatment of high-grade astrocytoma in children: Results of a randomized trial. J Neurooncol 7:165, 1989.
39. Vertosick FT, Selker RG: Brain stem and spinal metastasis of supratentorial glioblastoma multiforme: A clinical series. Neurosurgery 27:516, 1990.
40. Warnick RE, Edwards MSB: Pediatric brain tumors. Cur Probl Pediatr 21:129, 1991.
41. Weir B, Grace M: The relative significance of factors affecting postoperative survival in astrocytomas. Grades one and two. Can J Neurol Sci 3:47, 1976.
42. Bernstein M, Hoffman HJ, Holliday WC, et al.: Thalamic tumors in children. Long-term follow-up and treatment guidelines. J Neurosurg 61:649, 1984.
43. Page LK, Clark R: Gliomas of the septal area in children. Neurosurgery 8:651, 1981.
44. Gillet GR, Symon L: Hypothalamic glioma. Surg Neurol 28:291, 1987.
45. Wisoff JH, Abbott IR, Epstein F: Surgical management of exophytic chiasmatic-hypothalamic tumors of childhood. J Neurosurg 73:661, 1990.
46. Hoffman HJ, Becker L, Craven MA: A clinically and pathologically distinct group of benign brainstem gliomas. Neurosurgery 7:243, 1980.
47. Stroink AR, Hoffman HJ, Hendrick EB, et al.: Transependymal benign dorsally exophytic brainstem gliomas in childhood: Diagnosis and treatment recommendations. Neurosurgery 20:439, 1987.
48. Bloom HJG: Intracranial tumors: response and resistance to therapeutic endeavors, 1970–1980. Int J Radiat Oncol Biol Phys 8:1083, 1982.
49. Deutsch M: Radiotherapy for primary brain tumors in very young children. Cancer 50:2785, 1982.
50. Marsa GW, Probert JC, Rubenstein LJ, Bagshaw MA: Radiation therapy in the treatment of childhood astrocytic gliomas. Cancer 32:646, 1973.
51. Bamford FN, Jones PM, Pearson D, Ribeiro GG, Shalet SM, Bearwell CG: Residual disabilities in children treated for intracranial space-occupying lesions. Cancer 37:1149, 1976.
52. Danoff BF, Chowchock FS, Marquette C, et al.: Assessment of the long-term effects of primary radiation therapy for brain tumors in children. Cancer 18:1580, 1982.
53. Duffner PK, Cohen ME, Thompason PRM, Lansky SB: The long-term effects of cranial irradiation on the central nervous system. Cancer 56:1841, 1985.
54. Hochberg FH, Slotnick B: Neuropsychologic impairment in astrocytoma survivors. Neurology 30:172, 1980.
55. Kun LE, Mulhern RK, Crisco JJ: Quality of life in children treated for brain tumors: Intellectual, emotional and academic function. J Neurosurg 58:1, 1983.
56. Kun LE, Mulhern RK: Neuropsychologic function in children with brain tumors: II. Serial studies of intellect and time after treatment. Am J Clin Oncol 6:651, 1983.
57. Richard GE: Effects of irradiation on the hypothalamic and pituitary regions. In Gilbert HA, Kagan RA (eds): Radiation Damage to the Nervous System. New York, Raven Press, 1980, pp 175–180.
58. Shalet SM, Beardwell CG, Aarons BM, et al.: Growth impairment in children treated for brain tumors. Arch Dis Child 53:491, 1978.
59. Spunberg JJ, Chang CH, Goldman M, et al.: Quality of long-term survival following irradiation for intracranial tumors in children under the age of two. Int J Radiat Oncol Biol Phys 7:727, 1981.
60. Coulon RA, Till K: Intracranial ependymomas in children: A review of 43 cases. Childs Brain 3:154, 1977.

61. Kun LE, Kovnar KH, Sanford RA: Ependymomas in children. Pediatr Neurosci 14:57, 1988.

62. Goldwein JW, Glauser TA, Packer RJ: Recurrent intracranial ependymomas in children: Survival, patterns of failure, and prognostic factors. Cancer 66:557, 1990.

63. Healey EA, Barnes PD, Kupsky WJ, et al.: The prognostic significance of postoperative residual tumor in ependymoma. Neurosurgery 28:666, 1991.

64. Nazar GB, Hoffman HJ, Becker LE, et al.: Infratentorial ependymomas in childhood: Prognostic factors and treatment. J Neurosurg 72:408, 1990.

65. Salazar OM: A better understanding of CNS seeding and a brighter outlook for postoperatively irradiated patients with ependymomas. Int J Radiat Oncol Biol Phys 9:1231, 1983.

66. Waller KE, Wara WM, Sheline GE, et al.: Intracranial ependymomas: Results of treatment with partial or whole brain irradiation without spinal irradiation. Int J Radiat Oncol Biol Phys 12:1937, 1986.

67. Friedman HS, Oakes WJ: The chemotherapy of posterior fossa tumors in childhood. J Neurooncol 5:217, 1987.

68. Dohrman GJ, Farwell JR, Flannery JT: Oligodendrogliomas in children. Surg Neurol 10:21, 1978.

69. Mork SJ, Lindegaard K-F, Halvorsen TB, et al.: Oligodendroglioma: Incidence and biological behavior in a defined population. J Neurosurg 63:881, 1985.

70. Sutton LN, Pakcer RJ, Rorke LB, et al.: Cerebral gangliogliomas during childhood. Neurosurgery 13:124, 1983.

71. Berger MS, Kincaid J, Ojemann GA, Lettich E: Brain mapping techniques to maximize resection, safety, and seizure control in children with brain tumors. Neurosurgery 25:786, 1989.

72. Drake JM, Hendrick EB, Becker LE, Chuang SH, Hoffman HJ: Intracranial meningiomas in children. Pediatr Neurosci 12:134, 1985–1986.

73. Herz DA, Shapiro K, Shulman K: Intracranial meningiomas of infancy, childhood, and adolescence: Review of the literature and addition of 9 case reports. Childs Brain 7:43, 1980.

74. Wakai S, Arai T, Nagai M: Congenital brain tumors. Surg Neurol 21:597, 1984.

75. Vannucci RC, Baten M: Cerebral metastatic disease in childhood. Neurology 24:981, 1974.

Chapter 31

INTRAVENTRICULAR TUMORS

ROBERT A. SANFORD, M.D., and DAVID J. DONAHUE, M.D.

This chapter discusses tumors that arise within the ventricular system, a relatively uncommon group with distinct histology. Midline gliomas arising from central structures and invading the ventricles secondarily are not uncommon and tend to occur in the younger age groups. They are discussed in other chapters.

Regardless of origin, intraventricular tumors are relatively silent until they become large and/or obstruct the flow of cerebrospinal fluid (CSF), producing hydrocephalus and increased intracranial pressure. Unless cerebral parenchyma is invaded, the supratentorial tumors produce no focal deficit, going unrecognized until the symptoms and signs of intracranial hypertension, vomiting, headache, papilledema, and obtundation occur. False localizing signs of sixth nerve palsy or hemiparesis with uncal herniation develop late in the course. In the young child these tumors may not be appreciated until head enlargement is noted. Fourth ventricular tumors present with cerebellar findings in addition to intracranial pressure phenomena.

CHOROID PLEXUS TUMORS

The most common intraventricular tumors of childhood arise from the choroid plexus. Guerard,[1] in 1832, reported a tumor arising from the choroid plexus in a 3-year-old girl. Choroid plexus tumors are relatively common in the younger child (less than 2 years of age).[2]

Histologically, choroid plexus tumors are divided into a benign (choroid plexus papilloma) and malignant (choroid plexus carcinoma) type. Choroid plexus is derived embryologically from the ependymal lining of the neural tube.[3] The benign papilloma is difficult to distinguish histologically from normal choroid plexus architecture with its delicate papillary fronds bearing a layer of well-differentiated cuboidal to columnar epithelium, which lack cilia and blepharoplasts.[3] The distinguishing features denoting malignant choroid plexus carcinoma are focal invasion, dedifferentiation of cells, and marked nuclear pleomorphism.[4] Carcinomas tend to be larger at diagnosis than papillomas. They disseminate along CSF pathways early, an uncommon and late finding in the benign papilloma. Current antigen profiles are not reliable in distinguishing benign from malignant varieties.[5] Biochemical studies suggest that transthyretin may be a marker specific to choroid plexus tumors, helping to distinguish them from papillary ependymoma.[6, 7]

Grossly, choroid plexus tumors appear red to grayish with a smooth irregular surface, like the lobes of a cauliflower,[8] which may be appreciated on magnetic resonance imaging (MRI). These tumors are highly vascular and bleed profusely when they are torn or undergo biopsy. The macroscopic appearance of benign and malignant forms are indistinguishable, although at surgery the carcinoma is more friable, has smaller lobules, and is seen to be invasive.

The trigone of the lateral ventricle is the usual localization in children,[2, 4, 9–12] whereas fourth ventricular tumors are more typical in adults.[13] Third ventricular location is unusual.[14]

The computed tomographic (CT) scan appearance of the choroid plexus papilloma is usually a homogeneous, lobulated intraventricular mass that is markedly enhanced after intravenous infusion of iodinated contrast. The carcinoma may be more variegated in appearance both before and after contrast.[13] Cystic forms are more common in adults.[15]

MRI discloses vividly the anatomy, demonstrating the characteristic molding of tumor within the ventricle (Fig. 31–1). The sagittal and coronal views may show the characteristic egress of tumor through ventricular outlets.[16] Nonhomogeneity of signal noted on unenhanced T1- and T2-weighted images has been related to vascularity,[17] calcification, or old hemorrhage.[13] Gadolinium infusion produces intense enhancement.[17] In the past, angiography was utilized frequently for preoperative planning, but may be unnecessary if high-resolution MR readily identifies hypertrophied feeding

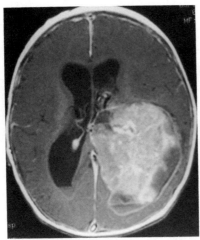

FIGURE 31–1. Large choroid plexus tumor as seen on enhanced MRI scan. Note smooth borders of the expansile lesion located intraventricularly. The tumor insinuates itself throughout the ventricular system via the intraventricular foramina.

arteries. The vascular supply may be anterior choroidal,[18] posterior choroidal, or lateral striate vessels.[5]

Prevention of intraoperative hemorrhage in young children with limited blood volume is critical for a successful outcome. This requires presurgical identification and early intraoperative control of the vascular pedicle, which is usually medial and inferior to the tumor with the venous drainage medial and posterior. Various surgical approaches are predicated on microsurgical technique, which allows interruption of the vascular supply before debulking. Recent reports describe temporal-occipital, posterior parietal, or superior parietal[2, 5, 9, 19] approaches for trigonal lesions. The tumor mass is usually large and firm, not lending itself to displacement at operation. Therefore, the approach needs to be individualized to achieve the least obstructed route to the vascular pedicle. On occasion the authors have even used an interhemispheric approach through a portion of the posterior corpus callosum.

The choroid plexus carcinoma (Fig. 31–2) is even more difficult to mobilize because of its invasive nature and increased vascularity associated with peritumor parasitized vascular supply. Because of the additional surgical risks of hemorrhage involved, the Toronto group recommends presurgical chemotherapy to reduce vascularity and facilitate gross total surgical resection.[20]

The most important determinant of long-term survival is complete resection. Complete surgical resection is curative for choroid plexus papilloma. The only long-term survivals in choroid plexus carcinoma have occurred after gross total resection and irradiation. The role of chemotherapy is unproven but seems promising.[20–22] Because confirmation of total excision is important, postoperative CT and/or MRI scan should be obtained within 48 hours of resection.[23] Spinal MRI is necessary to rule out subarachnoid seeding of tumor for both papilloma and carcinoma. All children need serial imaging to rule out recurrence.

SUBEPENDYMAL GIANT CELL ASTROCYTOMA

Subependymal giant cell astrocytomas (SGCA) arise from the head of the caudate near the foramen of Monro and are unique to patients with tuberous sclerosis (Bourneville's disease),[24, 25] first described in 1880.[26] Tuberous sclerosis, one of the phakomatoses, is inherited in a dominant fashion, and is usually clinically evident. However, spontaneous formes fruste do occur, and the diagnosis can remain unrecognized until symptoms and signs of increased intracranial pressure due to a subependymal giant cell astrocytoma arise. Intraventricular tubers (candlewax gutterings) as well as cortical tubers are nonprogressive hamartomatous lesions. Once the diagnosis of tuberous sclerosis is suspected, a baseline cranial CT is often obtained for evaluation of seizures and mental retardation or hydrocephalus secondary to obstruction of the foramen of Monro by a subependymal giant cell astrocytoma. Multiple, unenhancing calcifications of tubers lining the ventricular walls may be seen.[27] If small lesions are present at the foramen of Monro, there is significant chance of tumor progression (Fig. 31–3), warranting close follow-up. The senior author (RAS) presented five patients whose tumors were documented to progress at a slow rate over 3 to 5 years, eventually requiring surgical removal. The subependymal giant cell tumor tends to enhance with intravenous contrast on CT scan, helping to differentiate it from the more benign tumors.[27, 28] However, on MRI the more inert subependymal lesion may enhance with gadolinium,[29] whereas the small calcified lesion may be missed entirely, making CT the better study for serial follow-up. Dilated intratumoral vessels or hemorrhage strongly suggests subependymal giant cell tumor.[30]

Microscopic evaluation of subependymal giant cell astrocytomas reveals large cells with uniform nuclei and abundant homogeneous hyaline cytoplasm radiating around blood vessels.[3, 31] Mitotic activity varies and

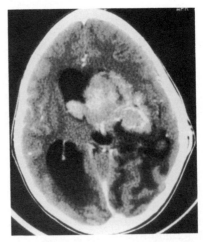

FIGURE 31–2. Choroid plexus carcinoma. Notice the irregular surface of the tumor and its tendency to invade brain parenchyma. Notice also evidence of prior resection attempt posterior to tumor. This patient eventually underwent a complete resection of her tumor.

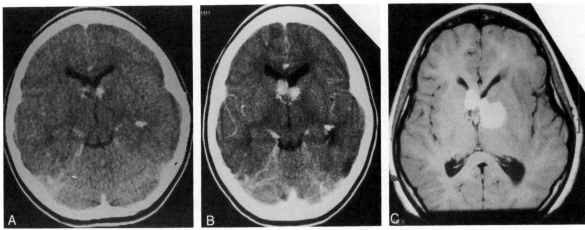

FIGURE 31–3. Serial enhanced CT scans of a patient with subependymal giant cell astrocytoma. *A,* 1985. *B,* Enhanced scan done in 1989. *C,* MRI of same patient, done in 1992. Note location of lesions near foramen of Monro and their progressive enlargement with time.

does not correlate with rate of tumor progression or survival.[24, 32] The tumors are vascular and well demarcated, and often have focal calcification.[3] Perhaps the occasional angiomatous appearance of the tumor accounts for clinical presentations of intratumoral hemorrhage[33] and the occasional encounter of brisk intraoperative bleeding.

The most common clinical presentation of SGCA to the neurosurgeon is at consultation for evaluation of unilateral or bilateral mass lesions noted on routine neuro-imaging of a child with tuberous sclerosis. Occurrence peaks at 8 to 18 years of age.[30] In the asymptomatic patient, tumor progression should be documented before surgical intervention since the rate of growth is slow. Functional status and quality of life issues need to be considered and discussed in cases of patients with limited life expectancy and asymptomatic patients. Serial radiologic studies are recommended at 12- to 18-month intervals (RAS).[30, 34] True malignant degeneration in these tumors has not been reported, and a slow rate of growth is the rule.

The other clinical presentation is that of increased intracranial pressure from hydrocephalus due to obstruction of the foramen of Monro. In the symptomatic patient, surgical resection should be considered at the time of diagnosis because ventriculomegaly facilitates surgical resection. Occasionally a ventricular CSF shunt can be avoided by complete tumor removal via the transcortical or transcallosal approach. We favor the transcallosal route because it facilitates identification of distorted anatomy, prevents cortical collapse when CSF is removed, and avoids cortical scar in an already epileptogenic brain. Preoperative cardiac evaluation is warranted because of potentially lethal arrhythmias from rhabdomyomas.[35]

In seven personal cases following gross total surgical resection, there has been no tumor regrowth, although two of the children now have progressive enlargement of untreated tumors in the opposite lateral ventricle. The benefit of standard irradiation of subependymal

giant cell astrocytoma has been suggested but not confirmed. J. Loeffler (personal communication) has utilized stereotaxic radiosurgery for small (<3 cm) subependymal tumors of the head of the caudate in children with tuberous sclerosis. We have similarly treated three biopsy-proven <3-cm subependymal giant cell astrocytomas in two children whose tumors had demonstrated progressive growth on serial CT scans. It is too early to tell whether this treatment will prove effective, but it appears reasonable for the asymptomatic patient with a high level of intellectual function.

SUBEPENDYMOMA

Scheinker, in his original description of subependymomas (1945),[36] suggested that the predominantly ectodermal elements were derived from subependymal glia. Interestingly, no mention of "mixed" or "pure" forms of this tumor was made in his original description. Subsequently, the subependymoma, or at least its "mixed" form, has come to be considered a variant of ependymoma.[37] The subependymoma usually occurs as an asymptomatic lesion in the fourth ventricle of older adults, but may arise in the walls of the third or lateral ventricles.[37] Most symptomatic childhood subependymomas arise in the fourth ventricle.[37–40] Supratentorial subependymomas in children are exceedingly rare; three case reports were found in our review of the literature.[41–43]

These tumors are firm and rubbery, forming smooth nodules continuous with the ventricular wall. They are avascular and generally discrete from adjacent brain parenchyma.[36, 44]

Microscopically, the "pure" form consists of nests of small glial cells interspersed among broad areas of glial fibers;[45] hypocellularity and a relatively avascular appearance characterize the "pure" form. The increased cellularity, ependymal rosette formation, and increased vascularity seen in the "mixed" form are more suggestive of ependymomas.[41] Most patients with "mixed" varieties[37] have a worse prognosis and are younger than those harboring the "pure" form.

The typical CT appearance of subependymomas is that of a nonspecific, homogeneous,[46] isodense intraventricular[41, 47] lesion which enhances faintly after intravenous infusion of contrast.[39, 48] Subependymomas may contain calcification[48] or gross cysts.[41] Radiographically they cannot be distinguished from ependymomas.[39, 41]

MRI appearance is also indistinguishable from that of the ependymoma, appearing isointense on T1-weighted and hyperintense on T2-weighted imaging.[49–51] Large tumors may display multicystic changes or small areas of hemorrhage. Lateral ventricular tumors tend to abut the septum pellucidum. Angiographic appearance is that of an avascular mass.

Complete excision, feasible in the supratentorial variety, especially when associated with the septum pellucidum,[52] is recommended.[44] The diagnosis of subependymoma should probably be reserved for the "pure" form mentioned above. The true subependymoma does not require irradiation[40, 44] unless recurrent or progressive tumor is demonstrated. "Mixed types" probably are more aggressive tumors. Some authors believe they should be treated and staged as ependymomas.[49]

COLLOID CYST

Colloid cysts of the third ventricle are extremely rare in young children and infants.[53, 54] Histogenesis remains unresolved, but most authors support neuroepithelial origin.[55] The anterior third ventricle location may produce obstruction of one or both foramina of Monro as well as the outlet of the third ventricle. The cyst wall is intimately associated with the tela choroidea of the third ventricular roof and may adhere to the choroid plexus.[55] Inflammatory changes of the thin connective tissue layer on the outside of the cyst wall[53] explain its tendency to adhere to surrounding structures such as the fornical pillars and choroid plexus. The cyst is lined with a single layer of low to high columnar or cuboidal epithelium, which is often ciliated. The cyst contains a mucoid substance that varies from gelatinous to firm in consistency.

The CT appearance of colloid cysts ranges widely from hypodense to isodense to hyperdense on CT.[56, 57] Increased density within the cyst correlates with high cholesterol content[56] and increased viscosity; lower density portends a more aqueous character.[58] Vessels in the cyst wall and adjacent choroid plexus may account for post-contrast enhancement.[57, 58] The MRI scan (Fig. 31–4) shows markedly increased signal within the cyst and is related to cholesterol content.[56]

As with other intraventricular tumors, the progressive signs of increased intracranial pressure are due to progressive hydrocephalus.[60] Although acute deteriora

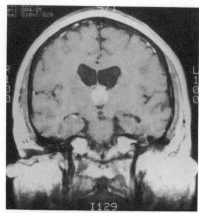

FIGURE 31–4. Typical appearance of a colloid cyst of the third ventricle occluding foramen of Monro and distending the third ventricle.

tion and death have been emphasized in the literature,[61] the more chronic complaints, such as headache and altered mental status, are the rule.

Many surgeons advocate treatment of all colloid cysts,[62] whereas others recommend serial follow-up of asymptomatic lesions less than 1.7 cm in diameter.[60] Small anterior third ventricle lesions rarely result in sudden death. The small cyst should be no more dangerous than the usual CSF ventricular shunt, which usually gives several days to months of prodromal symptoms,[61] allowing the forewarned patient and physician time to intervene. Simple shunting of the enlarged ventricles, leaving the cyst undisturbed, is not recommended[63] as the cyst is best removed at the time of ventriculomegaly and, if symptomatic, is presumed to be progressively enlarging.

Operative results have been excellent when resection, which is curative, is performed via the transfrontal or transcallosal approach. Surgical approaches to the anterior third ventricle have been exhaustively catalogued and described.[64] Vascular structures can be avulsed, and fornical damage can result from overzealous dissection, producing dissociative syndromes and memory deficits. Hydrocephalus may persist in spite of complete cyst removal, requiring CSF diversion.

Stereotactic aspiration, first described by Bosch,[65] has many advocates.[58, 62, 66] Mathiesen, et al,[68] suggest that colloid cysts frequently recur following stereotactic aspiration. The CT appearance may predict success as larger cysts are less likely to migrate away from the probing stylet and the hypodense ones contain easily aspirated, low-viscosity fluid.[58] Spillage of cyst contents can precipitate aseptic meningitis[55, 66, 67] whatever the method used for cyst drainage or removal.

CONCLUSION

Intraventricular tumors in children include the choroid plexus papillomas, choroid plexus carcinomas, subependymal giant cell astrocytomas, subependymo mas, and colloid cysts. Meningiomas are discussed elsewhere. They commonly present with hydrocephalus and manifestations of increased intracranial pressure. Magnetic resonance imaging facilitates the planning of the operative approach to these tumors. Gross total resection of even very large tumors is a realistic goal in most patients. Stereotactic resection and stereotactic radiosurgery may prove useful for treating patients with small progressive lesions or unresectable residual tumor. The benefits of adjunctive chemotherapy remain to be delineated.

REFERENCES

1. Guerard M: Tumeur fongeuse dans le ventricle droit du cerveu chez une petite fille de trois ans. Bull Soc Anat Paris 8:211, 1832.
2. Matson DD, Crofton FDL: Papilloma of the choroid plexus in childhood. J Neurosurg 17:1002, 1960.
3. Russell DS, Rubenstein LJ: Pathology of Tumors of the Nervous System, 4th ed. Baltimore, Williams & Wilkins, 1977.
4. Ho DM, Wong T, Liu H: Choroid plexus tumors in childhood: Histopathologic study and clinico-pathological correlation. Childs Nerv Syst 7:437, 1991.
5. Johnson DL: Management of choroid plexus tumors in children. Pediatr Neurosci 15:195, 1989.
6. Herbert J, Cavallaro T, Dwork AJ: A marker for primary choroid plexus neoplasms. Am J Pathol 136:1317, 1990.
7. Matsushima T, Inoue T, Takeshita I, et al.: Choroid plexus papillomas: An immunohistochemical study with particular reference to the coexpression of prealbumin. Neurosurgery 23:384, 1988.
8. Rubenstein LJ: Tumors of the central nervous system. In Firminger HI (ed): Atlas of Tumor Pathology, 2nd ed. Washington, D.C., Armed Forces Institute of Pathology, 1972, pp 257–262.
9. Spallone A, Pastore FS, Giuffre R, et al.: Choroid plexus papillomas in infancy and childhood. Childs Nerv Syst 6:71, 1990.
10. Ellenbogen RG, Winston KR, Kupsky WJ: Tumors of the choroid plexus in children. Neurosurgery 25:327, 1989.
11. McGirr SJ, Ebersold MJ, Scheithauer BW, et al.: Choroid plexus papillomas: Long-term follow-up results in a surgically treated series. J Neurosurg 69:843, 1988.
12. Rovit RL, Schechter MM, Chodroff P: Choroid plexus papillomas: Observations on radiographic diagnosis. Am J Roentgenol Rad Ther Nucl Med 110:608, 1970.
13. Coates TL, Hinshaw DB, Peckman N: Pediatric choroid plexus neoplasms: MR, CT, and pathologic correlation. Radiology 173:81, 1989.
14. Jooma R, Grant DN: Third ventricle choroid plexus papillomas. Childs Brain 10:242, 1983.
15. Gradin WC, Taylon C, Fruin AH: Choroid plexus papilloma of the third ventricle: Case report and review of the literature. Neurosurgery 12:217, 1983.
16. Hopper KD, Foley LC, Nieves NL, et al.: The intraventricular extension of choroid plexus papillomas. Am J Neuroradiol 8:469, 1987.
17. Goldberg HI: Extraaxial brain tumors. In Atlas SW (ed): Magnetic Resonance Imaging of the Brain and Spine. New York, Raven Press, 1991, pp 327–378.
18. Goldberg HI: The anterior choroidal artery. In Newton TH, Potts DG (eds): Radiology of the Skull and Brain: Angiography. St. Louis, CV Mosby, 1974, pp 1628–1658.
19. Gudeman SK, Sullivan HB, Rosner MJ, et al.: Surgical removal of bilateral papillomas of the choroid plexus of the lateral ventricles with resolution of hydrocephalus. J Neurosurg 50:677, 1979.
20. Pillay PK, Humphreys RP, St. Clair S, et al.: Choroid Plexus Carcinomas in Children: A Role for Preresection Chemotherapy. AANS Annual Meeting Program 484, 1992 (Abstract).
21. Allen J, Wisoff J, Helson L, et al.: Choroid plexus carcinoma: responses to chemotherapy alone in newly diagnosed young children. J Neurooncol 12:69, 1992.
22. Duffner PK, Cohen ME, Horowitz M, et al.: The treatment of

choroid plexus carcinoma in infancy with chemotherapy. Ann Neurol 26:460, 1989.
23. Sanford RA, Theofilos C, Muhlbauer MS, et al.: Radiological Assessment of Surgical Resection of Pediatric Brain Tumors. Scientific Program: American Association of Neurological Surgeons 431, 1992 (Abstract).
24. Shepherd CW, Scheithauer BW, Gomez MR, et al.: Subependymal giant cell astrocytoma: A clinical, pathological, and flow cytometric study. Neurosurgery 28:864, 1991.
25. Altermatt HJ, Scheithauer BW: Cytomorphology of subependymal giant cell astrocytoma. Acta Cytol 36:171, 1992.
26. Clifford RJ, Sharbrough FW, Cascino GD, et al.: Magnetic resonance image-based hippocampal volumetry: Correlation with outcome after temporal lobectomy. Ann Neurol 31:138, 1992.
27. Rieger E, Binder B, Starz I, et al.: Tuberous sclerosis complex: Oligosymptomatic variant associated with subependymal giant-cell astrocytoma. Pediatr Radiol 21:432, 1991.
28. Moran V, O'Keefe F: Giant cell astrocytoma in tuberous sclerosis: computed tomographic findings. Clin Radiol 37:543, 1986.
29. Wippold II FJ, Baber WW, Gado M, et al.: Pre- and postcontrast MR studies in tuberous sclerosis. J Comput Assist Tomogr 16:69, 1992.
30. Braffman BH, Bilaniuk LT, Naidich TP, et al.: MR imaging of tuberous sclerosis: Pathogenesis of this phakomatosis, use of gadopentetate dimeglumine, and literature review. Radiology 183:227, 1992.
31. Zulch KJ: Brain Tumors: Their Biology and Pathology. 3rd ed. Berlin, Springer-Verlag, 1986 pp 258–273.
32. Chow CW, Klug GL, Lewis EA: Subependymal giant-cell astrocytoma in children. An unusual discrepancy between histological and clinical features. J Neurosurg 68:880, 1988.
33. Waga S, Yamamoto Y, Kojima T, et al.: Massive hemorrhage in tumor of tuberous sclerosis. Surg Neurol 8:99, 1977.
34. Morimoto K, Mogami H: Sequential CT study of subependymal giant-cell astrocytoma associated with tuberous sclerosis. J Neurosurg 65:874, 1986.
35. Painter MJ, Pang D, Ahdad-Barmada M, et al.: Connatal brain tumors in patients with tuberous sclerosis. Neurosurgery 14:570, 1984.
36. Scheinker IM: Subependymoma: A newly recognized tumor of subependymal derivation. J Neurosurg 2:232, 1945.
37. Scheithauer BW: Symptomatic subependymoma. Report of 21 cases with review of the literature. J Neurosurg 499:689, 1978.
38. Kalfas IH, Hahn J: Symptomatic subependymoma in a 14-year-old girl, diagnosed by NMR scan. Childs Nerv Syst 2:44, 1986.
39. Stevens JM, Kendall BE, Love S: Radiological features of subependymoma with emphasis on computed tomography. Neuroradiology 26:223, 1984.
40. Rea GL, Akerson RD, Rockswold GL, et al.: Subependymoma in a 2 1/2 year old boy. J Neurosurg 59:1088, 1983.
41. Lobato RD, Sarabia M, Castro S, et al.: Symptomatic subependymoma: Report of four new cases studied with computed tomography and review of the literature. Neurosurgery 19:594, 1986.
42. Kazner E, Wende S, Grumme TH, Lankscha W, Stochdorf O: Computed tomography in intracranial tumours, New York, Springer, 1982, pp 119–129.
43. Changaris DG, Powers JM, Perot PL, et al.: Subependymoma presenting as subarachnoid hemorrhage. J Neurosurg 55:643, 1981.
44. Epstein F: Comment: Symptomatic subependymoma: Report of four new cases studied with computed tomography and review of the literature. Neurosurgery 19:594, 1986.
45. Lombardi D, Scheithauer BW, Meyer FB, et al.: Symptomatic subependymoma: a clinicopathological and flow cytometric study. J Neurosurg 75:583, 1991.
46. Matsumura A, Ahyai A, Hori A: Intracerebral subependymomas. Clinical and neuropathological analyses with special reference to the possible existence of a less benign variant. Acta Neurochir 96:15, 1989.
47. Sekiya T, Iwabuchi T, Suzuki S, et al.: Subependymoma of the septum pellucidum. MRI features and its usefulness in planning surgery. Neurol Med Chir (Tokyo) 30:874, 1990.
48. Artico M, Bardella L, Ciappetta P: Surgical treatment of subependymomas of the central nervous system. Report of 8 cases and review of the literature. Acta Neurochir 98:25, 1989.

49. Jooma R, Torrens MJ, Bradshaw J, et al.: Subependymomas of the fourth ventricle: Surgical treatment in 12 cases. J Neurosurg 62:508, 1985.

50. Spoto GP, Press GA, Hesselink JR, et al.: Intracranial ependymoma and subependymoma: MR manifestations. Am J Neuroradiol 11:83, 1990.

51. Atlas SW: Intraaxial brain tumors. In Atlas SW (ed): Magnetic Resonance Imaging of the Brain and Spine. New York, Raven Press, 1991, pp 223–326.

52. French JD, Bucy PC: Tumors of the septum pellucidum. J Neurosurg 5:433, 1948.

53. Zulch KJ: Brain Tumors: Their Biology and Pathology. 3rd ed. Berlin, Springer-Verlag, 1986, pp 437–440.

54. Buchsbaum HW, Colton RP: Anterior third ventricular cysts in infancy. J Neurosurg 26:264, 1967.

55. Russell DS, Rubinstein LJ: Pathology of Tumours of the Nervous System. 5th ed. Baltimore, Williams & Wilkins, 1989, pp 721–725.

56. Maeder PP, Holtas SL, Basibuyuk LN, et al.: Colloid cysts of the third ventricle: Correlation of MR and CT findings with histology and chemical analysis. Am J Neuroradiol 11:575, 1990.

57. Ganti SR, Antunes JL, Louis KM, et al.: Computed tomography in the diagnosis of colloid cysts of the third ventricle. Radiology 138:385, 1981.

58. Kondziolka D, Lunsford LD: Stereotactic management of colloid cysts: factors predicting success. J Neurosurg 75:45, 1991.

59. Atlas SW: Magnetic Resonance Imaging of the Brain and Spine. New York, Raven Press, 1991, pp 299–302.

60. Camacho A, Abernathey CD, Kelly PJ, et al.: Colloid cysts: Experience with the management of 84 cases since the introduction of computed tomography. Neurosurgery 24:693, 1989.

61. Ryder JW, Kleinschmidt-Demasters BK, Keller TS: Sudden deterioration and death in patients with benign tumors of the third ventricle area. J Neurosurg 64:216, 1986.

62. Hall WA, Lunsford LD: Changing concepts in the treatment of colloid cysts. J Neurosurg 66:186, 1987.

63. Carmel PW: Brain tumors of disordered embryogenesis. In Youmans JR (ed): Neurological Surgery, 3rd ed. Philadelphia, WB Saunders, 1990, pp 3223–3249.

64. Apuzzo MLJ (ed): Surgery of the Third Ventricle. Baltimore, Williams & Wilkins, 1987.

65. Bosch DA, Rahn T, Backlund EO: Treatment of colloid cysts of the third ventricle by stereotactic aspiration. Surg Neurol 9:15, 1978.

66. Musolino A, Fosse S, Munari C, et al.: Diagnosis and treatment of colloid cysts of the third ventricle by stereotactic drainage. Report on eleven cases. Surg Neurol 32:294, 1989.

67. Abenathey CD, Davis DH, Kelly PJ: Treatment of colloid cysts of the third ventricle by stereotaxic microsurgical laser craniotomy. J Neurosurg 70:525, 1989.

68. Mathiesen T, Grane P, Lindquist C, et al.: High recurrence rate following aspiration of colloid cysts in the third ventricle. J Neurosurg 78:748, 1993.

Chapter 32

OPTIC NERVE GLIOMAS AND OTHER TUMORS INVOLVING THE OPTIC NERVE AND CHIASM

DENNIS L. JOHNSON, M.D., and DAVID C. McCULLOUGH, M.D.

In the Martin and Cushing series of 2000 brain tumors, only 1 per cent were optic nerve gliomas.[1] Major pediatric neurosurgical centers report a higher incidence because 75 per cent of optic gliomas occur in the first decade of life. They make up 4 per cent of brain tumors seen at Children's Hospital National Medical Center, as compared with 3.6 per cent reported by Matson,[2] 4 per cent by Sayers,[3] and 6 per cent by Hoffman.[4]

PATHOLOGY

The tumors may be solid, gelatinous, or cystic. Tumors may appear as fusiform enlargement of the optic nerve, with secondary involvement of the chiasm, or may envelop primarily the chiasm and spread secondarily to the optic nerves or into the hypothalamus.

"Skip" lesions, or segmental nodules of glioma, may also be seen along the optic pathway[5-11] (Fig. 32–1). The microscopic appearance (Fig. 32–2) is that of a low-grade astrocytoma with simple bipolar, pilocytic astrocytes and numerous Rosenthal's fibers.[12-14] Evidence of histologic malignancy is extremely unusual in children but has been described in adults.[15-18] Malignant transformation of optic gliomas is uncommon.[4, 19-22]

BIOLOGIC BEHAVIOR

Since optic gliomas were first described in the early nineteenth century[23, 24] their management in children has been controversial. The controversy has stemmed from a poor understanding of the biologic behavior of the tumor. Martin and Cushing concluded that any

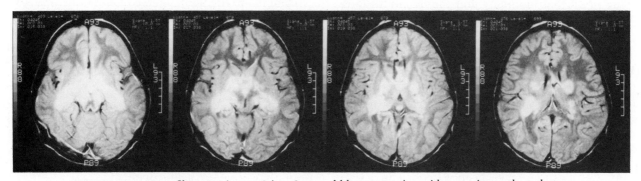

FIGURE 32–1. Neurofibromatosis type 1 in a 3-year-old boy presenting with precocious puberty but no detectable visual abnormalities.

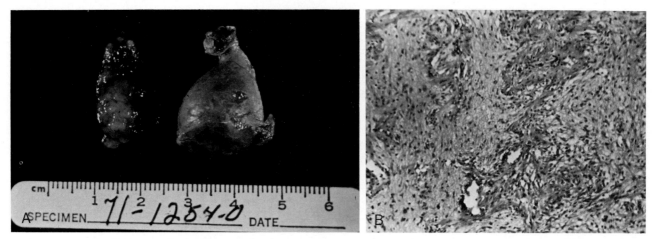

FIGURE 32–2. *A*, Optic glioma confined to optic nerve. *B*, Characteristic microscopic appearance, with bipolar, pilocytic astrocytes enmeshed in optic nerve.

treatment of optic gliomas was presumptuous.[1] Fowler and Matson reported that the biologic behavior of these tumors was difficult to predict.[25] Although some tumors progress inexorably despite aggressive treatment, many patients have survived over 20 years in spite of incomplete tumor removal and no radiation therapy.[2–4, 26–30] Taveras and colleagues reported cases of long-term survival with radiation therapy alone.[31] Spontaneous tumor regression and visual improvement also have been cited.

In 1969, the dilemma of optic pathway gliomas was heightened with the assertion of Hoyt and Baghadassarian that the biologic behavior of these tumors was not frankly neoplastic but rather hamartomatous.[27] In a long-term study of visual fields in nonirradiated and irradiated patients, Glaser and associates found no beneficial effect from radiation.[32] They also condemned surgical morbidity as unwarranted. In contrast, Hoffman[4] and others[29, 33–36] have documented the relentlessly aggressive biologic behavior of some optic gliomas—behavior that is at least slowed by radiation therapy.

Tissue culture studies have confirmed the neoplastic character of these tumors.[37] Although sometimes problematic, the biologic behavior of optic gliomas is usually indolent, and survival for longer than 10 years can be expected. Slow but progressive visual loss is the rule, but the protracted morbidity and the quality of long-term survival has not been well documented.

DIAGNOSTIC TESTS

Computed tomography (CT) and magnetic resonance imaging (MRI) provide accurate localization and narrow the spectrum of possible diagnoses. Optic gliomas are usually isodense, and many are enhanced by intravenous contrast material, especially the more posterior lesions. Calcifications have been described in lesions that involve the optic tract.[38] With modern neuro-imaging, there is seldom a need for plain skull x-ray films, which classically demonstrate a J-shaped sella; optic foraminal views showing an optic foramen >7 mm or a difference of more than 2 mm between the right and the left foramina;[2] tomography; arteriography; or pneumoencephalography. Visual evoked responses may help to document a change in an individual patient but have limited usefulness in screening or diagnosis.[39]

CLASSIFICATION, PRESENTATION, AND THERAPY

Optic pathway gliomas and other tumors from which they must be differentiated can be classified by anatomic location. The clinical presentation, differential diagnosis, treatment, and prognosis of tumors that are confined to (1) the optic nerve, (2) the optic nerve and chiasm, and (3) the chiasm and the hypothalamus are distinctly different.

TUMORS OF THE OPTIC NERVE

Presentation and Diagnosis

Tumors of the optic nerve commonly present in childhood, with proptosis, visual loss, papilledema, or optic atrophy.[40] The proptotic eye is displaced downward and outward. In the very young, visual loss may be manifested by strabismus, nystagmus, or both. Papilledema is seen more often than optic atrophy and is probably due to perineurial venous obstruction. These tumors are found in 10 to 15 per cent of asymptomatic children with neurofibromatosis type 1 when screened with CT or MRI scans (Fig. 32–3).[41, 42] Optic nerve meningiomas are also associated with neurofibromatosis 1. Although meningiomas are less commonly seen in children, they are more aggressive.[43, 44]

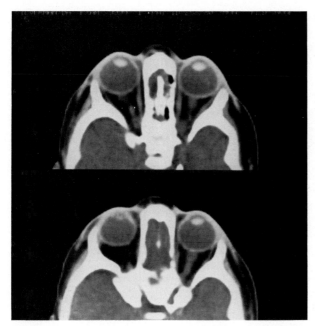

FIGURE 32-3. Optic nerve glioma with fusiform enlargement of both optic nerves in a 4-month-old infant with nystagmus.

Differential Diagnosis

The differential diagnosis in children with neurofibromatosis 1 who present with proptosis includes optic nerve gliomas, neurofibromas of the orbit, and congenital defects of the sphenoid wing. All three conditions may be found in the same patient. Optic gliomas may be seen in association with plexiform neurofibromas of the eyelid and glaucoma in this group of patients.[42] Disfiguring proptosis is usually caused by a diffuse neurofibroma that is virtually impossible to remove. Pulsating exophthalmos is more characteristic of congenital defects in the sphenoid bone. The diagnosis can usually be made on neuroradiologic grounds alone. In children who present with proptosis but without the stigmata of neurofibromatosis, other tumors must be considered. In the differential diagnosis (Table 32–1) are hemangioma, lymphoma, rhabdomyosarcoma, and metastasis from neuroblastoma, leukemia, or Ewing's sarcoma. Fibrous dysplasia, paranasal mucocele, and meningioma are rarely seen. Neuro-imaging narrows the diagnostic range in any given child.

Treatment

Optic gliomas limited to the intraorbital or intracranial optic nerve that do not include the chiasm and that are associated with loss of vision are resected. If the tumor is completely excised and the proximal cut end of the nerve is free of tumor, the tumor will not recur.[45, 46] The approach to children with impaired vision is more problematic. We recommend surgical resection in children younger than 5 years of age in whom acuity is impaired but cannot be quantitated and in whom visual fields cannot be accurately traced. In the older child with normal visual acuity or in the child with neurofibromatosis, the surgeon and family may wish to observe the lesion with careful follow-up by clinical examination (visual acuity and fields) and by MRI or CT at 6-month intervals. In a review of 623 cases of optic glioma, Alvord and Lofton found a 71 per cent progression rate in patients younger than 20 years.[45] Optic nerve gliomas may spread to the chiasm and even into the opposite nerve.[47, 48] Spinal metastases,[49] as well as leptomeningeal dissemination,[50] have also been described.

TUMORS OF THE OPTIC NERVE AND CHIASM

Presentation and Diagnosis

Tumors that involve the optic chiasm and the posterior optic nerve present more commonly with optic atrophy than with papilledema. Loss of visual acuity is not so profound as with the tumors that involve the nerve more anteriorly, but a visual field deficit can usually be identified in both eyes. CT demonstrates fusiform enlargement of one or both optic nerves and expansion of the optic chiasm (Fig. 32–4).

Differential Diagnosis

The diagnosis of optic nerve and chiasm glioma can be assured in the patient with von Recklinghausen's disease if fusiform enlargement of the optic nerve and

TABLE 32-1. DIFFERENTIAL DIAGNOSIS OF OPTIC GLIOMAS

Optic nerve glioma
  Hemangioma
  Lymphoma
  Rhabdomyosarcoma
  Metastases
    Neuroblastoma
    Leukemia
    Ewing's sarcoma
  Fibrous dysplasia
  Paranasal mucocele
  Meningioma
  Neurofibromatosis
    Orbital neurofibroma
    Congenital defect in sphenoid bone
Optic nerve and chiasm glioma
  Germinoma
  Sarcoidosis
Optic chiasm glioma extending into the hypothalamus
  Pituitary adenoma
  Craniopharyngioma
  Malignant astrocytoma
  Epidermoid and dermoid tumors
  Chordoma
  Colloid cyst
  Fibrous dyplasia
  Sarcoidosis
  Histiocytosis X
  Tuberculous granuloma
  Hemangioendothelioma

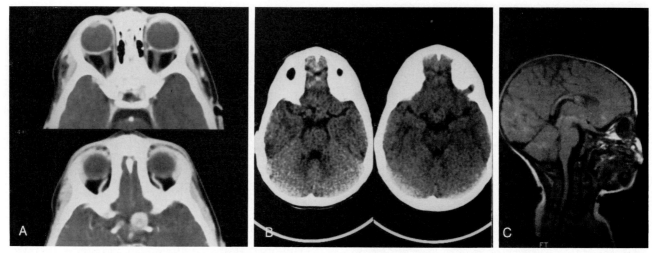

FIGURE 32–4. Optic nerve glioma extending into optic chiasm in a 7-month-old infant with spasmus nutans. *A*, With contrast enhancement. *B*, Without contrast enhancement. *C*, Sagittal magnetic resonance imaging (MRI) through optic nerve and chiasm tumor.

chiasm can be identified on CT. In the child without neurofibromatosis, germinoma and sarcoidosis should be considered in the differential diagnosis.

Clinical Prognosis and Therapy

Although many authors do not differentiate this group of tumors from neoplasms of the chiasm extending into the hypothalamus, tumors localized to the nerve and chiasm do not cause pituitary dysfunction, hydrocephalus, or clinical evidence of hypothalamic dysfunction. Tym reported four cases of optic glioma confined to the chiasm and optic nerve that were verified histologically.[51] All patients were alive and well 9 to 18 years following diagnosis. Three of the four patients had neurofibromatosis, and none received radiation therapy. Heiskanen and co-workers reported 14 patients, none of whom had undergone biopsy.[52] Follow-up was 4 to 18 years, with a mean of 10 years. Nine patients received radiation therapy. All but one was alive at follow-up, but two patients developed pan-

hypopituitarism following radiation therapy. Three patients received no radiation therapy, and visual acuity was "stable" in all survivors. Thirty per cent of these patients had neurofibromatosis. In the series of Hoyt and Baghadassarian,[27] nine patients had tumors confined to the optic nerve and chiasm. Thirty per cent of those patients had deterioration of vision, but there was no difference in the visual morbidity of patients who received radiation therapy and those who did not receive radiation therapy. All patients were alive at follow-up, but the length of follow-up was not well documented.

Children with optic gliomas confined to the chiasm should be observed carefully every 6 months for clinical or radiographic evidence of progression. Radiation therapy is reserved for patients with documented progression. Stabilization or improvement of vision can be expected with radiation therapy exceeding 4500 cGy.[53] Tumor control can usually be achieved with external beam radiation in patients with progressive disease.[54] Interstitial radiotherapy with ^{125}I seeds is an alternative for tumors less than 3 cm in diameter.[9]

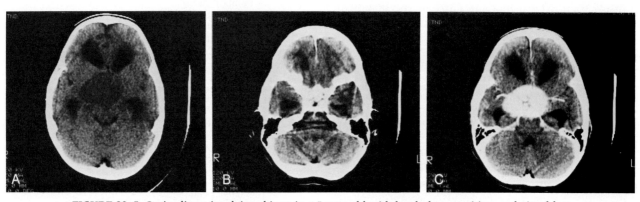

FIGURE 32–5. Optic glioma involving chiasm in a 5-year-old with headaches, vomiting, and visual loss in the right eye. *A*, Without contrast enhancement. *B*, With contrast enhancement. *C*, With contrast enhancement demonstrating hydrocephalus.

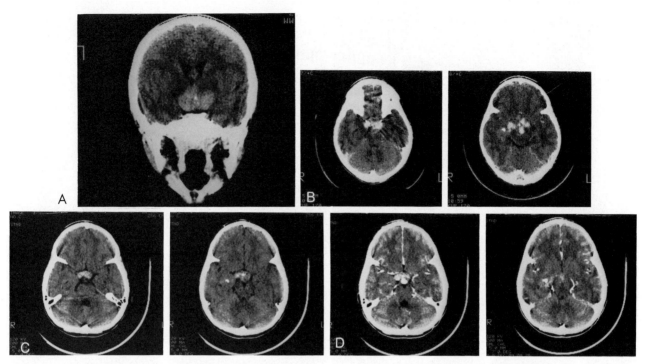

FIGURE 32–6. Optic chiasm—hypothalamus glioma in a 6-year old child with neurofibromatosis, right esotropia, and right hemianopsia. *A*, Coronal plane film before irradiation with contrast enhancement. *B*, Before irradiation with contrast enhancement. *C*, Without contrast enhancement, 3½ years after irradiation. *D*, With contrast enhancement, 3½ years after irradiation.

TUMORS OF THE OPTIC CHIASM EXTENDING INTO THE HYPOTHALAMUS

Presentation

Gliomas that originate primarily from the chiasm and extend posteriorly and superiorly into the hypothalamus present with symptoms and signs of increased intracranial pressure as well as hypothalamic dysfunction. Increased intracranial pressure is caused by hydrocephalus secondary to occlusion of the foramina of Monro. Headaches, vomiting, and obtundation are more commonly seen in this group. The tumor diffusely infiltrates the chiasm and the walls of the third ventricle as well as the hypothalamus, but it is not known to invade the dura. Signs of hypothalamic invasion include the diencephalic syndrome,[55] diabetes insipidus, anorexia, obesity, hypersomnia, and precocious puberty. Spasmus nutans (head bobbing, head tilt, and nystagmus) has been described in association with optic glioma,[47, 56] and in our experience, most of these infants have chiasmatic tumors extending into the hypothalamus. Suprasellar germinomas classically present with painless visual loss, diabetes insipidus, and hypopituitarism.[57] Hemiplegia has also been reported.[4, 58]

Diagnosis

Radiographically, these tumors in this location are often large, may be cystic, and are associated with ven-

triculomegaly (Figs. 32–5 and 32–6). In the patient with neurofibromatosis, the tumor is most probably an optic glioma. However, in the absence of neurofibromatosis, the differential diagnosis includes pituitary adenoma, craniopharyngioma (Fig. 32–7), germinoma (Fig. 32–8),[59] malignant astrocytoma (Fig. 32–9), metastatic medulloblastoma from the posterior fossa, epidermoid and dermoid tumors, chordoma, colloid cyst, fibrous dysplasia, sarcoidosis, histiocytosis X (Fig. 32–10), tuberculous granuloma, and hemangioendothelioma (see Table 32–1).

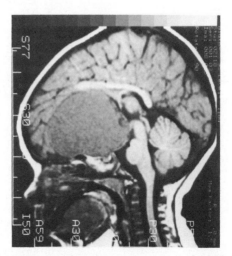

FIGURE 32–7. Craniopharyngioma in an 8-month-old infant who was blind at presentation.

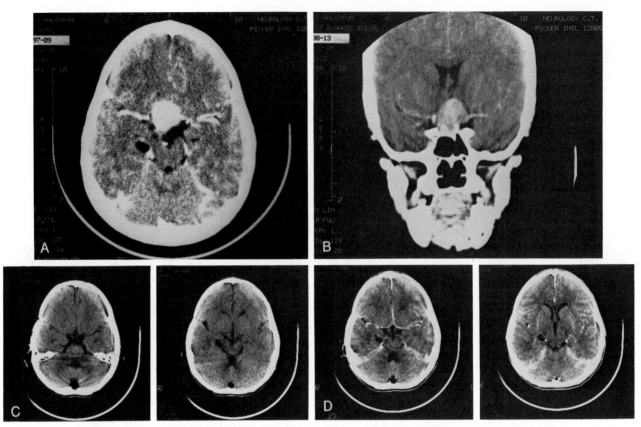

FIGURE 32–8. Germinoma in an 8-year-old boy with severe headaches, rapidly progressive visual loss, and long-standing emotional problems. *A*, Before irradiation. *B*, Before irradiation in coronal plane. *C*, Without contrast enhancement, 18 months after irradiation. *D*, With contrast enhancement, 18 months after irradiation.

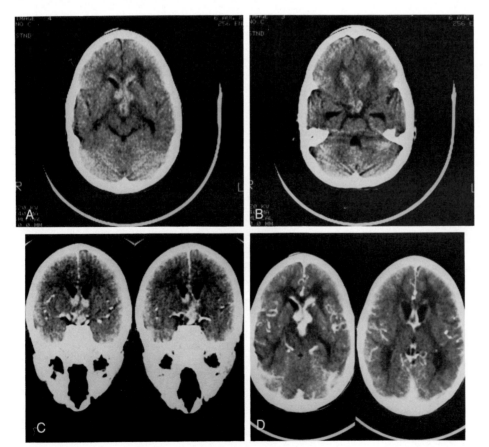

FIGURE 32–9. Malignant glioma in a 6-year-old boy with diabetes insipidus. *A* and *B*, Without contrast enhancement. *C*, Coronal view, with contrast enhancement. *D*, With contrast enhancement.

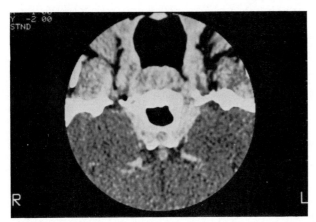

FIGURE 32–10. Histiocytosis X in a 17-year-old girl presenting with diabetes insipidus.

Clinical Prognosis and Therapy

Most authors do not separate optic chiasmatic–hypothalamic gliomas from other gliomas of the optic pathway. However, Heiskanen and colleagues reported five patients who would qualify for this group.[52] One patient died following ventriculography. Three patients died within 3 years of surgery, and one patient died 15 years after surgery and radiation therapy.

Lloyd reported 20 patients with tumors at this site.[24] Six patients died, and in the five on whom autopsy was performed, extension into the hypothalamus was confirmed. Visual acuity was decreased in all but one patient. Fourteen patients in this group received radiation therapy. Three of the patients who died had radiation therapy. The follow-up period varied from 2 to 13 years.

Hoyt and Baghadassarian reported a total of 19 patients with tumor extending into the hypothalamus.[27] Twenty-five per cent of those patients who were irradiated experienced deterioration of their visual acuity. Thirty-three per cent of those who were not treated with radiation deteriorated. Four of their patients died, but the follow-up of the other patients in this category is not documented.

Although reports generally express outcome as survival and overlook quality of life, the poor prognosis in this group has been confirmed by other authors.[29, 33, 34]

In light of the diverse differential diagnosis and the ominous natural history of optic chiasmatic-hypothalamic tumors, a surgical approach is germane. Indeed, surgical removal is possible for pituitary adenomas, craniopharyngiomas, epidermoid and dermoid tumors, colloid cysts, granulomas, and hemangioendotheliomas. Histiocytosis X is treated with low-dose radiation. In contrast, other suprasellar and sellar lesions are less amenable to treatment. Germinomas are responsive to radiation, although suprasellar germinomas carry a worse prognosis than those in the pineal region[4] and may recur outside the field of irradiation. A combination of surgical debulking and radiation therapy is the best treatment for progressive optic gliomas, malignant astrocytomas, and chordomas. Supervoltage radiation therapy with tumor doses of 5500 to 6000 cGy given over 6 to 6.5 weeks is administered with rotational fields.[34]

Recent reports suggest that chemotherapy has at least a palliative effect on optic gliomas. Rosenstock and associates reported 16 patients treated with vincristine and actinomycin D.[60] The diagnosis was confirmed by biopsy in 14 of the patients. Four children with recurrent disease who had previously been treated with radiation therapy were free of progression 13 to 115 months following chemotherapy. Three were still under treatment and seven were stable 1 to 16 months following chemotherapy. Two children developed progressive disease and were treated with radiation therapy.

Intellectual retardation and delayed endocrinopathies associated with radiation therapy are correlated with the age of the child at treatment.[34, 61–71] In children younger than 5 years of age, chemotherapy may delay tumor progression until an age when radiation would have less risk of disabling, long-term side effects. Moreover, Sayers has suggested that tumor growth may slow after the first 15 years of life.[3]

CONCLUSION

The presentation, treatment, and prognosis for tumors that involve primarily the nerve, the nerve and optic chiasm, and the optic chiasm extending into the hypothalamus are distinctive.

Tumors restricted to the nerve that present with visual loss should be resected. Children with neurofibromatosis who have no apparent visual loss may be observed by careful follow-up. Great care must be exercised in the follow-up of the very young child with no demonstrable visual loss but with a tumor confined to the optic nerve.

Tumors of the optic nerve and chiasm are more likely to present with visual field loss in both eyes. When the CT scan demonstrates fusiform enlargement of one or both optic nerves, including the chiasm, an optic glioma is most probably present. Since no beneficial effect of radiation therapy has yet been demonstrated in this group, radiation therapy should be reserved for clinical and radiographic progression. Visual acuity often remains stable over long periods and may even improve spontaneously.

In contrast, tumors that involve primarily the chiasm, with extension into the hypothalamus, present with signs of increased intracranial pressure and hypothalamic dysfunction. Even though the prognosis in this group of children is poor, a surgical approach is warranted. Benign lesions that may masquerade as optic gliomas can be removed, whereas more malignant tumors such as germinoma are responsive to radiation therapy. Since children younger than 5 years of age are not good candidates for radiation therapy, even if there is radiologic evidence of progression, chemotherapy may be a reasonable alternative.

Although the natural history of optic gliomas does not appear to be different in patients with neurofibromatosis, the differential diagnosis is more restricted. Furthermore, these patients tend to develop other tumors that confound long-term survival. Radiation therapy should be undertaken with considerable forethought.

REFERENCES

1. Martin P, Cushing H: Primary gliomas of the chiasm and optic nerves in their intracranial portion. Arch Ophthalmol 52:209, 1923.
2. Matson DD: Neurosurgery of Infancy and Childhood. Springfield, IL, Charles C Thomas, 1969, pp 436–448.
3. Sayers MP: Optic nerve gliomas. In McLaurin RL (ed): Pediatric Neurosurgery. Surgery of the Developing Nervous System. New York, Grune & Stratton, 1982, pp 513–522.
4. Hoffman HJ: Optic pathway gliomas. In Amador L (ed): Brain Tumors in the Young. Springfield, IL, Charles C Thomas, 1983, pp 622–633.
5. Condon JR, Rose FC: Optic nerve gliomas. Br J Ophthalmol 51:703, 1967.
6. Arkhangelsky VN: Neoplasms of the optic nerve. Ophthalmologica 151:260, 1966.
7. Chutorian AM, Schwartz JF, Evans RA, et al.: Optic gliomas in children. Neurology (Minneap) 14:83, 1964.
8. Jain NS: Optic gliomas. Br J Ophthalmol 45:54, 1961.
9. Mohadjer M, Etou A, Milios E, et al.: Chiasmatic optic glioma. Neurochirurgia (Stuttg) 34:90, 1991.
10. Myles ST, Murphy SB: Gliomas of the optic nerve and chiasm. Can J Ophthalmol 8:508, 1973.
11. Spender WH: Primary neoplasms of the optic nerve and its sheaths: Clinical features and current concepts of pathogenetic mechanisms. Trans Am Ophthalmol Soc 70:490, 1972.
12. Anderson DR, Spencer WH: Ultrastructural and histochemical observations of optic nerve gliomas. Arch Ophthalmol 83:324, 1970.
13. Verhoeff FH: Primary intraneural tumors (gliomas) of the optic nerve, a histologic study of eleven cases, including a case showing cystic involvement of the optic disc, with demonstration of the origin of cytoid bodies of the retina and cavernous atrophy of the optic nerve. Arch Ophthalmol 51:120, 1922.
14. Verhoeff FH: Tumors of the optic nerve. In Penfield W (ed): Cytology and Cellular Pathology of the Nervous System. Vol. 3. New York, Paul B. Hoeber, 1932, pp 1029–1039.
15. Brooks WH, Parker JC, Jr., Young AB, et al.: Malignant gliomas of the optic chiasm in adolescents. Clin Pediatr 15:557, 1976.
16. Harper CG, Stewart-Wynne EG: Malignant optic gliomas in adults. Arch Neurol 35:731, 1978.
17. Hoyt WF, Meshel LG, Lessel S, et al.: Malignant optic gliomas of adulthood. Brain 96:121, 1973.
18. Spoor TC, Kennerdell VS, Martinez AJ, et al.: Malignant gliomas of the optic pathway. Am J Ophthalmol 89:284, 1980.
19. Christensen E, Andersen SR: Primary tumors of the optic nerve and chiasm. Acta Psychiatr Neurol Scand 27:5, 1952.
20. Marshall D: Glioma of the optic nerve, as a manifestation of von Recklinghausen's disease. Am J Ophthalmol 37:15, 1954.
21. Oxenhandler DC, Sayers MP: The dilemma of childhood optic gliomas. J Neurosurg 48:340, 1978.
22. Wilson CB, Feinsod M, Hoyt WF, et al.: Malignant evolution of childhood chiasmal pilocytic astrocytoma. Neurology (Minneap) 26:322, 1976.
23. Hudson AD: Primary tumors of the optic nerve. R Lond Ophthalmol Hosp Rep 18:317, 1912.
24. Lloyd LA: Gliomas of the optic nerve and chiasm in childhood. Trans Am Ophthalmol Soc 71:488, 1973.
25. Fowler FD, Matson DD: Gliomas of the optic pathways in childhood. J Neurosurg 14:515, 1957.
26. Dodge HW, Love JG, Craig WM, et al.: Gliomas of the optic nerves. Arch Neurol Psychiatry 79:607, 1958.
27. Hoyt WF, Baghadassarian SA: Optic glioma of childhood. Br J Ophthalmol 53:793, 1969.
28. Miller NR, Iliff WJ, Green WR: Evaluation and management of gliomas of the anterior visual pathways. Brain 97:743, 1974.
29. Packer RJ, Savino PJ, Bilaniuk LT, et al.: Chiasmatic gliomas of childhood. A reappraisal of natural history and effectiveness of cranial irradiation. Childs Brain 10:393, 1983.
30. Tenny RT, Laws ER, Jr., Younge BR, et al.: The neurosurgical management of optic glioma. Results in 104 patients. J Neurosurg 57:452, 1982.
31. Taveras JJ, Mount LA, Wood EH: The value of radiation therapy in the management of glioma of the optic nerves and chiasm. Radiation 66:518, 1956.
32. Glaser JS, Hoyt WF, Corbett J: Visual morbidity with chiasmal glioma. Arch Ophthalmol 85:3, 1971.
33. Brand WN, Hoover SV: Optic gliomas in children: Review of 16 cases given megavoltage radiation therapy. Childs Brain 5:459, 1979.
34. Danoff BF, Kramer S, Thompson N: The radiotherapeutic management of optic nerve gliomas in children. Int J Radiat Oncol Biol Phys 6:45, 1980.
35. Eggers H, Jakobiec FA, Jones IS: Tumors of the optic nerve. Doc Ophthalmol 41:43, 1976.
36. MacCarty CS, Boyd AS, Jr., Childs DS: Tumors of the optic nerve and optic chiasm. J Neurosurg 33:439, 1970.
37. Martuza RL, Kornblith PL, Liszczak TM: Characteristics of human optic gliomas in tissue culture. J Neurosurg 46:78, 1977.
38. Fletcher WA, Imes RK, Hoyt WF: Chiasmal gliomas: Appearance and long-term changes demonstrated by computerized tomography. J Neurosurg 65:154, 1986.
39. Cohen ME, Duffner PK: Visual evoked responses in children with optic gliomas with and without neurofibromatosis. Childs Brain 10:99, 1983.
40. Walsh FB: The ocular signs of tumors involving the anterior visual pathways. Am J Ophthalmol 42:347, 1956.
41. Lewis RA, Gerson LP, Axelson KA, et al.: Von Recklinghausen neurofibromatosis: II. Incidence of optic gliomata. Ophthalmology 91:929, 1984.
42. Listernick R, Charrow J, Greenwald MJ, et al.: Optic gliomas in children with neurofibromatosis type 1. J Pediatr 114:788, 1989.
43. Karp LA, Zimmerman LE, Borit A, et al.: Primary intraorbital meningiomas. Arch Ophthalmol 91:24, 1974.
44. Walsh FB: Meningiomas, primary within the orbit and optic canal. In Smith JL (ed): Neuro-ophthalmology Symposium of the University of Miami and the Bascom Palmer Eye Institute. vol 5. St Louis, CV Mosby, 1970, pp 240–266.
45. Alvord EC Jr, Lofton S: Gliomas of the optic nerve or chiasm: outcome by patient's age, tumor site, and treatment. J Neurosurg 68:85, 1988.
46. Wright JE, McNab AA, McDonald WI: Optic nerve glioma and the management of optic nerve tumours in the young. Br J Ophthalmol 73:967, 1989.
47. Kelly TW: Optic glioma presenting as spasmus nutans. Pediatrics 45:295, 1970.
48. Rand CW, Irvine R, Reeves DL: Primary glioma of the optic nerve. Arch Ophthalmol 21:799, 1939.
49. Kocks W, Kalff R, Reinhardt V, et al.: Spinal metastasis of pilocytic astrocytoma of the chiasma opticum. Childs Nerv Syst 5:118, 1989.
50. Bruggers CS, Friedman HS, Phillips PC, et al.: Leptomeningeal dissemination of optic pathway gliomas in three children. Am J Ophthalmol 15:719, 1991.
51. Tym R: Piloid gliomas of the anterior optic pathways. Br J Surg 49:322, 1961.
52. Heiskanen O, Raitta C, Torsti R: Management and prognosis of gliomas of the optic pathways in children. Mod Probl Paediatr 18:216, 1977.
53. Bataini JP, Delanian S, Ponvert D: Chiasmal gliomas: results of irradiation management in 57 patients and review of literature. Int J Radiat Oncol Biol Phys 21:615, 1991.
54. Pierce SM, Barnes PD, Loeffler JS, et al.: Definitive radiation therapy in the management of symptomatic patients with optic glioma. Survival and long-term effects. Cancer 65:45, 1990.
55. DeSousa AL, Kalsbeck JE, Mealey J, Jr, et al.: Diencephalic syn-

drome and its relation to opticochiasmatic glioma: Review of twelve cases. Neurosurgery 4:207, 1979.

56. Albright AL, Sclabassi RJ, Slamovits TL, et al.: Spasmus nutans associated with optic gliomas in infants. J Pediatr 105:778, 1984.

57. Bowman CB, Farris BK: Primary chiasmal germinoma. A case report and review of the literature. J Clin Neuro-ophthalmol 10:9, 1990.

58. McCullough DC, Epstein F: Optic pathway tumors. A review with proposals for clinical staging. Cancer 56:1789, 1985.

59. Cohen DH, Steinberg M, Buchwald R: Suprasellar germinomas: Diagnostic confusion with optic gliomas. Case report. J Neurosurg 41:490, 1974.

60. Rosenstock JG, Packer RJ, Bilaniuk L, et al.: Chiasmatic optic glioma treated with chemotherapy. J Neurosurg 63:862, 1985.

61. Bamford FN, Jones PM, Pearson D, et al.: Residual disabilities in children treated for intracranial space-occupying lesions. Cancer 37:1149, 1976.

62. Brauner R, Malandry F, Rappaport R, et al.: Growth and endocrine disorders in optic glioma. Eur J Pediatr 149:825, 1990.

63. Hochberg FH, Slotnick B: Neuropsychologic impairment in astrocytoma survivors. Neurology 30:172, 1980.

64. Kun LE, Mulhern RK, Crisco JJ: Quality of life in children treated for brain tumors. Intellectual, emotional, and academic function. J Neurosurg 58:1, 1983.

65. Danoff BF, Cowchock FS, Marquette C, et al.: Assessment of the long-term effects of primary radiation therapy for brain tumors in children. Cancer 49:1580, 1982.

66. Eiser C: Intellectual abilities among survivors of childhood leukemia as a function of CNS radiation. Arch Dis Child 53:391, 1978.

67. Goff JR, Anderson HR, Jr., Cooper PF: Distractibility and memory deficits in long-term survivors of acute lymphoblastic leukemia. J Dev Behav Pediatr 1:158, 1980.

68. Hirsch JF, Renier D, Czernichow P, et al.: Medulloblastoma in childhood. Survival and functional results. Acta Neurol Chir 48:1, 1979.

69. Raimondi AJ, Tomita T: Advantages of "total" resection of medulloblastoma and disadvantages of full head postoperative radiation therapy. Childs Brain 5:550, 1979.

70. Shalet SM, Beardwell CG, Aarons BM, et al.: Growth impairment in children treated for brain tumours. Arch Dis Child 5:491, 1978.

71. Spunberg JJ, Chang CH, Goldman M, et al.: Quality of long-term survival following irradiation for intracranial tumors in children under the age of two. Int J Radiat Oncol Biol Phys 7:727, 1981.

Chapter 33

CRANIOPHARYNGIOMAS

HAROLD J. HOFFMAN, M.D., and JOHN R. W. KESTLE, M.D.

Craniopharyngioma is the most common nonglial tumor of childhood. In Matson's large series of brain tumors, craniopharyngiomas constituted 9 per cent.[1] At the Hospital for Sick Children, these tumors account for 6 per cent of brain tumors and 14 per cent of supratentorial tumors.[2] Despite their benign histologic appearance, many patients demonstrate a progressive deteriorating course despite treatment, and some die of their disease.[3] These extra-axial lesions insinuate themselves into adjacent neural structures, and total removal has been considered hazardous by some surgeons. The methods of management have been debated, and the proponents of radical removal, radiotherapy, or a combination of these modalities vigorously espouse their points of view.[1, 2, 4–16] At the Hospital for Sick Children, the goal for each patient is total removal of the lesion. We believe that this can be accomplished in the vast majority of children with craniopharyngiomas.

PATHOLOGY

Erdheim was the first to propose the well-accepted hypothesis that craniopharyngiomas arise from embryonic squamous cell rests of an incompletely involuted hypophyseal-pharyngeal duct.[17] These rests lie in the pituitary stalk, extending from the tuber cinereum to the pituitary gland. Therefore, the tumor is adherent to the tuber cinereum and can insinuate itself into the substance of the hypothalamus. Elsewhere, the tumor is covered by meninges and is easily separated from neural and vascular structures. Because of the infiltrative nature of the tumor in the tuber cinereum, concern has been expressed that surgical removal may leave nests of tumor cells behind in this region.[18] The nests of tumor seen in sections through the anterior hypothalamus are, in reality, fingers of tumor that have been sectioned transversely and thus appear to be isolated cell rests (Fig. 33–1). As pointed out by Sweet,[15] an intense astrogliosis is induced by the tumor in the tuber cinereum. The layer of gliosis separates the tumor from the functional hypothalamic neurons and provides a plane of separation when the tumor capsule is pulled off the brain in this region.

Grossly, the tumors are largely or partially cystic. Because of their location, craniopharyngiomas compress the optic chiasm anteriorly, the diaphragma sellae inferiorly, and the third ventricle superiorly; they may fill the anterior third ventricle and cause hydrocephalus. If the diaphragma sellae is deficient, the tumor can infiltrate the pituitary gland and expand the sella. The tumor may also extend posteriorly down the clivus, ventral to the pons. The solid portions of the tumor may contain small granular or large craggy foci of calcification (Fig. 33–2). The cystic portion contains yellow-green fluid in which glittering cholesterol crystals are seen.

The cyst walls are composed of columnar or stratified squamous epithelium resting on a collagenous basement membrane that separates the tumor from the surrounding meninges. In the solid portion, the epithelial elements are separated by loosely arranged stellate cells, giving rise to the "adamantinomatous" pattern.

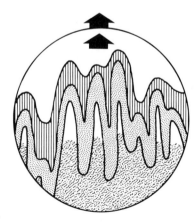

FIGURE 33–1. Diagrammatic representation of fingers of tumor surrounded by astrogliosis invading adjacent brain.

418

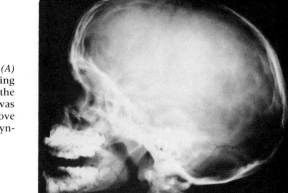
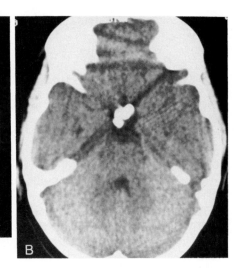

FIGURE 33–2. Skull film *(A)* and CT scan *(B)* demonstrating large focus of calcium within the sella. The tuberculum was drilled off in order to remove this portion of the craniopharyngioma.

Calcification of the keratin is common, and as the masses of keratin coalesce, large foci of calcification may occur.

CLINICAL FEATURES

Approximately half of all craniopharyngiomas occur in patients younger than 18 years of age.[19, 20] These tumors are rarely seen in patients younger than 5 years of age, although occurrences as early as the neonatal period have been reported.[21] The youngest child treated at the Hospital for Sick Children was 22 months old.[8] In most large series there is an equal proportion of the two sexes or a slight male predominance.

The time between onset of symptoms and diagnosis is usually short, with most patients being treated within a year.[9] The clinical findings at presentation in the patients treated at the Hospital for Sick Children since 1975 are outlined in Table 33–1 and discussed in detail below.[8]

TABLE 33–1. CLINICAL FINDINGS IN 50 CHILDREN WITH CRANIOPHARYNGIOMA

	N	%
Headache	34	68
Endocrinopathy	33	66
Short stature	20	40
Diabetes insipidus	12	24
Obesity	9	18
Hypothyroid	7	14
Delayed puberty	7	14
Precocious puberty	1	2
Visual disturbance	29	58
Poor acuity	21	42
Field cut	19	38
Diplopia	4	8
Nystagmus	2	4
Hydrocephalus	24	48

SYMPTOMS

Headache, the most common complaint on admission, was present in 34 (68 per cent) of the 50 children. Its duration could be ascertained in 25 patients and ranged from 2 weeks to 4 years (mean 37.8 weeks).

Symptoms or signs related to the endocrine system were common, being present in 33 patients (66 per cent). Seven patients had hypothyroidism as detected by preoperative screening tests (thyroxine <5 µg/dl), with a normal or low level of thyroid-stimulating hormone. Twenty patients were of short stature; at admission, this was either the major complaint or height was found to be below the third percentile for their age and sex. Twelve patients had diabetes insipidus at admission. Nine patients were obese, with weights above the 97th percentile for age and sex or with a history of recent excessive weight gain. Seven children displayed a delay in the appearance of secondary sexual characteristics, and one presented with precocious puberty at the age of 5 years.

Complaints related to vision were present in 29 children (58 per cent). Nineteen had a field defect, the most common being a bitemporal hemianopia (eight patients). Twenty-one children had decreased visual acuity in one or both eyes; four were blind in one eye. Four children complained of diplopia and two had see-saw nystagmus. Visual acuity showed a significant relationship to tumor location. Of the 25 patients with a prechiasmatic tumor, 15 (60 per cent) had a defect in visual acuity and 14 of them suffered a severe loss of vision (visual acuity $<20/60$); 12 (48 per cent) of these 25 children had a visual field defect. Of the 23 patients with a retrochiasmatic tumor, five (21.7 per cent) had impaired visual acuity and seven (30.4 per cent) had a visual field defect. The two patients with sellar tumors had normal acuity and normal visual fields.

PREOPERATIVE EVALUATION

All patients with a craniopharyngioma should be evaluated in detail by neuroradiologic, endocrinologic, ophthalmologic, and neuropsychological studies prior to surgery.

NEURORADIOLOGY

Plain Skull X-ray. These are abnormal in more than one half of children with craniopharyngioma. The most common finding is abnormal calcification in the suprasellar region. Enlargement of the sella may also be seen. Unless patients are referred with a plain skull film already done, it is not a regular part of the preoperative assessment.

Computed Tomography (CT). CT scanning is widely used for evaluating patients with craniopharyngioma, and all patients treated at the Hospital for Sick Children since 1975 have had a CT scan.[16] Typically there is a low-density cyst surrounded by a partially calcified contrast-enhancing capsule (Fig. 33–3). There may be an associated partially calcified contrast-enhancing solid tumor. Occasionally, solid tumors are seen without cyst formation (Fig. 33–4). Fine coronal images enhanced with intravenous contrast may show the relationship of the tumor to the surrounding vascular structures (Fig. 33–5), although this is better demonstrated on MRI. The main value of CT is in demonstrating calcification, which is not seen on MRI. This differentiates the craniopharyngioma from other suprasellar lesions.

Magnetic Resonance Imaging (MRI). MRI is now the investigation of choice. It is sensitive and has allowed for identification of small tumors in patients with no symptoms other than headache. It is better than CT scanning for demonstrating the relationship of the tumor to the surrounding structures (optic chiasm, carotid arteries, third ventricle) (Fig. 33–6). The sagittal format of the MRI nicely demonstrates the tumor centered in the suprasellar region and the direction of growth, which may be anterior, superior, posterior, or a combination of these (Fig. 33–7). Some degree of

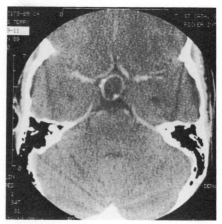

FIGURE 33–3. Axial CT scan demonstrating a low-density cystic craniopharyngioma with a partially calcified, contrast-enhancing capsule.

enlargement of the sella and/or blunting of the dorsum sellae may be seen.

ENDOCRINOLOGIC TESTING

Neuroendocrinologic testing performed preoperatively should include tests for diabetes insipidus, impairment of the pituitary-adrenal axis, and impairment of the pituitary-thyroid axis. Even patients with no symptoms referable to pituitary dysfunction should be tested because careful evaluation reveals some endocrine deficiency in most patients.[22]

Serum cortisol levels should be measured in the morning and in the evening. Impairment of adrenocorticotropic hormone may affect the absolute levels of serum cortisol, but may also be reflected only in a loss of the normal diurnal variation in serum cortisol levels. Because many of these patients have no adrenal reserve preoperatively, they must be given exogenous

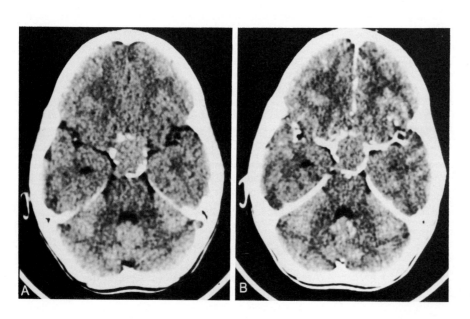

FIGURE 33–4. Axial CT scan of solid craniopharyngioma. Note the calcification (A) and enhancement (B) in the capsule.

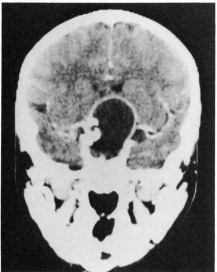

FIGURE 33–5. Coronal contrast-enhanced CT scan demonstrating the relationship of the tumor to surrounding vascular structures in a prechiasmatic tumor.

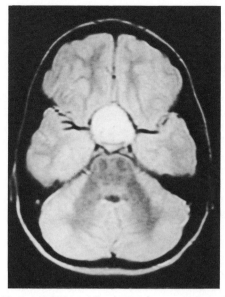

FIGURE 33–6. Axial T2-weighted MRI demonstrating relationship of tumor to anterior cerebral and middle cerebral vessels.

steroid supplements (dexamethasone, 0.2 mg/kg to a maximum of 10 mg, as a loading dose, then 0.1 mg/kg every 6 hours to a maximum of 4 mg, as maintenance) prior to any stressful procedure, such as angiography or surgery.

Thyroid function should be assessed with serum thyroxine (T_4) and triiodothyronine (T_3), or T_3 radioactive uptake levels. Patients with hypothyroidism should be given replacement therapy with L-thyroxine.

Assessment for diabetes insipidus includes question-

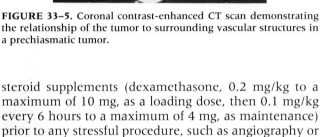

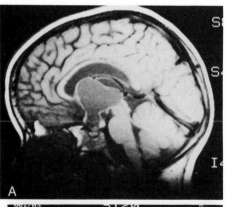

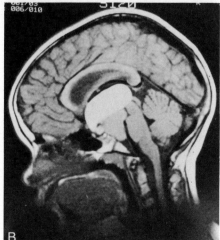

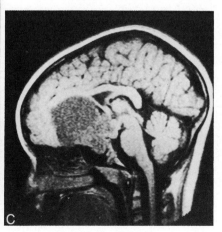

FIGURE 33–7. Sagittal MRI images demonstrating retrochiasmatic *(A and B)* and prechiasmatic *(C)* craniopharyngiomas.

ing the patient about urinary frequency, new onset of nocturia, or new onset of enuresis. Serum electrolytes should be checked and, of course, corrected if abnormal. Water deprivation with serial serum and urine osmolarities is the most sensitive test for confirming the presence of diabetes insipidus.

Serum growth hormone levels, and luteinizing hormone (LH) and follicle-stimulating hormone (FSH) levels in pubertal and postpubertal patients complete the endocrine work-up. The results of the preoperative endocrinology testing in the patients seen at the Hospital for Sick Children are outlined in Table 33–1.

OPHTHALMOLOGIC TESTING

All patients with a craniopharyngioma should have a thorough visual examination preoperatively. Visual acuity and tangent screen visual field testing are included in the preoperative assessment. The visual findings in the patients at the Hospital for Sick Children are outlined in Table 33–1.

NEUROPSYCHOLOGICAL TESTING

Patients with craniopharyngiomas may have distortion of the columns of the fornix resulting in memory difficulties. Furthermore, surgery for craniopharyngioma may disturb the fornices and result in a memory deficit. Consequently, neuropsychological testing prior to surgery is desirable in patients with craniopharyngioma.

SURGICAL CLASSIFICATION OF CRANIOPHARYNGIOMAS

It is useful in operative planning to divide patients according to the location of their craniopharyngioma.

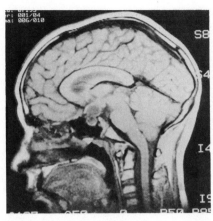

FIGURE 33–9. Sagittal T1-weighted MRI scan showing sellar craniopharyngioma with a small suprasellar extension. The tuberculum was drilled off via a subfrontal approach in order to remove the sellar component.

The three categories are sellar, prechiasmatic, and retrochiasmatic.[8]

Sellar tumors are the least common (4 per cent). They show no displacement of vessels and do not impinge on the optic apparatus (Fig. 33–8) unless there is suprasellar extension (Fig. 33–9).

The prechiasmatic tumors make up half of the total group. These extend anteriorly and present between the two optic nerves at operation (Fig. 33–7C and 33–10). They typically elevate the A1 segment of the anterior cerebral artery but do not usually displace the basilar artery. They impinge on the optic nerves, and these children frequently present with visual impairment.

The retrochiasmatic tumors extend posteriorly (Figs. 33–7A and B, and 33–11). They typically fill the third ventricle and encroach on the foramen of Monro causing hydrocephalus. As these tumors do not impinge on the optic apparatus, these patients rarely have visual

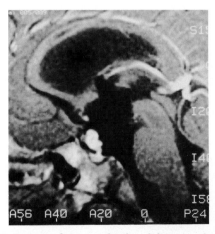

FIGURE 33–8. Sagittal T1-weighted gadolinium-enhanced MRI scan showing small sellar recurrence of craniopharyngioma, which was then removed via the transphenoidal route.

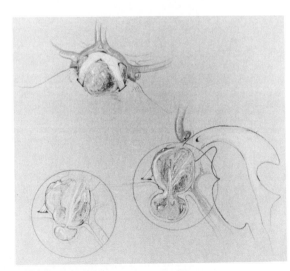

FIGURE 33–10. Diagrammatic representation of prechiasmatic craniopharyngioma presenting between the optic nerves.

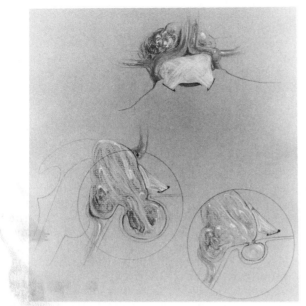

FIGURE 33-11. Diagrammatic representation of a retrochiasmatic craniopharyngioma.

complaints, but on examination they frequently have papilledema due to their hydrocephalus. They do not displace the anterior cerebral artery but may displace the basilar artery posteriorly from the clivus. The presenting features in the three categories of craniopharyngioma are outlined in Table 33-2.

INITIAL SURGICAL MANAGEMENT

Before the development of steroid therapy, the morbidity and mortality rates after surgical treatment of craniopharyngioma were prohibitive. By the early 1950s, with the advent of steroid therapy, Matson was able to remove craniopharyngiomas safely and totally;[12] however, few other surgeons were able to duplicate his results. Their failure to do so was a result of the commonly accepted view that there is no line of cleavage between tumor and adjacent brain and that forcible removal of the craniopharyngioma would severely damage the hypothalamus and optic apparatus. Radia-

tion therapy was (and still is) widely advocated for the treatment of craniopharyngioma.[4-6, 11, 13, 14, 23, 24] Over the past 15 years, however, an increasing number of reports have identified various complications of radiation therapy.[24-27] Furthermore, since irradiation does not necessarily prevent growth of a craniopharyngioma, we continue to see recurrent craniopharyngiomas in patients treated with biopsy or cyst aspiration and radiation therapy.[3, 28]

In 1976, Sweet showed that craniopharyngiomas are separated from functional brain by an intense astrogliosis, which provides a margin of safety between the tumor and functioning brain tissue.[15] It is this plane that has prompted some surgeons to advocate total removal as the procedure of choice.[8, 15] Others still recommend various combinations of biopsy, cyst aspiration, insertion of a drainage catheter, subtotal resection, and/or radiotherapy (interstitial or external beam).

Techniques for investigating and treating patients with craniopharyngiomas have changed radically in the past 15 years. Modern neuro-imaging tools allow earlier diagnosis of these lesions and better assessment of what surgery has accomplished. In situations in which tumor has been left behind, surgeons have been encouraged to reoperate on recurrent tumors when they are small and easily removed. The operating microscope has allowed visualization of important structures and performance of the delicate maneuvers necessary to separate the craniopharyngioma from the visual structures surrounding it. Surgical tools such as the ultrasonic aspirator, which can decompress solid craniopharyngiomas, and the laser, which can vaporize foci of tumor and even fragment pieces of calcium, have facilitated safe excision, rendering tumors formerly considered inoperable both safely accessible and totally removable. No longer are we satisfied with subtotal or partial removal of a craniopharyngioma. Large, solid, calcified tumors that were difficult to deal with can now be removed safely. At the Hospital for Sick Children, total excision of a craniopharyngioma whenever possible has been the goal of treatment.

HYDROCEPHALUS

Craniopharyngiomas may be large enough to obstruct the foramen of Monro and produce hydrocepha-

TABLE 33-2. SURGICAL CLASSIFICATION OF 50 CRANIOPHARYNGIOMAS

	PRECHIASMATIC	RETROCHIASMATIC	SELLAR
Number	25	23	2
Presentation			
Headache	Common	Common	Rare
Visual			
Field defect	12 (48%)	7 (30%)	0
Poor acuity	15 (60%)	5 (22%)	0
Endocrinopathy	Rare	Common	Common
Hydrocephalus	7 (28%)	17 (74%)	0
Surgical approach	Subfrontal	Subfrontal and pterional	Subfrontal through tuberculum or transsphenoidal

lus. In the past, a ventriculoperitoneal (VP) shunt was often inserted preoperatively. More recently we have found this unnecessary, as tumor removal will decompress the anterior third ventricle and re-establish cerebrospinal fluid (CSF) flow.

SURGICAL TECHNIQUE

Many surgical approaches to craniopharyngiomas have been described, including subfrontal, pterional, subtemporal, transcallosal, transsphenoidal and transpalatal. However, in order to remove the tumor totally, the surgeon must have easy access to both optic nerves and both internal carotid arteries as well as the overlying lamina terminalis. For sellar and prechiasmatic tumors, these criteria are met by the subfrontal approach alone. For retrochiasmatic tumors, the pterional approach, to allow access to the posterior portion of the tumor, is combined with the subfrontal approach.

Subfrontal Approach (Prechiasmatic and Sellar Tumors)

The patients are put in a supine position with the neck extended and the nose pointing directly upward in an anatomic position. A right-sided approach is preferred.

The incision in the scalp is made behind the hairline, and the unilateral frontal bone flap extends from the midline medially down to the supraorbital margin inferiorly, out to the pterion laterally and back to just in front of the coronal suture posteriorly (Fig. 33–12A). The dural opening is along the supraorbital ridge. Draining veins from the frontal pole to the superior sagittal sinus are coagulated and divided, and the olfactory tract is coagulated and divided just behind the olfactory bulb to avoid avulsion of the bulb from the cribriform plate.

The chiasmatic cistern is opened, and the frontal lobe is retracted off the chiasm and optic nerves, allowing full visualization of optic nerves, chiasm, and internal carotid artery. This brings the tumor into view. Tumor removal may be performed between the two optic nerves, between the carotid artery and optic nerve, or through the lamina terminalis. We usually begin the dissection between the two optic nerves. The tumor capsule is pierced with a fine needle, and the contents are aspirated. The capsule is then coagulated and incised, and any remaining fluid is removed. The solid contents of the tumor are then removed with the ultrasonic aspirator. Once the tumor is decompressed, traction is applied to the capsule, and the filamentous adhesions between the tumor and the adjacent structures are freed. The glial reaction surrounding tumor allows one to pull tumor capsule free of the anterior third ventricle (lamina terminalis) and the hypothalamus. If the diaphragma sellae is deficient, the craniopharyngioma will invade the pituitary gland, and traction on the tumor will free it from this structure as well. It may also be intimately adherent to the side of the sella, and as one pulls the tumor free, venous bleeding may occur from the cavernous sinus. This can be controlled easily with gentle pressure. With the tumor removed, there is a clear view of both optic nerves, both internal carotid arteries, and the intact membrane of Liliequist posteriorly.

For sellar tumors, the subfrontal approach is used. The dura over the tuberculum is opened and the tuberculum is drilled off, allowing access to the tumor in the sella.[29]

Extension to Pterional Approach (Retrochiasmatic Tumors)

In the case of a retrochiasmic tumor, the usual bone flap for a subfrontal approach is extended laterally to include the pterion and the anterior temporal bone.

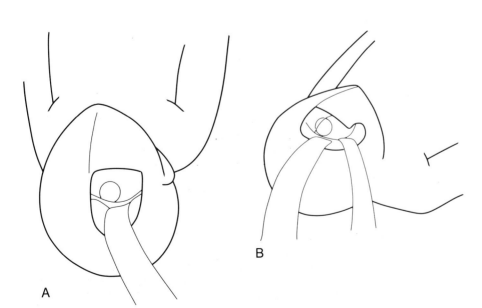

FIGURE 33–12. Diagrammatic representation of the operative approach for prechiasmatic *(A)* and retrochiasmatic *(B)* craniopharyngiomas.

The dural opening is extended laterally through the sylvian region and over the temporal pole. The frontal lobe is retracted upward and the temporal lobe is retracted posteriorly (Fig. 33–12B), bringing the bifurcation of the internal carotid artery and the optic nerve and chiasm into view. The optic nerve and chiasm are separated from the internal carotid artery, exposing the craniopharyngioma capsule. This is coagulated and incised, and the craniopharyngiomas contents are emptied by suction and the ultrasonic aspirator. With this done, the tumor typically collapses, allowing dissection and tumor removal between the optic nerve and carotid artery. As the chiasm moves back away from the tuberculum sellae, the tumor may also be extracted between the two optic nerves.

Retrochiasmatic tumors extend up into the floor of the third ventricle toward the foramen of Monro, and in removing them, it is helpful to open the lamina terminalis. This is done just below the A1 segment of the anterior cerebral artery. The craniopharyngioma capsule can be seen invaginating the thinned out floor of the third ventricle. Downward pressure may be applied on the floor of the third ventricle in order to displace the tumor downward so that it can be extracted from below. Rarely, if the floor of the third ventricle is extremely thinned out, some of the tumor can be extracted through it.

Large chunks of calcification may be problematic. It is occasionally necessary to fragment them in situ with the ultrasonic aspirator or the laser in order to get them out safely. Another option is to drill off the tuberculum,[29] which makes more room for them to be removed between the optic nerves. This is particularly useful for subchiasmatic calcification.

At the end of the procedure it is useful to introduce an angled mirror to inspect the inferior surface of the chiasm and the other areas of the tumor bed that cannot be directly visualized.

POSTOPERATIVE CARE

Postoperatively, the patient must be monitored closely. Surgical retraction of the frontal lobe may result in seizure activity, and prophylactic doses of phenytoin should be administered for a period of 7 to 10 days (5 to 7 mg/kg/24 hours). Preoperative doses of dexamethasone are continued for 48 to 72 hours postoperatively, at which point maintenance doses of cortisone (25 mg/m²/24 hours) are substituted. Eventually, the cortisone should be reduced to the lowest effective level, with a warning to the patient that an increase in dosage may be necessary to avoid possible addisonian crises during periods of stress or infection.

If the sphenoid sinus has been entered during a surgical approach through the tuberculum sellae, prophylactic antibiotics should be administered to prevent postoperative meningitis.

Total removal of a craniopharyngioma almost invariably leads to diabetes insipidus. This condition normally becomes manifest during the first 24 to 48 hours postoperatively. Treatment is now simple and effective. Desmopressin (DDAVP) is administered by nasal instillation in doses of 5 to 20 μg (contained in 0.05 to 0.2 cc) every 12 to 24 hours. This material is extremely effective for postoperative as well as long-term management.

Thyroid studies should be repeated after surgery. If there is evidence of hypothyroidism, thyroid treatment should be instituted. Similarly, gonadotropic hormones should be assessed in pubertal children, and appropriate replacement therapy should be started if the hormone levels are found to be depressed.

Finally, clinical monitoring of the patient's growth, together with growth hormone studies, should begin 6 months postoperatively. If growth slows or halts entirely, and if growth hormone levels are significantly depressed, replacement therapy is begun. However, in some cases, normal growth continues despite the absence of growth hormones. Therapeutic intervention in such cases is obviously unnecessary.

ASSESSMENT AND MANAGEMENT OF RESIDUAL TUMOR

Despite an intraoperative appearance of total removal, there may be residual craniopharyngioma identified radiologically. All patients should undergo plain and contrast-enhanced CT scanning within 24 hours of surgery. The patient is said to have had a total excision if the CT scan shows no evidence of enhancing tumor. Some residual calcium without any enhancement is allowed, and these patients are also classified as having had a total removal. If the intraoperative assessment by the surgeon was that he had performed a complete removal and the postoperative CT scan shows enhancing tumor left behind, a repeat craniotomy is recommended. If, on the other hand, there was tumor that could not be removed intraoperatively and the surgeon was aware of this, a repeat operation is not recommended, and it is in this group that postoperative radiation is used.

It is important that CT scanning be used for follow-up of patients with residual calcification, since MRI does not demonstrate calcification well.

RESULTS

From January 1, 1975, to December 31, 1989, 93 patients underwent surgical management of their craniopharyngioma at the Hospital for Sick Children. There were 50 patients who had their first microsurgical tumor removal at this hospital. Their results have recently been reviewed.[8]

Three patients have died in the follow-up period. One patient who was admitted cachectic and septicemic died of infection while in hospital. Two others died 9 years after surgery.

Over the follow-up period (1 to 14 years), 17 patients (34 per cent) have had tumor recurrence. Thirteen of these occurred in the 45 patients in whom total excision was thought to have been accomplished. Four of the recurrences occurred in the five patients who were known to have had a subtotal excision. The average time to recurrence was 2½ years. Ten of the recurrences were treated by surgery alone, six by surgery and radiotherapy, and one by radiotherapy alone.

The visual fields were unchanged or improved in 59 per cent of the patients. In 70 per cent of the group, visual acuity improved or did not change.

In all patients at follow-up, some form of hormone replacement was necessary: 93 per cent were using DDAVP, 89 per cent were using cortisone, 83 per cent were using thyroid replacement, 30 per cent were using sex hormone replacement, and 20 per cent were using growth hormone.

Twenty-seven patients in the series underwent psychometric evaluation. Twenty-six of the 27 had a full-scale intelligence quotient (IQ) within or above the range of normal. There were 16 children with memory impairment, but 14 of these were attending regular school and making satisfactory progress.

OTHER TREATMENT MODALITIES

RADIATION THERAPY

Radiation therapy has been demonstrated to have a destructive effect on craniopharyngiomas, even though the brain parenchyma would be expected to be harmed by doses high enough to affect the stratified squamous epithelium of the tumor. In the Cleveland Clinic series, 78 per cent of patients treated with subtotal resection alone have died, compared with 18 per cent of patients receiving postoperative radiation therapy.[30] Similar reductions in recurrence have been achieved by the ad-

dition of radiation therapy to subtotal resection in other series.[13]

However, radiation therapy does have risks. Calcification of the basal ganglia is commonly seen in patients irradiated for parasellar lesions. Furthermore, radiation therapy is not always effective, and craniopharyngiomas can continue their relentless growth despite radiation therapy. In such cases, the radiation therapy creates an intense reaction that makes any further surgery an impossibility.

The major risks are radiation necrosis of the brain and optic nerves.[18, 31, 32] This delayed reaction of the brain to radiation may result from too large a total dose, too short an interval between fractions, or too few fractions. Current recommendations are 5000 to 6000 rad given with rotating ports, 6 × 6 cm maximum, and no more than 200 rad per day. In addition to radiation necrosis, parasellar irradiation may give rise to meningeal sarcomas, meningiomas, and bilateral carotid occlusion.[25–27, 33] In children, exposure of the brain to radiation may lead to a decline in intellect. At the Hospital for Sick Children, radiotherapy is reserved for the adjuvant treatment of residual tumor that was found to be nonresectable at operation.

To avoid the complications of external beam radiation therapy, the intracystic injection of radioactive isotopes has been proposed.[5, 34] The radionuclide can be placed into the tumor cyst stereotactically or via an indwelling catheter connected to an Ommaya reservoir. These techniques have been shown to reduce the size of the cyst and to prevent further tumor growth. They are limited to use in tumors made up of one or two large cysts with a minor solid component.

Focused radiotherapy (gamma knife) has been reported by Steiner in 36 patients.[35] The solid portion of the tumor was treated with 20 to 50 Gy at the isocenter and 10 Gy at the periphery after the cystic portion had

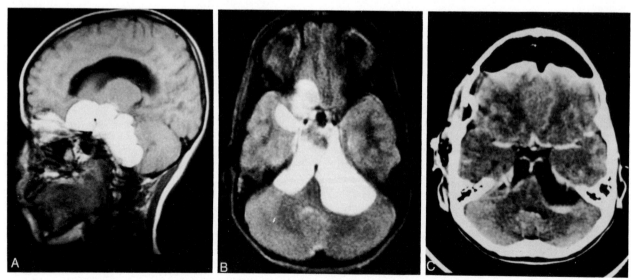

FIGURE 33–13. T1-weighted sagittal *(A)* and axial *(B)* MRI of a giant cystic craniopharyngioma extending into the posterior fossa. Most of the lesion was excised *(C)*, but portions of the cyst wall in the posterior fossa were filamentous and left behind. A catheter was left in the cyst for subsequent aspiration as necessary.

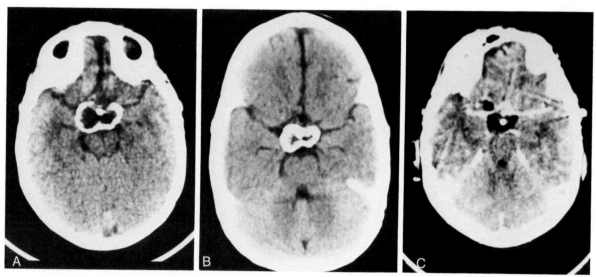

FIGURE 33–14. Axial CT scan showing recurrent craniopharyngioma *(A)* referred with a drainage catheter within the cystic tumor *(B)*. The tumor capsule has thickened considerably after 6 weeks of injection of bleomycin into the cyst. This made the previously fragile capsule thick so that it could be manipulated intraoperatively, allowing tumor removal *(C)*. Note remaining catheter in *C*.

been treated with intracystic Yttrium-90 or Phosphorus-30. At The Hospital for Sick Children, we have referred patients for gamma knife treatment who have a small intrasellar tumor recurrence.

INTRACYSTIC CATHETER PLACEMENT

Occasionally, a ventricular catheter is placed into a large tumor cyst and attached to a subcutaneous reservoir. This allows aspiration of the cyst fluid when compressive symptoms are evident. In rare instances, we have performed this procedure for huge lesions that could not be totally resected (Fig. 33–13). In one patient who was sent to us with such a catheter in place, we elected to inject bleomycin three times a week for 6 weeks. This technique, described by Takahashi,[36] thickened an otherwise fragile tumor capsule and made subsequent surgery for tumor removal easier (Fig. 33–14).

SUMMARY

Craniopharyngiomas are benign tumors arising from squamous cell rests in the pituitary stalk. They give rise to symptoms by compressing nearby neural structures. The goal of surgical therapy is total excision; this can be achieved in more than 60 per cent of patients with acceptable morbidity.

After presumed total excision, if there is obvious tumor left behind, reoperation is indicated to remove such residual tumor. If only a subtotal excision can be performed because of the nature of the tumor and its relationship to surrounding structures, postoperative radiation therapy should be carried out. Without such therapy, recurrence of symptoms will become evident within a matter of months.

REFERENCES

1. Matson DD: Neurosurgery of Infancy and Childhood. 2nd ed. Springfield, IL, Charles C Thomas, 1969, p 545.
2. Hoffman HJ: Supratentorial tumors in childhood. *In* Youmans J (ed): Neurological Surgery. 2nd ed. Philadelphia, WB Saunders Co., 1982, pp 2702–2732.
3. Grover WD, Rorke LB: Invasive craniopharyngioma. J Neurol Neurosurg Psychiatry 31:580, 1968.
4. Backlund EO: Studies on craniopharyngiomas. III. Stereotaxic treatment with intracystic Yttrium-90. Acta Chir Scand 139:237, 1973.
5. Backlund EO: Studies on craniopharyngiomas. IV. Stereotaxic treatment with radiosurgery. Acta Chir Scand 139:344, 1973.
6. Cavazzuti V, Fischer EG, Welch K, et al.: Neurological and psychophysiological sequelae following different treatments of craniopharyngioma in children. J Neurosurg 59:409, 1983.
7. Hoffman HJ, Chuang S, Ehrlich R, et al.: The microsurgical removal of craniopharyngiomas in childhood. *In* Chapman PH (ed): Concepts in pediatric neurosurgery, Vol. 6. New York, S Karger, 1985, pp 52–62.
8. Hoffman HJ, Da Silva M, Humphreys RP, Drake J, Smith M, Blaser S: Aggressive surgical management of craniopharyngiomas in children. J Neurosurg 76:47, 1992.
9. Hoffman HJ, Hendrick EB, Humphreys RP, et al.: Management of craniopharyngiomas in children. J Neurosurg 47:218, 1977.
10. Katz EL: The late results of radical excision of craniopharyngiomas. J Neurosurg 42:86, 1975.
11. Manaka S, Teramoto A, Takakura K: The efficacy of radiotherapy for craniopharyngioma. J Neurosurg 62:648, 1985.
12. Matson DD, Crigler JF: Management of craniopharyngioma in childhood. J Neurosurg 30:377, 1969.
13. Mori K, Handa H, Murata T, et al.: Results of treatment for craniopharyngioma. Childs Brain 6:302, 1980.
14. Pollack IF, Lunsford LD, Slamovits TL, et al.: Stereotaxic intracavity irradiation for cystic craniopharyngiomas. J Neurosurg 68:227, 1988.
15. Sweet WH: Radical surgical treatment of craniopharyngioma. Clin Neurosurg 23:52, 1976.
16. Yasargil MG, Gurcic M, Kis M, Siegenthaler G, Teddy P, Roth P: Total removal of craniopharyngiomas. J Neurosurg 73:3, 1990.
17. Erdheim J: Ober hypophysengangsyeschwulste und Hirncholesteatome. Sitzungsb Akad Wissensch 113:537, 1904.
18. Amacher AL: Craniopharyngioma: The controversy regarding radiotherapy. Childs Brain 6:57, 1980.

19. Bannr M, Hoare RD, Stanley P, et al.: Craniopharyngiomas in children. J Pediatr 983:781, 1973.
20. Bloom HJ: Tumors of the central nervous system. *In* Voute PA, et al. (eds): Cancer in Children, 2nd ed. New York, Springer-Verlag, 1986, pp 197–222.
21. Azar-Kia B, Kreskman VR, Schecter MM: Neonatal craniopharyngioma: Case report. J Neurosurg 42:91, 1975.
22. Thomsett MJ, Conte FA, Kaplan SL, et al.: Endocrine and neurologic outcome in childhood craniopharyngioma: Review of effect of treatment in 42 patients. J Pediatr 97:728, 1980.
23. Kramer S, Southard M, Mansfield CM: Radiotherapy in the management of craniopharyngiomas. Further experiences and late results. AJR 103:44, 1968.
24. Shillito J Jr: Treatment of craniopharyngioma. Clin Neurosurg 33:533, 1985.
25. Sogg RL, Donaldson SS, Yorke CH: Malignant astrocytoma following radiotherapy of a craniopharyngioma. Case report. J Neurosurg 48:622, 1978.
26. Ushio Y, Arita N, Yoshimine T, et al.: Glioblastoma after radiotherapy for craniopharyngioma: Case report. Neurosurgery 21:33, 1987.
27. Waga S, Handa H: Radiation-induced meningioma: With review of literature. Surg Neurol 5:215, 1976.
28. Fischer EG, Welch K, Skhillito J Jr, et al.: Craniopharyngiomas in children. Long-term effects of conservative surgical procedures combined with radiation therapy. J Neurosurg 73:534, 1990.
29. Patterson R, Danylevich A: Surgical removal of craniopharyngiomas by a transcallosal approach through the lamina terminalis and sphenoid sinus. Neurosurgery 7:111, 1980.
30. McMurray FG, Hardy RW, Dohn DF, et al.: Long-term results in the management of craniopharyngiomas. Neurosurgery 1:238, 1977.
31. D'Lorenzo N, Nolletti A, Palma L: Late cerebral radionecrosis. Surg Neurol 10:281, 1978.
32. Ross HS, Rosenbert S, Friedman AH: Delayed radiation necrosis of the optic nerve. Am J Ophthalmol 76:683, 1973.
33. Allen J: The effects of cancer therapy on the nervous system. J Pediatr 93:903, 1978.
34. Kobayashi T, Kageyama N, Ohara K: Internal irradiation for cystic craniopharyngioma. J Neurosurg 55:896, 1981.
35. Steiner L: Stereotactic radiosurgery with the cobalt-60 gamma unit in the treatment of intracranial tumors and arteriovenous malformations. *In* Schmidek HH, Sweet WH (eds): Operative Neurosurgical Techniques: Indications, Methods, and Results. Philadelphia, WB Saunders, 1988, 515–529.
36. Takahashi H, Nakazawa S, Shimura I: Evaluation of postoperative intratumoral injection of bleomycin for craniopharyngioma in children. J Neurosurg 62:120, 1985.

Chapter 34

PINEAL REGION TUMORS

MICHAEL S.B. EDWARDS, M.D. and JAMES E. BAUMGARTNER, M.D.

Pineal region tumors make up 0.4 to 1.0 per cent of brain tumors in adults[1] and 3 to 8 per cent of brain tumors in children.[2] While germinoma and astrocytoma account for 53 to 78 per cent of pineal region tumors, a wide variety of histologically distinct tumor types can be found in this region (Table 34–1).[2–4] The surgical experience in treating lesions in this location, prior to 1943, was disappointing, with mortality and morbidity rates in excess of 90 per cent.[5] Accordingly, treatment consisting of a shunting procedure followed by empiric radiation therapy became widely accepted.[6–8] Although this approach resulted in a 60 to 70 per cent 5-year survival and a 50 to 60 per cent 10-year survival, the results were generally best for older children, with most children under 6 years of age experiencing early tumor recurrence or death.[2, 7, 9] Recent surgical experience has been more favorable, with significantly lowered morbidity (10 to 27 per cent) and mortality (0 to 2 per cent).[2, 10–12] Therefore, modern treatment protocols are appropriately based on the tissue diagnosis at presentation.[2, 9, 11, 13–18]

HISTORY

Herophilus, an Alexandrian anatomist, first described the pineal gland more than 2300 years ago. He believed it was a valve that controlled the flow of memories from the rear brain ventricles, where they were stored, forward to the consciousness-serving portions of the brain.[19] The pineal body was considered by Descartes to be "the seat of the soul,"[20] and was labeled "the gland of mystery" by Cuneo and Rand.[21] Virchow is credited with the first description of pineal tumors in 1865.[22]

Surgery for pineal region tumors began early in this century. Horsley, in 1910, attempted to remove a pineal tumor using an infratentorial approach, but the patient developed "profound complications."[23] Krause, in 1913, successfully removed a pineal mass using a supracerebellar, infratentorial approach.[24] Puusep, in

1914, used a supracerebellar approach, which included dividing the right transverse sinus and the tentorium; however, the patient died.[25] Dandy, who advocated aggressive tumor removal, described a transcallosal operation in 1921,[26] but experienced seven perioperative deaths before successfully removing a pineal tumor in 1931.[27] In 1928, Max Peet successfully removed a pineal tumor using Dandy's approach, and the patient was alive when Kahn reported the case in 1937.[28] Van Wagenen used a lateral transventricular approach in 1931 to resect a pineoblastoma.[12] In spite of these rare successes, the early surgical experience was dismal. Russell and Sachs reviewed all cases reported before 1943 and found a 90 per cent operative mortality.[29]

TABLE 34–1. TUMORS OF THE PINEAL REGION

Tumors of germ cell origin
  Germinoma
  Nongerminoma germ cell tumors (NG-GCT)
    Teratoma
    Dermoid
  Nongerminoma malignant germ cell tumors (NG-MGCT)
    Choriocarcinoma
    Embryonal carcinoma
    Endodermal sinus tumor or yolk sac tumor
    Combinations of the above
Tumors of pineal parenchymal origin
  Pineocytomas
  Pineoblastomas
Mixed pineocytoma and pineoblastoma
Tumors of supporting (glial stroma) or adjacent tissues, and others
  Gliomas
  Ganglioneuroma and ganglioglioma
  Meningioma (neurofibromatosis type 2)
Non-neoplastic cysts and vascular lesions
  Arachnoid cysts
  Vascular lesions
    Aneurysm of vein of Galen
    Arteriovenous malformation
    Cavernous malformations
  Pineal cysts (benign or ependymal)

Adapted from Russell DS, Rubinstein LJ: Pathology of Tumours of the Nervous System. 4th ed. Baltimore, Williams and Wilkins, 1977, pp 284–295.

Cushing, in 1932, wrote, "I have never succeeded in exposing a pineal tumor sufficiently well to justify an attempt to remove it." He advocated a generous sub-temporal decompression followed by radiotherapy for "pineal tumor unverified." Cushing described his approach as a "therapeutic shot in the dark" but defended it on the grounds of the radiation sensitivity of pineoblastomas.[30] Torkildsen proposed a shunting procedure followed by radiation therapy in 1948. This became the standard treatment until the 1980s.[18]

However, some surgeons continued to attempt tumor resection. New operations were developed, including an occipital transtentorial approach by Poppen[31] and the supracerebellar infratentorial approach of Krause[32] as modified by Stein.[11] Improvement in microsurgical technique and neuroanesthesia have resulted in encouraging surgical results. Hoffman et al., in a series of 22 children undergoing surgery between 1975 and 1982, using the operating microscope and a trans-callosal approach, reported only one operative death.[33, 34] Stein, using his supracerebellar infratentorial approach in a series of 65 adult and pediatric patients, had an operative mortality rate of 2 per cent and a long-term morbidity rate of 2 per cent.[35] Edwards et al., in 1988, reported a series of 30 children with no operative mortality, a 27 per cent immediate morbidity, but only a 10 per cent long-term morbidity.[4]

CURRENT CONTROVERSIES

The current debate over the appropriate treatment of pineal region tumors in children can be divided into three questions:

1. Is tissue diagnosis necessary?
2. Is a radiation test dose (2000 cGy) followed by a repeat scan a rational first step in treatment?
3. With a diagnosis of germinoma, should focal or craniospinal radiation therapy be used?

We will address these topics in the following discussion.

PREOPERATIVE ASSESSMENT

PRESENTATION

The clinical manifestations of pineal region tumors are related to increased intracranial pressure from obstructive hydrocephalus, from pressure upon or infiltration of the midbrain tectum (Parinaud's syndrome), and, rarely, from tumor invasion of the hypothalamic-pituitary axis (diabetes insipidus).[2] Precocious puberty was first reported in association with a pineal tumor by Huebner in 1898.[36] This rare occurrence is thought to be caused by tumor secretion of human chorionic gonadotropin.[37] Presenting signs and symptoms from two large pediatric pineal series are summarized in Table 34–2.[2, 4]

TABLE 34–2. PRESENTING SIGNS AND SYMPTOMS IN CHILDREN WITH PINEAL REGION TUMORS

SYMPTOMS	EDWARDS ET AL.[4]	ABAY ET AL.[8]
Headache	25/33 (76)%	20/27 (74%)
Nausea/vomiting	13/33 (39%)	16/27 (59%)
Diplopia	4/33 (12%)	16/27 (59%)
Lethargy	7/33 (21%)	6/27 (22%)
Delayed menses	1/33 (3%)	1/27 (4%)
SIGNS		
Parinaud's syndrome	19/33 (58%)	12/27 (44%)
Papilledema	5/33 (15%)	24/27 (89%)
CN VI palsy	3/33 (9%)	3/27 (11%)
CN III palsy	1/33 (3%)	10/27 (37%)
Polyuria	2/33 (6%)	2/27 (7%)
Ataxia	6/33 (18%)	6/27 (22%)

CN = cranial nerves

In the pediatric population, males are 3.5 to 4 times more likely to develop pineal tumors than females. Most tumors present in the second decade, with an average age at presentation of 13 years.[2, 4]

NEURORADIOLOGY

Magnetic resonance (MR) imaging with multiplanar imaging and superior tissue contrast and resolution, has revolutionized the diagnosis and treatment of pineal region masses. Because of the large number of histologically distinct tumor types possible in this region and the variability of associated MR signal characteristics, MR imaging is rarely tumor histology-specific. However, some generalizations are possible: (1) Pineoblastomas and malignant teratomas (and some nongerminoma malignant germ cell tumors) tend to be large (>4 cm) and irregular in shape, whereas most other tumors tend to be round or ovoid and 2 to 3 cm in diameter. (2) Only dermoid (Fig. 34–1) and mature teratoma have a fat signal; fat signal is not seen in malignant teratoma. (3) Hemorrhage is found only in choriocarcinoma and appears to be closely associated with this tumor type. (4) Tumors originating from collicular plate or surrounding temporal lobes are probably gliomas or pineocytomas (Fig. 34–2). (5) Males with diabetes insipidus and Parinaud's syndrome usually have pineal tumors with subependymal metastasis or extension to the hypothalamus and are most often germinomas.[6]

Although gadolinium pentetic acid (DTPA)–enhanced MR imaging has not improved diagnostic specificity, it facilitates the detection of subependymal and "drop" spinal metastases in malignant pineal tumors, making tumor staging much more accurate.

Preoperative MR imaging of the entire neuraxis, with and without gadolinium, should be obtained to rule out metastasis and to avoid postoperative artifacts associated with surgery (e.g., blood in the subarachnoid space, which can mimic tumor).

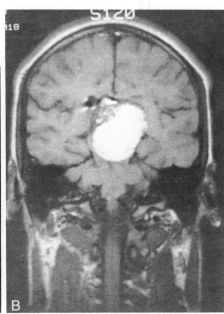
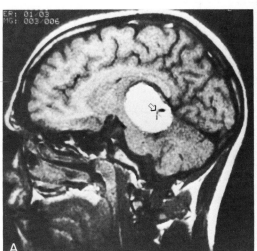

FIGURE 34–1. *A*, Gadolinium-enhanced , T1-weighted, parasagittal MR image (note fat signal, *arrow*), and *B*, gadolinium-enhanced, T1-weighted, coronal MR image of a pineal region dermoid. As this tumor is primarily supratentorial, it was approached via an occipital transtentorial route.

TUMOR MARKERS

Once the presence of a pineal region mass has been demonstrated radiographically, cerebrospinal fluid (CSF) (preferably obtained preoperatively, via lumbar puncture, ventriculostomy, or ventriculoperitoneal shunt) should be examined for cytology, and blood and CSF examined for "tumor markers." Positive CSF cytology confirms a malignant histology and can occasionally be diagnostic.

Specific types of germ cell tumors can manufacture biologic markers including alpha-fetoprotein (AFP), the beta subunit of human chorionic gonadotropin (hCG),[38] and placental alkaline phosphatase (PLAP).[39] Table 34–3 lists the reported associations between histology and tumor markers. Like MR imaging, tumor markers are suggestive but only occasionally diagnostic of tumor histology. HCG and AFP are particularly helpful in diagnosis and subsequent follow-up of nongerminoma germ cell tumors (NG-GCT). Elevated HCG is seen in choriocarcinoma and may be minimally elevated in germinoma and a benign suprasellar teratoma. In our experience, HCG is a less reliable marker than AFP. Elevated AFP, with or without elevated HCG, is

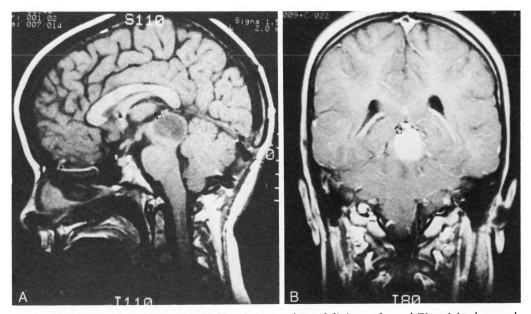

FIGURE 34–2. *A*, T1-weighted, midsagittal MR image, and *B*, gadolinium-enhanced, T1-weighted, coronal MR image of an anaplastic astrocytoma. Arrows point to tumor. The appearance is also consistent with a pineocytoma. Because this tumor is primarily infratentorial, it was approached via a supracerebellar infratentorial route.

TABLE 34–3. TUMOR MARKERS IN PATIENTS WITH PINEAL TUMORS

HISTOLOGY	AFP	HCG	PLAP
Germinoma	−	− / + *	+
Malignant teratoma	+ / −	+ / −	+ / −
Endodermal sinus tumor	+	−	+ / −
Pineocytoma	−	−	−
Undiff. germ cell tumor	+ / −	+ / −	+ / −
Pineocytoma/blastoma	−	−	−
Choriocarcinoma	−	+	+ / −
Embryonal cell tumor	+	+	+ / −
Teratoma	−	− /rare +	+ / −

AFP = Alphafetoprotein, HCG = human chorionic gonadotropin, PLAP = placental alkaline phosphatase.
  Data from Edwards MS, et al,[4] Shinoda J, et al,[39] and Washiyama K, et al.[40]
  *When HCG is elevated the levels are low and are believed to be due to syntrophoblastic cells within the germinoma.

evidence of a nongerminoma malignant germ cell tumor (NG-MGCT). Elevated AFP alone suggests an endodermal sinus tumor. Elevation of both AFP and HCG suggests embryonal carcinoma or malignant teratoma. However, some NG-MGCT do not produce any markers. Germinoma, the most common pineal region tumor, is not associated with elevations of AFP or HCG. PLAP was initially thought to be a specific serum and CSF marker for germinoma;[39] subsequent studies have shown this association to be strong but not always diagnostic (Table 34–3).[40] Dramatically elevated PLAP levels correlate more strongly with germinoma than do mildly elevated PLAP levels.

Some authors advocate following levels of melatonin (MLT) in patients with pineal region masses. Although increased levels of MLT have been reported in a patient with a pineocytoma,[41] the circadian rhythm of MLT secretion is usually normal or depressed in patients with pineal region masses.[9] In our experience, MLT determinations have not been useful in managing patients with pineal region tumors.

The growth regulatory polyamines, spermidine and putrescine, are both elevated during active cell growth. In some nonglial tumors, longitudinal studies have shown them to be sensitive markers of tumor activity and response to therapy.[42] Polyamines are also elevated in acute hydrocephalus. Preliminary studies indicate that polyamines, particularly putrescine, may be useful in follow-up of malignant childhood tumors including pineal germ cell tumors.[43] Further study is necessary to define the role of these markers in the treatment of pineal region tumors.

Both CSF and serum levels of tumor markers should be obtained preoperatively whenever possible. A CSF-to-serum gradient suggests that the neoplasm is intracranial. If the serum level exceeds the CSF levels, the possibility of metastasis or a primary extracranial germ cell tumor should be considered. Generally, lumbar CSF levels of tumor markers exceed ventricular CSF levels.[38] Tumor markers and cytology are extremely useful postoperatively in monitoring response to therapy and in identifying early tumor recurrence.[38–40, 42, 43]

Cytologic studies should be obtained no sooner than 2 weeks postoperatively, and specimens can be obtained via lumbar puncture or by a ventriculoperitoneal shunt tap. However, lumbar CSF is more sensitive in determining CSF dissemination. CSF cytologic findings need to be correlated with gadolinium DTPA MR imaging or metrizamide myelogram/computed tomography (CT) of the spine.

SURGICAL TREATMENT

IS TISSUE DIAGNOSIS NECESSARY?

Previous justifications for ''blind'' radiotherapy are based on a presumed high risk of biopsy and the high frequency of germinoma in the pineal region, an argument first outlined by Cushing.[30] Surgery has become much safer, and treatment options beyond test dose radiotherapy are now available. Tumor markers and MR data are suggestive, not diagnostic. The most compelling reason for obtaining tissue diagnosis is the need to base therapy on tumor histology. Avoidance of radiation for benign or radioresistant lesions in the developing brain is obviously desirable. Although most (70 to 86 per cent)[2, 4, 33] pineal region tumors of childhood are ultimately treated with radiation therapy, the variety of radiation therapy doses and distribution varies significantly based on histology and extent of disease. In our opinion, there is no justification for radiation and or chemotherapy without first obtaining a tissue diagnosis. (A possible exception is found in Japanese adolescent males with uniformly gadolinium-enhancing pineal region masses.)

VENTRICULOSTOMY VERSUS VENTRICULOPERITONEAL SHUNT

Because pineal region masses usually compromise the posterior third ventricle or the aqueduct of Sylvius, most patients present with some degree of hydrocephalus. If necessary, a shunt can be placed to divert CSF and obtain cytologic and CSF marker information. If MR images suggest that obstruction of the CSF pathways can be corrected surgically, ventriculostomy and definitive surgery should be pursued in a timely fashion. Particularly for benign and radiosensitive tumors, this approach may obviate shunt placement. In the case of malignant tumors and germinoma, ventriculoperitoneal shunts have been implicated as a conduit for tumor cells, allowing peritoneal seeding (an extremely rare occurrence). Although metastatic germinoma does respond to radiation and chemotherapy, the prognosis for extra-CNS metastatic malignant pineal region tumors has been generally dismal.[33, 40, 44] Attempts to block shunt-borne tumor metastasis with shunt filters have been complicated by an unacceptably high rate of shunt failure and revision, and are therefore not considered practical.[45, 46]

STEREOTACTIC VERSUS OPEN BIOPSY

Because pineal region tumors often have mixed histology and stereotactic biopsy is associated with significant sampling error, open biopsy is the preferred surgical approach. An open approach also allows a more extensive resection, if frozen-section pathology results support this option (i.e., dermoid, teratoma, cavernous malformation). Finally, the French experience with stereotactic biopsy of the pineal region in young children has been less than satisfactory, a high incidence of hemorrhage being associated with this approach (C. Motolese, personal communication).

When AFP is elevated, particularly with large tumors or when subarachnoid spread is documented, a CT-guided stereotactic biopsy may be a reasonable approach.

SURGICAL APPROACHES

Planning for surgical resection of pineal region tumors is based on tumor location as visualized on midsagittal and coronal MR images. If the majority of the tumor is located above the tentorium, an occipital transtentorial route is pursued (see Fig. 34–1). If the majority of the tumor is located below the tentorium, a supracerebellar infratentorial approach is favored (see Fig. 34–2). Patients are positioned prone in a Concorde-type position, with the head rotated 15 degrees away from the craniotomy side for the occipital transtentorial approach. A standard Concorde position is used for the supracerebellar infratentorial approach. Bolsters are used in older children. Three-point head fixation is preferred, using pediatric pins in children below the age of 6 years. Ventricular decompression is usually accomplished at operation by ventriculostomy. A ventriculoperitoneal shunt is usually reserved for hydrocephalus that persists postoperatively. Every effort should be made to achieve a watertight dural closure, as metastasis may be facilitated by tumor infiltration into the venous or lymphatic drainage of the soft tissues overlying the operative site.[44]

Supracerebellar Infratentorial Approach

After a generous midline suboccipital craniectomy, exposing the transverse sinuses and torcula and extending inferiorly but not including the foramen magnum, intracranial pressure is lowered using the ventriculostomy. Only enough CSF is drained to produce dural pulsations. Mannitol is not necessary if CSF drainage is employed, and its use may increase the risk of developing a subdural fluid collection postoperatively. The dura is opened in a "V" shaped fashion and reflected superiorly. The inferior dura is left intact, acting as a sling for the cerebellum. The cisterna magna is opened and CSF drained, allowing the cerebellum to fall away from the tentorium. Next, bridging veins over the dorsal surface of the cerebellar hemispheres and vermis are coagulated and divided with the aid of the operative microscope. The cerebellum is gently retracted inferiorly and the tentorium superiorly, using a self-retaining retractor; thus the arachnoid in the region of the quadrigeminal cisterns is exposed. This arachnoid is almost always thickened, probably as a reaction to the tumor, and must be divided sharply. Next the precentral cerebellar vein is coagulated and divided. At this point tumor is visualized and a tumor biopsy may be performed. If further tumor resection is planned, great care must be taken to preserve the deep venous structures, the vein of Galen, the basal vein of Rosenthal, and the internal cerebral veins, which are located superior and lateral to the tumor. These are generally displaced by, not enveloped by, tumor. If necessary, the anterior portion of the vermis can be divided to expose tumor lying in the inferior quadrigeminal cistern region.[11, 16]

Occipital Transtentorial Approach

A horseshoe-shaped flap is created, centered approximately 3 cm to the left or right of midline and based just below the level of the tentorium. A craniotomy or craniectomy is then created, exposing the transverse sinus from above. A dural flap is then reflected inferiorly toward the transverse sinus. With the operative microscope, bridging veins to the transverse sinus and tentorium are coagulated and divided, and the tentorium is exposed by gentle retraction of the occipital lobe with a self-retaining retractor. Good ventricular decompression is critical for safe occipital lobe retraction. A wedge of tentorium is then removed after the fourth cranial nerve is identified and thus avoided. Biopsy may be taken at this point. If further tumor removal is planned, great care must be taken to preserve the venous arch formed by the vein of Galen and the basilar veins of Rosenthal.[31] This arch is the limiting margin under which the operation is performed.[47] If necessary, the superior vermis can be retracted inferiorly following division of the precentral cerebellar vein to provide greater exposure inferiorly.[48]

BIOPSY VERSUS RADICAL RESECTION

As noted above, stereotactic biopsy seems reasonable in cases with elevated AFP, positive CSF cytology, and/or evidence of subependymal seeding or parenchymal or spinal drop metastasis. There is concern over possible sampling error with this procedure as 15 per cent of tumors are of mixed histology.[4] Also, nondiagnostic tissue can be obtained using this approach. If open biopsy is pursued in this setting, there is no evidence to suggest that more than a diagnostic biopsy is warranted.

For benign tumors, an attempt at gross total resection is justified, as this may be curative. Some authors advocate debulking encapsulated portions of more malignant tumors without evidence of metastatic spread.[16] The benefit of this approach over biopsy alone is uncertain, particularly as newer, more effective chemotherapeutic regimens become available.

PERIOPERATIVE CARE

All patients are treated with antibiotics (ceftizoxime and vancomycin), high-dose steroids, and relative fluid restriction intraoperatively. They are managed in a pediatric intensive care unit (ICU) postoperatively. If a ventriculostomy is in place, ICP is continuously monitored and CSF drained to maintain ICP in a normal range for age. Steroids are continued and tapered over 2 to 3 weeks. Antibiotics are used for 48 hours postoperatively in shunted patients or until the ventriculostomy is discontinued in patients without shunts.

Serum electrolytes and osmolarity are followed closely throughout hospitalization, and fluid management is adjusted to prevent hyponatremia and hypoosmolarity. Postoperative MR images (with and without contrast) are obtained within 48 hours of surgery.

POSTOPERATIVE CARE

All patients are followed postoperatively with serial MR images with and without gadolinium. Patients are restaged, as outlined above, at the completion of radiation therapy and/or chemotherapy, or when recurrence or progression is suspected.

Table 34–4 outlines the management of patients with pineal region tumors. Benign tumors are treated by surgery alone, and when complete resection is achieved, it is curative. Subtotally resected tumors must be followed closely with serial scans, as they may require additional surgery. Pineocytoma and low-grade astrocytomas are also treated with close observation following gross total resection.

Irradiation of the primary tumor site was used for nondisseminated tumors such as germinoma, subtotally resected pineocytomas, pineoblastoma, and intermediate- and high-grade astrocytomas that were negative for AFP and had negative CSF cytology. Close follow-up is imperative for the detection of recurrence and dissemination following radiation therapy. Five-year survival for germinoma treated with focal external radiation therapy (XRT) is greater than 85 per cent.[4, 33] Craniospinal radiation is not indicated for focal germinoma. Chemotherapy is extremely effective for disseminated germinoma. The effectiveness of chemotherapy

TABLE 34–4. TREATMENT PLAN FOR PINEAL REGION MASSES IN CHILDREN

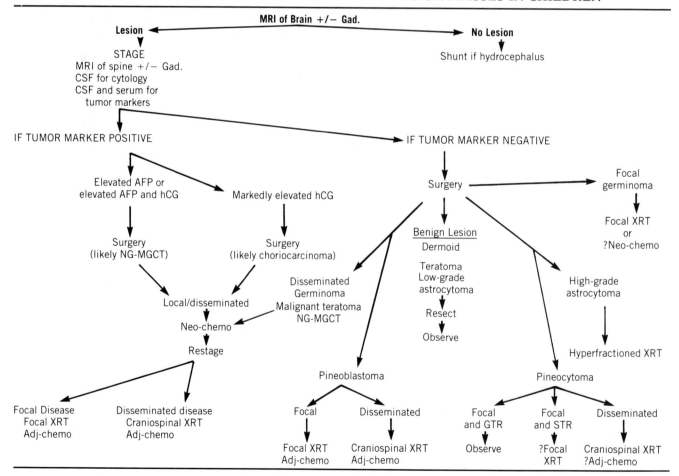

Gad. = Gadolinium DTPA; Neo-chemo = neoadjuvant chemotherapy; Adj-chemo = adjuvant chemotherapy; MRI = magnetic resonance imaging; CSF = cerebrospinal fluid; AFP = alpha-fetoprotein; hCG = human chorionic gonadotropin; NG-MGCT = nongerminoma malignant germ cell tumor; XRT = external radiation therapy; GTR = gross total resection; STR = subtotal resection.

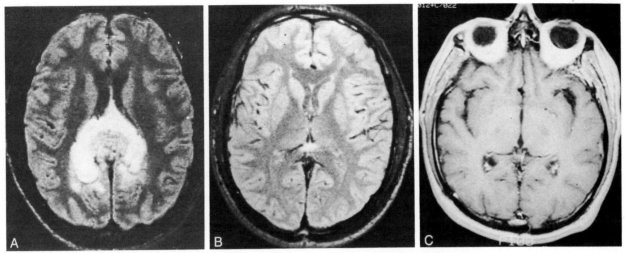

FIGURE 34–3. Gadolinium-enhanced, T1-weighted, axial MR images immediately preoperatively *(A)*, following two cycles of neoadjuvant chemotherapy *(B)*, and 3 years after operation *(C)*. Note mixed choriocarcinoma/embryonal cell carcinoma. The patient was treated with biopsy and neoadjuvant chemotherapy—eight cycles) followed by focal consolidation radiation therapy. Note the rapid response to chemotherapy.

as the only treatment for focal germinoma, obviating radiation therapy, is an interesting but unproven therapy currently in the early stages of testing (L Sutter, personal communication). Pineal region moderately anaplastic astrocytomas respond both clinically and radiographically following focal radiation therapy in more than 80 per cent of cases,[4] but long-term data are not yet available. The clinical course of pineocytomas and pineoblastomas and their response to radiation and chemotherapy are variable but generally poor.[4, 49]

Disseminated pineocytoma and pineoblastoma are treated with craniospinal XRT and adjuvant chemotherapy, but results are poor.[4, 49]

The UCSF experience in treating NG-MGCT with craniospinal radiation followed by chemotherapy was disappointing, with durable remissions in only one of eight treated patients. Results have been significantly improved by using neoadjuvant (induction) multi-drug chemotherapy (VBPE: vinblastine, bleomycin, cisplatin, etoposide) for NG-MGCT and disseminated germinoma (Fig. 34–3). Marked reduction of tumor bulk was observed on MR image by the second cycle of chemotherapy (6 weeks). Patients were treated with up to eight cycles of chemotherapy and then restaged. Radiation therapy (consolidation therapy) was given focally for residual local disease and craniospinal radiation administered only if there was evidence of disseminated disease at the completion of chemotherapy. Six of 10 patients treated on this protocol achieved prolonged tumor-free survival (median greater than 3 years).[50] Other investigators have also reported improved response and survival with NG-MGCT and disseminated germinoma using neoadjuvant chemotherapy protocols.[51, 52] We are currently treating choriocarcinoma with this protocol.

In patients with recurrent disease or tumors refractory to induction chemotherapy, a variety of methods to increase drug delivery are under investigation. Experience in three patients with recurrent disseminated intracranial germinoma who initially responded to systemic chemotherapy aided by mannitol blood-brain barrier disruption at recurrence have been encouraging. All three patients are alive 15 to 30 months after therapy (E. Neuwelt, personal communication). The use of high-dose chemotherapy with bone marrow rescue is also under investigation.

CONCLUSIONS

Tissue diagnosis is necessary for optimal treatment of pineal region tumors in children. Preoperative staging should include craniospinal MR imaging with and without gadolinium, CSF for cytology, and serum and CSF measurement of biologic tumor markers. The surgical approach is determined by preoperative MR imaging, and the extent of resection by the results of staging and intraoperative frozen section histopathology. There is no longer a role for the radiation test dose (2000 cGy) in the management of these tumors. Postoperative treatment is based on histopathology and extent of disease. Benign tumors are treated with surgery only, and nondisseminating focal tumors with surgery and focal radiation therapy. NG-MGCT are best treated with neoadjuvant chemotherapy followed by focal radiation therapy, which is for focal disease; craniospinal radiation therapy is reserved for disease that remains disseminated at the completion of induction chemotherapy.

REFERENCES

1. Russell DS, Rubinstein LJ: Pathology of Tumours of the Nervous System. 4th ed. Baltimore, Williams & Wilkins, 1977, pp 284–295.

2. Hoffman HJ, Yoshida M, Becker LE, et al.: Experience with pineal region tumors in childhood. Experiences at the Hospital for Sick Children. *In* Humphreys RP (ed): Concepts in Pediatric Neurosurgery 4. Basel, S Karger, 1983, pp 360–386.

3. Bloom HJG: Primary intracranial germ cell tumors. Clin Oncol 2:233, 1983.

4. Edwards MSB, Hudgins RJ, Wilson CB: Pineal region tumors in children. J Neurosurg 68:689, 1988.

5. Ventureyra ECG: Pineal region: Surgical management of tumours and vascular malformations. Surg Neurol 16:77, 1981.

6. Tien RD, Barkovich AF, Edwards MSB: MR imaging of pineal tumors. Am J Neuroradiol 11:557, 1990.

7. Dearnaly DP, O'Hern RP, Whittaker S, et al.: Pineal and CNS germ cell tumors: Royal Marsden Hospital experience 1962–1987. Int J Radiat Oncol Biol Phys 18:773, 1990.

8. Abay EO, Laws ER, Grado GL, et al.: Pineal tumors in children and adolescents: Treatment by shunting and radiotherapy. J Neurosurg 55:889, 1981.

9. Vorkapic P, Waldhauser F, Bruckner R, et al.: Serum melatonin levels: A new neurodiagnostic tool in pineal region tumors? Neurosurgery 21:817, 1987.

10. Neuwelt EA, Glasberg M, Frenkel E, et al.: Malignant pineal region tumors. A clinico-pathological study. J Neurosurg 51:597, 1979.

11. Stein BM: The infratentorial supracerebellar approach to pineal lesions. J Neurosurg 35:197, 1971.

12. Van Wagenen WP: A surgical approach for removal of certain pineal tumors: Report of a case. Surg Gynecol Obstet 53:216, 1931.

13. Chapman PH, Linggood RM: The management of pineal area tumors: A recent reappraisal. Cancer 46:1253, 1980.

14. Jamieson KG: Excision of pineal tumors. J Neurosurg 35:550, 1971.

15. Packer RJ, Sutton LN, Rosenstock JG, et al.: Pineal region tumors of childhood. Pediatrics 74:97, 1984.

16. Stein BM: Surgical treatment of pineal tumors. Clin Neurosurg 26:490, 1979.

17. Suzuki J, Iwabuchi T: Surgical removal of pineal tumors (pinealomas and teratomas). Experience in a series of 19 cases. J Neurosurg 23:565, 1965.

18. Torkildsen A: Should extirpation be attempted in cases of neoplasms in or near the third ventricle of the brain. Experiences with a palliative method. J Neurosurg 5:269, 1948.

19. Preslock JP: The pineal gland: Basic implications and clinical correlations. Endocr Rev 5:282, 1984.

20. Descartes R: Les passions de L'ame. 1649.

21. Cuneo HM, Rand CW: Pinealoma. *In* Cuneo HM, Rand CW (eds): Brain Tumors of Childhood. Springfield, Charles C Thomas, 1952, pp 70–91.

22. Virchow R: Vorlesungen uber pathologie: Die krankhaften geschwulste. Berlin, August Hirschwalk, 1864–1865, p 148.

23. Camins MB, Schlesinger EB: Treatment of tumours of the posterior part of the third ventricle and the pineal region: A long term follow-up. Acta Neurochir (Wien) 40:131, 1978.

24. Oppenheim H, Krause F: Operative erfolge bei geschwulsten der serhugel und vierhugelgegend. Berl Klin Wochenschr 50:2316, 1913.

25. Puusep L: Die operative entfernung einer zyswte der glandual pinealis. Neurol Centrabl 33:560, 1914.

26. Dandy WE: An operation for the removal of pineal tumors. Surg Gynecol Obstet 33:113, 1921.

27. Dandy WE: Operative experience in cases of pineal tumor. Arch Surg 33:19, 1936.

28. Kahn E: Surgical treatment of pineal tumors. Arch Neurol Psychiatr 38:833, 1937.

29. Russell WO, Sachs E: Pinealoma: A clinicopathologic study of seven cases with a review of the literature. Arch Pathol 35:869, 1943.

30. Cushing H: Pinealomas. *In* Intracranial Tumors. Notes Upon a Series of Two-Thousand Verified Cases with Surgical-Mortality Percentages Pertaining Thereto. Springfield, Ill, Charles C Thomas, 1932, pp 62–65.

31. Poppen JL: The right occipital approach to a pinealoma. J Neurosurg 25:706, 1966.

32. Krause F: Operative freilegugn der vierhugel, nebst beobachtungen uber hirndruck und dekopression. Zentraltbl Chir 53:2812, 1926.

33. Hoffman HJ, Otsubo H, Hendrick EB, et al.: Intracranial germ-cell tumors in children. J Neurosurg 74:545, 1991.

34. Hoffman HJ, Yoshida M, Becker LE, et al.: Experience with pineal region tumours in childhood. Neurol Res 6:107, 1984.

35. Stein BM: The suboccipital, supracerebellar approach to the pineal region. *In* Neuwelt EA (ed): Diagnosis and Treatment of Pineal Region Tumors. Baltimore, William & Wilkins, 1984, pp 213–222.

36. Huebner O: Tumor der glandula pinealis. Dtsch Med Wochenschr 24:214, 1898.

37. Cohen AR, Wilson JA, Sadeghi-Nejad A: Gonadotropin-secreting pineal teratoma causing precocious puberty. Neurosurgery 28:597, 1991.

38. Allen JC, Nisselbaum J, Epstein F, et al.: Alphafetoprotein and human chorionic gonadotropin determination in cerebrospinal fluid. An aid to the diagnosis and management of intracranial germ-cell tumors. J Neurosurg 51:368, 1979.

39. Shinoda J, Yamada H, Sakai N, et al.: Placental alkaline phosphatase as a tumor marker for primary intracranial germinoma. J Neurosurg 68:710, 1988.

40. Washiyama K, Houno M, Tanaka R: Placental alkaline phosphatase in cerebrospinal fluid of 26 patients with primary intracranial germ cell tumors [Abstract 28]. *In* Program and Abstracts of the Fourth International Symposium on Pediatric Neuro-Oncology. Tokyo, 1991, p 84.

41. Barber SG, Smith JA, Hughes RC: Melatonin as a tumour marker in a patient with pineal tumour. Br Med J 2:328, 1978.

42. Marton LJ, Edwards MSB, Levin VA, et al.: CSF polyamines: a new and important means of monitoring patients with medulloblastoma. Cancer 47:757, 1981.

43. Phillips PC, Kremzner LT, De Vivo DC: Cerebrospinal fluid polyamines: Biochemical markers of malignant childhood brain tumors. Ann Neurol 19:360, 1986.

44. Galassi E, Tognetti F, Frank F, et al.: Extraneural metastases from primary pineal tumors. Review of the literature. Surg Neurol 21:497, 1984.

45. Watterson J, Priest JR: Control of extraneural metastasis of a primary intracranial nongerminomatous germ-cell tumor. J Neurosurg 71:601, 1989.

46. Berger MS, Baumeister B, Geyer JR, et al.: The risks of metastases from shunting in children with primary central nervous system tumors. J Neurosurg 74:872, 1991.

47. Lapras C, Patet JD: Controversies, techniques and strategies for pineal tumor surgery. *In* Apuzzo MLJ (ed): Surgery of the Third Ventricle. Baltimore, Williams & Wilkins, 1987, pp 649–662.

48. Luo SQ, Li DZ, Zhang MZ, et al.: Occipital transtentorial approach for removal of pineal region tumors: Report of 64 consecutive cases. Surg Neurol 32:369, 1989.

49. D'Andrea AD, Packer RJ, Rorke LB, et al.: Pineocytomas of childhood. A reappraisal of natural history and response to therapy. Cancer 59:1353, 1987.

50. Edwards MSB, Ablin A, Wara W, et al.: Modern management of pineal-region tumors in children [Abstract 69]. *In* Program and Abstracts of the Fourth International Symposium of Pediatric Neuro-Oncology. Tokyo, 1991, p 85.

51. Allen JC, Kim JH, Packer RJ: Neoadjuvant chemotherapy for newly diagnosed germ-cell tumors of the central nervous system. J Neurosurg 67:65, 1987.

52. Kirkove CS, Brown AP, Symon L: Successful treatment of a pineal endodermal sinus tumor. Case report. J Neurosurg 74:832, 1991.

Chapter 35

TUMORS OF THE SKULL AND METASTATIC BRAIN TUMORS

TAE SUNG PARK, M.D., and BRUCE A. KAUFMAN, M.D.

Most pediatric skull lesions present as a mere "lump" or "bump" or after incidental discovery on a skull radiograph. Establishing the diagnosis often requires biopsy or excision of the lesion. The lesions are usually benign with respect to their potential for growth or risk of complications, but some have the potential for intracranial extension or have systemic manifestations. The most frequent lesions will be individually reviewed, and the less common ones summarized. Tumors metastatic to the brain are exceedingly rare and will be reviewed in the final section.

PRESENTATION AND EPIDEMIOLOGY

Many of the "lumps" will be discovered after minor and incidental trauma, but the two most common posttraumatic diagnoses follow an obvious injury. A calcified cephalohematoma can develop after birth trauma in the neonate, although this diagnosis accounted for 9 per cent of the "nontraumatic" lesions in one series.[1] The "growing fracture" occurs primarily in children less than 3 years old who sustain a linear skull fracture. Although unusual, it may develop in older children and adults and has even been reported in a neonate at birth.[2] The incidence of growing fractures, estimated to be about 1 per cent of all infant skull fractures, suggests that infants with skull fractures should routinely undergo follow-up for 3 to 6 months.[3]

Most of the nontraumatic lesions are benign processes (90 per cent according to Choux et al.,[4] and 75 per cent according to Ruge et al.[1]). The most common are epidermoid or dermoid cysts, accounting for between 30 and 60 per cent of all the lesions; of the two, epidermoids are much more frequent. Histiocytosis X lesions are the next most common (7 to 16 per cent). Occult dysraphic states (meningocele, encephalocele),

fibrous dysplasia, hemangiomas, and hamartomas each represent approximately 3 per cent of the total. True benign neoplasms of the skull, such as the osteoma, are rare. Primary malignant neoplasms, such as osteogenic sarcoma, are even more infrequent.

DIAGNOSTIC EVALUATION

The evaluation of both skull and intracranial lesions has paralleled advances in neuro-imaging. Angiography is rarely necessary. Although the plain radiograph remains helpful, computed tomography (CT) often gives more information on the extent of bone involved and the precise contours of a bony defect. Because of the lack of signal from bone, magnetic resonance imaging (MRI) is less helpful with isolated calvarial lesions, but is unsurpassed in defining any intracranial involvement. Since the more frequent lesions can have similar radiographic appearances, excisional biopsy of skull lesions is often the final diagnostic test and the definitive therapeutic maneuver.

For skull lesions, the radiographic evaluation will frequently begin with a plain radiograph, but the principles involved apply equally to the interpretation of CT scans.[5] The border of the lesion with the skull, or "zone of transition," should be analyzed first. With a zone of transition less than 3 to 5 mm on all borders, the lesion is likely to be a slow-growing one. Although a wide zone of transition would suggest a malignant tumor, this could also occur in an infectious or inflammatory process. Conversely, a narrow zone of transition can persist with malignant degeneration of a previously benign lesion.

The margin of the lesion should be assessed for sclerosis. Slow-growing lesions allow time for the surrounding bone to re-form, as with epidermoid or dermoid cysts. Faster-growing lesions, such as eosinophilic granuloma, do not allow for new bone formation at the margin.

The differential erosion of the inner or outer table of the skull can give some indication of the origin of the lesion. For example, eosinophilic granulomas and dermoids of the anterior fontanelle arise outside the calvarium and show more scalloping of the outer table. An enlarging arachnoid cyst or pacchionian granulation will preferentially remodel the inner table.

The use of CT versus MRI depends on the need to assess the intracranial compartment. In most lesions, CT gives an adequate definition of the underlying brain, but yields much more information on the extent of bone involvement.[6] CT with three-dimensional reconstruction can be helpful in defining those lesions involving the base of the skull and the orbit. MRI would be preferable in those cases in which high intracranial definition is needed, as is the case with suspected dermal sinus tracts, in defining direct extension of malignant tumors or suspected metastatic disease, and in the staging of histiocytosis X (Fig. 35–1).

TRAUMATIC SKULL LESIONS

CALCIFIED CEPHALOHEMATOMA

Subperiosteal hematoma in the neonate occurs most frequently in the parietal region, with its spread limited by cranial suture lines. Calcification beneath the elevated periosteum can begin within several weeks but usually resolves as the skull grows and remodels. In older lesions, diploic bone may develop between the outer table and the elevated periosteum.[7] Those that persist present as a nontender, firm, rounded, nonmobile mass. Plain radiographs may resemble fibrous dysplasia or meningiomas involving the skull. Treatment is unnecessary, but may be rendered for cosmetic reasons and involves reshaping of the calcified mass.

GROWING FRACTURES (LEPTOMENINGEAL CYSTS)

The pathophysiologic properties that lead to the enlargement of a skull fracture have been debated, but laceration of the dura at the site of injury appears to be a prerequisite. Pulsatile pressure, from an outpouching of arachnoid or underlying brain, gradually remodels the skull and enlarges the opening.[8] There may be primary injury to the underlying brain, with encephalomalacia and cyst formation, or injury secondary to herniation of cerebral tissue through the defect. Dysfunction of the underlying brain or the delayed onset of seizure activity may result. The growing fracture need not have a cyst associated with it, and when studied pathologically, many cysts do not have leptomeningeal elements.[9, 10]

Skull radiographs of growing fractures reveal an irregular, elliptical defect in the skull (Fig. 35–2). En-

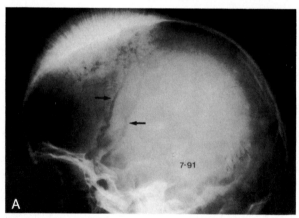
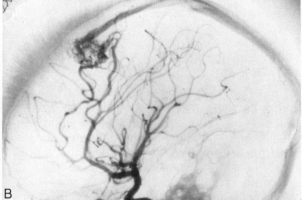
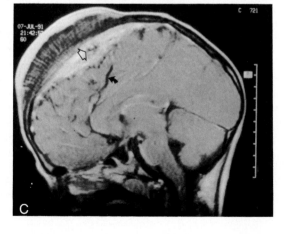

FIGURE 35–1. Meningioma. This ten-year-old boy presented with a large, nonmobile, nontender frontal calvarial mass and was neurologically normal. At surgery, the tumor was found to be invading the scalp and posterior sagittal sinus. *A,* The calvarial changes are obvious in this advanced case, with marked spiculation and thickening of bone and enlarged vascular grooves *(arrows).* *B,* Angiography documents the proximal occlusion of the sagittal sinus and an arteriovenous connection from the anterior cerebral artery into the sagittal sinus. *C,* MRI (TE 800, TR 22, 1.5 T, post Gd-DPTA). The sagittal image clearly defines the significant posterior extent of the tumor. The flow void of the large feeding vessel from the anterior cerebral artery *(curved arrow)* and the arteriovenous shunt *(hollow arrow)* are also seen. Coronal imaging (not shown) clearly demonstrated the lateral extent of the tumor.

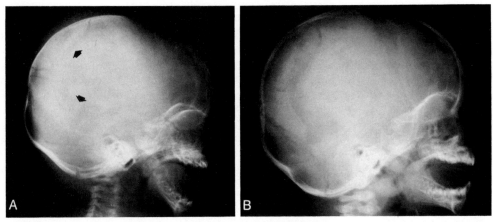

FIGURE 35–2. Growing skull fracture. *A*, Two-month-old child with posterior parietal comminuted skull fracture *(arrows)*. The inferior fracture line is poorly seen. *B*, Five months after injury the fractures have enlarged throughout their extent, with smooth remodeling of the margins.

largement of the fracture may be obvious if radiographs are compared to those from the time of the original injury. The bony margins are often sclerotic, and the edges scalloped, with the inner table eroded more than the outer table.[9, 10] A CT scan shows the bony defect and adequately identifies any underlying cerebral injury or herniation of tissue through the defect.[10]

Treatment requires operative exposure and closure of the dural defect. Frequently, the dural defect is larger than the calvarial defect, and the bone edges must be removed to expose the dura. If the cranial defect is large, autologous bone (e.g., split-thickness calvarium) can be used to perform a simultaneous cranioplasty.

CONGENITAL SKULL LESIONS

EPIDERMOID AND DERMOID TUMORS OF SKULL

Epidermoid and dermoid tumors are rare relative to all skull and brain tumors (epidermoid 0.3 to 1.8 per cent, dermoid 0.04 to 0.7 per cent).[11] Cranial dermoids are usually found around the orbits, around the anterior fontanelle, and along cranial sutures.[1] These tumors are cysts, with stratified keratinizing squamous epithelium forming the capsule of epidermoids, and additional dermal appendages such as hair follicles and sebaceous glands included in the wall of dermoids. These cysts are felt to arise from the ectopic inclusion of ectodermal elements during the later stages of neurulation and cranial development.

The tumor typically presents as a painless swelling in the subcutaneous tissue, covered with normal skin and fixed to the underlying tissue. Although usually small, these tumors can achieve a large size. Those arising in the orbit may also present with exophthalmos. The cysts will more frequently involve the outer table (87 per cent) but may erode both tables (56 per cent).[11]

The typical radiograph shows a rounded erosion of the bone with well-defined sclerotic margins (Fig. 35–

3). On CT scanning, the lesion is usually hypodense, but it can be isodense and have capsular calcification or enhancement.[11] There may be an increased T2 signal on MRI.[5] Any cutaneous stigmata suggesting intracranial involvement, such as a sinus tract, can be evaluated with either CT or MRI. Complete surgical excision of the capsule results in cure.

FIBROUS DYSPLASIA

In fibrous dysplasia, normal bone is replaced by fibrous tissue, composed of fibroblasts and collagen fiber bundles interspersed with trabeculae of immature bone.[12] This lesion is not hereditary and probably represents a developmental defect of mesenchymal tissue. It is usually detected in the first few decades of life and is most active during periods of bone growth and during puberty. Although progression usually ceases after puberty, continued growth into adulthood does occur.[13]

One bone is involved in 70 per cent of the cases

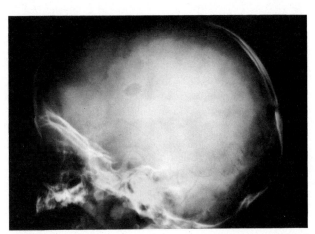

FIGURE 35–3. Epidermoid of skull. This epidermoid cyst has the typical appearance, a lytic lesion with sclerotic margins. Tangential views (not shown) revealed that only the outer table was involved.

(monostotic form), with cranial involvement in 10 to 27 per cent of these. The polyostotic form typically has an earlier age of onset, may be more quickly progressive, and has cranial involvement in 50 per cent of the cases.[14] When cutaneous pigmented lesions ("cafe au lait" spots) and endocrine dysfunction accompany the polyostotic form, it is termed Albright's syndrome.

The radiographic appearance varies depending on the amount of bone within the lesion. The more fibrous lesions may be radiolucent or have the more common ground-glass appearance, while the ossified lesions are sclerotic.[13, 15] The sclerotic form in the cranium usually involves the sphenoid bone or frontotemporal region. Growth can lead to facial disfigurement or compression of cranial nerves exiting their foramina.[14] Computed tomography is very good at defining the margins of the bony lesion, and with the increasing availability of three-dimensional reconstruction techniques, it is valuable in planning surgical and craniofacial procedures[15] (Fig. 35–4). CT can also help to differentiate these lesions from a meningioma or an expanding plexiform neurofibroma.

Surgery can be curative if the lesion can be completely excised, but the frequent involvement of the orbit and skull base often precludes total removal or requires extensive craniofacial procedures.[16] When cranial nerves are compressed or endangered, as with op-

tic canal compression, surgical debulking should be considered. Surgical remodeling of the bone may be performed in nonprogressing lesions in adults for cosmetic reasons.[17]

These lesions can undergo malignant degeneration into sarcomas, with osteogenic sarcoma being the most common type. The incidence of spontaneous degeneration has been estimated at 0.5 per cent, more commonly in the polyostotic form.[12] Radiation therapy used to treat the lesion primarily may increase the risk of malignant transformation to as much as 44 per cent.[18] The time to degeneration is variable, from several years to several decades, and the most frequent site of degeneration is the skull or femur.

NEUROFIBROMATOSIS

Less than 1 per cent of patients with neurofibromatosis (von Recklinghausen's disease) are found to have a congenital absence of the membranous portions of the sphenoid and adjacent bones. A progressive widening of the superior orbital fissure results in a large defect in the posterior superior portion of the orbit, ultimately causing a pulsatile exophthalmos with progressive proptosis. This condition must be distinguished from an exophthalmos resulting from a neurofibroma

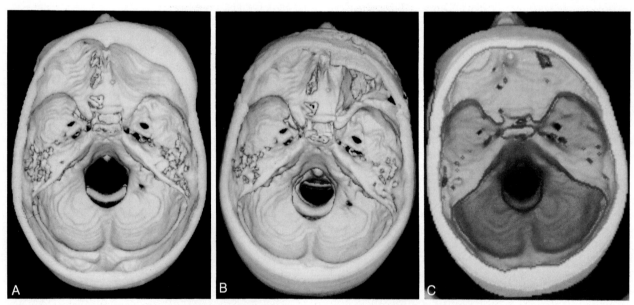

FIGURE 35–4. Fibrous dysplasia—three-dimensional CT reconstructions. *A,* Preoperative three-dimensional osseous surface CT reformation (method Vannier-Marsh*) of a 13-year-old boy with fibrous dysplasia affecting the right orbit, ethmoids, and frontal bone. The protrusion of the right frontal bone and thickening of the calvaria are evident. *Method is described in Marsh JL. Vannier MW: Three dimensional surface imaging from CT scans for the study of craniofacial dysmorphology. J Craniofac Genet Delev Biol 9:61, 1989.) *B,* One week following resection of the involved bone and reconstruction of the frontal bone and orbital roof with autologous split calvaria. The involved resected bone was discarded. *C,* Four years postoperatively, integration of the autogenous calvarial grafts into the calvaria and orbital roof is demonstrated.

(This case was provided by Dr. Jeffrey L. Marsh, Cleft Palate and Craniofacial Deformities Institute, St. Louis Children's Hospital, Washington University Medical Center, St. Louis, Missouri. The three-dimensional osseous CT reformations were produced in the Digital Imaging Laboratory, Mallinckrodt Institute of Radiology, St. Louis, Missouri, directed by Dr. Michael W. Vannier.)

of the trigeminal nerve or an enlarging optic glioma, both of which can occur in these patients.

Radiographically, the orbit appears "empty," because of the absence of sphenoid bone.[19] Again, CT scanning can define the margins of bony loss and the herniation of intracranial contents into the orbit. A collection of cerebrospinal fluid is frequently found over the temporal lobe.

Extracranial surgery to provide cosmetic changes has been done in the past. By the use of techniques of craniofacial reconstruction, however, reconstruction of the cranial vault and orbit with dural repair can be accomplished via an intracranial and mostly extradural approach.[20]

OTHER CONGENITAL LESIONS

Pacchionian granulations, particularly when they are large, can create defects in the overlying calvarium. These can be seen as small lucent areas on plain radiographs, often multiple and clustered around the sagittal sinus. The inner table and diploe are thinned or absent. No intervention is needed for these nonpathologic findings.

Parietal foramina, defects in the parietal bones just anterior to the lambdoid sutures, normally occur in pairs on either side of the sagittal suture, but can be unilateral. They have been seen in up to 60 per cent of the adult population and are usually no larger than a few millimeters in diameter, often with an emissary vein passing to the calvarium.[21] They can attain a very large size and may require a cranioplasty for cerebral protection. The smaller foramina require no treatment. However, the defect identified on radiographs must be distinguished from lesions that should be excised, i.e., histiocytosis X and epidermoid cysts.

Sinus pericranii represent an abnormal communication between the intracranial venous sinuses and extracranial venous cysts. These infrequent cysts are usually identified in the first three decades of life, but can present at any age. They are usually painless fluctuant masses.[22] They reduce in size and turgor with any decrease in venous pressure, as when the patient is standing, but a Valsalva maneuver or holding the head in a dependent position would increase venous pressure and increase the apparent size of the lesion.

Plain radiographs will reveal thinning of the bone, with a lucency at the site of communicating veins. CT scanning shows a soft tissue density that will enhance with intravenous contrast.[23] MRI can be expected to show some flow void in the defect, although turbulent flow may yield mixed signals, and intravenous gadolinium may give enhancement.[23] Where the defect in bone is larger, the differential diagnosis for these lesions would include meningoceles, dermoids, and eosinophilic granulomas.

Surgical excision is indicated to avoid gradual enlargement or accidental trauma resulting in bleeding. There are usually multiple channels through the skull that must be carefully occluded as the mass is reflected off the skull.

Aplasia cutis congenita, the congenital absence of skin and skin appendages, can occur anywhere on the body. Those lesions on the scalp are usually solitary, but 20 per cent will have a concurrent defect in the skull.[21] The dura may also be absent, leaving the arachnoid and brain exposed at the base of the lesion. The lesion is often found along suture lines, frequently at the vertex near midline.

Although many other congenital anomalies have been associated with aplasia cutis congenita, affected children may have normal findings on neurologic examination and normal development. Aplasia cutis congenita appears to occur spontaneously, but there is a form with autosomal dominance with incomplete penetrance and variable expression.[21] Teratogens have not been excluded as potential causes.

Clinical examination may be sufficient to plan treatment, as the absence of tissue is quite apparent. MRI can delineate abnormalities in the underlying brain. Since these lesions do not close spontaneously, reconstructive surgery to establish dermal closure is necessary, and cranioplasty with bone grafting may be necessary. Potential complications in this condition and its treatment include infection and hemorrhage from, or thrombosis of, the exposed sagittal sinus.

LYMPHOPROLIFERATIVE DISEASE

HISTIOCYTOSIS X

Histiocytosis X refers to a continuum of disease in which a proliferation of reticuloendothelial cells forms granulomatous lesions. At one end of the spectrum is diffuse systemic involvement (Letterer-Siwe disease), usually affecting young children and frequently progressive and fatal. At the other end are patients with a solitary granulomatous lesion (eosinophilic granuloma). Cases of cranial involvement, exophthalmos, and diabetes insipidus (Hand-Schüller-Christian disease) are intermediate. The constant feature among these states is the presence of Langerhans' histiocytes—hence the now preferred name Langerhans' cell histiocytosis. This group of diseases probably represents a disturbance of immunologic function, rather than a true neoplasm.

In all patients with histiocytosis X, there is a high incidence of head and neck lesions (83 per cent), with calvarial lesions the most common.[24] The calvarial lesions, slightly more common in the parietal and frontal regions, present as localized painful swellings that are immobile.[25] They appear "punched out" without sclerosis on plain radiographs, with a sharp demarcation and beveling of the adjacent skull (Fig. 35–5). The lesions do not invade the scalp, and although they frequently extend to the dura, intracranial extension is rare. After diagnosis, evaluation for additional intracranial disease should be undertaken.[26]

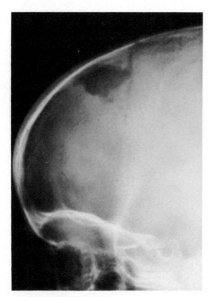

FIGURE 35–5. Eosinophilic granuloma. A lytic lesion of eosinophilic granuloma without a sclerotic margin is clearly seen (compare with Fig. 35–3).

The possibility of disseminated lesions requires the accurate diagnosis obtainable only with surgical excision. For skull lesions this is usually an excisional biopsy, using curettage for complete removal. If the diagnosis is confirmed, further evaluation is necessary to define the extent of active disease. This would include measurement of hematologic, immunologic, and liver functions, a skeletal survey (more sensitive than nuclear bone scan), a chest radiograph, and a careful examination for skin lesions. If any hematologic abnormalities are discovered, a bone marrow biopsy is necessary.

Multiple lesions can be treated with low-dose radiation (300 to 1000 rads), and multifocal disease requires chemotherapy. Disseminated disease is frequently fatal despite therapy. After surgical excision of a solitary lesion, continued follow-up is necessary, since up to one third of patients can later develop a new lesion after several years, particularly children less than 5 years of age.[25]

Leukemia involving the skull is much less frequent than leptomeningeal or cerebral infiltration. There can be multiple, poorly defined lucent areas, similar to neuroblastoma.

NEOPLASMS OF SKULL

Hemangiomas account for 3 to 5 per cent of calvarial masses.[1, 4] Usually seen in older children and adults, and most frequently located in the parietal region, they can be hard and painful. Pathologically, they are cavernous angiomas growing within the diploë. Forming a predominantly lytic lesion on plain radiographs, they have a classic "sunburst" appearance due to radiating bony spicules, a finding that may be more clearly developed in the older patient (Fig. 35–6).[27] Excision or curettage is usually curative.

Osteoma of the skull is uncommon (2/106 in combined series from Choux et al.[4] and Ruge et al.[1]). It presents as a firm nontender mass when arising from the calvarium or by causing painful sinus obstruction when in the paranasal sinuses. With routine radiography it is dense with sharp demarcation.[7] The smaller lesions can be ground down, whereas the larger ones may need resection and cranioplasty.

Aneurysmal bone cysts occur mainly in the long bones and spines of older children and adults, but rarely (3 to 6 per cent of all cysts) involve the calvarium.[27–29] Arising from within the diploë, symmetrical growth involves both tables of the skull.[30] In general, the plain radiographic appearance of aneurysmal bone cysts varies with the age of the lesion. Early, it is lytic; then multiple internal septa develop within a thin bony shell, and finally it becomes calcified.[31] CT reveals an enhancing multiloculated lesion with densities that reflect the varying amounts of fibrous tissue, bone, and vascular space.[32] Angiography in calvarial lesions rarely shows abnormal vascularity, but may be useful for preoperative embolization.[30, 32] Surgical excision is recommended because of the risk of extension or significant hemorrhage after incidental trauma.

Osteoblastoma is a rare skull tumor in young children. It may present as a tender or nontender mass, with a radiographic appearance that can vary from purely osteolytic to mixed with surrounding sclerosis.[33] Excision rather than simple curettage should be considered, as recurrence has been reported.[34]

Melanotic neuroectodermal tumor of infancy (progonoma) presents during the first year of life. It is thought to derive from neural crest cells.[35] In two thirds of cases, the tumor is located in the maxilla; in the remaining cases, tumor occurs in the skull, brain, and mandible. It simulates a malignant tumor with its rapid growth, but metastases are rare. On plain films and CT scans, there is marked spiculated bone formation. This can resemble osteogenic sarcoma.[36] The tumor can be completely cured with resection.[27]

Meningiomas are rare in children, and only a small fraction of these present as a primary skull mass. As in adults, they cause hyperostosis, and their treatment is total removal if possible.

Chondroma of the skull is rarely seen in the pediatric population and may be part of a generalized chrondromatosis (Ollier's disease). It occurs primarily at the skull base or paranasal sinuses.[37, 38] The tumors grow slowly and are usually confined by a capsule.[39] An attempt at surgical resection should be made, but location may make this impossible.

Chordomas rarely present in childhood; their incidence peaks between the third and sixth decades of life. In the pediatric patient the lesions are more commonly located in the skull base, and lower cranial nerve dysfunction and long tract signs are more frequent than in adults.[40] Metastases to the lung have also been reported more frequently in children.[40] CT will reveal bony de-

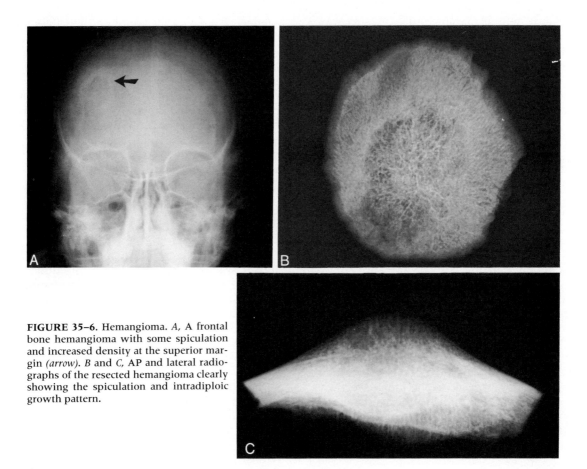

FIGURE 35–6. Hemangioma. *A,* A frontal bone hemangioma with some spiculation and increased density at the superior margin *(arrow). B* and *C,* AP and lateral radiographs of the resected hemangioma clearly showing the spiculation and intradiploic growth pattern.

struction and homogeneous enhancement, but MRI is much better at defining the tumor extent and extradural location. The location of this tumor makes complete surgical resection an extensive undertaking. The transoral approach, with or without mandibulotomy, has been reported with good results, but the patient must be followed for secondary instability of the upper cervical spine if it is not fused primarily.[41] Long-term survival for children with cranial chordomas treated with surgery and radiation approaches 50 per cent.[42] Residual disease can be treated with radiation therapy for control, but it is not curative.

Neuroblastoma, because of its relative frequency, is often seen metastatic to the facial bones, skull, and skull base. Skull metastases cause thickening of the bone with a "hair on end" appearance, due to spiculated bone within the lesion, and interspersed lytic areas (Fig. 35–7).[43]

Sarcomas involving the skull include rhabdomyosarcoma, osteogenic sarcoma, Ewing's sarcoma, fibrosarcoma, chondrosarcoma, and myxochondrosarcoma. *Osteogenic sarcoma* rarely presents as a primary skull tumor, but the incidence increases in the presence of fibrous dysplasia or Paget's disease, and after radiation therapy (as discussed earlier in this chapter).[6, 44] The primary lesions can vary from osteolytic to osteoblastic, but are typically lytic with a large zone of transition and no periosteal reaction. On MRI or CT, mineralization of tumor matrix in the presence of aggressive bony

destruction and soft tissue extension suggests the diagnosis.[44] Those tumors arising in areas of prior irradiation may be difficult to distinguish from radiation osteitis.[6] *Rhabdomyosarcomas* are the most common orbital neoplasm in children, but they also occur in the nasopharynx, paranasal sinuses, and middle ear. The incidence of direct meningeal extension has been reported to be as high as 35 per cent.[45] At presentation the CT

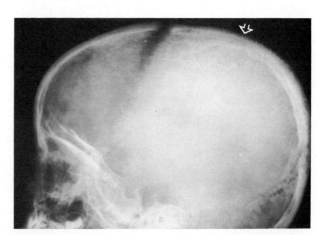

FIGURE 35–7. Neuroblastoma metastatic to skull. Extensive cranial involvement by metastatic neuroblastoma. The posterior parietal region shows multiple small lytic areas, with spiculation more apparent at the superior margin *(open arrow).* Splitting of the cranial sutures indicates associated increased intracranial pressure.

will show poorly defined margins and an extensive area of involvement.[46] *Ewing's sarcoma* accounts for 10 per cent of all primary bone tumors, but only 1 to 6 per cent of these sarcomas arise in the skull, usually on the frontal or parietal bone. It has also been reported to arise at the skull base in a child.[47] This tumor can also be metastatic to the skull.

METASTATIC BRAIN TUMORS

Only 6 to 12 per cent of children with malignant solid tumors will develop brain metastases, with the lower percentage occurring in the younger patients.[48–50] The tumors most frequently metastasizing are nephroblastoma (Wilms' tumor) and osteogenic and embryonal rhabdomyosarcoma.[48, 50] The propensity of each tumor type to metastasize varies considerably: Wilms' tumor, 13 per cent; osteogenic sarcoma, 8 to 14 per cent; rhabdomyosarcoma, 6 to 13 per cent; germ cell tumors, 50 per cent; neuroblastoma, 0 to 2.7 per cent. This correlates directly with each tumor's frequency of pulmonary metastasis; those with higher rates of pulmonary disease have higher rates of brain involvement. Neuroblastoma rarely spreads to the lung; direct invasion of the lung or penetration of the leptomeninges leads to brain metastasis in these patients. In general, brain metastasis has been reported to occur a median of 10 months after metastatic pulmonary disease is detected.[50]

The clinical presentation of a child with cerebral metastasis is somewhat different from that of an adult. The onset of symptoms is more abrupt, with acute or catastrophic neurologic symptoms in 20 per cent. These may be related to a relatively high rate of intratumoral hemorrhage. There is a higher incidence of seizures at initial presentation: 50 per cent in the group less than 15 years old.[50] Otherwise, symptoms and signs of increased intracranial pressure or focal deficits are noted.

The diagnostic evaluation and treatment approach is similar to that in adults. The survival of these children is seriously limited, however, probably because of the significant concurrent disseminated disease. With aggressive treatment, including surgery, radiation, and chemotherapy, extended survival has been reported.[51, 52]

Nephroblastoma, or *Wilms' tumor*, is one of the most common abdominal tumors of childhood, but frequently has pulmonary involvement at the time of diagnosis.[48, 53] Cerebral metastasis is present in up to 13 per cent of these patients at autopsy, but clinically it is much less frequently apparent.[48] The time from initial diagnosis to the discovery of cerebral metastasis has varied from 6 to 36 months.

Sarcoma patients can develop central nervous system metastasis, with a frequency of 7 per cent, and two thirds of these involve the brain.[49] Rhabdomyosarcoma and Ewing's sarcoma involve the lungs early and, as expected, have higher rates of cerebral metastasis. Recently, the more effective treatment of patients with

osteogenic sarcoma is extending their lives, permitting 45 per cent to develop pulmonary recurrences, and 13 per cent of those have brain disease. In these patients, the brain metastases are a very late sequela of their recurrent disease.[54]

Neuroblastoma is also one of the more frequently detected cerebral metastases, in spite of its low rate of metastasis, because it is the most common solid tumor in children. Metastasis to the brain is usually the result of direct extension from a contiguous involved structure, such as the spinal leptomeninges.[55]

CONCLUSIONS

Although the exact incidence of pediatric skull lesions is unknown, they are rather infrequent. The most common lesions are post-traumatic cephalohematomas and growing fractures, epidermoid cysts, and eosinophilic granulomas. Although plain radiographs and CT scans will help to distinguish between the more common lesions, biopsy is usually necessary. The pathologic finding will dictate the need for systemic evaluation, as with eosinophilic granuloma.

Metastatic tumors to the brain in children are rare, although with some tumor types the incidence may be as high as 12 per cent. The majority of children with cerebral metastasis will have pulmonary disease first or concurrently. The most common metastatic tumors are Wilms' tumor, embryonal rhabdomyosarcoma, osteogenic sarcoma, and neuroblastoma.

REFERENCES

1. Ruge JR, Tomita T, Naidich TP, et al.: Scalp and calvarial masses of infants and children. Neurosurgery 22:1037, 1988.
2. Moss SD, Walker ML, Ostergard S, et al.: Intrauterine growing skull fracture. Childs Nerv Syst 6:468, 1990.
3. Locatelli D, Messina AL, Bonfanti N, et al.: Growing fractures: An unusual complication of head injuries in pediatric patients. Neurochirurgia 32:101, 1989.
4. Choux M, Gomez A, Choux A, et al.: Diagnostic and therapeutic problems concerning tumors of the vault. Childs Brain 1:207, 1975.
5. Naidich TP: The neuro-imaging quiz. Pediatr Neurosci 13:223, 1987.
6. Lee YY, van Tassel P, Nauert C, et al.: Craniofacial osteosarcomas: Plain film, CT, and MR findings in 46 cases. AJR 150:1397, 1988.
7. Epstein JA, Epstein BS: Deformities of the skull surfaces in infancy and childhood. J Pediatr 70:636, 1967.
8. Scarfo GB, Mariottini A, Tomaccini D, et al.: Growing skull fractures: Progressive evolution of brain damage and effectiveness of surgical treatment. Childs Nerv Syst 5:163, 1989.
9. Lende RA, Erickson TC: Growing skull fractures of childhood. J Neurosurg 18:479, 1961.
10. Tandon PN, Banerji AK, Bhatia R, et al.: Cranio-cerebral erosion (growing fracture of the skull in children). Part II. Clinical and Radiological Observations. Acta Neurochir (Wien) 88:1, 1987.
11. Rubin G, Scienza R, Pasqualin A, et al.: Craniocerebral epidermoids and dermoids: A review of 44 cases. Acta Neurochir (Wien) 97:1, 1989.
12. Taconis WK: Osteosarcoma in fibrous dysplasia. Skeletal Radiol 17:163, 1988.
13. Davies ML, Macpherson P: Fibrous dysplasia of the skull: Disease activity in relation to age. Br J Radiol 64:576, 1991.

14. Sassin JF, Rosenberg RN: Neurological complications of fibrous dysplasia of the skull. Arch Neurol 18:363, 1968.
15. Mendelsohn DB, Hertzanu Y, Cohen M, et al.: Computed tomography of craniofacial fibrous dysplasia. J Comput Assist Tomogr 8(6):1062, 1984.
16. Chen YR, Noordhoff MS: Treatment of craniomaxillofacial fibrous dysplasia: How early and how extensive? Plast Reconstr Surg 86(5):835, 1990.
17. Munro IR: Discussion: Treatment of craniomaxillofacial fibrous dysplasia. How early and how extensive? Plast Reconstr Surg 86(5):843, 1990.
18. Slow IN, Stern D, Friedman EW: Osteogenic sarcoma arising in a preexisting fibrous dysplasia: Report of case. J Oral Surg 29:126, 1971.
19. Poole MD: Experiences in the surgical treatment of cranio-orbital neurofibromatosis. Br J Plast Surg 42:155, 1989.
20. Marchac D: Intracranial enlargement of the orbital cavity and palpebral remodeling for orbitopalpebral neurofibromatosis. Plast Reconstr Surg 73:534, 1984.
21. Kaplan SB, Kemp SS, Oh KS: Radiographic manifestations of congenital anomalies of the skull. Radiol Clin North Am 29(2):195, 1991.
22. Ohta T, Waga S, Handa H, et al.: Sinus pericranii. J Neurosurg 42:704, 1975.
23. Sadler LR, Tarr RW, Jungreis CA, et al.: Sinus pericranii: CT and MR findings. J Comput Assist Tomogr 14(1):124, 1990.
24. DiNardo LJ, Wetmore RF: Head and neck manifestations of histiocytosis X in children. Laryngoscope 99:721, 1989.
25. Rawlings CE, Wilkins RH: Solitary eosinophilic granuloma of the skull. Neurosurgery 15(2):155, 1984.
26. Moore JB, Kulkarni R, Crutcher DC, et al.: MRI in multifocal eosinophilic granuloma: Staging disease and monitoring response to therapy. Am J Pediatr Hematol Oncol 11(2):174, 1989.
27. Kozlowski K, Campbell J, McAlister W, et al.: Rare primary cranial vault and base of the skull tumors in children. Radiol Med 81:213, 1991.
28. Bilge T, Coban O, Ozden B, et al.: Aneurysmal bone cysts of the occipital bone. Surg Neurol 20:227, 1983.
29. Clavier E, Thiebot J, Godlewski J, et al.: Intracranial aneurysmal bone cyst: A rare CT appearance. Neuroradiology 30:269, 1988.
30. Luccarelli G, Fornari M, Savoiardo M: Ángiography and computerized tomography in the diagnosis of aneurysmal bone cyst of the skull. J Neurosurg 53:113, 1980.
31. Sherman RS, Soong KY: Aneurysmal bone cyst of temporal bone. Radiology 68:54, 1957.
32. Arthur RJ, Brunelle F: Computerized tomography in the evaluation of expansile lesions arising from the skull vault in childhood—a report of 5 cases. Pediatr Radiol 18:294, 1988.
33. Miyazaki S, Tsubokawa T, Katayama Y, et al.: Benign osteoblastoma of the temporal bone of an infant. Surg Neurol 27:277, 1987.
34. Cabezudo JM: Recurrent benign osteoblastoma of the parietal bone. (Letter) Neurosurgery 25:1012, 1989.
35. Walsh JW, Strand RD: Melanotic neuroectodermal tumors of the cranium in infancy. Childs Brain 9:329, 1982.
36. Jones HH, Parker BR, Ballerio CG, et al.: Case Report 617. Skeletal Radiol 19:527, 1990.
37. Wu WQ, Lapi A: Primary non-skeletal intracranial cartilaginous neoplasms: report of a chondroma and mesenchymal chondrosarcoma. J Neurol Neurosurg Psychiatry 33:469, 1970.
38. Bingas B: Tumours of the base of the skull. In Vinken PJ, Bruyn GW (eds): Handbook of Clinical Neurology, Vol 17. Amsterdam, North Holland Publishing, 1974, p 136.
39. Russell DS, Rubinstein LJ: Pathology of Tumours of the Nervous System. 5th ed. Baltimore, Williams & Wilkins, 1989, p 818.
40. Matsumoto J, Towbin RB, Ball WS: Cranial chordomas in infancy and childhood. A report of two cases and review of the literature. Pediatr Radiol 20:28, 1989.
41. Nagib MG, Wisiol ES, Simonton SC, et al.: Transoral labiomandibular approach to basiocciput chrodomas in childhood. Childs Nerv Syst 6:126, 1990.
42. Wold LE, Laws ER: Cranial chordomas in children and young adults. J Neurosurg 59:1043, 1983.
43. Zimmerman RA, Bilaniuk LT: CT of primary and secondary craniocerebral neuroblastoma. AJR 135:1239, 1980.
44. Kornreich L, Grunebaum M, Ziv N, et al.: Osteogenic sarcoma of the calvarium in children: CT manifestations. Neuroradiology 30:439, 1988.
45. Tefft M, Fernandez C, Donaldson M, et al.: Incidence of meningeal involvement by rhabdomyosarcoma of the head and neck in children: A report of the Intergroup Rhabdomyosarcoma Study (IRS). Cancer 42:253, 1978.
46. Scotti G, Harwood-Nash DC: Computed tomography of rhabdomyosarcomas of the skull base in children. J Comput Assist Tomogr 6:33, 1982.
47. Steinbok P, Flodmark O, Norman MG, et al.: Primary Ewing's sarcoma of the base of the skull. Neurosurgery 19:104, 1986.
48. Vannucci RC, Baten M: Cerebral metastatic disease in childhood. Neurology 24:981, 1974.
49. Kramer ED, Lewis D, Raney B, et al.: Neurologic complications in children with soft tissue and osseous sarcoma. Cancer 64:2600, 1989.
50. Graus F, Walker RW, Allen JC: Brain metastases in children. J Pediatr 103:558, 1983.
51. Deutsch M, Albo V, Wollman MR: Radiotherapy for cerebral metastases in children. Int J Rad Oncol Biol Phys 8:1441, 1982.
52. Takamiya Y, Toya S, Otani M, et al.: Wilms' tumor with intracranial metastases presenting with intracranial hemorrhage. Childs Nerv Syst 1:291, 1985.
53. Jaffe N: Metastases in malignant childhood tumors: The role of adjuvant therapy and the utility of multidisciplinary treatment. Semin Oncol 4:117, 1977.
54. Baram TZ, van Tassel P, Jaffe NA: Brain metastases in osteosarcoma: Incidence, clinical and neuroradiological findings and management options. J Neurol Oncol 6:47, 1988.
55. Dresler S, Harvey DG, Levisohn PM: Retroperitoneal neuroblastoma widely metastatic to the central nervous system. Ann Neurol 5:196, 1979.

Chapter 36

INTRAMEDULLARY TUMORS OF THE SPINAL CORD

FRED J. EPSTEIN, M.D., and JOHN RAGHEB, M.D.

Intramedullary spinal cord tumors are relatively uncommon neoplasms, accounting for only 6 per cent of central nervous system tumors of childhood.[1-6] They occur most frequently between the ages of 10 and 16 and are equally divided between the sexes. Because of the rarity of these tumors, individual neurosurgeons may have relatively little experience with surgical management and long-term follow-up of afflicted patients. For this reason, there has been little impetus to modify the traditional treatment of biopsy, dural decompression, and radiation therapy, despite the recognition that after a relatively short remission serious disability or death ensues.

Over the past several years, the senior author has operated on 156 intramedullary spinal cord tumors in children. In most cases, a gross total excision of the neoplasm was performed. It has become clear that this surgical philosophy is compatible with neurologic recovery and, in many cases, possible permanent cure. This chapter describes this large personal experience and includes references to older works that will further our understanding of these relatively uncommon tumors.

PATHOLOGY

Unlike adult intramedullary tumors, of which 50 per cent are ependymomas, approximately 58.7 per cent of pediatric intramedullary tumors are astrocytomas. Furthermore, in pediatric patients, "pure" intramedullary ependymomas represent only 28 per cent of all intramedullary lesions (excluding conus medullaris or filum terminale tumors that extend into the lumbar sacral subarachnoid space).

When evaluating intramedullary lesions in children, further diagnostic considerations include "cystic lesions" (hydromyelia, syringomyelia), which have a reported incidence of 4.7 per cent, and congenital tumors, with an incidence of 5.8 per cent. Additional lesions include metastatic medulloblastomas, among others (e.g., dermoid tumor, intramedullary lipoma).

There is a definite predisposition for the pediatric tumors to be rostrally located, compared with the adult tumors. A total of 46 per cent of pediatric intramedullary tumors are cervical and cervicothoracic, whereas in adults, only 28 per cent of these tumors occur in the cervical or cervicothoracic cord. Intramedullary tumors generally occupy many cord segments (average six), and rarely, the entire length of the spinal cord from the cervicomedullary junction to the conus medullaris is involved.

CLINICAL MANIFESTATIONS

Clinical symptoms are commonly present for months, or even years, prior to neurosurgical consultation. In some cases, the course may be punctuated by exacerbations and remissions that are possibly related to alterations in edema surrounding the neoplasm.[1, 2] On occasion, the onset of symptoms may be associated with a trivial spinal injury. It has been suggested that in rare cases, injury may precipitate peritumoral edema and may result in the relatively rapid progression of symptoms.[2, 7, 8]

In our experience, the most common early symptom was local pain along the spinal axis. Other symptoms included motor disturbance, radicular pain, paresthesia, dysesthesias, and, in rare instances, sphincter dysfunction.[9-12]

Weakness of the lower extremities was usually first manifested as an alteration of a previously normal gait. This was often extremely subtle and obvious only to the parent, who noted a tendency for the child to fall more frequently or to walk on the heels or the toes. In young children, there was commonly a history of being a "late walker," and in the youngest (younger than 2 years), there was often a history of motor regression (i.e., starting to crawl again instead of walking, or refusing to stand).

A total of 70 per cent of patients experienced severe pain along the spinal axis, which was secondary to distention of the dural tube and was most acute in the bony segments directly over the tumor. Characteristically, the pain was worse in the recumbent position, as venous congestion further distended the dural tube and resulted in typical night pains. It was common to discover that patients had a long-standing history of taking analgesics, including narcotics, after a nondiagnostic orthopedic evaluation.[1, 2, 9, 12, 13]

Radicular pain occurred in 10 per cent of patients and was usually limited to one or two cervical or lumbar dermatomes, similar to root pain from a variety of disease processes.[8]

Painful dysesthesias occurred in 10 per cent of patients and were generally described as painful hot or cold sensations in one or more extremities. In rare circumstances, this was the primary symptom and was not associated with objective signs of neurologic dysfunction.[1, 7, 14]

Paresthesias were occasionally associated with the dysesthetic pain, and both of these symptoms were more common with neoplasms in the cervical spinal cord than with those in the thoracic spinal cord.

Cervical Tumors

The most common early symptoms were nuchal pain and head tilt with torticollis. Mild upper extremity monoparesis was the next most common symptom and was often extremely subtle during the early stages of the illness. Very often, in young children, the first manifestation of weakness was switching "handedness" in right-handed and left-handed patients. Neoplasms in the caudal cervical spinal cord commonly caused weakness and atrophy of the intrinsic muscles of the hand, in contradistinction to tumors rostral to C5, which were less likely to cause significant weakness until relatively late in the clinical course. Interestingly, weakness of the lower extremities only evolved months or, rarely, 2 to 3 years after the first symptoms, and bowel and bladder dysfunction was rarely present at the time of primary diagnosis.[1, 2, 7–9, 15, 16]

Sensory abnormalities were generally limited to one upper extremity, and a discrete sensory level was only noted very late in the course of the disease, and then only in association with severe neurologic disability.[8, 9, 17]

In most patients, there was increased reflex activity in the lower extremities, with or without extensor plantar signs and clonus.

Thoracic Tumors

Mild scoliosis was the most common early sign of an intramedullary thoracic cord neoplasm. Pain and para-spinal muscle spasm commonly occurred before there were objective signs of neurologic dysfunction, and were commonly assumed to be secondary to the evolving scoliosis. Insidious progressive motor weakness in the lower extremities was first manifested by awkwardness and, only later, by frequent falls and an obvious limp. Early sensory abnormalities were uncommon, although dysesthesias and paresthesias were occasionally present. Increased reflexes and extensor plantar signs, with or without clonus, occurred relatively early in the neurologic course.

A presenting complaint of bowel and bladder dysfunction was most unusual and was diagnostic of neoplasm extending into the conus medullaris. In general, these symptoms evolved only late in the clinical course if the tumor was rostral to T10.[1, 2, 8, 9, 15, 16]

Hydrocephalus

Increased intracranial pressure may complicate the clinical manifestation of intramedullary tumors in as many as 12.5 per cent of patients. The computerized tomography (CT) scan may disclose a normal or markedly dilated ventricular system. Although the etiology of the increased pressure has not been established, some authors have noted a dense arachnoiditis at the outlets of the fourth ventricle, while others have maintained that the greatly elevated cerebrospinal fluid (CSF) protein level interferes with normal circulatory dynamics.[2, 15, 17]

Rarely, severely increased intracranial pressure in the absence of other neurologic signs may be the presenting sign of an intramedullary tumor. It must be suspected if the CSF protein level is markedly elevated in the absence of demonstrable intracranial pathology.

NEURODIAGNOSTIC STUDIES

Spinal cord tumors may be divided into two general categories: holocord and focal.

Holocord Astrocytomas

These neoplasms are almost invariably cystic, and the solid component of the neoplasm spans a variable length of the cord and is associated with huge, non-neoplastic rostral and caudal cysts that expand the central canal above and below the tumor.

Plain spinal x-ray films commonly disclose a diffusely widened spinal canal with relatively localized erosion or flattening of the pedicles. Whereas the former is secondary to long-standing expansion of the entire spinal cord, the latter occurs only adjacent to the solid component of the neoplasm.[1, 2, 15, 9–12]

Magnetic resonance (MR) scanning is now the diagnostic test of choice to image lesions of the spinal cord. MR provides exquisite anatomic detail of intramedullary spinal cord lesions without artifact from the surrounding bone. Solid and cystic components of intra-medullary tumors can be readily distinguished in most circumstances. Holocord tumors appear as areas of decreased signal on T_1-weighted MR within an expanded spinal canal with a variable pattern of enhancement (Figs. 36–1A-C, 36–2A,B). MR has almost entirely replaced myelography and has eliminated the confusion in distinguishing holocord tumors from hydromyelia in the presence of a widened spinal cord.

FOCAL TUMORS

Focal spinal cord neoplasms are generally 3 to 6 segments in length and are commonly associated with flattening of the pedicles immediately adjacent to the neoplasm on plain film. MR imaging readily visualizes focal areas of cord enlargement and differentiates cystic and solid components of the neoplasm.

TREATMENT

Elsberg[18] and Elsberg and Beer[19] first advocated radical removal of intramedullary tumors in classic reports in which a two-stage procedure was described. At the first surgery, a long, midline posterior myelotomy overlying the tumor was performed, following which the dura was not closed. One week later, the wound was reopened, and a large volume of tumor was extruded through the myelotomy, facilitating the establishment of a clear plane of cleavage and total tumor excision. Since that time, Elsberg's underlying thesis concerning the feasibility of total tumor removal has been established by many neurosurgeons, although utilization of the operating microscope and contemporary instrument systems has rendered a two-stage procedure unnecessary.

Surgical exploration is mandatory for any child with

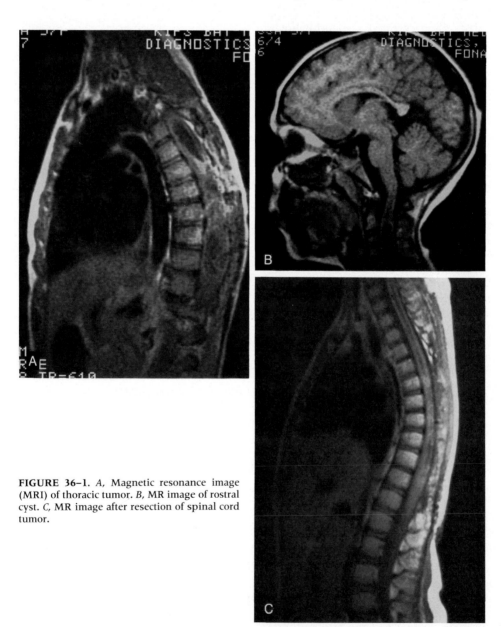

FIGURE 36–1. *A*, Magnetic resonance image (MRI) of thoracic tumor. *B*, MR image of rostral cyst. *C*, MR image after resection of spinal cord tumor.

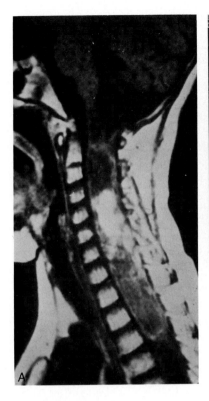
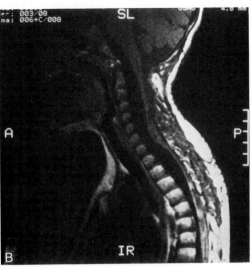

FIGURE 36–2. *A*, T_1-weighted MRI postgadolinium demonstrates a large focal cervicothoracic tumor with a rostral medullary cyst. *B*, MRI with gadolinium after gross total resection.

a progressively symptomatic intramedullary mass. There is no justification for giving radiation therapy without obtaining a definitive tissue diagnosis. Furthermore, in most situations, surgery should be directed toward total or radical removal of the tumor; there is no acceptable rationale for intending only to obtain a biopsy specimen and then "automatically" administering a full course of postoperative radiation therapy.

SURGERY

The contemporary neurosurgeon must have a clear understanding of the necessity of pursuing radical or even total excision when technically possible. Ependymomas are clearly demarcated from adjacent normal cord and, therefore, in most circumstances, may be totally extirpated. Astrocytomas have an interface between the tumor and the normal spinal cord that serves as a glia-tumor interface facilitating total removal.[10]

When dealing with an intramedullary congenital tumor (dermoid, epidermoid), it is safest to evacuate its contents while leaving intact the cyst wall, which is often inseparable from normal neural tissue.

It is desirable to carry out a limited laminectomy over the solid component of the neoplasm but not to unnecessarily extend it rostrally or caudally.

In our first surgical experience with "holocord" widening, a total laminectomy from C1 to T12 was carried out. It was subsequently recognized that it was not necessary to expose the spinal cord over the rostral and caudal cysts. For this reason, it was important to define

as accurately as possible the location of the solid component of the neoplasm vis-a-vis cysts.

Locating the solid component of the neoplasm has been greatly simplified by MR scanning with the addition of intravenous contrast. Occasionally, even with MR imaging, it may be impossible to locate the solid component of a holocord neoplasm, and in this situation, clinical findings may be helpful.

CLINICAL INDICATIONS OF TUMOR LOCATION IN THE PRESENCE OF HOLOCORD EXPANSION

In the presence of holocord widening associated with a cystic astrocytoma, it is the solid component of the neoplasm that is responsible for primary neurologic dysfunction, whereas the rostral and caudal cysts that expand the remainder of the spinal cord remain asymptomatic in the early stages of the disease.

Therefore, neurologic symptoms in one or both upper extremities in the presence of holocord widening suggests that the solid component of the neoplasm is within the cervical cord.

Conversely, progressive scoliosis, neurologic dysfunction, or both, limited to the lower extremities, are strongly suggestive of solid neoplasm within the thoracic cord, while bowel and bladder dysfunction indicate extension of the neoplasm into the conus medullaris.

In our experience, the presence of normal bowel and bladder function, and an expanded conus, are invariably associated with a cyst.

Spinal cord ependymomas do not adhere to this clinical pattern, as they may expand any length of the spinal cord, with a relative paucity of signs and symptoms referable to the segmental involvement. It is tempting to speculate that this is directly related to the primary anatomic location of the tumor in the region of the central canal, which causes very gradual compression of adjacent neural structures as the tumor increases in volume. This may be analogous to the rostral and caudal cystic components of the spinal cord astrocytomas, which are also in the region of the central canal and asymptomatic at the time of primary diagnosis. The origin of the solid component of the astrocytoma is probably relatively asymmetric and may cause symptoms as a result of both compression and infiltration of adjacent neural tissues.

SURGICAL INSTRUMENTATION

Spinal cord tumors are firm, often contain microscopic foci of calcium, and only rarely have a cleavage plane to facilitate an en bloc resection. In the majority of cases it is necessary to remove the tumor from inside out, until the almost invariably present glia-tumor interface is recognized as a change in color and consistency between the tumor and adjacent normal neural tissues.

In the past, neurosurgeons were limited to traditional suction-cautery techniques for removal of neoplasms. These techniques were often satisfactory for brain tumors; however, they were extremely hazardous with tumors of the spinal cord. This was because of the heat and movement transmitted through the tumor to the adjacent normal spinal cord, which was invariably firmly adherent to it. As a result of these technical limitations, there was a significant morbidity associated with intramedullary spinal cord surgery.

ULTRASONIC ASPIRATOR

The development and application of the Cavitron ultrasonic aspirator (CUSA) system was a significant improvement over the conventional systems and made a major contribution to spinal cord surgery.[9-12] It is important to describe briefly the CUSA in order to appreciate fully its impact on intramedullary spinal cord surgery.

The CUSA system incorporates three major systems at the handpiece to provide maximum efficiency in removing tissue. The three systems are:

1. Vibration. The surgical tip vibrates longitudinally, thereby fragmenting tissue in contact with its distal annular end. The level of vibration is adjustable.

2. Irrigation. Sterile irrigating solution is routed from an intravenous equipment source hanging from the console to the coaxial space between the outer surface of the surgical tip and the inner surface of the flue. The fluid exits near the tip, enters the operating field, and suspends the fragmented particles.

3. Suction. A suction pump contained in the console applies suction to the hollow surgical tip. Fluid and particulate matter are aspirated at the distal end of the tip and subsequently are deposited in a canister. The suction available at the tip is adjustable from 0 to 24 mm of mercury (0–24 mm Hg).

The ultrasonic dissecting system is capable of discrete removal of a broad range of tissue. It is important to emphasize that the primary value of ultrasonic dissection is the fragmentation of tissue by the vibrating tip of the handpiece. If it were possible to observe the operation of the instrument in slow motion, one would see the following: (1) tissue fragmentation within 1 mm of the vibrating tip, (2) suspension of fragmented tissue in the irrigation, (3) aspiration of the tissue-irrigation solution.

Because the suction removes an emulsion of tissue and irrigation solution, there is no movement of adjacent tissue. This is an important divergence from conventional suction-cautery technique in which there is a great deal of transmitted movement.

Laboratory studies of the CUSA system have demonstrated that normal electric conduction in neural tissue is maintained beyond a 1-mm radius of the vibrating instrument tip. For this reason, dissection with the ultrasonic instrument may be carried out immediately adjacent to vital structures with little attendant risk.[9-12]

LASER

The CUSA is the ideal instrument to rapidly debulk and remove all but residual fragments of spinal cord neoplasm. The neurosurgical laser is ideal for removing the residual fragments, as it may be employed with great precision along the length of the glia-tumor interface.

Although the laser may be employed in place of the CUSA, it is extremely tedious and time-consuming to use when the lesion is a voluminous intramedullary neoplasm. In addition, the resulting laser "char" makes it difficult to recognize the glia-tumor interface and mandates frequent interruptions of the ongoing dissection so that the blackened tissue can be gently removed with a small-caliber suction.

ULTRASONOGRAPHY

Ultrasound has become an essential adjunct in spinal cord tumor surgery. Ultrasonography prior to opening the dura is valuable in demonstrating adequate exposure of the expanded cord and in identifying the solid and cystic components of the tumor. Insight into the pathology of the lesion, which is important in planning surgical strategy, can be gleaned from the echo pattern of the tumor. Ependymomas usually appear as uniformly echogenic masses that are centrally located and symmetrically expand the spinal cord (Fig. 36–3). Astrocytomas and gangliogliomas have variable echo characteristics and can expand the cord asymmetrically. Ultrasound is also valuable in assessing the depth of

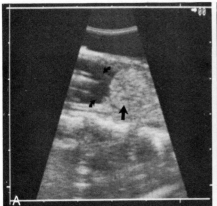
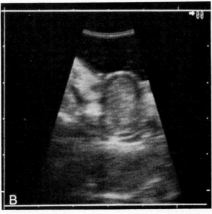
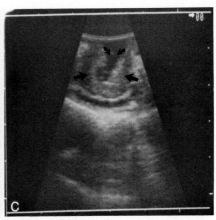

FIGURE 36–3. Intraoperative ultrasonography. *A*, Sagittal view prior to dural opening demonstrates solid tumor (large arrow) and polar cyst (small arrows). *B*, Transverse view. Solid tumor expands spinal cord and obliterates subarachnoid space. *C*, Transverse view, after resection. Note intramedullary cavity (curved arrows) and normal spinal cord (straight arrows).

resection vis-a-vis the anterior cord surface, in identifying and draining intratumoral cysts, and in identifying an enlarged ventral subarachnoid space. Occasionally, ultrasound may be useful in monitoring the depth and extent of tumor resection. Although helpful, it is unfortunately not entirely reliable because of artifact in the surgical bed.

SURGICAL TECHNIQUE

In patients who have not been previously operated on, an osteoplastic laminotomy is carried out. This permits replacement of the bone that is a nidus for subsequent osteogenesis and posterior fusion. Replacement of the bone may prevent the post-surgical evolution of spinal deformity and offer protection against future local trauma.

Even following careful consideration of the clinical and neuroradiologic examinations, it is not possible to be certain that the laminectomy is of sufficient length to expose the entirety of the solid component of the neoplasm. For this reason, transdural ultrasonography is utilized to define further the location of the tumor vis-a-vis the bone removal.

After laminectomy is carried out, the wound is filled with saline, and the head of the transducer probe is placed into gentle contact with the dura. Utilizing this technique, the spinal cord is viewed in both sagittal and transverse sections. The rostral and caudal limits of the tumor as well as the presence or absence of associated cysts are immediately obvious. Occasionally, an echogenic tumor provides a striking ultrasound image; however, most commonly, the solid component of the neoplasm is only manifest as a widened spinal cord.

If the laminectomy is not sufficiently long to expose the entirety of the solid component of the neoplasm, it is lengthened, segment by segment, until ultrasonography discloses that the entire tumor mass is exposed. Only at this juncture is the dura opened. This is limited to the area overlying the expanded spinal cord; it is not extended rostrally or caudally over the normal spinal cord. In addition, it is not necessary to open the dura widely over the rostral or caudal cyst, as these are easily drained as the solid component of the neoplasm is excised.

It is important to emphasize that the "swollen" spinal cord is commonly rotated and distorted, and it is essential that careful inspection identify normal landmarks prior to placing the myelotomy. Since the posterior median raphe is generally obliterated, the only sure way of recognizing the posterior midline is by identifying the dorsal root entry zones bilaterally. Rotation of the spinal cord may occasionally make this difficult, and even surprising, in terms of the distorted location of the midline. In any event, this is important, as otherwise it is possible that the myelotomy may be placed away from the median raphe and may sever multiple nerves along the dorsal root entry zone (Fig. 36–4A).

In the presence of holocord widening associated with rostral and caudal cysts, the ultrasound image will have clearly defined the junction of cyst and neoplasm over the rostral and caudal poles of the tumor. It is in the "junctional" regions that the midline myelotomy is started.

The carbon dioxide laser utilized at 6 to 8 watts is an ideal instrument for placing the myelotomy, as the cord is incised and hemostasis obtained simultaneously. Although neurosurgeons are loath to interrupt blood vessels on the surface of the spinal cord, it is tedious and time-consuming to preserve these vascular channels. They are not at all essential to the preservation of neurologic function and are almost inevitably disrupted during the course of the procedure, even if primarily preserved.

After the cyst is entered, inspection of the cavity identifies the rostral or caudal neoplasm that extends into it. In most cases, it is not necessary to extend the myelotomy over the cyst, since it is easily drained as either pole of the neoplasm is identified and removed. Because the cyst fluid is produced by the tumor, it is

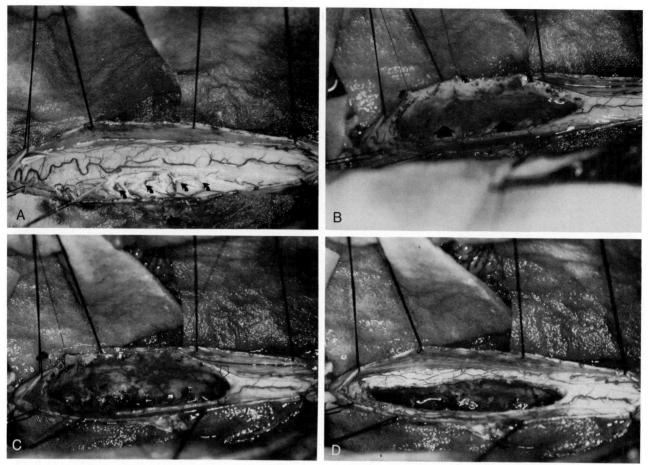

FIGURE 36–4. Operative exposure. *A,* Initial exposure of swollen spinal cord. Note rotation of cord with obliteration of normal landmarks. Dorsal roots (arrows) are exposed bilaterally to identify midline. *B,* Myelotomy completed. Pial traction sutures in place (small arrows). Tumor (large arrows) and caudal cyst (open arrows) exposed. *C,* Tumor resected. Note large intramedullary cavity with rostral and caudal cysts (open arrows). *D,* Pial sutures removed. Subarachnoid space re-expanded.

unlikely to reaccumulate following gross total excision of the neoplasm. After identifying the rostral and caudal cyst-tumor junctions, the myelotomy is continued over the midline of the cord between the previously placed incisions. Following completion of the myelotomy, there is usually 1 to 2 mm of white matter, overlying the neoplasm, that is removed with laser or bipolar cautery and a very fine suction. Most astrocytomas are gray or pink and may be distinguished from adjacent white matter.

At this juncture, it is essential that pia traction sutures be utilized to open the myelotomy incision and further expose the intramedullary tumor. It is satisfactory to utilize any fine suture material, and it is our practice simply to ''hang'' small clamps on the sutures rather than to suture the pia to adjacent tissues (Fig. 36–4*B*).

It must be emphasized that in the presence of an astrocytoma, there must be no effort to define a plane or cleavage around the tumor. These neoplasms must be removed from the inside out, until a glia-tumor interface is recognized by the change in color and con-

sistency of the adjacent tissues. There is rarely a true plane of dissection, and furtive efforts to define its presence result only in unnecessary retraction and manipulation of functioning neural tissue.

Ependymomas have a distinct plane of cleavage between the tumor and the adjacent neural tissue. Small tumors may occasionally be removed in one piece, whereas the more common bulky tumors must be excised bit by bit. In the latter cases, it is hazardous to attempt to carry out an en bloc excision, as there will invariably be excessive manipulation of adjacent neural tissue. In these cases, the centrum of the tumor must be debulked with the CUSA or the laser, following which the residual fragments may be removed along the cleavage plane. In all these cases, the entirety of the residual cavity is lined by normal-appearing white matter.

In the presence of cystic holocord neoplasms, tumor removal is initiated at either the rostral or the caudal pole of the neoplasm, in the region of the tumor-cyst junction.

As tumor excision continues, it is helpful to recognize

that the anterior extent of the neoplasm is only rarely ventral to the anterior wall of cyst. The bulk of the tumor is most often within the posterior two thirds of the spinal cord (as viewed in cross-section), and the general dimensions of the tumor may be roughly conceptualized following inspection of the rostral and caudal cysts (Fig. 36–4C).

The excision of the solid noncystic astrocytoma is initiated in the midportion rather than the rostral or caudal pole of the neoplasm. This is because there is no clear rostral or caudal demarcation of the tumor, as occurs when there are rostral and caudal cysts. In addition, the poles of the neoplasm are the least voluminous, and for this reason, removal of this part of the neoplasm may be the most hazardous because normal neural tissue may be easily disrupted.

The CUSA is utilized to remove the bulk of the neoplasm, following which the carbon dioxide laser is used to vaporize the visible remaining fragments. The dura is closed primarily, as it is unnecessary to utilize a dural substitute for decompression if tumor excision has been grossly complete (Fig. 36–4D).

IINTRAMEDULLARY LIPOMAS

Intramedullary lipomas are rare congenital tumors most commonly located in the thoracic spinal cord (Fig. 36–5). These tumors are not neoplasms, and they increase in size and in relation to fatty tissue elsewhere in the body. Myelopathic signs and symptoms evolve slowly and generally are first manifest during rapid growth spurts or after excessive weight gain.

The MRI scan is diagnostic of intramedullary lipomas. Therefore, there is usually no preoperative uncertainty as to the etiology of the lesion.

The goal of surgery is to carry out subtotal excision of the lipoma and a dural decompression. There must be no effort to excise this tumor totally, as it is intimately adherent and intertwined with adjacent functional neural tissue.

The carbon dioxide laser is an excellent instrument for debulking the lipoma, as the high water content of the fatty tissue is vaporized, thereby shrinking the mass. This is accomplished with no surgical trauma to adjacent tissue, as the tumor gradually "melts."

Debulking the lipoma often results in significant or complete neurologic recovery. This is often permanent, as the lipoma is unlikely to grow in the absence of alterations of body fat content.

EVOKED POTENTIAL MONITORING

Intraoperative somatosensory evoked potential (SSEP) monitoring can provide sensitive information regarding dorsal column function which can be updated every few seconds. This type of information has proved useful in many forms of spinal surgery, such as spinal instrumentation, but unfortunately has not

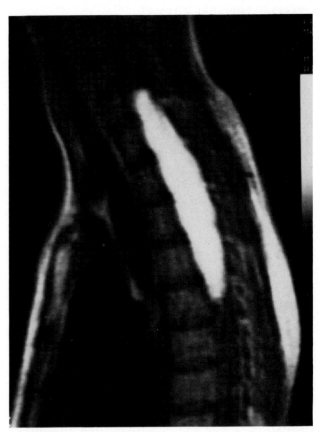

FIGURE 36–5. MR image of intramedullary lipoma. Increased signal on T1.

proved to be predictive of postoperative motor function, particularly in intramedullary spinal cord surgery. The recent development of motor evoked potentials (MEP) provides a means of monitoring corticospinal tract function in "real time." MEPs are generated by transcutaneous stimulation over motor cortex and then recorded over the spinal cord by means of subdural or epidural electrodes placed both rostral and caudal to the surgical site. These potentials are sensitive to anesthetic technique as well as surgical manipulation, and it is therefore best to have an experienced neurophysiologist in the operating room to monitor and interpret changes in these potentials.

We have found MEPs to be a reliable means of monitoring corticospinal tract function intraoperatively, and they have also allowed for more aggressive tumor resection. In cases in which the SSEPs decline in the presence of stable MEPs, it is the MEP that appears more predictive of overall postoperative outcome. MEPs have therefore allowed more aggressive tumor resection in situations in which surgery otherwise may have been stopped prematurely based on the SSEP data. The ultimate efficacy of intraoperative MEP as a predictor of postoperative motor function in spinal cord surgery is yet to be determined, but it appears that this technique will be of increasing importance in spinal cord surgery in the future.

POTENTIAL SURGICAL PITFALLS

MISSING ROSTRAL OR CAUDAL TUMOR FRAGMENT

In cases in which the entire spinal cord was expanded (holocord astrocytomas), it was a consistent finding that the neoplasm was associated with a rostral and a caudal cyst that extended up and down the central canal but did not contain neoplasm. In three patients, a large intratumor cyst was confused with a rostral cyst, and the tumor removal was prematurely terminated on the assumption that the superior part of the tumor had been removed. In these patients, the symptoms recurred 3 months, 6 months, and 18 months postoperatively as the cysts re-formed. The symptoms were rapidly evolving scoliosis in two patients, and paraspinal and cervical pain in one. In all patients, re-exploration disclosed only residual tumor that had been neglected as a direct result of misinterpreting a large tumor cyst for a rostral or caudal cyst. It is essential when cysts are identified over the poles of the tumor, that they be opened up widely enough to be certain that this is the cyst that is extending above or below the tumor, and not a cyst within the tumor. The former are lined by white matter, whereas cysts that occur within the neoplasm are lined by tumor tissue.

Intraoperative ultrasonography may also help to differentiate the rostral and caudal cysts from the intratumor cyst. The former symmetrically expand the cord, occupy two thirds of the diameter, and are smooth-walled. Intratumor cysts are eccentric and asymmetric, are of varying volume, and often have irregular walls (Fig. 36–6).

ANTERIOR SUBARACHNOID SPINAL FLUID LOCULATION

In several patients, there has been dramatic posterior extrusion of the spinal cord through the dural opening at some time during the tumor dissection. This was associated with a deterioration of evoked potentials, and the authors initially misinterpreted this as acute spinal cord swelling. The authors now recognize that it is not uncommon for cerebrospinal fluid to become loculated anterior to the spinal cord and to result in its posterior displacement. It is effectively dealt with by retraction of the lateral margin of the spinal cord and puncturing the cyst. It has been a consistent finding that this intraoperative problem has occurred only in patients who have had previous surgery and in whom there are dense adhesions between the lateral spinal cord and the dural tube. It seems that the anterior subarachnoid space does not communicate freely with the posterior subarachnoid space, and this may be responsible for the hydrodynamics that promote this intraoperative problem. One patient in this series had a huge tumor in the lower thoracic cord. Although the patient was neurologically stable immediately after surgery, one week later the patient became paraplegic. The

CT scan disclosed that the spinal cord had extruded from the spinal canal. During surgery, there was a huge anterior loculation of cerebrospinal fluid that had displaced the spinal cord posteriorly through the dural decompression, and the cord had become incarcerated on the rostral and caudal dura, with secondary infarction. Retrospectively, it was apparent that the dura had been excised at the time of the first operation, and it had not been closed at the time of the tumor resection. This permitted the trapped anterior subarachnoid compartment to displace the cord out of the spinal canal, with subsequent infarction. As a result of this experience, the authors do not leave the dura open under any circumstances, and if it has been previously excised, a suitable dural substitute is used.

POSTOPERATIVE NEUROLOGIC MORBIDITY RELATED TO SEGMENTAL LOCATION OF THE NEOPLASM

Postoperative neurologic morbidity may be correlated with the segments of the spinal cord that are involved with the neoplasm. Whereas an extensive dissection may be carried out with little risk in those segments of the spinal cord that are largely white matter, this does not seem to be the case in the lowest segments, where gray matter is most abundant.

Dissections within the cervical spinal cord are associated with little morbidity, though it is not uncommon to note some anterior horn cell dysfunction as manifested by atrophy of one or more muscle groups of an upper extremity. When this has occurred, it has been permanent.

Dissections extending from the junction of the cervical and thoracic regions to T9 are associated with remarkably little neurologic morbidity.

Tumors that are located in the lower spinal cord segments, from T9 to T12, have the greatest incidence of significant postoperative neurologic morbidity. This is because neoplasms in the conus medullaris or just above it compress or infiltrate gray matter, whereas tumors that occur in more rostral regions of the spinal cord compress white matter tracts. Therefore, the resultant signs and symptoms are based on pathologic anatomy and pathophysiology that is specific to the segmental location of the neoplasm.

Whereas an extensive intramedullary dissection may be carried out with relative impunity in white matter in the rostral cord, this is not the case in the gray matter in the region of the conus medullaris, and the surgeon must be aware of these technical limitations.

Significant preoperative sphincteric dysfunction suggests that the tumor is extending into the conus medullaris, as this rarely occurs if the tumor is rostral to T12. Conversely, the absence of bowel and bladder problems suggests that the tumor does not extend into the conus medullaris, though it may be symptomatically expanded by a caudal cyst.

If there is not preoperative bowel and bladder dysfunction, it will occur postoperatively when the conus medullaris is disrupted. Therefore, it is essential that

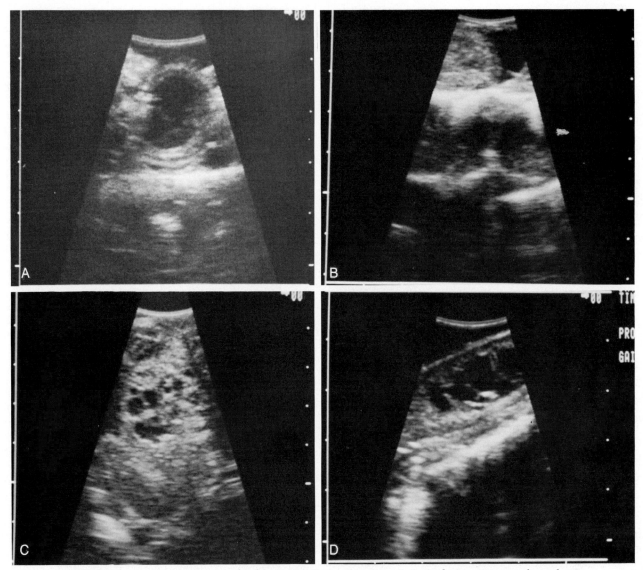

FIGURE 36–6. Ultrasonography of polar cyst. *A*, Transverse view. *B*, Sagittal view. Intramural cyst has "Swiss cheese" appearance. *C*, Transverse view. *D*, Sagittal view.

the myelotomy not be extended, as this invariably results in sphincter dysfunction that may be permanent.

Intraoperative ultrasonography is invaluable, as it clearly discloses the location of the conus medullaris, which may not be obvious to the surgeon as a result of distortion and rotation as well as superimposed neural elements.

It is important that the patient be advised that at least a temporary increase in neurologic dysfunction is to be expected with surgery in this area, and we would assume that long-term or permanent morbidity will also be significant.

DURAL SUBSTITUTES

In the course of operating on 78 patients who had undergone previous surgery, the authors have had the opportunity to re-explore a variety of dural substitutes (e.g., Gelfilm, Cargile membrane, cadaver dura, Silastic). Also, in many patients, the dura was simply left open.

It has been a consistent observation that all biologic material acts as a nidus for proliferation of fibrous tissue. At the time of re-exploration, there were dense adhesions between the spinal cord, the pseudodura that replaced the biologic membrane, and the deep muscle superficial to it. As a result, the dissection was invariably tedious and prolonged. In addition, the normal anatomic landmarks along the posterior surface of the spinal cord were distorted, and there were adhesions along the lateral margins of the cord, fixing it to the dural tube.

In patients in whom Silastic was used as a dural substitute, there were no adhesions and only minimal thickening of the leptomeninges immediately beneath the Silastic (Fig. 36–7).

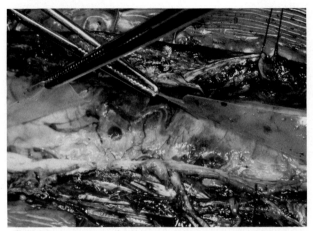

FIGURE 36–7. Silastic duraplasty. Note absence of adherence to spinal cord.

These observations are not intended to imply that the use of biologic materials is contraindicated or in any way deleterious to neurologic function. It is only suggested that in a patient in whom there is a likelihood of future surgery, Silastic will invariably facilitate the procedure, whereas the biologic materials will make it more difficult.

WOUND CLOSURE

Patients who have been previously irradiated are at high risk for wound dehiscence and cerebrospinal fluid fistula. In the first 14 previously irradiated patients operated on in this series, nine had problems with wound healing, and five developed meningitis. Since that experience, we have utilized plastic surgical expertise and muscle transposition from areas outside of the radiation fields. Although this is time-consuming, and the dissection is extensive, it has eliminated serious complications referable to wound healing. We view this as indispensable to procedures being carried out under these circumstances.

DISCUSSION

A number of important observations are clearly relevant in terms of understanding the biology of this group of neoplasms as well as recommending proper surgical management. It has been a consistent observation that in the presence of holocord expansion, the solid component of the astrocytoma is often limited to several segments usually visualized by MRI. Indeed, the actual location of the neoplasm may be in those segments of the spinal cord that correspond to the neurologic dysfunction. The lack of significant neurologic dysfunction relating to spinal segments that were distended with fluid is probably directly related to the anatomic location of the cyst within the center of the cord as compared with the solid component of the neoplasm, which was relatively diffuse.

The presence of cysts that were similar in appearance to those associated with cystic astrocytoma of the cerebellum suggests that many astrocytomas are congenital tumors that have their inception some time during gestation. The fluid produced by the tumor extends up and down the spinal cord in the region of least resistance, that is, the central canal.

One might also speculate that in some cases the classic symptoms of syringomyelia may, in fact, be a late manifestation of such a cyst in which the tumor has either involuted or is not anatomically obvious. Perhaps the centrally located cyst may gradually expand over many years and compress the surrounding cord. In this regard, it is significant that a few patients with holocord widening had exceedingly small neoplasms (between 1.5 and 3 cm) that were mistakenly diagnosed as syringomyelia or hydromyelia. Our experience would suggest that the presence of xanthochromic cyst fluid is pathognomonic of an associated neoplasm, whereas clear fluid is diagnostic of hydromyelia.

It is our perspective that the presence of a widened spinal cord from the cervicomedullary junction to the conus medullaris, which is associated with a relatively slowly evolving neurologic deficit, is indicative of a slowly growing tumor that may have a good long-term prognosis and should be treated aggressively.

Nevertheless, it must be emphasized that despite gross total tumor excisions, it would be naive to assume that residual tumor fragments were not commonly left in situ. The authors have hypothesized that in some patients the fragments may remain dormant or may involute in a way similar to what has been noted to occur in many astrocytomas of the cerebellum. However, whether or not this is reality or "wish-fulfillment" will only be known many years from now, following long-term follow-up and retrospective analysis.

In most cases of holocord tumor, the initial complaint was a weak arm, or a mildly weak leg, and associated pain somewhere along the spinal axis. The signs and symptoms were consistently relatively minor, when compared with the apparently diffuse nature of the pathologic process. It is perfectly understandable that neurosurgeons faced with this clinical dilemma have been most concerned about inflicting a greater neurologic deficit as a result of extensive dissection within a rather well-functioning spinal cord. This rationale has been used for a temporizing surgical approach, consisting of a limited laminectomy and biopsy and relying on radiation therapy to control tumor growth. Unfortunately, the natural history of these tumors, with radiation therapy, is slow deterioration and eventual severe neurologic disability or death.

The outcome following radical resection of these tumors was directly related to the patient's preoperative neurologic status. Although a transient increase in weakness or sensory loss was commonly present during the immediate postoperative period, only a few patients had a significant deficit following surgery. Patients with paraparesis or quadriparesis, who were ambulatory before surgery, had neurologic improvement over several weeks. The group with severe deficits preoperatively rarely made any significant improvement, although their downhill course abated.

There is no evidence that radiation cures benign astrocytomas of the spinal cord, and there is abundant evidence that it has a deleterious effect on the immature developing nervous system. Spinal cord neoplasms should be recognized as potentially excisable lesions, with radiation therapy being reserved for possible adjunctive use if there is a recurrence. At that time, it might be employed following a second radical surgical resection.[1, 5, 9–11, 15, 20, 21]

Intramedullary spinal cord astrocytomas are occasionally highly malignant. In these cases, the clinical course is rapid, and radical surgery has not significantly improved the dismal prognosis. Unlike cranial glioblastomas, those that occurred in the spinal cord disseminated over the entire neuraxis within 6 months of primary surgery.[22] For this reason, we now routinely employ total neuraxis irradiation in the presence of a malignant tumor.

Children who have undergone extensive laminectomy and, in addition, have denervation of the paravertebral muscles from tumor infiltration of anterior horn cells as well as operative muscle retraction, are at risk for developing severe spinal deformities as they pass through periods of rapid growth. Every effort should be made to replace the lamina whenever possible in the hope of limiting postoperative spinal deformity. Close collaboration with a pediatric orthopedic surgeon experienced with kyphoscoliosis is essential in following these patients.[23–25]

SUMMARY

The senior author has carried out gross total excision of intramedullary spinal neoplasms in 156 consecutive patients. This experience has led to the following conclusions:

1. Holocord widening occurs in 60 per cent of cases and is diagnostic of a cystic astrocytoma.

2. Radical tumor excision is compatible with partial or total recovery of neurologic function.

3. The success of surgery is directly related to the preoperative neurologic status of the patient. Paralysis or near paralysis was never improved, while mild to moderate preoperative neurologic dysfunction often improved.

4. While this experience has established the efficacy of radical surgery, there is no information to suggest the duration of remission or the likelihood of a permanent cure. This will become known only at the time of retrospective analysis, many years from now.

REFERENCES

1. Anderson FM, Carson MU: Spinal cord tumors in children. A review of the subject and representation of twenty-one cases. J Pediatr 43:190, 1953.
2. Arseni C, Horvath L, Issiescu D: Intraspinal tumors in children. Psychiatr Neurol Neurochir 70:123, 1967.
3. DeSousa AL, Kalseech JE, Mealey J, Jr., et al.: Intraspinal tumors in children: A review of 31 cases. J Neurosurg 51:437, 1979.
4. Garrido E, Stein BM: Microsurgical removal of intramedullary spinal cord tumors. Surg Neurol 7:214, 1977.
5. Hamby WB: Tumors in the spinal canal in childhood. J Neuropathol Exp Neurol 3:347, 1944.
6. Kernohan JW, Woltman HW, Adson AW: A review of 51 cases with an attempt at histological classification. Arch Neurol Psychiatry 25:679, 1931.
7. Goy AM, Pinto RS, Ragavendra BN, et al.: Intramedullary spinal cord tumors: MR imaging with emphasis on associated cysts. Radiology 161:381, 1986.
8. Richardson FL: A report of 16 tumors of the spinal cord in children: The importance of spinal rigidity as an early sign of disease. J Pediatr 57:42, 1960.
9. Epstein F: Spinal cord astrocytomas of childhood. In Symon L (ed): Advances and Technical Standards in Neurosurgery, Vol. 13. Vienna, Springer-Verlag, 1986.
10. Epstein F, Epstein N: Surgical management of "holo-cord" intramedullary spinal cord astrocytomas in children. J Neurosurg 54:289, 1981.
11. Epstein F, Epstein N: Surgical treatment of spinal cord astrocytomas of childhood: A series of 19 patients. J Neurosurg 57:685, 1982.
12. Epstein F, Ragavendra N, John R, et al.: Spinal cord astrocytomas of childhood, surgical adjuncts and pitfalls. In Humphreys RP (ed): Concepts in Pediatric Neurosurgery, Vol. 5. Basel, Karger, 1985, pp 224–238.
13. Reimer R, Onofrio BM: Astrocytomas of the spinal cord in children and adolescents. J Neurosurg 63:669, 1985.
14. Guidetta B: Intramedullary Tumors of the spinal cord. Acta Neurochir 17:7, 1967.
15. Coxe WS: Tumors of the spinal canal in children. Am Surg 27:62, 1961.
16. Rasmussen TB, Kernohan JW, Adson AW: Pathologic classification with surgical consideration of intraspinal tumors. Ann Surg 3:513, 1940.
17. Ingraham FD: Intraspinal tumors in infancy and childhood. Am J Surg 39:342, 1938.
18. Elsberg CA: Diagnosis and Treatment of Surgical Diseases of the Spinal Cord and Its Membranes. Philadelphia, W.B. Saunders Co., 1916, pp 288–289.
19. Elsberg CA, Beer R: The operability of intramedullary tumors of the spinal cord. A report of two operations with remarks upon the extrusion of intraspinal tumors. Am J Med Sci 142:636, 1911.
20. Grant FC, Austin GM: The diagnosis, treatment and prognosis of tumors affecting the spinal cord in children. J Neurosurg 13:535, 1956.
21. Greenwood J: Surgical removal of intramedullary tumors. J Neurosurg 26:276, 1967.
22. Eden K: Dissemination after gliomas of the spinal cord in the Leptomeninges. Brain 61:298, 1938.
23. Catell HS, Clark GL, Jr.: Cervical kyphosis and instability following multiple laminectomies in children. J Bone Joint Surg 49:713, 1967.
24. Shenkin HA, Alpers BJ: Clinical and pathological features of gliomas of the spinal cord. Arch Neurol Psychiatry 52:87, 1944.
25. Svien HJ, Thelen EP, Keith HM: Intraspinal tumors in children. JAMA 155:959, 1954.

Chapter 37

EXTRAMEDULLARY SPINAL TUMORS

RICHARD A. COULON, JR., M.D.

Spinal tumors can be divided anatomically by location into intramedullary and extramedullary lesions. As the name implies, intramedullary lesions encompass all tumors situated within the spinal cord parenchyma. This is a fairly restricted group with respect to pathology. Gliomas predominate. In contrast, extramedullary lesions include all tumors lying outside the spinal cord proper. This group, the subject of this chapter, constitutes a diverse collection of neoplasms including intradural/extramedullary and extradural lesions (Table 37–1).

Most published studies relating to spinal tumors in children cover the entire spectrum of neoplasms, both intramedullary and extramedullary. Non-neoplastic masses and developmental anomalies are often included.[1-13] Consequently, it is difficult to determine the true incidence of spinal canal tumors, let alone extramedullary lesions. Tumors of the nervous system in children are common and constitute approximately 20 to 23 per cent of all pediatric tumors.[14] Spinal canal tumors, however, are far less common than their intracranial counterparts. Intracranial to intraspinal ratios have been reported to range from 20:1 to 5:1.[15-18] Di Lorenzo et al.,[19] in an extensive review of the literature which included 56 of their own cases, accumulated data on 1234 patients. They identified a ratio of intracranial to intraspinal tumors of 6.7:1. Spinal canal tumors therefore account for about 12 to 15 per cent of all nervous system tumors. Sixty-eight per cent of the lesions reviewed by Di Lorenzo were extramedullary, 43 per cent were extradural, 24.4 per cent were intradural, and 1 per cent were intra-extradural. This preponderance of extramedullary lesions is consistent with the diverse nature and multiplicity of origin of these lesions.

CLINICAL FINDINGS

In the pediatric age group, the presentation of spinal canal lesions may be diverse. This is not because the presentation is different at different ages, but because age affects how the symptoms and signs are manifested.[20, 21] Infants do not speak and therefore cannot complain in the usual manner. Although toddlers are verbal, they are often unable to state their complaints clearly, and their statements are often misleading. It is only through astute parental observation that a concise history can be obtained. Partly for this reason and also because of difficulty in eliciting clear physical signs in the younger age groups, spinal canal tumors are frequently identified late in their course. It is also a contributing factor in their misdiagnosis. Erroneous diagnoses are noted in up to two thirds of reported cases.[18, 20]

The most common symptoms and signs of a spinal canal tumor are pain and motor weakness.[4, 6, 22–24] These

TABLE 37–1. EXTRAMEDULLARY TUMORS

A. Intradural
  1. Congenital tumors
     a. Epidermoid/dermoid
     b. Teratomas
  2. Meningeal tumors
     a. Meningiomas
  3. Nerve sheath tumors
     a. Schwannomas
     b. Neurofibromas
  4. Vascular tumors
     a. Hemangioblastomas
  5. Metastatic tumors
     a. Extraneural origin
        Leukemias
        Lymphomas
     b. Neural origin
        Gliomas
        PNET

B. Extradural
  1. Neural crest tumors
     a. Ganglioneuromas
     b. Ganglioneuroblastomas
     c. Neuroblastomas
  2. Soft tissue tumors
     a. Sarcomas
  3. Bone tumors
     a. Primary benign
        Osteoblastomas
        Aneursymal bone cysts
     b. Primary malignant
        Ewing's sarcomas
        Osteogenic sarcomas
        Chordomas
     c. Secondary (Metastatic)

symptoms may vary from case to case, depending upon the site of the lesion. Pain, usually spinal or radicular, is the most frequent initial symptom of extramedullary lesions. Radicular pain is common in extramedullary lesions but uncommon in intramedullary disease. It can serve as a point of differentiation between the two.[24, 25] Pain is usually manifested by decreased range of motion in the spine, paraspinal muscle spasm, or both. Pain frequently presents clinically as irritability in infants and toddlers, especially when they are lifted or manipulated. Lesions of the cauda equina may cause sciatic pain. Motor weakness is most commonly manifested as a gait disturbance involving one or both lower extremities. In young children, it may begin as a regression in attained ambulatory skills and progress to complete refusal to walk. Reflexes may be increased or decreased, depending upon the location of the lesion and the stage of cord compression.

Bladder and bowel complaints are next in frequency. In pretrained infants and toddlers, bladder and bowel complaints are nearly impossible to detect except in cases of frank retention. In older children, these complaints can present as regression in bladder and bowel control, incontinence, enuresis, urgency, dribbling, or constipation. Often these symptoms are mistaken for a behavioral problem.

Although sensory changes are not infrequent, they are more a sign than a symptom, especially at younger ages. Sensory changes are usually radicular in the early stages of extramedullary disease.[25] If cord compression occurs, the ipsilateral spinothalamic and corticospinal tract may be compromised early, and a Brown-Séquard syndrome may develop because of unilateral cord compression.[25] With time, a bilateral pattern may develop. The Brown-Séquard syndrome is more common in extramedullary than in intramedullary lesions. The former are more likely to exert unilateral external pressure on the cord. The latter disrupts the cord internally and tends to produce bilateral findings.

In addition to purely neurologic manifestations, there are often other factors that should suggest a spinal canal lesion. Any midline cutaneous marker overlying the spine could warn of a congenital lesion such as an epidermoid or dermoid tumor. Cutaneous lesions of the neurocutaneous syndromes should also suggest intraspinal disease (e.g., neurofibromas, schwannomas, and meningiomas). Spinal deformities including scoliosis, kyphosis, and the like, especially when associated with pain, are often warning signs of underlying spinal canal tumors.

DIAGNOSTIC STUDIES

PLAIN FILMS

Plain films reveal abnormalities in 50 to 60 per cent of extramedullary lesions.[4, 18, 26, 27] In intradural extramedullary lesions, scalloping of the posterior vertebral body, increased sagittal diameter of the spinal canal

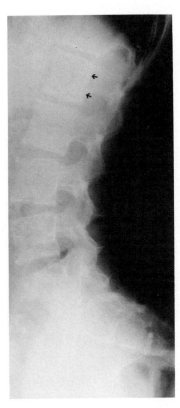

FIGURE 37–1. Lateral film of the lumbar spine. Scalloping of the posterior border of the L1 vertebral body *(arrows)*.

(Fig. 37–1), widening of the interpeduncular distance, and erosion of a pedicle (Fig. 37–2) are common plain film abnormalities. Enlargement of the neural foramina is a frequent finding in neurofibromas and schwannomas and usually indicates both intradural and extradural involvement (Fig. 37–3). Congenital tumors are often associated with characteristic vertebral anomalies and/or deformities. Extradural lesions are often related to paraspinous disease with direct extension into the spinal canal or metastatic disease that spreads to the spine. In the former, paraspinal masses are commonly visible along with secondary bony changes. In metastatic disease, frank destructive changes such as disruption of the vertebral body with or without fracture, absent pedicle, and others are present. Primary bone tumors can cause cord compression and are usually seen on plain films. Often the radiographic pattern is diagnostic.

TOMOGRAPHY

Tomography supplements plain film. Tomograms are helpful in more clearly identifying abnormalities that are obscured or poorly visualized because of overlying soft tissue or bone shadows.

MYELOGRAPHY

Myelography is useful in determining the presence or absence of spinal cord compression, the level of com-

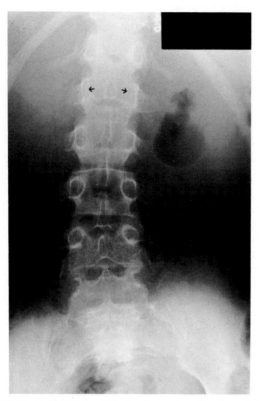

FIGURE 37–2. A-P film of the lumbar spine. Erosion of the L1 pedicles bilaterally *(arrows).*

pression, and the nature of the lesion, that is, whether it is intradural versus extradural or intramedullary versus extramedullary (Fig. 37–4). Myelography also provides an opportunity to remove spinal fluid for analysis. Myelography has disadvantages, however: (1) it is invasive; (2) it can be complicated by allergic reactions to the contrast medium; (3) it can cause neurologic deterioration; and (4) frequently it is technically difficult in young children and often requires general anesthesia. For these reasons, myelography has given way in recent years to CT scanning and magnetic resonance imaging (MRI).

COMPUTED TOMOGRAPHY (CT)

The CT scan is useful for showing changes in the spine and surrounding soft tissue if the level of the abnormality is known. It defines bony alterations that are subtle on plain film. It also defines the extent of these changes, delineates adjacent soft tissue masses, and indicates the degree to which they involve the spine and spinal canal. Unfortunately, CT scanning offers little insight into intraspinal disease. When CT scanning is used in conjunction with myelography, more information may be forthcoming, but it is of limited value (Fig. 37–5). MRI is the best noninvasive modality for identifying the extent of intraspinal disease.

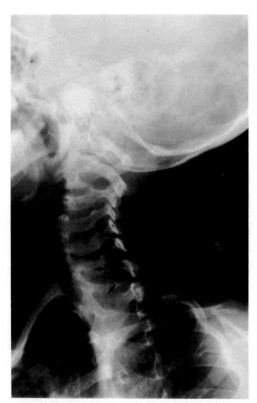

FIGURE 37–3. Oblique film of the cervical spine. Enlargement of the left C7 foramen *(arrows).*

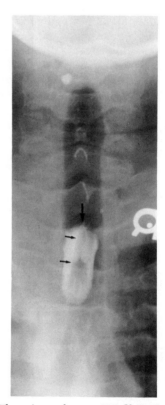

FIGURE 37–4. Thoracic myelogram (AP film). Complete obstruction to flow of contrast *(large arrow).* Deviation of the spinal cord to the right *(small arrows)* due to an extramedullary mass in the left spinal canal.

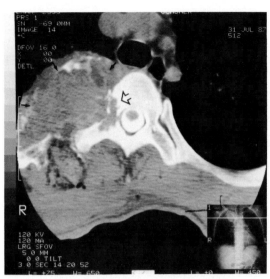

FIGURE 37–5. CT scan/myelogram axial projection. Paravertebral mass (*small arrows*) eroding the adjacent vertebral body, pedicle, and transverse process (*open arrow*). Contrast medium within the spinal subarachnoid space demonstrates the absence of intraspinal involvement.

MAGNETIC RESONANCE IMAGING (MRI)

Magnetic resonance imaging (MRI) is the most useful tool today to evaluate the spinal canal and its contents. Unlike the CT scan, it provides high-resolution views of the canal and its contents in multiple projections. Because MRI can produce clear sagittal pictures of the entire spine, it is an excellent screening modality. For the same reason, it can define the extent of a disease process that spans multiple levels. It can often define and differentiate extradural and intradural disease. If MRI has one disadvantage, it is its failure to clearly define bone. This does not mean that MRI will not reveal bony lesions, but that plain films, tomograms, and CT scanning are often better choices.

RADIONUCLEOTIDES

Isotope scans offer little today in the diagnosis of extramedullary lesions. They have been supplanted by the modern scanners. Radionucleotides, however, are still excellent for defining bony disease. Isotope scans often pick up abnormalities before they are apparent on plain films. They can also be superior screening tools. They are particularly useful in metastatic disease.

INTRADURAL EXTRAMEDULLARY TUMORS

CONGENITAL TUMORS

Epidermoid and Dermoid Tumors. These lesions are not true neoplasms but dysembryonic malformations. They are generally thought to arise from an in-

vagination or displacement of skin elements into the neural canal during development.[28–30] The characteristic of the lesion depends upon the timing. There are incidences, however, when these tumors are thought to arise iatrogenically from lumbar punctures.[31–35] Histologically, both lesions are lined by stratified squamous epithelium containing desquamated epitheleal cells and keratin. Dermoids differ from epidermoids in that they also contain hair follicles and sebaceous glands.

Dermoids appear more commonly in children. Epidermoids are more evenly distributed over all ages. Both are usually found in the lumbar region, followed by the thoracic and the cervical areas.[30] The majority are associated with some sort of midline cutaneous abnormality such as a hairy patch, port wine nevus, or dermal sinus. Dermal sinuses have been implicated in intraspinal infections.[10, 18, 36–39]

The clinical presentation is nonspecific unless there is a history of chronic recurring meningitis. Generally, lesions in the lumbar area present as low back pain or sciatic-type pain in the lower extremities. Lower-extremity motor and sensory changes and sphincter changes usually occur later. Lesions involving higher spinal segments can be extramedullary or intramedullary and more commonly present with motor, sensory, and sphincter changes.

Plain films frequently show bony changes common to all expanding lesions, i.e., bony erosion of the pedicles, widening of the interpeduncular distance, and scalloping of the posterior vertebral body. Spinal anomalies, particularly spina bifida, are frequently noted. Myelography will distinguish an intramedullary process from an extramedullary process. It will also show the presence of a partial or total block to contrast flow. Epidermoids are generally isointense with cerebrospinal fluid (CSF) on both CT and MRI scans (Fig. 37–6), making small lesions difficult to identify. Large lesions are more easily noted because of their mass effect. Dermoids almost always have the intensity of fat. They show low attenuation on CT scanning. On MRI, they have a high signal intensity on short TR/TE images. Occasionally, they may have low signal intensity on T1-weighted images on MRI and higher signal intensity on CT scanning. This results from secretions of sweat glands within the tumor.

Complete removal is the treatment of choice. If removal is not complete, the lesion is likely to recur. Although these lesions are usually easily removed, extensive adhesions may complicate surgery. This may be especially true if there have been previously associated infections.

Teratomas. Teratomas are lesions that contain elements of all three germ layers. Unlike epidermoid and dermoid tumors, these malformations may undergo malignant changes and become true neoplasms. Teratomas of the spine are divided into two groups, those located within the spinal canal and those located in the sacrococcygeal area. The latter, which rarely cause neurologic problems and are not generally considered true spinal lesions, are not discussed here.

Spinal teratomas constitute between 3 and 9 per cent

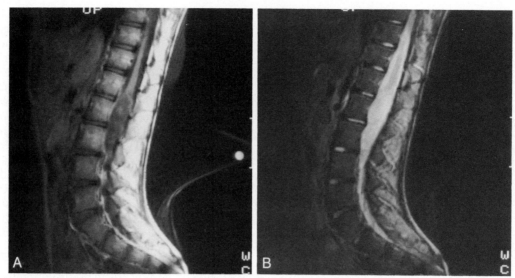

FIGURE 37–6. Noncontrast sagittal MRI scan of an upper lumbar canal epidermoid tumor. *A*, Short TR/TE weighted image (T1) showing the lesion to be near isodense to CSF. *B*, Long TR/TE image (T2) showing the lesion isodense to CSF.

of intraspinal tumors in children.[4, 18, 19, 26] They are thought to arise from germ cells displaced into the dorsal midline during migration from the yolk sac to the gonads.[40–43] They are primarily lesions of childhood. One third of diagnoses are made in children younger than age 5.[44] The tumors are most frequently found in the thoracolumbar and lumbar regions.[30] They are intradural and usually extramedullary but can be intramedullary. They may be cystic, solid, or a combination of both. They produce no specific symptoms.

Plain films usually show changes of a chronic expanding intraspinal mass. The spinal canal may be enlarged with erosion of adjacent pedicles and posterior vertebral bodies. The tumors may contain calcium. There may be associated bony anomalies such as spina bifida.[30] CT myelography will show a mass of multiple tissue densities, including calcium. MRI shows a similar pattern of multiple tissue signals that is often variable and may be cystic, partially cystic, or solid.

Treatment consists of surgical removal. At times, however, these lesions are extremely adherent to the spinal cord or the roots of the cauda equina, and removal may be difficult. Failure to attain complete removal will be followed by their recurrence.

MENINGEAL TUMORS

Meningiomas are rare in childhood. They account for about 2 per cent of all tumors found in childhood.[45] They make up 2 to 5 per cent of pediatric spinal canal tumors.[18, 46] Most present late, between the ages of 12 and 15.[46] As in adults, meningiomas are most common in the thoracic region but occur with less frequency (48 per cent versus 81 per cent in adults).[46, 47] They are usually intradural/extramedullary but rarely may be extradural.[48, 49] Pain is the most common presenting symptom; motor deficit usually occurs later. About 20

per cent of cases are associated with von Recklinghausen's disease.[46] Histologically, the tumors resemble adult lesions and are generally benign. Meningiomas as a group, however, appear to be more aggressive in children than in adults but rarely undergo malignant changes.[50]

Plain films are positive in about 20 per cent of cases and show changes consistent with an intraspinal mass.[46] Most commonly, the interpeduncular distance is increased or an adjacent pedicle is eroded. Myelography demonstrates an extramedullary mass with or without a block. On CT scan/myelography, meningiomas appear hypodense or isodense and enhance with contrast. On MRI, they have a relaxation time similar to that of cord parenchyma and appear homogeneous and isodense with the cord (Fig. 37–7). They enhance with contrast.[51]

Treatment is total excision if possible. The outlook is excellent, although recurrence rates of 20 per cent have been reported in children, reflecting the somewhat more aggressive nature of this lesion in childhood.[50]

NERVE SHEATH TUMORS

The origin of nerve sheath tumors is uncertain, and the terminology describing them is confusing. Classically, nerve sheath tumors are divided into two categories, schwannomas and neurofibromas.[52] Schwannomas are composed of Schwann cells, neurofibromas of a mixture of Schwann cells and fibroblasts with an abundance of collagen fibers. As a group, these tumors make up 9 to 10 per cent of all spinal canal tumors in childhood.[46, 53] They occur late in childhood, usually between ages 9 and 15.[46] They are uniformly distributed along the spine.[46] Pain is the presenting complaint in 80 per cent of patients, motor weakness in 20 per cent.[46] The duration of symptoms is 5 to 12 months,

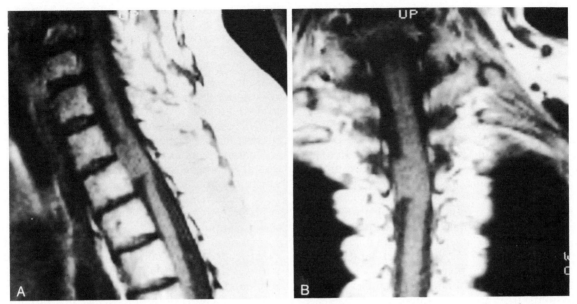

FIGURE 37–7. Noncontrast sagittal *(A)* and coronal *(B)* MRI scan of the thoracic spine. Both are short TR/TE weighted images (T1). The lesion is isodense to cord parenchyma.

considerably shorter than in adults.[46] On rare occasions, these lesions have presented as subarachnoid hemorrhage.[54–56] Approximately 25 per cent are associated with von Recklinghausen's disease.[46] They may be located intradurally (52 per cent), extradurally (29 per cent), or intradurally/extradurally as dumbbell tumors (19 per cent).[46] Rarely, they have been reported to be intramedullary or interosseous.[57, 58] These tumors are generally benign but can undergo malignant degeneration in 3 to 10 per cent of cases, becoming sarcomas.[59–61]

Plain films are abnormal in 70 per cent of patients, usually showing widening of the canal, scalloping of the posterior vertebral margin, and erosion of a pedicle. In dumbbell tumors, the vertebral foramen is usually enlarged and eroded. Myelography will show an intradural or extradural filling defect. CT scan/myelography reveals a mass that appears isodense or hypodense to skeletal muscle.[51] Generally, these tumors do not enhance with contrast. On MRI, they appear slightly hyperintense to skeletal muscle and show variable contrast enhancement on T1 sequence (Fig. 37–8). On T2

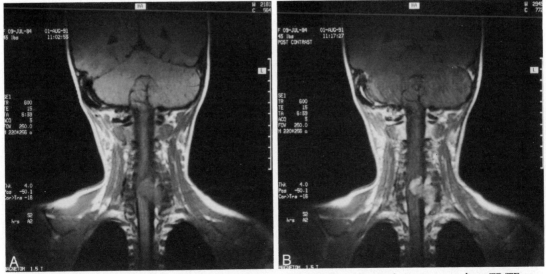

FIGURE 37–8. Coronal MRI scan precontrast *(A)* and postcontrast *(B).* Both images are short TR/TE-weighted images (T1). The lesion appears isodense to skeletal muscle precontrast and hyperintense following contrast injection.

sequence, they are hyperintense with respect to skeletal muscle.[51] Treatment consists of total removal when possible. Failure to do so will result in recurrence.

VASCULAR TUMORS

Hemangioblastomas. These benign lesions are uncommon, but when they occur they appear frequently in children. Hurt found that about 25 per cent were identified in patients under 21 years of age.[62] Hemangioblastomas are most prevalent in the cerebellum but are also seen in the spinal cord and medulla.[63] The majority of hemangioblastomas occur as isolated lesions. Ten to 20 per cent of all hemangioblastomas occur as a part of the Von Hippel–Lindau complex.[64] Approximately 50 per cent of spinal hemangioblastomas occur in conjunction with the Von Hippel–Lindau complex.[65] They may be multiple. Spinal lesions have a predilection for the cervical and dorsolumbar regions. Although some may appear intramedullary, they are usually attached to the pia. An accompanying syrinx is common. Others are located on spinal nerves, either adjacent to the cord or in the cauda equina. These lesions do not produce specific symptoms other than nerve root irritation or cord compression. Many are asymptomatic throughout life and are identified only at autopsy.[66, 67]

Myelography reveals a filling defect associated with enlarged surface vessels and widening of the cord shadow. Selective angiography shows a distinct homogeneous tumor blush. It can be distinguished from an arteriovenous malformation by the lack of the usual tangle of vessels and the absence of rapid shunting.[68] MRI shows a tumor nodule that is isodense and not clearly defined but becomes hyperintense with contrast. The accompanying syrinx is clearly seen if present. Feeding vessels are manifested as serpentine areas of flow void.[69]

Treatment is surgical removal. If these tumors are not removed completely, they will recur. In cases in which complete extrication is impossible, radiation therapy should be considered.[70]

METASTATIC DISEASE

Metastatic intradural extramedullary disease most commonly occurs via the spinal fluid pathways. Its origins may be neural or extraneural. Tumors that involve lymphoma and leukemia are the most likely extraneural source; tumors that involve the brain and spinal cord are the most likely neural source.[71]

Metastasis of Extraneural Sources

Leukemia. Leukemia is one of the more common systemic malignancies to involve the central nervous system in childhood. Central nervous system (CNS) involvement appears to be more common in acute myelogenous leukemia (AML) and may be present at or near initial diagnosis in up to 30 per cent of patients.[72] It appears early less commonly in acute lymphocytic leukemia (ALL). Without prophylactic treatment, however, 50 to 80 per cent of patients with ALL develop CNS disease at some time.[73-75] Prophylactic treatment will reduce the risk in ALL to 2 to 10 per cent. Its effects in AML are less clear.[76]

CNS leukemia presents as either parenchymal or meningeal disease or both.[77] Leukemic cells gain access to the parenchyma and meninges via their blood vessels. Spinal meningeal disease may involve the dura or the arachnoid primarily. A few cases of extradural disease have been reported.[78] Dural involvement may reach sufficient proportions to produce mass lesions. This is more common in AML. Hemorrhage can occur with formation of subdural hematoma. Arachnoid involvement leads to leukemic cell infiltrates within the CSF pathways as well as infiltrates within adjacent nerve roots and the spinal cord. With intraspinal mass formation or cord infiltration, symptoms of cord disease will appear. With meningeal disease only, symptoms of meningeal or nerve root irritation are more common. If the subarachnoid spaces become congested with leukemic infiltrates, hydrocephalus may occur.

Diagnosis is made by cytocentrifugation of the CSF. Malignant cells are usually present. Myelography, CT scan/myelography, and MRI may be helpful if a mass is present. The latter two diagnostic methods may show meningeal involvement with enhancement of the meninges or changes in the CSF signal.

Treatment usually involves combinations of radiation therapy and chemotherapy. Rarely is surgical intervention indicated unless acute cord compression is present.

Lymphoma. Lymphoma can involve the CNS as either a primary or a secondary lesion. Primary lesions are almost entirely limited to non-Hodgkin's lymphoma.[79] Both Hodgkin's and non-Hodgkin's lymphoma can involve the CNS secondarily,[73, 80] but the association with non-Hodgkin's lymphoma is more common. Involvement is usually extradural and involves secondary invasion of the epidural space from paravertebral lymph nodes or direct bony involvement.[80] The thoracic spine is usually involved.[80] Meningeal disease may occur, however. Symptoms will depend upon the location and type of involvement. The presence of CNS symptoms in a child with lymphomatous disease should be enough to cause suspicion of CNS disease.

Plain films may show a paravertebral mass or bone lesion with or without a fracture. In the presence of a mass encroaching upon the spinal canal, myelography will usually show the level of intraspinal disease. CT scan and MRI scan may be helpful not only to reveal the intraspinal lesion but to give a clear picture of bony and soft-tissue disease (Fig. 37–9).

Treatment usually is nonsurgical. Various combinations of radiation therapy and chemotherapy are used. Occasionally in cases of acute cord compression, decompression laminectomy may be indicated.

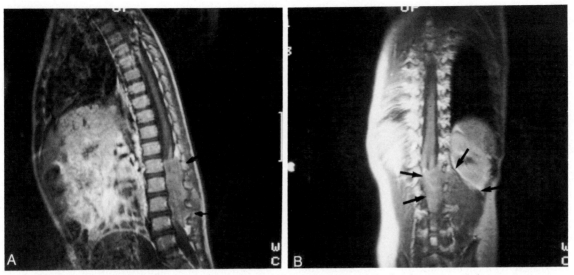

FIGURE 37–9. Noncontrast sagittal *(A)* and coronal *(B)* MRI Scan of the lumbar spine. Both images are short TR/TE-weighted images (T1) of a non-Hodgkin's lymphoma, which involves the paraspinal area and the spinal canal *(arrows)*.

Metastasis of Neural Origin

Primitive neuroectodermal tumors (PNET) are the most common neural tumors to spread in this manner. Within this group, medulloblastomas are the most common, followed by anaplastic astrocytomas and ependymomas.[81] Many other tumors have been implicated as a source, including germ cell tumors, oligodendrogliomas, benign cerebellar astrocytomas, pilocytic astrocytomas of the hypothalamus, choroid plexus papillomas, neuroblastomas, retinoblastomas, rhabdomyosarcomas, and others.[71, 82–88] Spinal cord tumors have also been associated with spinal subarachnoid spread, particularly myxopapillary ependymomas.

Within the PNET group, metastasis is frequently found at diagnosis of the primary lesion. Parker et al. noted that 49 per cent of the PNET reviewed had metastasized at diagnosis of the primary lesion.[81] Deutsch et al. noted that 44 per cent of the medulloblastomas they reviewed had metastases at that time.[89] Other tumors, notably anaplastic astrocytomas and ependymomas, appear more likely to have metastases at the time of relapse of the primary lesion or thereafter.[81]

Spread via the CSF pathways appears to be related to the proximity of the primary tumor to the subarachnoid space. Posterior fossa tumors as a group therefore metastasize more frequently than their supratentorial counterparts. This is the case with anaplastic astrocytomas. PNET, however, appear unaffected by location.[81] Surgery has also been implicated in spread. This may be a factor in certain tumors, but again the PNET appear to be unaffected, with 40 to 50 per cent spreading before surgery.[81]

Drop metastases are usually multiple. They are most common in the lumbar region. When located at higher levels, they are usually found dorsally; however, they may be ventral or may even encase the cord.[90] Pain, most commonly radicular, is usually the initial com-

plaint. Meningeal signs are common. Motor and sensory changes appear later.

Diagnosis is usually confirmed by myelography or MRI. CSF cytology is helpful when it is positive, but it can be falsely negative.[89] Myelography is usually definitive but can also result in false negatives.[81] MRI, which is noninvasive, appears to be useful and is likely to replace myelography as more experience with the procedure is gained (Fig. 37–10). Because MRI shows the entire spinal subarachnoid space and cord, it serves as an excellent screening test.

The presence of drop metastases usually indicates a

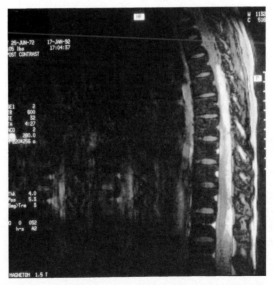

FIGURE 37–10. Noncontrast sagittal MRI scan of the thoracic spine. The image is a short TR/TE weighted image (gradient echo) showing extensive subarachnoid metastases from a posterior fossa ependymoma. The lesions appear hyperintense to both spinal cord and CSF.

poor prognosis. Treatment is generally nonsurgical unless the diagnosis is in doubt or a solitary lesion is producing acute cord compression with neurologic deterioration. Most cases are treated with combinations of radiation therapy and chemotherapy.

EXTRADURAL EXTRAMEDULLARY TUMORS

NEURAL CREST TUMORS

Tumors of neural crest tissue are common in childhood, accounting for about 10 to 20 per cent of all spinal tumors.[91–93] This group consists primarily of ganglioneuromas and neuroblastomas. The former is benign, the latter malignant. Between these extremes is the ganglioneuroblastoma. All three types of tumor commonly originate from the adrenal medulla or the paravertebral sympathetic chain. As a rule, they involve the spinal canal by direct extension although neuroblastomas may metastasize.

Ganglioneuromas. These benign tumors are less common then neuroblastomas and account for approximately 1 to 3 per cent of spinal lesions in childhood.[3, 18, 19] They are more common in older children and young adults.[94–96] Histologically, they are characterized by clumps of mature ganglion cells interposed among Schwann cells. They are well circumscribed and usually found in the posterior mediastinum but may also be located in the abdomen. They are slow-growing and often asymptomatic until they have reached large size. They rarely involve the spinal canal unless it is by direct extension.

Ganglioneuroblastomas. Some consider these tumors to represent a stage in the maturation of neuroblastomas.[97] They occur in young children, 0 to 6 years of age. Histologically, ganglioneuroblastomas are characterized by both mature ganglion cells and neuroblasts, with intermediate forms present. They are subclassified into immature and imperfect forms.[97, 98] These tumors are usually well circumscribed, but tissue invasion may be present. They are most frequently found in the posterior mediastinum and abdomen. Their behavior is unpredictable. Some act benign while others are frankly malignant, with metastases in up to 40 per cent of cases.[95] The spinal canal is rarely affected unless there is direct extension or metastasis to the vertebra.

Neuroblastomas. These malignant tumors constitute the extreme of the group. They are more common in younger children and are unusual after age 9.[97] Histologically, they are composed of dense sheets of neuroblasts with little interspersed stroma. They are friable, fairly circumscribed masses, with areas of invasion of surrounding tissue. Thirty-five to 40 per cent arise from the adrenal medulla. Other common locations are the sympathetic chain in the posterior mediastinum and the retroperitoneal space.[95, 97] Neuroblastomas are highly malignant but appear to have a better prognosis in children under 2 years of age. The tumor readily metastasizes, and most older children show spread at the time of diagnosis.[99–101] Liver, lymph nodes, and bone are the common sites. Neuroblastomas involve the spinal canal in 4 to 17 per cent of patients.[93, 102–104] Involvement is usually by direct extension or metastasis to the spine. Rarely, these lesions can arise directly within the spinal canal. These are usually congenital lesions.[16, 19, 105, 106]

This group of tumors can frequently be seen as a paraspinal mass on plain films of the chest and abdomen. Associated bony changes may be present, such as erosion of a pedicle or an adjacent neural foramen. Visible calcification may occur in as many as 50 per cent of cases.[71] Bone destruction secondary to bone marrow involvement can be seen. Although myelography may show an epidural mass with encroachment on the spinal canal, CT scan and MRI are the studies of choice. Both modalities will clearly define the extraspinal and intraspinal components of the mass and show bone metastases when they are present.

Treatment of ganglioneuromas is surgical removal, including a laminectomy if the spinal canal is involved. Ganglioneuroblastomas present a more perplexing problem because of their unpredictability. In the presence of cord compression, laminectomy is indicated. The use of radiation therapy and chemotherapy is less clear. Treatment of neuroblastomas is complex. If there is acute cord compression, laminectomy may be indicated. The principal treatment scheme, however, consists of radiation therapy and chemotherapy. The type and extent of these treatments depend upon the patient's age and the stage of the disease.

SOFT TISSUE TUMORS

The most common tumor to arise in the soft tissue surrounding the spine is the sarcoma. Rhabdomyosarcoma is probably the most common of this group.[107] Approximately one third of these lesions are located in the head and neck area. They tend to be parameningeal and may involve the base of the skull or the cervical spine. They may also arise in the retroperitoneal space or urogenital tract, especially in older children. These soft tissue tumors invade the spinal canal directly from their paraspinal position or gain access into the spinal subarachnoid spaces.[85] As noted earlier, neuroblastomas and Hodgkin's and non-Hodgkin's lymphoma can commonly involve paraspinal tissue and directly invade the spinal canal. ALL and AML can invade the epidural space, although this rarely happens. Ch'ien et al. noted that 0.7 per cent of patients with AML and 0.2 per cent of patients with ALL had this complication.[108] Malignant fibrous histiocytomas, malignant hemangiopericytomas, and embryonal mesenchymal tumors occasionally arise in the soft tissue adjacent to the spine and can invade the spine.

TUMORS OF THE BONY SPINE

Two varieties of tumor involve the bony spine, those arising from bone and those arising from metastasis to bone. Tumors arising from bone may be benign or malignant; tumors arising from metastasis to bone are by nature malignant. A multitude of tumors of bone may involve the spine, but they rarely affect the spinal cord. Most are uncommon in children.

Primary Benign Tumors

Osteoblastomas. Osteoblastoma is the only benign tumor that favors the spine in childhood.[109–112] About 40 per cent occur in the spine. About two thirds of all osteoblastomas occur in childhood, with a 2:1 predilection for males. Osteoblastomas may affect any portion of the vertebra, arising at any level; however, the lumbar and sacral areas are the more frequently involved areas. Pain, occasionally accompanied by scoliosis, is the most common symptom.[113, 114] The tumor appears on plain film as a radiolucent area containing areas of new bone formation at varying stages. A soft tissue component often extends beyond the host bone. Bone scanning may be helpful in locating the lesion but is of little help otherwise. CT scanning and MRI will permit visualization of the extent of the lesion, its soft tissue component, and the involvement of the spinal canal.[51] Treatment is surgical curettage with supplemental bone grafting if necessary. Cure is possible with total excision. Subtotal removal is associated with occasional remissions, but recurrence is more likely; radiation therapy should be considered in these cases. Rarely, osteoblastomas undergo malignant transformation.[115–117]

Aneurysmal Bone Cyst. Aneurysmal bone cysts are nontumorous growths characterized by widespread destruction of bone. They are not uncommon in the spine. The majority are recognized before the age of 20 years.[118–120] They may occur at any level of the spine and may affect any part of the vertebra although the posterior arch and body are most frequently involved. Spine pain is the usual presenting symptom, but radicular pain is also common. Cord compression can occur and may be sudden, associated with collapse of a vertebra or hemorrhage.[121] Radiographs show an expansile destructive process with a soft tissue mass extending beyond bone (Fig. 37–11). As the process matures, the lesion becomes more clearly demarcated.[122] CT scanning reveals a similar lytic expansile lesion with eggshell-like peripheral calcification. MRI shows the same basic pattern with variable signal intensities. Medium to high intensity is common on short TR/TE, but high intensity is usual on long TR/TE (Fig. 37–12). A fluid level is common within the tumor.[51]

Treatment consists of total en bloc resection if possible. If en bloc resection is impossible, surgical curettage should be performed. Recurrence most frequently occurs within a few months of incomplete resection and may require a repeat surgical procedure.[120] Recurrence rates appear higher in childhood than at other ages.[123] The use of radiation is controversial. Some believe it should be a primary treatment while others believe it should be reserved for cases of incomplete removal or recurrence.[119, 124]

Primary Malignant Tumors

Primary malignant tumors of the vertebral column are rare in childhood. Ewing's sarcoma is a common childhood tumor of bone, yet Savini et al. reported only

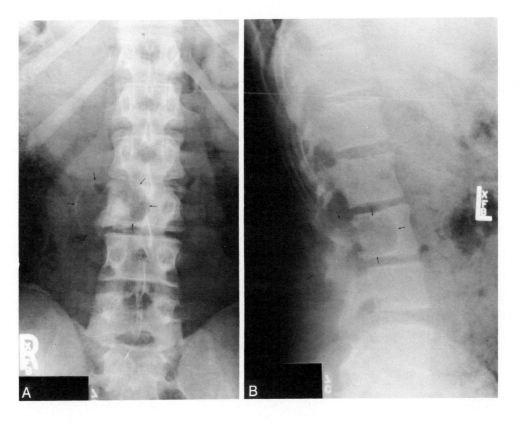

FIGURE 37–11. A-P *(A)* and lateral *(B)* films of the lumbar spine. Expansile changes in the L3 vertebra and an associated soft-tissue mass with a thinly calcified margin *(arrows)* due to an aneurysmal bone cyst.

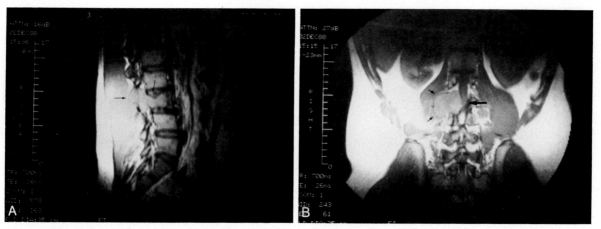

FIGURE 37–12. Noncontrasted sagittal *(A)* and coronal *(B)* MRI scan of the lumbar spine. Both images are short TR/TE-weighted images (T1). The lesion is delineated from adjacent bone and soft tissue *(small arrows).* Encroachment of the spinal canal is clearly visible on the coronal image *(B) (large arrow).*

7 of 217 cases (3.2 per cent) occurring as a primary spinal tumor in patients younger than age 16.[125] Similarly, they found that only 6 of 5000 (0.1 per cent) osteogenic sarcomas originated in the spine, and only one of these was in a child. Other tumors, the classic chondrosarcomas and mesenchymal chondrosarcomas, are even rarer.

Chordomas account for about 3 per cent of all primary bone tumors.[14, 126] They are relatively rare in childhood, with only 4 per cent occurring before age 20.[127] These tumors arise from notochordal remnants and most often affect the cranial base or the sacrococcygeal region. Although chordomas can occur anywhere along the spine, more than 50 per cent occur in the sacrococcygeal region.[128–131] They are slow-growing but invariably compress the spinal nerves or the cord and have been found to metastasize to varying degrees

(10 to 43 per cent), particularly to the lung, liver, lymph nodes, and adjacent tissues.[132–135] Radiographically, chordomas produce extensive bone destruction, usually over several vertebral segments. A paraspinal soft tissue mass is present. CT scanning demonstrates similar bony changes. It also offers the advantage of clearly showing the soft tissue mass, which frequently reveals areas of amorphous calcification scattered randomly and septated areas of low attenuation. The soft tissue mass will enhance with contrast.[136, 137] MRI exhibits a similar pattern but provides better contrast between the tumor mass and surrounding tissue, especially on long TR/TE images[138, 139] (Fig. 37–13). Treatment of choice is total excision. However, because of the nature of the tumor, total excision is often impossible and tumor recurrence is inevitable. Radiation therapy has been recommended in cases of incomplete removal as well as in recurrence. Although radiation therapy is not curative, it does slow down the tumor growth.[140–142] Chemotherapy has little value in the treatment of chordomas.

METASTATIC TUMORS

About 25 per cent of spinal tumors in children are secondary,[143] spreading to the spinal canal via adjacent soft tissue or metastasized to the vertebrae. Metastatic lesions are the less common of the two types of secondary tumors. In a series of 250 patients with secondary lesions of the spine, Torma noted only 11 per cent in the pediatric age group.[144] Most common were sarcomas, which comprised 77 per cent. In this group, Ewing's sarcoma comprised 33 per cent, followed by nonspecific sarcomas (26 per cent), osteogenic sarcomas (7 per cent), lymphosarcomas (7 per cent), and reticular sarcomas (4 per cent). Neuroblastomas accounted for 11 per cent. Neuroblastoma and Hodgkin's lymphoma, however, usually invade the canal and do not metastasize.[145] Ch'ien et al. noted similar tumor types.[108] Chondrosarcoma, synovial sarcoma, teratoma (ovar-

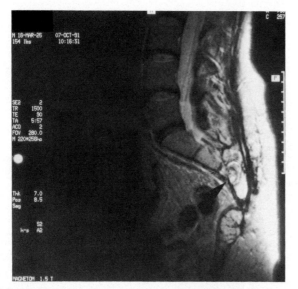

FIGURE 37–13. Noncontrast sagittal MRI scan of the sacral region. The image is a long TR/TE-weighted image (T2) that shows a mixed intensity mass involving the lower sacrum and sacral canal *(arrow).*

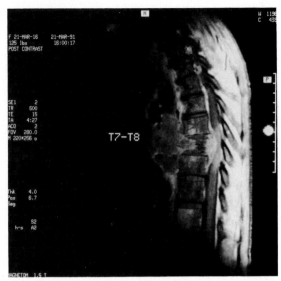

FIGURE 37–14. Noncontrast sagittal MRI scan of the thoracic spine. The image is a short TR/TE-weighted image (T1) of a large paraspinal metastatic mass (Ewing's sarcoma). There is secondary involvement of the adjacent vertebra and spinal canal with cord compression.

ian), rhabdomyosarcoma, embryonal cancer of the testes, renal cell carcinoma, teratocarcinoma, and Wilms' tumor have also been reported but occur infrequently.[144, 146, 147]

Sixty to 70 per cent of metastatic lesions are noted after diagnosis of the primary tumor.[143, 148] The spine appears to be the most common bony site; 80 per cent of bony metastases noted by Leeson et al. occurred there.[147] The thoracic spine was the most common region.[144] Symptoms are nonspecific, varying from spinal pain to varying degrees of cord compression, resulting from either extension of the tumor beyond the bone or pathologic fractures. Plain films demonstrate evidence of bony destruction. Myelography shows the presence or absence of a spinal block. CT scan/myelography exhibits the bony and soft tissue lesion and the degree of canal compromise. MRI appears to be the ideal study because it can scan the entire spine, recognize bone involvement before plain film, and show the extent of intraspinal disease[149–151] (Fig. 37–14). Treatment depends upon the histopathology of the primary lesion and the presence or absence of impending cord compression. Generally, most lesions are treated nonsurgically with radiation therapy or chemotherapy unless cord function is threatened.

CONCLUSION

As can be seen, extramedullary lesions are a diverse group. Treatment may be varied. Frequently therapy requires a multidisciplinary approach incorporating an orthopaedic surgeon, a medical oncologist, and others.

The standard surgical procedure is laminectomy. Occasionally, more radical approaches may necessitate internal fixation and fusion to treat spinal instability. Adjunct radiation therapy and/or chemotherapy may be required, and they frequently constitute the main management modalities in extramedullary lesions.

Extensive laminectomies in children, especially young children, should be avoided because they invariably result in a secondary spinal deformity, usually of a kyphotic type. This is particularly true in the cervical and thoracic regions. Radiation therapy can also adversely affect the growing spine. Stunting of growth or asymmetry of growth may follow, resulting in shortened stature in the former and spinal deformity, usually scoliosis, in the latter.

Adherence to the standard precautions so necessary in pediatric surgical procedures is always paramount. Adequate monitoring, a secure airway, meticulous attention to homeostasis, and temperature control are essential. The use of the operating microscope, Cusa, Laser, and intraoperative somatosensory evoked response may all be helpful but appear generally more appropriate for intramedullary lesions.

REFERENCES

1. Arseni MC, Ionesco S: Les compressions medullaires dues a des tumeurs intrarachidiennes. Etude clinico-statistique de 362 cas. J Chir 75:582, 1958.
2. Banna M, Greyspeerdt GL: Intraspinal tumours in children (excluding dysraphism). Clin Radiol 22:17, 1971.
3. Coxe WS: Tumors of the spinal canal in children. Am J Surg 27:62, 1961.
4. DeSousa AL, Kalsbeck JE, Mealey J Jr, et al.: Intraspinal tumors in children: A review of 81 cases. J Neurosurg 51:437, 1979.
5. Dodge HW Jr, Keith H, Campagna MJ: Intraspinal tumors in infants and children. J Intern Coll Surg. 26:199, 1956.
6. Farwell JR, Dohrmann GJ: Intraspinal neoplasms in children. Paraplegia 15:262, 1977–78.
7. Hamby WB: Tumors in the spinal canal in childhood. An analysis of the literature with report of a case. J Nerv Ment Dis 81:24, 1935.
8. Hamby WB: Tumors in the spinal canal in childhood. II. Analysis of the literature of a subsequent decade (1933–1942); report of a case of meningitis due to an intramedullary epidermoid communicating with a dermal sinus. J Neuropathol Exp Neurol 3:397, 1944.
9. Iraci G: Intraspinal tumors of infancy and childhood: A review of 19 surgically verified cases. J Pediatr Surg 1:534, 1966.
10. Matson D, Tachdjian MO: Intraspinal tumors in infants and children: Review of 115 cases. Postgrad Med 34:279, 1963.
11. Ross AT, Bailey OT: Tumors arising within the spinal canal in children. Neurology 3:922, 1953.
12. Svien HJ, Thelen EP, Keith HM: Intraspinal tumors in children. JAMA 155:959, 1954.
13. Till K: Observations on spinal tumours in childhood [abridged]. Proc R Soc Med 52:333, 1959.
14. Young JL Jr, Miller RW: Incidence of malignant tumors in U. S. children. J Pediatr 86:254, 1975.
15. Bailey P: Discussion in Spurling RG, Mayfield FH: Neoplasms of the spinal cord: A review of forty-two surgical cases. JAMA 107:928, 1936.
16. Grant FC, Austin GM: The diagnosis, treatment, and prognosis of tumors affecting the spinal cord in children. J Neurosurg 13:535, 1956.
17. Haft H, Ransohoff J, Carter S: Spinal cord tumors in children. Pediatrics 23:1152, 1959.
18. Matson DD: Primary intraspinal tumors. In Matson DD (ed): Neurosurgery of Infancy and Childhood. 2nd ed. Springfield, IL, Charles C Thomas, 1969, pp 647–688.

19. Di Lorenzo N, Giuffre R, Fortuna A: Primary spinal neoplasms in childhood: Analysis by 1234 published cases (including 56 personal cases) by pathology, sex, age and site. Differences from the situation in adults. Neurochirurgia 25:153, 1982.

20. Anderson FM, Carson MJ: Spinal cord tumors in children: A review of the subject and presentation of twenty-one cases. J Pediatr 43:190, 1953.

21. Mellinger JF: Tumors of the spinal cord. In Swaiman KF, Wright FS (eds): The Practice of Pediatric Neurology. Vol 2. St. Louis, CV Mosby Company, 1982, pp 864–870.

22. Arseni C, Horvath L, Iliescu D: Intraspinal tumours in children. Psychiatr Neurol Neurochir 70:123, 1967.

23. Kordás M, Paraiez E, Szenasy J: Spinal tumors in infancy and childhood. Zentrabl Neurochir 38:331, 1977.

24. Menkes JH: Tumors of the nervous system. In Menkes JH (ed): Textbook of Child Neurology. 3rd ed. Philadelphia, Lea & Febiger, 1985, pp 531–589.

25. Schliack H, Stille D: Clinical symptomatology of intraspinal tumors. In Vinken PJ, Bruyn GW (eds): Handbook of Clinical Neurology. Part I. Tumours of the spine and spinal cord. Vol 19. Amsterdam, North-Holland Publishing Company, 1976, pp 23–49.

26. Hendrick EB: Spinal cord tumors in children. In Youman JR (ed): Neurological Surgery. Vol 5. Philadelphia, WB Saunders Company, 1982, pp 3215–3221.

27. Jörgensen J, Oversen N, Poulsen JO: Intraspinal tumours in the first two decades of life. Acta Orthop Scand 47:391, 1976.

28. Bostroem E: Uber die pialem Epidermoide, Dermiode und Lipoma und dural Dermoide. Zentralbl Allg Path 8:1, 1897.

29. Leech RW, Olafson RA: Epithelial cysts of the neuraxis: Presentation of three cases and a review of the origins and classification. Arch Pathol Lab Med 101:196, 1977.

30. Takeuchi J, Ohta T, Kajikawa H: Congenital tumours of the spinal cord. In Vinken PJ, Bruyn GW (eds): Handbook of Clinical Neurology. Vol 19. Amsterdam, North Holland Publishing Company, 1975, pp 355–392.

31. Batnitzky S, Keucher TR, Mealey J Jr, et al.: Iatrogenic intraspinal epidermoid tumors. JAMA 237:148, 1977.

32. Gibson T, Norris W: Skin fragments removed by injection needles. Lancet 2:983, 1958.

33. Halcrow SJ, Crawford PJ, Craft AW: Epidermoid spinal cord tumour after lumbar puncture. Arch Dis Child 60:978, 1985.

34. Shaywitz BA: Epidermoid spinal cord tumors and previous lumbar punctures. J Pediatr 80:638, 1972.

35. Van Gilder JC, Schwartz HG: Growth of dermoids from skin implants to the nervous system and surrounding spaces of the newborn rat. J Neurosurg 26:14, 1967.

36. el-Gindi S, Fairburn B: Intramedullary spinal abscess as a complication of a congenital dermal sinus. Case report. J Neurosurg 30:494, 1969.

37. Matson DD, Jerva MJ: Recurrent meningitis associated with congenital lumbo-sacral sinus tract. J Neurosurg 25:288, 1966.

38. Walker AE, Bucy PC: Congenital dermal sinuses: A source of spinal meningeal infection and subdural abscesses. Brain 57:401, 1934.

39. Wright RL: Congenital dermal sinuses. Prog Neurol Surg 4:175, 1971.

40. Ashley DJB: Origin of teratomas. Cancer 32:390, 1973.

41. Chiquoine AD: The identification, origin, and migration of premordial germ cells in the mouse embryo. Anat Rec 118:135, 1954.

42. Newcastle NB, Francoeur J: Teratomatous cysts of the spinal canal: With sex chromatin studies. Arch Neurol 11:91, 1964.

43. Rosenbaum TJ, Soule EH, Onofrio BM: Teratomatous cyst of the spinal canal. J Neurosurg 49:292, 1978.

44. Naidich TP, McLone DG, Harwood-Nash DC: Spinal dysraphism. In Newton TH, Potts DG (eds): Modern Neuroradiology. Vol 1. CAT of the Spine and Spinal Cord. San Anselmo, CA, Claradel Press, 1983, pp 299–353.

45. Merten DF, Gooding CA, Newton TH, et al.: Meningiomas of childhood and adolescence. J Pediatr 84:696, 1974.

46. Fortuna A, Nolletti A, Nardi P, et al.: Spinal neurinomas and meningiomas in children. Acta Neurochir 55:329, 1981.

47. Nitter K: Spinal meningiomas, neurinomas, and neurofibromas and hourglass tumors. In Vinked PJ, Bruyn GW (eds): Handbook of Clinical Neurology. Vol 20. Amsterdam, North Holland Publishing Company, 1976, pp 77–322.

48. Kaya U, Özden B, Turantan MI, et al.: Spinal epidural meningioma in childhood: A case report. Neurosurgery 10:746, 1982.

49. Motomochi M, Makita Y, Nabeshima S, et al.: Spinal epidural meningioma in childhood. Surg Neurol 13:5, 1980.

50. Deen HG Jr, Scheithauer BW, Ebersold MJ: Clinical and pathological study of meningiomas of the first two decades of life. J Neurosurg 56:317, 1982.

51. Barkovich AJ: Neoplasms of the spine. In Barkovich AJ (ed): Contemporary Neuroimaging. Vol I. Pediatric Neuroimaging. New York, Raven Press, 1990, pp 273–291.

52. Russell DS, Rubinstein LJ: Tumors of the nerve roots and peripheral nerves. In Russell DS, Rubinstein LJ (eds): Pathology of the Nervous System. London, Arnold Ltd., 1971, pp 284–304.

53. Koos W, Laubichler W, Sorgo G: Statistical studies on spinal tumors in childhood and adolescence. Neuropaediatrie 4:273, 1973.

54. Grollmus J: Spinal subarachnoid hemorrhage with schwannoma. Acta Neurochir 31:253, 1975.

55. Halpern J, Feldman S, Peysere E: Subarachnoid hemorrhage with papilledema due to a spinal neurofibroma. Arch Neurol Psychiatr 79:138, 1958.

56. Prieto A Jr, Cantu RC: Spinal subarachnoid hemorrhage associated with neurofibroma of the cauda equina. J Neurosurg 27:63, 1967.

57. Cantore C, Ciapetta P, Delfini R: Intramedullary spinal neurinomas. Report of two cases. J Neurosurg 57:143, 1982.

58. Lesoin F, Delansheer E, Krivosic I, et al.: Solitary intramedullary schwannomas. Surg Neurol 19:51, 1983.

59. Canale D, Bebin J, Knighton RS: Neurologic manifestations of von Recklinghausen disease of the nervous system. Confin Neurol 24:359, 1964.

60. Hosoi K: Multiple neurofibromatosis (von Recklinghausen's disease) with special reference to malignant transformation. Arch Surg 22:258, 1931.

61. Stout AP: Tumors of the peripheral nerves. In Stout AP (ed): Atlas of Tumor Pathology. Fascicle 6. Bethesda, MD, Armed Forces Institute of Pathology, 1949, pp 9–32.

62. Hurth M, Andre JM, Djindjian R: Les hemangioblastomes intrarachidiens. Neurochirurgie 21(Suppl 1):1, 1975.

63. Rubinstein LJ: Tumors and malformations of the blood vessels. In Rubinstein LJ (ed): Tumors of the Central Nervous System. Fascicle 6. Atlas of Tumor Pathology, Second Series. Bethesda, MD, Armed Forces Institute of Pathology, 1972, pp 235–256.

64. Raney RB, Courville CB: Multiple hemangioblastomas of the central nervous system: Review of the literature and report of a case. Bull Los Angeles Neurol Soc 2:104, 1937.

65. Melmon KL, Rosen SW: Lindau's disease—review of the literature and study of a large kindred. Am J Med 36:595, 1964.

66. Horton WA, Wong V, Eldridge R: Von Hipple-Lindau disease: Clinical and pathological manifestations in nine families with 50 affected members. Arch Intern Med 136:769, 1976.

67. Kendall B, Russell J: Haemangioblastomas of the spinal cord. Br J Radiol 39:817, 1966.

68. Di Chiro G, Doppman JL: Differential angiographic features of hemangioblastomas and arteriovenous malformations of the spinal cord. Radiology 93:25, 1969.

69. Sato Y, Waziri M, Smith W, et al.: Hipple-Lindau disease: MR imaging. Radiology 166:241, 1988.

70. Sung DK, Chang CH, Harisiadis L: Cerebellar hemangioblastomas. Cancer 49:553, 1982.

71. Pascual-Castroviejo I: Pathology of spinal cord tumors in children. In Pascual-Castroviejo I (ed): Spinal Tumors in Children and Adolescents. New York, Raven Press, 1990, pp 11–34.

72. McElwain TJ, Clink HM, Jameson B, et al.: Central nervous system involvement in acute myelogenous leukemia. In Whitehouse JMA, Kay HE (eds): Central Nervous System Complications of Malignant Disease. London, Macmillan, 1979, pp 91–96.

73. Brett EM: Neurological aspects of childhood reticuloses and some other medical diseases. In Brett EM (ed): Pediatric Neurology. London, Churchill Livingstone, 1983, pp 568–581.

74. Evans AE, Gilbert ES, Zandstra R: The increasing incidence of central nervous system leukemia in children (Children's Cancer Study Group A). Cancer 26:404, 1970.
75. Pinkel D: Treatment of acute leukemia. Pediatr Clin North Am 23:117, 1976.
76. Dahl GV, Simone JV, Hustu HO, et al.: Preventive central nervous system irradiation in children with acute nonlymphocytic leukemia. Cancer 42:2187, 1978.
77. Mellinger JF: Central nervous system involvement in childhood lymphoblastic leukemia. In Swaiman KF, Wright FS (eds): The Practice of Pediatric Neurology. Vol 2. St. Louis, C. V. Mosby Company, 1982, pp 871–880.
78. Lo WD, Matthay KK, Kushner J: Spinal cord compression in a child with acute lymphoblastic leukemia. Am J Pediatr Hematol Oncol 7:373, 1985.
79. Henry JM, Heffner RR Jr, Dillard SH, et al.: Primary malignant lymphomas of the central nervous system. Cancer 34:1293, 1974.
80. Whisnant JP, Siekert RG, Sayr GP: Neurologic manifestations of the lymphomas. Med Clin North Am July:1151, 1956.
81. Packer RJ, Siegel KR, Sutton LN, et al.: Leptomeningeal dissemination of primary central nervous system tumors of childhood. Ann Neurol 18:217, 1985.
82. Arseni C, Horvath L, Carp N, et al.: Spinal dissemination following operation on cerebral oligodendroglioma. Acta Neurochir 37:125, 1977.
83. Erlich SS, Davis RL: Spinal subarachnoid metastasis from primary intracranial glioblastoma multiforme. Cancer 42:2854, 1978.
84. McLaughlin JE: Juvenile astrocytomas with subarachnoid spread. J Pathol 118:101, 1976.
85. Raney RB: Spinal cord "drop metastases" from head and neck rabdomyosarcoma: Proceedings of the Tumor Board of Children's Hospital of Philadelphia. Med Pediatr Oncol 4:3, 1978.
86. Shapiro K, Shulman K: Spinal cord seeding from cerebellar astrocytomas. Childs Brain 2:177, 1976.
87. Tarlov IM, Davidoff LM: Subarachnoid and ventricular implants in ependymal and other gliomas. J Neuropathol Exp Neurol 5:213, 1946.
88. Tomita T: Asymptomatic leptomeningeal dissemination of tumor to the spinal cord: Report of three cases. Neurosurgery 14:323, 1984.
89. Deutsch M, Reigel DH: The value of myelography in the management of childhood medulloblastoma. Cancer 45:2194, 1980.
90. Stanley P, Senac MO Jr, Segall HD: Intraspinal seeding from intracranial tumors in children. AJR 144:157, 1985.
91. Dargeon HW: Neuroblastoma. J Pediatr 61:456, 1962.
92. Koop CE, Kiesewetter WB, Horn RC: Neuroblastoma in childhood: Survival after major surgical insult to the tumor. Surgery 38:272, 1955.
93. Le Pintre J, Schweisguth O, Labrune M, et al.: Les neuroblastomes en sablier. Etuse de 22 cas. Arch Fr Pediatr 66:829, 1969.
94. Ringertz N, Lidholm SO: Mediastinal tumors and cysts. J Thorac Surg 31:458, 1956.
95. Stout AP: Ganglioneuroma of the sympathetic nervous system. Surg Gynecol Obstet 84:101, 1947.
96. Stowens D: Neuroblastoma and related tumors. Arch Pathol 63:451, 1957.
97. Russell DS, Rubinstein LJ: Peripheral tumors of the neurone series. In Russell DS, Rubinstein LJ (eds): Pathology of the Nervous System. London, Arnold Ltd., 1971, pp 305–333.
98. Feigin I, Cohen M: Maturation and anaplasia in neuronal tumors of the peripheral nervous system; with observations on the glial-like tissue in ganglioneuroblastoma. J Neuropathol Exp Neurol 36:748, 1977.
99. deLorimier AA, Bragg KU, Linden G: Neuroblastoma in childhood. Am J Dis Child. 118:441, 1969.
100. Evans AE, D'Angio GJ, Koop CE.: Diagnosis and treatment of neuroblastoma. Pediatr Clin North Am 23:161, 1976.
101. Gross RE, Farber S, Martin LW: Neuroblastoma sympatheticum. A study of 217 cases. Pediatrics 23:1179, 1959.
102. King D, Goodman J, Hawk T, et al.: Dumbbell neuroblastomas in children. Arch Surg 110:888, 1975.
103. Phillips R: Neuroblastoma. Hunterian Lecture. Ann R Coll Surg Engl 12:29, 1952.
104. Traggis DG, Filler RM, Druckman H, et al.: Prognosis for children with neuroblastoma presenting with paralysis. J Pediatr Surg 12:419, 1977.
105. Fortner J, Nicastri A, Murphy ML: Neuroblastoma: Natural history and results of treating 133 cases. Ann Surg 167:132, 1968.
106. Haden MA, Keats TE: Congenital intraspinal neuroblastoma with intraspinal calcification in the neonatal period: Report of a case with a 32-year follow-up. Pediatr Radiol 13:335, 1983.
107. Maurer HM: The Intergroup Rhabdomyosarcoma Study: Update, November 1978. Natl Cancer Inst Monogr 56:61, 1981.
108. Ch'ien LT, Kalwinsky DK, Peterson G, et al.: Metastatic epidural tumors in children. Med Pediatr Oncol 10:455, 1982.
109. Crabbe WA, Wardill JC: Benign osteoblastoma of the spine. Br J Surg 50:571, 1963.
110. Lichtenstein L: Benign osteoblastoma. Cancer 9:1044, 1956.
111. Marsh BW, Bonfiglio M, Brady LP, et al.: Benign osteoblastoma: Range of manifestations. J Bone Joint Surg 57A:1, 1975.
112. McLeod RA, Dahlin DC, Beabout JW: The spectrum of osteoblastoma. AJR 126:321, 1976.
113. Akbarnia BA, Rooholamini SA: Scoliosis caused by benign osteoblastoma of the thoracic or lumbar spine. J Bone Joint Surg 63A:1146, 1981.
114. Mehta MH, Murray RO: Scoliosis produced by painful vertebral lesions. Skeletal Radiol 1:223, 1977.
115. Merryweather R, Middlemiss JH, Sanerkin NG: Malignant transformation of osteoblastoma. J Bone Joint Surg 62B:381, 1980.
116. Schajowicz F, Lemos C: Malignant osteoblastoma. J Bone Joint Surg 58B:202, 1976.
117. Seki T, Fukuda H, Ishii Y, et al.: Malignant transformation of benign osteoblastoma. A case report. J Bone Joint Surg 57A:424, 1975.
118. Dábska M, Buraczewsky J: Aneurysmal bone cyst. Pathology, clinical course and radiologic appearance. Cancer 23:371, 1969.
119. Hay MC, Paterson D, Taylor TK: Aneurysmal bone cysts of the spine. J Bone Joint Surg 60B:406, 1978.
120. Tillman BP, Dahlin DC, Lipscomb PR, et al.: Aneurysmal bone cyst: An analysis of ninety-five cases. Mayo Clin Proc 43:478, 1968.
121. Shacked I, Tadmor R, Wolpin G, et al.: Aneurysmal bone cyst of a vertebral body with acute paraplegia. Paraplegia 19:294, 1981.
122. Mirra JM: Bone Tumors: Diagnosis and Treatment. Philadelphia, JB Lippincott Company, 1980.
123. Lichtenstein L: Aneurysmal bone cyst: Observations on fifty cases. J Bone Joint Surg 39A:873, 1957.
124. Nobler MP, Higinbotham NL, Phillips RF: The cure of aneurysma bone cyst. Irradiation superior to surgery in an analysis of 33 cases. Radiology 90:1185, 1968.
125. Savini R, Giunti A, Boriani S: Benign and malignant spinal tumors. In Bradford DS, Hensinger RM (eds): The Pediatric Spine. New York, Thieme, 1985, pp 131–154.
126. Dahlin DC: Bone Tumors. General Aspects and Data on 6221 Cases. Springfield, IL, Charles C Thomas, 1978.
127. Sundaresan N, Galicich JH, Chu FCH, et al.: Spinal chordomas. J Neurosurg 50:312, 1979.
128. Mindell ER: Chordoma. J Bone Joint Surg 63A:501, 1981.
129. O'Neill P, Bell BA, Miller JD, et al.: Fifty years of experience with chordomas in southeast Scotland. Neurosurgery 16:166, 1985.
130. Utne JR, Pugh DG: The roentgenologic aspects of chordoma. Am J Roentgenol 74:593, 1955.
131. Volpe R, Mazabraud A: A clinicopathologic review of 25 cases of chordoma (a pleomorphic and metastasizing neoplasm). Am J Surg Pathol 7:161, 1983.
132. Huvos AG: Bone Tumors. Philadelphia, WB Saunders Company, 1979.
133. Kamrin RP, Potanos JN, Pool JL: An evaluation of the diagnosis and treatment of chordoma. J Neurol Neurosurg Psychiatry 27:157, 1964.
134. Sibley RK, Day DL, Dehner LP, et al.: Metastasizing chordoma

in early childhood: A pathological and immunohistochemical study with review of literature. Pediatr Pathol 7:287, 1987.

135. Want CC, James AE Jr: Chordoma: Brief review of the literature and report of a case and widespread metastases. Cancer 22:162, 1968.

136. Krol G, Sundaresan N, Deck M: Computed tomography of axial chordomas. J Comput Assist Tomogr 7:286, 1983.

137. Meyer JE, Lepk RA, Lindfors KK, et al.: Chordomas: Their CT appearance in the cervical, thoracic, and lumbar spine. Radiology 153:693, 1984.

138. Petterson H, Hudson T, Hamlin D, et al.: Magnetic resonance imaging of sacrococcygeal tumors. Acta Radiol (Diagn) (Stockh) 26:161, 1985.

139. Rosenthal DI, Scott JA, Mankin HJ, et al.: Sacrococcygeal chordoma: Magnetic resonance imaging and computed tomography. AJR 145:143, 1985.

140. Amendola BE, Amendola MA, Oliver E, et al.: Chordoma: Role of radiation therapy. Radiology 158:839, 1986.

141. Cummings BJ, Hodson DI, Bush RS: Chordoma: The results of megavoltage radiation therapy. Int J Radiat Oncol Biol Phys 9:633, 1983.

142. Pearlman AW, Friedman M: Radical radiation therapy of chordoma. AJR 108:332, 1970.

143. Baten M, Vannucci RC: Intraspinal metastatic disease in childhood cancer. J Pediatr 90:207, 1977.

144. Törmä T: Malignant tumours of the spine and the spinal extradural space. A study based upon 250 histologically verified cases. Acta Chirurg Scand 225 (Suppl):1, 1957.

145. Howman-Giles RB, Gilday DL, Ash JM: Radionuclide skeletal survey in neuroblastoma. Radiology 131:497, 1979.

146. Bever CT Jr, Koenigsberger MR, Autunes JL, et al.: Epidural metastasis by Wilms' tumor. Am J Dis Child 135:644, 1981.

147. Leeson MC, Makley JT, Carter JR: Metastatic skeletal disease in the pediatric population. J Pediatr Orthop 5:261, 1985.

148. Lewis DW, Packer RJ, Raney B, et al.: Incidence, presentation, and outcome of spinal cord disease in children with systemic cancer. Pediatrics 78:438, 1986.

149. Godersky JC, Smoker WRK, Knutzon R: Use of magnetic resonance imaging in the evaluation of metastatic spinal disease. Neurosurgery 21:676, 1987.

150. Kamholtz R, Sze G: MRI of spinal metastasis. MRI Decisions 4:2, 1990.

151. Sarpel S, Sarpel G, Yu E, et al.: Early diagnosis of spinal-epidural metastasis by magnetic resonance imaging. Cancer 59:1112, 1987.

Chapter 38

PHAKOMATOSES:
Surgical Considerations

LUIS SCHUT, M.D., ANN-CHRISTINE DUHAIME, M.D.,
and LESLIE N. SUTTON, M.D.

Phakomatoses, or neurocutaneous syndromes, are a group of genetic disorders having in common neurologic, ocular, and dermatologic manifestations. The term "phakomatosis" was used by van der Hoeve in 1923 to link various conditions in which birthmarks, eye lesions, and tumors are found.[1] Since that time, the list of syndromes showing these features has lengthened, as has our understanding of the genetics and pathophysiology of each entity. In the past several years, advances in molecular biologic techniques as well as neuro-imaging have increased our ability to classify, diagnose, and predict the progression of these disorders.

The phakomatoses are of interest to the neurosurgeon for several reasons. First, clues to the genesis, etiology, and biology of central nervous system (CNS) neoplasms can be garnered from the study of diseases in which they can be predicted to occur at a high frequency. Second, indications and goals for surgery may be different in a case of a neurocutaneous disorder than in a sporadic case. Finally, an understanding of the natural history and genetics of the disease is critical to the care of the patient as well as the family. This is particularly true in children, as these diseases tend to be progressive, and the diagnosis of a neurocutaneous disorder may not be obvious unless a high index of suspicion is maintained. Nearly 10 per cent of all pediatric astrocytomas alone have been found to be associated with neurocutaneous syndromes, a statistic that emphasizes the importance of their recognition.[2]

THE NEUROFIBROMATOSES

The term "multiple neurofibromatosis" was introduced by Frederick Daniel von Recklinghausen in 1882 to describe two patients with cutaneous neurofibromas which he believed might be comprised of nervous elements.[3] It is now known that neurofibromatosis consists of at least two distinct disorders, which bear some superficial resemblances but are genetically and clinically distinct. The neurofibromatoses are the most common of the phakomatoses, affecting approximately 100,000 people in the United States.[4] About half the cases appear to be due to new mutations. Neurofibromatosis 1 (NF1), also known as peripheral or von Recklinghausen's neurofibromatosis, is the more common of the two. It is one of the most frequent autosomal dominant disorders found in humans, occurring with an incidence of 1 in 3000 people.[5, 6] In recent years, the gene coding for neurofibromatosis 1 has been localized to the long arm of chromosome 17.[7, 8] Neurofibromatosis 2 (NF2), which occurs in about 1 in 50,000 individuals, has been genetically localized to the long arm of chromosome 22, although other genes may also be involved.[9, 10] It is also known as central neurofibromatosis, or bilateral acoustic neurofibromatosis (BANF). The two types of neurofibromatosis have in common some cutaneous manifestation and a predisposition toward central nervous system tumors, but have many other clinical features which distinguish them from one another. Both types appear to be characterized by a disorder of neuroectodermal and mesodermal tissues in which dysplasia and neoplasia occur. Since many of the affected tissues—including nerve cells, glia, Schwann cells, melanocytes, and some visceral or endocrine organs—are derived from the embryonic neural crest, it has been postulated that the neurofibromatoses represent disorders of neural crest differentiation and regulation. The "neurocristopathy" theory is an attempt to relate the findings in this disease to abnormalities in migration, cell regulation, and cell-to-cell interactions among tissues derived from the embryonic neural crest.[11–13] Abnormalities in growth factors have also been postulated as contributing to the findings in these disorders.[14, 15] More recently, molecular genetic techniques have provided important clues as to why patients with these disorders are predisposed to central nervous system tumors, with the identification of various tumor suppressor genes and oncogenes that may be affected by the underlying genetic abnormality.[16–19] It is expected that many new insights will be gained in the upcoming years that will shed light on the mechanisms of tumor formation both in NF patients and in the general population.

DERMATOLOGIC, OPHTHALMOLOGIC, AND SKELETAL MANIFESTATIONS

Neurofibromatosis 1 (NF1)

Penetrance of the clinical features in NF1 may be variable, and this is particularly true in children because the cutaneous stigmata often occur later in life. The most common cutaneous finding is the cafe-au-lait spot. In prepubertal children this is considered diagnostic when five or more spots of at least 0.5 cm in diameter can be found.[20, 21] In adults, six spots of at least 1.5 cm are needed to solidify the diagnosis, along with at least one of the other characteristic findings or a positive family history (Table 38–1).[4]

Other dermatologic manifestations of NF1 include axillary or inguinal freckling and subcutaneous neuro-

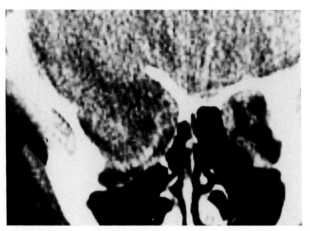

FIGURE 38–1. Congenital dysplasia of the sphenoid wing (coronal CT scan).

fibromas. The latter are benign tumors containing Schwann cells, fibroblasts, and collagen.[22] In children, they are usually sessile, subcutaneous masses, but increase in size and number with puberty and pregnancy and often become pedunculated. These tumors can undergo malignant degeneration into a malignant schwannoma or neurogenic sarcoma in 2 to 29 per cent of patients, most often in the adult population.[23]

Congenital neurofibromas are often of the plexiform type and have a propensity for the periorbital region. They are progressive and usually highly vascular lesions that present an enormous cosmetic and surgical challenge. Staged subtotal resections may be of some benefit, but the lesions are not curable and recurrence is the rule.[24, 25] It should be kept in mind that pigmented plexiform neurofibromas of the neck or trunk that extend into the midline may also extend to involve the intraspinal compartment.[26]

Ophthalmologic manifestations that may be present early in life include Lisch nodules, orbital osseous dysplasia, and buphthalmos. Lisch nodules are gelatinous, hamartomatous elevations of the iris and can be seen grossly or by slit-lamp examination. They do not interfere with vision. The nodules are present in more than 90 per cent of patients with NF1 and are usually present by puberty.[27] One of the characteristic dysplastic lesions in the disorder, sphenoid dysplasia leading to pulsatile exophthalmos, may be the presenting sign of NF1 in an infant or young child. The bony defect is easily distinguished from other forms of proptosis by CT scan (Fig. 38–1) and may be corrected by reconstructive surgery, most often using rib grafts. Buphthalmos, or "ox eye," may also be seen early in life. This is an enlargement of the globe resulting from glaucoma that is usually unilateral. This finding commonly occurs in patients with facial involvement and, when seen in combination with an asymmetric facial hypertrophy and plexiform neurofibroma of the eyelid, is known as François syndrome.[28] Preservation of useful vision in the involved eye is particularly important, since visual pathway tumors may compromise the opposite eye in the future.

TABLE 38–1. DEFINITIONS OF NEUROFIBROMATOSIS 1 AND NEUROFIBROMATOSIS 2

I. Neurofibromatosis 1 may be diagnosed in Caucasians when two or more of the following are present:

    Six or more cafe-au-lait macules whose greatest diameter is more than 5 mm in prepubescent patients and more than 15 mm in postpubescent patients.

    Two or more neurofibromas of any type *or* one plexiform neurofibroma.

    Freckling in the axillary *or* inguinal region.

    A distinctive osseous lesion as sphenoid dysplasia *or* thinning of long-bone cortex, with or without pseudoarthrosis.

    Optic glioma.

    Two or more Lisch nodules (iris hamartomas).

    A parent, sibling, or child with neurofibromatosis 1 on the basis of the previous criteria.

II. Neurofibromatosis 2 may be diagnosed when one of the following is present:

    Bilateral 8th cranial nerve masses seen by MRI with gadolinium.

    A parent, sibling, *or* child with neurofibromatosis 2 and either unilateral 8th cranial nerve mass or any one of the following:

        Neurofibroma

        Meningioma

        Glioma

        Schwannoma

        Posterior capsular cataract or opacity at a young age.

From Nance WE, Bailey BJ, Broaddus WC, et al.: NIH Consensus Development Conference Statement: Acoustic Neuroma. Neurofibromatosis Res Nwltr 8(1–2):1–8, 1992.

Optic gliomas are the most common intracranial tumor in NF1 and may be confined to the optic nerve itself, presenting as proptosis or visual loss. These will be discussed further below.

Skeletal lesions may be present at birth and include congenital bowing and pseudoarthrosis, most often affecting the tibia. Tibial pseudoarthrosis is often resistant to treatment, requiring amputation in up to 80 per cent of patients.[29] Segmental hypertrophy of the extremities and vertebral scalloping in association with tumors or meningoceles may occur.[30] Lateral thoracic meningoceles are characteristic of NF1 and may mimic a spinal neoplasm, from which they can be differentiated by myelography. These usually require no specific treatment.[31]

The most common skeletal manifestation of NF1 is scoliosis, which may be present in more than half of all patients.[29] This usually presents during late childhood and may be related to mesodermal dysplasia or neurogenic factors. A severe kyphoscoliosis of the cervicothoracic region is particularly characteristic and requires early aggressive surgical treatment if severe deformity and neurologic compromise are to be avoided.[32] Multiple procedures, including anterior and posterior fusions and internal fixation, may be needed to achieve solid arthrodesis in patients with scoliosis, because of its extraordinary tendency toward rapid progression. Preoperative evaluation should always include spinal cord imaging to identify intraspinal neoplasms, which will be discussed further below.[33–36] The use of MRI-compatible spinal instrumentation should be encouraged, since new lesions requiring radiographic evaluation are likely to develop in time.

Neurofibromatosis 2 (NF2)

Patients with central neurofibromatosis may also have dermal and plexiform neurofibromas and cafe-au-lait spots, although these are less common than in NF1. Lisch nodules and optic nerve gliomas may occur, though they are rare. However, juvenile posterior subcapsular cataracts are common, being found in up to 85 per cent of adults with NF2. These lesions may require intervention to preserve vision, and patients should undergo regular examinations to permit early diagnosis.[4]

NF2 patients have a high risk of multiple spinal neurofibromas, which may be associated with both skeletal and neurologic manifestations. These lesions will be discussed in more detail below.

CENTRAL NERVOUS SYSTEM (CNS) MANIFESTATIONS

Neoplasms of the brain, spinal cord, cranial nerves, nerve roots, and meningeal coverings all occur with increased frequency in the neurofibromatoses. In general, NF1 is associated with intracranial, spinal, and peripheral tumors arising from astrocytic or neuronal origins (e.g., gliomas, astrocytomas, neurofibromas, and dysplasias), whereas NF2 produces tumors of the coverings of the nervous system (e.g., schwannomas, meningiomas, and ependymomas).[4] Estimates of the frequency of CNS tumors in children with NF range from less than 5 per cent to 14 per cent.[37, 38] These disorders are sufficiently common that a careful history and physical examination pertinent to the diagnosis of NF should be a routine part of the work-up of any child with a CNS tumor, particularly in those types less common in childhood, such as meningiomas or acoustic neuromas.

While the two types of neurofibromatosis have some overlap in tumors to which a patient is predisposed, distinct differences in frequencies distinguish one disorder from the other. In NF1, anterior visual pathway tumors have been estimated to occur in 5 to 15 per cent of patients. With routine screening of patients with MRI, this frequency may be even higher. Whereas the mean age of patients with tumors confined to the optic nerve is in the early twenties, chiasmatic tumors occur most often in the first decade of life. When symptomatic, such tumors may be the first manifestation of NF in a young child, presenting variably with visual complaints, headache, hydrocephalus, endocrine disturbance, or other neurologic signs or symptoms.[39]

MRI has now become the test of choice for evaluating visual pathway tumors in NF. Biopsy is often unnecessary when the MRI is typical, but unusual lesions can be approached stereotactically or directly, usually via the pterional approach. Although many of these lesions are indolent and produce minimal symptoms, more extensive surgery may be indicated for debulking of a large lesion with symptomatic mass effect and can be approached either pterionally or transcallosally, depending on the size, symptoms, and location of the tumor. Aggressive surgery of some lesions may result in visual compromise, hypothalamic damage, or other neurologic complications. Patients with significant clinical or radiographic progression of optic pathway tumors also can be treated with chemotherapy, particularly if they are younger than 5 years of age, and with radiation if they are older. Each modality carries its own risks and benefits, and there is at present no clear agreement as to the optimal treatment algorithm.[40–45]

The management of tumors confined to the optic nerve depends in part on the degree of functional vision as well as associated proptosis. The natural history of these lesions is not entirely clear, and consensus as to appropriate management, ranging from surgery to radiation to observation, is yet to be attained.[46]

The pathognomonic feature of neurofibromatosis 2 is the presence of bilateral acoustic neuromas. Other intracranial tumors characteristic of NF2 include schwannomas of other cranial nerves and meningiomas, which may be multifocal. Acoustic tumors occur in more than 95 per cent of patients with the disorder and usually present in adolescence. Acoustic neuromas may occur, though rarely, in NF1 as well. The lesions are best imaged with MRI with gadolinium enhancement.

The management of acoustic neuromas in neurofibromatosis has been controversial. The goal of management is to preserve maximal function, and the role and timing of surgery has been much discussed. Some authors advocate early aggressive treatment of these lesions as the approach with the highest chance of preserving long-term function of the facial or even acoustic nerves. Others have stressed the indolent growth rate of many of these lesions and have advocated that surgery be reserved for large tumors causing brainstem compression or progressive hearing or cranial nerve dysfunction, since surgery often results in loss of these functions, which, when bilateral, is extremely debilitating.[47–50] More recently, the role of radiosurgery has been considered, as a theoretic manner in which the lesions could be reduced or eliminated with a possibly lower acute morbidity.[51, 52] At the present time, management is determined on an individual basis.[4]

Although specific frequencies may differ between the two NF types, gliomas of all grades can occur in the cerebrum, brainstem, and spinal cord, as can ependymomas, meningiomas, schwannomas, and neurofibromas. A change in school performance, personality, or neurologic findings in a child with NF, or a new complaint of pain, orthopaedic deformity, or bowel and bladder patterns, should prompt a search for a new or changing lesion. In planning management, special care is taken to preserve as much neurologic function as possible, since the progression of the disease may result in further compromise of a complementary nervous system region in the future. In addition, the long-term risks of therapy known to increase the chance of second tumors, such as radiation and chemotherapy, may influence the ultimate prognosis in a child treated for a neoplasm who is already predisposed to oncogenesis.

The CNS in neurofibromatosis 1 is characterized pathologically by disorganization and the presence of hamartomas, heterotopias, and low-grade neoplasms. Such abnormal architecture may result in the syndromes of aqueductal stenosis, syringomyelia, and central precocious puberty. The latter condition can be treated medically.[53] Macrocephaly may be seen in three fourths of patients with NF1.[54] The relatively high incidence of intellectual handicap (approximately one third), including hyperactivity, behavioral disturbance, and learning disability, probably reflects the intrinsic cerebral disorganization characteristic of NF1 and seen on MRI as areas of abnormal signal intensity.[38, 55] (Fig. 38–2). The brains of patients with NF2 do not show this marked disorganization, and cognitive function in patients with NF2 is generally normal.[56]

The use of MRI, particularly with contrast, has proved valuable in the evaluation of these patients, for it has demonstrated in vivo the extraordinary and previously unsuspected range of abnormalities in the NF central nervous system. However, many completely asymptomatic lesions are also found, raising the dilemma of how to manage incidentally found focal brain and spinal cord lesions. Most centers follow the policy of watchful waiting in the management of the many "bright spots" seen on MRI, assuming that these represent hamartomas or low-grade neoplasms. Changes in symptoms, signs, size, or enhancement pattern of these lesions may warrant biopsy and institution of ap-

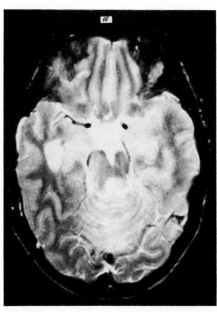

FIGURE 38–2. Multiple areas of abnormal signal intensity in a patient with NF 1 seen on T2-weighted magnetic resonance imaging.

propriate therapy for those found to be more biologically aggressive.

In patients with neurofibromatosis, special considerations for management of some problems may be needed because of the extent and natural history of the nervous system involvement. An example of this is multiple spinal neurofibromas, which can occur in both NF1 and NF2, where complete excision is not possible (Fig. 38–3). When multiple pedunculated dumbbell tumors are found on screening studies but the patient is asymptomatic, as is common in NF2, no intervention is needed. However, if myelopathy or radiculopathy develops, surgical debulking of the symptomatic lesion is warranted, with consideration given to early stabilization in order to prevent the progressive deformity to which these children are predisposed. As mentioned above, when intervention is needed because of scoliosis rather than myelopathy, as often happens in the setting of multiple plexiform intra- and paraspinal plexiform neurofibromas (most commonly seen in NF1), early spinal instrumentation and stabilization may offer the best chance of limiting progressive neurologic compromise.

Other spinal manifestations of NF can present a formidable challenge to the neurosurgeon and the orthopaedic surgeon. Large intrathoracic or intra-abdominal neurofibromas or ganglioneuromas may extend into the spinal canal, requiring staged anterior and posterior resections and stabilization. As mentioned above, scoliosis in patients with NF may require aggressive intervention because of its tendency toward relentless progression. Intramedullary astrocytomas and ependymomas occur with increased frequency in NF, and also may be associated with severe spinal deformity, which may be exacerbated if radiation therapy is required. Early stabilization should be considered in these cases

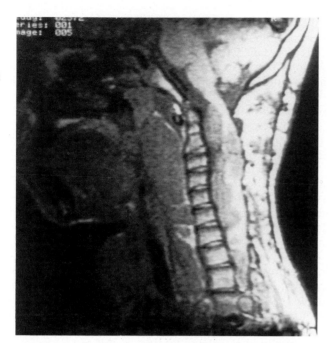

FIGURE 38–3. Multiple spinal neurofibromas in a child with NF 1.

as well. Finally, patients known to have intraspinal neurofibromas of the cervical region with encroachment on the intrathecal space should be handled with extra caution during intubation and positioning for any type of surgery, and preoperative awake flexion and extension testing may be useful.

OTHER NEOPLASMS

Tumors of other neural crest cell derivatives that occur in association with NF1 include pheochromocytoma and neuroblastoma. The former may influence anesthetic management and should be kept in mind during preoperative evaluation or if hypertension is discovered. Neurofibromas and gangliogliomas may arise from the visceral neural plexus. Non-neural crest tumors that occur more commonly than would be expected include leukemia, sarcoma, and Wilms' tumor, and NF1 is considered to be the most common single gene defect associated with childhood cancer.[57]

GENETIC COUNSELING

Diagnostic criteria for the two neurofibromatoses have recently been updated by a National Institutes of Health Conference Panel (see Table 38–1).[4] With these guidelines, the diagnosis of NF usually can be made in a patient and family members on clinical grounds. However, phenotypic variability, paucity of clinical signs in early childhood, and a high spontaneous mutation rate complicate clinical diagnosis. While essentially all affected offspring of a parent with neurofibromatosis 1 can be distinguished from unaffected siblings

by the presence of the criterion number of cafe-au-lait spots by the age of 5 years, other situations exist in which the diagnosis may be equivocal.[4, 38] Direct genetic analysis of NF1 and NF2 is likely to become the standard of diagnosis, and these techniques also should be applicable to prenatal testing.[56]

PROGNOSIS

Although the neurosurgeon often sees patients who have the more severe manifestations of the neurofibromatoses, population-based studies can provide a more balanced view of lifetime risk of complications. In one such study, approximately 3 per cent of patients with NF1 had moderate to severe retardation, and an additional 30 per cent had mild cognitive deficits. About 7 per cent had skeletal deformity requiring surgery; just over 1 per cent had severe plexiform neurofibromas of the head and neck; and nearly 16 per cent had treatable complications such as aqueductal stenosis, endocrine tumors, and spinal neurofibromas. Only 5 per cent had CNS tumors or malignant tumors.[38] A similar study showed comparable complication rates, but a higher incidence of mental retardation, which was usually mild (45 per cent), and a significant frequency of depression and anxiety.[55]

In both the neurofibromatoses, penetrance is high, but in NF2 there is less variability among affected individuals. An MRI with gadolinium at puberty in at-risk individuals will usually make the diagnosis, and the prognosis for the individual patient depends on rate of growth of acoustic neuromas, disabilities associated with these tumors or their treatment, and presence and extent of other tumors such as meningiomas and schwannomas. It may be that future interventions will be aimed at the underlying genetic abnormality that predisposes patients to the formation of tumors, and that in this way the prognosis will be improved.[16]

TUBEROUS SCLEROSIS

Although tuberous sclerosis (TS) is inherited as an autosomal dominant trait, the majority of cases are thought to be sporadic.[58, 59] Linkage analysis appears to show genetic heterogeneity in tuberous sclerosis, with different families having the responsible gene localized to chromosome 9, 11, and possibly a third locus.[60, 61] Next to neurofibromatosis 1, it is the phakomatosis most likely to be seen by the neurosurgeon and has a prevalence of about 1 in 10,000 to 12,000 children.[58, 62] Also known as Bourneville's disease, tuberous sclerosis most often becomes manifest in childhood with progressive symptoms involving the skin, viscera, and nervous system.

The most typical early skin lesions are the so-called "ash leaf spots." These are small, hypopigmented areas that often have an ash leaf or thumb print shape with one end rounded and the other tapered. The spots are usually present at birth and may be accentuated in pale individuals by ultraviolet light. In a few patients, ash leaf spots first appear later in childhood.[63]

Facial angiofibromas, or "adenoma sebaceum," appear in a butterfly distribution by middle childhood and occur in 90 per cent of patients with tuberous sclerosis. When severe, the raised nodules may obscure vision and may bleed when traumatized. These lesions can be treated with shave excision or with the carbon dioxide laser.[64]

Other skin manifestations of TS include cafe-au-lait spots, areas of subependymal fibrosis (shagreen, or sharkskin, patches), which are most often located in the lumbosacral area, and subungual fibromas of the fingers and toes, presenting by adolescence.

The eye lesions of TS consist of hamartomas in the retina which are most often asymptomatic (Fig. 38–4). Hamartomas may also be found in the visceral organs. The lungs may show cystic or "honeycomb" changes. Angiomyolipomas of the kidneys are benign tumors occurring in a high percentage of patients with TS. When large, they may interfere with renal function. Cardiac rhabdomyomas occur in as many as half the patients and sometimes prompt the diagnosis of TS in infancy. They may be associated with arrhythmias, and a cardiac evaluation may be advisable prior to surgery. These lesions often regress spontaneously.[65, 66]

It is the CNS lesion, however, that most often brings the patient with TS to medical attention, and the disease is described classically as including the triad of characteristic skin lesions, seizures, and mental retardation. The pathologic substrate of the neurologic symptoms and that for which the disease is named is the subependymal nodule or "tuber." These benign hamartomatous lesions are multiple and occur in the lining of the lateral and third ventricles. They can be seen on CT scan, MRI, or sometimes by ultrasonography at birth.[67, 68] The tubers are usually calcified, protrude into the ventricle ("candle guttering"), and do not enhance with contrast material. Pathologically, the subependymal lesions consist of glial nodules. Cortical tubers are similar lesions that occur at the brain surface and are believed to represent aberrant populations of cells that failed to migrate or differentiate properly.[69] Abnormal cell surface factors may play a role in the formation of these lesions. Low-density areas in the cortex and in white matter are seen on CT scan in patients with tuberous sclerosis and have been attributed to demyelination.[70] Uncalcified tubers may also appear as hypodense areas and can be differentiated from demyelination, when indicated, by MRI.[71]

The presence of subependymal and subpial tubers illustrates the intrinsic disorganization of the brain in tuberous sclerosis, which most likely accounts for the tendency toward slow intellect and seizures. As would be predicted, these two clinical features are not entirely independent. While 80 per cent of TS patients with seizures develop them by age 5, those who have onset of seizures before age 2 have a higher incidence of retardation. Conversely, patients without seizures are likely to be intellectually normal.[62] When seizures present very early in life as infantile spasms, the diagnosis of TS may be missed unless carefully sought, because of the paucity of associated findings at this age.[72]

Perhaps with greater frequency than was previously recognized, patients may have a single prominent cortical tuber that corresponds to a seizure focus.[73] Biopsy of cortical tubers is not routinely necessary, since unlike the subependymal nodules, these lesions are not associated with tumor formation. However, resection may be indicated in cases of intractable seizures. Because of the diffuse nature of the disease, improved control and not elimination of the seizures is the goal of surgery. Nonetheless, a significant improvement in quality of life may be obtained by a resection of a epileptogenic tuber and surrounding cortex in selected patients.[74]

The characteristic brain tumor in tuberous sclerosis is the subependymal giant cell tumor, which is reported to occur in 7 to 23 per cent of patients.[70] These lesions are believed to arise from a subependymal tuber and nearly always occur at the foramen of Monro. Pathologically, these are usually giant cell astrocytomas, though other histologic types have also been described.[67, 75–78] Tumors usually present with headache or other indications of increased intracranial pressure when hydrocephalus develops from ventricular obstruction. CT scans show an isodense soft tissue mass associated with calcification that enhances brightly with contrast material (Fig. 38–5). Tubers may also enhance on MRI with gadolinium.[79] While an enhancing mass in a patient with TS must be considered a tumor, when asymptomatic, the mass may be observed by follow-up with serial scans, with surgery reserved for symptomatic lesions.[77]

Most giant cell tumors can be approached transcallosally. Although the intense vascularity of some tumors may limit resection, the ultrasonic aspirator may be extremely useful in reducing the mass of the tumor. Large vessels often occur on the ventricular surface and at the site of attachment of the tumor to the lateral ventricular wall. Therefore, if the intraventricular portion of the tumor can be debulked internally, with care

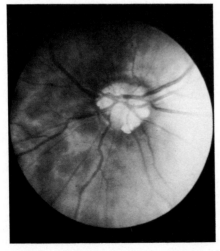

FIGURE 38–4. Retinal hamartoma in tuberous sclerosis.

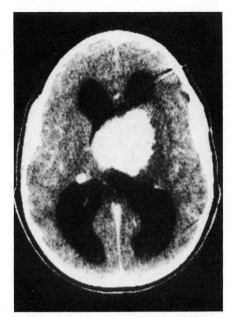

FIGURE 38–5. Enhanced CT scan showing intraventricular tumor in tuberous sclerosis.

taken to protect the normal ependymal surface and choroid plexus, this problem may be minimized. The goal of surgery is to establish free communication between the anterior and posterior compartments of the lateral ventricles, and between the lateral and third ventricles, thus relieving obstruction. In some cases, shunting may also be necessary, but if communication has been established, a single shunt, rather than multiple shunts into various compartments, will suffice.

These tumors tend to grow slowly and behave in a benign fashion, but they may recur and cause progressive symptoms. Radiation therapy has been used to control tumor growth but has met with limited success.[76] Reoperation may be indicated for progressive disease. Interestingly, the usual histologic features of malignancy, such as cellular atypia, mitosis, and necrosis, do not predict outcome in this tumor type.[80]

STURGE-WEBER SYNDROME

This disorder, also known as encephalotrigeminal angiomatosis, is classified with the phakomatoses because of involvement of the skin, eyes, and nervous system. However, it is unlike the other syndromes in that it occurs sporadically, and the genetic influences remain unknown. One theory suggests that Sturge-Weber syndrome, along with other birth defects involving the skin, represents lethal genes that survive by mosaicism.[81]

The characteristic skin lesion in the Sturge-Weber syndrome is a facial port-wine stain, or nevus flammeus, which is present at birth. Only those nevi that include the ophthalmic trigeminal distribution (i.e., the upper eyelid and forehead) are associated with this syn-

drome. This group comprises about 40 per cent of all children with facial port-wine stains.[82] The facial nevus can be treated by means of laser therapy.[83] Eye findings in this syndrome include unilateral glaucoma, which is the most common and may be difficult to treat, as well as buphthalmos and retinal angiomas.[84, 84]

The brain lesion associated with this disorder is an ipsilateral pial venous angiomatous malformation that most often involves the occipital or parieto-occipital lobe. Pathologically, the lesion is characterized by calcification in the outer cortical zone of the brain parenchyma surrounding the abnormal vessels. Microscopic intravascular calcifications are also seen. Radiographically, cortical calcifications in this syndrome can be discerned on plain skull films as wavy double lines, the so-called "tram track" sign. CT scan is even more sensitive in demonstrating the vascular malformation, particularly in infants in whom calcification may be minimal. Surrounding brain atrophy can also be seen by CT (Fig. 38–6). Arteriography shows a lack of cortical vein visualization beneath the affected cortex, enlargement of the deep draining veins, and in some cases nonfilling of the sagittal sinus.[86] MRI with gadolinium shows the venous congestion, angiomatous changes, and parenchymal alterations even before calcification occurs.[87] Cerebral blood flow as seen by SPECT scanning is decreased adjacent to the lesion.[88]

The disease is characterized clinically by seizures, hemiparesis, hemiatrophy, visual field defects, and sometimes retardation. Seizures usually begin in infancy and early childhood. As with tuberous sclerosis, early seizure onset is correlated with poor prognosis for intellectual development. The progression of neurologic problems is typically described as stepwise, with each prolonged seizure episode followed by an incomplete recovery to baseline. It has been proposed that sequen-

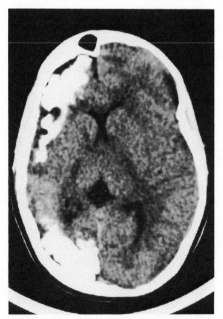

FIGURE 38–6. Unenhanced CT scan in a patient with Sturge-Weber syndrome.

tial cortical vessel thrombosis may explain the clinical deterioration as well as the angiographic findings.[86]

Treatment for the Sturge-Weber syndrome historically has been medical, with control of seizures the goal. Antiplatelet medications have also been suggested as a preventive measure for presumed cortical thrombosis, but outcome comparisons with the variable natural history of the disease are difficult to assess. Medical control of seizures may become more difficult with time, and refractoriness to maximum medications may occur.

In light of the poor outlook for patients with large lesions and early onset of seizures, with respect to both seizure control and neurologic function, early aggressive surgery has been proposed by some authors.[89] Hemispherectomy, hemidecortication, and lobectomy have been performed for this condition. These procedures seem to be tolerated best with respect to preservation of function when they are done in the first few months of life. Good seizure control, minimal hemiparesis, and normal intelligence have been reported, but the ability to prevent deterioration has not been universal.[84, 90, 91] These aggressive procedures are not without risk, especially in very young infants, and the role of surgery in the management of Sturge-Weber disease remains controversial.

VON HIPPEL–LINDAU DISEASE

Cerebellar and other CNS hemangioblastomas, angiomatosis retinae, and various visceral cysts and tumors constitute the syndrome known as Von Hippel–Lindau disease. Although isolated cerebellar hemangioblastomas in children have been reported,[92] the disease usually presents in adulthood. It is transmitted as an autosomal dominant trait with variable penetrance, with a gene locus on the short arm of chromosome 3.[93] A positive family history is found in about 20 per cent of patients. The diagnosis is made by the presence of two or more separate characteristic lesions in a given individual or by a single lesion with a positive family history.[94]

The retinal hemangiomas in Von Hippel–Lindau disease occur in 60 per cent of patients.[59, 95] They appear as small vascular blotches with a feeding artery and draining vein. Because of an abnormal absence of tight junctions in the capillaries of the angioma, leakage of blood into and beneath the retina can occur. Retinal detachment and visual loss may result, and this sometimes is the presenting symptom of the disease.[96] The retinal lesions can be treated with the laser or other forms of coagulation therapy. Glaucoma may also occur in association with angiomatosis retinae.[95] Because of these problems, it is recommended that at-risk children undergo ophthalmologic examination by the age of 2 years.[97]

The most common visceral lesions in Von Hippel–Lindau disease are pheochromocytoma and renal cysts and tumors. Pheochromocytoma may be bilateral, and

hypertension in a patient with the syndrome is highly suggestive. The work-up includes measurements of 24-hour urine catecholamines and careful body CT scan or MRI, including the course of the sympathetic chain in the abdomen and thorax.[98] Nuclear medicine studies may also be useful in the work-up of pheochromocytoma in children.[99]

The renal lesions in Von Hippel–Lindau disease occur in two thirds of patients and range from simple cysts to malignant hypernephroma. The risk of malignant progression of a cystic kidney lesion increases with age, and renal cell carcinoma is present in 25 to 38 per cent of all patients.[94] It is the leading cause of death in Von Hippel–Lindau disease. Interestingly, the gene deletion responsible for sporadic renal cell carcinoma is also located on 3p.[100] Management of the kidney lesions in VHL is controversial, ranging from conservative approaches to bilateral prophylactic nephrectomies; routine surveillance of patients and at-risk relatives is recommended.[101]

Other visceral lesions include angiomas, cysts, and adenomas of the pancreas, liver, spleen, lung, epididymis, and ovary. These lesions are usually asymptomatic.

The most characteristic CNS lesion in Von Hippel–Lindau disease is the cerebellar hemangioblastoma. These lesions occur in 35 to 60 per cent of patients and are usually said to be more common in males.[95, 97] When the same tumor occurs sporadically, it is usually in the older individual, whereas it is most common in young adults when associated with Von Hippel–Lindau disease. These are benign tumors characterized histologically by abundant capillaries, reticulin stroma, and "pseudoxanthoma" cells. They are cystic in 60 per cent of patients. An increased hematocrit is frequently seen in association with hemangioblastomas and is presumed to be a consequence of an erythropoietic factor elaborated by the tumor. Hematocrits tend to return to normal after tumor removal.

On CT scan, hemangioblastomas appear as cystic or isodense lesions that are well delineated and enhance uniformly in the solid portion with contrast material. Multiple lesions may be present, and angiography has been reported to be more sensitive in finding accessible asymptomatic lesions, which the surgeon can then remove prophylactically during an operation for larger symptomatic lesions.[102] More recently, MRI with gadolinium has shown CNS lesions, which are often multiple, in 72 per cent of patients with the disease, although 41 per cent of patients with CNS tumors were asymptomatic.[97] Lesions are seen most often in the cerebellum, spinal cord, and brainstem, with predilection for the craniocervical junction and conus medullaris.[102]

Complete resection of a hemangioblastoma is curative. In cystic lesions, the mural nodule must be removed, or the cyst will recur. Radiation therapy for subtotally removed or recurrent lesions has been reported to be beneficial.[103]

Lesions in the spinal cord are often associated with a syrinx cavity. These tend to be located dorsally in the cord and can usually be removed surgically. Patients with multiple lesions that are asymptomatic are generally treated conservatively. However, if an accessible lesion can be removed with little risk during an operation for a symptomatic lesion, this may be warranted. As more data with serial MRI in Von Hippel–Lindau patients with asymptomatic lesions become available, a better understanding of the natural history and risks of deterioration should become available.

Since the condition is progressive, patients with Von Hippel–Lindau disease should undergo screening on a routine basis including MR imaging of the neuraxis, CT or MRI of the viscera, specifically kidney, ophthalmologic examinations, renal function tests, and measurement of urinary VMA. Genetic counseling and routine screening of adult relatives who are at risk should also be part of the treatment plan.

ATAXIA-TELANGIECTASIA

Also known as Louis-Bar syndrome, after the description by Denise Louis-Bar in 1941,[104] ataxia-telangiectasia is a fascinating disorder that links genetics, neurologic degeneration, immunology, aging, and cancer. It is unique among the phakomatoses in that it is transmitted as an autosomal recessive trait, with a gene locus on the long arm of chromosome 11.[105] The disease itself is rare, occurring in two to three per 100,000 births, but with a gene frequency estimated to occur in at least one per cent of the population.[106] For this reason, ataxia-telangiectasia has generated much interest among epidemiologists, geneticists, oncologists, and others seeking to understand the relationship between a faulty gene and the occurrence of more common degenerative and malignant diseases in the population at large.

As with many neurocutaneous disorders, the characteristic external lesions are not usually present at birth. The first to appear are the conjunctival telangiectasias. These are bilateral and become progressively more pronounced throughout childhood.[107] Finer telangiectasias appear over the ears, neck, face, and antecubital and popliteal fossae and increase with exposure or irradiation. Premature graying and thinning of the hair, loss of skin elasticity and subcutaneous fat, and seborrheic dermatitis are manifestations akin to accelerated aging and have been described as progeric.

These and other features of the disease are thought to be consequences of the underlying genetic abnormality in ataxia-telangiectasia. The chromosomes of patients with the disease show increased rates of spontaneous breakage and are more sensitive to agents inducing chromosomal instability. It is thus classified, along with several other conditions, among the so-called clastogenic disorders, which are hypothesized to result from a defect in DNA repair. Other related characteristic features of the disease include immunodeficiency, radiation sensitivity, and an increased incidence of neoplasia. The immune disorder includes impaired synthesis of immunoglobulins A and E (IgA and IgE), with an increased incidence of recurrent sinopulmo-

nary infections, which are the most common cause of death.[108] Radiosensitivity has led to fatalities in patients with ataxia-telangiectasia treated with conventional doses of radiation.[109] Subclinical radiosensitivity may occur in heterozygotes. Some estimates place the frequency of ataxia-telangiectasia carriers as high as 1 in 60 in the population, and suggest that screening for carriers could permit higher doses of radiation therapy to be given without increased risk of toxicity in the remaining population of patients requiring radiation therapy for malignancy.[110]

The increased risk of cancer in homozygotes, both lymphoreticular malignancies and solid tumors, has been well documented and has been estimated to occur in 10 to 38 per cent of ataxia-telangectasia patients.[107, 111] The association between malignancy and immunodeficiency is seen in other disorders, such as the acquired immunodeficiency syndrome (AIDS), but the molecular genetic underpinnings of this dual susceptibility are yet to be determined.[111] Next to infection, malignancy is the most common cause of death in ataxia-telangiectasia. The cancer risk of a heterozygote with the gene has been estimated to be several times that of the normal population and may account for a large proportion of cancer deaths in younger individuals in the population at large.[106]

A persistence of fetal proteins in the serum is another characteristic of ataxia-telangiectasia. This feature has been hypothesized to result from a defect in differentiation of specific cell populations, but its exact cause remains unknown. An elevated serum level of alpha-fetoprotein is present in essentially all patients with the disease but is not found in heterozygotes.[112]

The principal neurologic manifestations of the disorder are ataxia and choreoathetosis Affected children appear normal in infancy. Ataxia usually becomes obvious by age 2, as mobility increases, along with a cerebellar type of dysarthria. Athetosis occurs a bit later. Intellect is preserved, but development may plateau as a child becomes progressively disabled. However, intelligence may be superficially masked by the characteristic dull, sad-looking face that is also thought to be a manifestation of the cerebellar disorder. The personality has been described as placid. Disturbances of eye movement are manifestations of oculomotor apraxia. The children have a characteristic posture, with a tendency to hunch and drop the head. Strength, however, remains normal until late in the disease. Reflexes become absent in adolescence, and toes remain downgoing. Sensation is usually normal, although peripheral neuronal degeneration has been reported.[107, 108, 113, 114]

The major neuropathologic feature of ataxia-telangiectasia is atrophy of the cerebellum with diffuse cell loss, which is most marked in the vermis. Reactive gliosis is present. Brainstem and spinal demyelination, cell loss, and gliosis are also found. CT scan shows a nonspecific pattern of cerebellar atrophy.

The prognosis in ataxia-telangiectasia is poor. Most patients are wheelchair-bound by adolescence. Although survival beyond the teens was formerly considered rare, more recent reports document longer survival.[111] Supportive care, physical therapy, and prevention and treatment of infections have been the mainstays of therapy, as no specific intervention has yet been found for the underlying genetic lesion.

INCONTINENTIA PIGMENTI

Also known as Bloch-Sulzberger syndrome, this rare disorder has been postulated to be transmitted by an x-linked dominant gene.[115] There is a strong female predominance in the disease. Affected patients present at infancy with the first of three stages of skin changes, which is characterized by vesiculobullous lesions affecting the trunk, extremities, and scalp but sparing the face. It is accompanied by peripheral eosinophilia. The second stage, usually lasting for several months, is marked by verrucous lesions in a similar distribution. In the third stage, tan or gray macules in a whorled or streaked pattern appear. These generally resolve at puberty.

A variety of ocular findings have been reported, including intraocular masses described as pseudogliomas, optic atrophy, and uveitis.[116] Developmental defects of teeth and bones are sometimes found, suggesting a disorder of ectodermal derivatives. The CNS is involved in about half the patients, with symptoms including seizures, ataxia, and mental retardation, the last being reported in about 15 per cent.[117] As in other phakomatoses, early seizure onset is correlated with a poor intellectual outcome.

CT scan in incontinentia pigmenti may show various patterns of brain atrophy and areas of low density.[116] Pathologically, the brain shows the effects of acute hemorrhagic encephalopathy and atrophy, as well as some features suggestive of abnormal migration of fetal nervous elements.

The disease progression in incontinentia pigmenti is variable, with some patients dying in early childhood and others having a more benign course characterized by typical skin lesions but only mild CNS involvement.

PROTEUS SYNDROME

One of the more recently described phakomatoses, proteus syndrome, by its choice of name implies a varied clinical presentation.[118] Manifestations include hemihypertrophy, macrodactyly, pigmented nevi, scoliosis, ocular hamartomas, and a characteristic "cerebroid" gyriform pattern to the palmar or plantar skin.[118, 119] It was probably this condition, not neurofibromatosis, that was manifested in the famous "elephant man," James Merrick.

SUMMARY

A working familiarity with the phakomatoses is essential for the neurosurgeon encountering young patients and their families. Complete care and planning for the future are greatly aided when the neurosurgeon is prepared for the development of new clinical manifestations of the disorder. Pertinent questions and examinations for cutaneous stigmata, careful family history, and ophthalmologic consultation when appropriate should be a routine part of the evaluation of all children with CNS tumors. Application of molecular genetic techniques to the study of these disorders offers an opportunity to greatly augment knowledge of the basic causes of neoplasia. Advances in molecular genetics and neuro-imaging will continue to enhance our understanding of these disorders with respect to diagnosis, screening, natural history, and new approaches to therapy in the years to come.

REFERENCES

1. Van der Hoeve J: Eye diseases in tuberous sclerosis of the brain and in von Recklinghausen disease. Trans Ophthalmol Soc UK 43:534, 1923.
2. Kibirige M, Birch J, Campbell R, et al.:A review of astrocytoma in childhood. Pediatr Hematol Oncol 6(4):319, 1989.
3. von Recklinghausen F. Uber die Multipen Fibrome der Haut Une Ihre Beziehung Zuden Multiplen Neuromen. Berlin, A Hirschwald, 1882.
4. Mulvihill J, Parry D, Sherman J, et al.: Neurofibromatosis 1 (von Recklinghausen disease) and neurofibromatosis 2 (bilateral acoustic neurofibromatosis). An update. Ann Intern Med 113:39, 1990.
5. Crowe F, Schull J, Need J: A Clinical, Pathological and Genetic Study of Multiple Neurofibromatosis. Springfield, IL, Charles C Thomas, 1956.
6. Riccardi V, Eichner J: Neurofibromatosis: Phenotype, Natural History, and Pathogenesis. Baltimore, MD, Johns Hopkins University Press, 1986.
7. Menon A, Gusella J, Seizinger B: Progress toward the isolation and characterization of the genes causing neurofibromatosis. Cancer Surv 9(4):689, 1990.
8. Collins F, O'Connell P, Ponder B, Seizinger B: Progress toward identifying the neurofibromatosis (NF1) gene. Trends Genet 5(7):217, 1989.
9. Fontaine B, Rouleau G, Seizinger B, et al.: Molecular genetics of neurofibromatosis 2 and related tumors (acoustic neuroma and meningioma). Ann NY Acad Sci 615:338, 1991.
10. Neurofibromatosis Conference Statement. National Institutes of Health Consensus Development Conference. Arch Neurol 45:575, 1988.
11. Boland R: Neurofibromatosis—the quintessential neurocristopathy: Pathogenetic concepts and relationships. In Riccardi VM, Mulvihill JJ (eds): Neurofibromatosis (von Recklinghausen's Disease). Advances in Neurology, Vol 29. New York, Raven Press 1981, pp 67–75.
12. Jones M: The neurocristopathies: reinterpretation based upon the mechanism of abnormal morphogenesis. Cleft Palate J 27(2):136, 1990.
13. Weston J: The regulation of normal and abnormal neural crest cell development. In Riccardi V, Mulvihill J (eds): Neurofibromatosis (von Recklinghausen's Disease). Advances in Neurology, Vol 29. New York, Raven Press, 1981, pp 77–95.
14. Kanter W, Eldridge K, Fabricant R, et al.: Central neurofibromatosis with bilateral acoustic neuroma: Genetic, clinical and biochemical distinctions from peripheral neurofibromatosis. Neurology 30:851, 1980.
15. Kessler J, Cochard P, Black I: Neural crest differentiation and response to nerve growth factor in murine embryos. In Riccardi V, Mulvihill J (eds): Neurofibromatosis (von Recklinghausen's Disease). Advances in Neurology, Vol 29, New York, Raven Press, 1981, pp 115–123.
16. McDonald J, Dohrmann G: Molecular biology of brain tumors. Neurosurgery 23(5):537, 1988.

17. Steck P, Saya H: Pathways of oncogenesis in primary brain tumors. Curr Opin Oncol 3(3):476, 1991.
18. O'Connell P, Cawthon R, Viskochil D, et al.: The NF1 translocation breakpoint region. Ann NY Acad Sci 615:319, 1991.
19. Knudson AJ: Nakahara memorial lecture. Hereditary cancer, oncogenes, and anti-oncogenes. Int Symp Princess Takamatsu Cancer Res Fund 20:15, 1989.
20. Crowe F, Schell W: Diagnostic importance of cafe-au-lait spots in neurofibromatosis. Arch Intern Med 91:758, 1953.
21. Whitehouse D: Diagnostic value of the cafe-au-lait spot in children. Arch Dis Child 41:316, 1966.
22. Rubinstein L: Tumors of the Central Nervous System. Washington, DC, Armed Forces Institute of Pathology, 1972.
23. Hope DG, Mulvihill JJ: Malignancy in neurofibromatosis. In Riccardi VM, Mulvihill JJ (eds): Neurofibromatosis (von Recklinghausen's Disease). Advances in Neurology, Vol. 29. New York, Raven Press, 1981, pp 35–56.
24. Zimmerman R, Bilaniuk L, Metzger R, et al.: Computed tomography of orbital facial neurofibromatosis. Radiology 146:113, 1983.
25. Dufresne C, Hoopes J: Pseudomalignancies. Clin Plast Surg 14(2):367, 1987.
26. Riccardi V: Von Recklinghausen neurofibromatosis. N Engl J Med 305:1617, 1981.
27. Lewis R, Riccardi V: Von Recklinghausen neurofibromatosis: Incidence of iris hamartomas. Ophthalmology 88:348, 1982.
28. Francois J: Ocular aspects of the phakomatoses. In Vinken PJ, Bruyn GW (eds): Handbook of Clinical Neurology, Vol. 14. New York, American Elsevier, 1972, pp 619–667.
29. DiSimone R, Berman A, Schwentker E: The orthopedic manifestation of neurofibromatosis. A clinical experience and review of the literature. Clin Orthop 230:277, 1988.
30. Salerno N, Edeiken J: Vertebral scalloping in neurofibromatosis. Radiology 97:509, 1970.
31. Robinson R: Intrathoracic meningocele and neurofibromatosis. Br J Surg 51:432, 1964.
32. Chaglassian J, Riseborough E, Hall J: Neurofibromatosis scoliosis: Natural history and results of treatment in thirty-seven cases. J Bone Joint Surg 58:695, 1976.
33. Sirois J, Drennan J: Dystrophic spinal deformity in neurofibromatosis. J Pediatr Orthop 10(4):522, 1990.
34. Shufflebarger H: Cotrel-Dubousset instrumentation in neurofibromatosis spinal problems. Clin Orthop 245:24, 1989.
35. Holt J: Neurofibromatosis in children. Am J Roentgenol 130:615, 1978.
36. Betz R, Iorio R, Lombardi A, et al.: Scoliosis surgery in neurofibromatosis. Clin Orthop 245:53, 1989.
37. Blatt J, Jaffe R, Deutsch M, Adkins J: Neurofibromatosis and childhood tumors. Cancer 57:1225, 1986.
38. Huson S, Compston D, Harper P: A genetic study of von Recklinghausen neurofibromatosis in southeast Wales. II. Guidelines for genetic counselling. J Med Genet 26:712, 1989.
39. Lewis R, Gerson L, Axelson K, et al.: Von Recklinghausen's neurofibromatosis. II. Incidence of optic gliomata. Ophthalmology 91:929, 1984.
40. Easley J, Scharf L, Chou J, Riccardi V: Controversy in the management of optic pathway gliomas. Twenty-nine patients treated with radiation therapy at Baylor College of Medicine from 1967 through 1987. Neurofibromatosis 1(4):248, 1988.
41. Petronio J, Edwards M, Prados M, et al.: Management of chiasmal and hypothalamic gliomas of infancy and childhood with chemotherapy. J Neurosurg 74(5):701, 1991.
42. Kovalic J, Grigsby P, Shepard M, et al.: Radiation therapy for gliomas of the optic nerve and chiasm. Int J Radiat Oncol Biol Phys 18(4):927, 1990.
43. Rodriguez L, Edwards M, Levin V: Management of hypothalamic gliomas in children: An analysis of 33 cases. Neurosurgery 26(2):242, 1990.
44. Pierce S, Barnes P, Loeffler J, et al.: Definitive radiation therapy in the management of symptomatic patients with optic glioma. Survival and long-term effects. Cancer 65(1):45, 1990.
45. Packer R, JG R, Bilaniuk L, et al.: Chiasmatic hypothalamic/thalamic gliomas in childhood: Efficacy of treatment with chemotherapy alone. Ann Neurol 16(3):402, 1984.
46. Duffner P, Cohen M: Isolated optic nerve gliomas in children

with and without neurofibromatosis. Neurofibromatosis 1(4):201, 1988.
47. Kemink J, LaRouere M, Kileny P, et al.: Hearing preservation following suboccipital removal of acoustic neuromas. Laryngoscope 100(6):597, 1990.
48. Maniglia A, Fenstermaker R, Ratcheson R: Preservation of hearing in the surgical removal of cerebellopontine angle tumors. Otolaryngol Clin North Am 22(1):211, 1989.
49. Martuza R, Eldridge R: Neurofibromatosis 2 (bilateral acoustic neurofibromatosis). N Engl J Med 318(11):684, 1988.
50. Martuza R, Ojemann R: Bilateral acoustic neuromas. Clinical aspects, pathogenesis and treatment. Neurosurgery 10:1, 1982.
51. To S, Lufkin R, Rand R, et al.: Volume growth rate of acoustic neuromas on MRI post-stereotactic radiosurgery. Comput Med Imaging Graph 14(1):53, 1990.
52. Sawaya R: Neurosurgery issues in oncology. Curr Opin Oncol 3(3):459, 1991.
53. Laue L, Comite F, Hench K, et al.: Central precocious puberty and neurofibromatosis: Treatment with luteinizing hormone-releasing hormone analogue. Am J Dis Child 139:1097, 1985.
54. Weichert K, Dire M, Benton C, et al.: Macrocranium and neurofibromatosis. Radiology 107:163, 1973.
55. Samuelsson B, Samuelsson S: Neurofibromatosis in Gothenburg, Sweden. I. Background, study design and epidemiology. Neurofibromatosis 2(1):6, 1989.
56. Pulst S: Prenatal diagnosis of the neurofibromatoses. Clin Perinatol 17(4):829, 1990.
57. Meadows A, Coutifaris C, Obringer A, Zackai E: Variable expression of the neurofibromatosis gene: Considerations in diagnosis and treatment of children with cancer. Presented at International Society of Pediatric Oncology, XIIth meeting, Marseilles, France, 1981.
58. Sampson J, Scahill S, Stephenson J, et al.: Genetic aspects of tuberous sclerosis in the west of Scotland. J Med Genet 26(1):28, 1989.
59. Martuza R: Neurofibromatosis and other phakomatoses. In Wilkins R, Rengachary S (eds): Neurosurgery. New York, McGraw-Hill, 1982, pp 511–521.
60. Haines J, Amos J, Attwood J, et al.: Genetic heterogeneity in tuberous sclerosis. Study of a large collaborative data set. Ann N Y Acad Sci 615:256, 1991.
61. Kandt R, Pericak-Vance M, Hung W, et al.: Linkage studies in tuberous sclerosis. Chromosome 9? 11? or maybe 14! Ann N Y Acad Sci 615:284, 1991.
62. Wiederholt W, Gomez M, Kurland L: Incidence and prevalence of tuberous sclerosis in Rochester, Minnesota, 1950 through 1982. Neurology 35:600, 1985.
63. Oppenheimer E, Rosman N, Cooling E: The late appearance of hypopigmented maculae in tuberous sclerosis. Am J Dis Child 139:408, 1985.
64. Bellack G, Shapshay S: Management of facial angiofibromas in tuberous sclerosis: Use of the carbon dioxide laser. Otolaryngol Head Neck Surg 94:37: 1986.
65. Smythe J, Dyck J, Smallhorn J, Freedom R: Natural history of cardiac rhabdomyoma in infancy and childhood. Am J Cardiol 66(17):1247, 1990.
66. Watson G: Cardiac rhabdomyomas in tuberous sclerosis. Ann NY Acad Sci 615:50, 1991.
67. Legge M, Sauerbrei E, MacDonald A: Intracranial tuberous sclerosis in infancy. Radiology 153:667, 1984.
68. Stricker T, Zuerrer M, Martin E, Boesch C: MRI of two infants with tuberous sclerosis. Neuroradiology 33(2):175, 1991.
69. Huttenlocher P, Heydeemann P: Fine structure of cortical tubers in tuberous sclerosis: A Golgi study. Ann Neurol 16:595, 1984.
70. Fitz C: Tuberous sclerosis. In Hoffman HJ Epstein F (eds): Disorders of the Developing Nervous System: Diagnosis and Treatment. Boston, MA, Blackwell Scientific Pub, 1986, pp 625–634.
71. Curatolo P, Cusmai R, Pruna D: Tuberous sclerosis: Diagnostic and prognostic problems. Pediatr Neurosci 12:123, 1985–86.
72. Riikonen R, Simell O: Tuberous sclerosis and infantile spasms. Dev Med Child Neurol 32(3):203, 1990.
73. Cusmai R, Chiron C, Curatolo P, et al.: Topographic comparative study of magnetic resonance imaging and electroencephalography in 34 children with tuberous sclerosis. Epilepsia 31(6):747, 1990.

74. Bye A, Matheson J, Tobias V, Mackenzie R: Selective epilepsy surgery in tuberous sclerosis. Aust Paediatr J 25(4):243, 1989.
75. Boesel C, Paulson G, Kosnick F, Earle K: Brain hamartomas and tumors associated with tuberous sclerosis. Neurosurgery 4:410, 1979.
76. Kapp J, Paulson G, Odom G: Brain tumors with tuberous sclerosis. J Neurosurg 26:191, 1967.
77. McLaurin R, Towbin R: Tuberous sclerosis: Diagnostic and surgical considerations. Pediatr Neurosci 12:43, 1985–86.
78. Tsuchida T, Kamata K, Kawamata M, et al.: Brain tumors in tuberous sclerosis. Report of 4 cases. Childs Brain 8:271, 1981.
79. Martin N, Debussche C, De Broucker T, et al.: Gadolinium-DPTA enhanced MR imaging in tuberous sclerosis. Neuroradiology 31(6):492, 1990.
80. Shepherd C, Scheithauer B, Gomez M, et al.: Subependymal giant cell astrocytoma: A clinical, pathological, and flow cytometric study. Neurosurgery 28(6):864, 1991.
81. Happle R: Lethal genes surviving by mosaicism: A possible explanation for sporadic birth defects involving the skin. J Am Acad Dermatol 16(4):899, 1987.
82. Enjolras O, Riche M, Merland J: Facial port-wine stains and Sturge-Weber syndrome. Pediatrics 76:48, 1985.
83. Paller A: The Sturge-Weber syndrome. Pediatr Dermatol 4(4):300, 1987.
84. Venes J: Sturge-Weber syndrome. In Hoffman H, Epstein F (eds): Disorders of the Developing Nervous System: Diagnosis and Treatment. Boston, MA, Blackwell Scientific Publications, 1986, pp 617–623.
85. Iwach A, Hoskins H, Hetherington JJ, Shaffer R: Analysis of surgical and medical management of glaucoma in Sturge-Weber syndrome. Ophthalmology 97(7):904, 1990.
86. Garcia J, Roach E, McLean W: Recurrent thrombotic deterioration in the Sturge-Weber syndrome. Childs Brain 8:427, 1981.
87. Sperner J, Schmauser I, Bittner R, et al.: MR-imaging findings in children with Sturge-Weber syndrome. Neuropediatrics 21:146, 1990.
88. Chiron C, Raynaud C, Dulac O, et al.: Study of the cerebral blood flow in partial epilepsy of childhood using the SPECT method. J Neuroradiol 16(4):317, 1989.
89. Ogunmekan A, Hwang P, Hoffman H: Sturge-Weber-Dimitri disease: Role of hemispherectomy in prognosis. Can J Neurol Sci 16(1):78, 1989.
90. Hoffman H, Hendrick E, Dennise M: Hemispherectomy for Sturge-Weber syndrome. Childs Brain 5:233, 1978.
91. Ito M, Sato K, Ohnuki A, Uto A: Sturge-Weber disease: Operative indications and surgical results. Brain Dev 12(5):473, 1990.
92. Pasztor A, Sztenak L, Dobronyi I, et al.: Angioblastoma of the posterior fossa in three children. J Pediatr Neurosci 1:281, 1985.
93. Maher E, Bentley E, Yates J, et al.: Mapping of the von Hippel-Lindau disease locus to a small region of chromosome 3p by genetic linkage analysis. Genomics 10(4):957, 1991.
94. Cohen M, Duffner P: Von Hippel-Lindau disease. In Hoffman H, Epstein F (eds): Disorders of the Developing Nervous System: Diagnosis and Treatment. Boston, MA, Blackwell Scientific Publications, 1986, pp 625–634.
95. Hubschmann O, Vijayanathan T, Countee R: Von Hippel-Lindau with multiple manifestations: Diagnosis and management. Neurosurgery 8:92, 1981.
96. Jakobiec F, Font R, Johnson F: Angiomatosis retinae: An ultrastructural study and lipid analysis. Cancer 38:2042, 1976.
97. Filling-Katz M, Choyke P, Oldfield E, et al.: Central nervous system involvement in von Hippel-Lindau disease. Neurology 41(1):41, 1991.
98. Stein P, Black H: A simplified diagnostic approach to pheochromocytoma. A review of the literature and report of one institution's experience. Medicine (Baltimore) 70(1):46, 1991.
99. Khafagi F, Shapiro B, Fischer M, et al.: Phaeochromocytoma and functioning paraganglioglioma in childhood and adolescence: Role of iodine-131 metaiodobenzylguanidine. Eur J Nucl Med 18(3):191, 1991.
100. van der Hout A, van der Vlies P, Wijmenga C, et al.: The region of common allelic losses in sporadic renal cell carcinoma is bordered by the loci D3S2 and THRB. Genomics 11(3):537, 1991.
101. Lamiell J, Salazar F, Hsia Y: von Hippel-Lindau disease affecting 43 members of a single kindred. Medicine (Baltimore) 68(1):1, 1989.
102. Seeger J, Burke D, Knake J, Gabrielsen T: Computed tomographic and angiographic evaluation of hemangioblastomas. Radiology 138:65, 1981.
103. Sung D, Chang C, Harisiadis L: Cerebellar hemangioblastoma. Cancer 49:553, 1982.
104. Louis-Bar D: Sur un syndrome progress if comprenant des telangiectasies capillaires cutanees et conjunctivals symmetrique, a disposition naevoide et des troubles cerebelleux. Confina Neurol 4:32, 1941.
105. Foroud T, Wei S, Ziv Y, et al.: Localization of an ataxia-telangiectasia locus to a 3-cM interval on chromosome 11q23: Linkage analysis of 111 families by an international consortium. Am J Hum Genet 49(6):1263, 1991.
106. Swift M, Sholman L, Perry M, Chase C: Malignant neoplasms in the families of patients with ataxia-telangiectasia. Cancer 76:209, 1976.
107. Logan W: Ataxia-telangiectasia. In Hoffman H, Epstein F (eds) Disorders of the Developing Nervous System: Diagnosis and Treatment. Boston, MA, Blackwell Scientific Publications, 1986, pp 635–651.
108. Hosking G: Ataxia-telangiectasia. Annotations. Dev Med Child Neurol 24:77, 1982.
109. Taylor A, Harnden D, Arlett C, et al.: Ataxia-telangiectasia: A human mutation with abnormal radiation sensitivity. Nature 258:427, 1975.
110. Gatti R, Boder E, Vinters H, et al.: Ataxia-telangiectasia: An interdisciplinary approach to pathogenesis. Medicine (Baltimore) 70(2):99, 1991.
111. Morrell D, Cromartie E, Swift M: Mortality and cancer incidence in 263 patients with ataxia-telangiectasia. J Natl Cancer Inst 77:89, 1986.
112. Waldmann T, McIntire K: Serum alpha-fetoprotein levels in patients with ataxia-telangiectasia. Lancet ii:212, 1972.
113. Boder E, Sedgwick R: Ataxia-telangiectasia. A familial syndrome of progressive cerebellar ataxia, oculocutaneous telangiectasia and frequent pulmonary infection. Pediatrics 21:526, 1958.
114. Kwast O, Ignatowicz R: Progressive peripheral neuron degeneration in ataxia-telangiectasia: an electrophysiological study in children. Dev Med Child Neurol 32(9):800, 1990.
115. Crolla J, Gilgenkrantz S, de Grouchy J, et al.: Incontinentia pigmenti and X-autosome translocations. Non-isotopic in situ hybridization with an X-centromere-specific probe (pSV2X5) reveals a possible X-centromeric breakpoint in one of five published cases. Hum Genet 81(3):269, 1989.
116. Avrahami E, Harel S, Jurgenson U, Cohn D: Computed tomographic demonstration of brain changes in incontinentia pigmenti. Am J Dis Child 139:372, 1985.
117. O'Brien J, Feingold M: Incontinentia pigmenta. A longitudinal study. Am J Dis Child 139:711, 1985.
118. Samlaska C, Levin S, James W, et al.: Proteus syndrome. Arch Dermatol 125(8):1109, 1989.
119. Burke J, Bowell R, O'Doherty N. Proteus syndrome: Ocular complications. J Pediatr Ophthalmol Strabismus 25(2):99, 1988.

Chapter 39

POSTSURGERY MANAGEMENT OF BRAIN TUMORS

ROGER J. PACKER, M.D.

Surgery, although of extreme importance and probably the single most significant factor affecting outcome for children with brain tumors, is only the first step in the treatment of many childhood brain tumors. Optimal management of patients with primary central nervous system (CNS) tumors requires a multidisciplinary, comprehensive approach. More than one half of all children with brain tumors can now be expected to be alive and free of disease 5 years following diagnosis, many apparently cured of their illness after the appropriate use of surgery, radiotherapy, and chemotherapy. However, such therapies can also cause significant neurologic sequelae, and their use requires an understanding of the biology of the tumor, its pattern of growth, the extent of the tumor at time of diagnosis, the tumor's probable response to each modality of therapy, and the possible toxicities of treatment. This chapter reviews general aspects of postsurgical management of children with brain tumors and how comprehensive treatment approaches can be applied to improve outcome for patients with brain tumors.

GENERAL ASPECTS OF POSTSURGICAL TREATMENT

POSTSURGICAL STAGING STUDIES

A major advance in the management of childhood brain tumors has been the understanding that even within histologic categories of CNS malignant tumors, subgroups of patients exist who require different management.[1-3] This overall approach has been used for many years with regard to other childhood tumors, especially the leukemias. However, such substratifica-

tion has only recently gained acceptance in childhood brain tumors. The vast majority of parameters utilized to determine risk are based on clinical factors.[2, 3] As the biology of childhood brain tumors is better elucidated, no doubt classification and stratification of patients will change. Factors that will probably be of some usefulness in the future include immunohistochemical tumor profiles, cytogenetic results, and molecular genetic findings. At the present time, separation of patients into risk groups is based on a variety of factors including: (1) symptoms at the time of diagnosis, (2) the age of the patient at the time of diagnosis, (3) the histologic features of the tumor, and (4) the results of postsurgical evaluations for the extent of residual disease at the primary tumor site and at distant CNS sites. This stratification can be used in some tumors to determine the need for a particular type of therapy. It is also crucial for the appropriate evaluation of the efficacy of the newer forms of treatment.

DISEASE AT THE PRIMARY TUMOR SITE

Assessment of the extent of residual disease at the primary disease site, after surgery, has been objectively possible only since the introduction of computed tomography (CT) in the mid-1970s.[4] The advent of magnetic resonance imaging (MRI) has furthered our ability to evaluate the extent of disease and in many cases has supplanted CT.[5] Neurosurgical determination of residual disease is helpful, but it is not totally reliable.

In some tumors (ependymomas, craniopharyngiomas, low-grade gliomas, and perhaps primitive neuroectodermal tumors), the amount of postoperative residual disease seems to be an extremely important determinant of outcome. In other tumor types, the significance of small amounts of residual disease remains unclear. Improvements in neuro-imaging techniques have dramatically changed the way disease can be evaluated. With these changing techniques, there has to be a continual re-evaluation of the significance of findings. Clearly, with MRI small residual masses are now seen that were never seen on CT. It remains unclear how significant these small residual lesions are, especially if other forms of treatment are to be used, and if CT data concerning the significance of persistent disease can be directly applied to MR findings.

Another confounding factor is the distinction between residual disease and postoperative change. Large residual lumps of disease (usually greater than 1.5 cm^2 in area) are most commonly accepted as evidence of residual disease. Newer computerized techniques to determine the volumetric size of tumors also may make the determination of residual mass more objective. However, enhancement at the rim of the postoperative bed is more difficult to evaluate, as such enhancement may represent either residual tumor or postoperative damage to the surrounding brain. There is some experimental evidence to suggest that enhancement on CT seen within the first 48 to 72 hours postsurgery represents residual tumor, as there has not been enough time for neovascularization to occur in damaged brain within the operative bed.[6] However, this has not been conclusively shown, and series that have been purported to support this contention have included only a handful of patients. Making distinctions even more difficult is the fact that almost all studies, to date, have been based on CT, and it is not clear whether CT findings can be directly applied to MRI. In general, the postoperative MRI will be more informative than the postoperative CT. In infiltrating lesions, the extent of disease as shown on MRI is much greater than that appreciated on CT.[7, 8] However, especially on T2-weighted images, postoperative damage is extremely well visualized, and distinction from residual small amounts of tumor is virtually impossible.[9]

The postoperative surgical impression remains a valuable adjunct in the evaluation of residual disease. In patients with posterior fossa tumors, infiltration within the brainstem or cerebral peduncle, which is obvious to the surgeon, may be poorly seen on CT. On MRI, this is less a problem, but it does occur at times. At the present time, it would seem that either CT or MRI can be used in the postoperative evaluation of many pediatric extra-axial lesions, such as primitive neuroectodermal tumors/medulloblastomas (PNETs/MBs). However, for intra-axial lesions, such as brainstem gliomas, MRI is clearly the procedure of choice.[7] In those institutions where postoperative MRI is not readily available, CT is still useful. The neuro-imaging technique chosen must be interpreted in the context of the findings at the time of surgery. Although the data are less than definitive, it would seem that the scans should be performed within 48 to 72 hours of surgery to avoid some of the difficulties in separating residual tumor from postoperative changes.

DISEASE DISTANT FROM THE PRIMARY SITE

Primary CNS tumors in children are much more likely to disseminate to distant neuroaxis sites than are tumors in adults.[10, 11] Leptomeningeal disease at the time of diagnosis occurs in as many as 10 per cent of all children with CNS tumors and is especially common in patients with PNETs/MBs (including those occurring in the posterior fossa and in other sites within the nervous system) and in germ cell tumors. In the vast majority of patients, such dissemination is asymptomatic at the time of diagnosis or is overshadowed by symptoms caused by the tumor at the primary disease site. Failure to diagnose dissemination may result in disease relapse in untreated areas and increased neurologic morbidity.

Prior to the advent of MRI, the combination of cerebrospinal fluid cytologic examination and myelography was the optimal means of evaluating the extent of disease. Although there is often reluctance to perform myelography in the postoperative period, in most cases this procedure can be done effectively and safely. If cerebrospinal fluid cytologic examination alone is used to determine the extent of disease, almost 50 per cent of patients with documented lump subarachnoid disease will be incorrectly considered to have no disease spread. The early experience with spinal MRI was disappointing. Only large areas of subarachnoid disease could be visualized. With the introduction of paramagnetic agents, such as gadolinium, spinal MRI has become a viable alternative to myelography.[12] However, to be as sensitive as myelography, enhanced spinal MRI must be performed in multiple planes, and noncontiguous transverse images of the spine must be obtained (especially through the cauda equina region). With the wider use of enhanced spinal MRI, it has become relatively clear that, if performed correctly, enhanced MRI is as sensitive as myelography, if not more so, in the detection of leptomeningeal disease spread. However, local meningeal postoperative irritation and postoperative blood clots can mimic leptomeningeal tumor. The significance of all postoperative changes seen on enhanced spinal MRI in children with central nervous system tumors has not been shown conclusively.

Since leptomeningeal disease is probably the single most significant risk factor in stratifying patients with malignant primary central nervous system tumors, appropriate evaluation must be performed. The combination of enhanced spinal MRI performed in multiple planes and lumbar cerebrospinal cytologic examination is probably the best initial screening test. This combination of tests should be performed in all patients with tumors known to frequently disseminate through the neuroaxis (such as PNETs/MBs, germ cell tumors, and posterior fossa malignant gliomas or ependymomas) within 10 to 14 days following surgery. In patients with spinal subarachnoid lump disease, no further evaluation is indicated. In equivocal cases, myelography followed by CT can be a useful adjunct. In patients whose tumors are at lower risk for leptomeningeal dissemination (cortical anaplastic gliomas and low-grade ependymomas), all that is probably warranted is enhanced spinal MRI. In patients at very low risk for leptomeningeal dissemination, no surveillance testing seems indicated.

The significance of tumor cells found in the cerebrospinal fluid during the first 10 to 14 days postoperatively is unclear, as it is conceivable that these cells were shed at the time of surgery and are not representative of preoperative disseminated disease. In those patients with a normal neuro-imaging study of the spine and positive cytology, a repeat spinal tap at 21 days is indicated. If the repeat cerebrospinal fluid is still positive for tumor cells, this should be taken as proof of disseminated disease.

OTHER SURVEILLANCE STUDIES

The need for other tests to assess the extent of disease postoperatively is less well established. Bone scans and bone marrow aspirates have been recommended for all children with PNETs/MBs of the posterior fossa, but the yield is low and their need inconclusive. If these tests are to be used, they should probably be reserved for those children under 3 years of age at diagnosis, who are most likely to have bone disease at the time of diagnosis. Tumor markers, such as the polyamines, seem better suited to follow the course of illness than to determine the extent of disease at the time of diagnosis.[13, 14]

RADIOTHERAPY

Radiotherapy increases the duration of survival and the rate of cure for children with many types of CNS malignancies.[15, 16] Radiotherapy for children with brain tumors is primarily delivered by external beam techniques, utilizing photon beam irradiation produced by linear accelerators (x-rays) or cobalt teletherapy equipment (gamma-irradiation). For some types of CNS tumors that rarely spread outside their primary site, local radiotherapy results in long-term tumor control. Doses in the 5000 to 5500 cGy range, delivered as 180 to 200 cGy per dose per day, once daily, have been most successfully used and do not cause a high incidence of radionecrosis to the surrounding normal brain. However, for those types of childhood CNS tumors that frequently disseminate to the neuroaxis, including most of the malignant childhood brain tumors, local radiotherapy alone infrequently results in long-term disease control. Craniospinal radiotherapy, in doses between 3600 and 4000 cGy, supplemented with local radiotherapy to a total dose of 5000 to 5500 cGy at the primary tumor site, has resulted in improved tumor control (Table 39–1). In the majority of cases, this extensive neuroaxis irradiation is given "presymptomatically" in an attempt to eradicate tumor that, although not measurable, is believed to have disseminated prior to diagnosis.

Whole-brain irradiation has been incriminated as causing significant neurocognitive and neuroendocrinologic sequelae.[17, 18] However, without such therapy, the chance for disease control in tumors such as PNETs/MBs and anaplastic gliomas of the posterior fossa is markedly lessened. It is not known what total dose or volume of irradiation is "safe" in a child of any age, and it is unlikely that a totally safe dose exists within the ranges needed to control tumor. Age clearly does seem to be a crucial factor, as younger children are prone to suffer more severe sequelae, believed to be due primarily to their more immature central nervous system.

Various means have been employed in an attempt to increase the efficacy of radiotherapy while not increasing its toxicity. Agents that enhance radiotherapy have not yet been shown to be of increased efficacy. The direct implantation of radioactive substances into the tumor (brachytherapy) may be used in the future for tumors with low proclivities to disseminate to the neuroaxis.[19] Stereotactic radiosurgery, whereby a large dose of radiation is delivered in a single session to a stereotactically defined intracranial volume, is a technique that has been available since the 1950s. This delivery form of radiotherapy has been shown to be effective for other types of intracranial lesions, most notably small arteriovenous malformations, but has not gained widespread use in pediatric brain tumors. There has been recent increased interest in the utilization of this technique, especially for small extracranial or extra-axial lesions. A modification of this technique, util

TABLE 39–1. POSTOPERATIVE TREATMENT OF CHILDHOOD TUMORS

TYPE	LOCAL RADIOTHERAPY	CRANIOSPINAL PLUS LOCAL RADIOTHERAPY	ADJUVANT CHEMOTHERAPY
PNET		X	X (in certain subsets of patients)
Low-grade glioma	? (in subtotally resected tumors)		
Anaplastic glioma of cortex	X		X
Aplastic glioma of posterior fossa		X	?
Brainstem gliomas	X		
Low-grade ependymomas	X		?
Anaplastic ependymomas		X	?
Germ cell tumors		X	?
Craniopharyngiomas	X (in subtotally resected tumors)		

izing fractionated stereotactic radiation treatments, is now being explored in the treatment of some intra-axial intracranial lesions, including those occurring in childhood.

The use of hyperfractionated radiotherapy, whereby radiotherapy is delivered in lower individual doses two or more times daily, has been recently applied to the management of pediatric brain tumors.[20] In theory, the use of this treatment allows the delivery of higher doses of radiotherapy without increasing the risk of normal tissue damage. Preliminary results in various series treating children with extensive brainstem gliomas suggest that doses of radiotherapy between 6480 cGy and 7800 cGy have been relatively well tolerated. However, these higher dosage regimens have not yet been shown to improve survival.[21] Although no patient in a pediatric series, to date, has developed lethal radiation necrosis, there does seem to be an increased incidence of local intralesional cystic/necrotic change. In addition, since the number of patients in series reported who have survived 5 years is relatively small, the long-term safety of these regimens remains unproven. There is some enthusiasm to attempt these regimens in other childhood brain tumors, especially tumors that are more rapidly dividing than brainstem gliomas, such as PNETs/MBs.

CHEMOTHERAPY

Initially employed almost exclusively in children with recurrent disease, chemotherapy has recently been shown to play a significant role in the management of newly diagnosed patients with PNETs/MBs of the posterior fossa and anaplastic gliomas of childhood when given with and after radiotherapy (see Table 39–1).[3, 22, 23] Retrospective multicenter trials have shown that certain subsets of children with PNETs/MBs of the posterior fossa and cortical anaplastic gliomas seem to benefit from the addition of lomustine (CCNU), vincristine, and prednisone after radiotherapy.[3, 23] Trials with other drug combinations, especially those utilizing platinum compounds, have also suggested benefit.[3] Various chemotherapeutic approaches are now being actively evaluated in newly diagnosed patients, including: (1) the use of multi-agent chemotherapy in an attempt to overcome tumor heterogeneity in both cellular make-up and response to treatment, and (2) preradiation chemotherapy, in an attempt to overcome microvascular changes caused by radiation that might adversely affect delivery of the drug to the tumor site and potentiate the effects of radiotherapy.[24–26]

As experience with chemotherapeutic agents has grown and more effective drugs or drug regimens are developed, chemotherapy has been increasingly used in very young children with brain tumors. This is the group of patients most likely to have severe irreversible brain damage after radiotherapy. However, the safety of most drugs as regards the immature brain has not been established. Actinomycin D and vincristine have been successfully used in children under 5 years of age

with chiasmatic gliomas to at least delay the need for radiotherapy. Other combinations, including the combination of vincristine and carboplatin, may be even more useful. MOPP chemotherapy, which is composed of nitrogen mustard, vincristine, procarbazine, and prednisone, has been shown to be somewhat effective against a variety of brain tumors in children under 3 years of age.[27] The most impressive results have been shown in children with PNETs/MBs. More recently, cycles of cisplatinum and etoposide, alternating with cycles of cyclophosphamide and vincristine, have shown efficacy in a wide variety of infant brain tumors. These and other cisplatinum-containing drug regimens have at least delayed the need for immediate radiotherapy in children under 3 years of age with a variety of malignant brain tumors. It is still unclear which tumors in these very young children respond best to chemotherapy, as some tumors, such as brainstem gliomas, which are highly resistant to chemotherapy in older patients, have been reported to respond well to various drug regimens in infants. An important, and controversial, issue is whether chemotherapy alone can be used to treat some infants with malignant brain tumors. There is some evidence to suggest that patients treated with chemotherapy who have complete radiographic disappearance of tumor can be safely observed by follow-up after completion of the chemotherapeutic regimens.[27] Radiotherapy is then delayed until there is evidence of tumor regrowth.

SURVEILLANCE TESTING FOR RECURRENT DISEASE

The frequency with which children should be re-evaluated for disease recurrence and the means that should be employed in these evaluations constitute a gray area in the postsurgical management of children with brain tumors.[28] Asymptomatic local disease does recur, and it seems logical, although unproven, that treating recurrence earlier will improve outcome. It has been recommended that neurologic clinical evaluation and some type of neuro-imaging procedure (either CT or MRI) be performed at regular intervals after diagnosis, more frequently in malignant lesions and less frequently in slower-growing tumors. Once again, MRI has essentially supplanted CT in these evaluations. The need for routine surveillance of the spine in patients with malignant CNS tumors remains controversial. Isolated leptomeningeal disease relapse does occur, but in the vast majority of patients it is symptomatic at the time of relapse. As experience grows with enhanced spinal MRI, it seems that this technique can be used in patients at highest risk for isolated leptomeningeal disease relapse. This is especially true for those patients undergoing newer treatment trials utilizing reduced doses of radiotherapy in an attempt to reduce treatment-related sequelae.

A possible schema for surveillance based on the growth pattern of central nervous system tumors is

TABLE 39–2. PROPOSED SCHEDULE OF SURVEILLANCE STUDIES FOR CHILDREN WITH BRAIN TUMORS

TUMOR TYPE	3 mo*	6 mo	9 mo	12 mo	18 mo	24 mo	30 mo	36 mo	42 mo	48 mo
PNET	CT	CT; M^B	CT^A	CT; M^B	CT	CT; M^B	CT	CT; M^B		CT (yearly, thereafter)
Low-grade glioma		CT or NMRI			CT or NMRI		CT or NMRI		CT or NMRI	(yearly, thereafter, if residual disease)
Anaplastic glioma	CT	CT; M^B	CT^A	CT; M^B	CT	CT; M^B	CT	CT		CT (yearly, thereafter)
Brainstem glioma	NMRI	NMRI	NMRI	NMRI	NMRI	NMRI	NMRI	NMRI	NMRI	NMRI (yearly, thereafter)
Ependymoma	CT^A	CT; M^B	CT^A	CT; M^B	CT	CT; M^B	CT	CT; M^B	CT	CT (yearly, thereafter)
Germ cell tumor	CT^A	CT; M^B, TM	CT^A	CT; M^B, TM	CT	CT; m^B, TM	CT	CT; M^B, TM	CT	CT (yearly, thereafter)

*Time noted either after diagnosis or after completion of initial treatment staging studies.

^{A}Only if residual local disease is present.

^{B}Only if initial myelogram is positive or if malignant cells are found in cerebrospinal fluid.

M, myelogram; TM, tumor markers (see text).

outlined in Table 39–2. Cerebrospinal fluid markers, such as the polyamines for patients with PNETs/MBs and human chorionic gonadotrophin (hCG) and alpha-fetoprotein for patients with mixed germ cell tumors, may also be useful adjuncts in the follow-up of patients for disease recurrence.

LONG-TERM SEQUELAE

It is now recognized that survivors of childhood brain tumors may have significant neurologic, cognitive, and endocrine residual deficits.[9, 17, 29, 30] Many of these deficits are believed to be related to treatment, although other factors, including the patient's preoperative status and postoperative course, have an impact on outcome, especially as regards intellectual function.

Early reports suggested that most children who had survived primary brain tumors and received whole-brain radiotherapy were retarded.[17, 29, 31] More recent studies have suggested that most of these patients have normal intelligence but may have significant learning disabilities.[18] In addition, radiation-related cognitive changes are not static but may progress over time, with the full extent of deficits not being evident until three or more years after treatment. Based on available information, it seems that all survivors of childhood CNS malignancies should undergo a complete neuropsychological evaluation within the first year of diagnosis, to assess intellectual abilities and design appropriate educational programs. In children who have received whole-brain irradiation, testing should be repeated at yearly intervals for at least the first 3 years after diagnosis.

The detrimental effects of treatment on endocrine function are even more poorly characterized than are intellectual deficits.[17, 29, 30] Biochemical growth hormone insufficiency occurs in 67 to 100 per cent of children who have received whole-brain irradiation, and decreased growth velocity occurs in over half of these patients. Thyroid and gonadotropin function are more variably impaired. Endocrine deficits may also occur in patients treated with local radiotherapy, espe-

cially in patients with posterior fossa tumors, since radiation portals for posterior fossa tumors usually include the posterior portion of the hypothalamus. Linear growth needs to be carefully followed in children with all forms of brain tumors, and in any child with decelerated linear growth, endocrine evaluation is indicated. Similarly, gonadotropin evaluation should be performed in any patient with delayed puberty. Thyroid function studies are indicated, on at least a yearly basis for the first 3 years after treatment, in any child who received whole-brain irradiation or local irradiation that involved the hypothalamus.

The evaluation for thyroid dysfunction is complicated by the possible occurrence of transient thyroid dysfunction in patients following cranial irradiation. It has recently been shown that some children and adults will show temporary laboratory evidence of hypothyroidism within the first year following radiotherapy; however, thyroid levels will spontaneously return to normal. The significance of such transient changes is unclear.

POSTSURGICAL TREATMENT OF SPECIFIC TUMOR TYPES

Other chapters have dealt with the treatment of individual childhood tumors in more detail. The general principles of postoperative treatment described previously will be applied to briefly summarize postsurgical treatment for the more common forms of primary CNS tumors.

PRIMITIVE NEUROECTODERMAL TUMORS/MEDULLOBLASTOMAS (PNETS/MBS)

Although PNETs/MBs may occur in any region of the central nervous system, the most extensive studies on the efficacy of antineoplastic treatment have been performed in children with posterior fossa lesions.[32–35] Disagreement exists regarding whether posterior fossa

PNETs (also known as medulloblastomas) should be categorized and treated differently from PNETs in the pineal region (pineoblastomas) or cerebral cortex (central neuroblastomas). Until tumor-specific markers become available, such controversies cannot be settled, and for this review, all PNETs will be considered as a single entity.[33-36]

After complete postoperative staging, including enhanced spinal MRI and/or myelography, most patients with PNETs/MBs can be stratified into two major risk groups.[1, 3, 37] It is still unsettled whether the size of the primary tumor at the time of surgery or the amount of residual disease after surgery is the more important determinant of outcome. The Chang staging system has been most widely utilized to characterize the local extent of posterior fossa tumors at the time of diagnosis.[38] This is an intraoperative staging system that has been modified (in part) to be used in combination with neuroradiographic findings. T_1-T_2 Chang posterior fossa PNETs/MBs are less than 3 cm in diameter and do not cause hydrocephalus, whereas T_3-T_4 Chang tumors cause internal hydrocephalus, infiltrate the brainstem, and/or locally disseminate. Outcome of patients with T_1-T_2 is better than those of patients with T_3-T_4 lesions. Multiple single-institution studies have reported that total surgical resection of PNETs/MBs improves survival.[39, 40] However, multivariate analysis, taking into account other factors including the original size of the tumor, the histologic features of the tumor, and the age of the patient, have failed to statistically confirm the association between extent of resection (total versus partial) and outcome. However, these studies do confirm that patients who undergo only a biopsy rarely survive. Since pineal region tumors and, to a lesser extent, cortical PNETs/MBs are less amenable to surgical resection than posterior fossa lesions, and dissemination to other sites in the central nervous system occurs readily, especially with the pineal PNETs/MBs, most PNETs/MBs outside the posterior fossa will fall into the poor-risk group.

Recently, the significance of all of these staging factors has been questioned by an international study performed by the International Society of Pediatric Oncology. In this study, accepted risk factors were not clearly associated with outcome. However, the results of this most recent study are confounded by the fact that staging was incomplete in many patients and that the overall survival for both groups of patients was somewhat lower than that from other contemporary series.

All patients with PNETs/MBs who are older than 3 years of age at the time of diagnosis, independent of risk factors, should be treated with craniospinal and supplemental local radiotherapy.[41-43] As many as 60 per cent of patients with favorable-risk characteristics can be expected to be alive and free of disease 5 years following diagnosis with such treatment. A reduction in the dose of whole-brain irradiation therapy may be possible in this "average"-risk group.[44] However, a recent study attempting to decrease the dose of craniospinal irradiation from 3600 to 2340 cGy demonstrated a higher leptomeningeal disease relapse rate in children with the lower dose of radiotherapy. Further trials are planned in which those children receiving lower-dose radiotherapy will also be given chemotherapy in an attempt to improve the efficacy of the low-dose radiotherapy given to the craniospinal axis. Such reduction trials should be done as part of prospective randomized trials evaluating both tumor control and long-term sequelae. The addition of chemotherapy has not been shown to be of benefit, as yet, in patients with so-called average-risk disease. However, the overall survival in patients with average-risk disease is no better and possibly worse than survival rates reported in recent studies utilizing adjuvant chemotherapy in patients with poor-risk disease. This raises the question whether all patients with PNETs/MBs should receive chemotherapy.

In children with poor-risk factors, the 5-year survival rate after radiotherapy alone is less than 40 per cent. In a nationwide trial, the use of adjuvant chemotherapy with CCNU, vincristine, and prednisone was shown to be of some benefit. Children with locally extensive PNETs/MBs (Chang T_3-T_4) had a 59 per cent 5-year disease-free survival rate after treatment with radiotherapy plus chemotherapy as compared to 41 per cent after treatment with radiotherapy alone.[1] Other drug combinations used both prior to and after chemotherapy have also shown efficacy in preliminary treatment trials.[45, 46] In one study, the use of adjuvant vincristine during radiotherapy and CCNU, vincristine, and cisplatinum after radiotherapy demonstrated a 5-year actuarial disease-free survival rate of over 85 per cent.[3] Based on available information, it seems that all poor-risk patients should be considered candidates for adjuvant chemotherapy, once again preferably as part of a prospective, randomized treatment trial.

In children who are under 3 years of age at diagnosis with PNETs/MBs, because of the potential detrimental effects of radiotherapy, treatment with chemotherapy alone or chemotherapy followed at a later time by radiotherapy should be strongly considered. Trials using various types of chemotherapy have shown that disease in 30 to 50 per cent of children with PNETs/MBs under the age of 3 years can be controlled with chemotherapy alone for a 12- to 18-month period. Children who have no residual disease postoperatively and no evidence of leptomeningeal dissemination seem to fare the best with chemotherapy alone.

EPENDYMOMAS

The factors predictive of outcome and the optimal postsurgical management of children with ependymomas are far from established.[47-49] Survival rates of 10 to 70 per cent with similar means of treatment have been reported. Ependymomas have a variable tendency to seed the neuroaxis. Anaplastic lesions are more likely to disseminate than are tumors arising in the posterior fossa. However, based on available information, it seems that the extent of CNS disease in all children with ependymomas should be completely evaluated; all patients should undergo postoperative myelography or enhanced spinal MRI.

The value of radiotherapy in low-grade lesions is inconclusive, but in nonrandomized, retrospective series, reported survival rates are higher for children who have received local radiotherapy than for those treated with surgery alone. The best survival rates for children with anaplastic ependymomas are in those who have received craniospinal plus supplemental radiotherapy to the primary tumor site. However, when patients are matched for other risk factors, it is unclear whether the routine use of craniospinal radiotherapy in patients with nondisseminated disease is of benefit.[50, 51] Chemotherapy is not of proven efficacy for children with ependymomas of any histologic subtype, but should be considered as part of any randomized treatment trials. Cisplatinum drugs have shown some efficacy in children with recurrent ependymomas and may be useful in newly diagnosed patients.

BRAINSTEM GLIOMAS

Local radiotherapy is of transient benefit in over 80 per cent of children with brainstem gliomas but results in long-term disease control in probably fewer than 20 per cent of patients. In patients with exophytic lesions, especially at the cervicomedullary junction where they may be amenable to radical surgical resections, the role of radiotherapy is unclear.[52–54]

Recent work suggests that patients with brainstem gliomas can be stratified on the basis of clinical, radiographic, and pathologic findings into two major risk groups (Table 39–3).[52] As many as 60 per cent of patients in the average risk group will be alive and free of disease 5 years after diagnosis, after treatment with conventionally fractionated doses of radiotherapy (total dose in the 5000 to 5500 cGy range). Since children with one or more unfavorable criteria will rarely survive longer than 18 months following diagnosis after similar radiotherapy, more aggressive treatment regimens, even if they are potentially more neurotoxic, should be strongly considered for those children with poor-risk factors.

The preliminary results of trials utilizing higher doses of radiotherapy in hyperfractionated treatment regimens suggest possible benefit. In one report, over 40 per cent of patients (both adults and children) with brainstem gliomas treated with 7200 cGy of radiotherapy were alive and free of progressive disease 5 years following diagnosis.[55] However, as experience grows with hyperfractionated radiation regimens, this apparent survival advantage becomes less clear.[21]

Chemotherapy has yet to be shown to be of benefit in children with brainstem gliomas.[56, 57] Children with brainstem gliomas can develop clinically significant leptomeningeal spread early in the course of illness, and such dissemination may become an increasing problem when local disease control of malignant lesions improves.[58] However, since local disease control is so poor, extensive evaluation for dissemination at diagnosis is not warranted in children with brainstem gliomas.

LOW-GRADE GLIOMAS

The value of either radiotherapy or chemotherapy has not been well established in patients with low-grade gliomas.[57, 59, 60] There is no evidence that the addition of such therapy after these lesions have been grossly resected, as in patients with cerebellar astrocytomas, is of any benefit.[61, 62] Reported 5-year survival rates for children with tumors that were partially resected, in nonrandomized series, are higher in patients who had received radiotherapy than in patients treated with surgery alone. However, 10- and 20-year survival rates are similar in irradiated and nonirradiated patients. When possible, a period of observation is probably indicated in those children with low-grade partially resected lesions, since for poorly understood reasons, some partially resected lesions do not grow for years, if at all. In those patients who show clinical or radiographic progression of lesions, radiotherapy is then probably indicated, if further surgery seems unlikely to be of benefit.

In young children, especially those younger than 5 years of age, local radiotherapy can cause significant long-term neuropsychological deficits.[57, 63] Treatment with actinomycin D and vincristine has been shown to be of at least short-term benefit in children with progressive chiasmatic gliomas and has delayed the need for radiotherapy.

TABLE 39–3. STRATIFICATION OF CHILDREN WITH BRAINSTEM GLIOMAS

	AVERAGE RISK (ALL OF THE BELOW)	POOR RISK (ANY OF THE BELOW)
Clinical findings at diagnosis	No cranial nerve deficits	Cranial nerve deficits
CT findings	Isodense or mixed-density mass on unenhanced CT; variable enhancement; may be exophytic; localized lesion	Hypodense mass on CT; minimal enhancement after contrast; entire brainstem involved
Histology	Low-grade glioma	Anaplastic glioma

ANAPLASTIC GLIOMAS OF THE CEREBRUM

The best results, to date, in children with anaplastic cerebral gliomas have occurred after treatment with local radiotherapy and chemotherapy. The primary disease site is the most common site of disease failure, and at present, extensive evaluation for disease dissemination at diagnosis does not seem warranted in patients with anaplastic gliomas. However, as with patients who have brainstem gliomas, disease dissemination does occur and may be of greater concern if local disease control can be improved.

Although radiotherapy is of at least transient benefit

in most patients, fewer than 15 per cent of patients with anaplastic gliomas have long-lasting disease control after radiotherapy alone. Recently, a 40 per cent 5-year survival rate has been reported after treatment with radiotherapy, followed by CCNU and vincristine.[23] Randomized treatment trials, attempting to confirm the benefit of this drug regimen and evaluating potentially more effective combinations, are under way. In the future, increased local radiotherapy, such as brachytherapy or stereotactic radiosurgery, may be of some benefit for newly diagnosed patients.[19] However, there is concern that such localized treatment will fail to control at the edge of the primary lesion. In addition, the utilization of higher doses of chemotherapy coupled with either hematopoietic growth factors or autologous bone marrow rescue is being evaluated.[64]

ANAPLASTIC GLIOMAS OF THE POSTERIOR FOSSA

Anaplastic gliomas of the posterior fossa frequently disseminate to the neuroaxis, and complete postoperative staging, including enhanced spinal MRI or myelography, is indicated in all patients.[65] Craniospinal radiotherapy with supplemental local radiotherapy seems to result in the best disease control.[65, 66] Based on information obtained from treatment trials for children with anaplastic cortical gliomas, adjuvant chemotherapy should be explored in this group of patients.

GERM CELL TUMORS

Germ cell tumors in childhood occur primarily in the pineal or suprasellar region. Germinomas and mixed germ cell tumors (including embryonal cell carcinomas) make up the majority of tumors. Both tumor types readily disseminate to the neuroaxis, and a full extent of disease evaluation, including spinal MRI or myelography, is indicated in all patients at the time of diagnosis.

Five-year survival rates as high as 80 per cent are reported in patients with germinomas after treatment with craniospinal radiotherapy supplemented with local radiotherapy. Recently, there has been an attempt to reduce the dose of craniospinal radiation in children with localized germinomas by using preradiation chemotherapy (high-dose cyclophosphamide).[25, 67] Chemotherapy may also be of benefit in children with disseminated disease at the time of diagnosis.

Patients with mixed germ cell tumors rarely experience long-term disease control after craniospinal radiotherapy and local radiotherapy.[68, 69] Alternative means of treatment should be explored in these patients. One potentially beneficial approach is coupling craniospinal and local radiotherapy with chemotherapy of proven benefit in non–central nervous system germ cell tumors. Trials utilizing preradiation cisplatinum-based chemotherapy, followed by radiation therapy and more adjuvant therapy, are currently under way for these tumors.

CRANIOPHARYNGOMAS

The appropriate treatment for craniopharyngiomas is controversial.[70–72] However, it does seem that the addition of local radiotherapy in children with partially resected tumors is of benefit. Chemotherapy has no proven role in this tumor. Since disease recurrence is almost exclusively at the primary disease site in patients with craniopharyngiomas, evaluation for disease disseminated at the time of diagnosis is not warranted.

CHOROID PLEXUS CARCINOMAS

Choroid plexus carcinomas are extremely difficult tumors to treat. There is recent evidence to suggest that the most important single determinant of outcome is the extent of resection. Postoperative imaging of the primary site and for leptomeningeal disease is indicated in all patients.

In patients without any residual disease, observation alone is a reasonable option. The efficacy of postoperative radiotherapy or chemotherapy is unproven. However, patients who have residual disease postsurgery have a highly unfavorable prognosis and are candidates for treatment trials utilizing chemotherapy and/or radiotherapy.

REFERENCES

1. Allen JC: Childhood brain tumors. Current status of clinical trials in newly diagnosed and recurrent disease. Pediatr Clin North Am 32:633, 1985.
2. Packer RJ, Savino PJ, Bilaniuk LT, et al.: Chiasmatic gliomas of childhood: A reappraisal of natural history and effectiveness of cranial irradiation. Childs Brain 10:393, 1983.
3. Packer RJ, Sutton LN, Goldwein JW, et al.: Outcome of children with medulloblastoma/primitive neuroectodermal tumor (MB/PNET) in the computed tomographic era: Improved survival with the use of adjuvant chemotherapy. J Neurosurg 74:433, 1991.
4. Segall MD, Batzinsky S, Zee C-S, et al.: Computed tomography in the diagnosis of intracranial neoplasms in children. Cancer 56:1748, 1985.
5. Packer RJ, Batzinsky S, Cohen ME: Magnetic resonance imaging in the evaluation of intracranial tumors of childhood. Cancer 56:1767, 1985.
6. Cairncross JG, Pexam JHW, Rothbone MP, et al.: Postoperative contrast enhancement in patients with brain tumors. Ann Neurol 17:570, 1985.
7. Packer RJ, Zimmerman RA, Leurson T, et al.: Nuclear magnetic resonance imaging in the evaluation of brainstem gliomas of childhood. Neurology 35:397, 1985.
8. Packer RJ, Zimmerman RA, Sutton LN, et al.: Magnetic resonance imaging (MRI) of the posterior fossa and upper cervical cord. Pediatrics 76:84, 1985.
9. Packer RJ, Zimmerman RA, Bilaniuk LT: Magnetic resonance imaging (MRI) in the evaluation of treatment-related central nervous system (CNS) damage. Cancer 58:33, 1986.
10. Packer RJ, Siegel KR, Schut L, et al.: Central nervous system spread of childhood brain tumors at diagnosis or at initial disease recurrence. In Chapman PH (ed): Concepts in Pediatric Neurosurgery. Vol. 6. New York, S Karger, 1985, pp 16–25.
11. Packer RJ, Siegel KR, Sutton LN, et al.: Leptomeningeal dissemination of primary central nervous system tumors of childhood. Ann Neurol 18:271, 1985.

12. Kramer ED, Rafto S, Packer RJ, Zimmerman RA: Comparison of myelography with computed tomography follow-up versus magnetic resonance imaging for subarachnoid metastatic disease in children. Neurology 41:46, 1991.

13. Edwards MSB, Davis RL, Laurent JP: Tumor markers and cytologic features of cerebrospinal fluid. Cancer 56:1773, 1985.

14. Phillips PC, Kremzner LT, DeVivo DC: Cerebrospinal fluid polyamines and childhood primary brain tumors. Ann Neurol 14:373, 1983.

15. Bouchard J, Pierce CB: Radiation therapy in the management of neoplasms of the central nervous system, with a special note in regard to children. Twenty years experience, 1939–1958. Am J Roentgenol 84:610, 1960.

16. Kun LE: Principles of radiation therapy. In Cohen ME, Duffner PK (eds): Brain Tumors of Children. Principles of Diagnosis and Treatment. International Review of Child Neurology series. New York, Raven Press, 1984, pp 47–70.

17. Duffner PK, Cohen ME, Thomas PRM, et al.: The long-term effects of cranial irradiation in the central nervous system. Cancer 56:1841, 1985.

18. Packer RJ, Sposto R, Atkins TA, et al.: Quality of life in children with primitive neuroectodermal tumors (medulloblastoma)—PNET-MB. Pediatr Neurosc 13:169, 1987.

19. Gutin PM, Phillips TL, Wara WW, et al.: Brachytherapy of recurrent malignant brain tumors with removable high-activity iodine-125 sources. J Neurosurg 60:61, 1984.

20. Shin K, Muller P, Geggree P: Superfractionation radiation therapy in treatment of malignant astrocytoma. Cancer 52:2040, 1983.

21. Barkovich AJ, Krishner J, Kun LE, et al.: Brainstem gliomas: A classification system based on magnetic resonance imaging. Pediatr Neurosurg 16:73, 1991.

22. Edwards MS, Levin VA, Wilson CB: Brain tumor chemotherapy. An evaluation of agents in current use for phase II and III trials. Cancer Treat Rep 64:1179, 1980.

23. Sposto R, Ertel IM, Jenkin RDT, et al.: The effectiveness of chemotherapy for treatment of high-grade astrocytoma in children: Results of a randomized trial. J Neurooncol 7:165, 1989.

24. Allen JC, Nelson L, Jereb B: Pre-radiation chemotherapy for newly diagnosed childhood brain tumors—a modified phase II trial. Cancer 52:2001, 1983.

25. Allen JC, Walker R, Kim JH: Pre-radiation chemotherapy for newly diagnosed central nervous system germinoma—an attempt to reduce radiotherapy dose while increasing survival. Ann Neurol 18:404, 1985.

26. Bleyer W, Milstein J, Balias F, et al.: Eight-drugs-in-one-day chemotherapy for brain tumors. A new approach and rationale for pre-radiation chemotherapy. Med Pediatr Oncol 11:213, 1983.

27. Van Eys J, Cangir A, Coady D, et al.: MOPP regimen as primary chemotherapy for brain tumors in infants. J Neurooncol 3:237, 1984.

28. Kun LE, D'Souza B, Tefft M: The value of surveillance testing in childhood brain tumors. Cancer 56:1818, 1984.

29. Danoff BF, Cowchock FS, Marquette C, et al.: Assessment of the long-term effects of primary radiation therapy for brain tumors in children. Cancer 49:1580, 1982.

30. Sheline GE: Irradiation injury of human brain. A review of clinical experience. In Gilbert HA, Kagan AK (eds): Radiation Damage to the Nervous System. A Delayed Therapeutic Hazard. New York, Raven Press, 1980, pp 39–59.

31. Raimondi AJ, Tomita T: The advantages of total resection of medulloblastoma and disadvantages of whole brain postoperative radiation therapy. Childs Brain 5:50, 1979.

32. Cushing H: Experience with cerebellar medulloblastoma. A critical review. Acta Pathol Microbiol Scand 7:1, 1930.

33. Rorke LB: Classification and grading of childhood brain tumors: Overview and statement of the problem. Cancer 56:1848, 1985.

34. Rorke LB: The cerebellar medulloblastoma and its relationship to primitive neuroectodermal tumors. J Neuropathol Exp Neurol 42:1, 1983.

35. Rorke LB, Gilles FH, Davis RL, et al.: Revision of the World

36. Rubinstein LJ: Editorial. J Neurooncol 3:195, 1984.

37. Packer RJ, Sutton LN, Rorke LB, et al.: Prognostic significance of cellular differentiation in primitive neuroectodermal tumors (medulloblastoma) of childhood. J Neurosurg 61:296, 1984.

38. Chang CH, Houseplan EM, Herbert C: An operative staging system and megavoltage radiotherapeutic technique for cerebellar medulloblastoma. Radiology 93:1351, 1969.

39. Norris DG, Bruce DA, Byrd RI, et al.: Improved relapse-free survival in medulloblastoma utilizing modern techniques. Neurosurgery 9:661, 1981.

40. Park TS, Hoffman HJ, Hendrich E, et al.: Medulloblastoma: Clinical presentation and management. Experience at the Hospital for Sick Children, Toronto, 1950–1980. J Neurosurg 58:543, 1983.

41. Jereb B, Krishnaswasmi S, Ried A, et al.: Radiation for medulloblastoma adjusted to prevent recurrence to the cribriform plate region. Cancer 54:602, 1984.

42. Landberg TC, Lindgren ML, Cavallin-Stahl EK, et al.: Improvement in the radiotherapy of medulloblastoma, 1946–1975. Cancer 45:670, 1980.

43. McFarland DR, Horowitz H, Saenger EL, et al.: Medulloblastoma. A review of prognosis and survival. Br J Radiol 42:198, 1969.

44. Tomita T, McLone DG: Medulloblastoma in childhood: Results of radical resection and low-dose neuroaxis radiation therapy. J Neurosurg 64: 38, 1986.

45. McIntosh S, Chen M, Sartain PA, et al.: Adjuvant chemotherapy for medulloblastoma. Cancer 56:1316, 1985.

46. Packer RJ, Siegel KR, Sutton LN, et al.: Efficacy of combination chemotherapy with cis-platinum (CPDD), lomustine (CCNU), and vincristine (VCR) in children with primitive neuroectodermal tumors—medulloblastoma (PNET-MB) of children. Ann Neurol 18:394, 1985.

47. Fokes EC, Jr., Earle KM: Ependymomas: Clinical and pathological aspects. J Neurosurg 30:585, 1969.

48. Kernohan JW, Fletcher-Kernohan EM: Ependymomas: A study of 109 cases. A Res Nerv and Ment Dis Proc 16:182, 1973.

49. Pierre-Kahn A, Hirsch JF, Roux FX, et al.: Intracranial ependymomas in childhood—survival and function results of 47 cases. Childs Brain 10:145, 1983.

50. Goldwein JM, Corn BJ, Finlay JL, et al.: Is craniospinal irradiation required to cure children with malignant (anaplastic) intracranial ependymomas. Cancer 67:2766, 1991.

51. Salazar OM, Casto-Via M, Van Houtte D, et al.: Improved survival in cases of intracranial ependymoma after radiation therapy. Late report and recommendations. J Neurosurg 59:652, 1983.

52. Albright AL, Guthkelch AN, Packer RJ: Prognostic factors in pediatric brainstem gliomas. J Neurosurg 65:751, 1986.

53. Hoffman JH, Becker L, Craven MA: A clinically and pathologically distinct group of benign brainstem gliomas. Neurosurgery 7:243, 1980.

54. Panitch MS, Berg BO: Brainstem tumors of childhood and adolescence. Am J Dis Child 119:465, 1970.

55. Edwards MSB, Wara WM, Urtasan RC, et al.: Hyperfractionated radiation therapy for brainstem gliomas: A phase I-II trial, J Neurosurg 70:691, 1989.

56. Fulton DS, Levin VA, Wara WW, et al.: Chemotherapy of pediatric brainstem tumors. J Neurosurg 54:715, 1981.

57. Levin V, Edwards M, Wara W, et al.: 5-Fluorouracil and 1-(2-chloroethyl)-3-cyclohexyl-1-nitrosourea (CCNU) followed by hydroxyurea, misonidazole, and irradiation for brainstem gliomas. Pilot study of the Brain Tumor Research Center and the Children's Cancer Group. Neurosurgery 14:679, 1984.

58. Packer RJ, Allen J, Deck M, et al.: Brainstem glioma: Clinical manifestations of meningeal gliomatosis. Ann Neurol 14:177, 1983.

59. Fazekas JT: Treatment of grade 1 and 2 brain astrocytomas. The role of radiotherapy. Int J Radiat Oncol Biol Phys 2:661, 1977.

60. Leibel SA, Sheline GE, Wara WW, et al.: The role of radiation therapy in the treatment of astrocytoma. Cancer 35:1551, 1975.

61. Gjerris F, Klinken L: Long-term prognosis in children with benign cerebellar astrocytoma. J Neurosurg 49:179, 1978.

62. Griffin RW, Beaufait D, Blasko JC: Cystic cerebellar astrocytoma in childhood. Cancer 44:276, 1979.

63. Rosenstock JC, Packer RJ, Bilaniuk L, et al.: Chiasmatic optic glioma treated with chemotherapy: A preliminary report. J Neurosurg 63:863, 1985.

64. Finlay JL, August C, Packer RJ: High-dose multi-agent chemotherapy followed by bone marrow rescue for malignant astrocytoma of childhood and adolescence. J Neurooncol 9:239, 1990.

65. Packer RJ, Sutton LN, Rorke LB, et al.: Oligodendrogliomas of the posterior fossa in childhood. Cancer 56:195, 1985.

66. Salazar OM: Primary malignant cerebellar astrocytoma in children. A signal for postoperative craniospinal irradiation. Int J Radiat Oncol Biol Phys 7:1661, 1981.

67. Wara WW, Jenkins RDT, Evans A, et al.: Tumors of the pineal and suprasellar regions: Children's Cancer Study Group treatment results, 1960–1975. Cancer 43:689, 1979.

68. Packer RJ, Stutton LN, Rorke LB, et al.: Intracranial embryonal cell carcinoma. Cancer 54:142, 1984.

69. Packer RJ, Sutton LN, Rosenstock JG, et al.: Pineal region tumors of childhood. Pediatrics 74:97, 1984.

70. Bruce DA, Schut L, Rorke LB: Craniopharyngiomas in a capsule. *In* Epstein F, Hoffman HJ, Raimondi AJ (eds): Concepts in Pediatric Neurosurgery Vol. 1. New York, S Karger, 1981, pp 29–35.

71. Cavazzuti V, Fischer EG, Welsh K, et al.: Neurological and psychological sequelae following different treatments of craniopharyngiomas in children. J Neurosurg 59:409, 1983.

72. Hoffman HJ, Henrich EG, Humphreys RP: Management of craniopharyngiomas in children. J Neurosurg 47:218, 1977.

INFECTIONS

Chapter 40

SUPPURATIVE CENTRAL NERVOUS SYSTEM INFECTIONS

WILLIAM R. CHEEK, M.D.

CRANIAL AND INTRACRANIAL INFECTIONS

The treatment of suppurative cranial and intracranial infections continues to be a challenge, although the overall incidence of these disorders in the United States has undoubtedly decreased since the advent of antibiotics. Improved diagnostic methods and more sophisticated techniques of culturing purulent material have influenced certain aspects of management and have improved results.[1] The importance of early recognition of these infections cannot be overemphasized; the basic therapeutic principles of identification of the infectious agent and the administration of appropriate antibiotics in amounts sufficient to achieve systemic sterilization must be observed.

BRAIN ABSCESS

Brain abscess, fortunately, is not common in children. A busy neurosurgical service will see only one to three brain-abscess patients in the pediatric age group in a year.[2–7] The development of antibiotics appears to have decreased the incidence of brain abscess,[8, 9] but agreement on this point is not universal.[2, 7, 10] The reduction in incidence is logically attributed to a decrease, due to the use of antibiotics, in the number of patients with sinusitis, mastoiditis, and otitis,[11] all of which are frequently associated with the development of brain abscess. Significant reduction in intracranial complications secondary to otitic infection following the development of antibiotics has been well documented by Proctor;[12] however, the incidence of brain abscess increased in his series relative to the total incidence of complications.

There are a variety of causes of brain abscesses: (1) contiguous infection, such as sinusitis or mastoiditis, by direct extension or propagation through venous channels; (2) direct introduction via penetrating wounds; (3) hematogenous spread from a distant focus of infection or hematogenous origin without known infection elsewhere, as is frequently the case with congenital heart disease; (4) intracranial abscess formation as a result of an infected dermoid tumor in the frontal lobe or the cerebellum.

The pathologic characteristics of the mature lesion in children do not differ significantly from those in adults. Initially, the organism produces an inflammatory reaction consisting of congestion and an outpouring of polymorphonuclear leukocytes, toxic changes in the neurons, and perivascular infiltration of the polymorphonuclear leukocytes. Next, the involved tissues become necrotic, and necrosis is accompanied by liquefaction and pus formation. The brain then attempts to wall off the necrotic purulent material; since fibroblasts in the brain arise from the vessels, this reaction occurs most effectively in the gray matter, where the fibroblasts are most common. This wall, composed of fibroblasts, capillaries, and collagen, is similar to granulation tissue elsewhere in the body and becomes thicker and more fibrous as collagen deposition increases. Edema and swollen glial elements appear in the brain tissue surrounding the capsule.

As the lesion matures over the space of a few weeks, astrocytes proliferate and produce a gliotic zone external to the fibrous capsule (Fig. 40–1). Grant[13] in a clinical study of patients with brain abscess during the pre-antibiotic era, demonstrated the presence of a capsule in every patient after a period of 6 weeks. Brain abscesses in children tend to be larger lesions character-

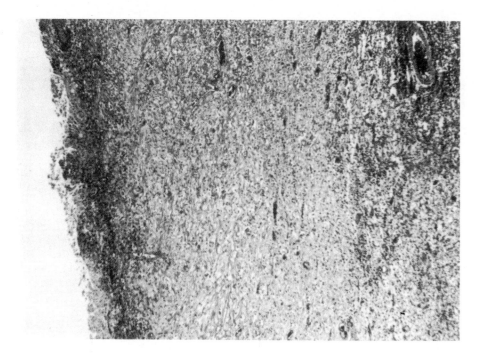

FIGURE 40–1. Photomicrograph of a section of the wall of a brain abscess, showing the different layers. To the left is that portion of the lining next to the cavity ($\times$ 50).

ized by thinner walls and the presence of more edema in the surrounding brain tissue than is the case in adults.[2] Pathologic differences have not been documented.[14]

Brain abscess is a rare occurrence in infants and, prior to the development of antibiotics, was always fatal.[15] More recent reports by Munslow, Stovall, Price, et al.[16] and Hoffman, Hendrick, and Hiscox[17] have shown gram-positive organisms to be the cause of these large lesions, but the source is unknown. Infants are believed to be susceptible to gram-negative brain abscess because the M-fraction of immunoglobulins does not cross the placenta. Because infants do not develop paranasal sinuses and mastoid air cells until the age of one year, infection in these areas is not a source of brain abscess in young infants. Idriss, Gutman, and Kronfol[4] have reported meningitis to be frequently associated with these abscesses. The failure of the infection to become well encapsulated, together with the dearth of clinical signs, accounts for the larger size of the lesion when the diagnosis is made.[16, 17] The rare disorder of pyocephalus in newborns is secondary to cerebral abscess 50 per cent of the time.[18]

The incidence of brain abscess in the past has been stated to be 4 to 7 per cent in children with congenital heart disease.[19–21] The early correction of congenital cardiac lesions in recent years has undoubtedly played a role in reducing the incidence in these children. A child with congenital heart disease and symptoms of stroke should be evaluated for possible brain abscess.[22] Brain abscesses from this source almost never occur in infants under 2 years of age. Tetralogy of Fallot that has not been totally corrected surgically is the most common underlying cardiac anomaly.[8, 21, 23, 24] A right-to-left shunt is always present, causing bypass of the pulmonary bed and allowing circulating bacteria direct access to the cerebral circulation. Although the majority of these children are cyanotic, the first reported cure was that of a girl with noncyanotic disease.[25] Decreased oxygen saturation to the brain and focal encephalomalacia may set the stage for focal infection,[8] but since these conditions occur with other diseases such as sickle cell disease, which has no particular propensity to brain abscess,[26] the right-to-left shunt is the primary etiologic factor. Studies of the acute bacteremia support this reasoning.[27] Brain abscess has also occurred in children with right-to-left shunt caused by arteriovenous aneurysm.[28, 29] Subacute bacterial endocarditis is rarely a factor in brain abscess.

Infective endocarditis is associated with neurologic complications in as many as 40 per cent of patients.[30] Infected emboli may result in mycotic aneurysm, meningitis, or brain abscess. Of these, brain abscess occurs only rarely, although microscopic, multiple abscesses are a common autopsy finding.[31]

Neutropenia and/or immunosuppression may result from a number of causes, most of them iatrogenic. The development of intracranial infection following transplantation poses a daunting challenge to both the neurosurgeon and the transplant team. In a large series of heart transplants and heart-lung transplants followed at the University of Pittsburgh, intracranial infection occurred in 13/417 patients (3.1 per cent). Mortality (77 per cent) was related to the presence of extensive multisystem infectious complications.[32]

Nocardia is a frequent offender in the abscesses found in chronically immunosuppressed patients.[32–34] Less often, Listeria is the organism identified and has been reported in children with leukemia.[35] Mycotic abscesses have occurred in leukemic children treated with amphotericin and may present a formidable problem, particularly if multiple.[36]

A rising incidence of acquired immunodeficiency syndrome (AIDS) among teenagers is to be expected given the increase of HIV infection in this age group. Until recently, AIDS in children was found almost exclusively in those with hemophilia or transplacental infection. In adults and older teens, Toxoplasma encephalitis is the most frequent neuropathologic complication; however, fungal and tuberculous abscesses are reported. In one study, central nervous system tuberculosis was reported to occur in three patients with AIDS and seven patients with AIDS-related complex followed for 48 months.[37, 38] Nine of these patients were intravenous drug users. The clinical spectrum included meningitis in two patients, multiple cerebral abscesses in one, and tuberculomas in four.

The evolution of an abscess in immunosuppressed animals has been divided into three stages based on histologic evaluation: cerebritis stage (1 to 11 days), early-capsule stage (12 to 17 days), and late-capsule stage (18 days and later).[39] These authors found a significant delay in the evolution of experimental alpha streptococcus brain abscess. Histologically, abscesses in the immune-suppressed animals were characterized by a decrease and delay in collagen formation, a reduction in polymorphonuclear leukocytes and macrophages, longer persistence of bacterial organisms, and an increase in gliosis. Schroeder et al. found a similar delay in collagen deposition in rats with *Staphylococcus aureus* brain abscess treated with short-term dexamethasone.[40] This was manifested as a thinner capsule in the early capsule stage. However, at 12 to 18 days after inoculation, there was no difference in abscess wall thickness between the control and experimental groups. Therapeutic doses of dexamethasone had little effect on mortality rates, incidence of abscess formation, or intensity of inflammatory response in the experimental animals.

Opportunistic infections are only rarely seen in infants and young children with HIV infection.[41] The authors of this article postulate that one of the reasons that opportunistic infections are so rare is that in the older child and, particularly, in the adult, they are principally reactivation infections. Common bacterial infections occur early and often in childhood AIDS, but the central nervous system infections are uncommon.[42, 43]

Abscess may form in any area of the brain, but only rarely are they located in the brainstem.[44, 45] Hematogenous lesions are usually located in the distribution of the middle cerebral artery,[2, 46, 47] while those secondary to otitic or sinus infection are invariably in adjacent areas of the brain, that is, the temporal lobe and cerebellum or the frontal lobe, respectively.[2, 6, 48] Direct penetration of the dura can be caused by many types of wounds, and the abscess may not form for such a prolonged period that the initial injury will be unknown or forgotten.[49] Minor wounds around the eye should be examined carefully since puncture of the orbital roof in a child requires little force.[50, 51]

Clinical Features

Awareness of brain abscess as a possibility is extremely important,[10] since early diagnosis is the best way to achieve low morbidity and mortality. The clinical picture in infants consists of an enlarging head and full fontanelle without localizing neurologic signs. Fever is seldom present, but should such a lesion exist, the peripheral white blood cell count will be 18,000/mm³ or greater.[4, 17] Infants usually do not have a history of infection.

In older children, the presence of cyanotic heart disease or a history of one of the following conditions should alert the physician to the possibility of brain abscess: (1) purulent infection such as sinusitis, mastoiditis, or chronic otitis media (Fig. 40–2); (2) penetrating head wound, even in the remote past;[49, 51] (3) nasal or occipital dermal sinus tract; (4) esophageal stricture and subsequent dilations.[52] The primary infection may have been treated with antibiotics and no longer be present. Fever is usually a symptom at some phase of the illness[4, 46, 53] and should suggest the possibility of brain abscess. The interval between the primary infection and abscess formation may be of many months' duration but is usually 1 to 4 weeks.[6, 8] The early symptoms are those common to many infectious processes: malaise, fever, irritability, lethargy, and anorexia. Although these symptoms are usually present at some stage in the illness,[3, 47] their absence does not rule out brain abscess. By the time a child with a brain abscess is hospitalized, the peripheral white blood cell count is usually greater than 10,000/mm³ and the sedimentation rate is almost always elevated.[4, 12, 26, 46] Blood cultures are invariably negative.[4, 47]

Neurologic signs and symptoms are related to increased intracranial pressure and secondary to focal effects of the mass. Headache, vomiting, and diminished level of consciousness are the most common symptoms.[2, 4, 7, 8, 11, 46, 47] Because of the frequent presence of

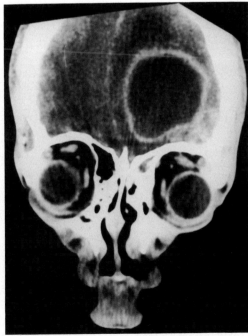

FIGURE 40–2. CT scan showing left frontal abscess and associated left frontal sinusitis.

considerable cerebral edema adjacent to the lesion and the relatively late stage of the disease at which the child is first seen, coma may deepen rapidly. The level of consciousness is particularly related to outcome in patients with brain abscess, and if it is deteriorating, examination and diagnostic tests must be performed on an emergency basis.[4, 46, 54] These symptoms may be present regardless of the location of the lesion and may be the only symptoms. Focal neurologic symptoms may be noted in more than half the patients,[8, 26, 46] and seizures may occur in 20 to 50 per cent.[47, 54, 55] Specific neurologic findings are related to location of the abscess and usually are not pronounced.

Partial aphasia, mild or moderate hemiparesis, and partial visual-field defects are the most common localizing signs. The seizures may have a lateralizing feature. Careful search must be made for foci of infection in the ears, paranasal sinuses, and the chest; the scalp must be inspected for a sinus tract. Lumbar puncture should not be performed in a patient with symptoms suggestive of brain abscess as any information obtained would not be diagnostic for brain abscess. Cultures will be negative unless the capsule has ruptured into the cerebrospinal fluid. Protein, sugar, and cell count can be normal,[7, 8] and any abnormal findings have no characteristic pattern.[26, 56] The risk of herniation with this procedure is too great to justify its use.[6, 7, 47, 57, 58]

Diagnosis

Following the history and examination, skull roentgenograms will facilitate the search for evidence of recent or old head trauma, signs of increased intracranial pressure, or the presence of gas within the brain (Fig. 40–3).[59, 60] Computed tomography (CT) with bone and soft-tissue windows may show this same type of information, but a fracture may be missed. Appropriate plain x-ray films to localize a focus of infection in the sinuses, chest, or mastoids should be obtained. If the patient's condition permits, an electroencephalogram will frequently show characteristic delta waves in the area of the abscess[5, 8, 47, 61] and can be helpful in distinguishing brain abscess from encephalopathy, encephalitis, or cerebral infarction.

Prior to the advent of CT scanning, angiography and air studies were the ultimate localization procedures.[7, 8, 11] Mass effect from vessel displacement was the usual finding in angiograms of patients with brain abscess, but in a small percentage, increased vascularity in the capsule could been seen.[62]

A CT scan is currently the most readily available definitive diagnostic procedure. With this test an abscess can be diagnosed and localized with a high degree of accuracy[63, 64] in less than 30 minutes. In addition, multiple abscesses and daughter abscesses can be seen clearly[63–65] and the amount of edema assessed. The fact that the evolution from cerebritis to abscess formation can be followed[63] facilitates the timing of the surgery. The CT scan should be performed with and without intravenous contrast material (Fig. 40–4). In all patients the CT scan shows decreased attenuation in the lesion area without contrast enhancement, and in 80 to 90 per cent it shows a ring with enhancement on the initial study.[62, 66] The correlation of this ring with capsule formation is not yet completely known.[67, 68]

Recent clinical data show that administration of steroids to a patient whose lesion is in the cerebritis stage may result in definite reduction in contrast enhancement. Contrast enhancement in well-encapsulated lesions is not reduced.[69] Increased uptake of contrast material by the ependyma may indicate the presence of ventriculitis and signal the need for appropriate therapy.[62] Magnetic resonance imaging (MRI) can now be done in many centers for diagnosing brain abscess. It should be performed with and without enhancement. This technique outlines areas of edema particularly well (Fig. 40–5).

Real-time ultrasonography is also useful in neonates with open fontanelles;[70, 71] it can be done easily and quickly in the nursery and repeated as necessary in assessing progress.[72] CT and MRI scanning should be done immediately on any child in whom brain abscess is a possibility or on any infant with an enlarging head and full fontanelle. Either CT scanning or MRI can be used to follow the progress of a brain abscess as reflected by the size of the ring enhancement.

Treatment

In the main, treatment of brain abscess still consists of surgery for diagnostic culture and therapeutic evacuation of the purulent material[73, 74] followed by administration of systemic antibiotic therapy appropriate to the organisms cultured. If diagnosed during the cerebritic stage, the disease may be cured by antibiotic therapy.[75] Cure of abscess has been reported increasingly in the last few years without surgery,[76–80] but this mode of therapy must be used with caution and only while carefully monitoring with CT or MRI in a hospital setting.[81] With these cautions in mind, cure of multiple

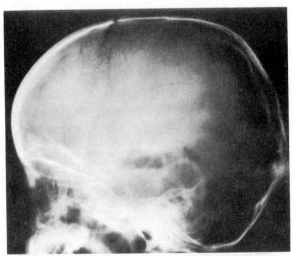

FIGURE 40–3. Lateral skull x-ray film of a 3-year-old boy with gas in a right temporal lobe abscess due to *Clostridium perfringens.* Pieces of pencil were found in the abscess.

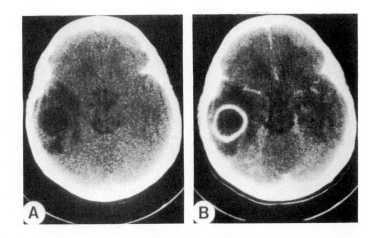

FIGURE 40–4. CT scan in a 10-year-old boy. *A,* Before contrast injection. *B,* After contrast injection. Note edema surrounding the abscess and typical ring enhancement after contrast injection.

abscesses without surgical diagnosis can now be accomplished in some cases.[77, 82–85] Clinical and experimental evidence in the past has shown the relative ineffectiveness of antibiotics in killing bacteria in suppurative lesions even though apparently adequate levels of drugs are present.[86, 87] Recent experience at Texas Children's Hospital and other institutions indicates that it is possible to cure a significant percentage of patients with brain abscess without surgery (Fig. 40–6). The organisms should be cultured for optimal antibiotic therapy, and aspiration of the lesion may be required[78, 88] even if reduction of mass effect is not considered critical. In cases in which positive cultures can be obtained from blood or sinus drainage, direct aspiration may be unnecessary.

Surgical treatment is required with (1) a stuporous or comatose patient, (2) deteriorating neurologic status, (3) marked mass effect on CT scan or MRI, (4) failure of lesions to improve with 1 to 2 weeks of antibiotic therapy, or (5) the need to obtain organisms for culture. There are three surgical options—catheter drainage, single or multiple tapping, and excision.

Catheter drainage is the oldest successful method and has been used with good results.[13, 89–91] It consists of making a burr hole over the most insensitive portion of the cortex where the abscess is superficial, opening the dura, and making a small cortical incision. The abscess is palpated with a brain cannula and punctured with a small soft catheter (No. 10 F) over a stylet. The catheter is anchored loosely with a suture through the scalp. Pus usually flows spontaneously from the tube. Gentle aspiration with a syringe can be performed at the operating table and saline irrigation used to help empty the cavity. Instillation of local antibiotics is unnecessary if the organism is sensitive to an antibiotic that perfuses well into the brain from the blood.[92] The catheter is left in place for about 7 days until drainage ceases and is then removed. This method is best suited for supratentorial lesions that are relatively near the surface.

Tapping is usually done through a burr hole also and has been a useful method since Dandy first described it in 1926.[93] It is preferred for evacuating deep collections or those in sensitive areas,[94, 95] as well as those in children with congenital heart disease.[26] With the sophisticated methods of localization and follow-up currently available (CT and MRI) and antibiotic therapy, tapping is the treatment of choice for any brain abscess requiring surgery.[96, 97] The procedure can sometimes be per-

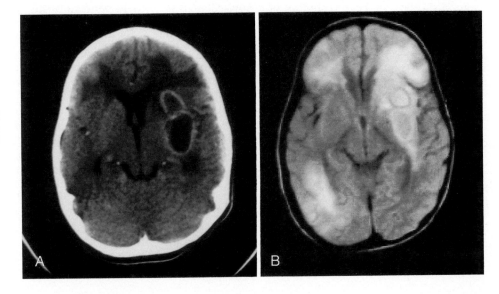

FIGURE 40–5. CT scan (*A*) and magnetic resonance image (*B*) made within 24 hours on a brain abscess patient. Note areas of edema.

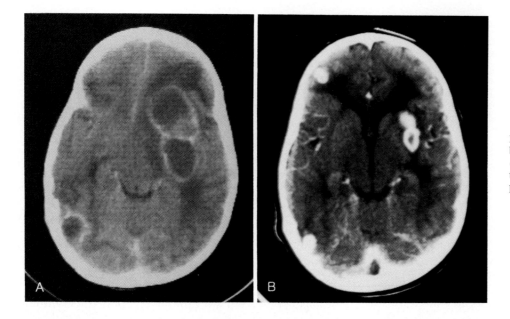

FIGURE 40–6. CT scans of multiple brain abscesses at time of diagnosis (*A*) and after 2 months of antibiotic therapy (*B*). No surgical drainage was performed.

formed under local anesthesia, and a single aspiration is frequently all that is required.[47, 93] Every child should be followed up with a CT scan or MRI. Tapping may be repeated should material re-accumulate. Current stereotaxic techniques together with intraoperative ultrasound make extremely accurate placement of the cannula or catheter possible even for lesions in deep or critical areas.[98–100]

Excision of the entire abscess is best accomplished after encapsulation, but removal of deep lesions or those in critical areas of the cortex is not advisable. Except in abscesses containing gas, the advantages of excision over the other two methods are open to serious question.[55, 57, 101, 102] Excision allows removal of the gas-containing lesion as well as identification and closure of any extracranial communication.[103] Damage to surrounding brain from the dissection may increase morbidity;[95] certainly if excision is carried out, dissection must be done carefully to cause only minimal trauma to the surrounding brain. Surrounding white matter should not be resected as was advised in the past.[104] Every effort should be made to avoid spillage of the abscess contents into either the subarachnoid space or the ventricular system.

Excision is performed in the manner usual for removing a mass lesion. The bone opening is centered over the most superficial part of the abscess, and a cortical incision is made through the closest silent area. The capsule can be palpated with a blunt cannula to localize the lesion if intraoperative ultrasound is not available. Intraoperative ultrasound helps in localizing the abscess and directing a cannula into its center. The lesion is resected intact if possible.

If the lesion is large, deflating it by aspiration prior to removal may be advisable to decrease trauma to the surrounding brain. When resection is completed, the area is irrigated copiously with saline, and the wound closed as it would be following removal of any intracranial mass. No drain is left in the brain. Good results can

be achieved by resection, but atrophy on follow-up CT scan has been reported, as well as an increase in epilepsy.[2, 7, 105, 106] Any focus of infection elsewhere must be eradicated as soon as possible by appropriate therapy.

Regardless of the surgical treatment contemplated, as soon as the possibility of a brain abscess arises, the patient should be started on dexamethasone, to reduce cerebral edema, and antibiotics. With appropriate antibiotic coverage, dexamethasone can be given in the usual doses without increasing the risk of spreading the infection. If the organism is unknown prior to surgery because a culturable focus of infection such as mastoiditis or sinusitis is not present, antistaphylococcal penicillin and chloramphenicol may each be started in doses appropriate to the treatment of meningitis. Other regimens such as those employing cephalosporins along with metronidazole (Flagyl) may be used as long as all the suspected organisms are covered. Pretreatment with antibiotics probably accounts for some of the 15 to 40 per cent of sterile cultures of abscess contents, but is still mandatory.[6, 47, 55, 95] When laboratory information is available regarding organism sensitivities, the antibiotic regimen can be altered appropriately. If a high rate of positive findings is expected, material from the abscess must be cultured meticulously for aerobes, anaerobes, and fungi as soon as possible. Systemic antibiotics should be continued for 3 to 6 weeks, depending on clinical response. With intensive antibiotic therapy, rupture of the abscess into the ventricular system need not be fatal; however, rupture can be avoided if the abscess is drained early. Treatment of brain abscess fails because of late recognition and inadequate antibiotic therapy.[101] Anticonvulsant medication should be given to all patients.

Results

The long-term results cannot be expected to be as good in infants as in older children. The enormous size of abscesses in infants and relatively poor host resistance make for greater brain damage; additionally, almost all of these infants have hydrocephalus.[16, 17, 107] Early recognition and referral for neurosurgical treatment improve the prognosis.[76, 108] Mortality in older children can be reduced to nearly zero with early diagnosis, intensive antibiotic therapy, and treatment, if indicated, with surgical drainage or excision. The neurosurgeon must be prepared to perform emergency surgery if the level of consciousness is poor or deteriorating, since the death rate in comatose patients is high.[2, 109] This approach will also decrease morbidity, which tends to be greater in children than in adults.[110, 111]

One must remember that every brain abscess causes some degree of destruction of brain tissue. An increasing number of survivors experience seizures as time passes (up to 72 per cent). The seizures are not related to age, site of abscess (except for the cerebellum), or residual neurologic deficit. The presence or absence of seizures preoperatively does not necessarily predict that a patient will develop seizures postoperatively.[112] The interval between treatment and seizure development is longest in children who are under 10 years of age. The seizures usually occur infrequently and can be controlled by anticonvulsant medication, which should be given prophylactically to all patients.[21, 113, 114] A follow-up electroencephalogram in brain-abscess patients with seizures almost invariably shows a localized sharp and slow wave complex.

SUBDURAL EMPYEMA

Subdural empyema of the intracranial space is an uncommon disorder that occurs principally in children and adolescents. The incidence is approximately one-fifth that of brain abscess.[115] It is usually secondary to paranasal sinus or middle-ear infection, but may also be a complication of purulent scalp infection or osteomyelitis of the skull or may be secondary to hematogenous infection in a subdural hematoma. The pathway from contiguous infection is usually retrograde through infected venous channels or a bone defect. The collections are located most often over the frontoparietal convexities and may involve the interhemispheric space; spread to the posterior fossa is rare.[116]

These lesions may become very large before they are diagnosed. In patients with subdural empyema who also have meningitis, brain abscess, or extradural abscess, the prognosis worsens. Signs and symptoms consist of headache, vomiting, signs of infection, and nuchal rigidity.[117] The history may be as long as 6 months. Sedimentation rate and peripheral white blood cell count are elevated. Infants have increasing head size and bulging fontanelles; seizures are common.[118] Focal signs may develop late in the disease process, often accompanied by a deteriorating level of consciousness, indicating the need for rapid institution of treatment. If symptoms are suggestive of subdural empyema, spinal puncture should not be done because of the danger of precipitating brain herniation. The fluid will not be of diagnostic value, showing only elevated protein and pleocytosis, usually of lymphocytes.

The diagnosis of a subdural collection can be made by CT scanning or MRI. CT findings may be subtle early in the disease and may not be diagnostic.[119–121] An interhemispheric spread should be noted, as should the presence of a brain abscess. The empyema can be seen as an extracerebral mass and any interhemispheric spread can be observed (Fig. 40–7). The injection of contrast medium enhances the cortical membrane (Fig. 40–8) on a CT and MRI.[121] Infratentorial empyemas are, fortunately, rare, representing as little as 3 per cent of all subdural empyemas. These subdural collections are particularly difficult to identify by means of computerized tomography.[122, 123] It would appear that MR imaging is the diagnostic study of choice whenever an intracranial infection is suspected.

The early differentiation between a sterile subdural effusion and subdural empyema in infants with *Haemophilus* type B meningitis may be difficult. It has been suggested that the presence of *Haemophilus influenzae* capsular antigen, when combined with computerized tomography, not only allows accurate identification of empyema when present, but accurately predicts whether or not a fluid collection has a high probability of becoming infected.[124] This finding, based on a study of 52 patients with meningitis complicated by subdural fluid collection, may prove of great value in reducing the morbidity of this complication. Plain skull roentgenograms may reveal sinusitis, mastoiditis, or skull osteomyelitis.

Treatment consists of an antibiotic regimen similar to that for brain abscess, and administration of local antibiotics is usually not necessary.[115] The patient is given steroids to control increased intracranial pressure and anticonvulsants to prevent seizures. A focus of infection identified elsewhere should be eradicated as soon as possible.[125]

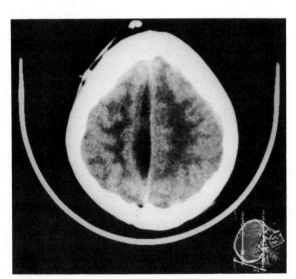

FIGURE 40–7. MRI showing interhemispheric spread of subdural empyema.

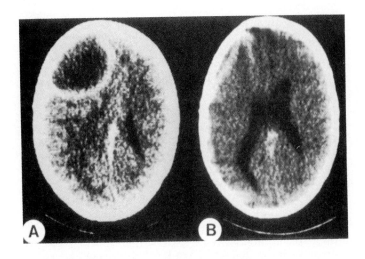

FIGURE 40-8. CT scan of patient with subdural empyema. *A,* Preoperative scan with contrast enhancement. *B,* Ten days after surgery, with contrast enhancement.

Virtually all cases of subdural empyema must be surgically drained.[118, 121, 126–129] Evacuation and irrigation through multiple burr holes are adequate if the pus is thin and there is no interhemispheric collection. If the pus is thick or an interhemispheric collection is present, a craniotomy should be performed and the infected material removed as completely as possible. Drains are usually not necessary, but irrigating catheters may be left in the subdural space for a few days.

At the time of surgery, pus should be taken in an airtight container directly to the bacteriology laboratory for Gram's stain and culture. Isolation of anaerobic organisms is particularly important since these bacteria are frequently present in paranasal sinus infection.[130] Mortality was formerly 40 per cent,[131] but widespread use of CT and MRI scanning for early diagnosis has reduced it to 10 to 13 per cent.[127, 129, 132] A few cases diagnosed early have been reported cured with antibiotics alone.[133, 134]

Complications such as cortical thrombophlebitis, brain abscess, and meningitis decrease the success rate. Early diagnosis and therapy, along with meticulous attention to bacteriologic studies, should improve the prognosis. After surgery, a follow-up CT scan should be obtained to rule out the presence of an intracerebral abscess not seen on the initial examination. Seizure incidence in long-term survivors is about 26 per cent;[135] anticonvulsants should be continued for at least 2 years after surgery. If no seizures have occurred after this time and if electroencephalography shows no epileptogenic focus, the patient can be taken off anticonvulsant medication on a trial basis.

EPIDURAL ABSCESS

Epidural intradural abscess is almost always secondary to or associated with another infection such as mastoiditis, sinusitis, postoperative flap infection, or osteomyelitis of the skull. It may also result from infection of compound wounds of the head. A purulent extradural collection without osteomyelitis of the skull is rare.[136] Increased intracranial pressure from this lesion alone is uncommon as the mass effect is usually not great, but it can be associated with subdural empyema or brain abscess, both of which must be ruled out in all patients by CT or MRI scanning. Epidural abscess serves as a focus of infection and may cause septicemia, which cannot be successfully treated until the epidural infection is eradicated. Plain skull roentgenograms often show osteomyelitis or air in the subdural space.[136]

The patient frequently manifests few specific clinical signs except those due to infection, such as fever or malaise. The number of peripheral white blood cells is increased. Local findings of scalp redness, swelling, and tenderness, together with focal headache secondary to sinus infection, mastoiditis, or skull osteomyelitis, are usually present. If neurologic signs and symptoms do occur, they usually appear late in the course of the disease and when a large lesion is present.

Therapy consists of evacuation of the epidural collection through burr holes or by craniectomy if osteomyelitis is present. All epidural granulations should be removed as thoroughly as possible.[136] A catheter drain may be left in the epidural space for the first few days and is desirable if the cavity is large. The bone should be treated as described in the following section. Associated sinusitis or brain abscess must be treated promptly.

In patients with frontal sinusitis and associated epidural abscess, the latter can sometimes be adequately drained through an opening made in the posterior sinus wall during surgical exploration of the sinus. The antibiotics used in the initial treatment of brain abscess should be started when epidural abscess is first thought to be present. Cultures for aerobes, anaerobes, and fungi should be done carefully so that appropriate drugs can be selected. Follow-up CT or MRI scans until the patient recovers will allow monitoring of the progress of the lesion and detection of the presence of the more serious brain abscess or subdural empyema.[137]

OSTEOMYELITIS OF THE SKULL

Osteomyelitis of the skull is most commonly a complication of a compound skull wound following either surgery or trauma. It may also occur in the frontal bone

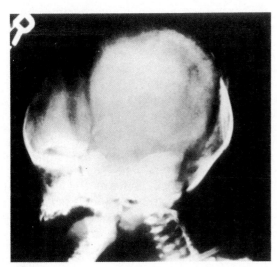

FIGURE 40–9. Typical "moth-eaten" appearance of osteomyelitis of the skull.

secondary to sinus infection or in the parietal and temporal bones from ear infection.[138] Osteomyelitis may develop in the skull of a newborn as a complication of an infected scalp wound from use of forceps or secondary to intrauterine monitoring.[139–141] Rarely, it occurs opportunistically in a child with a suppressed immune mechanism and may be due to fungus.[142]

Clinical signs consists of local heat, swelling, tenderness, and redness. In the postsurgical period, poor healing of the suture line or a draining sinus of the wound may signal the problem. The patient may not have fever.[143] If the infection is severe, the patient will have high fever and suffer prostration, and peripheral white blood cells will be elevated. In this last situation, blood cultures are indicated. *Staphylococcus aureus* is the organism most commonly associated with postsurgical and post-traumatic wounds. The disease may progress rapidly if an epidural abscess is also present.[138] Meningitis almost never occurs unless the dura is open from previous surgery or has been lacerated from a compound wound.

X-ray examination of the skull may show no change for the first 10 to 14 days. Then, the classic picture is of a "moth-eaten" appearance (Fig. 40–9). Radionuclide scan with technetium-labeled organic phosphate[144] shows changes as soon as the infection is present; scalp artifact is not a problem with current scintillation cameras. CT scanning can detect bony changes and determine whether any intracranial collection of pus is present.

Treatment consists of debridement of the area and antibiotic therapy, usually for a prolonged period.[145] In a postsurgical wound, the bone flap must be removed while preserving the pericranium. Poorly vascularized and infected bone surrounding the craniotomy must be removed back to a well-vascularized bone margin. It is rarely necessary to remove bone other than that already devitalized, that is, the flap or the sequestrum, if surgical treatment is prompt and antibiotic therapy adequate. Infected granulation tissue should be curetted away and any epidural abscess treated as described above with care taken not to penetrate the dura. The removal of any infected granulation tissue attached to the skull and producing bone destruction should stop the process, making removal of the underlying bone unnecessary (Fig. 40–10). The wound is copiously irrigated with saline solution throughout the procedure and is closed in one layer with nylon or stainless steel sutures. A drain may be left in place for 24 hours. Administration of local antibiotics is not usually indicated. These same principles are used in treating skull osteomyelitis arising from other causes. Early debridement should resolve the process rapidly. Cranioplasty should be delayed for at least 6 months.

SPINAL INFECTIONS

Although infections involving the spine are not common in children,[146] they do occasionally occur, involving the bony structures, the intervertebral discs, the spinal canal, or the spinal cord. A spinal infection may be suppurative or not; symptoms may be nonspecific unless direct or indirect involvement compromises neural function. Diagnosis has been made easier by modern imaging techniques, but the clinician must be alert to the possibility of spinal infection. Surgical therapy is not always required.

FIGURE 40–10. Ten-day-old girl with extensive staphylococcal osteomyelitis of the skull. *A,* Before debridement. Note forceps pointing to infected granulations. *B,* After debridement. Well-vascularized bone was preserved. The wound subsequently healed without incident.

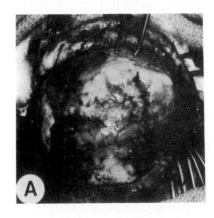
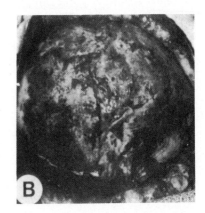

Spinal Cord Abscess

Abscess in the spinal cord occurs much more rarely than brain abscess. By 1977, only 15 cases in children had been reported.[147] Spinal cord abscess may occur from direct spread, as in the case of a dermal sinus tract. More frequently, it is metastatic from hematogenous or lymphatic routes.[148] On occasion, no primary source can be determined. Spinal cord abscess is usually single but may be multiple. It occurs most frequently in the thoracic cord but may be at any level and may involve the entire length of the cord.

The pathology is similar to that of brain abscess, and histologic findings depend upon the stage of the disease. The most common organisms recovered are Staphylococcus and Streptococcus, but many others, including fungi, have been cultured. Occasionally, multiple organisms are found, and sterile abscesses have also been reported.[147] The cerebrospinal fluid (CSF) findings are usually nonspecific, but organisms are sometimes found, especially if there is an associated meningitis. Abscesses arising from contiguous spread are almost always at the adjacent level of the cord.

Signs and symptoms depend on the level, size, and chronicity of the lesion. There are usually signs of infection, such as fever and elevated peripheral white blood cell count; indications of a primary infection elsewhere, such as mastoiditis or endocarditis, may be present, or the child may have the symptoms of meningitis, such as headache, vomiting, and nuchal rigidity. Some children experience prolonged backache before the onset of other symptoms.

In all cases treated surgically, paraparesis or paraplegia had developed before diagnosis. This complication may occur suddenly; if paralysis is complete, and especially if the onset was rapid, the prognosis is worse. If spinal cord abscess is suspected, a magnetic resonance imaging (MRI) scan of the spine should be carried out immediately. A CT myelogram should be performed if MRI scanning is not available. Surgical exploration should then be performed as an emergency measure.

Laminectomy is done at the appropriate level followed by aspiration of the cord at its widest point, using a 25-gauge needle inserted into the midline of the dorsal aspect of the cord. When pus is recovered, a dorsal midline myelotomy is made, just large enough to evacuate the purulent material. Cultures are sent for aerobes, anaerobes, and fungi. The wound is copiously irrigated with Ringer's solution and closed in the usual fashion. If the cavity is extensive, a drain can be left in place and brought out through the wound; the drain is removed in 24 to 48 hours.

Appropriate antibiotics are administered intravenously, and treatment should proceed as it would for brain abscess. Prior to the development of antibiotics, only two of nine children with this diagnosis survived, but from 1948 to 1977, in all six cases reported, children with spinal cord abscess survived. With the clinician's alertness to the possibility of spinal cord abscess, current diagnostic imaging techniques, prompt surgical drainage, and adequate antibiotic therapy, the prognosis should continue to improve.

Spinal Epidural Abscess

Although spinal epidural abscess is rare in children,[149, 150] it is a most important spinal infection from the neurosurgical standpoint. It occurs most frequently in the midthoracic or lower lumbar region.[151] The pus collects dorsally since the dura adheres ventrally to the posterior longitudinal ligament from C1 to S2.[149] Staphylococcus aureus is the most common causative organism,[150] although many others have been cultured. The organism spreads into the epidural space hematogenously, except in cases of osteomyelitis of the vertebra or those in which there is a penetrating wound.[149] An antecedent infection may have been present in the latter case or a history of trauma may be obtained.[150]

Rankin and Flothow[152] described the classic symptomatic progression in 1946; spinal ache followed by root pain, impaired cord function, and finally paraplegia. This course is generally invariable in adults, but children often demonstrate no clear-cut syndrome.[150] Fever and irritability are usually present. A child will sometimes limp.[151] Rigidity of the spinal column and evidence of pain on movement are common in infants, and lower extremity weakness or paralysis is usually present before the diagnosis is made. Back pain may not be present in older children,[150] but hip pain can be prominent.[61] Sufficient radicular inflammation may cause abdominal pain and spinal ileus mimicking an acute abdomen.[158] Peripheral white blood cell count may be increased and the sedimentation rate elevated. Blood cultures are frequently negative.

Once the epidural abscess is suspected, the work-up should progress on an emergency basis. Plain radiographs are nonrevealing except rarely, when associated osteomyelitis of the vertebra is present.[149] MRI scanning should now be the imaging procedure of choice in cases suspected of this diagnosis. Spinal CT scanning may establish the diagnosis,[154] but intrathecal contrast injection should be used if there is any question, especially in the presence of a neurologic deficit.[155] The agent may have to be introduced via cisternal or C1–C2 puncture because of the level of the abscess. Direct puncture of the abscess by spinal needle may yield pus for culture. Spinal fluid findings are nondiagnostic. When the diagnosis of spinal epidural abscess is established, surgical decompression should be carried out immediately,[149, 151, 156–158] unless an absolute contraindication exists.

Results are best in those patients with a slow course and if surgery is done before significant neurologic deficit occurs. A limited laminectomy[150] is the procedure of choice in a child since it may not lead to the development of kyphoscoliosis later. In many cases the pus can be removed by irrigation of the epidural space through a limited opening.[159] If adequate evacuation of pus cannot be accomplished in this way and if multiple laminae must be removed, an en bloc removal of the laminae is advised, with debridement of the epidural space and replacement of the laminae as described by Hulme and Dott.[160]

A drain should be left in the epidural space for 24 to 48 hours. Cultures for aerobes, anaerobes, fungi, and tuberculosis should be obtained at the operating table. Following surgery, appropriate intravenous antibiotics must be continued until the child is afebrile, the peripheral white blood cell count normal, and the sedimentation rate less than 20 mm/hr; these changes will take several weeks. Local irrigation with antibiotics after surgery is unnecessary. With early diagnosis and surgical drainage before serious deficit occurs, the prognosis should be good in most cases.[158]

SPONDYLITIS

Pyogenic vertebral osteomyelitis is no longer common in children.[161, 162] Characteristically caused by *Staphylococcus aureus*, it produces suppurative destruction of the vertebral body and can involve vertebrae at any level. Radiographic changes occur within two weeks of onset. Thoracic and lumbar lesions cause abdominal symptomatology and pain,[161] while the initial symptom in cervical disease may be torticollis.[163] Spondylitis is not of neurosurgical interest unless a collection of epidural pus produces cord compression. Treatment should be under the guidance of an orthopedic surgeon.

Because tuberculous spondylitis continues to be seen occasionally in the United States, the causative organism of spondylitis in a child must be established by blood culture or biopsy of the lesion. If *Staphylococcus aureus* or other pathogens cannot be cultured, a skin test for tuberculosis, a chest x-ray, and sputum and urine samples for AFB smear and culture should be obtained.

Tuberculous spondylitis in children frequently causes cord compression,[164] producing partial or complete paraplegia. Diagnosis of epidural involvement and accurate localization is now readily accomplished with CT scanning.[165] MRI scanning should be diagnostic as well. Early operation via an anterior approach[162, 164] is probably advisable in all cases but especially in those with neurologic involvement.

Posterior decompression, i.e., laminectomy, is contraindicated since tuberculosis of the spine is an anterior disease. Laminectomy can increase spinal deformity and instability[162] and can aggravate the neurologic deficit. Any surgical exploration should be under the supervision of an orthopedic surgeon as fusion will almost certainly be required for stabilization (Fig. 40–11). Neurologic deficit tends to occur slowly over a long period of time; hence, recovery of function is usually good and may continue to improve for up to 24 months after surgery.[164]

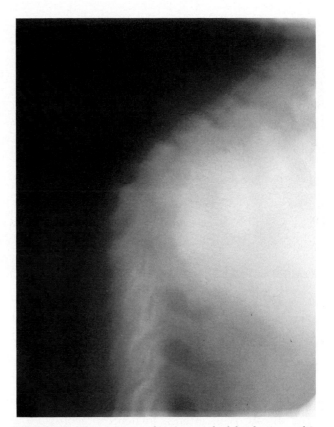

FIGURE 40–11. Tomogram showing marked kyphosis resulting from tuberculous spondylitis.

DISCITIS

Discitis is an inflammation of the intervertebral disc without suppuration. Children with discitis have low-grade fever, an elevated sedimentation rate, spinal pain, and radiographic changes, which consist of a narrowing of the disc space along with irregularity and haziness of the vertebral end-plate (Fig. 40–12). There may be a history of previous infection or trauma. Young children will refuse to walk or even sit if the pain is severe enough. Older children frequently complain of back or lower extremity pain, but abdominal pain[166] is also common. Discitis is most commonly located in the lumbar spine, followed by the thoracic spine and, rarely, the cervical area.[166, 167]

The cause of discitis is debatable, although bacterial infection is most likely. The blood supply to the intervertebral disc is abundant below the age of 20 years[168] and may be responsible for the hematogenous spread of bacteria to the discs of children. Many cases have yielded positive cultures from biopsy, either open or needle, but not the majority.[169] The organism cultured is usually *Staphylococcus aureus*, although unusual causes have been found.[170, 171] Some clinicians advise reserving biopsy for those cases that do not respond to routine treatment or in which tuberculosis may be present.[172, 173]

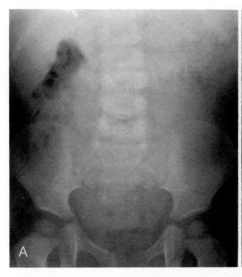
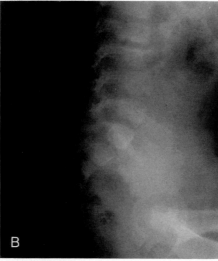

FIGURE 40–12. Anteroposterior (A) and lateral (B) radiographs showing typical changes of discitis at L2–L3.

The diagnosis is based on the clinical symptoms noted above and on imaging changes. CT scan has been useful in evaluating early or atypical cases.[174] MRI findings have been well documented[172] and are diagnostic (Fig. 40–13). Treatment consists primarily of bed rest and immobilization. Antistaphylococcal drugs may hasten clinical improvement.[167]

The disease is of interest to neurosurgeons in the differential diagnosis of other spine disorders that might produce cord compression, i.e., tumor or epidural abscess. The prognosis is usually good, with significant spine deformity a rare occurrence.[146, 169, 173]

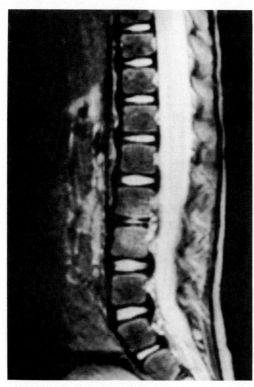

FIGURE 40–13. MRI showing typical disc narrowing and epidural inflammatory changes of discitis.

CONGENITAL DERMAL SINUS

These tubular tracts are dysraphic defects that communicate from the spine to the deeper layers, sometimes all the way to the spinal cord. They are discussed in detail elsewhere in this volume. For this section, it is important to emphasize the following: (1) The skin opening is in the midline and may be tiny and difficult to see. Although it can occur from the upper cervical region to the midsacrum, it is most commonly found in the lumbar or lumbosacral area. (2) Intraspinal infectious complications can be severe and produce permanent neurologic sequelae. (3) The lesion should be excised in toto as soon as it is diagnosed.[175]

REFERENCES

1. Small M, Dale B: Intracranial suppuration 1968–1982, a 15 year review. Clin Otolaryngol 9:315, 1984.
2. Arseni C, Horvath L, Dumitrescu L: Cerebral abscesses in children. Acta Neurochir 14:197, 1966.
3. Beller AJ, Sahar A, Praiss I: Brain abscess. J Neurol Neurosurg Psychiatry 3:757, 1973.
4. Idriss ZH, Gutman LT, Kronfol NM: Brain abscesses in infants and children. Clin Pediatr 17:738, 1978.
5. Loeser E, Scheinberg L: Brain abscesses: A review of 99 cases. Neurology 7:601, 1957.
6. Samson DS, Clark K: A current review of brain abscess. Am J Med 54:201, 1973.
7. Wright RL, Ballantine HT: Management of brain abscess in children and adolescents. Am J Dis Child 114:113, 1967.
8. Matson DD, Salam M: Brain abscess in congenital heart disease. Pediatrics 27:772, 1961.
9. McClelland CJ, Craig B, Crockard HA: Brain abscesses in Northern Ireland. J Neurol Neurosurg Psychiatry 41:1043, 1978.
10. Chalstrey S, Pfleiderer G, Moffat DA: Persisting incidence and mortality of sinogenic cerebral abscess: A continuing reflection of late clinical diagnosis. J R Soc Med 84:193, 1991.
11. Matson D: Brain abscess. In Matson DD (ed): Neurosurgery of Infancy and Childhood. Springfield, IL, Charles C Thomas, 1969, pp 708–715.
12. Proctor CA: Intracranial complications of otitic origin. Laryngoscope 76:288, 1966.
13. Grant F: The mortality from abscess of the brain. JAMA 99:550, 1932.

14. Friede R: Developmental Neuropathology. New York, Springer-Verlag, 1975, pp 175–176.
15. Sanford H: Abscess of the brain in infants under 12 months of age. Am J Dis Child 35:256, 1928.
16. Munslow RA, Stovall VS, Price RD, et al.: Brain abscess in infants. J Pediatr 51:74, 1957.
17. Hoffman HJ, Hendrick EB, Hiscox JL: Cerebral abscess in early infancy. J Neurosurg 33:172, 1970.
18. Izquierdo JM, Sanz F, Coca JM, et al.: Pyocephalus of the newborn child. Child's Brain 4:129, 1978.
19. Maronde R: Brain abscess and congenital heart disease. Ann Intern Med 33:602, 1950.
20. Newton E: Hematogenous brain abscess in cyanotic congenital heart disease. Q J Med 25:201, 1956.
21. Taussig HB, Crocetti A, Eshaghpour E, et al: Long-time observations on the Blalock-Taussig Operation III: Common complications. Johns Hopkins Med J 129:274, 1971.
22. Kurlan R, Griggs RC: Cyanotic congenital heart disease with suspected stroke: Should all patients receive antibiotics? Arch Neurol 40:209, 1983.
23. Chakraborty RN, Bidwai PS, Kak VK, Banjaree AK, et al: Brain abscess in cyanotic congenital heart disease. Indian Heart J 41:190, 1989.
24. Tyler HR, Clark DB: Incidence of neurologic complication in congenital heart disease. Arch Neurol Psychiatry 77:17, 1957.
25. Smolik EA, Blattner R, Heys FM: Brain abscess associated with congenital heart disease. JAMA 130:145, 1946.
26. Raimondi AJ, Matsumoto S, Miller RA: Brain abscess in children with congenital heart disease. J Neurosurg 23:588, 1965.
27. Wood WB, Smith MR, Perry WD, et al: Studies on the cellular immunology of acute bacteremia. J Exp Med 94:521, 1951.
28. Dove AM, Fan LL, Wood BP: Radiological cases of the month. Pulmonary arteriovenous malformation presenting with brain abscess. Am J Dis Child 144:1045, 1990.
29. Meachan WF, Scott H: Congenital pulmonary arteriovenous aneurysm complicated by Bacteroides abscess of the brain. Ann Surg 147:404, 1958.
30. Ting W, Silverman N, Levitsky S: Valve replacement in patients with endocarditis and cerebral septic emboli. Ann Thorac Surg 51:18, 1991.
31. Lerner PI: Neurologic complications of infective endocarditis. Med Clin North Am 69:385, 1985.
32. Hall WA, Martinez AJ, Dummer JS, et al.: Central nervous system infections in heart and heart-lung transplant recipients. Arch Neurol 46:173, 1989.
33. Fried J, Hinthorn D, Ralstin J, et al.: Cure of brain abscess caused by Nocardia asteroides resistant to multiple antibiotics. South Med J 81:412, 1988.
34. Raby N, Forbes G, Williams R: Nocardia infection in patients with liver transplants or chronic liver disease; radiologic findings. Radiology 174:713, 1990.
35. Hutchinson RJ, Heyn R: Listerial brain abscess in a patient with leukemia: Successful nonsurgical treatment. Clin Pediatr 22:312, 1983.
36. Foreman NK, Mott MG, Parkyn TM, Moss G: Mycotic intracranial abscesses during induction treatment for acute lymphoblastic leukemia. Arch Dis Child 63:436, 1988.
37. Bishburg E, Sunderam G, Reichman LB, Kapila R: Central nervous system tuberculosis with the acquired immunodeficiency syndrome and its related complex. Ann Intern Med 105:210, 1986.
38. Moskowitz LB, Hensley GT, Chan JC, et al.: The neuropathology of acquired immune deficiency syndrome. Arch Pathol Lab Med 108:867, 1984.
39. Obana WG, Britt RH, Placone RC, et al.: Experimental brain abscess development in the chronically immunosuppressed host. Computerized tomographic and neuropathological correlations. J Neurosurg 65:382, 1986.
40. Schroeder KA, McKeever PE, Schlaberg DR, Hoff JT: Effect of dexamethasone on experimental brain abscess. J Neurosurg 66:264, 1987.
41. Civitello LA: Neurologic complications of HIV infection in children. Pediatr Neurosurg 17:104, 1991–92.
42. Belman AL, Diamond G, Dickson D, et al.: Pediatric AIDS: Neurologic syndromes. Am J Dis Child 142:29, 1988.
43. Bernstein LJ, Krieger BZ, Novick BE, et al.: Pediatr Infect Dis 4:472, 1985.
44. Danziger J, Allen KL, Block S: Brain stem abscess in children. J Neurosurg 40:391, 1974.
45. Robert CM Jr, Stern WE, Brown WJ, et al.: Brain stem abscess treated surgically. Surg Neurol 3:153, 1975.
46. Eberhard SJ: Diagnosis of brain abscess in infants and children: A retrospective study of 26 cases. N C Med J 30:363, 1969.
47. McGreal D: Brain abscesses in children. Can Med Assoc J 86:261, 1962.
48. Shaw MD, Russell JA: Cerebellar abscess: A review of 47 cases. J Neurol Neurosurg Psychiatry 38:429, 1975.
49. Mikhael MA, Mattar AG: Case report: Chronic graphite granulomatous abscess simulating a brain tumor. J Comput Assist Tomogr 1:713, 1977.
50. Fanning WL, Willett LR, Phillips CF, et al.: Puncture wound of the eyelid causing brain abscess. J Trauma 16:919, 1976.
51. Miller CF, Brodkey JS, Colombi BJ: The danger of intracranial wood. Surg Neurol 7:95, 1977.
52. Kolter R, Schild JA, Holinger PH: Delayed CNS complications. Laryngoscope 85:1379, 1975.
53. Torales A, Franco FR, Calderson E: Intracranial abscesses in children. Bol Med Hosp Infant Mex 35:33, 1978.
54. Snyder BD, Farmer TW: Brain abscess in children. South Med J 64:687, 1971.
55. von Alphen HAM, Dreissen JJR: Brain abscess and subdural empyema. J Neurol Neurosurg Psychiatry 39:481, 1976.
56. DeVio D: Cerebral abscess in children. Dev Med Child Neurol 13:800, 1971.
57. Morgan H, Wood MW, Murphy F: Experience with 88 consecutive cases of brain abscess. J Neurosurg 38:698, 1973.
58. Nielsen H: Cerebral abscess in children. Neuropediatrics 14:76, 1983.
59. Norrell H, Howieson J: Gas-containing brain abscess. Am J Roentgenol 109:273, 1970.
60. Russel JA, Taylor J: Circumscribed gas-gangrene abscess of the brain. Br J Surg 50:434, 1963.
61. Donowitz LG, Cole W, Lohr JA: Acute spinal epidural abscess presenting as hip pain. Pediatr Infect Dis 2:44, 1983.
62. Nielsen H, Gyldensted C: Computed tomography in the diagnosis of cerebral abscess. Neuroradiology 12:1201, 1977.
63. New PFJ, Davis K, Ballantine HT: Computed tomography in cerebral abscess. Radiology 121:641, 1976.
64. Zimmerman RA, Patel S, Bilaniuk LT: Demonstration of purulent bacterial intracranial infections by computed tomography. Am J Roentgenol 127:155, 1976.
65. Stephanov S: Experience with multiloculated brain abscesses. J Neurosurg 49:199, 1978.
66. Price H, Danziger A: The role of computerized tomography in the diagnosis and management of intracranial abscess. Clin Radiol 29:571, 1978.
67. Enzemann DR, Britt R, Yeager AS: Experimental brain abscess evolution; computed tomographic and neuropathologic correlation. Radiology 133:113, 1979.
68. Garvey G: Current concepts of bacterial infections of the central nervous system: Bacterial meningitis and bacterial brain abscess. J Neurosurg 59:735, 1983.
69. Britt RH, Enzmann DR: Clinical stages of human brain abscesses on serial CT scans after contrast infusion. J Neurosurg 59:972, 1983.
70. Gray PH, O'Reilly C: Neonatal Proteus mirabilis meningitis and cerebral abscess: Diagnosis by real-time ultrasound. J Clin Ultrasound 12:441, 1984.
71. Lam AH, Berry A, de Silva M, et al.: Intracranial Serratia infection in preterm newborn infants. Am J Neurol Radiol 5:447, 1984.
72. Nielsen HC, Shannon K: Use of ultrasonography for diagnosis and management of neonatal brain abscesses. Pediatr Infect Dis 2:460, 1983.
73. Bruszkiewicz J, Doron Y, Peyser E, et al.: Brain abscess and its surgical management. Surg Neurol 18:7, 1982.

74. Wong TT, Lee LS, Wang HS, Shen EY, et al.: Brain abscesses in children—a cooperative study of 83 cases. Child's Nerv Syst 5:19, 1989.

75. Heineman HS, Braude AJ, Osterholm JL: Intracranial suppurative disease. JAMA 218:1542, 1971.

76. Berg B, Franklin G, Cunco R, et al.: Neurosurgical cure of brain abscess: Early diagnosis and follow-up with computerized tomography. Ann Neurol 3:474, 1978.

77. Boom WH, Tuazon CU: Successful treatment of multiple brain abscesses with antibiotics alone. Rev Infect Dis 7:189, 1985.

78. George B, Roux F, Pillon M, et al.: Relevance of antibiotics in the treatment of brain abscesses. Report of a case with eight simultaneous brain abscesses treated and cured medically. Acta Neurochir 47:285, 1979.

79. Keren G, Teyrel DL: Nonsurgical treatment of brain abscesses: Report of two cases. Pediatr Infect Dis 3:331, 1984.

80. Vaquero J, Cabezudo JM, Leunda G: Nonsurgical resolution of a brain stem abscess: Case report. J Neurosurg 53:726, 1980.

81. Kobrine AI, David DO, Rizzoli HV: Multiple abscesses of the brain: Case report. J Neurosurg 54:93, 1981.

82. Barsoum AH, Lewis H, Cannillo KL: Nonoperative treatment of multiple brain abscesses. Surg Neurol 16:283, 1981.

83. Basit AS, Ravit B, Banerji AK, Tandon PN: Multiple pyogenic brain abscesses: An analysis of 21 patients. J Neurol Neurosurg Psychiatry 36:591, 1989.

84. Maniglia AJ, Goodwin WJ, Arnold JE, Ganz E: Intracranial abscesses secondary to nasal, sinus and orbital infections in adults and children. Arch Otolaryngol Head Neck Surg 115:1424, 1989.

85. Rennels MB, Woodward C, Robinson WL, et al.: Medical cure of apparent brain abscesses. Pediatrics 72:220, 1983.

86. Black P, Graybill R, Charache P: Penetration of brain abscesses by systematically administered antibiotics. J Neurosurg 38:705, 1973.

87. Smith MR, Wood WB: An experimental analysis of curative action of penicillin in acute bacterial infections. J Exp Med 103:509, 1956.

88. Burke LP, Ho U, Cerullo LJ, et al.: Multiple brain abscesses. Surg Neurol 16:452, 1981.

89. Macewen W: Pyogenic Infective Diseases of the Brain and Spinal Cord. Glasgow, James Maclehose & Sons, 1893.

90. Mount L: Conservative surgical therapy of brain abscesses. J Neurosurg 7:385, 1960.

91. Selker R: Intracranial abscess: Treatment by continuous catheter drainage. Child's Brain 1:368, 1975.

92. Fischer EG, McLennon J, Suyuki Y: Cerebral abscesses in children. Am J Dis Child 135:746, 1981.

93. Dandy W: Treatment of chronic abscess of the brain by tapping. JAMA 87:1477, 1926.

94. Ballantine HT Jr, White JC: Brain abscess. N Engl J Med 148:14, 1953.

95. Jooma O, Pennybacker JB, Tutton GK: Brain abscess: Aspiration, drainage, or excision. J Neurol Neurosurg Psychiatry 14:308, 1951.

96. Coin CG, Hucks-Follis AG, Mehegan CC: Computed tomographically guided percutaneous transmoid drainage of a cerebellar abscess. Surg Neurol 20:387, 1983.

97. Hirsch JF, Roux FX, Sante-Rose C, et al.: Brain abscess in childhood. A study of 34 cases treated by puncture and antibiotics. Child's Brain 10:251, 1983.

98. Broggi G, Franzini A, Peluchetti D, et al.: Treatment of deep brain abscesses by sterotactic implantation of an intracavity device for evacuation and local application of antibiotics. Acta Neurochir 76:94, 1985.

99. Walsh PR, Larson SJ, Rytell MW, et al.: Sterotactic aspiration of deep cerebral abscesses after CT-directed labeling. Appl Neurophysiol 43:205, 1980.

100. Wild AM, Xuereb JH, Marks PV, Gleave JR: Computerized tomographic stereotaxy in the management of 200 consecutive intracranial mass lesions. Analysis of indications, benefits and outcome. Br J Neurosurg 4:407, 1990.

101. Garfield J: Management of supratentorial intracranial abscess. Br Med J 2:7, 1969.

102. Liske E, Weikers NJ: Changing aspects of brain abscesses. Neurology 14:294, 1964.

103. Young RF, Frazee J: Gas within intracranial abscess cavities: An indication for surgical excision. Ann Neurol 16:35, 1984.

104. Le Beau J: Radical surgery and penicillin in brain abscess. J Neurosurg 3:359, 1946.

105. Aebi C, Kaufmann F, Schaad UB: Brain abscess in childhood—long-term experiences. Eur J Pediatr 150:282, 1991.

106. Rousseaux M, Lesoin F, Destee A, et al.: Long-term sequelae of hemispheric abscesses as a function of the treatment. Acta Neurochir 74:61, 1985.

107. Butler NR, Barrie H, Paine KWE: Cerebral abscess as a complication of neonatal sepsis. Arch Dis Child 32:461, 1951.

108. Sutton DL, Ouvrier RA: Cerebral abscess in the under-6-month age group. Arch Dis Child 58:901, 1983.

109. Yang Y: Brain abscess: A review of 400 cases. J Neurosurg 55:794, 1981.

110. Carey ME, Chou S, French LA: Long-term neurological residual in patients surviving brain abscess with surgery. J Neurosurg 34:652, 1971.

111. Nielsen H, Harmsen A, Gyldensted C: Cerebral abscess. A long-term follow-up. Acta Neurol Scand 67:330, 1983.

112. Legg NJ, Gupta PC, Scott DF: Epilepsy following cerebral abscess. Brain 96:259, 1973.

113. Buonaguro A, Colangelo M, Daniele B, Cantone G, et al.: Neurological and behavioral sequelae in children operated on for brain abscess. Child's Nerv Syst 5:153, 1989.

114. Kerr FWL, King RB, Meagher JN: Brain abscess: A study of 47 consecutive cases. JAMA 168:868, 1958.

115. Bhandari YS, Sankari NBS: Subdural empyema: A review of 37 cases. J Neurosurg 32:35, 1970.

116. Pathak A, Sharma BS, Mathuriya SN, Khosla VK, et al.: Controversies in the management of subdural empyema. A study of 41 cases with review of literature. Acta Neurochir 102:25, 1990.

117. McLaurin R: Subdural infection. In Gurdjian ES (ed): Cranial and Intracranial Suppuration. Springfield, IL, Charles C Thomas, 1969, pp 73–88.

118. Rao S, Dinakar I: Subdural empyema in infants. Indian J Pediatr 38:358, 1971.

119. Moseley IF, Kendall B: Radiology of intracranial empyemas, with special reference to computed tomography. Neuroradiology 26:333, 1984.

120. Renaudin JW, Frazee J: Subdural empyema—importance of early diagnosis. Neurosurgery 7:477, 1980.

121. Wackym PA, Canalis RF, Feuerman T: Subdural empyema of otorhinological origin. Laryngol Otol 104:118, 1990.

122. Borovitch B, Johnston E, Spagnuoloa E: Infratentorial subdural empyemas: Clinical and computerized tomography findings. Report of three cases. J Neurosurg 72:299, 1990.

123. Morgan DW, Williams B: Posterior fossa subdural empyema. Brain 108 (Part 4):983, 1985.

124. Suchet I, Horwitz T, Kitay S, Cruz RM: The predictive value of computed tomography and Haemophilus influenzae capsular antigen in subdural fluid collections. Clin Radiol 39:265, 1988.

125. Hoyt DJ, Fisher SR: Otolaryngologic management of patients with subdural empyema. Laryngoscope 101:20, 1991.

126. Bannister G, Williams B, Smith S: Treatment of subdural empyema. J Neurosurg 55:82, 1981.

127. Hockley AD, Williams B: Surgical management of subdural empyema. Child's Brain 10:294, 1983.

128. Khan M, Griebel R: Subdural empyema: A retrospective study of 15 patients. Can J Surg 27:283, 1984.

129. Smith HP, Hendrick EB: Subdural empyema and epidural abscess in children. J Neurosurg 58:392, 1983.

130. Yoshikawa TT, Chow A, Guze LB: Role of anaerobic bacteria in subdural empyema: Report of 4 cases and review of 327 cases from the English literature. Am J Med 58:99, 1975.

131. Glasauer FE, Coots D, Levy LF, et al.: Subdural empyema in Africans in Rhodesia. Neurosurgery 3:385, 1978.

132. Zimmerman RD, Leeds N, Danziger A: Subdural empyema: CT findings. Radiology 150:417, 1984.

133. Mauser HW, Ravijst RA, Elderson A, et al.: Nonsurgical treatment of subdural empyema: Case report. J Neurosurg 63:128, 1985.

134. Rosazza A, de Tribolet N, Deonna T: Nonsurgical treatment of interhemispheric subdural empyemas. Helv Paediatr Acta 34:577, 1979.

135. Hitchcock E, Andreadis A: Subdural empyema: A review of 29 cases. J Neurol Neurosurg Psychiatry 27:422, 1964.
136. Woodhall BL: Osteomyelitis and epi-, extra- and subdural abscesses. In Clinical Neurosurgery. Vol. 16. Baltimore, Williams & Wilkins, 1967, pp 239–255.
137. Weingarten K, Zimmerman R, Becker RD, Heier LA, et al.: Subdural and epidural empyemas: MR imaging. Am J Roentgenol 152:615, 1989.
138. French LA, Chou SN: Osteomyelitis of the skull and epidural space. In Gurdjian ES (ed): Cranial and Intracranial Suppuration. Springfield, IL, Charles C Thomas, 1969, pp 59–72.
139. Brook I: Osteomyelitis and bacteremia caused by Bacteroides fragilis: A complication of fetal monitoring. Clin Pediatr 19:639, 1980.
140. Listinsky JL, Wood BP, Ekholm SE: Parietal osteomyelitis and epidural abscess: A delayed complication of fetal monitoring. Pediatr Radiol 16:150, 1986.
141. Overturf G, Balfour G: Osteomyelitis and sepsis: Severe complications of fetal monitoring. Pediatrics 55:244, 1975.
142. Reinig JW, Hungerford GD, Mohrmann ME, et al.: Case report 268. Diagnosis: Cryptococcal osteomyelitis of the calvaria. Skeletal Radiol 11:221, 1985.
143. Matson D: Osteomyelitis. In Matson DD (ed): Neurosurgery of Infancy and Childhood. Springfield, IL, Charles C Thomas, 1969, pp 701–704.
144. Humphreys RP, Gilday DL, Ash JM, et al.: Radiopharmaceutical bone scanning in pediatric neurosurgery. Child's Brain 5:249, 1979.
145. Bullitt E, Lehman R: Osteomyelitis of the skull. Surg Neurol 11:163, 1979.
146. La Rocca H: Spinal sepsis. In Rothman RH, Simeone FA (eds): The Spine. Philadelphia, WB Saunders, 1982, pp 757–774.
147. Menezes AH, Graf C, Perret GE: Spinal cord abscess: A review. Surg Neurol 8:461, 1977.
148. Arty PK: Abscess within the spinal cord: Review of literature and report of three cases. Arch Neurol Psychol 51:533, 1944.
149. Enberg RN, Kaplan R: Spinal epidural abscess in children. Clin Pediatr 13:247, 1974.
150. Fischer EG, Greene CS, Winston KR: Spinal epidural abscess in children. Neurosurgery 9:257, 1981.
151. Baker C: Primary spinal epidural abscess. Am J Dis Child 121:337, 1971.
152. Rankin RM, Flothow PG: Pyogenic infection of the spinal epidural space. West J Surg 54:320, 1946.
153. Tyson GW, Grant A, Strachan WE: Spinal epidural abscess presenting as acute abdomen in a child. Br J Surg 66:3, 1979.
154. Leys D, Lesoin F, Viaud C, et al.: Decreased morbidity from acute bacterial spinal epidural abscesses using computed tomography and nonsurgical treatment in selected patients. Ann Neurol 17:350, 1985.
155. Burke DR, Brant-Zawadski M: CT of pyogenic spine infection. Neuroradiology 27:131, 1985.
156. Dei-Anang K, Hase U, Schurmann K: Epidural spinal abscesses. Neurosurg Rev 13:285, 1990.
157. Phillips GE, Jefferson A: Acute spinal epidural abscess. Observations from fourteen cases. Postgrad Med J 55:712, 1979.
158. Verner EF, Musher DM: Spinal epidural abscess. Med Clin North Am 69:375, 1985.
159. DeVilliers JC, Cluvier P: Spinal epidural abscess in children. S Afr J Surg 16:149, 1978.
160. Hulme A, Dott N: Spinal epidural abscess. Br Med J 1:64, 1954.
161. Bolivar R, Kohl S, Pickering LK: Vertebral osteomyelitis in children: Report of four cases. Pediatrics 62:549, 1978.
162. La Rocca H: Pyogenic spondylitis. In Rothman RH, Simeone FA (eds): The Spine. Philadelphia, WB Saunders, 1982, pp 758–765.
163. Visudhiphan P, Chiemchanya A, Somburanasin R, et al.: Torticollis as the presenting sign in a cervical spine infection and tumor. Clin Pediatr 21:71, 1982.
164. Bailey HL, Gabriel M, Hodgson AR, et al.: Tuberculosis of the spine in children. J Bone Joint Surg 54:1633, 1972.
165. La Berge JM, Brant-Zawadski M: Evaluation of Pott's disease with computed tomography. Neuroradiology 26:429, 1984.
166. Galil A, Gorodischer R, Bar-Ziv J, et al.: Intervertebral disc infection (discitis) in childhood. Eur J Pediatr 139:66, 1982.
167. La Rocca H: Intervertebral disc space inflammation in children. In Rothman RH, Simeone FA (eds): The Spine. Philadelphia, WB Saunders, 1982, pp 776–767.
168. Doyle JR: Narrowing of the intervertebral disc space in children. J Bone Joint Surg 42A:1191, 1960.
169. Spiegel PG, Kenglia KW, Isaacson AS, et al.: Intervertebral disc space inflammation in children. J Bone Joint Surg 54A:284, 1972.
170. Claesson B, Flasen E, Kjellman B: Kingella kingae infections: A review and a presentation of data from ten Swedish cases. Scand J Infect Dis 17:233, 1985.
171. Diament MJ, Weller M, Bernstein R: Candida infection in a premature infant presenting as discitis. Pediatr Radiol 12:96, 1982.
172. Du Lac P, Panuel M, Devred P, Bollini G, et al.: MRI of disc space infection in infants and children. Report of 12 cases. Pediatr Radiol 20:175, 1990.
173. Scoles P, Quinn TP: Intervertebral discitis in children and adolescents. Clin Orthop 162:31, 1982.
174. Berger P: Childhood discitis: Computed tomographic findings. Radiology 149:701, 1983.
175. Cheek WR, Laurent JP: Dermal sinus tracts. In Chapman PH (ed): Concepts in Pediatric Neurosurgery. Vol 6. Basel, S Karger, 1985, pp 63–75.

PART VI

VASCULAR DISEASES

Chapter 41

ISCHEMIC STROKES AND MOYAMOYA SYNDROME

R. MICHAEL SCOTT, M.D., and KENNETH L. RENKENS, Jr., M.D.

In this chapter, the major causes of ischemic stroke in children are reviewed, with special attention directed to those of neurosurgical importance, including moyamoya syndrome. Causes of hemorrhagic stroke, such as aneurysm and arteriovenous malformation (AVM) rupture, and other hematologic disorders are discussed in other chapters in this text and will not be reviewed here.

HISTORY

The first generally acknowledged report of stroke in children was by Thomas Willis in 1667.[1] Multiple reports of "pediatric hemiplegia" were subsequently presented in the latter part of the nineteenth century without regard for etiology. Osler,[2] Sachs and Peterson,[3] and Freud[4] all reported series of pediatric patients with strokes. In a landmark paper in 1927, Ford and Schaffer[5] described the etiology, outcome, and quality of survival in a series of children with strokes and began the modern era of the evaluation of the child with stroke.

INCIDENCE

The general incidence of stroke in children is not known with certainty. A survey in a Rochester, Minnesota, population of children younger than 15 years of age detected an incidence of cerebrovascular disease, including both ischemic stroke and subarachnoid or intracerebral hemorrhage, of 2.52 per 100,000 population.[6] Banker's pediatric autopsy series reported that 8.7 per cent of the patients had died of complications of cerebrovascular disease,[7] but the most common cause of death was hemorrhage secondary to bleeding

from an AVM rather than occlusive cerebrovascular disease. A recent Japanese series of ischemic cerebrovascular disease in children under age 16, excluding moyamoya syndrome, calculated a rate of 0.2/100,000 per year.[8]

NEONATAL STROKES

The etiology of fixed neurologic deficits noted at birth or detected shortly thereafter has been disputed for many years. Suggested etiologies have included perinatal asphyxia and trauma, as well as in utero arterial occlusions probably secondary to embolization.[9] Other possible etiologies for this so-called hemiplegic cerebral palsy include disseminated intravascular coagulation, respiratory distress syndrome, infection, and congenital heart disease. Clinically, these children are often hypotonic at presentation but may also have "brainstem" symptoms including hypotension, apnea, and bradycardia. CT scanning may not detect the presence of a perinatal or neonatal stroke until the second week of life,[10] but MRI diagnosis should be more suggestive of infarct earlier in its course.

ARTERIOSCLEROSIS

Premature cardiac or cerebrovascular atherosclerosis may be an occasional etiologic factor in a child presenting with stroke. The most common laboratory findings in this group of children are low levels of high-density lipoprotein cholesterol (C-HDL) and high levels of triglycerides, with the mechanism of cerebrovascular atherosclerosis thought to be related to lipoprotein-mediated endothelial damage and thrombus formation.[11]

515

A more unusual cause is homocystinuria,[12] atherosclerosis being caused by homocystine-related endothelial cell injury and cell detachment. The treatment in both syndromes is directed toward correcting the metabolic abnormalities by appropriate dietary measures and the administration of antiplatelet and cholesterol-lowering agents, although there are no controlled studies on the efficacy of any of these medications in children.

CEREBRAL ARTERITIS

Stroke in children may occur from cerebral arteritis due to a variety of causes: (1) collagen vascular disease, particularly lupus erythematosis,[13] and (2) following infections or sepsis of any type, including such unusual infections as cat scratch disease[14] or *Mycoplasma* upper respiratory tract infections.[15] In such cases that occurred following primary herpes or varicella-zoster virus infection, hemiplegia occurred 3 to 8 weeks following the infection.[16] CT scans show areas of infarction, typically in the basal ganglia or internal capsule, and cerebral arteriography demonstrates segmental arteritis, often in the middle cerebral artery. It is possible that the virus or infecting agent enters the cerebral arterial walls via the sympathetic or trigeminal nervous system leading to endothelial wall damage, subsequent stenosis, and thrombosis.[17] Treatment of these children is directed toward the underlying cause of the arteritis, with steroids often prescribed empirically in hopes of reducing the inflammatory component of the demonstrated arterial changes.

FIBROMUSCULAR DYSPLASIA

Fibromuscular dysplasia has been implicated as the cause of an ischemic stroke occurring in a child.[18] There is controversy regarding the appropriate treatment of this syndrome in adults, but most authorities favor medical treatment with antiplatelet agents. Rarely, surgery to dilate the stenotic segment of the internal carotid may be indicated;[19] extracranial to intracranial bypass[20] and balloon catheter angioplasty[21] have also been proposed.

SICKLE CELL ANEMIA

Strokes occur in approximately 20 per cent of patients with sickle cell disease, and children with this illness have a high risk for cerebral infarction. In one third of such patients, neurologic symptoms have their onset before the age of 5 years. Strokes usually occur because of progressive occlusive disease of the major vessels of the circle of Willis—probably as a result of intravascular sickling in the vasa vasorum of these arteries, leading to arterial wall damage and stenosis,[22] or as a result of reduction in brain capillary flow as a direct consequence of sickling. Typically, the strokes in children with SS disease are marked by acute hemiparesis and seizures, and long-term neurologic deficits, mental retardation, or both often occur. Although there seems to be no predictive factor indicating the sickler at risk to develop stroke,[23] an initial stroke is followed by a subsequent one in two thirds of patients, with 80 per cent of the repeated strokes occurring within 3 years of the first stroke. Hyperventilation may trigger stroke by inducing cerebral arteriolar constriction and a decrease in cerebral blood flow, and those factors known to induce sickling, such as fever, infection, dehydration, and surgery, may also lead to stroke in susceptible patients.

Treatment includes increasing intravascular volume with fluids, correction of metabolic acidosis, administration of oxygen, and transfusion of packed red cells. Heparinization has been advocated but is unproven. Hypertransfusion to decrease the level of hemoglobin S to less than 30 per cent has been reported to stop the progression of intracranial stenoses and to reduce the incidence of stroke recurrence,[24] although this therapy risks such effects as progressive iron accumulation in body tissues and sensitization to red cell antigens.

CARDIAC DISEASE

Strokes may occur in children either with congenital or acquired heart disease.[25] In children with left-to-right shunts, emboli from bacterial endocarditis may lead to acute stroke, although this cause of stroke in children is becoming less frequent with the widespread use of prophylactic antibiotics in children at risk. Mycotic aneurysms may occur in these children as well; their diagnosis and treatment are discussed elsewhere in this text. Stroke may also occur in this group of children because of the combination of dehydration, fever, and polycythemia, with vascular thromboses occurring most often in the distribution of the middle cerebral artery territory. Mitral valve prolapse has also been reported as a cause of stroke in children,[26] although the incidence and the cause of stroke in patients so affected remain unclear.

MISCELLANEOUS CAUSES OF ISCHEMIC STROKE IN CHILDREN

There is an extensive literature on idiopathic brainstem infarction in children.[27] Most of the children are males, and arteriography will frequently reveal an occlusion of the vertebral or basilar artery without obvious cause. The treatment of and prognosis for these children are not clear from the literature, but most authorities recommend antiplatelet medication such as aspirin following idiopathic infarction. Other syndromes associated with ischemic cerebral infarction in children include chronic nephrotic syndrome,[28] the

MELAS syndrome (mitochondrial myopathy, encephalopathy, lactic acidosis, and stroke),[29] non–central nervous system cancer,[30] and vasoconstrictor drugs such as phenylpropanolamine[31] and cocaine.[32]

EXTRACRANIAL ARTERIAL DISSECTION

Dissection of the carotid or vertebral arteries may occur spontaneously or secondary to trauma,[33] with ischemic deficits resulting from emboli from the site of dissection or reduced cerebral blood flow from the narrowed vessel caliber. The site of carotid dissection is most commonly between C2 and the skull base; in children, the vessel is most commonly injured at this site by contusion or puncture from a sharp object such as a pencil entering the open mouth. The development of symptoms may occur hours or days following the trauma, with the injury presumably leading to dissection in the vessel wall, development of thrombus, and finally, cerebral embolization leading to symptoms. There may be a history of headache; facial, neck, or scalp pain; and Horner's syndrome noted by the patient's family or examiner, resulting from injury to the sympathetic plexus around the internal carotid artery. Onset may be spontaneous and unrelated to trauma, but this is rare in children. The diagnosis should be suspected if a neurologic deficit develops in a child who has a history of trauma, but who has a normal CT or a CT abnormality that does not account for the clinical deficit. Standard or MRI angiography establishes the diagnosis, demonstrating a tapering stenosis (the so-called "string" sign) or a focal area of narrowing frequently associated with an aneurysmal pouch above the tightest area of stenosis in the affected vessel. Vertebral artery dissection in children occurs in most cases without a clear etiology; signs and symptoms are similar to those expected in an adult—headache, vomiting, dysarthria, and other lower brainstem and cerebellar-related symptomatology. Horner's syndrome may occur because of lateral medullary ischemia or infarction. Cases have been reported in association with direct extracranial vertebral artery trauma due to atlantoaxial subluxation.[34]

The treatment of such dissections remains controversial, but since the evidence seems to point clearly to thrombus formation and subsequent embolization as the cause of neurologic symptoms, we favor the use of anticoagulation with heparin initially and then conversion to sodium warfarin (Coumadin) for a period of 6 months. Follow-up angiography frequently discloses healing of the dissection (Fig. 41–1). Recurring symptoms during or after treatment may necessitate surgical therapy such as direct carotid or vertebral artery surgery with resection and grafting of the injured section of vessel or extracranial to intracranial arterial bypass and ligation of the internal carotid or vertebral artery.[35] Surgery is rarely required in the treatment of children with these syndromes.

MIGRAINE

Migraine is usually a benign disease in children, but there are reports of infarcts, documented by CT, occurring in children with variants of the classic disorder, particularly in the vertebrobasilar distribution.[36] The etiology of these permanent deficits is unknown but is presumably related to changes in caliber of reactive vessels, leading to ischemia and infarction during the migraine attack.

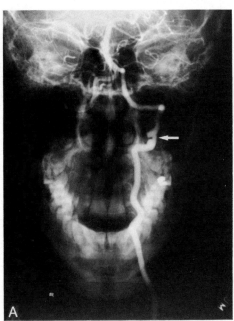
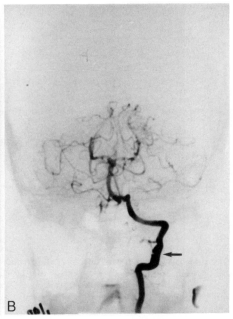

FIGURE 41–1. *A,* Left vertebral arteriogram of a 7-year-old black male, with onset of classic posterior circulation TIAs following mild head trauma. A web-like stenosis in the artery at C2-C3 can be seen associated with a poststenotic aneurysmal dilatation of the vessel. *B,* Repeat vertebral arteriogram 6 months later showing healing of the aneurysm and partial resolution of the stenosis while on Warfarin (Coumadin) anticoagulation. (Radiographs courtesy of Dr. Dennis Johnson, Washington, DC.)

MOYAMOYA SYNDROME

Moyamoya syndrome is a chronic occlusive cerebrovascular disease characterized by progressive stenosis of the proximal intracranial internal carotid and its branches, with concomitant enlargement of tiny subsidiary and proximal penetrating arteries at the base of the brain to form the so-called moyamoya vessels. These unusual, dilated vessels are a source of collateral flow to the ischemic brain distal to the stenotic process (Fig. 41–2). The word "moyamoya" in Japanese means "something hazy, like a puff of cigarette smoke drifting in the air" and was the term used by Suzuki in 1969 to describe the angiographic appearance of the dilated collateral vessels seen in this disorder.[37] The disease, which was initially described in Japan, is now recognized worldwide, with about half of the case reports in the literature occurring in other cultures.[38]

The etiology of the disorder is unknown. There is a familial incidence in Japan of 7 per cent,[39] and the disease has occurred in identical twins.[40] A distinction is made in the Japanese literature between "moyamoya disease," which by definition requires the presence of the classic arteriographic picture in the absence of any known cause, and the syndromic variants.[41] This distinction seems less important in the Western Hemisphere, since the clinical course of the arterial process appears unrelated to its associations. The syndrome is associated with hereditary diseases such as neurofibromatosis[42–44] and sickle cell anemia.[22, 45] It occurs following infectious diseases of the central nervous system, including tuberculous meningitis[46] and leptospirosis;[47] following radiation to the brain;[48, 49] in Fanconi's anemia,[50] Down's syndrome,[51, 52] connective tissue diseases,[53–55] and renal artery stenosis with hypertension;[56] and in patients with type I glycogenosis,[57] craniopharyngioma,[58] and optic glioma.[59] Ten of our last 15 patients had preexisting or concomitant medical conditions, including previous surgery for congenital heart disease, previous cranial radiation, renal artery stenosis with hypertension, giant intracranial aneurysm with hemorrhage, and congenital urogenital syndromes with extensive reconstructive surgery. The common factor in all patients with the moyamoya syndrome is a progressive occlusive process of the supraclinoid carotid artery and its bifurcation, with the gradual development of the moyamoya collateral pathways and the inevitable development of symptoms of cerebral ischemia.

The posterior circulation becomes involved in many cases as the disease progresses.[60] The histopathologic findings are nonspecific and include intimal hyperplasia and disordered or redundant internal elastic lamina in the stenotic proximal vessels. The moyamoya vessels themselves can be normal or can show attenuation of the elastic lamina, fibrin deposition with resultant thrombi, and microaneurysm formation. No inflammatory cells are usually present. Immunohistochemical staining of dura and superficial temporal artery from patients with moyamoya syndrome have demonstrated a probable increase in the amount of basic fibroblast growth factor (FGF) in these tissues, and Hoshimaru and colleagues have suggested that basic FGF may play a role in the development of the arterial wall changes seen in these patients.[61]

The most common clinical presentation in children is recurrent episodes of cerebral ischemia and stroke, as opposed to the adult presentation of intracranial hemorrhage, which can be intraventricular, intracerebral, or subarachnoid.[62] Headache, stroke, and seizures were the most characteristic presenting signs and symptoms in series of children from both Japan and the Western Hemisphere.[63, 64] In 13 of our patients with moyamoya syndrome who were younger than 12 years of age, 12 of the 13 patients had a combination of strokes and TIAs at presentation; only one patient had TIAs only.

The diagnostic evaluation of these children begins with a CT scan, which in some cases may demonstrate the blush of the enlarged moyamoya vessels on contrast enhancement[65] or, most commonly, small infarcts in various distributions. MRI will confirm these findings, with high-quality MRI angiography being virtually diagnostic, demonstrating signal intensity changes in the circle of Willis corresponding to the arteriographic changes, and demonstrating punctate signal changes due to the moyamoya vessels themselves throughout the basal ganglia in advanced cases (see below). The electroencephalogram (EEG) shows interesting changes during and after hyperventilation, termed the "rebuild-up phenomenon." During hyperventilation, there is a build-up of high-voltage slow waves that disappear after termination of hyperventilation; 20 to 60 seconds later there is a return of high-voltage slow waves. Karasawa and associates attributed these changes to the vasoconstrictive effect of hyperventilation on cerebral blood flow in the normal vessels over the cortical surface.[66] The second slow wave effect is thought to be due to ischemia in the brain, secondary to a "steal" from the deep moyamoya collateral vessels

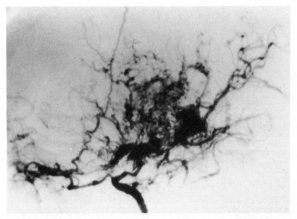

FIGURE 41–2. Left internal carotid arteriogram demonstrating advanced moyamoya changes. There is severe stenosis of the intracranial internal carotid artery, with an enlarged meningohypophyseal trunk and ophthalmic artery—both of which supply leptomeningeal collateral to the involved hemisphere. Extensive basal moyamoya changes collateralize the middle cerebral circulation. The ophthalmic–middle meningeal anastomosis is probably incidental.

to the now dilated cortical vessels following the termination of hyperventilation. Although other tests have been proposed to evaluate these children, such as radioisotope scanning[67] and cerebral blood flow studies,[68] including single photon emission computed tomographic scans (SPECT) and positron emission tomographic scanning (PET), cerebral angiography remains the definitive diagnostic test. It is important that the arteriographer study all circulations, including the external carotid system, in order to determine the presence and location of preexisting collateral flow and to determine whether surgical therapy might be helpful.

The angiographic progression of moyamoya syndrome has been well described in the literature and has been divided into six stages by Suzuki[37] (Fig. 41–3). Matsushima and Inaba[69] correlated the angiographic staging proposed by Suzuki with clinical presentations and noted that the symptoms occur when there is an imbalance between the spontaneously developing collaterals from the moyamoya vasculature, skull base, dura, and leptomeninges and the degree of brain ischemia caused by the proximal occlusive disease process. The rate of progression is difficult to predict, but it is generally thought that the syndrome has a progressive phase, during which the occlusions occur and the collaterals develop, and a stable phase when all collaterals are fully developed, the occlusive process is completed, and ischemic attacks disappear. Clinical disease progression may be erratic and episodic, with neurologic events and deficits building up over decades, or fulminant, with multiple bilateral strokes occurring within a period of several months.[70] Prognosis has been felt to be related to age of onset of symptoms, with a poorer prognosis related to onset in patients under 6 years of age.[67] In our personal series, the patient's prognosis has been heavily influenced by neurologic status and degree of cerebral infarction on CT or MRI scanning at time of diagnosis and surgical treatment, rather than by age. Of children presenting at age 4 or under, all patients with bilateral infarcts at initial diagnosis were developmentally delayed at long-term follow-up (mean 4.5 years). Children older than 4 years at diagnosis were similarly developmentally delayed if they either had suffered bilateral strokes by the time of diagnosis or had preexisting neurologic syndromes related to tumor surgery and/or radiation. Angiographically, prognosis appears directly related to the extent of proximal occlusive disease, with extension into the proximal posterior cerebral arteries and bilateral or dominant hemisphere disease carrying a relatively poor prognosis—although this is not always the case.

No medical therapy (e.g., steroids, vasodilators, low-molecular-weight dextran, antiplatelet agents, and anticoagulants) has been proved to be an effective treatment in this condition. The stenoses continue to progress, albeit at an unpredictable rate in a given patient, and medications do not seem to affect this process; however, antiplatelet agents such as aspirin appear to be important in reducing the incidence of symptoms in many of these children, probably because of the many small thromboses and subsequent embolizations that must be occurring distal to the moyamoya stenoses. We have noted in several patients, preoperatively and postoperatively, that TIAs were favorably affected by aspirin intake, and we believe that it is an important adjunct in the treatment of this syndrome.

Surgical procedures to treat moyamoya syndrome, with the exception of attempts to denervate the cerebral vasculature proposed by Suzuki and colleagues,[62] have been designed to augment transdural collaterals that are already part of the ongoing moyamoya process. Superficial temporal to middle cerebral artery bypass, initially carried out by Yasargil in a child with moyamoya syndrome,[71] can effectively increase hemisphere

FIGURE 41–3. The angiographic stages of moyamoya disease, according to Suzuki. As the internal carotid stenosis progresses to occlusion, the external carotid collateral becomes the dominant source of hemisphere blood flow. (Reprinted by permission of the publisher from The Moyamoya Syndrome and the neurosurgeon by HA Krayenbuhl, Surgical Neurology, vol 4, p 359. Copyright 1975 by Elsevier Science Publishing Co., Inc.)

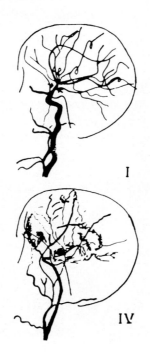
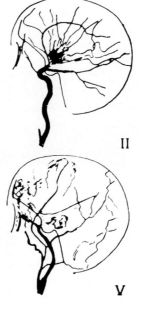
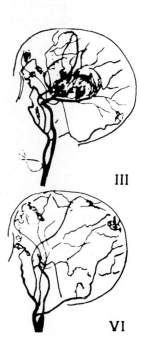

I   II   III

IV   V   VI

collateral flow.[30, 72, 73] However, there are significant technical problems in carrying out this procedure in children. The donor and recipient vessels are often extremely small, preexisting leptomeningeal collateral flow may be disturbed when the middle cerebral branch is temporarily occluded, and extensive opening of the dura, necessary to find a suitable recipient vessel, may disturb preexisting transdural collateral.

Other operative techniques have depended on the natural tendency of the ischemic brain to form collateral flow from any available source. The encephalomyosynangiosis (EMS), described by Henschen,[74] involves the placement of the inner surface of the temporalis muscle directly on the brain surface, following an extensive temporal craniotomy. No series describing this procedure in patients with moyamoya syndrome treated in the Western Hemisphere has been published, although recent reports from Japan have documented improved clinical status and dramatic postoperative angiographic results.[75–77] Complications related to the procedure include transient focal seizures and chronic subdural hematomas; the alteration in skull configuration following the relocation of the temporalis may be disfiguring. The large skin incision and dural flap required for the procedure have the potential to interrupt a

number of preexisting collaterals to the brain from the dura, and we believe that this procedure has limited application in the treatment of children with moyamoya syndrome.

It is apparent from the literature that a less dramatic stimulus than the EMS can induce collateral vessels in the appropriate patient. Ausman and co-workers noted this process in a patient in whom the bone flap was not replaced following a bypass from the superficial temporal artery (STA) to the middle cerebral artery (MCA).[78] Spetzler and colleagues[79] noted multiple transdural collaterals occurring 6 weeks after an intact superficial temporal artery was sutured to the arachnoid in a patient with no satisfactory recipient vessel at the time of the intended STA-MCA anastomosis. Matsushima and colleagues[80] transposed the intact superficial temporal artery with a strip of attached galea to a linear dural opening beneath an elliptical craniotomy in hopes of promoting transdural collateral formation, naming their procedure "encephalo-duro-arterio-synangiosis (EDAS)." Subsequent papers by Matsushima and co-workers[69, 77] have demonstrated dramatic enlargement of the donor vessel, increased transdural collateral formation, and other favorable changes such as a decrease in moyamoya vessels and increased middle

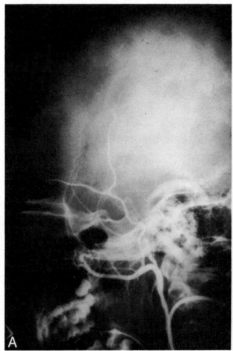
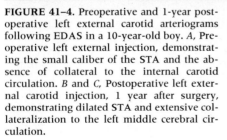
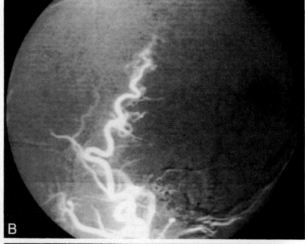
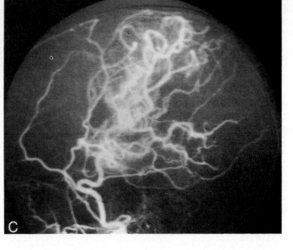

FIGURE 41–4. Preoperative and 1-year postoperative left external carotid arteriograms following EDAS in a 10-year-old boy. *A*, Preoperative left external injection, demonstrating the small caliber of the STA and the absence of collateral to the internal carotid circulation. *B* and *C*, Postoperative left external carotid injection, 1 year after surgery, demonstrating dilated STA and extensive collateralization to the left middle cerebral circulation.

cerebral artery filling. Clinical and EEG improvement was also noted, although intellectual function appeared unchanged.

The advantages of this surgical technique are that (1) it is simple, (2) there is no temporary occlusion of middle cerebral artery branches, (3) there are multiple donor arteries available, including the occipital artery and both divisions of the superficial temporal artery, and (4) the craniotomy can be planned to avoid disruption of preexisting transdural collaterals. In Matsushima's original description of the procedure, the arachnoid membrane was left intact, but we as well as others[63, 81, 82] have found that failure to open the arachnoid beneath the donor vessel may hinder the development of collaterals. We have modified Matsushima's procedure by using fine microscissors and jeweller's forceps to open the arachnoid in a linear fashion over the surface of the brain where the donor vessel will lie, and then suturing the vessel's soft tissue cuff directly to the pia with a number of interrupted 10-0 monofilament nylon sutures.[83] Postoperative arteriograms have demonstrated a highly satisfactory increase in transdural collateral flow to the operated hemisphere (Fig. 41–4). These children can be observed adequately by follow-up with MRI angiography after a postoperative arteriographic baseline, usually obtained at one year postoperatively, has been established (Fig. 41–5), and MRI angiography will probably become utilized more widely in the postoperative management of these children. SPECT and/or PET scanning may also be helpful in following the course of the patient's disease following diagnosis and treatment, although the long-term implications of the results of these studies have not been established. Matsushima and colleagues have recently suggested that STA-MCA anastomosis combined with EMS may be superior to EDAS in the development of collateral circulation and postoperative clinical improvement,[76] but the technical challenges of this procedure in small children nevertheless remain formidable.

Meticulous anesthetic management is extremely important when any neurosurgical procedure is carried out in a child with moyamoya syndrome. The anesthesiologist should be made aware that hyperventilation during induction and in the course of the procedure must be specifically avoided because of its potential to constrict already maximally dilated collateral vasculature and thereby worsen neurologic deficits in these children who already have compromised cerebral flow.[84] The children must be kept volume-repleted, and transfusions should be avoided, since a lower hematocrit is probably safer from a rheologic standpoint than a high one. The patients should have adequate pain medication and sedation postoperatively to avoid crying and hyperventilation.

REFERENCES

1. Willis T: Pathologiae Cerebri et Nervosi Generis Specimen. In quo Agitur de Morbis Convulsivis, et de Scorbuto. Oxonii, excedebat Guil Hall, impensis Ja, Allestry, 1667, p 49.
2. Osler W: The Cerebral Palsies of Children: A Clinical Study from the Infirmary of Nervous Diseases. Philadelphia, Blakiston & Co., 1889, pp 1–55.
3. Sachs B, Peterson F: A study of cerebral palsies of early life, based upon an analysis of one hundred and forty cases. J Nerv Ment Dis 17:295, 1890.
4. Freud S: Die Infantile Cerebrallahmung. Vienna, Holder, 1897.
5. Ford FR, Schaffer AJ: The etiology of infantile acquired hemiplegia. AMA Arch Neurol Psychiatry 18:323, 1927.
6. Schoenberg BS, Mellinger JF, Schoenberg DG: Cerebrovascular disease in infants and children: A study of incidence, clinical features, and survival. Neurology 28:763, 1978.
7. Banker BQ: Cerebral vascular disease in infancy and childhood. I. Occlusive vascular diseases. J Neuropathol Exp Neurol 20:127, 1961.
8. Satoh S, Shirane R, Yoshimoto T: Clinical survey of ischemic cerebrovascular disease in children in a district of Japan. Stroke 22:586, 1991.
9. Barmada MA, Mossy J, Schuman RM: Cerebral infarcts with arterial occlusion in neonates. Ann Neurol 6:495, 1979.
10. Mannino FL, Trauner DA: Strokes in neonates. J Pediatr 102:605, 1983.
11. Daniels SR, Bates S, Lukin RR, et al.: Cerebrovascular arteriopathy (arteriosclerosis) and ischemic childhood stroke. Stroke 13:360, 1982.
12. Brattstorm LE, Hardebo JE, Hultberg BL: Moderate homocysteinemia. A possible risk factor for arteriosclerotic cerebrovascular disease. Stroke 15:1012, 1984.
13. Moore P, Cupps TR: Neurological complications of vasculitis. Ann Neurol 14:155, 1983.
14. Selby G, Walker GL: Cerebral arteritis in cat-scratch disease. Neurology 29:1413, 1979.
15. Maytal J, Resnick TJ: A TIA-like syndrome associated with Mycoplasa pneumoniae infection. Pediatr Neurol 1:308, 1985.
16. Bodensteiner JB, Hille MR, Riggs JE: Clinical features of vascular thrombosis following varicella. Am J Dis Child 146:100, 1992.
17. Editorial: Cerebrovascular complications of primary herpes varicella-zoster infection. Lancet 339:1449, 1992.
18. Llorens-Terol J, Sole-Llenas J, Tura A: Stroke due to fibromuscular hyperplasia of the internal carotid artery. Acta Paediatr Scand 72:299, 1983.

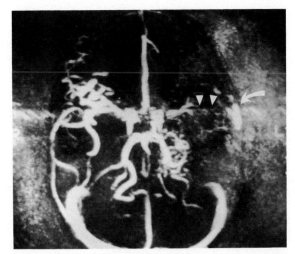

FIGURE 41–5. MRI angiogram demonstrating moyamoya changes restricted to left side (same case as in Fig. 41–4). The study demonstrates absence of a continuous linear signal from the left middle cerebral artery, indicating reduced or absent flow in the vessel *(arrowheads)*; there are also changes in the left distal posterior cerebral artery beginning at the posterior temporal artery origin. Strictly unilateral moyamoya changes are rare, and this study is shown to demonstrate the contrast between normal and abnormal sides. The bright signal on the surface of the left hemisphere *(curved arrow)* is from the dilated superficial temporal artery seen 1 year following an EDAS procedure and depicted in Figure 41–4.

19. Ojemann RG, Crowell RM: Surgical Management of Cerebrovascular Disease. Baltimore, Williams & Wilkins, 1983, pp 107–110.

20. Stephens HW, Jr: Microvascular anastomosis and carotid artery ligation for fibromuscular hyperplasia and carotid artery aneurysm. In Fein JM, Reichman OH (eds): Microvascular Anastomosis for Carotid Ischemia. New York, Springer-Verlag, 1974, pp 307–316.

21. Mullen S, Duda EE, Patronas NJ: Some examples of balloon technology in neurosurgery. J Neurosurg 52:321, 1980.

22. Stockman JA, Nigro DO, Mishkin MM, et al.: Occlusions of large cerebral vessels in sickle cell anemia. N Engl J Med 287:846, 1972.

23. Powars D, Wilson B, Imbus C, et al.: The natural history of stroke in sickle cell disease. Am J Med 65:461, 1978.

24. Russell MO, Goldberg HI, Hodson A, et al.: Effect of transfusion therapy on arteriographic abnormalities and recurrence of stroke in sickle cell disease. Blood 63:162, 1984.

25. Chugani HT, Menkes JH: Neurologic manifestations of systemic disease. In Menkes MD (ed): The Textbook of Child Neurology. Philadelphia, Lea & Febiger, 1985, pp 720–763.

26. Rice CPG, Boughner DR, Stiller C, et al.: Familial stroke syndrome associated with mitral valve prolapse. Ann Neurol 7:130, 1980.

27. Curless RG: Idiopathic ischemic infarction of the brain stem in children. Childs Nerv Syst 7:305, 1991.

28. Igarashi M, Roy S, Stapleton FB: Cerebrovascular complications in children with nephrotic syndrome. Pediatr Neurol 4:362, 1988.

29. Pavlakis SG, Phillips PC, DiMauro S, et al.: Mitochondrial myopathy, encephalopathy, lactic acidosis and stroke-like episodes (MELAS). Ann Neurol 16:481, 1984.

30. Packer RJ, Rorke LB, Lange BJ, et al.: Cerebrovascular accidents in children with cancer. Pediatrics 76:194, 1985.

31. Forman H, Levin S, Stewart B, et al.: Cerebrovasculitis and hemorrhage in an adolescent taking diet pills containing phenylpropanolamine: Case report and review of the literature. Pediatrics 83:737, 1989.

32. Klonoff DC, Andrews BT, Obana WG: Stroke associated with cocaine use. Arch Neurol 46:986, 1989.

33. Ojemann RG, Crowell RM: Surgical Management of Cerebrovascular Disease. Baltimore, Williams & Wilkins, 1983, pp 111–121.

34. Fraser RAR, Zimbler S: Hindbrain stroke in children caused by extracranial vertebral artery trauma. Stroke 6:153, 1975.

35. Gratzl O, Schmeidek P, Steinhoff H: Extra-intra-cranial arterial bypass in patients with occlusion of cerebral arteries due to trauma and tumor. In Handa H (ed): Microneurosurgery. Baltimore, University Park Press, 1980, pp 68–80.

36. Dunn DW: Vertebrobasilar occlusive disease and childhood migraine. Pediatr Neurol 1:252, 1985.

37. Suzuki J, Takaku A: Cerebrovascular "moyamoya" disease. A disease showing net-like vessels of brain. Arch Neurol 20:288, 1969.

38. Suzuki J, Kodama N: Moyamoya disease—a review. Stroke 14:104, 1983.

39. Kitahara T, Ariga N, Yamaura A, et al.: Familial occurrence of moyamoya disease: Report of three Japanese families. J Neurol Neurosurg Psychiatry 42:208, 1979.

40. Yamada H, Nakamura S, Kageyama N: Moyomoya disease in monovular twins. J Neurosurg 53:109, 1980.

41. Matsushima T, Inoue T, Natori Y, et al.: Does "unilateral" moyamoya disease exist? Clinical features of six children with unilateral occlusion or stenosis of the ICA associated with surrounding moyamoya vessels. Neurosurg, in press.

42. Lamas E, Diez Lobato R, Caballo A, et al.: Multiple intracranial arterial occlusions (moyamoya disease) in patients with neurofibromatosis. One case report with autopsy. Acta Neurochir 45:133, 1978.

43. Salyer WR, Salyer DC: The vascular lesions of neurofibromatosis. Angiology 25:510, 1974.

44. Taboada D, Alonso A, Moreno J, et al.: Occlusion of the cerebral arteries in von Recklinghausen's disease. Neuroradiology 18:281, 1979.

45. Seeler RA, Royal JE, Powe L, et al.: Moyamoya in children with sickle cell anemia and vascular occlusion. J Pediatr 93:808, 1978.

46. Metthew NT, Abraham J, Chandy J: Cerebral angiographic features in tuberculous meningitis. Neurology 20:1015, 1970.

47. Ximin L, Zuzhong R, Zhuan C, et al.: Moyamoya disease caused by leptospiral cerebral arteritis. Chinese Med J 93:599, 1980.

48. Rajakulasingam K, Cerullo LJ, Raimondi AJ: Childhood moyamoya syndrome. Postradiation pathogenesis. Childs Brain 5:467, 1979.

49. Servo A, Puranen M: Moyamoya syndrome as a complication of radiation therapy. J Neurosurg 48:1026, 1978.

50. Cohen N, Berant M, Simon J: Moyamoya and Fanconi's anemia. Pediatrics 65:804, 1980.

51. Pearson E, Lenn NJ, Cail WS: Moyamoya and other causes of stroke in patients with Down's syndrome. Pediatr Neurol 1:174, 1985.

52. Outwater EK, Platenberg RC, Wolpert SM: Moyamoya disease in Down's syndrome. AJNR 10:S23, 1989.

53. Ferris FJ, Levine HL: Cerebral arteritis: Classification. Radiology 109:327, 1973.

54. Silverstein A, Hollin S: Occlusion of the supraclinoid portion of the internal carotid artery. Neurology 13:679, 1963.

55. Trevor RP, Sondheimer FK, Fessel WJ, et al.: Angiographic demonstration of major cerebral vessel occlusion in systemic lupus erythematosus. Neuroradiology 4:202, 1972.

56. Ellison PH, Largent JA, Popp AJ: Moyamoya disease associated with renal artery stenosis. Arch Neurol 38:467, 1981.

57. Sunder TR: Moyamoya disease in a patient with type I glycogenosis. Arch Neurol 38:251, 1981.

58. Tsuji N, Kuriyama T, Iwamoto N, et al.: Moyomoya disease associated with craniopharyngioma. Surg Neurol 21:588, 1984.

59. Okuno T, Prensky AL, Gado M: The moyomoya syndrome associated with irradiation of an optic glioma in children: Report of two cases and review of the literature. Pediatr Neurol 1:311, 1985.

60. Miyamoto S, Kikuchi H, Karasawa J, et al.: Study of the posterior circulation in moyamoya disease. J Neurosurg 61:1032, 1984.

61. Hoshimaru M, Takahashi JA, Kikuchi H, et al.: Possible roles of basic fibroblast growth factor in the pathogenesis of moyamoya disease: an immunohistochemical study. J Neurosurg 75:267, 1991.

62. Suzuki J, Takaku A, Kodama N, et al.: An attempt to treat cerebrovascular "moyamoya" disease in children. Childs Brain 1:193, 1975.

63. Olds MV, Griebel RW, Hoffman HJ, et al.: The surgical treatment of childhood moyamoya disease. J Neurosurg 66:675, 1987.

64. Yamashiro Y, Takahashi H, Takahashi K: Cerebrovascular moyomoya disease. Eur J Pediatr 142:44, 1984.

65. Takahashi M, Miyauchi T, Kowada M: Computed tomography of moyamoya disease: Demonstration of occluded arteries and collateral vessels as important diagnostic signs. Radiology 134:671, 1980.

66. Karasawa J, Kikuchi H, Takahashi N, et al.: Electroencephalographic study of "moyamoya" disease in children: Pre- and postsurgical EEG changes and its pathophysiology (in Japanese). Rinsho Noha 22:527, 1980.

67. Maki Y, Nakada Y, Nose T, et al.: Clinical and radiologic follow-up study of "moyamoya." Childs Brain 11:155, 1984.

68. Takeuchi S, Tanaka R, Ishii R, et al.: Cerebral hemodynamics in patients with moyamoya disease. A study of regional cerebral blood flow by the Xe-133 inhalation method. Surg Neurol 23:468, 1985.

69. Matsushima Y, Inaba Y: The specificity of the collaterals to the brain through the study and surgical treatment of moyamoya disease. Stroke 17:117, 1986.

70. Scott RM: Surgical treatment of moyamoya syndrome in children. In Chapman PH (ed): Concepts in Pediatric Neurosurgery. Vol. 6. New York, S Karger, 1985, pp 198–212.

71. Krayenbuhl HA: The moyamoya syndrome and the neurosurgeon. Surg Neurol 4:353, 1975.

72. Boone SC, Sampson DS: Observations on Moyamoya disease: Case treated with superficial temporal middle cerebral artery anastomosis. Surg Neurol 9:189, 1978.

73. Karasawa J, Kikuchi H, Furuse S, et al.: Treatment of moyamoya disease with STA-MCA anastomosis. J Neurosurg 49:679, 1978.

74. Henschen C: Operative revaskularisation des zirkulatorisch ges-

chadigten Gehirns durch Auflage gestielter, Muskellappen (Encephalo-Myo-Synangiose). Langenbecks Arch Chir 264:392, 1950.

75. Kobayaski K, Takeuchi S, Tsuchida T, et al.: Encephalo-myo-synangiosis (EMS) in moyamoya disease with special reference to postoperative angiography. Neurol Med Chir (Tokyo) 21:1229, 1981.

76. Matsushima T, Inoue T, Suzuki SO, et al.: Surgical treatment of moyamoya disease in pediatric patients—comparison between the results of indirect and direct revascularization procedures. Neurosurgery 31:401, 1992.

77. Matsushima Y, Inaba Y: Moyamoya disease in children and its surgical treatment. Childs Brain 11:155, 1984.

78. Ausman JI, Moore J, Chou SN: Spontaneous cerebral revascularization in a patient with STA-MCA anastomosis. J Neurosurg 44:84, 1985.

79. Spetzler RF, Roski RA, Kopaniki DR: Alternative superficial temporal artery to middle cerebral artery revascularization procedure. Neurosurgery 7:484, 1980.

80. Matsushima Y, Fukai N, Tanaka K, et al.: A new surgical treatment of moyamoya disease in children. A preliminary report. Surg Neurol 15:313, 1981.

81. Cahan LD: Failure of encephalo-duro-arterio-synangiosis procedure in moyamoya disease. Pediatr Neurosci 12:58, 1985–86.

82. Matsushima T, Fukui M, Kitamura K, et al.: Encephalo-duro-arterio-synangiosis in children with moyamoya disease. Acta Neurochir (Wien) 104:96, 1990.

83. Rooney CM, Kaye EM, Scott RM, et al.: Modified encephaloduroarteriosynangiosis as a surgical treatment of childhood moyamoya disease: Report of five cases. J Child Neurol 6:24, 1991.

84. Sumikawa K, Nagai H: Moyamoya disease and anesthesia. Anesthesia 58:204, 1983.

ACKNOWLEDGMENTS: The authors wish to acknowledge the help of Drs. Patrick Barnes and Roy Strand in the Department of Neuroradiology at the Children's Hospital, Boston, and Dr. Samuel Wolpert in the Department of Neuroradiology at the Boston Floating Hospital for their expert neuroradiologic evaluation of these patients over the past two decades.

Chapter 42

VASCULAR MALFORMATIONS OF THE BRAIN

ROBIN P. HUMPHREYS, M.D.

The Report of the Joint Committee for Stroke Facilities explained in two papers the ischemic and hemorrhagic stroke problems to which a child may fall victim.[1] Much of the documentation concerned literature reports of known and less common circumstances of cerebrovascular disorders in children. Not unexpectedly, many of the etiologies of childhood stroke are idiosyncratic to that age group, and the causes in some instances differ dramatically from the stroke insult in adults.

Intracranial arterial aneurysm and arteriovenous malformation (AVM) are collectively, though not exclusively, the most common causes of spontaneous subarachnoid hemorrhage/intraventricular hemorrhage (SAH/IVH). In adults, a ruptured saccular aneurysm would be 6.5 times more likely than an AVM to account for that hemorrhage.[2] It is a moot point whether the ratio is reversed in children. Hourihan and associates,[3] in a review of 167 patients aged 20 years and younger, note that in twice as many, SAH was caused by aneurysm rather than AVM. Their paper includes the work of other authors studying the problem of pediatric SAH.[2, 4, 5] In a total review of 478 such patients, ruptured aneurysm accounts for 40 per cent of children's SAH and AVM for 26 per cent; no lesion was defined in 31 per cent. That such has been cumulative experience might appear to be at odds with the results of the Cooperative Study, in which 33 per cent of AVMs associated with hemorrhage occurred before age 20 years. This finding contrasts with that of only 1.5 per cent of intracranial aneurysms becoming symptomatic in that same period.[2, 6]

The material to be reviewed in this chapter is taken from the experience at The Hospital for Sick Children (HSC), Toronto, from 1949 to 1989.[7] This hospital serves as a widespread referral base exclusively for the care of children up to age 18 years; the statistics reflect the general population needs. With regard to SAH as

the presenting symptom, 26 children with ruptured intracranial aneurysm presented with SAH during that time period. This contrasts with 104 children who bled from their AVM and presented as SAH/IVH. In my opinion, rupture of an AVM is almost four times more likely to be the cause of the SAH/IVH than is a burst aneurysm.[7]

One might expect that these two vascular lesions, allegedly related to some congenital malfeasance, would be more flamboyant and detected during childhood and adolescent years. Such does not appear to be the circumstance for at HSC, there has been no case of an incidental aneurysm or AVM defined by arteriography or computed tomography (CT) performed for other reasons. Nor have there been many children with a conglomerate of vascular problems. The Cooperative Study contains 37 patients with coexisting angioma malformations and one or more aneurysms.[6] Hayashi and co-workers reviewed 73 patients with AVM associated with aneurysm and noted that only two patients were below the age of 10 years.[8] Ostergaard has recently added two more children with saccular aneurysm attendant to the AVM.[9] In the HSC series, there were no children with an admixture of aneurysm and AVM, but there was one child who had bilateral symmetric internal carotid artery aneurysms and another with a pontine AVM in association with a facial, orbital, and dural vascular malformation. A third child had an extensive spinal cord AVM associated with a small and similar lesion in the right temporal lobe.[10]

Most series of AVM note a common age of presentation at 20 to 40 years.[11-15] The fact that most lesions become symptomatic during this time span suggests a latency in the malformation's usual evolution.[6] While there is a certain age bias in the reporting of series from predominantly adult units, we have observed that of the approximately 10,000 cerebral arteriograms performed in our hospital for whatever reason, not one incidental aneurysm nor AVM has been uncovered, although three of the AVMs to be reported were incidental necropsy findings in children.[16]

Matson declared the AVM "the most frequent abnormality of intracranial circulation in childhood," and reported on his experience with 34 patients.[17] Since then, a number of reports have examined the problem of symptomatic AVM in children under 19 years of age.[3, 5, 18–26] This chapter will consider 132 children with AVM of the brain who were admitted to HSC from 1949 to 1989. We are excluding children with cavernous and venous malformations from this particular review; they will be discussed subsequently. The 132 patients reported comprise 128 studied for specific neurologic symptoms, three who died of other causes and whose AVM was discovered unruptured at necropsy, and one girl whose pontine AVM was detected in follow-up study of an extensive cranial-orbital vascular malformation.

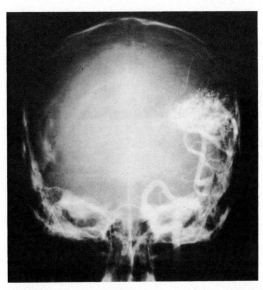

FIGURE 42–1. In this AP carotid injection, a large dominant hemisphere AVM extends in a wedge toward the lateral ventricle, where it picks up supply from the posterior choroidal vessels.

ARTERIOVENOUS MALFORMATIONS OF THE BRAIN

EMBRYOGENESIS AND PATHOLOGY

The classic AVM is presumed to represent a structural defect in the formation of the primitive arteriolar-capillary network normally interposed between brain arteries and veins. The stimulus, timing, and early architectural deficiencies in such malformations are not entirely clear. Padget believed that most of the malformations occur before the 40-mm embryo length, that is, before the arterial walls thicken, notwithstanding that it is after this time when the late histologic changes in the walls of the vessels convert them into the final adult form.[27]

The pathologic analysis of resected AVM specimens does not provide much additional information about the causation of AVM. The tangled arteriovenous communications, because of their low resistance, attract exaggerated blood flow. Given enough time, the malformations do have the capacity to expand their bulk by enlarging and increasing the tortuosity of the feeding and draining channels. The number of fistulous connections, however, probably does not change, and some lesions (such as those of the brainstem) may always remain small.[28]

The conglomeration of turgid, tortuous vessels covered by opacified and thickened arachnoid on the brain's surface is easily recognizable as the classic AVM. Sometimes the malformation is hidden in a sulcus or the subcortical tissues and served by a straightened, dilated anomalous artery, which acts as its only surface hallmark. The nearby cerebral convolutions show variable degrees of atrophy, and there may be local rusty staining from previous hemorrhage. The tough texture of the adjacent gray and white matter is due to gliosis, which permits dissection of the lesion through this relatively inert tissue.

Although some malformations are globular in shape, most describe a course to the subjacent ventricle in an inverted wedge-shaped fashion (Fig. 42–1). The component vessels show variation in their numbers, their caliber, and the thickness of their walls. Venous tortuosity, intimal thickening, arteriolization of veins, and evidence of hemorrhage and neuronal loss are indicative of the long-standing hemodynamic consequences within the malformation. In almost all circumstances there is microscopic evidence of previous hemorrhage, with hemosiderin-laden macrophages.[29, 30] Elastic and muscle fibers in the arteries are altered; the media varies in thickness, and substantial thinning of some vessels can result in aneurysmal dilatation of the structure.[30–32] However, those vessels with marked saccular dilatations are venous in origin.[29] Even the knowledge that some arteries show focal absence of elastic lamina does not isolate the primary vascular fault.

Given that the stage may be set by 60 days gestation for maldevelopment of a portion of the cerebrovascular tree, it is remarkable that the typical AVM does not declare itself except with symptoms. Although ruptured AVM is the most common cause of hemorrhagic stroke in children, most AVMs become symptomatic between 20 and 40 years of age.[6] Nor has there been any convincing evidence concerning the cause—hypertension, strenuous activity and head trauma—of bleeding from a malformation.[29] It is tempting to believe, therefore, that whatever the early embryologic fault, there are substantial postnatal and delayed factors that influence the development and declaration of the cerebral AVM.

NATURAL HISTORY

The criteria for patient selection for AVM therapy are still the subject of controversy. Understandably, matched trials of nonsurgical and surgical management programs for patients with cerebral AVM have not been reported. Whereas there might have been a certain conservatism expressed in earlier writings,[33-38] it is now recognized that with advances in surgical and anesthetic technology, the indications for and success with surgery have broadened. Some argue that the current improved results depend more importantly on the selection criteria and only marginally on surgical technique.[37] The matter is now further complicated by additional treatment options—proton-beam irradiation, stereotactic cryosurgery, and various forms of endovascular embolization.

The natural history of AVMs in the pediatric population is not well understood. In our present series, 79 per cent of the lesions presented with hemorrhage, a rate that is higher than that reported for adults.[6, 12] By defining our pediatric population as patients to age 18 years, we do not imply that there are differences between AVMs in patients of 17 versus 20 years of age, but rather between the *populations* of children and adults. Celli et al. reported a hemorrhage rate of over 80 per cent for AVM less than 2 cm in diameter.[39] Mori et al. concluded that the prognosis was less favorable in children with AVMs in comparison to adults, and they described a higher mortality rate in younger patients due to hemorrhage.[24] Gerosa et al. reported that the primary hemorrhage was fatal in 5.4 per cent of their patients, but that rebleeding occurred in 29 per cent and it carried a grim prognosis.[20]

The higher mortality rate from AVM hemorrhage in children (25 per cent over our entire series) may be due to several factors. First, there is a higher incidence of AVM location in the posterior cranial fossa, where the effects of hemorrhage are more critical. A significant difference was found in comparison between the number of children with posterior fossa AVM in our series (31 of 132) and the general adult series of Jomin et al. (8 of 150).[7, 15] Similarly, infratentorial AVMs were present in only 32 of 453 patients in the Cooperative Study; again this difference was significant. We believe that the hemodynamic compressive or hemorrhagic effects of a critically located infratentorial AVM lead to an earlier symptomatic onset when compared to most supratentorial malformations. Second, hemorrhage from a pediatric AVM may be more severe than in adults. Celli et al. stated that cerebral hemorrhages in children show more violent and massive bleeding, demonstrated by a higher frequency of intraparenchymal and intraventricular hemorrhage.[39] There is no evidence to suggest that the vessels of a "younger" AVM are more fragile than in the adult. The Cooperative Study reported an adult mortality rate from hemorrhage between 6 and 10 per cent.[6] Finally, there is some evidence that the smaller AVM is more inclined to hemorrhage than that which is larger.[11, 40] It is an observation that children's vascular malformations tend to be small rather than large and are secreted in unusual and/or awkward locations.

A large series of adult patients with AVM have indicated that the risk for re-hemorrhage is 2 to 4 per cent per year independent of prior hemorrhage.[11, 13, 14, 41-44]

Risk estimates were provided by large series of patients managed conservatively. The lack of prior large pediatric AVM series and the small number of patients *without* resection in our series prohibit a reasonable estimate of the rebleeding risk in children.

INITIAL CLINICAL ASSESSMENT

Symptoms

The symptoms of a cerebral AVM, whenever they appear, are representative of the structural defects in the vessels of the malformation, and the sump effect of the direct arteriovenous shunting. A greater percentage of children (than adults) experience hemorrhage as their first symptom, whereas relatively larger numbers of adults display the presumed ischemic symptoms of headache, dementia, and slowly progressive neurologic dysfunction. It is not always clear at operation or on histopathologic examination of excised tissues just where the hemorrhage originated. Certainly, there are deficiencies in some vessel walls possibly making them liable to rupture, yet others of the abnormal channels are thickened.[30] It appears to be true that it is the smaller AVMs that bleed and that generally there is less violent parenchymal disruption following AVM hemorrhage than with burst aneurysms.[39]

Spontaneous subarachnoid or, more frequently, intracerebral/intraventricular bleeding is the most common cause of symptoms experienced by children. In our review, 104 patients (104/132 = 79 per cent) experienced spontaneous intracranial hemorrhage as determined by the syndrome of headache, with bloody spinal fluid or blood clot recognized on CT or recovered at operation or autopsy (Table 42–1). The ictus is often explosive, when the previously well child screams out about sudden headache. It has again been confirmed that a surprising number of AVMs bleed during periods of quietude or even sleep.[2] Not surprisingly, therefore, the subarachnoid grading reflects the critical nature of the child at the time of first assessment (Table 42–2). Altered consciousness, meningism, and appropriate lateralized motor and sensory signs are present.

Epilepsy, which presumably results from gliosis of brain because of chronic ischemia adjacent to the arte-

TABLE 42–1.   ARTERIOVENOUS MALFORMATIONS: MODE OF PRESENTATION (HOSPITAL FOR SICK CHILDREN SERIES)

SYMPTOM	NO. OF PATIENTS
Hemorrhage	104
Chronic epilepsy	16
Delayed development/ischemia	5
Congestive heart failure	2
Headache	1
Incidental*	4
Total	132

*Three cases at postmortem and one as a result of craniofacial evaluation for complex facial vascular malformation.

TABLE 42–2.   ADMISSION SUBARACHNOID HEMORRHAGE (SAH) GRADE VERSUS LONG-TERM CLINICAL OUTCOME (n = 102)

SAH GRADE	NUMBER OF PATIENTS		
	Normal	Neurologic Deficit	Dead
I	11	3	1
II	15	4	2
III	22	5	1
IV	9	6	3
V	1	0	19

riovenous shunt, occurs as a presenting symptoms in 20 to 67 per cent of adult patients with AVM.[16, 17, 40, 45, 46] The proper management for a patient who has had one or two convulsions from an AVM and exclusive of frank SAH challenges treatment decisions. Recent reports indicate, however, that better than 70 per cent of patients with epilepsy related to AVM will remain seizure-free (or "nearly so") when the associated epileptogenic tissue is excised.[45] Sixteen of our patients presented with "chronic" seizures.

Of the remaining 12 children who had neither hemorrhage nor epilepsy in their profile, five had presenting symptoms of delayed development or signs of cerebral ischemia, two of congestive heart failure, one of chronic headache, and four of incidental malformations (see Table 42–1).

Investigations

When a child is seen with a typical headache-hemorrhage ictus, the surgeon should proceed directly with computed tomography (CT) and cerebral arteriography. The CT head scan will outline the blood clot and calcification if present and, on enhanced study, may detail the dilated feeding and draining vascular channels and large blood-containing varices. It will thus provide a clue to the site and side of the brain to be studied first with cerebral arteriography.

By means of selective internal carotid and vertebral artery injections, the numbers and location of the arterial feeders can be examined by arteriography. The numbers of arterial contributors can be determined by properly timed sequential films processed with subtraction techniques. Seldom is a malformation served by only one arterial channel. There may be only one *major* artery contributing to the lesion, but the surgeon should anticipate any number of minor vessels coming from pial or deep perforating sources.

On the other hand, the venous drainage in a child's AVM is frequently through a solitary channel by either a large cortical vein or the deep venous system, and it is usually precisely defined on arteriography. The overall architecture of the lesion is carefully studied on the arteriogram and its operability thus determined.

Some vascular malformations are angiographically "cryptic" and are thus not demonstrated on angiography.[47] These lesions, often in the distribution of the middle cerebral artery, are usually small, and there is evidence of a recent or old hemorrhagic history. Meticulous processing of the pathologic material uncovers the vascular malformation. There were five such cases in the present series. Hence, close follow-up must be maintained for all children with an intracerebral hemorrhage small enough to be treated conservatively; these patients may harbor an occult malformation.

As a rule, 90 per cent of the malformations found are supratentorial, most frequently within the distribution of the middle cerebral artery.[6, 32] However, any intracranial artery can be associated with the malformation, and in the HSC study, 24 per cent of the lesions were found below the tentorium.[48]

PREOPERATIVE MANAGEMENT

Inasmuch as the presenting symptom of 79 per cent of the lesions in children is spontaneous intracranial hemorrhage, urgent neurodiagnostic assessments and operative care are usually undertaken to identify and release the associated clot. As AVM surgery can be tedious and protracted, it is desirable, whenever circumstances permit, to plan the malformation excision as an elective procedure. Thus, if only subarachnoid hemorrhage occurred, or if the intracerebral hemorrhage is small and the patient's condition stable, interval surgery may be staged after a few days' wait. During that time, the child is monitored appropriately. Cerebral vasospasm is seldom a problem in children with AVMs, but rebleeding during the interval often is. Thus antispasm, antihypertensive pharmacologic measures are not required. If the operation can possibly be delayed for 3 to 7 days after the hemorrhage, the surgeon will be rewarded with a properly prepared patient whose relaxed brain contains a liquefying hematoma.

There is not the same urgency for the 21 per cent of patients whose presenting symptom is other than spontaneous hemorrhage. This group has been investigated in a traditional fashion for headaches, seizures, and developmental delay, and the malformation has been discovered during the testing or even during elective surgery. The clinical challenge will be to determine in advance whether surgical obliteration of the malformation will influence the headache, seizure, or developmental problem and whether, therefore, it should even be undertaken.[37, 49]

SURGERY

The ideal treatment for a brain AVM is total excision.[17, 28] Excision has now been achieved in almost all eloquent regions of brain (motor, basal ganglia, brainstem) as well as in less critical areas. Thus, except for lesions that penetrate the brainstem or basal ganglia, it is not so much the anatomic location of the lesion in a child that restrains the surgeon as it is the lesion's size. As large, lush, and thirsty AVMs are not common in children, and as it is usually the small malformations that produce hemorrhage, then paradoxically it may be the small, awkwardly positioned AVM that will present the greatest challenge to the surgeon.[40] Lesions that are about 1.0 cm across and located adjacent to or within a ventricle or positioned deeply along the medial face of the hemisphere can be difficult to isolate, particularly if the malformation lies between the surgical approach and the hemorrhage.

Moreover, the lateral hemispheral AVM may not always be found classically curled on the cortex. Instead, it may be hidden subcortically and bear as its only surface landmark an unusually straightened feeding artery running a nonanatomic course, or a red draining vein striking out toward an adjacent venous sinus. The most reliable surface markings are the veins because, regardless of their origin, all at some point cross the surface.[50]

Surgical management of a child with an AVM requires all of the major anesthetic and pharmacologic techniques currently available. Curiously, AVMs are less likely to bleed spontaneously during surgery from their original site of hemorrhage than are aneurysms, and thus the various vascular coils and varices can be gently manipulated aside. When bleeding does occur, it tends to be less torrential than with aneurysm rupture, and the bleeding usually represents transgression into the malformation itself. This bleeding can be controlled with gentle packing while the dissection proceeds at a more remote site.

The operating microscope is often though not always an ally, and it may be a disadvantage to the surgeon working upon large-convexity or cerebellar lesions. In these circumstances, the surgeon may lose sight of the perimeter of the AVM when working with the lowest magnifications. Magnifying loupes and a fiberoptic headlight can thus provide more mobility, permitting the surgeon to stay at the margin of the malformation, in its glial plane. A parenchymal clot, if present, can create much autodissection of the AVM. After the clot is removed, the surgeon will recognize the AVM hanging like a chandelier from the wall or roof of the clot cavity. Sometimes, however, the clot can be located "downstream" from the AVM, which often is isolated before the hematoma is reached.

The dissection proceeds with microinstruments in an organized circumferential fashion about the malformation, preserving until the end one or two major draining veins. As a rule, the feeding and draining vessels run a straight course to and from the malformation but become coiled within it. These vessels can be freed by dissection along the long axis and isolated with a blunt hook before the bipolar coagulation forceps are applied. It is not unusual for an accompanying artery or vein to be hidden immediately deep to the vessel about to be severed, and manipulation with the blunt hook will bring this surreptitious neighbor into view for coagulation too. Such is frequently the case with the major draining vein, which may obscure otherwise inconsequential arteries running beneath it or feeding it.[50] Most AVMs describe a wedge or torpedo profile toward the adjacent ventricle, and the surgeon should not be content that a total excision has been achieved until the ventricular wall has been visualized and, if necessary, the choroid plexus is detached from the choroidal vessels at the apex of the lesion. Once the malformation dissection has been completed, bleeding will cease in its bed and the brain is considerably relaxed. If operation has been decided upon, the surgeon should be satisfied with nothing less than total excision, even if two stages are necessary to achieve it. Proximal vessel ligation can be dangerous and is an inadequate solution; subtotal excision is messy, and the shunt remains served by newly recruited contributors.

The embolization of particulate material into the feeding channels of AVMs has been advocated during the past 20 years. Although staged embolization and resection have been reported to be of benefit for large AVMs,[51] no children in our series had such large lesions amenable to this type of therapy. It often happens that those lesions that could be treated with endovascular obliteration are also those most accessible for operative excision. Intravascular embolization was used in only two of our patients and failed in one of them.

One patient in our series with an AVM of the hypothalamus was referred for stereotactic radiosurgery. The role of radiosurgery for treating AVMs in children remains to be defined, although encouraging results in carefully selected patients have been reported.[52]

POSTOPERATIVE CARE AND RESULTS

The experienced surgeon who attempts total excision of the malformation will usually know if that goal has been achieved at the conclusion of the first craniotomy. If a deliberate decision has been made to stage the procedure, with a second attempt planned after an interval, the surgeon should discontinue the first procedure when the operative region is neither bleeding nor swelling. The child is then allowed to recover and, if necessary, undergo further study with repeat arteriography. One or two strategically placed metallic hemostatic clips will permit identification of the area of surgery and serve as coordinates for the further radiologic and surgical examination of the malformation that remains.

Whether one or two procedures are required to obliterate the lesion, the surgeon cannot be satisfied that total excision has been achieved until postoperative arteriography confirms it. The study will also show a diminished size of the proximal contributing arteries. If there is residual malformation, reoperation becomes necessary to excise the remaining lesion. A residual lesion can be responsible for continued bleeding in the bed of the malformation, which tends to arise from tiny "coils" of vessels lying within the adjacent brain white matter. These can usually be easily circumscribed and excised.

Thereafter, the child's convalescence depends only on rehabilitation needs, if any. The degree of their motor, speech, and cerebellar recovery can be remarkable.

Prophylactic anticonvulsant medication will usually be required for 6 to 24 months following AVM excision.

In the HSC series, 128 patients were treated (four children with incidental malformations have been excluded). Twenty-seven children received nonsurgical treatment and 13 died of hemorrhage. There were 105 patients who were operated upon and underwent any one or combination of the following: complete or incomplete AVM removal, obliteration of feeders, evacuation of hematoma, or shunting procedures. In 60 patients, the malformation was completely removed at the first operation, and in another 10 at a second procedure. Thirteen patients in the group treated by surgery died (12 per cent mortality), all of whom were grade 4 or 5 at the time of first assessment. All patients who died suffered hemorrhage; thus the mortality from the bleed, regardless of the method of treatment, is 25 per cent.[7]

A chronic seizure disorder was the reason for neurologic evaluation in 16 patients. All but one of these children were operated upon, and three had lingering postoperative epilepsy. Fourteen patients had acute seizures, most related to their hemorrhages, and only one (7 per cent) had lingering postoperative epilepsy. Paradoxically, six patients who had been operated upon who did not have any seizure disturbances before surgery were subject to this malady during the follow-up period. All these patients had intracerebral clots.

Except for those patients with incidental malformations and those who have died, there are 103 children available for follow-up examination 9 months to 30 years after treatment. One of these patients died suddenly at home 5 years after "total" resection of his AVM. Neither the completeness of resection nor the ultimate cause of death is known. Of the remaining 102 patients, 69 (67 per cent) are neurologically normal. A fixed neurologic deficit persisted in 28 patients (27 per cent). Progressive mental status deterioration occurred in another five, and one patient has had persistent chronic headache.

Nonoperative management was performed in 27 children. In 13 patients, death followed hemorrhage, either prior to surgical intervention or in children to whom surgery offered no chance for clinical recovery. Of eight children still living who are being observed by follow-up and have their AVMs intact, six are normal, one has a seizure disorder, and one has a persistent neurologic deficit.

CONCLUSION

Hemorrhagic stroke, at least in this review, is more likely to be due to bleeding from an arteriovenous malformation than a ruptured intracranial aneurysm. This process, which also distinguishes the child from the adult, is characterized by a number of other differentiations. More children bleed from their malformations and fewer suffer chronic seizures than do adults. In that regard, there are remarkable similarities between the HSC review and that of Gerosa et al.[20] The latter authors also indicate that 28 per cent of children suffer overt repeat hemorrhage, and the HSC study concludes that the mortality rate from any hemorrhage is 25 per cent. As with intracranial aneurysms, AVMs in children can be scattered throughout the brain, often in awkward locations. There are an unusual number (24 per cent) located below the tentorium. Wherever possible, total excision of the malformation must be attempted, with the expectation that the child's brain vasculature may be resilient to operative intrusion. Seventy per cent of children receiving surgical care can be expected to be neurologically intact after surgery. The surgical mortality of 4 per cent is influenced by the severity of the SAH/IVH, as all patients were clinical grades 4 or 5. Hence, with regard to arteriovenous malformations, Matson's exhortation is still valid, 24 years later.[17]

THE ANGIOMATOUS MALFORMATIONS

The identification and clinical impact of the angiomatous malformations of the brain—cavernous and venous—have been increasingly appreciated with the advent of modern neuroimaging. Many of these lesions are being clearly defined by computed tomography or magnetic resonance imaging, which tests have been obtained in children with headaches, seizure disorders, or an overt neurologic ictus of other types, or for clinically unrelated reasons.[53] When one of these lesions is detected, its number, size, and anatomic location have to be carefully evaluated with regard to relevance to the patient's symptoms. The subsequent management decisions may be difficult indeed.

CAVERNOUS ANGIOMAS

That diagnostic imaging has influenced the detection of cavernous angiomas of the brain in both children and adults is confirmed in recent papers.[54, 55] These lesions, which account for 8 to 16 per cent of all cerebrovascular malformations, are found most frequently in the cerebral hemispheres when they occur intracranially.[54] They appear as a dark blue or purple lobulated mass which, although unencapsulated, is well circumscribed. The surrounding brain is frequently stained by old hemorrhage. Scott theorizes that growth of the cavernous angioma is possibly due to rupture with hemorrhage from these thin-walled vessels, with repeated re-endothelialization of hemorrhagic cavities, growth of new blood vessels as part of the organization of the hematomas, and the laying down of additional fibrous scar.[55] Perhaps this potential for multiple and varying areas of biologic change accounts for the occasional difficulty in obtaining a complete excision of this angioma.

Unlike traditional cerebral AVMs, the natural history and risk factors for cerebral cavernous angiomas are not yet known. A recent review suggests that continuing symptoms developed in 40 per cent of patients and that hemorrhage recurs in 8 per cent.[56] A pattern of inheritance exists as autosomal dominant for the familial form of cavernous angioma.

The cavernous angioma typically comes to attention because of hemorrhage, seizure, or progressive neurologic deficit. With the exception of those lesions in the brainstem, most episodes of bleeding from the cavernous malformation are minor, and indeed some may be undetected. This is especially the case for lesions within the centrum semiovale of non-eloquent brain. Fatal hemorrhage has been reported, but usually from an angioma lying within the posterior fossa.[54] The chronic irritative effect of hemosiderin is the likeliest explanation for those angiomas that produce seizures, for which a focal event appears to be the most frequent pattern. Occasionally a cavernous angioma may mimic a neoplasm by producing a progressive neurologic deficit, especially in the case of the cystic or extracerebral malformations, each of which may progressively enlarge like a neoplasm.[54]

Historically, cerebral arteriography has been the only modality with which this lesion has been defined—and poorly at that (Fig. 42–2). The majority of cavernous angiomas do not demonstrate any abnormal vasculature, whereas a small number will show a capillary blush or early draining vein. MRI is now the study of choice to identify the cavernous angioma, which has a central core of mixed signal intensity surrounded by a rim of hypointense signal produced by hemosiderin.[54]

There is no standard treatment for children with a defined cavernous angioma, who usually declare their lesion with overt symptoms requiring remedial action.[55] For children who have bled, the angioma is best excised early, when the hematoma bed can facilitate the surgical definition and the malformation can be completely excised. If a convulsion has been responsible for the child's assessment, the focal lesion and the surrounding hemosiderin-stained brain are excised; at this early stage a more formal seizure operation is not required. One cannot be as ambitious for those angiomas lying within brainstem or within the basal ganglia—especially if they are large. Each patient's treatment must be individualized as to the risk of future bleeding or seizure recurrence. Moreover, if the patient is asymptomatic—whether the lesions are single or multiple—one is disinclined to recommend therapy.

Like cerebral AVMs in children, the small cavernous angioma may be difficult to localize at operation, especially if it lies subcortical. Stereotactic CT guidance can be an excellent identifier of the covert lesion and thus permit the surgeon to make a safe, judicious entry through cortex to the malformation. At that point, the lesion is easily circumscribed, and bleeding from disrupted vessels is seldom a problem. The brainstem angioma will be more difficult to isolate and totally remove. Laser dissection and vaporization of the mass can be of assistance in some cases. Once the angioma is excised, the vast majority of patients are completely relieved of their symptoms.[54, 55]

VENOUS ANGIOMAS

Of all vascular malformations of the brain, the venous angioma is the most common, yet paradoxically it is the least likely to cause symptoms.[57, 58] This type of angioma is composed of dilated medullary veins separated by normal-appearing neural parenchyma.[54] The

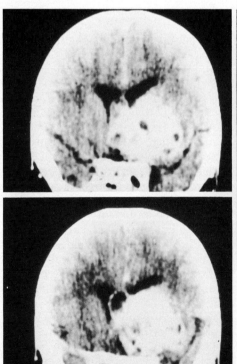

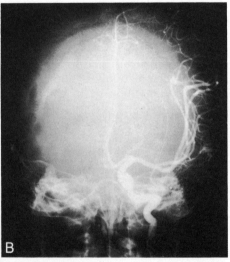

FIGURE 42–2. *A,* The enhanced CT scan coronal image outlines a large, biopsy-proven cavernous angioma lying within the left basal ganglia. *B,* Remarkably, there is little vascular abnormality apart from vessel shifts on the carotid arteriogram (same case as *A*).

veins of the angioma drain centripetally into venous channels around which they are arranged, and the angioma must thus be regarded as a "physiologically competent anomaly of venous drainage."[54]

The latter must be the principle that governs the clinical evaluation of patients with these lesions. Rigamonti et al. suggest that the venous malformation is "frequently associated with other, more symptomatic conditions and is often erroneously identified as the source of the symptoms."[58] Hence, recurring headache can probably be attributed to a different cause; similarly, the patient with a seizure disorder must be studied carefully before the angioma is tagged as the responsible factor.

While spontaneous hemorrhage is a feared complication of this malformation, the real threat is unknown. Studies of appropriate brain specimens show a general absence of hemosiderin-laden macrophages in parenchyma surrounding a venous angioma; these changes are more commonly found with the AVM or cavernous angioma.[59] This suggests that the venous angioma poses an insignificant risk of bleeding.[53] When hemorrhage does occur, it more commonly occurs in the posterior fossa. If hematoma must be evacuated, that alone should be the goal of operation, and the surgeon should resist the temptation to take any vessels.

The arteriographic features of this type of angioma are well established. Enlarged medullary veins converge into a central draining channel that reaches either the superficial drainage system or, less commonly, the deep venous collecting system. The caput medusae appearance with normal arterial and capillary phases is always demonstrated. If an early draining vein is noted, the lesion is much more likely to be a traditional AVM.[58] Most venous angiomas can be diagnosed on infused CT scan, on which a linear or curvilinear enhancing pattern is noted in the medullary substance of the hemisphere.[58] The MRI appearance is again of a linear area of hypointensity on T1- and T2-weighted images.[60]

With regard to the defined venous angioma, the present consensus is that as the malformation represents an anomalous but competent venous drainage pattern, all other avenues of investigation must be exhausted to explain the patient's symptoms before the angioma is treated.[53, 54, 58] The majority of these lesions are asymptomatic or of minor consequence only. In those situations in which the angioma is thought to be "symptomatic," high-field MRI is required to rule out underlying pathology. If present, that pathology should be treated independent of the angioma.[58] Occasionally it may be necessary to evacuate the hematoma created by a venous angioma, and only clot removal should be attempted. Obliteration of any of the major draining veins is to be avoided.

REFERENCES

1. Gold AP, Challenor YB, Gilles FH, et al.: Report of the Joint Committee for Stroke Facilities. IX. Strokes in children (Part I). Stroke 4:835, 1973.
2. Locksley HB: Report on the Cooperative Study of Intracranial Aneurysms and Subarachnoid Hemorrhage. Section V, Part I. Natural history of subarachnoid hemorrhage, intracranial aneurysms and arteriovenous malformations. Based on 6,368 cases in the Cooperative Study. J Neurosurg 25:219, 1966.
3. Hourihan M, Gates PC, McAllister VL: Subarachnoid hemorrhage in childhood and adolescence. J Neurosurg 60:1163, 1984.
4. Laitinen L: Arteriella aneuryusm med subarachnoidal-blodning hos barn. Nord Med 71:329, 1964.
5. Sedzimir CB, Robinson J: Intracranial hemorrhage in children and adolescents. J Neurosurg 38:269, 1973.
6. Perret G, Nishioka H: Report on the Cooperative Study of Intracranial Aneurysms and Subarachnoid Hemorrhage. Section VI. Arteriovenous malformations. An analysis of 545 cases of craniocerebral arteriovenous malformations and fistulae reported to the Cooperative Study. J Neurosurg 25:467, 1966.
7. Kondziolka D, Humphreys RP, Hoffman HJ, et al.: Arteriovenous malformations of the brain in children: A forty year experience. Can J Neurol Sci 19:40, 1992.
8. Hayashi S, Arimoto T, Itakura T, et al.: The association of intracranial aneurysms and arteriovenous malformations of the brain. Case report. J Neurosurg 55:971, 1981.
9. Ostergaard JR: Association of intracranial aneurysm and arteriovenous malformation in childhood. Neurosurgery 14:358, 1984.
10. Hoffman HJ, Mohr G, Kusunoki T: Multiple arteriovenous malformations of spinal cord and brain in a child. Case report. Childs Brain 2:317, 1976.
11. Graf CJ, Perret GE, Torner JC: Bleeding from cerebral arteriovenous malformations as part of their natural history. J Neurosurg 58:331, 1983.
12. Guidetti B, Delitala A: Intracranial arteriovenous malformations. Conservative and surgical treatment. J Neurosurg 53:149, 1980.
13. Heros RC, Korosue K, Diebold PM: Surgical excision of cerebral arteriovenous malformation: Late results. Neurosurgery 26:578, 1990.
14. Itoyama Y, Uemura S, Ushio Y, et al.: Natural course of unoperated intracranial arteriovenous malformations: study of 50 cases. J Neurosurg 71:805, 1989.
15. Jomin M, Lesoin F, Lozes G: Prognosis for arteriovenous malformations of the brain in adults based on 150 cases. Surg Neurol 23:362, 1985.
16. Harwood-Nash DC, Fitz CR: Neuroradiology in Infants and Children. Vol 3. St Louis, C.V. Mosby Co., 1976, pp 907, 913–939, 1164.
17. Matson DD: Neurosurgery of Infancy and Childhood. 2nd ed. Springfield, IL, Charles C Thomas, 1969, pp 749–766.
18. Amacher AL, Allcock JM, Drake CG: Cerebral angiomas: The sequelae of surgical treatment. J Neurosurg 37:571, 1972.
19. Bruce DA, Schut L: Arteriovenous malformations in children. Childs Brain 8:232, 1981.
20. Gerosa MA, Cappellotto P, Licata C, et al.: Cerebral arteriovenous malformations in children (56 cases). Childs Brain 8:356, 1981.
21. Kelly JJ Jr, Mellinger JF, Sundt TM Jr: Intracranial arteriovenous malformations in childhood. Ann Neurol 3:338, 1978.
22. Laine E, Dhellemmes P, Clarisse C: Supratentorial arteriovenous malformations in children except aneurysm of the vein of Galen. Childs Brain 8:63, 1981.
23. Monges J, Jaimovich R, Cragnaz RJ: Vascular malformations in children. Bol Asoc Argentina Neurocir 30:41, 1981.
24. Mori K, Murata T, Hasimoto N, et al.: Clinical analysis of arteriovenous malformations in children. Childs Brain 6:13, 1980.
25. So SC: Cerebral arteriovenous malformations in children. Childs Brain 4:242, 1978.
26. Tiyaworabun S, Kramer HH, Lim DP, et al.: Cerebral arteriovenous malformations in children: Clinical analysis and followup results. Childs Brain 8:232, 1981.
27. Padget DH: The cranial venous system in man in reference to development, adult configuration and relation to the arteries. Am J Anat 98:307, 1956.
28. Drake CG: Cerebral arteriovenous malformations: Considerations for and experience with surgical treatment in 166 cases. Clin Neurosurg 26:145, 1979.
29. McCormick WF: Pathology of vascular malformations of the brain. In Wilson CB, Stein BM (eds): Intracranial Arteriovenous Malformations. Baltimore, Williams & Wilkins, 1984, pp 44–63.

30. Takashima S, Becker LE: Neuropathology of cerebral arteriovenous malformations in children. J Neurol Neurosurg Psychiatry 43:380, 1980.

31. Northfield DWC: The Surgery of the Central Nervous System: A Textbook for Postgraduate Students. Oxford, Blackwell Scientific Publications, 1973, pp 402–420.

32. Russell DS, Rubinstein LJ: Pathology of Tumors of the Nervous System. 4th ed. London, Edward Arnold Publishers Ltd, 1977, pp 136–138.

33. Forster DMC, Steiner L, Hakanson S: Arteriovenous malformations of the brain. A long-term clinical study. J Neurosurg 37:562, 1972.

34. Schatz SW, Botterell EH: The natural history of arteriovenous malformations. In Milliken C (ed): Cerebrovascular Disease. Proceedings of the Association of Research in Nervous and Mental Diseases, Vol 41. Baltimore, Williams & Wilkins, 1974, pp 180–187.

35. Svien JA, McRae JA: Arteriovenous anomalies of the brain. Fate of patients not having definitive surgery. J Neurosurg 23:23, 1965.

36. Troupp H, Marttila I, Halonen V: Arteriovenous malformations of the brain: Prognosis without operation. Acta Neurochir 22:125, 1970.

37. Troupp H: Arteriovenous malformations of the brain. What are the indications for operation? In Morley TP (ed): Current Controversies in Neurosurgery. Philadelphia, WB Saunders Co, 1967, pp 210–216.

38. Pellettieri L, Carlsson C-A, Grevsten S, et al.: Surgical versus conservative treatment of intracranial arteriovenous malformations. Acta Neurochir (Suppl) 29:1, 1980.

39. Celli P, Ferrante L, Palma L, et al.: Cerebral arteriovenous malformations in children. Clinical features and outcome of treatment in children and in adults. Surg Neurol 22:43, 1984.

40. Waltimo O: The relationship of size, density, and localization of intracranial arteriovenous malformations to the type of initial symptom. J Neurol Sci 19:13, 1973.

41. Fults D, Kelly DL: Natural history of arteriovenous malformations of the brain: A clinical study. Neurosurgery 15:658, 1984.

42. Crawford PM, West CR, Chadwick DW, et al.: Arteriovenous malformations of the brain: Natural history in unoperated patients. J Neurol Neurosurg Psychiatry 49:1, 1986.

43. Ondra SL, Troupp H, George ED, et al.: The natural history of symptomatic arteriovenous malformations of the brain: A 24-year follow-up assessment. J Neurosurg 73:387, 1990.

44. Wilkins RH: Natural history of intracranial vascular malformations. A review. Neurosurgery 16:421, 1985.

45. LeBlanc R, Feindel W, Ethier R: Epilepsy from cerebral arteriovenous malformations. Can J Neurol Sci 10:91, 1983.

46. Mohr JP: Neurological manifestations and factors related to the therapeutic decisions. In Wilson CB, Stein BM (eds): Intracranial Arteriovenous Malformations. Baltimore, Williams & Wilkins, 1984, pp 1–11.

47. Cohen HCM, Tucker WS, Humphreys RP, et al.: Angiographically cryptic histologically verified cerebrovascular malformations. Neurosurgery 10:704, 1982.

48. Humphreys RP: Infratentorial arteriovenous malformations. In Edwards MSB, Hoffman HJ (eds): Cerebrovascular Disease in Childhood and Adolescence. Baltimore, Williams & Wilkins, 1988, pp 309–320.

49. Wilson CB, Sang UH, Dominque J: Microsurgical treatment of intracranial vascular malformations. J Neurosurg 51:446, 1979.

50. Stein BM: General techniques for the surgical removal of arteriovenous malformations. In Wilson CB, Stein BM (eds): Intracranial Arteriovenous Malformations. Baltimore, Williams & Wilkins, 1984, pp 143–155.

51. Spetzler RF, Martin NA, Carter LP, et al.: Surgical management of large AVMs by staged embolization and operative excision. J Neurosurg 67:17, 1987.

52. Lunsford LD, Kondziolka D, Flickinger JC, et al.: Stereotactic radiosurgery for arteriovenous malformations of the brain. J Neurosurg 75:512, 1991.

53. Malik GM, Morgan JK, Ausman JI: Venous angiomas. In Wilkins RH, Rengachary SS (eds): Neurosurgery Update II. New York, McGraw-Hill, Inc, 1991, p 134.

54. McCormick PC, Michelsen WJ: Management of cavernous and venous malformations. In Barrow DL (ed): Intracranial Vascular Malformations. Neurosurgical Topics. American Association of Neurological Surgeons, Park Ridge, IL, 1990, p 197.

55. Scott RM, Barnes P, Kupsky W, et al.: Cavernous angiomas of the central nervous system in children. J Neurosurg 76:38, 1992.

56. Robinson JR, Little JR, Awad I: Natural history of cavernous angioma. Stroke 21:171, 1990. (Abstract)

57. Sarwar M, McCormick WF: Intracerebral venous angioma: Case report and review. Arch Neurol 35:323, 1978.

58. Rigamonti D, Spetzler RF, Medina M, et al.: Cerebral venous malformations. J Neurosurg 73:560, 1990.

59. McCormick WF: The pathology of vascular ("arteriovenous") malformations. J Neurosurg 24:807, 1966.

60. Michels LG, Bentson JR, Winter J: Computed tomography of cerebral venous angiomas. J Comput Assist Tomogr 1:149, 1977.

Chapter 43

INTRACRANIAL HEMORRHAGE DUE TO NONSTRUCTURAL CAUSES

JOAN VENES, M.D.

The operative technique used in the treatment of nonstructural intracranial hemorrhage does not differ from that for intracranial hemorrhage from a structural cause. What is perhaps the greatest difference is the necessity for the neurosurgeon to work closely with his colleagues in other disciplines, who, among other things, have made such rapid advances in the correction of the various coagulopathies that operative intervention, when indicated, is not only a safe but also a reasonable decision. The aim of this chapter is not to lay out specific plans of management for each condition reviewed. That is very much a case-by-case decision, and advances in hematology are so rapid that specific solutions might be quickly outdated. However, the neurosurgeon must recognize the risks, benefits, and prognoses associated with care of these children. Thus, the aim of this chapter is to familiarize the neurosurgeon with these rather uncommon problems so that he or she might more effectively interact with the nonsurgical disciplines involved in the determination of treatment.

IDIOPATHIC THROMBOCYTOPENIC PURPURA (ITP)

ITP is a hemorrhagic disorder of childhood that usually occurs following viral infection and runs a benign, self-limited course.[1] There were no cases of intracranial hemorrhage in one series of 350 cases[2] and only five in another large series of 413 cases.[3] However, although rare, intracranial hemorrhage accounts for almost all the mortality seen with ITP. In pregnant women with ITP it has been suggested that fetal scalp blood platelet counts be done early in labor and cesarean section be performed for those infants at high risk for bleeding.[4, 5]

In the child for whom surgical intervention is deemed mandatory, the use of dexamethasone and platelet replacement allows the performance of a safe operation, but close cooperation between the neurosurgeon and hematologist is essential to a satisfactory outcome.

NEONATAL ALLOIMMUNE THROMBOCYTOPENIA (NAT)

NAT results from the formation of a maternal antibody to paternal antigen on fetal platelets. Intracranial hemorrhage, which may be antenatal, occurs in approximately 15 to 20 per cent of infants with this form of thrombocytopenia.[6] In families with an affected infant, 75 per cent of subsequent infants are affected.

In cases in which there is a known history of NAT, several methods of management have been proposed. In a small study, Bussel et al. reported the administration of intravenous gamma globulin with or without dexamethasone to seven pregnant women.[6] All seven treated fetuses had platelet counts above 30×10^9/liter (n = 97) at birth, and none had an intracranial hemorrhage. In contrast, all seven of the untreated siblings had lower platelet counts and three had intracranial hemorrhages. Mild intrauterine growth retardation was noted in one treated infant, but all seven were developing normally 2 months to 4 years following treatment. Cordiocentesis followed by fetal platelet transfusions in affected fetuses has been suggested,[7] particularly in those infants known to be at high risk.[8] Several cases have been reported documenting that the conservative approach of elective cesarean section alone may not prevent intracranial hemorrhage in utero or postnatally.[9-11]

We do not yet have enough information concerning the incidence of the disorder or the efficacy of treatment to allow a decision as to whether screening of all first pregnancies is indicated. The prognosis for newborns with this condition and intracranial hemorrhage is poor, with only a rare unimpaired survivor. The decision as to whether surgical intervention should be attempted must be made in cooperation with the neonatologist, hematologist, and informed parents.

HEMOPHILIA

Hemophilia is an X-linked coagulation disorder due to deficiency of factor VIII (hemophilia A) or factor IX (hemophilia B). It occurs in moderate-to-severe form in 1 of 8000 live male births.[12]

Intracranial hemorrhage in the newborn or young infant is uncommonly the presenting event in previously undiagnosed hemophilia and is usually preceded by a history of trauma, which may be minimal, such as the use of forceps during delivery. In a retrospective study of 71 patients with CNS hemorrhage occurring in a population of 2500 hemophiliacs, only three occurred during the newborn period.[13] However, in cases of confirmed carriers, prenatal diagnosis may be justified to allow choice of the least traumatic delivery method.[14] The finding of prolongation of partial thromboplastin time (PTT) in the preoperative work-up of the infant with intracranial hemorrhage should always be viewed with concern that an inherited coagulopathy is a contributing factor.[15] Other inherited disorders of coagulation include homozygous protein C deficiency,[16] factor V[17] and factor X[18] deficiency. Prompt consultation with a hematologist is necessary before surgical intervention.

Minor head trauma is such a frequent occurrence in children that it may be overlooked. Indeed, even when a history of head trauma can be elicited, there may be no apparent direct relationship between the event and the onset of symptoms. The complaint of headache unrelieved by simple measures or accompanied by a change in sensorium is an absolute indication for computed tomography (CT) in the child with known coagulopathy. Once the diagnosis of intracranial hemorrhage is suspected, the hematologist must be consulted. Fujino et al. have recommended that replacement therapy be initiated at the earliest stage in cases of minor subarachnoid hemorrhage following trauma.[19] Eyster and co-workers also propose early intervention and suggest that therapy be maintained for 10 to 14 days.[13]

In those cases in which the diagnosis of hemophilia has not been confirmed, fresh frozen plasma can be used until the diagnosis of specific factor deficiency can be made and treatment with the appropriate concentrate in its most acquired immunodeficiency syndrome (AIDS)–virus–free form can be given.[14] Every effort should be made to manage the patient conservatively. The child will need to be closely monitored in an intensive care unit with close cooperation between the neurosurgeon and the hematologist. Craniotomy in these children is not technically different from that in other children with intracranial hemorrhage, with similar morbidity and mortality. However, in approximately 10 per cent of hemophiliacs, the presence of an inhibitor to the missing procoagulant makes correction of the clotting deficiency more difficult.

VITAMIN K DEFICIENCY

Vitamin K deficiency in the newborn period is a rare event in this country, given the widespread use of neonatal prophylaxis. On occasion, intracranial hemorrhage may be the initial event in the presentation of this disorder. A prolonged prothrombin time (PT), partial thromboplastin time (PTT), and test for elevated serum bilirubin should be done in all infants presenting with unexplained intracranial hemorrhage. However, direct tests for vitamin K deficiency are difficult. Cholestatic liver disease should be suspected when unexplained vitamin K deficiency occurs early in infancy. Kurzel has reported a case of fetal hepatotoxicity associated with prolonged PT and PTT and resulting in intracranial hemorrhage at delivery.[20] In that instance, the mother had taken excessively high doses of acetaminophen during pregnancy, resulting in maternal hepatic dysfunction. Other maternal drugs that predispose to vitamin K deficiency are the antituberculous and some antiepileptic agents.[21]

Vitamin K_1 and fresh frozen plasma will generally return the PT and PTT to normal within 12 to 18 hours, but once again if surgical intervention is required, there must be close cooperation between pediatrician and surgeon to ensure optimal timing of surgery. Other causes of hepatocellular injury leading to coagulopathy are viral infection, metabolic disorders, and hypoxic insult. The patient may be severely jaundiced, and disseminated intravascular coagulation may be present, further exacerbating the coagulation defect. Once again a multidisciplinary approach is an absolute necessity in decision-making related to surgical intervention.

DISSEMINATED INTRAVASCULAR COAGULATION (DIC)

In addition to underlying liver disease (mentioned above), DIC may be initiated by head trauma, sepsis, neonatal asphyxia, and some forms of cancer. The abnormally heightened activation of extrinsic or intrinsic coagulation cascades, accompanied by platelet aggregation, produces widespread intravascular clotting. Procoagulants are depleted, and widespread conversion of fibrinogen to fibrin is consistently the end result.[22] Thrombocytopenia is often but not always present. PT and PTT are elevated while all individual factors are depressed. Low fibrinogen concentration plus elevation of fibrin split (degradation) products are the most common findings. Attention to the underlying cause is, of course, critical to a successful outcome, but when life-threatening intracranial hemorrhage supervenes, correction of the bleeding diathesis becomes paramount. Heparin has been suggested for treatment of this disorder[23] but is contraindicated in the face of intracranial hemorrhage. Antithrombin III has been used with success in the treatment of children in whom malignancy underlies the condition.[24]

EXTRACORPOREAL MEMBRANE OXYGENATION (ECMO)

ECMO plays an increasingly important role in the management of infants and children with respiratory insufficiency of variable etiology. Some of the more common conditions treated with this modality are diaphragmatic hernia, meconium aspiration, and sepsis. More recently, ECMO has been shown to be of value in the treatment of children with both pulmonary hypertension and low cardiac output following operation for congenital heart disease.[25] The pathogenesis of intracerebral hemorrhage in the infant undergoing ECMO is not well understood. In one study of 21 infants, the data suggested an increase in cerebral blood flow velocity and vasodilation of the cerebral vessels at high cardiopulmonary bypass flows.[26] In another study,[27] the records of ten infants treated with ECMO complicated by hemorrhagic brain lesions were reviewed. ECMO requires the permanent ligation of the right common carotid artery and jugular vein and systemic heparinization. Seven (70 per cent) of the hemorrhages occurred on the side opposite carotid ligation and three were on the same side. One patient sustained a right temporal hemorrhage following cannulation of the left carotid artery. This study also suggests that alterations in cerebrovascular hemodynamics accompanying carotid ligation and reperfusion may contribute to the hemorrhagic event, although the significant lateralization noted by these authors remains to be demonstrated in other studies.

One thing is unfortunately painfully clear in the management of these infants, and that is the uniformly poor prognosis among those undergoing ECMO who sustain an intracranial bleed.[28–30] Although reanastomosis of the carotid artery may be useful in the prevention of stroke later in life, it would not affect outcome in these cases. In making the decision whether surgery for evacuation of the hematoma is indicated, it is important to consider that a number of the hemorrhages occur at a site of an infarction.

PRIMARY THALAMIC HEMORRHAGE IN THE FULL-TERM NEWBORN

Intraventricular hemorrhage (IVH) in the full-term newborn is uncommon. In a study of 19 full-term infants with IVH,[31] thalamic hemorrhage was documented in 12 infants (63 per cent). The majority of these infants had predisposing factors for cerebral venous infarction such as sepsis, cyanotic congenital heart disease, and coagulopathy. The incidence of cerebral palsy was higher in those infants with thalamic hemorrhage as a source of the intraventricular hemorrhage. An earlier report of this phenomenon in four healthy full-term infants who developed thalamic/intraventricular hemorrhage did not include a long enough follow-up to document the occurrence of cerebral palsy.[32] The authors of that series comment that "neurodevelopmental outcome was fairly good." Nevertheless, it behooves the neurosurgeon caring for infants shunted for hydrocephalus resulting from thalamic/intraventricular hemorrhage to have a high index of suspicion for the occurrence of neurodevelopmental problems.

An unusual cause of thalamic/intraventricular hemorrhage in a full-term neonate was reported by Wehberg and colleagues.[33] In that instance the 3-year-old sibling knelt on the infant's abdomen accidentally while getting into bed. Within 18 to 20 hours the infant became irritable, began vomiting, and eventually developed opisthotonus. CT demonstrated the hemorrhage, and he later required shunting for hydrocephalus. His outcome was satisfactory. Although the epidemiology of IVH in the full-term infant has been carefully studied, the pathogenesis is not well understood. One study postulates a rapid rise in central venous pressure as the inciting factor.[34] This would certainly be consistent with the events in this case.

CARDIOVASCULAR DISEASE

The dramatic advances in the recognition and repair of congenital heart defects make cerebral hemorrhage and/or ischemic stroke a rare event in these children. As recently as 1975, Humphreys and the group at Toronto Hospital for Sick Children reported on 16 intracranial hemorrhages, 14 of them fatal, in children who had congenital heart defects corrected surgically.[35] In 12 of these, the neurologic deficit was noted when the child awakened from anesthesia. The recent advances in both anesthetic and operative techniques related to the correction of congenital heart defects would render the accumulation of such an experience in one institution highly improbable today.

Nevertheless, intracranial hemorrhage still occurs from time to time in the management of children with congenital heart disease and must be addressed with a team approach to decision-making. Young et al. reported on four infants with coarctation of the aorta, moderate hypertension, and intracranial hemorrhage and commented on the usual association of this complication with more severe elevations of blood pressure.[36] Glauser, in discussing the neuropathologic lesions found in hypoplastic left heart syndrome, notes that cerebral necrosis is probably the initiating factor in major intracranial hemorrhage.[37] Ten of 40 infants undergoing autopsy had major intracranial hemorrhage, and of these, eight died within four days of surgery. In comparison with the nonhemorrhagic groups in whom death occurred, these infants had had cardiac surgery and/or hypoxic-ischemic episode and/or a low platelet count and/or low diastolic blood pressure and/or hyperglycemia. He postulated that cerebral necrosis due to hyperglycemia-enhanced hypoxia-ischemia was followed by reperfusion with capillary leakage due to thrombocytopenia. He also noted that a duration of cardiopulmonary bypass longer than 40 minutes was associated with a higher incidence of acquired neuropathology. If at all possible, careful neuro-imaging to determine the extent of neuropathology accompanying hemorrhage should be done prior to lifesaving neurosurgical intervention in this group. Evidence of widespread hypoxic-ischemic lesions accompanying the hemorrhage must give one pause in considering surgical intervention.

CANCER

In a review of the experience at Children's Hospital of Philadelphia over a 4-year period, Packer and colleagues report on 26 children with systemic malignancies who presented with cerebrovascular accidents.[38] Cerebrovascular accidents were causally related to DIC (8 patients), chemotherapy (8 patients), metastatic tumor (3 patients), and thrombocytopenia (3 patients), and in one patient fungal meningitis was thought to be the inciting event. The authors note that it is possible to delineate three major neuropathologic categories:

1. Vascular thrombosis due either to DIC or to acute arterial or sagittal sinus thrombosis secondary to L-asparaginase. All children in this group had leukemia.
2. Acute neurologic dysfunction in children with osteogenic sarcoma treated with high-dose methotrexate.
3. Obtundation, seizures, and focal neurologic deficits in patients with neuroblastoma metastatic to the torcular region.

Although thrombocytopenia is a frequent occurrence in the treatment of children with cancer, it uncommonly results in intracranial hemorrhage. The child most at risk is the leukemic patient in whom the white blood cell count is extremely high.[39, 40] These children are invariably thrombocytopenic with increased vascular fragility resulting from leukemic infiltration of blood vessel walls. This constellation of events, once a fairly common terminal event, is rarely seen today. Further complicating management in these desperately ill children is the fact that in over half the cases in which hemorrhage occurs it is multifocal.[41]

Acute promyelocytic leukemia is a rare form of leukemia in children. These children have been reported to be at higher risk for intracerebral hemorrhage[42] related to the release of a poorly characterized "procoagulant" factor as tumor cell lysis occurs, either spontaneously or as a result of treatment. At times the resulting DIC and intracranial hemorrhage may be the presenting features of the disease. As with other forms of childhood cancer, earlier diagnosis and aggressive management have significantly decreased the occurrence of this often fatal complication.

As with intracranial hemorrhage due to coagulopathy from other causes, the management decisions in the treatment of the child with hemorrhage associated with cancer demand a multidisciplinary approach involving parents or other caregivers and, when appropriate, the child. Although a sense of urgency should underlie any discussion in this situation, there is little to be gained by intervening surgically in anything other than the most optimal circumstances obtainable. The ethical issues that may surface in the management of these children are best addressed before a catastrophic event such as intracranial hemorrhage makes such discussion unreasonably hurried.

SYSTEMIC LUPUS ERYTHEMATOSUS (SLE)

Although thrombocytopenia is estimated to occur in 75 per cent of patients with SLE, SLE presenting as intracranial hemorrhage is extremely rare. Usually rash, arthritis, and fever are the presenting symptoms. Initial central nervous system (CNS) presentation occurs in less than 15 per cent of children. The more common manifestations of CNS involvement are seizures, headache, psychiatric dysfunction, hemiplegia or paraplegia, cranial nerve palsies, aseptic meningitis, and papilledema.[43] Recently, Cunningham and Conway reported the case of a 12-year-old previously healthy young girl who presented with fever and mental status changes.[44] Initial laboratory tests demonstrated thrombocytopenia and CT revealed a large intracranial hemorrhage, but at operation there was no evidence of vascular malformation or vasculitis. Subsequent laboratory tests revealed fluorescent nuclear antibody 3+ in a speckled gray pattern, total complement CH50 of 139 (normal 150 to 250), positive extractable nuclear antigen (ENA), 2+ Coombs, and negative lupus anticoagulant. These authors suggest that a work-up for SLE be considered in any patient with intracranial hemorrhage secondary to thrombocytopenia of unknown cause.

SUBSTANCE ABUSE

The spread of drug abuse to the school-age population suggests that a toxicology screen be done in any patient with nonhypertensive stroke. In one study of 72 patients 15 to 45 years of age who were hospitalized for nontraumatic intracerebral hemorrhage, five cases (7 per cent) were associated with sympathomimetic drug abuse.[45]

In a large study among patients 15 to 44 years of age (47 per cent less than 35 years old) with drug-related strokes, intracerebral hemorrhage was the most common form (34 per cent), followed by thrombosis (27 per cent), subarachnoid hemorrhage (25 per cent), and cerebral embolism (14 per cent). Seventy-one per cent of strokes occurring within 6 hours of drug use were hemorrhagic, and 73 per cent of these had a peripheral (lobar) location.[46] The greatest risk appears to be within 6 hours of drug use if infectious endocarditis is excluded. All forms of stroke are seen when cocaine and amphetamines are used, either alone or in combination with heroin. Strokes in heroin users were exclusively associated with infectious endocarditis. Hemorrhage in this latter condition results from rupture of a mycotic aneurysm.

Phenylpropanolamine is a drug widely used for a variety of conditions. Adolescents, in particular, use the drug for its effect as an anorexiant. This drug can be obtained over the counter and has been reported to cause intracerebral hemorrhage in an adolescent following the ingestion of an overdose of diet pills.[47]

CAVERNOUS ANGIOMA

Finally, it must be kept in mind that unexplained intracerebral hemorrhage does not equate with nonstructural hemorrhage. Angiographically occult vascular malformations are now identifiable with magnetic resonance imaging techniques. Commonly, these are cavernous angiomas. Once thought to be relatively benign in regard to recurrent hemorrhage, these lesions have been demonstrated to cause recurrent hemorrhage and persistent neurologic deficits.[48] The management of these lesions is discussed in Chapter 42. The evaluation of any child with nontraumatic, nonstructural intracranial hemorrhage, with or without associated coagulopathy, requires magnetic resonance imaging studies of the highest quality to rule out this treatable lesion.

REFERENCES

1. Hoyle D, Darbyshire P, Eden OB: Idiopathic thrombocytopenia in childhood—Edinburgh experience 1962–1982. Scott Med J 31:174, 1986.
2. Lusher JM, Iyer R: ITP in children. Semin Thromb Hemost 3:175, 1977.
3. McClure PD: ITP in children: Diagnosis and management. Pediatrics 55:68, 1975.
4. Kelton JG: Management of pregnant patient with idiopathic thrombocytopenic purpura. Ann Intern Med 99:796, 1983.
5. Scott JR, Cruikshank DP: Fetal platelet counts in the obstetric management of immunological thrombocytopenia. Am J Obstet Gynecol 136:495, 1980.
6. Bussel JB, Berkowitz RL, McFarland JG, et al.: Antenatal treatment of neonatal alloimmune thrombocytopenia. N Engl J Med 319:1374, 1988.
7. Murphy MF, Pullon HW, Metcalfe P, et al.: Management of fetal alloimmune thrombocytopenia by weekly in utero platelet transfusion. Vox Sang 58:45, 1990.
8. Mueller-Eckhardt D, Kiefel V, Grubert A, et al.: Three hundred forty-eight cases of suspected neonatal alloimmune thrombocytopenia. Lancet i:363, 1989.
9. Sia CG, Amigo NC, Harper RG, et al.: Failure of cesarean section to prevent intracranial hemorrhage in siblings with isoimmune neonatal thrombocytopenia. Am J Obstet Gynecol 153:79, 1985.
10. Morales WJ, Stroup M.: Intracranial hemorrhage in utero due to isoimmune neonatal thrombocytopenia. Obstet Gynecol 65(3 Suppl):20S, 1985.
11. Sadowitz PD, Balcom R: Intrauterine intracranial hemorrhage in an infant with isoimmune thrombocytopenia. Clin Pediatr (Phila) 24:655, 1985.
12. Stevenson AC, Kerr CB: On the distribution of frequencies in mutation to genes determining harmful traits in man. Mut Res 4:339, 1967.
13. Eyster ME, Gill FM, Blatt PM, et al.: Central nervous system bleeding in hemophiliacs. Blood 51:1179, 1978.
14. Kletzel M, Miller CH, Becton DL, et al.: Post-delivery head bleeding in hemophilic neonates. Causes and management. Am J Dis Child 143:1107, 1989.
15. Bray GL, Luban NL: Hemophilia presenting with intracranial hemorrhage. An approach to the infant with intracranial bleeding and coagulopathy. Am J Dis Child 141:1215, 1987.
16. Tarras S, Gadia C, Meister L, et al.: Homozygous protein C deficiency in a newborn. Clinicopathological correlation. Arch Neurol 45:214, 1988.
17. Whitelaw A, Haines ME, Bolsover W, Harris E: Factor V deficiency and antenatal intraventricular hemorrhage. Arch Dis Child 59:997, 1984.
18. deSousa D, Clark T, Bradshaw A: Antenatally diagnosed subdural hemorrhage in congenital factor X deficiency. Arch Dis Child 63:1168, 1988.
19. Fujino H, Kuwabara T, Yamashita T, et al.: Intracranial hemorrhage in hemophilia of children. Childs Brain 11:213, 1984.
20. Kurzel RB: Can acetaminophen excess result in maternal and fetal toxicity? South Med J 83:953, 1990.
21. Billman DO: Neonatal bleeding disorders. In Donn SM, Faix RG (eds): Neonatal Emergencies. New York, Futura Publ, 1991, p 438.
22. Corrigan JJ, Jr.: Activation of coagulation and disseminated intravascular consumption in the newborn. Am J Pediatr Hematol Oncol 1:245, 1979.
23. Gobel U, von Voss H, Jurgens H, et al.: Efficiency of heparin in the treatment of newborn infants with respiratory distress syndrome and disseminated intravascular coagulation. Eur J Pediatr 133:47, 1980.
24. Hanada T, Abe T, Takita H: Antithrombin III concentrates for treatment of disseminated intravascular coagulation in children. Am J Pediatr Hematol Oncol 7:3, 1985.
25. Klein MD, Shaheen KW, Whittlesey GC, et al.: Extracorporeal membrane oxygenation for the circulatory support of children after repair of congenital heart disease. J Thorac Cardiovasc Surg 100:498, 1990.
26. Van de Bor M, Walther FJ, Gangitano ES, et al.: Extracorporeal membrane oxygenation and cerebral blood flow velocity in newborn infants. Crit Care Med 18:10, 1990.
27. Mendoza JC, Shearer LL, Cook LN: Lateralization of brain lesions following extracorporeal membrane oxygenation. Pediatrics 88:1004, 1991.
28. Glass P, Miller M, Short B: Morbidity for survivors of extracorporeal membrane oxygenation: neurodevelopmental outcome at one year. Pediatrics 83:72, 1989.
29. Lillehei CW, O'Rourke PP, Vacanti JP, et al.: Role of extracorporeal membrane oxygenation in selected pediatric respiratory problems. J Thorac Cardiovasc Surg 98:968, 1989.
30. Weber TR, Connors RH, Tracy TF Jr, et al.: Prognostic determinants in extracorporeal membrane oxygenation for respiratory failure in newborn. Ann Thorac Surg 50:720, 1990.
31. Roland Eh, Floodmark O, Hill A: Thalamic hemorrhage with intraventricular hemorrhage in the full-term newborn. Pediatrics 85:737, 1990.
32. Trounce JO, Dodd KL, Fawer CL, et al.: Primary thalamic haemorrhage in the newborn: A new clinical entity. Lancet i:190, 1985.
33. Wehberg K, Vincent M, Garrison B, et al.: Intraventricular hemorrhage in the full-term neonate associated with abdominal compression. Pediatrics 89:327, 1992.

34. Lacey DJ, Terplan K: Intraventricular hemorrhage in full-term neonates. Pediatrics 75:714, 1983.

35. Humphreys RP, Hoffman HJ, Mustarde WT, et al.: Cerebral hemorrhage following heart surgery. J Neurosurg 43:671, 1975.

36. Young RSK, Leberthson RR, Lalneraitis EL: Cerebral hemorrhage in neonates with coarctation of the aorta. Stroke 13:491, 1982.

37. Glauser TA, Rorke LB, Winberg PM, et al.: Acquired neuropathologic lesions associated with hypoplastic left heart syndrome. Pediatrics 85:991, 1990.

38. Packer RJ, Rorke LB, Lange BJ, et al.: Cerebrovascular accidents in children with cancer. Pediatrics 76:194, 1985.

39. Creutzig U, Ritter J, Budde M, et al.: Early deaths due to hemorrhage and leukostasis in childhood acute monocytic leukemia. Associations with hyperleukocytosis and acute monocytic leukemia. Cancer 60:3071, 1987.

40. Renaudin JW, George RP: Coagulopathies causing intracranial hemorrhage. In Wilkins RH, Rengachary SS (eds): Neurosurgery. New York, McGraw-Hill, 1985, pp 1518–1520.

41. see No. 43.

42. Packer RJ: Cerebrovascular accident related to cancer. In Edwards MSB, Hoffman HJ (eds): Cerebral Vascular Disease in Children and Adolescents. Baltimore, Williams & Wilkins 1989, p 430.

43. King K, Kornreich H, Bernadin B, et al.: The clinical spectrum of SLE in childhood. Arthritis Rheum 20:287, 1977.

44. Cunningham S, Conway EE Jr.: Systemic lupus erythematosus presenting as an intracranial bleed. Ann Emerg Med 20:810, 1991.

45. Toffol GJ, Biller J, Adams HP Jr.: Nontraumatic intracerebral hemorrhage in young adults. Arch Neurol 44:485, 1987.

46. Kaku DA, Lowenstein DH: Emergence of recreational drug abuse as a major risk factor for stroke in young adults. Ann Intern Med 113:821, 1990.

47. Forman HP, Levin S, Stewart B, et al.: Cerebral vasculitis and hemorrhage in an adolescent taking diet pills containing phenylpropanolamine: Case report and review of the literature. Pediatrics 83:737, 1989.

48. Tung H, Giannotta SL, Chandrasoma PT, Zee CS: Recurrent intraparenchymal hemorrhages from angiographically occult vascular malformations. J Neurosurg 73:174, 1990.

Chapter 44

INTERVENTIONAL NEURORADIOLOGY

MICHEL E. MAWAD, M.D.

Interventional neuroradiologic procedures have rapidly been accepted as a form of or an adjunct to other therapies in the successful treatment of vascular malformations and neoplasms of the head and neck. Significant progress has been made in the understanding of central nervous system vascular disease processes and their repercussions on brain development and the hemodynamics of cerebrospinal fluid. Similarly, important technical advances have been achieved in the field of microcatheters and embolic devices, allowing for the treatment of lesions that heretofore have been considered technically inaccessible or beyond the realm of endovascular treatment. However, our knowledge of the natural history of many of the vascular dysplasias afflicting both adults and children remains limited and affects our ability to determine the indications for treatment particularly in the asymptomatic patient.

The ideal and most effective endovascular treatment is that which is fully integrated with the other therapeutic modalities such as surgery or radiosurgery. The successful outcome of any combined treatment depends heavily on a close cooperation between the interventional neuroradiologist, the neurosurgeon, the radiation therapist, and the anesthesiologist within the framework of a team approach.

METHODOLOGY

A wide variety of delivery systems is available in the form of coaxial catheters that are typically positioned in the internal carotid or vertebral arteries. In the pediatric age group these coaxial delivery catheters range in size from 4 to 6 French, depending on the size of the patient and that of the femoral artery.

Smaller microcatheters necessary to access the small branches of the internal carotid, external carotid or vertebral arteries are introduced through the coaxial guiding catheter. These microcatheters are usually of variable stiffness and can be advanced in the intracranial circulation over a flexible guidewire[1, 2] (Tracker-18 catheter, Target Therapeutics), or they can be carried by the blood flow[3] to a close proximity with the vascular lesion (Magic catheter, Balt Extrusion; Mini Torquer catheter, Ingenor).

Modified thrombolysis microcatheters have been developed with added side holes for the purpose of effectively delivering thrombolytic agents such as Urokinase or recombinant tissue plasminogen activator (r-TPA) inside a blood clot.

The embolic materials used vary with the type of vascular lesion being embolized and the goal of the devascularization procedure.

Two categories of embolic agents are currently being used in the treatment of vascular neoplasms or arteriovenous malformations (AVMs): particulate emboli and liquid adhesives.

The particulate emboli most widely used are polyvinyl alcohol (PVA)[4] in the powder form ranging in size from 50 to 1000 μm (Contour Emboli, Interventional Therapeutics Company). They produce vascular thrombosis associated with an inflammatory reaction that is not permanent. Other particulate emboli used are Gelfoam powder (Upjohn) and Microfibrillary Collagen (Medchem Products).

The liquid adhesive most commonly used in the treatment of AVMs and arteriovenous fistulas (AVFs) is *N*-butyl-2-cyanoacrylate[5] (NBCA, Tri-Point Medical), which polymerizes on contact with blood. Its polymerization time can be prolonged by the admixture of oily iodinated contrast medium such as iophendylate (Pantopaque, Lafayette Pharmacal). When properly used, NBCA allows excellent penetration of the nidus of the AVM/AVF and thus permanent occlusion.

Traumatic or spontaneous direct AVFs are best

treated utilizing detachable latex or silicone balloons.[6] The balloon is mounted on a flexible soft microcatheter and detached across the fistula using a valve system that varies according to the manufacturer. The goal of the treatment is to occlude the fistula while preserving the parent artery. Complete occlusion of the parent artery as a means of treatment is reserved for those instances in which preservation of the vessel is not possible.

Platinum microcoils,[7] with or without Dacron fibers, are embolic devices used for the occlusion of fistulas or vessels. They are pushed into the desired site of occlusion through a microcatheter or they can be injected with a syringe.

Guglielmi detachable coils[8, 9] (GDC, Target Therapeutics) are the newest embolic device used primarily at the present time for the electrocoagulation of aneurysms. A 0.5-milliampere DC current is used to produce electrothrombosis of the aneurysm and the controlled detachment of the platinum coil from the stainless steel delivery wire.

NOMENCLATURE AND INDICATIONS FOR TREATMENT

The indications for treatment of CNS vascular malformations rely on a thorough understanding of their pathology and natural history.

As mentioned earlier, our knowledge of the natural history of certain vascular malformations is limited and somewhat hinders our ability to set comprehensive indications for treatment. Conversely, the adjunct of magnetic resonance imaging (MRI) to computed tomographic (CT) scanning and cerebral angiography has added valuable information in the characterization of vascular malformations, particularly malformations that are angiographically occult.

Arteriovenous malformations (AVMs) are vascular malformations[10] with identifiable feeding arteries, an intervening nidus, and draining veins resulting in rapid arteriovenous shunting. AVMs can be solitary or multiple, particularly in the pediatric age group. They can be associated with direct *arteriovenous fistulas* (AVFs) within the nidus proper. These same fistulas can exist alone, without the coexistence of an AVM. The ideal treatment of an AVM is endovascular obliteration of the nidus using the liquid adhesive NBCA. If complete cure is not achieved, the endovascular treatment is followed by surgical excision or radiosurgery, depending on the size or location of the remaining nidus.

Cavernous vascular malformations[11, 12] or cavernomas are made of capillary or venous sinusoidal channels filled with clotted blood and not containing intervening neural or glial tissue. They are occult at angiography and do not produce any arteriovenous shunting. They have a rather diagnostic appearance on MRI and can be familial, especially when they are multiple. They can produce repetitive episodes of parenchymal or intraventricular hemorrhage, and when accessible, they should be removed surgically. The effectiveness of radiosurgery on these cavernous lesions is not widely accepted, although it has been tried on deep lesions that have produced prior cerebral hemorrhage.

Venous angiomas[11, 12] are not vascular malformations, but rather an anomalous venous drainage of a certain region of the brain, either superficial or, more often, deep. They have a characteristic appearance on CT, MRI, and angiography and are easily recognizable. The venous channels constituting the angioma and the corresponding large draining vein are histologically normal. Since surgical excision of venous angiomas may deprive adjacent brain from its venous drainage, operation should be carefully considered. In the rare instances when bleeding occurs as the result of a venous angioma, surgical intervention should be strictly limited to the evacuation of the hematoma.

Dural arteriovenous fistulas in the pediatric age group are usually acquired, with arterial blood supply usually arising from both meningeal branches of the external carotid system, as well as pial branches of the internal carotid or vertebral arteries. They are often associated with significant dysplastic dilatation of the draining veins. Their endovascular treatment is often difficult and palliative at best.

Vascular malformations of the vein of Galen[13–15] have been subdivided by Lasjaunias et al. into vein of Galen aneurysmal malformation (VGAM) and vein of Galen aneurysmal dilatation (VGAD). The VGAM is divided into two different types: *choroidal* VGAM, whereby the feeding anterior and posterior choroidal arteries supply fistula(s) located in the velum interpositum, and *mural* VGAM, whereby the feeding collicular and posterior choroidal arteries supply fistula(s) located in the wall of the median vein of the prosencephalon (MVP). Both types of VGAM drain into the embryonic precursor of the vein of Galen, which is the MVP. This dilated vein does not drain normal brain and does not communicate with normal cerebral veins. VGAD is simply a dilated vein of Galen, which drains a deep AVM of the brain or the superior aspect of the cerebellum. Here the dilated vein of Galen receives venous tributaries draining the deep AVM and adjacent normal structures. The dilatation of the vein of Galen is secondary to an acquired stricture of the venous outflow.

SPINAL AVMs/AVFs[16, 17]

Spinal vascular malformations are divided into several groups according to the location of the arteriovenous shunt, the origin of the feeding arteries, and the nature of the venous drainage. The three major categories include: intramedullary AVMs, perimedullary AVFs, and dural AVFs. The vast majority of spinal vascular malformations in the pediatric age group are of the intramedullary AVM type. They consist of a nidus located within the substance of the spinal cord supplied by either radiculomedullary or radiculopial branches and draining into medullary veins. These lesions are often located in the cervical or upper thoracic spinal cord and present with either a catastrophic intramedullary hemorrhage or a progressive myelopathy. Dural AVFs are rare in the pediatric age group; they usually present in the fifth or sixth decade and are more common in men. In addition to MRI and water-soluble myelography, spinal arteriography is essential for the characterization of spinal vascular malformations and for determining the optimal modality of their treatment.

ENDOVASCULAR TREATMENT

The ideal treatment of an AVM is its elimination, either by surgical excision or by radiosurgery. When possible, endovascular devascularization is performed as a preliminary step prior to either of these two therapeutic modalities to improve their results. In a small number of AVMs (about 10 per cent in our material), embolization therapy suffices as the sole and definitive treatment, resulting in complete and permanent obliteration of the vascular malformation. The liquid adhesive NBCA[18, 19] is the ideal embolic agent to use to obtain permanent obliteration of the nidus and, therefore, cure of the lesion. A small flow-guided catheter is utilized to achieve superselective catheterization of the nidus and deposition of the liquid adhesive with minimal or no reflux of the embolic mixture into the feeding pedicle or the draining vein. If, during the embolization, the nidus is obliterated, a small amount of glue can be deposited into the proximal draining vein to ensure elimination of the arteriovenous shunting.

In cases of large but surgically accessible AVMs for which surgical excision is contemplated as the form of treatment, staged embolization procedures using NBCA are performed to reduce the size of the vascular malformation, decrease the arteriovenous shunting, and allow for complete surgical removal. The goal of the endovascular treatment remains always to deeply penetrate the nidus with the liquid adhesive. The embolization procedures are staged and separated by intervals of time ranging in duration from 6 to 8 weeks. The purpose of staging the treatment sessions is to avoid rapid changes of the hemodynamics in the cerebral circulation and potential cerebral hemorrhage.

Deep AVMs that are not surgically accessible or are too large to be completely cured by endovascular therapy alone can be effectively treated by a combination of embolization procedure(s) followed by focused radiation therapy (Fig. 44–1). The same technique of deep penetration of the nidus with liquid adhesive is used as a preliminary adjunct to radiation therapy. When the deep AVM is large, the embolization procedures are staged over a period of time. The focused radiation therapy can be performed using either a gamma knife apparatus or a linear accelerator. Focused radiation therapy as the sole treatment of AVMs or when combined with endovascular therapy has the major drawback of the latency of its results, which varies from 18 to 36 months. During this period of time,

the patient is not completely protected from the risk of hemorrhage. In addition, a series of follow-up imaging studies such as MRI, preferably combined with magnetic resonance angiography, are necessary to assess the progression of the obliteration of the AVM. Ultimately, a follow-up conventional angiogram at about 24 months following the radiation treatment is necessary to verify the obliteration of the vascular malformation or its lack thereof. The endovascular treatment of VGAM and VGAD[20] has been established by Lasjaunias based on anatomic and embryologic observations made by Raybaud. The indications for treatment remain complex and beyond the scope of this chapter; they take into consideration the cardiac function of the child or newborn, the size of the ventricular system, the neurologic development of the child, and a close scrutiny of the anatomy of the malformation including its arterial feeders and the complexity of its venous drainage. When the endovascular treatment becomes indicated, the ideal technique consists of direct injection of pure NBCA via an arterial approach into one or several of the fistulas draining into the dilated vein of Galen. The direct transtorcular or retrograde transjugular venous approach using thrombogenic coils is reserved as an alternative second best treatment, to be given only when the intra-arterial injection of NBCA is not possible.

Pediatric spinal AVMs presenting with intramedullary hemorrhage or a progressive myelopathy are treated with surgical resection, embolization alone, or a combination of endovascular treatment followed by surgical resection. Once again, the ideal endovascular treatment of these difficult lesions is adequate and deep penetration of the nidus using NBCA. The nidus is selectively accessed through a radiculomedullary or radiculopial artery by means of a microcatheter, allowing for selective deposition of the liquid adhesive in the intramedullary vascular lesion (Fig. 44–2). Careful and exhaustive spinal angiography is performed prior to the embolization to better delineate the normal arterial spinal axis of the spinal cord and to avoid inadvertent escape of the embolic material into normal vessels. Occasionally, particulate emboli such as PVA are used in the embolization of spinal vascular malformations as a preoperative devascularization procedure or as a palliative measure. Recanalization of the vascular malformation remains the major disadvantage of particulate emboli.

CONCLUSION

Endovascular therapeutic procedures have become one of many important tools the neurosurgeon has at his disposal to treat cerebral and spinal vascular malformations in the pediatric age group. The interventional neuroradiologist has and must become an important member of an interdisciplinary team evaluating patients with vascular malformations and offering an intelligent course of treatment. This may include endo-

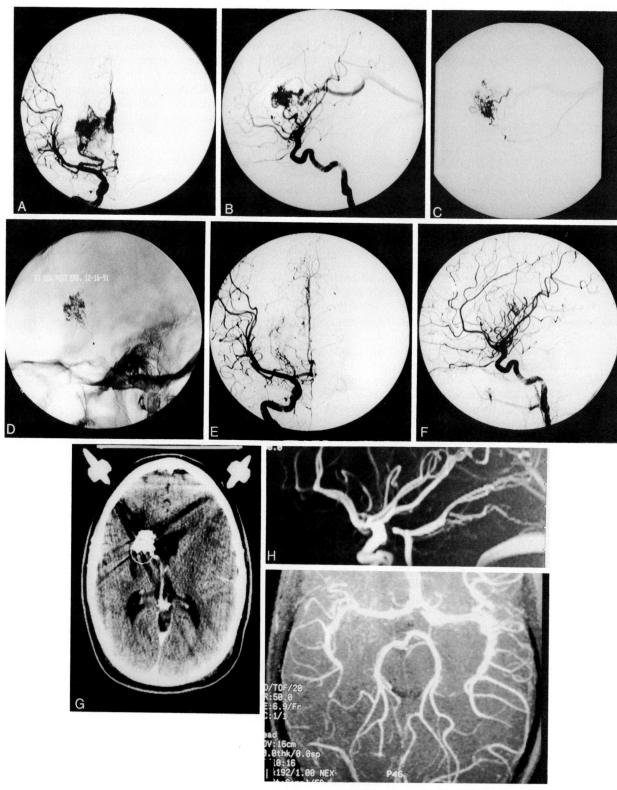

FIGURE 44–1 *See legend on opposite page*

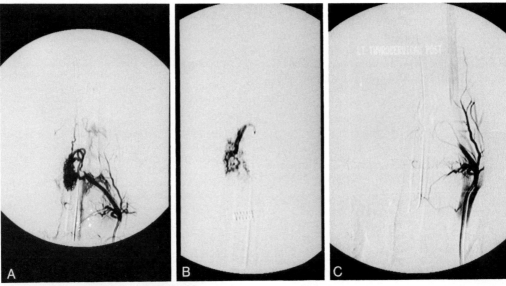

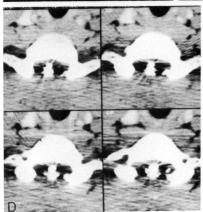

FIGURE 44–2. Juvenile intramedullary arteriovenous malformation of the cervical spinal cord treated by endovascular approach. *A,* Pre-embolization selective arteriogram of the thyrocervical trunk showing the glomus-type intramedullary arteriovenous malformation, supplied by cervical radiculomedullary branches of the left thyrocervical trunk. *B,* Superselective injection of the radiculomedullary branches feeding the arteriovenous malformation with good delineation of the intramedullary nidus. *C,* Postembolization left thyrocervical trunk arteriogram showing complete obliteration of the intramedullary vascular malformation and absence of arteriovenous shunting. *D,* Postembolization noncontrast axial CT studies of the cervical spine, showing the radiopaque cast of *N*-butyl-cyanoacrylate within the intramedullary arteriovenous malformation. The laminectomy defects relate to a prior unsuccessful surgical attempt at resecting the vascular malformation.

FIGURE 44–1. Deep arteriovenous malformation of the basal ganglia treated by a combination of embolization and stereotactic radiation therapy. *A* and *B,* AP and lateral views of the right internal carotid arteriogram showing the deep basal ganglionic arteriovenous malformation supplied by large lenticulostriate branches and draining into the deep venous system. *C,* Superselective arteriogram of the deep lenticulostriate feeder, using a flow-guided microcatheter. Note the selective opacification of the nidus of the vascular malformation and the early draining deep internal cerebral vein. *D,* Lateral view of the skull showing the radiopaque cast of *N*-butyl-cyanoacrylate selectively embolized in the nidus of the arteriovenous malformation. *E* and *F,* Postembolization AP and lateral views of a right internal carotid arteriogram shows almost complete obliteration of the vascular malformation and significant reduction in the degree of arteriovenous shunting. *G,* Postcontrast axial CT of the brain obtained during a localization study for subsequent stereotactic radiation therapy treatment of the residue of the arteriovenous malformation. *H* and *I,* Follow-up magnetic resonance angiographic studies of the head 6 months after the combined embolization/radiation treatment showing complete obliteration of the vascular malformation.

vascular therapy alone, surgical resection, focused radiation therapy, or any combination of these three therapeutic modalities. The continuing advances in the development of microcatheters, guidewires, and embolic materials and devices have opened new horizons in the management of cerebral and spinal vascular conditions.

REFERENCES

1. Wolpert SM, Kwan ESK, Heros D, Kasdon DL, Hedges TR: Selective delivery of chemotherapeutic agents with a new catheter system. Radiology 166:547, 1988.
2. Kikuchiy, Stroyher CM, Boyer M: New catheter for endovascular interventional procedures. Radiology 165:870, 1987.
3. Dion JE, Duckwiler GR, Lylyk P, Vinuela F, Bentson J: Progressive suppleness pursil catheter: a new tool for super-selective angiography and embolization. AJNR 11:657, 1989.
4. Scialfa G, Scotti G: Superselective injection of polyvinyl alcohol microemboli for the treatment of cerebral arteriovenous malformations. AJNR 6:957, 1985.
5. Brothers MF, Kaufman JCE, Fox AJ, Deveikis JP: N-Butyl-2 Cyanoacrylate substitute for IBCA in interventional neuroradiology. Histopathologic and polymerization time studies. AJNR 10:777, 1989.
6. Debrun G, Lacour P, Caron J: Detachable balloon and calibrated leak balloon techniques in the treatment of cerebral vascular lesions. J Neurosurg 49:635, 1978.
7. Hilal SK, Khandji AG, Chi TL, Stein BM, Bello JM, Silver AJ: Synthetic fiber coated platinum coils successfully used for endovascular treatment of arteriovenous malformations, aneurysms and direct arteriovenous fistulas of CNS. AJNR 9:1030, 1988.
8. Guglielmi G, Vinuela F, Sepetka I, et al.: Electrothrombosis of saccular aneurysms via endovascular approach. Part I: Electrochemical basis, technique and experimental results. J Neurosurg 75:1, 1991.
9. Guglielmi G, Vinuela F, Dion J, Duckwiler G: Electrothrombosis of saccular aneurysms via endovascular approach. Part II: Preliminary clinical experience. J Neurosurg 75:8, 1991.
10. McCormick WF: The pathology of vascular ("arteriovenous") malformations. J Neurosurg 24:807, 1966.
11. McCormick WF: Pathology of vascular malformations of the brain. In Wilson CB, Stein BM (eds): Intracranial Arteriovenous Malformations. Baltimore, Williams & Wilkins, 1984, pp 44–63.
12. McCormick WF: The pathology of angiomas. In Fein JM, Flamm ES (eds): Cerebrovascular Surgery, Vol IV. New York, Springer-Verlag, 1985, pp 1073–1095.
13. Lasjaunias P, Terbrugge K, Piske R, Lopez-Ibor L, Manelfe C: Dilatation de la veine de Galien. Formes anatomo-cliniques et traitements endovasculaires a propos de 14 cas explores et/ou traites entre 1983 et 1986. Neurochirurgie 133:315, 1987.
14. Raybaud C, Strother C, Hald J: Aneurysms of the vein of Galen: Embryologic considerations and anatomical features relating to the pathogenesis of the malformation. Neuroradiology 31:109, 1989.
15. Lasjaunias P, Garcia-Monaco R, Rodesch G, Terbrugge K: Deep venous drainage in great cerebral vein (vein of Galen) absence and malformations. Neuroradiology 33:234, 1991.
16. Rosenblum B, Olfield EH, Doppman JL, Dichiro G: Spinal arteriovenous malformations: a comparison of dural arteriovenous fistulas and intradural AVMs in 81 patients. J Neurosurg 67:795, 1987.
17. Riche MC, Modenesi-Freitas J, Djindjian M: Arteriovenous malformations of the spinal cord in children. A review of 38 cases. Neuroradiology 22:171, 1982.
18. Pelz DM, Fox AJ, Vinuela F, et al.: Preoperative embolization of brain AVMs with Isobutyl-2-cyanoacrylate. AJNR 9(4):757, 1988.
19. Debrun G, Vinuela F, Fox AJ, et al.: Embolization of cerebral arteriovenous malformations with bucrylate: experience in 46 cases. J Neurosurg 56:615, 1982.
20. Lasjaunias P: Arteriovenous fistulas of the brain. In Berenstein A, Lasjaunias P (eds): Surgical Neuro-Angiography, Vol IV. New York, Springer-Verlag, 1992, pp 270–308.

PART VII

APPLICATION OF NEWER TECHNOLOGIES

Chapter 45

SURGICAL TREATMENT OF EPILEPSY

WARWICK J. PEACOCK, M.D., and STEVEN N. ROPER, M.D.

Epilepsy is the most common neurologic disorder of childhood, and despite the potential for surgical management, it is only recently that surgical methods have been used in its treatment. The first surgical resection on an adult patient suffering from seizures was performed in 1886 by Sir Victor Horsley.[1] Operative surgery for intractable epilepsy was almost exclusively reserved for adults in whom temporal lobectomy became the most common procedure. Protocols for the selection, investigation, and treatment of candidates for surgery have been designed for adults with little thought for the needs of children.[2] Since the evolution of the new subspecialties of pediatric neurology and pediatric neurosurgery, those treating childhood seizures have become reluctant to watch the inevitable intellectual deterioration or arrest in development of children suffering from intractable seizures. It has become clear that the first few years of life constitute a critical period for brain maturation and also a time of maximal plasticity during which functional recovery from structural damage can occur.

During the first 8 years of life, the degree of connectivity between neurons in the brain increases enormously, as a result of dendritic branching and dendritic spine formation. Huttenlocher[3, 4] has shown that synaptic density reaches a maximum by about the eighth year and then, by a process of selective elimination of synapses, synaptic density is reduced and a plateau is reached by about the 14th year. Axonal growth cones, which will form the presynaptic terminals, navigate toward their specific synaptic site, apparently dependent upon appropriate electrical fields.[5] Frequent seizure activity may well interfere with this accurately guided migration, resulting in either incorrect or reduced synapse formation. As a full complement of anatomically correct synapses is the substrate for psychomotor development, the interference due to seizure activity may be the cause of the developmental arrest and mental retardation associated with early-onset intractable seizures. The fact that frequent epileptogenic activity may interfere with maturation in young children is the single most important concept involved in surgical considerations.

The greater degree of plasticity in the young brain is another important factor. Structural damage in the developing brain is associated with a much greater degree of functional recovery than would be found with a similar lesion in an adult. Villablanca performed left-sided hemispherectomies in kittens and adult cats. Although the kittens made a complete functional recovery, in the adult cats a noticeable hemiparesis persisted. He showed that in the cats that had undergone hemispherectomy as kittens, the remaining right hemisphere had connections with both sides of the brainstem and spinal cord, whereas in the cats who had undergone hemispherectomy as adults, the unusually great number of ipsilateral connections were not present.[6–8] Similarly, if the hemisphere dominant for speech is removed before the age of about 8 to 9 years, the remaining hemisphere has the ability to compensate and speech will return. However, speech is unlikely to recover if the dominant hemisphere is removed after about the age of 9 years.[9–14]

Because intractable seizures during the first 4 years of life may interfere with cerebral maturation and because marked plasticity is a feature during this time period, it is clearly wiser to perform the surgery as early as is reasonably possible. According to adult protocols, a certain minimum waiting period is advised, usually 2 to 3 years.[15, 16] In a child aged 3 months with the Sturge-Weber syndrome, who is having 60 seizures per day despite carefully planned anticonvulsant medication, waiting would be most inappropriate. It has been shown that in this situation the only hope of preventing severe mental retardation is to operate as soon as the seizures have been found to be unresponsive to

547

medication.[17] In adults with temporal lobe epilepsy, a seizure frequency of only one to two seizures per month may be sufficient for surgical consideration. Because of this low frequency, proving that the seizures are intractable despite the use of all available anticonvulsants may take a prolonged period of time; it may require months to decide that one drug has failed before switching to another. However, in young children the seizure frequency is often 40 to 100 seizures per day, and the repertoire of anticonvulsant medications available for many of the childhood seizure syndromes is limited. Therefore, establishing intractability may only require a few weeks.[18] In addition, if a structural abnormality such as cortical dysplasia,[15] Rasmussen's encephalitis,[19, 20] the Sturge-Weber syndrome,[17] or diffuse unihemispheral cystic gliosis is found, unresponsiveness to anticonvulsant medications is almost inevitable.

ETIOLOGIC FACTORS IN CHILDHOOD EPILEPSY

GENETIC FACTORS

Although tuberous sclerosis is the only pediatric epileptic syndrome to have a clearly Mendelian dominant type of inheritance pattern, an inherited predisposition is suspected in many other forms of childhood epilepsy.

INTRAUTERINE INSULTS

Because the histopathologic picture often appears identical no matter what the cause, it is frequently difficult to identify the etiologic factor in intrauterine insults. Metabolic, infective, traumatic, and vascular disorders may induce the structural changes that predispose to seizure activity. Neuroblasts migrate from the germinal layer which lines the ventricular wall out to the cortical surface between the 8th and the 20th weeks of intrauterine life. Defects of migration lead to the formation of gray matter heterotopias and cortical dysplasia.[21] Cortical dysplasia is characterized by the presence of bizarrely shaped cells that are incorrectly aligned with each other in a nonlaminated cortex with a poorly defined gray/white matter junction. Cortical dysplasia is frequently found to be the cause of infantile spasms.[22]

PERINATAL FACTORS

Although insults to the brain sustained in the perinatal period (for example, anoxic-ischemic insults and cortical contusions) often lead to hydrocephalus, cerebral palsy, and mental retardation, seizure disorders are a less common end result.

INFECTIOUS AND INFLAMMATORY CAUSES

Herpes encephalitis may produce focal cortical damage leading to surgically treatable epilepsy, but bacterial meningitis is more likely to produce diffuse cortical damage. Therefore, when epilepsy results from bacterial meningitis, surgical management is unlikely to be feasible. Rasmussen's encephalitis is a chronic progressive encephalitis restricted to one hemisphere which ultimately becomes atrophic.[19, 20] There is some debate as to whether a viral or autoimmune process is causative. In many countries, neurocysticercosis is a common cause of seizures in childhood.

VASCULAR ABNORMALITIES

Infarction in the territory of the middle cerebral artery is a relatively common finding in children with the infantile hemiplegia seizure syndrome. A wedge-shaped defect involving the frontal, parietal, and temporal lobes is characteristically seen on computed tomography (CT) and magnetic resonance imaging (MRI) scans. The cerebral abnormality found in the Sturge-Weber syndrome is a pial angiomatosis, which may involve the entire cortical surface of one hemisphere or only part of its surface. The underlying cortex is dysplastic and undergoes atrophy and calcification during the first few years of life. Arteriovenous malformations are occasionally found to be the cause of seizures in children.

TRAUMA

Cortical contusions or lacerations sustained as a result of closed head injury or depressed skull fracture may lead to cortical scarring and produce a focal cause of seizures.

NEOPLASMS

Low-grade astrocytomas, gangliogliomas, ganglioneuromas, and hamartomas are well described as treatable causes of childhood epilepsy, especially in the temporal lobe. Although there is much evidence to suggest that complete tumor removal alone is sufficient not only to cure the tumor but also to eliminate the seizures, debate continues as to whether tissue surrounding the tumor should be excised as well.

FEBRILE SEIZURES

The large percentage of patients with temporal lobe epilepsy who report febrile seizures in childhood raises the possibility that there is a causal relationship between the two conditions. A recent, prospective study, however, has failed to demonstrate such a causal relationship.[23] At this time, it seems that both conditions may be manifestations of an underlying defect that predisposes a patient to seizures.

PEDIATRIC SEIZURE TYPES

The International League Against Epilepsy (ILAE) has established a standardized classification of seizure types.[24] It consists of (1) partial seizures—which include simple partial, complex partial, and partial seizures with secondary generalization, and (2) generalized seizures—which include absence, atypical absence, myoclonic, clonic, tonic, tonic-clonic, and atonic seizures. Partial seizures are those in which the first clinical manifestations can be localized to a single hemisphere with a corresponding localization on electroencephalography (EEG). Generalized seizures have clinical onsets that suggest activation of both hemispheres. Complex seizures cause an alteration in consciousness, whereas simple seizures do not. Symptomatic seizures have a discernible underlying structural defect, whereas idiopathic seizures have no such defect. These definitions are, of course, dependent on the current state of our ability to detect these defects.

Several seizure types are seen frequently when dealing with surgical treatment of childhood epilepsy. Infantile spasms are described in the section on West's syndrome. They are classified as generalized seizures. However, as has been shown with current techniques, a subset of these patients can be defined with localized, structural deficits whose seizures can be cured or greatly improved by resection of the cortical abnormality. Simple partial seizures create the greatest problem when they affect the primary motor cortex. Epilepsia partialis continua is a continual maintenance of this type of seizure. It is seen most frequently in cases of Rasmussen's encephalitis. Complex partial seizures occur in the pediatric age group just as in adults and most commonly involve the temporal lobe. "Drop attacks" deserve special mention as they constitute the most common indication for corpus callosotomy. These injurious episodes involve loss of postural control to the point that the patient falls or is propelled to the ground. They may result from atonic seizures, tonic seizures, or episodes of myoclonus followed by atonia. Currently it is difficult to tell if all types of drop attacks respond equally to callosal sectioning, but improved attention to these details in surgical series should make this information available in the near future. Status epilepticus is the continuation of any seizure beyond 30 minutes, without regaining consciousness during this time. In rare instances, these episodes are not controlled even by high doses of intravenous barbiturates, and under these conditions surgical intervention may be indicated if the epileptogenic region is clearly documented.[25]

SEIZURE SYNDROMES OF CHILDHOOD THAT MAY BENEFIT FROM SURGERY

Although many pediatric seizure types such as petit mal or benign rolandic seizures are unlikely ever to benefit from surgery, there are certain seizure syndromes that result from a focal abnormality which can be resected. In others, the bilateral spread of seizure activity, which is essential for the manifestation of the clinical seizure, can be prevented by dividing the corpus callosum. A brief description of the childhood seizure syndromes that may benefit from surgery follows.

HEMICONVULSIONS, HEMIPLEGIA, EPILEPSY SYNDROME (INFANTILE HEMIPLEGIA SEIZURE SYNDROME)

This syndrome is characterized by the onset of a seizure involving the face, arm, and leg on one side during the first 2 years of life.[26, 27] Following the seizure, a permanent hemiplegia is noted to affect the side involved by the seizure. Eventually chronic seizures persist. In most cases they are complex partial seizures, but simple partial and secondarily generalized seizures also occur. Up to 80 per cent of the patients become mentally retarded.[26] The chronic seizures are often difficult to control, and surgical therapy may be indicated. Hemispherectomy is the appropriate procedure.

STURGE-WEBER SYNDROME

The Sturge-Weber syndrome, or encephalo-trigeminal-angiomatosis, is defined by a facial nevus, leptomeningeal angiomatosis, seizures, hemiplegia, and mental retardation.[28] Glaucoma is also seen in a significant number of cases. The "port wine stain" of the face usually involves the ophthalmic branch of the trigeminal nerve but may have a wider distribution. The leptomeningeal angiomatosis may cover an entire hemisphere or may be more localized. With time the abnormal vessels calcify, producing the characteristic "train track" appearance on plain radiographs. Seizures almost always begin in the first year of life and are frequently refractory to medical therapy. Progressive hemiparesis soon follows, often accompanied by hemianopsia. Hemispherectomy is the most common surgical procedure for these intractable cases although focal cortical resections have been described in cases with more limited cortical involvement.[17] Some familial clustering has been reported, but no clear genetic pattern of transmission has been determined.[29]

TUBEROUS SCLEROSIS

Tuberous sclerosis is a neurocutaneous syndrome with an autosomal dominant inheritance pattern.[30] It is a disorder of cellular migration and differentiation that affects the brain, retina, skin, kidneys, and lungs. Major diagnostic features of the syndrome include cortical tubers, subependymal nodules, giant cell astrocytomas in the brain, retinal hamartomas, facial angiofibromas (adenoma sebaceum), ungual fibromas, and multiple angiolipomas of the kidneys. Other frequent findings are hypomelanotic skin macules (including "ash-leaf spots") and rhabdomyomas of the heart. Neurologic manifestations of tuberous sclerosis include seizures, mental retardation, and motor deficits. Seizures occur in up to 92 per cent of these patients and usually present in the first year of life.[31] The seizures are most commonly focal motor seizures and infantile spasms. Older children often display complex partial and generalized tonic-clonic seizures. Cortical tubers are seen most clearly on MRI scans.[32] In some intractable cases, the area of epileptogenesis can be localized to a particular tuber. These patients are candidates for surgical resection of the tuber for seizure control. Although many tubers are evident by visual appearance and firm textures, intraoperative ultrasonography is also valuable in defining the extent of the lesion at surgery. Pathologic examination of the tubers shows disruption of the normal cortical cytoarchitecture, decreased myelination, giant neurons and astrocytes, and cells of indeterminate origin, which show immunohistologic markers for both neurons and astrocytes.[33] The frequent occurrence of multiple widespread lesions throughout the brain makes these patients challenging management problems.

Hemimegalencephaly/Epidermal Nevus Syndrome

Hemimegalencephaly is a rare congenital anomaly characterized by the diffuse enlargement of an entire cerebral hemisphere,[34] which is associated with seizures, hemiparesis, and mental retardation. These patients frequently have facial hemihypertrophy ipsilateral to the enlarged hemisphere. The seizures usually occur in the first months of life, and a large proportion are infantile spasms.[35] Many of these patients develop a neurocutaneous disorder termed the epidermal nevus syndrome. In addition to brain findings, there are skin lesions in the form of raised ovoid or linear plaques, and the eyes and musculoskeletal system may also be involved.[35] When surgery is indicated for intractable seizures, hemispherectomy is almost always the required procedure. The increased volume of the hemisphere makes functional hemispherectomy slightly awkward but otherwise presents no significant problems. Pathologic study of the involved hemisphere reveals gyral abnormalities, such as pachygyria or polymicrogyria, heterotopic gray matter, disordered cortical cytoarchitecture, and giant neurons and astrocytes.[36] The etiology of the syndrome is unknown, and no genetic transmission has been identified.

West's Syndrome

West's syndrome is defined by a specific seizure type (infantile spasms), hypsarrhythmia on EEG, and mental retardation. Infantile spasms usually start between 3 and 7 months of age and in most cases will resolve or change into other seizure types by 3 years.[37] The spasms consist of a sudden flexion or extension of the neck, trunk, and extremities. Mixed flexor-extensor spasms are the most common, but pure flexor or extensor spasms do occur.[38] The spasms occur in clusters and often begin on arousal from sleep. A high-amplitude, chaotic pattern called hypsarrhythmia is the most common EEG finding, although variants of the pattern may also be seen. In the symptomatic group, i.e., with seizures secondary to a detectable brain abnormality, the prognosis without surgery is almost uniformly poor including a 20 per cent mortality rate (over a 3- to 19-year follow-up period).[39] These patients develop mental retardation and other refractory seizure disorders, most commonly the Lennox-Gastaut syndrome. Adrenocorticotropic hormone (ACTH) is the most effective medical therapy, although its exact mechanism of action is still unknown. Etiologies are numerous and include dysgenetic, hypoxic-ischemic, infectious, hemorrhagic, traumatic, and metabolic mechanisms. Although the seizures are classified as generalized, a zone of cortical abnormality can be identified based on EEG, MRI, and positron emission tomography (PET) in some patients with intractable seizures. Surgical resection has produced good to excellent results.[40] These cases dramatically emphasize the fact that a focal cortical abnormality can produce an ictal phenomenon that appears generalized. The majority of the surgical cases have required tailored parieto-occipito-temporal resections.[41]

Lennox-Gastaut Syndrome

The Lennox-Gastaut syndrome is also strongly age-related, with a peak incidence between 1 and 7 years of age. It is defined by multiple seizure types including drop attacks, a slow spike and wave pattern on EEG, and mental retardation. It is often preceded by earlier seizures, with up to 25 per cent of patients having had infantile spasms earlier in life.[37] The constellation of seizure types is varied, but tonic or atonic drop attacks, atypical absence, and myoclonic seizures occur most commonly. The characteristic interictal EEG recording consists of diffuse slow spike and wave complexes that occur at a rate of 1 to 3 Hz. Mental retardation forms a prominent part of the clinical picture with up to 72 per cent of symptomatic cases being severely retarded.[42] Etiologies are numerous and include many of the factors listed in the section on West's syndrome. The prognosis is poor, especially in symptomatic cases.

Rasmussen's Encephalitis

Rasmussen's encephalitis is a chronic progressive inflammatory disease of unknown etiology involving one cerebral hemisphere.[19, 20] The syndrome consists of intractable simple partial motor seizures with episodes of epilepsia partialis continua. Generalized tonic-clonic seizures also occur sometime in the course of the disease in over half of the patients. The average age of seizure onset is about 6 years with a range from 14 months to 14 years. Progressive hemiplegia and mental deterioration occur over months to years associated with radiologic evidence of atrophy in the involved hemisphere. Anticonvulsant medication has been of little, or only temporary, help in controlling the seizures. Although the clinical course is usually characteristic, a biopsy with histologic evidence of perivascular lymphocytic cuffing is reassuring prior to resective surgery. Repeated limited cortical resections are not advisable. It is preferable to wait until a significant hemiplegia has developed with loss of digital dexterity in the affected hand before performing a hemispherectomy.

PRESURGICAL EVALUATION

HISTORY AND PHYSICAL EXAMINATION

The perinatal history is important in searching for a possible etiology. A precise developmental history, both before and after the onset of seizures, is essential for counseling the family and for establishing realistic expectations for improvement once the seizures are controlled. A family history is always important when dealing with a population that includes genetically transmitted conditions such as tuberous sclerosis. An accurate description of seizure types, duration, and frequency is essential, and factors that ameliorate and exacerbate the seizures should be discussed. A record of previous and current anticonvulsant regimens is necessary to confirm intractability. Neurologic deficits should be noted, and it should be borne in mind that a waxing and waning hemiparesis may actually be a Todd's paralysis in a patient who is in a postictal state most of the time.

A number of the syndromes associated with childhood epilepsy involve other organ systems, especially the skin. All patients with tuberous sclerosis should be evaluated for cardiac rhabdomyomas prior to major surgery.

ELECTROENCEPHALOGRAPHY (EEG)/TELEMETRY

The EEG and telemetry set the foundation for the physiologic evaluation of the patient. Detailed records of both the ictal and interictal states are required. Epileptiform abnormalities in pediatric patients are frequently widespread and multifocal. It is the nonepileptiform abnormalities on EEG that become most helpful in defining the zone of cortical abnormality. These include a focal "burst-suppression" pattern, amplitude attenuation across all frequencies, attenuation of faster frequencies, and polymorphic delta activity.[2] Injection of sodium thiopental induces increased beta activity in surrounding normal cortex and helps to more clearly define the abnormal areas by their impaired beta activation.[2, 40] In patients with drop attacks it is important to correlate EEG, telemetry, and electromyelogra-

phy (EMG) in order to define the physiologic process resulting in the falls.

EVOKED POTENTIALS

Both somatosensory and visual evoked potentials are performed to demonstrate physiologic disturbances in areas of cortical abnormality, but also to test the functional integrity of the opposite hemisphere. Severe dysfunction of the "good" hemisphere may preclude a satisfactory surgical result. Visual evoked potentials are sometimes useful in demonstrating a hemianopsia in uncooperative or very young patients.

NEUROPSYCHOLOGIC EVALUATION

The value of neuropsychologic evaluation in selection and prognostication in the surgical treatment of temporal lobe epilepsy is well established.[43] A number of older children benefit from this process. However, the majority of the younger, more severely affected patients do not function at a level suitable for this type of investigation, and their cognitive testing is incorporated within their developmental evaluations.

STRUCTURAL IMAGING

Many children with intractable seizures have structural lesions that can be seen on CT and/or MRI. The most recent MRI scanners are now able to demonstrate cortical dysgenesis seen in agyria-pachygyria, polymicrogyria, and heterotopic gray matter. The corpus callosum is also clearly seen with MRI. Areas of structural abnormality may correlate with those of functional abnormality to define the area in need of resection.

FUNCTIONAL IMAGING

PET has proved to be of value in the investigation of patients with uncontrollable epilepsy.[40] With use of 2-deoxyglucose, focal cerebral metabolic rates are measured. Areas of focal interictal hypometabolism have been shown to correlate well with the zone of cortical abnormality defined by electrocorticography[40] and histopathologic findings.[44]

Single photon emission computed tomography (SPECT) is another way to image functional activity of the brain based on regional blood flow. In adult series, ictal and early postictal SPECT shows focal areas of increased blood flow that correlate with the site of the initiation of the seizure in temporal lobe epilepsy.[45, 46] Interictal SPECT studies have been less promising.

CHRONIC INTRACRANIAL RECORDING/ELECTROCORTICOGRAPHY

In adult epilepsy surgery, in which temporal lobectomy is the most common procedure performed, definition of the area of epileptogenesis often requires the recording of multiple seizures directly from the surface of the brain or via depth electrodes. This is due, in part, to the fact that the location of the hippocampus, deep in the mesial temporal lobe, frequently renders surface recordings inadequate. A number of pediatric epilepsy centers also rely on chronic recordings from either epidural or subdural grids to help define the area of resection.[47–49] There is no question that in some cases this is absolutely necessary. The advantages of chronic recording are (1) it provides a better spatial resolution than scalp electrodes can provide, and (2) it provides the ability to map eloquent brain regions that may be in close proximity to the area in question over multiple testing sessions.

Chronic recordings from implanted electrodes are used less frequently in children than in adults for a number of reasons. The first is because the complication rate of chronic recordings is higher in children than in adults.[47–49] Second, nonepileptiform EEG abnormalities are more useful in children than in adults for defining the zone of cortical abnormality.[40] These areas are often relatively large and can be localized well on scalp EEG. Because they are present in the interictal state, more accurate spatial resolution can then be achieved by intraoperative electrocorticography (ECoG). The same interictal findings listed above for scalp EEG are also used in ECoG to define the abnormal region. A fast-acting barbiturate, such as sodium thiopental, is given intraoperatively to define areas with a loss of beta activation. The additional information obtained from PET scanning also helps to define the abnormal area metabolically without the need for chronic recordings.

SURGICAL TECHNIQUES

HEMISPHERECTOMY

Walter Dandy was the first surgeon to remove a cerebral hemisphere in 1928 from an adult patient with a diffuse right-sided glioma.[50] Ten years later, Kenneth McKenzie performed a right-sided hemispherectomy on a young woman with intractable seizures.[51] It was not until 1950, when Roland Krynauw described his results with 12 children on whom he had performed cerebral hemispherectomies for the infantile hemiplegia seizure syndrome, that a surgical procedure was used for a specifically pediatric seizure disorder.[52] Not only did he note that seizure control was excellent following the procedure, but he was impressed with the degree of functional recovery and the reduction in the aggressive behavior frequently associated with this type of epilepsy.

The number of hemispherectomies grew rapidly until reports of late hemorrhagic complications began to appear in the medical literature. Acute large bleeds into the hemicranial space were reported in 15 to 20 per cent of cases, as well as chronic superficial cerebral hemosiderosis, which was believed to be due to repeated small hemorrhages from a subdural membrane that had formed a lining of the space.[53, 54] Despite the fact that with persistent seizures the outcome from the infantile hemiplegia syndrome was extremely poor, the procedure fell into dispute. A few centers continued to perform hemispherectomy without encountering hemorrhagic complications.

Rasmussen noted that when large but subtotal hemispheral resections had been performed, late hemorrhagic complications did not occur.[55] Thereafter, he devised an ingenious technique, which he called functional hemispherectomy, whereby only the central area and temporal lobe were removed but all projection and commissural fibers from the remaining parts of the hemisphere were divided, achieving the same degree of seizure control without leaving a large space with its associated risks.

Hemispherectomy is considered only for a patient who is having uncontrollable seizures with a unilateral hemiparesis including loss of digital dexterity in the affected hand. The seizures may be partial involving the hemiparetic limbs, secondarily generalized, or primarily generalized. Epileptogenic activity should only arise from the affected hemisphere, and the hemisphere ipsilateral to the hemiplegia should appear normal on structural and functional testing. Even when speech is localized in the abnormal hemisphere, if the resection is performed before the age of 8 or 9 years, speech recovery is likely.[9–14]

The most common causes of the hemiplegia hemiseizure syndrome include infarction in the territory supplied by the middle cerebral artery, Rasmussen's encephalitis, the Sturge-Weber syndrome, hemimegalencephaly, and cortical dysplasia.[17, 19, 20, 56] It must be borne in mind that with the congenital anomalies and cerebral infarction, functional recovery from the hemiplegia is frequently so well developed by the time surgery is undertaken that little change is noted in the affected limbs following hemispherectomy.

The technique of the classic anatomic hemispherectomy requires a carefully planned stepwise approach. After induction of endotracheal general anesthesia and the establishment of wide-bore venous and arterial access lines, the entire scalp is shaved. With the patient supine the head is turned so that the sagittal plane is completely horizontal and placed on a soft circular head support with the dependent ear carefully protected. The incision is made from the hairline anteriorly in the midline back to the external occipital protuberance, and a second incision is made from the midpoint of the midline incision down to the zygomatic arch in front of the ear. It is wise to use an osteoplastic flap hinged on the temporalis muscle, with the bone flap extending from the midline to the floor of the temporal fossa and as far anteriorly and posteriorly as the scalp flaps allow. The dura is opened with a transverse incision across the middle of the exposure from frontal to occipital poles. One lower release incision is made down to the temporal pole and two in the upper part of the dura.

The procedure is carried out in three steps: arterial

ligation, venous obstruction, and hemispheral dissection. Elevation of the frontal lobe and retraction of the temporal pole permits the olfactory tract to be identified and divided. Posterior to this point, the optic nerve is seen, and after opening the overlying arachnoid, one exposes the internal carotid artery. The middle cerebral artery is then followed laterally in the opened sylvian fissure so that it, or its main branches, can be ligated between two hemoclips, either just proximal or distal to the trifurcation, thus sparing the lenticulostriate vessels which supply the corpus striatum. Next, the anterior bridging veins from the superomedial border of the frontal lobe which drain into the superior sagittal sinus are coagulated and divided. Retraction of the frontal lobe laterally from the falx permits the two anterior cerebral or pericallosal arteries to be be seen curving around the genu of the corpus callosum. At the genu, the anterior cerebral artery is clipped and divided while the contralateral vessel is carefully preserved. After the bridging veins from the inferolateral border of the temporal lobe have been coagulated and divided, the temporal lobe can be elevated to expose the posterior cerebral artery as it runs from the posterior margin of the midbrain across the free edge of the tentorium onto the medial surface of the occipital lobe, where it is clipped and divided. At this point the hemisphere often appears to subside as almost all the arterial inflow has been interrupted. All remaining bridging veins can now safely be interrupted without fear of congestion.

With gentle lateral retraction of the frontal and parietal lobes, the entire superior surface of the corpus callosum can be cleared. The corpus callosum is then divided from the genu to the rostrum, providing access to the anterior horn, body, and posterior horn of the lateral ventricle. Care must be taken posteriorly to avoid damage to the vein of Galen. A plane is now established between the caudate nucleus and the corpus callosum to allow lateral dissection over the lentiform nucleus to the insula. The plane is extended anteriorly to free the frontal lobe. Posteriorly, the roof of the temporal horn is opened to its anterior extent. Subpial dissection is used to remove the medial structures including the amygdala and hippocampus. In this way the hemispherectomy is performed en bloc. However, if the hemisphere is bulky, as is the case with hemimegalencephaly, or if the tissue is particularly firm, it is wise to first remove the frontal and parietal lobes and then to continue with the occipitotemporal resection. There is then less risk of tearing a medial bridging vein, which may be difficult to reach at that stage of the procedure. The cortex of the insular region is removed. Careful bipolar coagulation of any bleeding point is performed with repeated irrigation of the cavity.

The dura should be closed in a watertight fashion, and at least six to eight pairs of dural tack-up sutures are used to hold the dura up against the inner surfaces of the bone flap. The bone flap is secured and the scalp incision closed. If epidural hemostasis has been difficult to achieve, an epidural drain may be useful for 24 hours. It is also worthwhile to leave a subdural drain in place for 3 to 4 days to remove any blood products or particulate matter. This may prevent the development of a subdural membrane with its associated risks of late hemorrhage and hemosiderosis. The placement of a subdural to peritoneal shunt may also prevent the formation of a subdural membrane by constantly removing thrombin, the presence of which induces subdural membrane formation. However, since a percentage of these patients will inevitably develop shunt complications, the shunt is probably best avoided, unless there is clear evidence of persistently elevated intracranial pressure.

In order to avoid complications that arise from subdural membrane formation, Adams[57] described a technique of dural plication whereby a large portion of the remaining subdural space is obliterated by tacking the dura medially and creating a large epidural space. This technique does not seem to have achieved much popularity. Hoffman believes that hemidecortication is a reasonable alternative to hemispherectomy as this technique avoids entering the ventricular system.[58]

Rasmussen's functional hemispherectomy is used in some centers.[19, 20] A shorter midline incision is used with the same lateral extension. The bone flap extends from the midline down to the temporal floor but is not so wide as the one used for the classic anatomic hemispherectomy. The central cortex to be removed includes the pre- and postcentral gyri plus the adjacent 2 cm of the frontal and parietal lobes. A transverse suprasylvian subpial dissection gives protection to the branches of the middle cerebral artery. The two vertical incisions extend from the sylvian fissure to the midline and through to the medial surface anterior and posterior to the genu and splenium of the corpus callosum respectively after entering the body of the lateral ventricle. A standard temporal lobectomy is also performed with removal of the amygdala and hippocampus. A circumferential incision is made through the remaining frontal and occipital ventricular wall out to the pia so that the projection fibers passing from the corona radiata into the internal capsule can be divided in the remaining frontal and occipital lobes. These two portions will still have an intact arterial supply and venous drainage.

Seizure control with both the anatomic and functional hemispherectomy is excellent, but the latter should be associated with a lower complication rate.

FOCAL, LOBAR AND MULTILOBAR RESECTIONS

When an epileptogenic focus outside the temporal lobe does not involve the entire hemisphere, a focal, lobar or multilobar resection may bring about seizure control. In the majority of these patients there is no neurologic deficit, and so the primary sensorimotor cortex should be carefully preserved. The speech areas must also be protected especially in children over the age of 7 years, in whom speech mapping during awake surgery on the dominant hemisphere is important. However, at UCLA the majority of children undergoing focal resections have been under the age of 5 years, and awake surgery with local anesthesia is not only inappropriate, but usually unnecessary in this group.

Preoperative investigations will have localized the

epileptogenic focus as being in front of or behind the central area, but more precise localization is necessary at the time of surgery using somatosensory evoked potentials and ECoG. The exposure provided by the craniotomy should include the central area to facilitate cortical mapping. The pre- and postcentral gyri can be tentatively localized based on two anatomic facts. First, they are the two most parallel gyri running upward and backward from the sylvian fissure to the superomedial border. The central sulcal artery curves upward from the sylvian fissure and then runs superficially along the lower part of the central sulcus before disappearing into its depths. A strip of eight electrodes or a grid of 20 electrodes is placed across the central area at least 2.5 cm above the sylvian fissure for recording evoked potentials produced by stimulating the contralateral median nerve. The somatosensory cortex representing the arm can be identified.

Once the sensorimotor cortex has been clearly defined, ECoG can be performed using the 20-electrode grid. ECoG spikes may be limited to the area delineated by scalp EEG, CT and MRI, and PET. In children, however, ECoG spiking may be more widespread than the needed resection. Under those circumstances, nonepileptiform EEG abnormalities may prove more reliable than spike waves for localization. Polymorphic delta activity, amplitude attenuation, and attenuation of beta activity have proved to be extremely useful EEG patterns for demarcating a focus for resection. Intravenous boluses of sodium thiopental may be helpful in highlighting the attenuation of beta activity if necessary.

At UCLA this method has proved successful in identifying a focal area of cortical dysplasia, usually in the parieto-occipito-temporal region, in a group of young children with intractable infantile spasms.[40] Following the resection, in many cases, the seizures have been controlled.

TEMPORAL LOBECTOMY

Temporal lobectomy, the most common surgical procedure for epilepsy in adults,[59] is also performed in older children and teenagers. It has provided excellent results in well-selected pediatric populations, with 78 per cent of patients either becoming seizure-free or having only auras.[60] The procedure in children is the same as for adults, but the smaller brain size must be taken into account in younger children.

The patient is placed in the supine position with padding beneath the ipsilateral shoulder. It may be performed in rigid head fixation or on a well-padded support. The head is positioned with the face tilted slightly upward, with the sagittal plane approximately 30 degrees from the horizontal plane with the vertex tilted slightly upward. This orientation provides easy access to the mesial temporal structures. A routine frontotemporal question-mark incision is used with a hinged or free frontotemporal bone flap while care is taken to give good exposure of the posterior and inferior temporal region. The dural incision is based on the pterion, and posterior relaxing incisions are made as needed.

Upon opening the dura, one can identify the sylvian fissure; the superior, middle, and inferior temporal gyri; and the vein of Labbe. Small bridging veins over the temporal pole can be coagulated and cut. The posterior limit of the lobectomy is then determined. In adults, this posterior limit is 4.5 cm from the temporal tip along the middle temporal gyrus in the dominant hemisphere and 5.5 cm from the tip in the nondominant hemisphere. The extent of the resection must be reduced proportionately in younger children.

Next, a pial incision is made over the superior temporal gyrus parallel to the sylvian fissure beginning posteriorly and continuing around the temporal pole. The superior temporal gyrus is dissected off the sylvian fissure in a subpial fashion. Retraction and coagulation of the pia over the fissure must be kept to a minimum. This dissection stops at the limen insulae, the inferior and deep limit of the insular cortex. The posterior dissection is performed at right angles to the first incision through the superior, middle, and inferior temporal gyri, proceeding through the underlying white matter until the temporal horn is entered. A small cottonoid is placed in the ventricle to prevent blood from entering. The dissection is continued through the white matter between the roof of the temporal horn and the limen insulae, and is carried anteriorly past the pes hippocampi and through the lateral portion of the amygdala to meet the incision over the temporal pole. At this stage the temporal horn has been completely unroofed. The inferior dissection is continued through the basal portion of the inferior temporal gyrus and the fusiform gyrus, stopping at the collateral sulcus. Working within the temporal horn, the dissection is taken through the collateral eminence down to and through the pia of the collateral sulcus anteriorly until it meets the earlier incisions over the temporal pole. The lateral temporal lobe is now removed en bloc.

The resection of the mesial temporal structures is carried out under loupe or microscopic magnification. This begins by identifying the fimbria in the choroidal fissure and gently freeing it from the choroid plexus using a small ball hook. A subpial resection of the hippocampus is performed medial to the hippocampal fissure. The hippocampal arteries from the posterior cerebral artery are visualized in the hippocampal fissure, coagulated, and transected. The pia of the fissure is then cut. Next, the subpial resection is carried out over the subiculum and parahippocampal gyrus just lateral to the edge of the tentorium. The pia is divided and the dissection carried forward to include the lateral portion of the amygdala and the uncus and the mesial temporal structures are removed en bloc. Small portions of the lateral amygdala and the uncus may remain and can be removed piecemeal with gentle suction. The structures of the ambient cistern are easily identifiable through the pia. The wound is closed in the standard fashion.

CORPUS CALLOSOTOMY

Corpus callosotomy is undertaken not to resect an epileptogenic region but to limit the generalization of seizures when no discrete region can be found. Understandably, the procedure rarely produces a seizure-free state.[61] Drop attacks are the seizure type most amenable to treatment by corpus callosotomy.[62] Because of a reduction in postoperative cognitive deficits, many centers perform corpus callosotomy as a two-stage procedure. They first section the anterior two thirds of the callosum and reoperate to section the posterior one third if the seizure control from the first operation is unsatisfactory. However, if the patient is severely retarded, the corpus callosum can be divided in a single procedure without significant risk of creating a cognitive deficit.

The patient is placed in the supine position with the head held in a neutral position by rigid fixation. The head end of the table is raised to provide access to the anterior portion of the corpus callosum and then lowered during the operation to give exposure to the more posterior portion. Using an L-shaped scalp incision over the nondominant frontal lobe, a 4 × 6 cm free bone flap is made that crosses midline and is located with two thirds of the flap anterior to the coronal suture. The dural flap is U-shaped and based along the superior sagittal sinus. A careful dissection of bridging veins along the sagittal sinus may facilitate retraction of the medial frontal lobe. Careful attention is required to avoid excessive retraction of the supplementary motor area and the cingulate gyrus. The microscope is required for the rest of the operation. Working along the falx, the callosomarginal arteries are identified and protected, and the cingulate gyri are teased apart, exposing the pericallosal arteries and the corpus callosum. While gentle suction or the ultrasonic aspirator is applied, the dissection of the callosum is performed in the midline and carried forward to the genu. The division of the rostrum proceeds inferiorly until the A2 branches of the anterior cerebral arteries are seen coursing anteriorly and upward. Next, the body of the callosum is divided working posteriorly. If a two thirds section is desired, the posterior limit can be determined by measuring the length of the callosum on sagittal MRI and measuring the appropriate length intraoperatively. An intraoperative lateral skull x-ray may be helpful in determining the extent of callosal section.[63] The callosotomy is completed by dissection through the splenium, which is considerably thicker than the body. The wound is closed in the standard fashion.

SUMMARY AND CONCLUSIONS

Until recently, few children with intractable seizures were referred for surgical treatment because it was believed that most childhood seizure disorders would resolve spontaneously. Because clinical observation was the only method available for assessment, it was only the passage of time that revealed which children would suffer the effects of intractable epilepsy. With the recent introduction of EEG video telemetry, magnetic resonance imaging, and positron emission tomography, it has become possible to identify patients in whom there is a single resectable focus causing their seizures. It has been shown that in some babies, a focal area of hypometabolism may be responsible for a generalized seizure disorder such as infantile spasms. With resection of this focus, seizures have been controlled.

Although this new approach is offering hope for children with epilepsy and their families, much research needs to be done to answer the many challenging questions that have been presented by epilepsy surgery. Does seizure control following surgery always lead to neurodevelopmental progress and psychosocial adjustment? What is the optimal timing of surgery for each seizure type? With carefully planned large long-term studies, a greater understanding of neural development and plasticity will be achieved and a clearer insight established into the process of epileptogenesis.

REFERENCES

1. Horsley V: Brain surgery. Br Med J 2:670, 1886.
2. Shewmon DA, Shields WD, Chugani HT, Peacock WJ: Contrasts between pediatric and adult epilepsy surgery: Rationale and strategy for focal resection. J Epilepsy 3(Suppl):141, 1990.
3. Huttenlocher PR: Synaptic density in human frontal cortex—developmental changes and effects of aging. Brain Res 163:195, 1979.
4. Huttenlocher PR, de Courten C, Garey LJ, Van der Loos H: Synaptogenesis in human visual cortex—evidence for synapse elimination during normal development. Neurosci Lett 33:247, 1982.
5. Baumbach HD, Chow KL: Visuocortical epileptiform discharges in rabbits: Differential effects on neuronal development in the lateral geniculate nucleus and superior colliculus. Brain Res 209:61, 1981.
6. Villablanca JR, Burgess JW, Benedetti F: There is less thalamic degeneration in neonatal-lesioned cats after cerebral hemisperectomy. Brain Res 368:211, 1986.
7. Villablanca JR, Burgess JW, Olmstead CE: Recovery of function after neonatal or adult hemispherectomy in cats. I. Time course, movement, posture and sensorimotor tests. Behav Brain Res 19:205, 1986.
8. Villablanca JR, Gomez-Pinilla F: Novel crossed corticothalamic projections after neonatal cerebral hemispherectomy. A quantitative autoradiography study in cats. Brain Res 410:219, 1987.
9. McFie J: The effects of hemispherectomy on intellectual functioning in cases of infantile hemiplegia. J Neurol Neurosurg Psychiatry 24:240, 1961.
10. Basser LS: Hemiplegia of early onset and the faculty of speech with special reference to the effects of hemispherectomy. Brain 85:427, 1962.
11. Carlson J, Netley C, Hendrick EB, Pritchard JS: A reexamination of intellectual disabilities in hemispherectomized patients. Trans Am Neurol Assoc 93:198, 1968.
12. Smith A, Sugar O: Development of above normal language and intelligence 21 years after cerebral hemispherectomy. Neurology 25:813, 1975.
13. Smith A: Dominant and nondominant hemispherectomy. In Smith WL (ed): Drugs, Development and Cerebral Function. Springfield, IL, Charles C Thomas, 1972, pp 37–68.
14. Hillier WF Jr: Total left cerebral hemispherectomy for malignant glioma. Neurology 4:718, 1954.
15. Andermann F: Identification of candidates for surgical treatment of epilepsy. In Engel J (ed): Surgical Treatment of Epilepsy. New York, Raven Press, 1987, pp 51–70.
16. Hopkins A: The management of epilepsy uncontrolled by anticonvulsant drugs—surgery and other treatments. In Hopkins A (ed): Epilepsy. New York, Demos, 1987, pp 283–299.
17. Hoffman HJ, Hendrick EB, Dennis M, Armstrong D: Hemisperectomy for Sturge-Weber syndrome. Childs Brain 5:233, 1979.

18. Holmes G: Diagnosis and Management of Seizures in Children. Philadelphia, WB Saunders, 1987.
19. Rasmussen T, Olszewski J, Lloyd-Smith D: Focal seizures due to chronic localized encephalitis. Neurology 8:433, 1958.
20. Rasmussen T, Andermann F: Update on the syndrome of "chronic encephalitis" and epilepsy. Cleve Clin J Med 56(Suppl 2):s181, 1989.
21. Barth PG: Disorders of neuronal migration. Can J Neurol Sci 14:1, 1987.
22. Farrell MA, DeRosa MJ, Curran JG, Secor DL, Cornford ME, Comair YG, Peacock WJ, Shields WD, Vinters HV: Neuropathologic findings in cortical resections (including hemispherectomies) performed for the treatment of intractable childhood epilepsy. Acta Neuropathol 83:246, 1992.
23. Verity CM, Golding J: Risk of epilepsy after febrile convulsions: a national cohort study. Br Med J 303:1373, 1991.
24. Commission on classification and terminology of the International League Against Epilepsy 1981 Proposal for revised clinical and electroencephalographic classification of epileptic seizures. Epilepsia 22:489, 1981.
25. Gorman DG, Shields WD, Shewmon DA, Chugani HT, Finkel R, Comair YG, Peacock WJ: Neurosurgical treatment of refractory status epilepticus. Epilepsia 33(3):546, 1992.
26. Aicardi J, Amsili J, Chevrie JJ: Acute hemiplegia in infancy and childhood. Dev Med Child Neurol 11:162, 1969.
27. Roger J, Lob H, Tassinari CA: Status epilepticus. *In* Vinken PJ, Bruyn GW (eds): Handbook of Neurology. Vol 15, The Epilepsies. Amsterdam, North-Holland, 1974.
28. Sturge WA: A case of partial epilepsy, apparently due to a lesion of one of the vasomotor centres of the brain. Trans Clin Soc London 12:162, 1879.
29. Berg BO: Current concepts of neurocutaneous disorders. Brain and Development 13,1:9, 1991.
30. von Recklinghausen F: Ein Herx von einem Neugeborenen welches mehrer Theils nach aussen, Theils nach den hohlen prominierende Tumoren (Myomen) trug. Verh Ges Geburtsh 25 Marz. Monatsschr Geburtskd 220:1, 1862.
31. Gomez MR (ed): Tuberous Sclerosis: Neurologic and Psychiatric Features. 2nd ed. New York, Raven Press, 1988, pp 21–36.
32. McMurdo SK, Moore SG, Brant-Zawadski M, et al.: Magnetic imaging of intracranial tuberous sclerosis. AJNR 8:77, 1987.
33. Richardson EP: Pathology of tuberous sclerosis. Neuropathologic aspects. Ann NY Acad Sci 615:128, 1991.
34. Feld M, Gruner J, Heuyer G: Heterotopies volimineuses et malformations de l'hemisphere droite. Hydrocephalie avec lesions destructives de l'hemisphere gauche, seules cliniquement traduites. Rev Neurol 92:26, 1955.
35. Pavone L, Curatolo P, Rizzo R, et al.: Epidermal nevus syndrome: A neurologic variant with hemimegalencephaly, gyral malformation, mental retardation, seizures, and facial hemihypertrophy. Neurology 41:266, 1991.
36. Robain O, Floquet C, Heldt N, Rozenberg F: Hemimegalencephaly: A clinicopathological study of four cases. Neuropathol Appl Neurobiol 14:125, 1988.
37. Lombroso CT: A prospective study of infantile spasms: Clinical and therapeutic correlations. Epilepsia 24:135, 1983.
38. Kellway P, Hrachovy RA, Frost JD, Zion T: Precise characterization and quantification of infantile spasms. Ann Neurol 6:214, 1979.
39. Riikonen R: A long-term follow-up study of 214 children with the syndrome of infantile spasms. Neuropediatrics 13:14, 1982.
40. Olson DM, Chugani HT, Shewmon DA, Phelps ME, Peacock WJ: Electrocorticographic confirmation of focal positron emission tomographic abnormalities in children with intractable epilepsy. Epilepsia 31:731, 1990.
41. Shields WD, Shewmon DA, Chugani HT, Peacock WJ: The role of surgery in the treatment of infantile spasms. J Epilepsy 3(Suppl):321, 1990.
42. Chevrie JJ, Aicardi J: Childhood epileptic encephalopathy with slow spike-wave. A statistical study of 80 cases. Epilepsia 13:259, 1972.
43. Rausch R: Psychological evaluation. *In* Engel J Jr (ed): Surgical Treatment of the Epilepsies. New York, Raven Press, 1987.
44. Chugani HT, Shields WD, Shewmon DA, Olson DM, Phelps ME, Peacock WJ: Infantile spasms: I. PET identifies focal cortical dysgenesis in cryptogenic cases for surgical treatment. Ann Neurol 27:406, 1990.
45. Newton MR, Berkovic SF, Austin M, Rowe CC, Bladin PF, Lee KJ, McKay WJ: The postictal switch: rapid changes in cerebral blood flow after focal seizures shown by HMPAO SPECT. J Nucl Med 31:711, 1990.
46. Shen W, Lee BI, Park HM, Siddiqui AR, Wellman HH, Worth RM, Markand ON: HIPDM-SPECT brain imaging in the presurgical evaluation of patients with intractable seizures. J Nucl Med 31:1280, 1990.
47. Goldring S: Pediatric epilepsy. Epilepsia 28(suppl 1):82, 1987.
48. Resnick TJ, Duchowny MS, Deray MJ, Alfonso I: Subdural electrode recording in the preoperative evaluation of partial seizures in children. Ann Neurol 22:415, 1987.
49. Wyllie E, Luders H, Morris HH, et al.: Subdural electrodes in the evaluation for epilepsy surgery in children and adults. Neuropediatrics 19:80, 1988.
50. Dandy WE: Removal of right cerebral hemisphere for certain tumors with hemiplegia. Preliminary report. JAMA 90:823, 1928.
51. McKenzie KG, Cited by Williams DJ, Scott JW: The functional responses of the sympathetic nervous system of man following hemidecortication. J Neurol Psychiatry 2:315, 1938.
52. Krynauw R: Infantile hemiplegia treated by removing one cerebral hemisphere. J Neurol Neurosurg Psychiatry. 3:243, 1950.
53. Oppenheimer DR, Griffith HB: Persistent intracranial bleeding as a complication of hemispherectomy. J Neurol Neurosurg Psychiatry 29:229, 1966.
54. Griffith HB: Cerebral hemispherectomy for infantile hemiplegia in the light of the late results. Ann R Coll Surg 41:183, 1967.
55. Rasmussen T: Hemispherectomy for seizures revisited. Can J Neurol Sci 10:133, 1983.
56. Wilson PJE: Cerebral hemispherectomy for infantile hemiplegia. Brain 93:147, 1970.
57. Adams CB: Hemispherectomy—a modification. J Neurol Neurosurg Psychiatry 46:617, 1983.
58. Villamure JG: Hemispherectomy techniques. *In* Luders H (ed): Epilepsy Surgery. New York, Raven Press, 1991, pp 569–578.
59. Cahan DH, Sutherling W, McCullough AM, Rauch R, Engel J, Crandall PH: Review of the 20-year UCLA experience with surgery for epilepsy. Cleve Clin Q 41:313, 1984.
60. Meyer FB, Marsh WR, Laws ER, Sharbrough FW: Temporal lobectomy in children with epilepsy. J Neurosurg 64:371, 1986.
61. Fuiks KS, Wyler AR, Hermann BP, Somes G: Seizure outcome from anterior and complete corpus callosotomy. J Neurosurg 74:573, 1991.
62. Oguni H, Olivier A, Andermann F, Comair J: Anterior callosotomy in the treatment of medically intractable epilepsies: a study of 43 patients with a mean follow-up of 39 months. Ann Neurol 30:357, 1991.
63. Awad IA, Wyllie E, Luders H, Ahl J: Intraoperative determination of the extent of corpus callosotomy for epilepsy: two simple techniques. Neurosurgery 26:102, 1990.

Chapter 46

SPASTICITY

BRUCE B. STORRS, M.D.

Spasticity is a disabling component of many nervous system diseases of children. Spasticity is best defined as a velocity-dependent increase in resistance to passive stretch seen in concert with the other components of the upper motor neuron syndrome.[1-3] Hyperreflexia, weakness, motor control deficits, and posture-regulating deficits routinely accompany clinical spasticity.

HISTORY

Spasticity has been a topic of medical interest for more than 100 years and was the topic of much of the work that formed the beginnings of neurology in North America.

Following the initial description of the spasticity associated with cerebral palsy by Little in 1864,[4] British and continental neurologists published numerous articles on the subject of spasticity. Many of the great names in neurology used spasticity as the topic for their early works. Marie,[5] Jendrassik,[6] Gowers,[7, 8] Wallenberg,[9] and Strumpell[10] all published articles between 1884 and 1888 on spasticity.

In 1888, William Osler presented his series of 151 patients with cerebral palsy in three lectures delivered at the Philadelphia Infirmary for Nervous Diseases.[11] This material was presented later the same year as the keynote address at the third American Clinical Congress, the meeting that established American neurology as an entity.

In 1904, Charles Sherrington presented the Silliman lectures, a series of three lectures at Yale University. This material was published later the same year as the monograph "The Integrative Action of the Nervous System."[12] In this work Sherrington described the production of spasticity in animals by making an upper motor neuron lesion and the effective amelioration of the spasticity by performing a posterior rhizotomy. The basis for this famous monograph was published some 6 years earlier.[13]

The sectioning of posterior roots has been performed in humans for the control of pain since 1888,[14] and as a result of the work of Sherrington, the suggested extension of the indications for rhizotomy to include spasticity was made by Munro in 1904.

Otfrid Foerster reported on 159 surgically treated cases of spasticity in 1913.[15] In this report he detailed the treatment of spasticity by the sectioning of posterior lumbar rootlets with good results. The operative morbidity and mortality were surprisingly low.

Surgical treatments of spasticity introduced since Foerster include lesion-making in the spinal nerve roots,[16, 17] spinal cord with myelotomy[18-20] or dorsal root entry zone lesions,[21] electrodes for the stimulation of the spinal cord and cerebellum[22-24] either in a subdural or epidural location,[25-30] and refinements in the technique of sensory rootlet section.[31-34]

Medical therapies for the management of spasticity have included neurolytic agents, e.g., phenol,[35-37] alcohol,[38] spinal cord barbotage with iced saline, intrathecal opiates,[39, 40] broad-action neuromuscular agents such as benzodiazepine,[41] dantrolene,[42] neuromuscular blockade with botulin toxin,[43, 44] and specific modulators of spinal cord function such as baclofen.[45-51]

EFFECTS OF SPASTICITY

In children, spasticity occurs in several distinct clinical settings, each requiring an individual clinical approach. Spasticity is recognized as the common mediator of severe disability in many childhood conditions including cerebral palsy, traumatic encephalopathy, spinal cord injury,[52] congenital anomalies of the nervous system,[53, 54] degenerative spinal and cerebral diseases, and the hereditary spasticities. Amelioration of spasticity in those individuals adversely affected is an important clinical goal. The disabling effects of spasticity are seen in several areas of functional impairment. Muscle tone abnormalities coupled with the intrinsic weakness and primary motor control difficulties of the upper motor neuron syndrome lead to clumsiness and slowness of physical activity. Spasticity frequently leads to shortening of muscle length and resultant joint contracture. Progressive joint deformity may produce subluxation and eventually dislocation. Adduction contractures in the lower extremities produce the typical scissoring gait and, when severe, may preclude ambulation. Spasticity of the gastrocnemius and soleus may produce progressive flexion contracture of the foot with a toe-toe gait and decreased foot balance area, which compounds the existing balance disturbance.[55] Similar disabilities are seen in the upper extremities in patients with quadrispastic involvement.

Spasticity of the major trunk musculature often produces significant problems in trunk alignment and head position with predictable impact on cranial-sensory input as well as expressive output.

Functional effects on activities of daily living are seen in almost all patients with spasticity. In the mildest cases, loss of speed and dexterity may be the main disability and can be compensated for with a slower schedule. In more severe cases, however, actual limitation of activities may occur, and the patient may require assistance to perform the most basic of activities. Functional improvement in this group of patients is of great value.

FORMS OF SPASTICITY

The spasticity associated with cerebral palsy is the most common form seen in childhood and has the longest history of therapeutic intervention. This treatment forms the basis for the treatment of spasticity in other conditions.

Cerebral palsy is an inclusive term that describes a clinical entity of nonprogressive static encephalopathy predominantly affecting the motor system. The incidence of spasticity is approximately 2/1000 live births. The initial presentation of cerebral palsy in the young infant is usually not one of spasticity, but rather of decreased tone and persistent abnormal reflexes. However, by the age of 6 months, spasticity emerges as a common clinical presentation and is often the reason for the initial investigation of the nervous system.

Spasticity may also be associated with other pathologic entities seen in pediatric neurosurgery. Spasticity is not infrequently seen in patients with spinal cord pathologies such as spinal cord tumor, tethered spinal cord, syringohydromyelia, lipomyelomeningocele, diastematomyelia, and secondary tethering of the spinal cord with myelomeningocele. In obvious contradistinction to cerebral palsy, these are congenital structural lesions that have associated physical findings or medical or surgical history that point in the direction of the cause of the spasticity.

Spasticity following spinal cord injury is a well-recognized entity. Fortunately, spinal cord injury in childhood is relatively uncommon when compared to the young adult and adult population. The numbers of patients in the pediatric age group seen with spasticity secondary to spinal cord injury is relatively small. Trauma to the brain, however, is a significant cause of spasticity in childhood and may be seen in the clinical settings of accidental and intentional injuries. Recovery from these acute traumatic cerebral and spinal lesions is unpredictable, making permanent surgical solutions less attractive.

EVALUATION OF TREATMENT

In the evaluation of patients relative to a treatment plan, several important factors must be included in the decision-making. The first and most important is to make, as firmly as possible, a correct diagnosis of the patient's condition in order to make accurate predictions regarding success and eventual outcome for the patient. It is especially important to separate the progressive degenerative diseases of the nervous system from those of a static nature. Once the diagnosis of the basic underlying pathology has been secured, the second order of business is to establish the functional disability that is attributable to the spasticity, and although this may seem relatively straightforward, in a patient with multiple disabilities it is often difficult to assign a relative importance to the different components of the disability.[56] For example, in the patient with cerebral palsy, there will often be the coexistence of persistent primitive posturing, cerebellar deficit, primary muscular weakness, variable intellectual handicap, and fixed joint contracture, as well as an element of spasticity. A comprehensive evaluation of the patient's needs should be performed and not just a physical examination documenting the presence of spasticity.[57] In many cases, although the spasticity may indeed be demonstrable on examination, the contribution of spasticity to the whole disability picture is small, and the elimination of spasticity may provide limited or no functional advantage to the patient. It is in these patients that intervention should be withheld. The converse is also true. In the patient in whom it is determined that, in spite of multiple disability-producing factors, the reduction of spasticity will produce valuable increases in functional level, intervention may be advisable even though significant additional disabling factors may be present which, at the present time, are not correctable.

Objective tests of function are important in the evaluation process as well as in the assessment of results of therapy. Goniometric measurement of joint excursion is important and highly reproducible; evaluation of spasticity may be performed by use of the Ashworth scale (Table 46–1), a commonly used instrument with a high interrater reliability.[58]

Evaluation of the functional impact of spasticity requires estimation of ease of performance and quality of performance. Evaluation of the ease of assumption of postures (e.g., long sitting, half kneeling and side sit-

TABLE 46–1. ASHWORTH SCALE

GRADE	
1 =	No increased tone.
2 =	Slightly increased tone, manifested by a catch and release or minimal resistance when the affected part is moved in flexion or extension.
3 =	Marked increase in tone through most of range of motion, but affected parts are easily moved.
4 =	Considerable increase in tone: passive movement is difficult.
5 =	Affected parts rigid in flexion and extension.

ting) required in ambulation or transfer can be performed by use of the Assistance Scale (Table 46–2), a five-level objective score for the assumption and maintenance of posture.

Specific measures of childhood performance in the activities of daily living, mobility, and bowel-bladder function may be assessed by the WEEFIM (Functional Index Measure). Motor performance may be assessed by the Tufts Assessment of Motor Performance (TAMP.)[59] Recording of examinations on videotape allows for education of examiners and valuable future comparisons.

It is important that patients with cerebral palsy be evaluated by a team of health care professionals who are experienced in the evaluation of children with spasticity and can make the long-range determinations necessary for appropriate therapy plans. This team would typically consist of a pediatric neurosurgeon, a pediatric orthopaedist, a pediatric physiatrist, experienced physical, occupational, and speech therapists, a communications specialist for augmentative communication, a social worker, a neuropsychologist, and a nurse.

The evaluation of the patient with cerebral palsy should be conducted in an atmosphere of attempting to decrease the patient's disability and increase his functional level rather than a clinical setting in which the patient is examined to see whether he or she qualifies for a particular procedure or technique. Patients with cerebral palsy and their families are, as a rule, generally health conscious and sophisticated concerning medical and physical therapy systems. To subject the patient and the family to a contest type atmosphere to select "candidates" for surgery, while it may provide some positive benefit for the patient on whom you decide to

TABLE 46–2. ASSISTANCE SCALE

GRADE	
5 =	Maintains independently without assistance.
4 =	Maintains with unilateral upper extremity support or requires intermittent contact by therapist for balance only.
3 =	Maintains with bilateral upper extremity support or requires constant contact by therapist for balance only.
2 =	Full external support of one person.
1 =	Cannot be placed.

perform some surgery, is detrimental to the 80 per cent of patients for whom surgery is not the appropriate therapy and adds an additional unnecessary psychological burden. It is more appropriate, in the multidisciplinary setting, to evaluate the patient's abilities and disabilities and to present a unified treatment plan to maximize the patient's abilities, including such simple things as a change in the patient's seating or positioning, a change in the patient's education or therapy prescription, counseling, and ancillary services that may positively influence the patient's life.

TREATMENT

The techniques available for the treatment of spasticity in children are numerous. Physical therapy, occupational therapy, assistive devices, and augmentative communication devices play a major part in the treatment of spasticity in children. Drug therapy—given orally, intravenously, and intrathecally—has met with significant success in the management of spasticity.[60] Orthopaedic intervention has long been the mainstay of surgical treatment for progressive spasticity and remains the most effective treatment for fixed joint deformity. Orthopaedic intervention is the procedure of choice in patients with severe involvement and movement disorders (e.g., athetosis, chorea, and dystonia) and may be the procedure of choice in those patients with a single level of involvement. The advent of new treatments for spasticity has had little effect on the frequency of orthopaedic intervention. However, the quality of the result measured in functional gain is markedly enhanced by the combination of orthopaedic techniques and methods directed at the primary reduction of spasticity.

Selective posterior rhizotomy (SPR) is a safe predictable operation that provides reduction of spasticity in 95 per cent of patients with limited risks of additional sensory deficit. SPR is not indicated in patients with movement disorders or multiple severe fixed joint contractures.

Longitudinal or Bischoff's myelotomy may offer a solution in some patients with spinal cord injury.[61, 62] "T" myelotomy may offer some advantage over the straight longitudinal myelotomy in the management of spasticity.[63]

Drug therapy in spasticity is based on two effects.[64, 65] Therapy using the benzodiazepines takes advantage of both a receptor-specific effect and a secondary global reduction in sensory input through mild sedation. This approach is generally inappropriate in children. Drugs developed from the investigation of specific spinal cord receptors in spasticity such as the GABA-B agonist baclofen[66] have found a place in the management of spasticity of both spinal and cerebral origin. Baclofen may be effective in oral form in some children with spasticity. Usually, however, the oral doses of baclofen required to produce an effect may be too high, and sedation and severe muscular weakness may accompany the reduction in spasticity and become unwanted side effects in children. Intrathecal baclofen has been used for many years on an experimental basis to treat spasticity of spinal origin with good results in patients with spinal cord injuries and, to a lesser degree, patients with multiple sclerosis. Intrathecal baclofen has been used more recently in clinical trials with children having spasticity of presumed cerebral origin (cerebral palsy) with good results.

One of the significant advantages to intrathecal baclofen is that the response to the drug may be demonstrated prior to operative intervention and placement of the subcutaneous constant infusion pump. A test dose is administered to appropriately selected patients by lumbar puncture and injection of a single dose of intrathecal baclofen, 25 to 100 micrograms. A delayed onset of effect is seen in responders after approximately 2 hours and lasts approximately 8 hours. Patients who have a favorable response may elect to proceed with the placement of an intrathecal catheter and a subcutaneous pump for constant infusion. The concentration or rate of delivery of baclofen is adjusted until the desired result is achieved. The problems associated with the intrathecal administration of baclofen by pump fall into two general categories: drug-related (such as allergy, tachyphylaxis, and toxicity) and delivery-system–related (such as component failure and infection). The patient receiving intrathecal baclofen may require a "drug holiday" or temporary change to a different drug, such as intrathecal morphine, when tachyphylaxis occurs with baclofen. Double-blind studies have demonstrated a significant effect of intrathecal baclofen on spasticity of spinal origin. Continuations of these double-blind studies are currently being carried out in patients with cerebral palsy.

SELECTIVE POSTERIOR RHIZOTOMY

Selective posterior rhizotomy provides the permanent alleviation of spasticity in patients with cerebral palsy. It is a safe and predictable procedure. The procedure is performed today much the same as when initially reported by Otfrid Foerster in 1913. Modern improvements are the addition of intraoperative electrophysiologic testing,[67] improved sensitivity in patient selection, and improved postoperative rehabilitation. Application of SPR to properly selected patients with spasticity will result in dramatic reduction in spasticity and appropriate functional gains over time.[68]

Patient selection for SPR involves several important points. Patients with cerebral palsy and a history of prematurity who have functionally disabling spastic diplegia without significant athetosis, chorea, dystonia, persistent pathologic reflexes, or fixed joint contractures have the best result following SPR. Patients who have spasticity as a result of postnatal insult (e.g., meningitis, near drowning, or head injury) have a much less predictable functional outcome. Patients with quadrispastic cerebral palsy often have associated movement disorders and persistent pathologic reflexes

that limit their functional gains. Fixed joint contractures may be seen in all patient groups and are a significant obstacle to functional gains. Rhizotomy will produce marked reduction in spasticity, but fixed contracture must be addressed by timely orthopaedic surgical techniques if full functional gains are to be accomplished. Access to competent rehabilitation services is a necessary part of the postoperative treatment. In the absence of children's services, surgery is ill advised as the functional gains will surely be disappointing for all concerned.

A comprehensive evaluation of the patient's medical condition must be included in the therapeutic decision-making process. Patients with cerebral palsy often have a history of bronchopulmonary dysplasia requiring pretreatment with bronchodilators and increased pulmonary toilet. Children with cerebral palsy may have shunting systems for hydrocephalus secondary to intraventricular hemorrhage. Assessment of the shunting system should be performed prior to surgery. The ability to protect the airway and velopharyngeal competence also should be assessed prior to surgery. Epilepsy is not an infrequent co-morbidity with cerebral palsy and requires specific perioperative attention.

Operative Procedure

Patients are anesthetized in the standard fashion and given a short-acting muscle relaxant. These agents last approximately 20 minutes and will allow ease in positioning the patient as well as in the initial opening and laminectomy or laminotomy. The bladder is catheterized. Patients are placed prone on a prepared surgical bolster. It is important to remember that patients with cerebral palsy often have some contractures in the upper extremities, and under the action of pharmacologic paralysis it is possible to hyperabduct the arm and cause brachial plexus stretch injury. The arms are best left down at the side. Silver/silver chloride gel surface electrodes are placed over the appropriate muscle groups to be tested during intraoperative monitoring, usually the medial hamstrings, gastrocnemius and soleus, tibialis anterior, quadriceps femoris, and the adductor magnus.

Reference electrodes and ground electrodes are also placed. Attention to padding and proper protection of the eyes and skin are of course paramount in the prone position. Exposure and draping of the patient is performed to allow visualization of the lower extremities, and this will permit the operator or electrophysiologist to assess the presence or absence of twitch in the muscles and to assess the quality of muscular movement in the lower extremities if that is desired.

The technique for exposure of the sensory rootlets varies somewhat from operator to operator. Some operators prefer to make a single-level laminectomy or laminotomy to visualize the conus medullaris and then to separate out the rootlets. Others elect to do a laminotomy of the entire lumbar spine from L2 through S1 for visualization of exit foramina of all the nerve roots. The potential advantage of doing a single-level laminectomy is the length of the skin incision and the amount of bony removal necessary.[69, 70] The disadvantages are the potential for surgical trauma to the conus medullaris and possible confusion regarding the stimulation and identification of the nerve rootlets in a confined space. The advantage to the larger laminotomy is that all of the lumbar nerve roots and upper sacral roots can be viewed exiting their appropriate foramina and identified. Anomalies of the cauda equina (e.g., recurrent and conjoined roots and intraspinal dorsal root ganglia) are much easier to identify with the larger exposure. Additional incidental pathology such as tethered cord secondary to lipoma of the filum terminale or inclusion dermoid from remote lumbar punctures are best treated through the larger exposure. The obvious disadvantage to the more extensive exposure is that more bone removal is required with a longer skin incision and potentially more blood loss, although in experienced hands blood loss is nil even for the more extensive exposure. There is no evidence that stability of the spine is affected in any way by either procedure. Attempts to create an animal model of scoliosis by sectioning all of the dorsal rootlets along one side of the spine intradurally have failed. It was found that the only way to produce scoliosis was to produce either anterior horn cell injury or anterior root injury over multiple levels at the same time as a dorsal rhizotomy is performed.[71] Long-term clinical studies during follow-up of children with multiple-level laminectomies have borne out this experimental evidence.

Once the appropriate area is exposed, the multiple-level laminotomy can be performed quickly and bloodlessly by means of the air-driven craniotome. A useful technique is to (1) separate the ligamentum flavum from the lowermost lamina, (2) make a small entry into the spinal canal through the ligament into the epidural space bilaterally, (3) use the smallest craniotome attachment, (4) advance through the number of levels required bilaterally, and (5) lift off the bone plate as a single unit. This plate may then be replaced at the end of the procedure if desired. Once the laminar plate has been removed, the dura is opened and the nerve rootlets are identified. In the multilevel laminectomy, the last large nerve root exiting the foramina is always S1, and this should be confirmed by stimulation. Typically, the S2 nerve root on stimulation will produce a flexion of the toes, and the S1 nerve root will produce a plantar flexion of the foot. A distinction may be made between the two in this manner, and the appropriate count of the nerve roots may be made. Occasionally, developmental anomalies in the lumbar plexus may be encountered such as conjoined nerve root, intraspinal dorsal root ganglion, and aberrant and recurrent nerve roots, and these should be recognized for what they are and for the potential difficulties they may cause in interpretation of stimulation. Dorsal and ventral nerve roots are easily separated by visual inspection in most cases and then confirmed by stimulation. The ventral root has a much lower threshold to stimulation than the dorsal root. On rare occasions there may be duplication or absence of either root, and in these cases electrophysiology is indispensable.

The technique for intraoperative stimulation varies from center to center, and in fact there is even disagreement about whether electrophysiologic monitoring is necessary.[72] The argument against electrophysiologic monitoring is that it does not appear to influence the results and it is technically demanding and requires additional monitoring equipment. The argument for electrophysiologic monitoring is that if properly used, it allows absolute identification of motor and sensory roots. It allows the subgrouping of sensory rootlets into patterns of behavior that may be used as criteria for sectioning the roots, and it allows the investigation of anomalies of the lumbosacral plexus. The standard electrophysiologic techniques used in dorsal rhizotomy for cerebral palsy are necessary in more complex procedures such as selective posterior rhizotomy for spasticity in patients with myelomeningocele and in the investigation and treatment of patients with bladder spasticity.

One of the scientifically based methods for using electrophysiologic monitoring to select appropriate nerve rootlets for sectioning that has given excellent results is the "H" reflex recovery curve technique. This basically involves re-creating the "H" reflex by a direct stimulation of the dorsal rootlet with recording over the subserved muscle group. The rootlet is stimulated with a bipolar electrode with the cathode in the more central position, and recordings are made from over the muscle group using skin electrodes. The threshold of response is identified, and when this electrical threshold is reached, repetitive stimulation of the dorsal rootlet is used at a rate of 20 cycles per second. In the usual age group treated with selective posterior rhizotomy, this produces the maximum separation between the first stage response and the second stage response.[73] With the two pairs of stimuli applied with a 20 cycle per second rate or a 50 millisecond interval, the ratio of the amplitudes of the two "H" responses is measured. Two basic groups of fibers are identified: (1) fibers that have no decrement or have an incremental response, and (2) fibers that have a decremental response. In the standard "H" reflex recovery curve using a transcutaneous stimulus to the posterior tibial nerve, patients with spasticity will demonstrate a failure to decrement,[74–76] and this basic information was used in establishing this technique. When the fibers that do not decrement are identified, these fibers are sectioned. No attempts are made to spare a certain number of fibers or to spare fibers at a certain level. All fibers that meet the electrophysiologic criteria of incremental response or failure to decrement are sectioned.[77]

It is important that, prior to any electrophysiologic testing, any muscle relaxant used should be pharmacologically fully reversed. Even though the clinical period of activity is past and the "train of four" has returned, there may remain a significant effect on the more sensitive "H" reflex recovery curve. "Normal" transcutaneous nerve conduction responses may be obtained (e.g., "train of four") with only 30 per cent of the muscle receptors free of blocking agent. Direct stimulation of the rootlets with recording is much more sensitive to neuromuscular blockade, and a false decremental response may be seen.

It is important that this electrophysiologic testing be carried out at threshold and not at supramaximal stimulus levels. Stimulus frequencies are also critical to proper separation of response groups and reduction of artifact. As the voltage increases or the power increases, there is a significant amount of recruitment, and in fact volume conduction may be seen in non-neural structures such as the filum terminale. This volume conduction is responsible for much of the "spread" of activity seen in other techniques and is a source of intraoperative confusion. It is important that the "H" reflex recovery curve be conducted at the minimal setting that produces an electrical response in the muscle.

RESULTS OF TREATMENT

Results of treatment for spasticity may be judged in several ways. Objective measurements of spasticity on physical examination, such as the Ashworth Scale, provide valuable scalar information. The Ashworth Scale, which has been used for many years, has the advantages of being easily taught and having a relatively high interrater reliability.[78, 79] Application of Ashworth Scale studies to patients before and after treatment for spasticity provides valuable objective information. For example, Ashworth Scale determinations before and after selective posterior rhizotomy demonstrate that 95 per cent of the patients will have the reduction of at least one Ashworth Scale grade in spasticity postoperatively.[80] Approximately 50 per cent will have reduction of more than two grades. A reduction of one grade is believed to be a statistically significant improvement. The use of the myometer, a hand-held device to quantitate resistance to passive stretch, has been useful in some hands and has provided acceptable interrater reliability. Goniometric examinations of hip abduction and knee extension as well as ankle extension have been useful and have a concordant interrater reliability that allows them to be useful. Attempts to use a computerized kinesiometer, while reproducible and worthwhile in adults, have been of limited usefulness in children.

More importantly, evaluations of joint function, joint mobility, and true functional change in the patient are more worthwhile evaluators of success in the treatment of spasticity. Initial experiences with gait analysis have proved this technique to be valuable in assessing joint motion during activity and gait-specific actions such as heel and toe strike, the phasing of gait and indirect measurement of gait efficiency, stride length and cadence.[81]

The WEEFIM is a functional scale that evaluates activities of daily living, bowel and bladder, and mobility. The scale has a high interrater reliability and, when applied in the pre- and post-rhizotomy setting, demonstrates a significant improvement in 95 per cent of patients. The actual type of improvement—whether it be activities of daily living, bowel and bladder, or mobility—depends on the individual patient. Global WEE-FIM improvements are seen in almost all patients.

The use of an assistance scale in evaluating particular postures may be useful, particularly in those postures that are relatively stereotyped such as half kneeling, long sitting, and side sitting. The assistance scale measures the amount of assistance needed by the subject to assume and maintain the posture. There are obviously some educational or trainability factors involved; however, in a patient seen by the same physical therapist over multiple examinations, the reliability of these observations increases. Occupational therapy measures to assess improved function in the upper extremities have also been used, such as manual dexterity tests and ability to perform rapid alternating movements. Ease of speech and breath control may also show considerable improvement with alleviation of spasticity.

The goal of treatment of spasticity is to afford the patient enhanced functional potential. In order that interventions be efficient and goal directed, a team of providers is necessary to address the many facets of abilities and disabilities. This team must have at their disposal the full range of services and techniques to handle the changing needs of children with spasticity. No single approach or technique is suitable for all patients. Recognizing that the patients' needs will change over time as influenced by growth, development and the nature of their condition will allow the team to provide timely and appropriate intervention.

REFERENCES

1. Young RR: The physiology of spasticity and its response to therapy. Ann NY Acad Sci 531:146, 1988.
2. Katz RT: Management of spasticity. Am J Phys Med Rehabil 67(3):108, 1988.
3. Delwaide PJ: Spasticity: from pathophysiology to therapy. Acta Neurochir (Wien) 39(Suppl):91, 1987.
4. Little J: Obstetrical Society's Transactions Vol. 3, 1862.
5. Marie P: Arch de Physiologie, 1885.
6. Jendrassik P: Arch de Physiologie, 1885.
7. Gowers WR: Diseases of the Nervous System. London, 1887, vol. 2.
8. Gowers WR: On birth palsies. Lancet i:1888.
9. Wallenberg E: Ein Beitrag zur Lehre von der Cerebralen Kinderlahmungen. Jahrbuch fur Kinderheilkunde, 1886.
10. Strumpell K: Ueber die Acute Encephalitis der Kinder. Jahrbuch fur Kinderheilkunde, 1886.
11. Osler W: The Cerebral Palsies of Children. London, H.K. Lewis, 1889.
12. Sherrington CS: The Integrative Action of the Nervous System. New York, Charles Scribner's Sons, 1906.
13. Sherrington CS: Decerebrate rigidity and reflex coordination of movements. H Physiol (Lond) 22:319, 1898.
14. Abbe R: Resection of the posterior roots of spinal nerves to relieve pain, pain reflex, athetosis and spastic paralysis—Dana's operation. Med Rec 79:377, 1911.
15. Foerster O: On the indications and results of the excision of posterior spinal nerve roots in men. Surg Gynecol Obstet 16:463, 1913.
16. Kasdon DL, Lathi ES: A prospective study of radiofrequency rhizotomy in the treatment of post-traumatic spasticity. Neurosurgery 15:526, 1984.
17. Sindou M, Mertens P, Jeanmonod D: Microsurgical ablative procedures in the peripheral nerves and dorsal root entry zone for relief of focal spasticity in the limbs. Stereotact Funct Neurosurg 54–55:140, 1990.

18. Bischoff W: Die longitudinale Myelotomie. Zentralbl Neurochir 11:79, 1951.

19. Fogel JP, Waters RL, Mahomar F: Dorsal myelotomy for relief of spasticity in spinal injury patients. Clin Orthop 192:137, 1985.

20. Putty TK, Shapiro SA: Efficacy of dorsal longitudinal myelotomy in treating spinal spasticity: a review of 20 cases. J Neurosurg 75(3):397, 1991.

21. Sindou M, Jeanmonod D: Microsurgical DREZ-otomy for the treatment of spasticity and pain in the lower limbs. Neurosurgery 24(5):655, 1989.

22. Vodovnik L, Bowman BR, Winchester P: Effect of electrical stimulation on spasticity in hemiparetic patients. Int Rehabil Med 6(4):153, 1984.

23. Maiman DJ, Myklebust JB, Barolat-Romana G: Spinal cord stimulation for amelioration of spasticity: experimental results. Neurosurgery 21(3):331, 1987.

24. Feinstein B, Gleason CA, Libet B: Stimulation of locus coeruleus in man. Preliminary trials for spasticity and epilepsy. Stereotact Funct Neurosurg 52(1):26, 1989.

25. Penn RD, Myklebust BM, Gottlieb GL, Agarwal GC, Etzel ME: Chronic cerebellar stimulation for cerebral palsy. Prospective and double blind studies. J Neurosurg 53:160, 1980.

26. Vodovnik L, Bowman BR, Hufford P: Effects of electrical stimulation on spinal spasticity. Scand J Rehabil Med 16(1):29, 1984.

27. Barolat-Romana G, Myklebust JB, Hemmy DC, Myklebust B, Wenninger W: Immediate effects of spinal cord stimulation in spinal spasticity. J Neurosurg 62(4):558, 1985.

28. Gottlieb GL, Myklebust BM, Stefoski D, Groth K, Kroin J, Penn RD: Evaluation of cervical stimulation for chronic treatment of spasticity. Neurology 35(5):699, 1985.

29. Bajd T, Gregoric M, Vodovnik L, Benko H: Electrical stimulation in treating spasticity resulting from spinal cord injury. Arch Phys Med Rehabil 66(8):515, 1985.

30. Broseta J, Garcia-March G, Sanchez-Ledesma MJ, Barbera J, Gonzalez-Darder J: High-frequency cervical spinal cord stimulation in spasticity and motor disorders. Acta Neurochir (Wien) 39(Suppl):106, 1987.

31. Fasano VA, Broggi G, Barolat-Romana G, Sguazzi A: Surgical treatment of spasticity in cerebral palsy. Childs Brain 4:289, 1978.

32. Laitinen LV, Nilsson S, Mortamis J: Selective posterior rhizotomy for treatment of spasticity. J Neurosurg 58:895, 1983.

33. Peacock WJ, Arens LJ: Selective posterior rhizotomy for the relief of spasticity in cerebral palsy. S Afr Med J 62:119, 1982.

34. Sindou M, Keravel Y: Microsurgical procedures in the peripheral nerves and the dorsal root entry zone for the treatment of spasticity. Scand J Rehabil Med 17(Suppl):139, 1988.

35. Keenan MA, Todderud EP, Henderson R, Botte M: Management of intrinsic spasticity in the hand with phenol injection or neurectomy of the motor branch of the ulnar nerve. J Hand Surg (Am) 12:734, 1987.

36. Petrillo CR, Knoploch S: Phenol block of the tibial nerve for spasticity: a long-term follow-up study. Int Disabil Stud 10(3):97, 1988.

37. Morrison JE Jr, Hertzberg DL, Gourley SM, Matthews DJ: Motor point blocks in children. A technique to relieve spasticity using phenol injections. AORN J 49(5):1346, 1349, 1989.

38. Chabal C, Jacobson L, White J: Electrical localization of spinal roots for the treatment of spasticity by intrathecal alcohol injection. Anesth Analg 68(4):527, 1989.

39. Erickson DL, Blacklock JB, Michaelson M, Sperling KB, Lo JN: Control of spasticity by implantable continuous flow morphine pump. Neurosurgery 16(2):215, 1985.

40. Erickson DL, Lo J, Michaelson M: Control of intractable spasticity with intrathecal morphine sulfate. Neurosurgery 24(2):236, 1989.

41. Lossius R, Dietrichson P, Lunde PK: Effect of clorazepate in spasticity and rigidity: a quantitative study of reflexes and plasma concentrations. Acta Neurol Scand 71(3):190, 1985.

42. Ketel WB, Kolb ME: Long-term treatment with dantrolene sodium of stroke patients with spasticity limiting the return of function. Curr Med Res Opin 9(3):161, 1984.

43. Das TK, Park DM: Botulinum toxin in treating spasticity. Br J Clin Pract 43(11):401, 1989.

44. Snow BJ, Tsui JK, Bhatt MH, Varelas M, Hashimoto SA, Calne DB: Treatment of spasticity with botulinum toxin: a double-blind study. Ann Neurol 28(4):512, 1990.

45. Penn RD, Kroin JS: Continuous intrathecal baclofen for severe spasticity. Lancet ii:125, 1985.

46. Bovier P, Cambier J, Morselli PL: [Double-blind study of progabide in spasticity.] Etude en double-aveugle du progabide dans la spasticite. Therapie 40(3):181, 1985.

47. Hankey GJ, Stewart-Wynne EG, Perlman D: Intrathecal baclofen for severe spasticity. Med J Aust 145(9):465, 1986.

48. Penn RD, Kroin JS: Long-term intrathecal baclofen infusion for treatment of spasticity. J Neurosurg 66(2):181, 1987.

49. Mery JP, Kenouch S: Oral baclofen may be effective in patients with spasticity due to spinal cord injury or disease. (Letter) Am J Kidney Dis 10(4):326, 1987.

50. Penn RD: Intrathecal baclofen for severe spasticity. Ann NY Acad Sci 531:157, 1988.

51. Penn RD: Intrathecal baclofen for spasticity of spinal origin: seven years of experience. J Neurosurg 77(2):236, 1992.

52. Barolat G: Surgical management of spasticity and spasms in spinal cord injury: an overview. J Am Paraplegia Soc 11(1):9, 1988.

53. Park TS, Cail WS, Maggio WM, Mitchell DC: Progressive spasticity and scoliosis in children with myelomeningocele. Radiological investigation and surgical treatment. J Neurosurg 62(3):367, 1985.

54. Storrs BB: Selective posterior rhizotomy for treatment of progressive spasticity in patients with myelomeningocele. Preliminary report. Pediatr Neurosci 13(3):135, 1987.

55. Young RR, Wiegner AW: Spasticity. Clin Orthop 219:50, 1987.

56. Price R, Bjornson KF, Lehmann JF, McLaughlin JF, Hays RM: Quantitative measurement of spasticity in children with cerebral palsy. Dev Med Child Neurol 33(7):585, 1991.

57. Lehmann JF, Price R, de Lateur BJ, Hinderer S, Traynor C: Spasticity: quantitative measurements as a basis for assessing effectiveness of therapeutic intervention. Arch Phys Med Rehabil 70(1):6, 1989.

58. Ashworth B: Preliminary trial of carisoprodol in multiple sclerosis. Practitioner 192:540, 1964.

59. Haley SM, Ludlow LH: Applicability of the hierarchical scales of the Tufts Assessment of Motor Performance for school-aged children and adults with disabilities. Phys Ther 72(3):191, 1992.

60. Albright AL, Cervi A, Singletary J: Intrathecal baclofen for spasticity in cerebral palsy. JAMA 265(11):1418, 1991.

61. Putty TK, Shapiro SA: Efficacy of dorsal longitudinal myelotomy in treating spinal spasticity: a review of 20 cases. J Neurosurg 75(3):397, 1991.

62. Fogel JP, Waters RL, Mahomar F: Dorsal myelotomy for relief of spasticity in spinal injury patients. Clin Orthop 192:137, 1985.

63. Cusick JF, Larson SJ, Sances A: The effect of T-myelotomy on spasticity. Surg Neurol 6(5):289, 1976.

64. Delwaide PJ: Electrophysiological analysis of the mode of action of muscle relaxants in spasticity. Ann Neurol 17(1):90, 1985.

65. Basmajian JV, Shankardass K, Russell D: Ketazolam once daily for spasticity: double-blind cross-over study. Arch Phys Med Rehabil 67(8):556, 1986.

66. Latash ML, Penn RD, Corcos DM, Gottlieb GL: Short-term effects of intrathecal baclofen in spasticity. Exp Neurol 103(2):165, 1989.

67. Fasano VA, Broggi G, Barolat-Romana G, Sguazzi A: Electrophysiological assessment of spinal circuits in spasticity by direct dorsal root stimulation. Neurosurgery 4:146, 1979.

68. Peacock WJ, Staudt LA: Selective posterior rhizotomy: evolution of theory and practice. Pediatr Neurosurg 17:128, 1991–92.

69. Barolat G: Dorsal selective rhizotomy through a limited exposure of the cauda equina at L-1. Technical note. J Neurosurg 75(5):804, 1991.

70. Lazareff JA, Mata-Acosta AM, Garcia ML: Limited selective posterior rhizotomy for the treatment of spasticity secondary to infantile cerebral palsy: a preliminary report. Neurosurgery 27(4):535, 1990.

71. Alexander MA, Bunch WH, Ebbesson SO: Can experimental dorsal rhizotomy produce scoliosis? J Bone Joint Surg (Am) 54(7):1509, 1972.
72. Cohen AR, Webster HC: How selective is selective posterior rhizotomy? Surg Neurol 35(4):267, 1991.
73. Mayer RF, Mosser RS: Excitability of motoneurons in infants. Neurology 19:932, 1969.
74. Angel RW, Hoffman WW: The H reflex in normal, spastic and rigid subjects. Arch Neurol 8:591, 1963.
75. Futagi Y, Abe J, Tanaka J, Okamoto M, Ikoma H: Recovery curve of the H-reflex in normal infants, central coordination disturbance cases and cerebral palsy patients within the first year of life. Brain Dev 10:8, 1988.
76. Futagi Y, Abe J: H-reflex study in normal children and patients with cerebral palsy. Brain Dev 7:414, 1985.
77. Storrs BB, Nishida T: Use of the H reflex recovery curve in selective posterior rhizotomy. Pediatr Neurosci 14:120, 1988.
78. Bohannon RW, Smith MB: Interrater reliability of a modified Ashworth scale of muscle spasticity. Phys Ther 67(2):206, 1987.
79. Bohannon RW: Variability and reliability of the pendulum test for spasticity using a Cybex II isokinetic dynamometer. Phys Ther 67(5):659, 1987.
80. Storrs BB, Gabler-Spira D, Dias L, Nishida T: Selective posterior rhizotomy—a review of 100 cases. Concepts Pediatr Neurosurg 10:179, 1990.
81. Cahan LD, Adams JM, Perry J, Beeler LM: Instrumented gait analysis after selective dorsal rhizotomy. Dev Med Child Neurol 32(12):1037, 1990.

Chapter 47

STEREOTACTIC NEUROSURGERY

MARION L. WALKER, M.D., JOSEPH PETRONIO, M.D., and
CAROLYN MARIE CAREY, M.D.

Computed tomographic (CT)–guided stereotactic neurosurgery has evolved rapidly since its introduction on a widespread basis in the late 1970s following the development of stereotactic systems such as the Brown-Roberts-Wells (BRW) CT Stereotactic frame at the University of Utah.[1-4] The application of this technology to children soon followed.[5-11] Technical advances in surgical instrumentation, neuro-imaging, and computer hardware and software[12] have extended this technology to increasingly larger neurosurgical applications such as laser surgery,[13-16] stereotactic localization and excision of mass lesions,[3, 4, 17, 18] brachytherapy,[19-21] stereotactic radiosurgery,[22-28] neural transplantation,[29] and neuroendoscopy.[30-33] Stereotactic technology is certainly far beyond the point of being used for needle biopsy only.

Newer applications of stereotactic technology are rapidly approaching. Within a few years we will see frameless stereotaxy on a widespread basis. However, this chapter will draw mostly from the experiences of the past. We will discuss the role of stereotactic neurosurgery in children and discuss our experience using this technology in a purely pediatric population. Table 47–1 lists some of the advantages of stereotactic neurosurgery in the pediatric age group.

TABLE 47–1. ADVANTAGES OF STEREOTACTIC NEUROSURGERY IN CHILDREN

Ease of use
Accurate diagnosis
Controlled situation in the operating room
Multiple trajectories and biopsies possible
Phantom base for accuracy
Applicable in the posterior fossa
Minimal risk/few complications

PATIENT SELECTION

Almost any intracranial procedure can be performed using stereotactic techniques.[4, 18] Most, however, still are best performed in more standard ways. Stereotactic needle biopsy is indicated in patients for whom a tissue diagnosis is needed before definitive treatment, either surgical or nonsurgical, can be implemented.[34] Stereotactic guidance is indicated for the precise placement of craniotomy bone flaps over small cortical or subcortical lesions in eloquent brain areas.[35, 36] Stereotactic techniques may be used to define the limits of a lesion prior to surgical excision.

Feeding vessels in vascular lesions can be targeted with stereotactically guided craniotomies.[3, 4] CT-guided placement for shunts is usually worth the trouble only for precise catheter placement into small fluid spaces (e.g., loculated ventricular cysts, tumor cysts, slit ventricles).

On the pediatric neurosurgical service at the University of Utah/Primary Children's Medical Center, we have used CT stereotactic neurosurgery for a variety of intracranial procedures, including needle biopsy, guided craniotomy, neuroendoscopy, and shunt placement.

NEEDLE BIOPSY

Needle biopsy, as opposed to open craniotomy, still has an important place in neurosurgical patient management.[3-5, 37] It appears, however, that needle biopsy may be more commonly indicated in adult patients than in children, especially in tumor management. Adults have a much higher incidence of high-grade gliomas, and biopsy may play an important role in surgical decision-making.

Gross total excision should be attempted in most tumors of childhood,[38, 39] and so biopsy alone has a less important role in the decision-making process. Needle biopsy in children is indicated when tissue diagnosis is important and craniotomy may be contraindicated, or when the results of biopsy may preclude craniotomy (e.g., lymphoma).

We feel needle biopsy is contraindicated in pineal lesions. Although we have obtained biopsies from eight pineal lesions, these biopsies were obtained early in our series. The chance of a sampling error is high with pineal region tumors unless the entire tumor is examined pathologically. Since the tumor type may have a large influence on treatment decisions, it is best to avoid potential sampling errors that may occur with a needle biopsy. Open surgical excision is the preferred treatment for pineal region tumors whenever possible.[40, 41]

CRANIOTOMY

Stereotactically guided craniotomy facilitates precise placement of the bone flap and helps to define the limits of the intracranial procedure.[3, 4, 18, 42, 43] The closer the lesion is to the cortical surface, the more critical the placement of the craniotomy flap becomes, especially in eloquent brain areas. Stereotactic placement of bone flaps can be done quickly and precisely using the BRW system, especially when combined with the Stereotactic One software (see below).

The limits of the lesion can be defined stereotactically prior to craniotomy. The margins of the tumor, arteriovenous malformation (AVM), or other lesion can be mapped and the operative approaches defined using the precision of stereotactic techniques. Precise points, such as the feeding vessels of AVMs, can be identified and approached. Smaller craniotomies can be done, if appropriate.

NEUROENDOSCOPY

Neuroendoscopy is a rapidly developing and important area of neurosurgery. It has special applications in pediatric neurosurgery, particularly ventriculoscopy.[31–33] (See Chapter 48.) We have found that stereotactic techniques have important applications in ventriculoscopy. Rigid ventriculoscopes are easily adapted to the BRW system, allowing precise placement of the ventriculoscope into small intracranial cavities or ventricles. Flexible scopes can be placed stereotactically through a peel-away trocar while the advantages of the flexible scope are maintained. Our experience has included shunt placement, communication of intraventricular cysts, communicating isolated ventricles, and third ventriculoscopy.

With the arrival of frameless stereotaxy, we will be able to use ventriculoscopes that can be pointed at the target without the external BRW head ring. The computer will show the CT or magnetic resonance (MR)

image located at the intracranial end of the ventriculoscope as well as the direction of the passage. This will allow much more precise placement of cyst wall openings and help to eliminate the confusion caused by distorted anatomy.

MATERIALS/EQUIPMENT

We have used stereotactic techniques in 110 children over the past 10 years (1982 to 1992). The ages ranged from 4 months to 18 years. The median age was 9.1 years. Figure 47–1 shows the localization of the stereotactic procedures. The general principles involving the use of neurosurgical stereotactic instruments will be the same regardless of the manufacturer. Differences do exist, but it is not our purpose here to discuss all of the various CT stereotactic systems. Our experience is with the BRW CT stereotactic frame, and this chapter will focus on its use.

There are several important modifications to the usual technique of stereotactic surgery used in adults when applied to children.[10, 11] Obviously, the older the child, the more the technique becomes like that used in adult patients. The usual modifications for children are the use of general anesthesia, application of the base ring after intubation, use of the pediatric fixation pins, avoidance of overtightening the pins, and minimizing pressure during drilling (Table 47–2).

We have always used general anesthesia for stereotactic neurosurgical cases. This is especially important in younger children when cooperation is important.

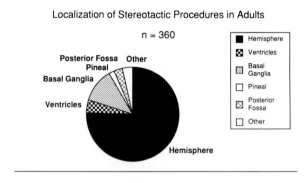

Localization of Stereotactic Procedures in Adults

n = 360

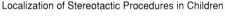

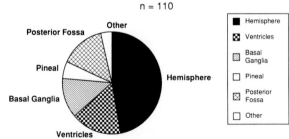

Localization of Stereotactic Procedures in Children

n = 110

FIGURE 47–1. Comparison of stereotactic procedures in adults versus children. (From the Department of Neurosurgery, University of Utah/Primary Children's Medical Center.)

TABLE 47–2. MODIFICATIONS OF TECHNIQUE FOR STEREOTACTIC NEUROSURGERY IN CHILDREN

General anesthesia
Apply base ring after intubation
Use pediatric fixation pins
Avoid overtightening pins
Minimize pressure during drilling

The base ring of the BRW frame is applied after intubation is complete, so that it does not interfere with normal induction and intubation.

The pediatric fixation pins are 1.5 cm longer than the standard BRW fixation pins (Fig. 47–2), allowing the frame to be used in younger children. There is no hard rule as to when the pediatric pins should be used, but we tend to use them for children under 10 years of age. However, if the patient's head size allows use of the adult pins, there is no contraindication to their use at any age. Care must be exercised when tightening the pins in infants. The pins are sharp and will penetrate bone, dura, and the cortical surface if tightened too much. We tighten the pins by fingertip control only in children under 2 years of age.

The next point is obvious but needs to be stated: avoid too much pressure when drilling with a twist drill. In fact, there is really no advantage to using a twist drill as opposed to using a pediatric perforator (7 mm). The larger opening from the perforator can still be made through a small incision and gives adequate exposure to make a controlled dural opening and allow for cortical entry without bleeding. If a twist drill is used, avoid excessive pressure in younger children. A thin skull, further thinned by intracranial hypertension, can be perforated easily with just a twist or two of

the drill. Be cautious, plunging may lead to unnecessary complications.

One of the more commonly asked questions regarding the use of stereotactic frames in pediatric neurosurgery is about the size and age of the child. Is there a limit to how young or how small a child may be before application of this technology is not practical? In general, stereotactic neurosurgery can be considered at any age. However, a very young child with open sutures and a thin skull is at risk both from penetration of the dura with the fixation pins and from movement of the head in the frame if the head is not secure. With caution, we have used the BRW stereotactic frame in several children under one year of age, the youngest being 4 months (Fig. 47–3). When using the frame in infants, be sure to have the fixation pins enter the skull on an oblique angle to avoid penetrating too deep. The skull must be tightly secured by the frame, but caution has to be used to avoid overtightening the pins. If there is significant hydrocephalus, cyst accumulation, or the risk of significant loss of CSF during the procedure, the BRW frame is contraindicated. The skull may collapse inward with the loss of CSF, dislodging the pins.

STEREOTACTIC INSTRUMENTS

Stereotactic instruments are varied, depending on the particular needs. The most commonly used instrument is probably the biopsy needle, and we prefer the Nashold side-cutting needle. A variety of biopsy needles are available, including a straight open-ended needle,

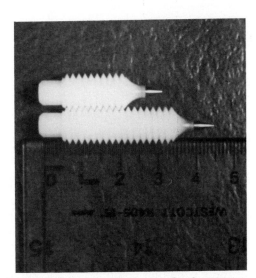

FIGURE 47–2. Adult and pediatric pins for the BRW stereotactic system. The pediatric pins are 1.5 cm longer.

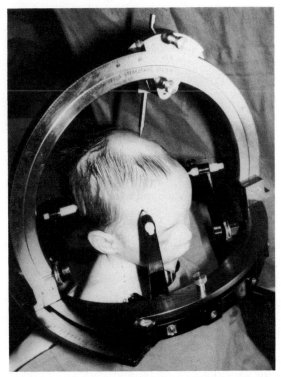

FIGURE 47–3. A 4-month-old infant in the BRW frame with entry point defined.

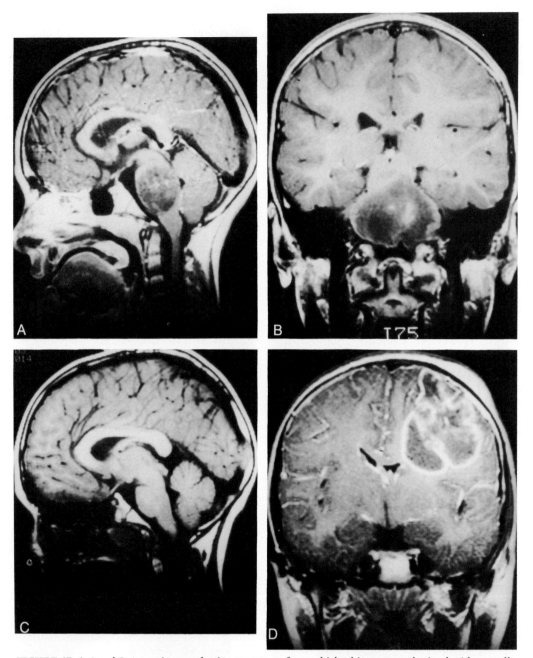

FIGURE 47–4. *A* and *B*, A pontine anaplastic astrocytoma from which a biopsy was obtained with a needle without the outer sleeve. Seventeen months later, the patient presented with headache, vomiting, and hemiparesis. The pons shows no tumor recurrence *(C)*, but there is seeding along the biopsy track *(D)*. Biopsy of the hemisphere lesion showed a glioblastoma.

which is especially useful for aspiration. Other instruments include scissors, grasping forceps, needles, ventriculoscopes, and laser fibers.

The outer sleeve for the biopsy needle should always be used. Seeding of tumor along the track is possible if the needle is used without the outer sleeve. We have seen this in one case. Biopsy of a malignant pontine glioma without the use of the outer sleeve resulted in seeding along the biopsy track, which was detected 17 months later (Fig. 47–4).

Standard BRW

One of the strong advantages of the BRW stereotactic system is the ability to use the phantom base ring to check all coordinates before the actual procedure is done (Fig. 47–5). This adds a considerable margin of safety. A small dedicated laptop computer, complete with software, comes with the system. The target and entry point must be chosen and all rods marked by means of the CT scanner computer. If the entry point

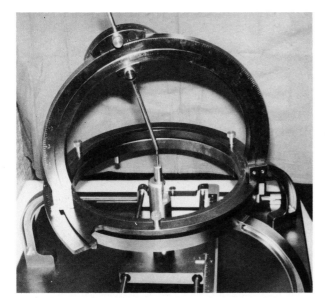

FIGURE 47–5. The phantom base ring allows the surgeon to check all coordinates and settings prior to starting surgery.

and target are on different CT slices, the rods must be marked separately on each CT scan level.

STEREOTACTIC ONE

Stereotactic One is a proprietary software program available for either the IBM compatible or the Macintosh personal computer. The data tape from the stereotactic CT scan is read into the computer in the operating room through a tape drive (Fig. 47–6). Once the data are in the operating room computer, Stereotactic One is used to mark the rods and to pick the entry point and the target. The program shows the projected pass through the brain, allowing the surgeon to pick a

new trajectory if needed. Multiple targets may be chosen. This software makes the use of the BRW frame much easier and simpler and truly saves time, since the rods are marked automatically and there is no need to mark each CT scan level if multiple trajectories are chosen.

COMPLICATIONS

Several potential complications may occur from stereotactic surgery (Table 47–3). Careful preoperative planning is necessary. Care must be taken to perform the biopsy on the correct lesion when more than one are present. Although it is rarely necessary, preparations should always be made for an emergency craniotomy. Fortunately, complications are rare in children. Table 47–4 lists some practical suggestions for avoiding complications in stereotactic surgery. Table 47–5 tabulates the complications in our series of 110 patients.

In our series there were no deaths. Death is certainly a potential risk but appears to be more likely in the adult population, probably due to the nature of the lesions undergoing biopsy.[34]

CT stereotactic biopsy appears to have a low morbidity in children, owing partly to the nature of the lesions seen in the pediatric age group. We experienced two cases of transient increase in neurologic deficit following needle biopsy (1.8 per cent). One case was complicated by a transient sixth nerve palsy following a pontine tumor biopsy, the other by a transient hemiparesis following biopsy of a tumor in the region of the basal ganglia. Both patients returned to their preoperative state within 24 hours.

Infection is also a potential complication. Fortunately, this seems to be rare. We experienced no infections in 110 stereotactic procedures. This includes all procedures, whether they involved needle biopsy only or open prolonged stereotactically guided craniotomy.

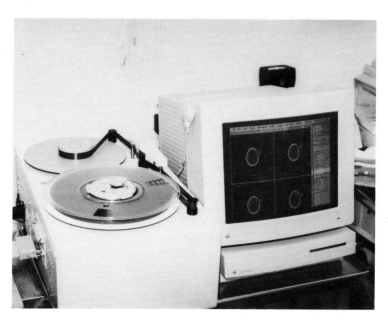

FIGURE 47–6. A reel-to-reel tape drive allows the CT scan data tape to be read directly into a personal computer for use with the Stereotactic One software.

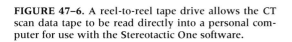

TABLE 47–3.   POTENTIAL COMPLICATIONS OF STEREOTACTIC NEUROSURGERY

Death
Infection
Bleeding
Biopsy of the wrong lesion
Unprepared for an emergency craniotomy
Tissue sample size
False-positive/false-negative diagnosis

TABLE 47–5.   COMPLICATIONS OF STEREOTACTIC NEUROSURGERY IN 110 PEDIATRIC PATIENTS

Death	0
Transient deficit	2
Infection	0
Bleeding	2
Seeding of tumor	1
False-positive	0
False-negative	4

Although a small amount of bleeding occasionally is seen at the biopsy site, significant post-biopsy bleeding is unusual, especially in children. We experienced two cases of bleeding (1.8 per cent) in our series. Neither case was complicated by a neurologic deficit. The bleeding was noted on routine follow-up CT scans.

Another potential complication is a false-positive or false-negative diagnosis obtained by needle biopsy. This sometimes can be attributed to the small tissue sample size. Undoubtedly, the pathologist would like to have as much tissue as possible. However, experience with needle biopsy will increase the confidence level of the pathologist. The usual problem is not the size of the sample but the location of the biopsy. One should always try to obtain the biopsy from the enhancing portion of the lesion if possible. Biopsies from a necrotic area will often be nondiagnostic. Likewise, the periphery of low-grade lesions may yield reactive or nondiagnostic tissue. We have experienced this four times in our series (3.6 per cent).

CONCLUSION

Stereotactic neurosurgery appears to be safe in the pediatric patient. This technology has an important place in the armamentarium of the pediatric neurosurgeon. Many applications have been developed since the early days of needle biopsy only. It appears that stereotactic techniques can be used in very young children and complications are few.

Soon we will see frameless stereotaxy and newer applications of this technology to children; 3-D digitizers will define stereotactic space with the use of CT and/or MRI images. This will allow real-time visualization of images during stereotactic neurosurgical procedures, increasing accuracy and safety.

TABLE 47–4.   AVOIDING COMPLICATIONS IN STEREOTACTIC NEUROSURGERY

Be sure the lesion is not an arteriovenous malformation!
Avoid the sylvian fissure
Do not cross two arachnoid planes
Plan a perpendicular trajectory if possible
Use a burr hole instead of a twist drill if more than one biopsy target is planned
Obtain biopsy from the enhancing area, not the necrotic center
Use both the outer cannula and the inner needle

REFERENCES

1. Brown RA: A computerized tomography-computer graphics approach to stereotactic localization. J Neurosurg 50:715, 1979.
2. Gildenberg PL: The history of stereotactic neurosurgery. Neurosurg Clin North Am 1:765, 1990.
3. Heilbrun MP, Roberts TS, Apuzzo MLJ, Wells TH, Sabshin JK: Preliminary experience with the Brown-Roberts-Wells (BRW) computerized tomography stereotaxic guidance system. J Neurosurg 59:217, 1983.
4. Heilbrun MP, Brockmeyer DL, Sunderland P: Stereotactic neurosurgery for mass lesions of the cranial vault. *In* Apuzzo MLJ (ed): Brain Surgery: Complication Avoidance and Management. New York, Churchill Livingstone, 1992, pp. 390–405.
5. Davis DH, Kelly PJ, Marsh WR, Kall BA, Goerss SJ: Computer-assisted stereotactic biopsy of intracranial lesions in pediatric patients. Pediatr Neurosci 14:31, 1988.
6. Finizio FS, Frank F, Ricci R, Ruggiero G: Contribution of stereotactic techniques to the diagnosis and treatment of cerebral tumors in childhood (tumors of the pineal region excluded). J Neuroradiol 15:353, 1988.
7. Broggi G, Franzini A, Migliavacca F, Allegranza A: Stereotactic biopsy of deep brain tumors in infancy and childhood. Childs Brain 10:92, 1983.
8. Godano U, Frank F, Fabrizi AP, Ricci RF: Stereotactic surgery in the management of deep brain lesions in infants and adolescents. Childs Nerv Syst 3:85, 1987.
9. Schmitt HP, Wowra B, Sturm V: Diagnostic value of the stereotactic approach to focal lesions in the deep brain of children and adolescents. Brain Dev 10:305, 1988.
10. Storrs BB, Walker ML: Use of a CT-guided stereotaxic apparatus in pediatric neurosurgery. Concepts Pediatr Neurosurg 5:214, 1985.
11. Pattisapu JV, Walker ML, Heilbrun MP: Stereotactic neurosurgery in children. Pediatr Neurosci 15:62, 1989.
12. Kall BA: The impact of computer and imaging technology on stereotactic surgery. Appl Neurophysiol 50:9, 1987.
13. Abernathey CD, Davis DH, Kelly PJ: Treatment of colloid cysts of the third ventricle by stereotaxic microsurgical laser craniotomy. J Neurosurg 70:525, 1989.
14. Kelly PJ, Alker GJ, Goerss S: Computer-assisted stereotactic laser microsurgery for the treatment of intracranial neoplasms. Neurosurgery 10:324, 1982.
15. Kelly PJ, Kall BA, Goerss S, Earnest F: Computer-assisted stereotaxic laser resection of intra-axial brain neoplasms. J Neurosurg 64:427, 1986.
16. Kelly PJ, Kall BA, Goerss SJ: Computer-interactive stereotactic resection of deep-seated and centrally located intraaxial brain lesions. Appl Neurophysiol 50:107, 1987.
17. Kelly PJ, Alker GJ: A stereotactic approach to deep-seated central nervous system neoplasms using the carbon dioxide laser. Surg Neurol 15:331, 1981.
18. Apuzzo MLJ, Chandrosoma PT, Cohen D, Zee C, Zelman V: Computed imaging stereotaxy: Experience and perspective related to 500 procedures applied to brain masses. Neurosurgery 20:930, 1987.
19. DeRiu PL, Rocca A: Interstitial irradiation therapy of supratentorial gliomas by stereotaxic technique. Long term results. Ital J Neurol Sci 9:243, 1988.

20. Coffey RJ, Friedman WA: Interstitial brachytherapy of malignant brain tumors using computed tomography-guided stereotaxis and available imaging software: Technical report. Neurosurgery 20:4, 1987.
21. Sapozink MD, Moeller JM, McDonald PN, Heilbrun MP: Improved precision of interstitial brain tumor irradiation using the BRW CT stereotaxic guidance system. Int J Radiat Oncol Biol Phys 13:1753, 1987.
22. Winston KR, Lutz W: Linear accelerator as a neurosurgical tool for stereotactic surgery. Neurosurgery 22:454, 1988.
23. Larson DA, Gutin PH, Leibel SA, Phillips TL: Stereotaxic irradiation of brain tumors. Cancer 65:792, 1990.
24. Lunsford LD, Kondziolka D, Bissonette DJ, Maitz AH, Flickinger JC: Stereotactic radiosurgery of brain vascular malformations. Neurosurg Clin North Am 3:79, 1992.
25. Lunsford LD, Kondziolka D, Flickinger JC: Stereotactic radiosurgery: current spectrum and results. Clin Neurosurg 38:405, 1992.
26. Kondziolka D, Lunsford LD, Flickinger JC: Stereotactic radiosurgery in children and adolescents. Pediatr Neurosurg 16:219, 1990.
27. Friedman WA: LINAC radiosurgery. Neurosurg Clin North Am 1:991, 1990.
28. Coffey RJ, Lunsford LD: Stereotactic radiosurgery using the 201 cobalt-60 source gamma knife. Neurosurg Clin North Am 1:933, 1990.
29. Fazzini E, Dwork AJ, Blum C, Burke R, Cote L, Goodman R, Jacobs TP, Naini AB, Pezzoli G, Pullman S: Stereotaxic implantation of autologous adrenal medulla into caudate nucleus in four patients with parkinsonism. One year follow-up. Arch Neurol 48:813, 1991.
30. Zamorano L, Chavantes C, Dujovny M, Malik G, Ausman J: Stereotactic endoscopic interventions in cystic and intraventricular brain lesions. Acta Neurochir (Wien) 54(Suppl):69, 1992.
31. Hor F, Desgeorges M, Rosseau GL: Tumor resection by stereotactic laser endoscopy. Acta Neurochir (Wien) 54(Suppl):77, 1992.
32. Hellwig D, Bauer BL, List-Hellwig E, Mennel HD: Stereotactic-endoscopic procedures on processes of the cranial midline. Acta Neurochir (Wien) 53(Suppl):23, 1991.
33. Hellwig D, Bauer BL: Endoscopic procedures in stereotactic neurosurgery. Acta Neurochir (Wien) 52(Suppl):30, 1991.
34. Chandrasoma PT, Smith MM, Apuzzo MLJ: Stereotactic biopsy in the diagnosis of brain masses: comparison of results of biopsy and resected surgical specimen. Neurosurgery 24:160, 1989.
35. Hariz MI, Fadstad H: Stereotactic localization of small subcortical brain tumors for open surgery. Surg Neurol 28:245, 1987.
36. Moore MR, Black PM, Ellenbogen R, Gall CM, Eldredge E: Stereotactic craniotomy: Methods and results using the Brown-Roberts-Wells stereotactic frame. Neurosurgery 25:572, 1989.
37. Kelly PJ, Daumas-Duport C, Kispert DB, Kall BA, Scheithauer BW, Illig JJ: Imaging-based stereotaxic serial biopsies in untreated intracranial glial neoplasms. J Neurosurg 66:865, 1987.
38. Sanford RA, Kun LE, Langston JW, Kovnar EH: Pitfalls in the management of low-grade gliomas. Concepts Pediatr Neurosurg 11:133, 1991.
39. Sanford RA, Duffner P, Krischer J, Kun LE, Burger PC: Effect of gross total resection on malignant brain tumors of infancy. Presented at 60th Annual Meeting, American Association of Neurological Surgeons, 1992. San Francisco, CA; American Association of Neurological Surgeons.
40. Bruce DA, Schut L, Sutton LN: Pineal region tumors. In McLaurin R, JL Venes, L Schut, F Epstein (eds): Pediatric Neurosurgery: Surgery of the Developing Nervous System. Philadelphia, WB Saunders, 1989, pp. 409–416.
41. Bruce JN, Stein BM: Pineal tumors. Neurosurg Clin North Am 1:123, 1990.
42. Apuzzo MLJ, Sabshin JK: Computed tomographic guidance stereotaxis in the management of intracranial mass lesions. Neurosurgery 12:277, 1983.
43. Kelly PJ: Stereotactic craniotomy. Neurosurg Clin North Am 1:781, 1990.

Chapter 48

VENTRICULOSCOPY

MARION L. WALKER, M.D., JOSEPH PETRONIO, M.D., and
CAROLYN MARIE CAREY, M.D.

Both the history and the future of ventriculoscopy are intimately linked to the management of hydrocephalus. While early ventriculoscopists sought merely to visually inspect the ventricular system or make crude attempts at controlling hydrocephalus, such as fulguration or avulsion of the choroid plexus,[1, 2] they were hindered by inferior equipment and inconsistent results.[3] Although technologic improvements in optical systems, neuroradiologic imaging, and computer-assisted stereotactic techniques have greatly improved the available equipment, the resurgence in popularity of ventriculoscopy is predicated largely upon the shortcomings of currently available techniques for cerebrospinal fluid (CSF) shunting.[4–14] Its ultimate utility in the armamentarium of the pediatric neurosurgeon will be determined to the point that it represents a more effective and cost-efficient means of managing hydrocephalus.

PROBLEMS WITH SHUNTS

With the development of valved shunt systems,[15] ventriculo-extracranial shunts became the standard treatment for all types of hydrocephalus. Despite decades of experience and refinement, the long-term morbidity and mortality rates associated with shunt systems are significant. Common shunt problems include all too frequent system malfunctions due to obstruction of the ventricular catheter,[4–6] valve failure,[4] and blockage or lack of absorption of CSF distally.[6–8] Additional problems relating to the site of distal drainage include abdominal, vascular, or pleural complications,[9] bacteremia, "shunt nephritis," or foreign body reactions.[16] Despite modern surgical techniques and antibiotics, infection rates may be as high as 8 per cent,[10, 11] with an associated 6 per cent mortality rate.[10]

Even when functional, shunts may be problematic because of their failure to drain at physiologic pressures. Complications from overdrainage include extra-axial collections and hematomas, low-pressure syndromes,[8, 12] and the slit-ventricle syndrome.[7, 13] While the lives of many have been spared and their quality of life has been improved with valved shunting systems, these ongoing difficulties prompt a continued search for better shunt systems or alternative therapies such as endoscopy.

HISTORY OF VENTRICULOSCOPY

V. L. l'Espinasse was the first to inspect in vivo the ventricles of a hydrocephalic child.[17] Using a cystoscope designed for the adult bladder, he was able to fulgurate the choroid plexus bilaterally in two infants. Despite the fact that one child lived for 5 years following the procedure, this success remained largely unnoticed.

Dandy utilized a primitive instrument that was similar in appearance to a funnel that emitted light reflected from a head mirror in attempting to coagulate the choroid plexus and reduce CSF production.[1, 18] He believed that the procedure was only partially successful, and he resorted to removing the choroid plexus in the standard fashion—by avulsing it with alligator forceps.

Shortly thereafter Mixter,[19] using a small urethroscope and a flexible sound, performed the first endoscopic third ventriculostomy in a 9-month-old girl with noncommunicating hydrocephalus. Although Fay and Grant,[20] Putnam,[21] and Scarff[2, 22, 23] continued to perform ventriculoscopy, it gradually fell from favor. In its nascent stages, the cerebral endoscope was primarily used to inspect the ventricles or crudely extirpate or fulgurate the choroid plexus.[2]

In the late 1940s and 1950s, Hopkins devised a means of forming a coherent (i.e., image-transmitting) fiberoptic bundle, using a solid rod lens system instead of a series of glass lenses in air.[24] This concept permitted the introduction of beams through a much smaller tel-

572

escape and formed the foundation for the entire flexible endoscopy industry.[24] Light could also be transmitted through an incoherent (nonimage-transmitting) fiber bundle, and Guiot utilized the reflective properties of a quartz rod to transmit light from an external source and photograph in color the inside of a lateral ventricle.[25]

Ventriculoscopy has had a poor reputation, owing in part to the optically inferior and bulky equipment of the pioneer ventriculoscopists. Modern equipment is safe and allows surgical procedures to be effectively performed with the instrument.[3]

INDICATIONS FOR VENTRICULOSCOPY

Ventriculoscopy has been performed for both diagnostic and therapeutic goals (Table 48–1). Diagnostic objectives include both anatomic surveillance and biopsy of lesions, whereas therapeutic interventions include cyst or hematoma aspiration, tumor resection, catheter placement, catheter and/or foreign body retrieval, and restoration or establishment of pathways for CSF flow or communication.

ANATOMIC INSPECTION

Direct inspection of the ventricular system has been used by some authors[26] to determine the etiology of hydrocephalus, whether postinflammatory or congenital. As described in the work of Fukushima et al.,[26] direct inspection of the ventricular system can be utilized alone in diagnosing intraventricular tumors such as pinealomas, or as a prelude to a definitive open approach. In addition, direct endoscopic inspection has been utilized to diagnose intraventricular spread of tumor.[27] Current magnetic resonance imaging capabilities probably leave little role for endoscopic inspection alone for diagnosis in the pediatric population.

BIOPSY

Endoscopy has been successfully performed for biopsy of intraparenchymal tumors,[28] intraventricular

TABLE 48–1. SUMMARY OF REPORTED INDICATIONS FOR VENTRICULOSCOPY

Diagnostic indications
  Anatomic inspection
  Biopsy
Therapeutic indications
  Cyst or hematoma aspiration
  Tumor resection
  Catheter placement or foreign body retrieval
  CSF communication
    Multicompartmental hydrocephalus
    Arachnoid cysts
    Unilateral hydrocephalus
    Third ventriculocisternostomy

tumors,[3, 26, 29–31] thalamic tumors,[29] pineal region tumors,[26, 29] and hypothalamic tumors.[32] In a series of 67 endoscopic cases published in 1978, Fukushima reported using a flexible endoscope and cup-shaped probe in 27 attempted tumor biopsies, including lateral ventricular tumors (n = 9), third ventricular tumors (n = 6), pineal region tumors (n = 4), and thalamic tumors (n = 2).[29] A useful histologic diagnosis was obtained in only 11 of 27 cases. Unsuccessful or nondiagnostic biopsies were attributed to the small, solitary biopsy specimens taken because of extensive gliosis or the perceived risk of hemorrhage. Apuzzo and co-workers reported 28 cases in which computed tomographic (CT)–guided stereotactic endoscopy was successfully utilized for biopsy of deep-seated brain masses.[33] Powell and colleagues reported on 11 patients with colloid cysts of the third ventricle who underwent diagnostic ventriculoscopy.[3] In their series, the diagnosis was correctly established endoscopically in five patients, and a CT diagnosis was confirmed in an additional five patients.

Obvious advantages of endoscopic biopsy include a significantly smaller and less traumatic surgical approach to deep lesions than with craniotomy,[31] direct visual inspection and confirmation of the biopsy target,[14, 33] and the ability to visually check for post-biopsy bleeding.[31]

CYST OR HEMATOMA ASPIRATION

Endoscopy has been successfully utilized for both aspiration of cysts[28, 30, 31] and evacuation of intracerebral hematomas.[28, 31] In the former case, both tumor-related cysts and abscess cavities have been aspirated endoscopically.[28, 31] It is technically feasible to endoscopically obtain a biopsy from the walls of tumor-associated cysts or abscesses as well as place catheters for instillation of radioisotopes, antibiotics, or percutaneous aspiration.[28] The suction-aspiration capabilities of the endoscope, as well as the potential for delivery of coagulating current or laser irradiation, also make it well suited, in theory, for evacuation of intraparenchymal or intraventricular hematomas.[31] Several authors report over 50 per cent effectiveness in evacuating intracranial hematomas, often sparing patients open procedures.[28, 31]

TUMOR RESECTION

Although large, solid, and vascular tumors may be difficult or impossible to remove endoscopically, currently available technology renders certain lesions such as the colloid cyst amenable to safe and effective endoscopic fulguration or resection. For example, Powell et al. successfully performed ventriculoscopic drainage in 5 of 6 attempted cases of colloid cyst of the third ventricle.[3] Using either a 25-gauge spinal needle or a 16-gauge Touhy spinal needle to aspirate colloid cysts under endoscopic visualization, they then withdrew the needle and passed a coagulating probe down the cannula.[3] Alternatively, the endoscopic rongeurs were used for lesions too viscous to aspirate.[3] Irrigation can be utilized with either warm Ringer's lactate[3] or normal saline. Fukushima et al. successfully performed endoscopic drainage and aspiration of tumor-related cysts in four patients in their series of 37 tumors treated endoscopically.[26]

Apuzzo and co-workers report the successful adaptation of CT-guided stereotactic technology to the endoscopic biopsy of intraventricular tumors, including craniopharyngiomas and ependymomas.[30] In addition, they believe that cyst puncture, aspiration, and excision under direct vision are potentially safe and effective in managing colloid cysts of the third ventricular region.

Endoscopic techniques may be safely utilized for biopsy of solid intraventricular tumors or attempted resection of small, poorly vascularized or cystic intraventricular tumors. The advantages in this situation include a limited and relatively atraumatic transcortical path to deep-seated lesions, lower overall morbidity than with open craniotomy, and the ability to enhance stereotactic procedures with direct visualization of the target lesion.

Catheter Placement or Foreign Body Retrieval

Several authors report endoscopic placement of catheters, whether in cysts[28, 30, 31] or in the ventricular system. Consistent and precise placement of a ventricular catheter at the time of shunt insertion has been shown to result in a lower long-term morbidity and a lower rate of shunt revision. Kleinhaus and co-workers successfully used an endoscope to fenestrate multicompartmental hydrocephalus and place a single ventricular catheter in a child with posthemorrhagic hydrocephalus.[34] At Primary Children's Medical Center of the University of Utah, we have successfully used the ventriculoscope to remove retained ventricular catheters from two patients and a foreign body (shotgun pellet) from a third.

Cerebrospinal Fluid Communication

Despite the previous indications for ventriculoscopy, it is the management of hydrocephalus and associated conditions that attracts pediatric neurosurgeons. In order to better delineate the clinical utility of ventriculoscopic surgery in the pediatric population, especially as it relates to the management of hydrocephalus and associated conditions, we retrospectively reviewed the cases of all children undergoing ventricular endoscopy at Primary Children's Medical Center of the University of Utah. Since July, 1987 we have performed 70 ventriculoscopic procedures on 50 children, ranging in age from 3 days to 18 (median, 2.68) years at the time of initial intervention.

The indications for endoscopic intervention in hydrocephalus are classified into four categories (Table 48–

TABLE 48–2. SUMMARY OF ENDOSCOPIC PROCEDURES FOR CSF COMMUNICATION PERFORMED AT PRIMARY CHILDREN'S MEDICAL CENTER—UNIVERSITY OF UTAH SINCE JULY, 1987

INDICATIONS	NO. OF PATIENTS	NO. OF PROCEDURES
Multicompartmental hydrocephalus	17	35
Unilateral	6	11
Bilateral	11	24
Unilateral hydrocephalus (isolated lateral ventricle)	9	10
Arachnoid cysts	14	15
Third ventriculostomy	10	10
Obstructive hydrocephalus	4	4
Slit-ventricle syndrome	6	6

2): multicompartmental hydrocephalus (unilateral or bilateral), unilateral hydrocephalus or an isolated lateral ventricle, focal arachnoid cysts, and noncommunicating hydrocephalus treated with third ventriculostomy.

Multicompartmental Hydrocephalus

The presence of septations or cystic areas within the ventricular system, as seen in infants with posthemorrhagic or postinfectious hydrocephalus, often prevents adequate drainage by conventional CSF shunts.[35] Such cases often require multiple shunts and/or blind fenestrations of the septa by multiperforated shunt tubes; even then, decompression might be incomplete,[36–39] with long-term mortality rates as high as 70 per cent.[39]

Kleinhaus et al. reported in a single case successful fenestration of loculated cyst collections in a child with postinfectious multicompartmental hydrocephalus.[34] The largest group of patients treated endoscopically at Primary Children's Medical Center of the University of Utah included those with unilateral or bilateral multicompartmental hydrocephalus, usually secondary to severe intraventricular hemorrhage of prematurity or recurrent ventriculitis. In this group of patients, 35 ventriculoscopic procedures were performed in 17 patients, usually for fenestration of multiple synechiae or septations. This group had the highest failure rate when measured in terms of the radiographic recurrence of loculated collections and the need for additional ventricular catheters and complex shunts. Although unilateral or focal compartmentalizations were associated with a more favorable outcome following ventriculoscopic fenestration, only 8 of 18 patients were believed to have had a "satisfactory" or "good" outcome when measured in terms of radiographically demonstrable reduction in ventricular size and clinical stability (Fig. 48–1).

Although success with endoscopic fenestration of multicompartmentalized ventricles has been sporadic, in some cases, especially with unilateral disease, it has been useful in reducing the number of ventricular cath-

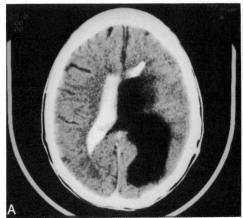
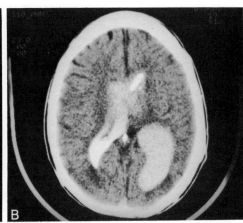

FIGURE 48–1. Axial iohexol CT-ventriculogram of a patient with unilateral multicompartmental hydrocephalus before (A) and after (B) ventriculoscopic fenestration.

eters and in simplifying or eliminating complex "Y-ed" or "T-ed" shunts. Surgical failures are probably related to the nature of the disease process itself; that is, treating inflammatory and reactive processes in the CNS with surgical lysis is probably suboptimal.

Arachnoid Cysts

Previous authors reported successful endoscopic fenestration of loculated CSF collections into the ventricular system or subarachnoid space.[40] In our experience, a favorable result with ventriculoscopic fenestration was obtained with the 15 procedures performed on 14 patients with focal arachnoid cysts, including cysts of the septum pellucidum (n=5), suprasellar cistern (n=3), interhemispheric fissure (n=2), and lateral ventricles (n=4). In this group, a "satisfactory" or "good" outcome was obtained in 9 of 14 patients treated endoscopically, including complete shunt independence in 9 of 14 patients (Fig. 48–2).

Heilman and Cohen reported on eight patients with isolated CSF cavities (six with hydrocephalus and a loculated cyst and two with trapped lateral ventricles)

treated by fenestration of the cyst wall or septum pellucidum, using a "saline torch"; all patients in this series underwent fenestration and shunt insertion.[40] Fukushima et al. treated six patients with fenestration of the septum pellucidum, including two with tumors obliterating the foramen of Monro and one with a cyst of the septum pellucidum.[26] Both groups concurred that fenestration is simple, safe, and effective and might allow simplification of some shunt systems and elimination of shunts in others.

Unilateral Hydrocephalus (Isolated Lateral Ventricle)

Since 1977, we have performed a total of ten endoscopic procedures on nine patients with unilateral hydrocephalus at Primary Children's Medical Center-University of Utah. In this group the surgical goal was usually fenestration of the septum pellucidum to establish a pathway for CSF flow between the two lateral ventricles (Fig. 48–3). This group included patients with anterior third ventricular tumors, such as chiasmal/hypothalamic gliomas or craniopharyngiomas, causing obstruction at the foramen of Monro. Satisfac-

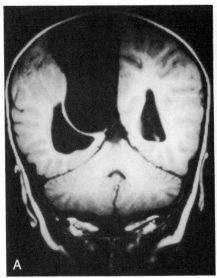
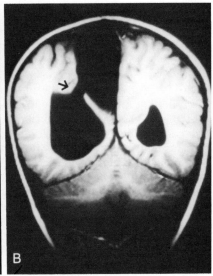

FIGURE 48–2. Coronal T1-weighted MR images of a loculated interhemispheric arachnoid cyst before (A) and after (B) ventriculoscopic fenestration. Note the large fenestration into the occipital horn of the lateral ventricle (arrow).

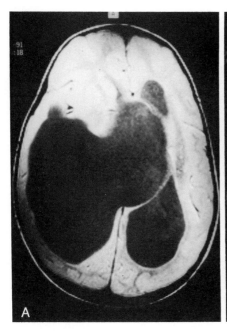 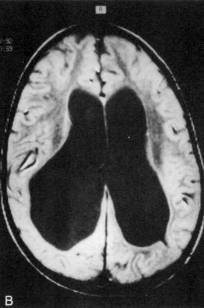

FIGURE 48–3. Axial T1-weighted MR images of a child with unilateral hydrocephalus before (A) and after (B) ventriculoscopic fenestration.

tory or good results were obtained in seven of nine children, with three of nine remaining completely shunt-independent (see Fig. 48–3).

Third Ventriculostomy

HISTORY OF THIRD VENTRICULOSTOMY

Before CSF shunting became commonplace, the most common operation for relief of obstructive hydrocephalus was third ventriculostomy.[41] In 1922, Dandy initially described a frontal craniotomy, elevation of the frontal lobe, sectioning of an optic nerve, and perforation of the lamina terminalis and floor of the third ventricle.[1] A high operative mortality rate and the necessity of sectioning the optic nerve caused him to adopt a less risky subtemporal approach.[42]

Mixter was the first to perform an endoscopic third ventriculostomy using a urethroscope directed into the third ventricle and a flexible sound for fenestration under visual guidance.[19] However, the procedure never became popular because of the cumbersome size and poor illumination with existing instrumentation. Since the early work by Dandy and Mixter, several authors[43–48] have reported successful fenestrations of the third ventricle. Scarff[49] later added an additional posterior midline opening into the interpeduncular cistern between and slightly behind the mamillary bodies; endoscopy still had an unacceptably high mortality rate, estimated to be as high as 30 per cent, due to intracranial complications such as hemorrhage.[22]

McNickle[50] introduced a percutaneous method of performing a third ventriculostomy that reduced the morbidity associated with craniotomy and improved the success rate to 71 per cent, compared with Dandy's 39 per cent. Subsequent experience with both craniotomy and percutaneous third ventriculostomy met with discouragingly inconsistent results (Table 48–3), and

with the introduction of valvular shunting devices,[15] impetus for refinement of third ventriculostomy was lost.

Initial attempts with a ventriculoscope proved less successful.[24, 51, 52] Some authors argued that ventriculoscopic fenestration failed to identify the position of important extra-ependymal structures and thereby offered no less risk of damage to important structures.[53]

INDICATIONS

CSF absorption mechanisms are usually intact in patients with acquired hydrocephalus.[14, 54, 55] As a result, several methods of "internal shunting" have been ex-

TABLE 48–3. SUMMARY OF REPORTED PERCUTANEOUS THIRD VENTRICULOSCOPIC PROCEDURES

AUTHOR	YEAR	NO. CASES	OPERATIVE MORTALITY (%)	SUCCESS RATE (%)
McNickle	1947	7	0	71
Forjaz et al.	1968	15	20	67
Perlman	1968	1	0	100
Raimondi	1972	3	0	0
Guiot	1973	14	0	64
Pierre-Kahn et al.	1975	44	7	64
Poblete and Zamboni	1975	10	0	70
Hoffman	1976	11	0	27
Sayers and Kosnick	1976	46	4	89
Ziedses des Plantes and Crezee	1978	61	0	15
Vries	1978	5	0	20
Hoffman et al.	1980	22	0	45
Jones	1990	24	0	50
Summary		263	3.5	52.5

Adapted with permission from Hoffman HJ, Harwood-Nash D, Gilday DL: Percutaneous third ventriculostomy in the management of non-communicating hydrocephalus. Neurosurgery 7:313, 1980.

plored, including third ventriculostomy by open craniotomy[1, 42, 48] using subfrontal[1, 41, 45, 56–59] or subtemporal[42, 46, 60] approaches, percutaneous techniques, including ventriculoscopic,[19, 51, 53, 61, 62] free-hand,[19, 43, 50–52, 61–63] or stereotactic[14, 53, 64–67] techniques, aqueductal reconstruction,[9, 68–70] and Torkildsen's ventriculocisternostomy.[71, 72] Despite inconsistent results with many of these procedures, they were often successful in managing obstructive hydrocephalus in the subgroup of patients with nontumoral late-onset aqueductal stenosis of adolescence or adulthood.

Patterson and Bergland noted that if third ventriculostomy fails to relieve hydrocephalus, the usual cause is an incompetent subarachnoid space.[73] Even Dandy[74] noted that the procedure seemed to work best in those patients with acquired aqueductal stenosis and tumors and not in children with congenital hydrocephalus.

Jones et al. treated 24 patients, including five patients with myelomeningocele and one with postmeningitic hydrocephalus, with endoscopic third ventriculostomy.[75] While their overall success rate was 50 per cent, they reported success in three of five patients with congenital hydrocephalus secondary to myelomeningocele. There is no consensus as to the utility of third ventriculostomy in the treatment of obstructive hydrocephalus secondary to myelomeningocele. While most reports suggest that third ventriculostomy alone in myelomeningocele patients is insufficient,[75] several groups report more favorable results, including shunt independence,[45, 50, 52, 62, 76, 77] as well as a significant reduction in shunt revision rates when shunt insertions are accompanied by ventriculostomy.[62, 77] Moreover, even in patients who required shunts, evidence exists to support the fact that conversion to a communicating hydrocephalus will make them less likely to have the massive and acute intracranial pressure rises than if the hydrocephalus had remained noncommunicating when shunt malfunction occurred.[7] Guiot et al. performed posterior third ventricular perforation in five patients with obstructive hydrocephalus and showed that third ventriculostomy could safely and easily be performed by stereotactic means.[44]

The potential advantages of endoscopic third ventriculostomy include a smaller risk of damage to vessels and neural tissue under direct vision, less cumbersome technical requirements than with open procedures, and the ability to directly visualize the ventriculostomy site as opposed to free-hand or stereotactic techniques.[52] Direct endoscopic visualization of the fenestration eliminates the need for intra- or postoperative radiopaque contrast ventriculography, which is used in blind techniques and has been linked with adhesive arachnoiditis[78–81] and delayed closure of the third ventriculostomy. In addition, successful third ventriculostomy eliminates the problems associated with mechanical shunting devices.[53] Overdrainage syndromes do not occur with third ventriculostomy, and third ventriculostomy is never "outgrown." According to Hoffman et al., ". . . a good lesion will not block or occlude, and by a single procedure the patient is cured of his hydrocephalus for life."[53]

At Primary Children's Medical Center-University of Utah, we have treated 10 patients since 1987 with ventriculoscopic fenestration of the lamina terminalis or floor of the third ventricle. Four patients were treated primarily with third ventriculostomy following the diagnosis of noncommunicating hydrocephalus. To date, two of four have remained shunt-independent with stable ventricular size on CT. Six patients with clinical and radiographic evidence of slit-ventricle syndrome were treated with ventriculoscopic third ventriculostomy in an attempt to improve cerebral compliance and functionally convert a noncommunicating hydrocephalus to a communicating form. In this group, only two of six have remained shunt-independent postoperatively, and an additional two of six report reduction in the frequency and severity of their headaches. Several groups continue to gather data and experience on the utility of endoscopic third ventriculostomy as an initial therapy for the noncommunicating hydrocephalus associated with myelomeningocele and other forms of congenital hydrocephalus as well as in patients with intractable headaches secondary to slit-ventricle syndrome.

TECHNICAL CONSIDERATIONS

PATIENT SELECTION

Ventricular Size

Because of the risk of damage to extraependymal structures with inadvertent penetration of the ependyma, ventricular size is a significant consideration in the selection of patients for endoscopy.[3, 53, 75] Jones et al. felt that as a prerequisite for third ventriculostomy, a patient should have a sufficiently dilated third ventricle, which they arbitrarily defined as greater than 1.0 cm in the bicoronal diameter.[75] Hoffman et al. believed that the third ventricle should be grossly dilated as a prerequisite to third ventriculostomy.[53] Consequently, ventricular drainage should not be performed preoperatively if ventriculostomy is being considered.[3, 53]

For patients who fail to meet this criterion for ventricular size, we have resorted to a preliminary externalization of any existing shunts, followed by gradual elevation of the drainage bag in an attempt to enlarge the ventricular system. Alternatively, we have performed stereotactic placement of the endoscope at the target of fenestration in patients with small ventricles or complex ventricular anatomy. In patients with myelomeningocele who are being evaluated for possible endoscopic third ventriculocisternostomy, the size of the massa intermedia is of paramount importance.

Etiology of Hydrocephalus

Despite extensive variability in the literature with percutaneous third ventriculoscopy (see Table 48–3), it is the patient with late-onset hydrocephalus secondary to aqueductal stenosis who has been most successfully treated in terms of shunt independence.[75] This is probably because CSF absorption mechanisms are usually intact in patients with acquired hydrocephalus.[14, 54, 55] Some authors believe that infantile forms of aqueductal stenosis are not amenable to treatment[14] with fenestration of the third ventricle, citing reports that the peripheral subarachnoid pathways may not have developed.[42, 54, 55] Noncommunicating hydrocephalus of other origins, including myelomeningocele and central nervous system (CNS) tumors, has also been successfully treated endoscopically.[75] Completely accurate patient selection will not be possible until a means is available to assess the resorptive capacity of the subarachnoid space preoperatively.[52]

INSTRUMENTATION

Rigid Versus Flexible Endoscopes

Improvement in the quality of available endoscopes has been a significant factor in the resurgence of interest in neuroendoscopy. Currently both rigid and flexible or steerable endoscopes are available for use in ventriculoscopy (Fig. 48–4). Rigid endoscopes have traditionally had superior optical properties as well as multiple ports for suction-irrigation, passage of biopsy forceps, sounds, or laser fibers. They can be more difficult to maneuver through a large ventricle or cyst when inserted through a standard burr hole. The use of flexible or steerable endoscopes has been reported by several authors to reduce the potential risk to brain tissue.[26, 27, 29] In addition, they tend to be more maneuverable,[26, 27] but they suffer in terms of optical properties and image quality when compared with rigid endoscopes.

The imminent availability of disposable scopes will prove invaluable in guaranteeing maximal sterility as well as in providing a convenient aid for such endoscopic procedures as catheter placement.

LASERS

Conventional electrocautery,[29] as well as more innovative forms of delivering cautery current such as a "saline torch," is available for endoscopic use.[40] Both the argon and neodymium-yttrium-aluminum-garnet (Nd:YAG) laser systems are ideally suited to neuroendoscopy because of their wavelengths, tissue absorption, and hemostatic properties. Argon or Nd:YAG laser energy can be endoscopically delivered through currently available fiberoptic delivery systems. As a result, both laser coagulation and vaporization of tissue are possible through the endoscope.[30, 31]

STEREOTACTIC ENDOSCOPY

Endoscopy and stereotaxy are indeed complementary. Several authors have documented the feasibility and wisdom of CT- or MR-guided stereotactic localization for endoscopic procedures.[14, 28, 30, 33, 64] Stereotactic technology permits precise localization in endoscopic procedures; this has proved invaluable, in our experience, in patients with small ventricles in which inadvertent penetration through the ependymal lining could prove disastrous (see *Complications of Ventriculoscopy* below) or in patients with complex ventricular anatomy such as multicompartmentalization. In addition, Apuzzo and co-workers believed that endoscopic technology enhances the spectrum and safety of diagnostic and therapeutic endeavors at a stereotactic target point.[30, 33] For example, in performing stereotactic third ventriculostomies, Kelly reports endoscopically inspecting the target in the floor of the third ventricle before and after fenestration with a leukotome.[14, 64] With the imminent availability of frameless stereotaxy and virtual reality, dynamic localization will be possible, permitting the endoscopist to navigate through complex ventricular or parenchymal structures with great facility.

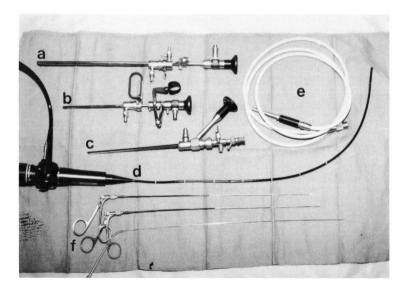

FIGURE 48–4. Endoscopic equipment utilized at Primary Children's Medical Center of the University of Utah, including rigid endoscopes (a–c), flexible or steerable endoscope (d), fiberoptic illumination system (e), and biopsy forceps and probes (f).

OPERATIVE TECHNIQUE

For most endoscopic procedures a standard burr hole provides sufficient exposure. The exact location of the burr hole depends on the specific endoscopic target. For routine endoscopic access to the frontal horn and foramen of Monro, we place a 14.0-mm burr hole at the coronal suture in the midpupillary line;[3, 52] in infants, this usually can be modified to the lateral aspect of the anterior fontanelle. For access to the septum pellucidum, the burr hole is often placed lower on the convexity to generate a more horizontal trajectory. Stereotactic placement of the endoscope permits selection of an entry point that is safest and most convenient. The dura must usually be opened widely, often to the limits of the burr hole. The lateral ventricle is tapped initially with a ventricular needle and subsequently with a standard vascular introducer to dilate a transcortical track. The telescope sheath with its stylet in place is advanced into the lateral ventricle down the track of the ventricular needle and introducer.

PERIOPERATIVE MANAGEMENT

Although some individuals have used postoperative intracranial pressure monitoring,[75] we have not found this to be necessary. We routinely utilize postoperative external ventricular drainage since it permits drainage of potentially irritating blood from the ventricles and provides access to the ventricular system for postoperative ventriculography. Because of the potential for neurologic sequelae, especially in cases of third ventriculostomy, in which complications such as hemorrhage, hemiplegia, and hypothalamic instability have been reported,[62] we have traditionally placed all endoscopy patients in the intensive care unit postoperatively.

IMAGING

Several imaging modalities are available for evaluating patients before or after ventriculoscopic surgery. Ventriculography with nonionic water-soluble contrast media such as iohexol (see Fig. 48–1) or radioisotope is often useful.[75]

Radionuclide scintiventriculography at 1-, 6-, 24-, and 48-hour intervals following injection of 500 microcuries of indium-labeled diethylenetriaminepenta-acetic acid (DTPA)[14, 64] has been useful in demonstrating communication between the third ventricle, interpeduncular cistern, and peripheral subarachnoid convexity in patients undergoing endoscopic third ventriculocisternostomy.[14] In this case, flow of radioisotope from the third ventricle into the interpeduncular cistern should occur by 6 hours, with flow over the convexities and along the sagittal sinus by 24 to 72 hours.[14]

Serial CT scans are useful postoperatively to evaluate ventricular size and to check for clinically significant intraventricular bleeding. Experience has shown that ventricular size does not always return to normal following successful endoscopic procedures for CSF communication, including third ventriculocisternostomy.[14, 53, 67] Despite large ventricular size, successfully treated children may have normal intellectual function and complete reversal of any signs or symptoms of hydrocephalus.[53]

At Primary Children's Medical Center of the University of Utah we have begun using magnetic resonance imaging (MRI) flow studies[83–85] to demonstrate CSF flow through ventriculoscopic fenestrations. MR images will often demonstrate a flow-void in the floor of the third ventricle.[75] In addition, flow-sequence sagittal MR images[14, 64] or cinematography[83–85] can be utilized to demonstrate patency of a third ventriculocisternostomy or other fenestrations.

COMPLICATIONS OF VENTRICULOSCOPY

Although many complications have been reported with ventriculoscopy, currently available equipment renders it effective and safe in experienced hands.[14, 26, 29, 82] A definite ''learning curve'' exists for technical proficiency; since most neurosurgeons have had relatively little training in endoscopy, they are both unfamiliar with the anatomy as seen through the endoscope and initially awkard at maneuvering about. As a result of inexperience or inability to recognize normal or pathologic anatomy, potentially disastrous complications are possible. This includes inadvertent penetration through the ependyma into paraventricular structures such as the hypothalamus, internal capsule, or basal ganglia, as well as injury to major vascular structures including the basilar or posterior cerebral arteries as well as smaller perforating vessels in the interpeduncular cistern. Reported complications include death, hemiparesis, hypothalamic injury, intraoperative bradycardia, infection, and subdural hematoma.[14, 62, 75] Jones et al. reported four aborted endoscopic third ventriculostomies, owing to poor visibility secondary to bleeding, altered anatomy (including a large massa intermedia or absence of a corpus callosum in one case each), and intraoperative bradycardia.[75] Overall the morbidity and mortality rates for endoscopic procedures by experienced surgeons are lower than respective open procedures.[14, 82]

The augmentation of endoscopic procedures with stereotactic localization further reduces the incidence of complications. In his 1991 series of stereotactic third ventriculostomies, Kelly reported no deaths and a morbidity rate of only 5 per cent.[14] Further developments in the technology of frameless stereotaxy as well as virtual reality will enable the neurosurgeons to maneuver through even the most complex or distorted intraventricular anatomy with confidence and further reduce morbidity and mortality.

SUMMARY

Endoscopy has been shown to be a potentially safe and effective tool in the surgical repertoire of the pediatric neurosurgeon and can be utilized for both diagnostic and therapeutic objectives. Its chief advantage in the management of focal cerebral or intraventricular lesions is based on the potential for reduction in surgical trauma, especially along the path to a deep-seated cerebral lesion.[31] This theoretic advantage must be viewed in light of the suspected pathology at hand and the relative risks and benefits of an endoscopic versus an open approach. It is in the management of hydrocephalus and its associated conditions that ventriculoscopy is likely to find the most utility, either in eliminating the need for CSF shunting devices or in reducing their complexity.

REFERENCES

1. Dandy WE: An operative procedure for hydrocephalus. Bull Johns Hopkins Hosp 33:189, 1922.
2. Scarff JE: The treatment of nonobstructive (communicating) hydrocephalus by endoscopic cauterization of the choroid plexuses. J Neurosurg 33:1, 1970.
3. Powell MP, Torrens MJ, Thomson JL, et al.: Isodense colloid cysts of the third ventricle: A diagnostic and therapeutic problem resolved by ventriculoscopy. Neurosurgery 13:234, 1983.
4. Forrest DM, Cooper DGW: Complications of ventriculo-atrial shunts. A review of 455 cases. J Neurosurg 29:506, 1968.
5. Hayden PW, Shurtleff DB, Stuntz TJ: A longitudinal study of shunt function in 360 patients with hydrocephalus. Dev Med Child Neurol 25:334, 1983.
6. Illingsworth RD, Logue V, Symon L, et al.: The ventriculocaval shunt in the treatment of adult hydrocephalus. Results and complications in 101 patients. J Neurosurg 35:681, 1971.
7. Hyde-Rowan MD, Rekate HL, Nulsen FE: Reexpansion of previously collapsed ventricles: The slit ventricle syndrome. J Neurosurg 56:536, 1982.
8. Jackson IJ, Snodgrass SR: Peritoneal shunts in the treatment of hydrocephalus and increased intracranial pressure. A 4-year survey of 62 patients. J Neurosurg 12:216, 1955.
9. Bryant MS, Bremer AM, Tepas JJ III, et al.: Abdominal complications of ventriculoperitoneal shunts. Case reports and review of the literature. Am Surg 54:50, 1988.
10. George R, Leibrock L, Epstein M: Long-term analysis of cerebrospinal fluid shunt infections. A 25-year experience. J Neurosurg 51:804, 1979.
11. Renier D, Lacombe J, Pierre-Kahn A, et al.: Factors causing acute shunt infection. Computer analysis of 1174 operations. J Neurosurg 61:1072, 1984.
12. Gruber R: Should "normalisation" of the ventricles be the goal of hydrocephalus therapy. Z Kinderchir 38 (Suppl 2):80, 1983.
13. Reddy K, Fewer HD, West M, et al.: Slit-ventricle syndrome with aqueduct stenosis: third ventriculostomy as definitive treatment. Neurosurgery 23:756, 1988.
14. Kelly PJ: Stereotactic third ventriculostomy in patients with nontumoral adolescent/adult onset aquaductal stenosis and symptomatic hydrocephalus. J Neurosurg 75:865, 1991.
15. Nulsen FE, Spitz EB: Treatment of hydrocephalus by direct shunt from ventricle to jugular vein. Surg Forum 2:399, 1952.
16. Gower DJ, Lewis JC, Kelly DL Jr: Sterile shunt malfunction. A scanning electron microscopic perspective. J Neurosurg 61:1079, 1984.
17. L'Espinasse VL: Neurological Surgery, 2nd ed. Philadelphia, Lea & Febiger, 1943, p. 442.
18. Iizuka J: Development of a stereotaxic endoscopy of the ventricular system. Confin Neurol 37:141, 1975.
19. Mixter WJ: Ventriculoscopy and puncture of the floor of the third ventricle. Boston Med Surg J 188:277, 1923.
20. Fay T, Grant FC: Ventriculoscopy and intraventricular photography in internal hydrocephalus. Report of a case. JAMA 80:461, 1923.
21. Putnam TJ: Treatment of hydrocephalus by endoscopic coagulation of the choroid plexus. Description of a new instrument and preliminary report of results. N Engl J Med 210:1373, 1934.
22. Scarff JE: Endoscopic treatment of hydrocephalus: Description of a ventriculoscope and preliminary report of cases. Arch Neurol Psychiatry 35:853, 1936.
23. Scarff JE: Third ventriculoscopy as the rational treatment of obstructive hydrocephalus. (Abstract) J Pediatr 6:870, 1935.
24. Griffith HB: Technique of fontanelle and persutural ventriculoscopy and endoscopic ventricular surgery in infants. Childs Brain 1:359, 1975.
25. Guiot G, Rougerie J, Fourestier M, et al.: Une nouvelle technique endoscopique: Explorations endoscopiques intracraniennes. La Presse Med 71:1225, 1963.
26. Fukushima T, Ishijima B, Hirakawa K, et al.: Ventriculofiberscope: A new technique for endoscopic diagnosis and operation. Technical note. J Neurosurg 38:251, 1973.
27. Oka K, Ohta T, Kibe M, et al.: A new neurosurgical ventriculoscope—technical note. Neurol Med Chir (Tokyo) 30:77, 1991.
28. Hellwig D, Bauer BL: Endoscopic procedures in stereotactic neurosurgery. Acta Neurochir (Wien) 52(Suppl):30, 1991.
29. Fukushima T: Endoscopic biopsy of intraventricular tumors with the use of a ventriculofiberoscope. Neurosurgery 2:110, 1978.
30. Apuzzo MLJ, Chandrasoma PT, Zelman V: Computed tomographic guidance stereotaxis in the management of lesions of the third ventricular region. Neurosurgery 15:502, 1984.
31. Auer LM, Holzer P, Ascher PW, et al.: Endoscopic neurosurgery. Acta Neurochir (Wien) 90:1, 1988.
32. Tabarin A, Corcuff J-B, Dautheribes M, et al.: Histiocytosis X of the hypothalamus. J Endocrinol Invest 14:139, 1991.
33. Apuzzo MLJ, Chandrasoma PT, Cohen D, et al.: Computed imaging stereotaxy: Experience and perspective related to 500 procedures applied to brain masses. Neurosurgery 20:930, 1987.
34. Kleinhaus S, Germann R, Sheran M, Shapiro K, Boley SJ: A role for endoscopy in the placement of ventriculoperitoneal shunts. Surg Neurol 18:179, 1982.
35. Kalsbeck JE, DeSousa AL, Kleinman MB, et al.: Compartmentalization of the cerebral ventricles as a sequela of neonatal meningitis. J Neurosurg 52:547, 1980.
36. Albanese V, Tomasello F, Sampaolo S: Multiloculated hydrocephalus in infants. Neurosurgery 8:641, 1981.
37. Rhoton AL Jr., Gomez MR: Conversion of multilocular hydrocephalus to unilocular. J Neurosurg 36:348, 1972.
38. Salmon JH: Isolated unilateral hydrocephalus following ventriculo-atrial shunt. J Neurosurg 32:219, 1970.
39. Shultz P, Leeds NE: Intraventricular septations complicating neonatal meningitis. J Neurosurg 38:620, 1973.
40. Heilman CB, Cohen AR: Endoscopic ventricular fenestration using a "saline torch." J Neurosurg 74:224, 1991.
41. Scarff JE: Treatment of hydrocephalus: An historical and critical review of methods and results. J Neurol Neurosurg Psychiatry 26:1, 1963.
43. Forjaz S, Martelli N, Latuf N: Hypothalamic ventriculostomy with catheter. J Neurosurg 29:655, 1968.
44. Guiot G, Derome P, Hertzog E, et al.: Ventriculocisternostomie sous controle radioscopique pour hydrocephalie obstructive. Presse Med 76/40:1923, 1968.
45. Vries JK: Endoscopy as an adjunct to shunting for hydrocephalus. Surg Neurol 13:69, 1980.
46. Voris HC: Third ventriculostomy in treatment of obstructive hydrocephalus in children. Arch Neurol Psych 65:265, 1951.
47. White J: Drainage of the third ventricle by transfrontal approach in obstructive hydrocephalus. Yale J Bio Med 11:431, 1938.
48. Stookey B, Scarff JE: Occlusion of the aqueduct of Sylvius by neoplastic and non-neoplastic processes with a rational surgical treatment for relief of the resultant obstructive hydrocephalus. Bull Neurol Inst NY 5:348, 1936.
49. Scarff JE: Third ventriculostomy by puncture of the lamina terminalis and the floor of the third ventricle. J Neurosurg 24:935, 1966.

50. McNickle HF: The surgical treatment of hydrocephalus. A simple method of performing third ventriculostomy. Br J Surg 334:302, 1947.

51. Guiot G: Ventriculo-cisternostomy for stenosis of the aqueduct of Sylvius. Acta Neurochir (Wien) 28:275, 1973.

52. Vries JK: An endoscopic technique for third ventriculostomy. Surg Neurol 9:165, 1978.

53. Hoffman HJ, Harwood-Nash D, Gilday DL: Percutaneous third ventriculostomy in the management of noncommunicating hydrocephalus. Neurosurgery 7:313, 1980.

54. Dandy WE, Blackfan KD: Internal hydrocephalus. An experimental, clinical and pathological study. Am J Dis Child 8:406, 1914.

55. Dandy WE, Blackfan KD: Internal hydrocephalus. Second paper. Am J Dis Child 14:424, 1917.

56. Guillaume J, Mazars G: Indications etresultats dela ventriculostomie sus-optique dans l-hydrocephalie de l'adulte. Rev Neurol 82:421, 1950.

57. Morello G, Migliavacca F: Third ventriculostomy (Stookey and Scarff operation) in the treatment of benign aqueductal stenosis. Acta Neurochir 7:417, 1959.

58. Scarff JE: Treatment of obstructive hydrocephalus by puncture of the lamina terminalis and floor of the third ventricle. J Neurosurg 8:204, 1951.

59. White JC, Michelsen JJ: Treatment of obstructive hydrocephalus in adults. Surg Gynecol Obstet 74:99, 1942.

60. Volkel JS, Voris HC: Third ventriculostomy in obstructive hydrocephalus: Long-term arrest in 4 cases. J Neurosurg 24:568, 1966.

61. Pierre-Kahn A, Renier D, Bombois B, et al.: Place de la ventriculo-cisternostomie dans le traitement des hydrocephalies non communicantes. Neurochirurgie 21:557, 1975.

62. Sayers MP, Kosnik EJ: Percutaneous third ventriculostomy: Experience and technique. Childs Brain 2:24, 1976.

63. Jaksche H, Loew F: Burr hole third ventriculo-cisternostomy. An unpopular but effective procedure for treatment of certain forms of occlusive hydrocephalus. Acta Neurochir 79:48, 1986.

64. Kelly P, Goerss S, Kall B, et al.: Computed tomography based stereotactic third ventriculostomy: Technical note. Neurosurgery 18:791, 1986.

65. Poblete M, Zamboni R: Stereotaxic third ventriculostomy. Confin Neurol 37:150, 1975.

66. Ziedses des Plantes BG, Crezee P: Transfrontal perforation of the lamina terminalis. Neuroradiology 16:51, 1978.

67. Musolino A, Soria V, Munari C, et al.: La ventriculocisternostomie stereotaxique dans le traitement de l'hydrocephalie obstructive triventriculaire. A propos de 23 cas. Neurochirurgie 34:361, 1988.

68. Backlund EO, Grepe A, Lunsford D: Stereotaxic reconstruction of the aqueduct of Sylvius. J Neurosurg 55:800, 1981.

69. Dandy WE: The diagnosis and treatment of hydrocephalus resulting from strictures of the aqueduct of Sylvius. Surg Gynecol Obstet 31:340, 1920.

70. Leksell L: Surgical procedure for atresia of aqueduct of Sylvius. Acta Psychiatr Neurol 24:559, 1949.

71. Torkildsen A: New palliative operation in cases of inoperable occlusion of the sylvian aqueduct. Acta Chir Scand 82:117, 1939.

72. Paine KWE, McKissock W: Aqueduct stenosis. Clinical aspects, and results of treatment by ventriculocisternostomy (Torkildsen's operation). J Neurosurg 12:127, 1955.

73. Patterson RH, Bergland RM: The selection of patients for third ventriculostomy based on experience with 33 operations. J Neurosurg 29:252, 1968.

74. Dandy WE: Diagnosis and treatment of strictures of the aqueduct of Sylvius (causing hydrocephalus). Arch Surg 51:1, 1945.

75. Jones RFC, Stening WA, Brydon M: Endoscopic third ventriculostomy. Neurosurgery 26:86, 1990.

76. Brocklehurst G: Transcallosal third ventriculochiasmatic cisternostomy: A new approach to hydrocephalus. Surg Neurol 2:109, 1974.

77. Natelson SE: Early third ventriculostomy in myelomeningocele infants: Shunt independence. Childs Brain 8:321, 1981.

78. Howland WJ, Curry JL: Experimental studies of Pantopaque arachnoiditis. Radiology 87:253, 1966.

79. Irstam L, Rosencrantz M: Water-soluble contrast media and adhesive arachnoiditis. Acta Radiol 15:1, 1974.

80. Johnson AJ, Burrow EH: Thecal deformity after lumbar myelography with iophendylate (Myodil) and meglumine iothalamate (Conray 280). Br J Radiol 51:196, 1978.

81. Manwaring KH, Rekate H, Kaplan A: Hydrocephalus management by endoscopy. (Abstract) Ann Neurol 26:488, 1989.

82. Hirsch JF: Percutaneous ventriculocisternostomies in noncommunicating hydrocephalus. Monogr Neural Sci 8:321, 1982.

83. Enzmann DR, Pelc NJ: Normal flow patterns of intracranial and spinal cerebrospinal fluid defined with phase-contrast cine MR imaging. Radiology 178:467, 1991.

84. Kahn T, Muller E, Lewin JS, et al.: MR measurement of spinal CSF flow with the RACE technique. J Comput Assist Tomogr 16:54, 1992.

85. Nitz WR, Bradley WG, Watanabe AS, et al.: Flow dynamics of cerebrospinal fluid: Assessment with phase-contrast velocity MR imaging performed with retrospective cardiac gating. Radiology 183:395, 1992.

Chapter 49

PEDIATRIC NEUROANESTHESIA

ROBERT CREIGHTON, M.D., and M. ELIZABETH McLEOD, M.D.

General anesthesia for the pediatric neurosurgical patient imposes special problems for the anesthesiologist. The age range for this patient population lies between the premature neonate and the 16-year-old young adult. Often the problems associated with an altered neurophysiology are complicated by those associated with neonatal anesthesia.

NEUROPHYSIOLOGY

In the infant the skull is not a rigid, essentially closed container. The sutures are not fused, and the fontanelles are open. The presence of an open fontanelle not only increases cranial compliance, but also provides a means of assessing intracranial pressure (ICP) noninvasively by direct application of a transducer.[1] In the older child, as in the adult, the skull is considered a rigid nonexpansile container in which the pressure depends on the total volume of brain substance, interstitial fluid, cerebrospinal fluid (CSF), and blood. A review of the pressure-volume intracranial compliance curve demonstrates that with initial volume changes in one compartment, compensation is possible, and only a small change in pressure results.[2] This is achieved by displacement of CSF into the relatively distensible spinal dural sac as well as by changes in the volume of the intracranial vascular bed.[3] Once the limit of compensation is reached, a small change in intracranial volume will result in a more dramatic change in intracranial pressure. Since access to the ventricular system is normally not available, the control of ICP by the anesthesiologist usually depends on alterations in cerebral blood volume and on the volume of intracellular and interstitial fluid.

In children, the cerebral blood flow (CBF) and cerebral metabolic rate ($CMRO_2$) are significantly higher, while cerebrovascular resistance is lower.[4] Changes in cerebral blood flow, when associated with changes in cerebral blood volume, can produce rapid alterations in ICP. Normally, CBF is controlled by $Paco_2$, Pao_2, and mean arterial pressure. In the normal adult, cerebral blood flow remains relatively constant between mean arterial pressures of 50 to 150 torr, provided changes are not abrupt.[2] This autoregulation, however, can be abolished by trauma, acidosis, and certain drugs.[5] In the neonate with birth asphyxia or respiratory distress syndrome, it has been shown that autoregulation may be entirely absent, and as a result, the cerebral circulation becomes pressure passive.[6] This can increase the risk of hemorrhage into the brain tissue and ventricles if wide swings in arterial pressure occur.

In man, the $Paco_2$ is the most important regulator of cerebrovascular resistance and cerebral blood flow. Indeed, a linear relationship exists so that over the range of 15 to 76 torr for each torr change in $Paco_2$, the cerebral blood volume changes 0.041 ml/100 gm/min.[7] Thus, hyperventilation plays an important role in the management of the patient with raised ICP, and end-tidal CO_2 measurement is an important component of patient monitoring. Except at extremes, arterial oxygen tension has little influence on cerebral blood flow.

ICP can also be reduced by a reduction of the cerebral interstitial volume with diuretics. Osmotic agents, in particular mannitol, are effective in lowering ICP.[8] This is achieved by an increase in plasma osmolality and withdrawal of fluid from intracellular and interstitial spaces. This action may result in transient increases in cerebral blood volume and ICP prior to the onset of diuresis, and these increases may be deleterious prior to craniotomy in the patient with raised ICP. Nonosmotic diuretics (e.g., furosemide, in doses of 1 mg/kg) will reduce ICP without producing significant changes in serum osmolality or electrolytes.[9, 10] The combination of mannitol 1 gm/kg and furosemide 0.7 mg/kg has been shown to produce a greater and more prolonged drop in ICP than either agent alone.[11]

The role of steroids remains controversial. In the elective situation, when dexamethasone therapy precedes the surgical treatment of tumors or vascular lesions, experimental evidence suggests that steroids should be of value.[12] The head-injured patient who is treated after the insult is less likely to derive the same benefit.

ANESTHETIC DRUGS

INTRAVENOUS AGENTS

Barbiturates reduce ICP.[13] Thiopentone decreases both cerebral blood flow and metabolism in a dose-dependent manner and thus is an ideal induction agent for the patient with raised ICP.

Propofol, which can be used as both an induction and a maintenance agent is reported to decrease CBF and metabolism.[14] During propofol anesthesia in baboons, autoregulation was preserved.[15] However, falls in mean arterial pressure after rapid bolus doses may result in falls in cerebral perfusion pressure, and so it is recommended that the dose of this agent be reduced in brain-injured patients.[16]

Diazepam produces decreases in both CBF and oxygen consumption.[17]

Midazolam maleate, like diazepam, decreases CBF and metabolism[18] and may prove useful in neuroanesthesia because of its short duration of action.

Narcotics are useful for the maintenance of anesthesia in pediatric neurosurgical patients, although, because of the danger of respiratory depression, they are rarely used for premedication. Intravenous morphine has little effect on CBF, and autoregulation remains intact.[19] Fentanyl in combination with droperidol results in small decreases in ICP,[20] making both neuroleptanesthesia and neuroleptanalgesia useful techniques. Alfentanil and sufentanil may be less appropriate for neuroanesthesia than fentanyl. Alfentanil has been shown to produce an increase in CSF pressure in patients with brain tumors.[21] Sufentanil, which did not increase CBF in healthy volunteers,[22] did produce increases in anesthetized animals.[23]

The neuromuscular blocking drugs have little effect on cerebral circulation. Succinylcholine produces clinically insignificant changes in ICP.[24] Pancuronium and atracurium in the presence of halothane have been shown to have no effect on CBF, ICP, or $CMRO_2$, although at sub-MAC (minimal anesthetic concentration) of halothane, the EEG arousal effects of atracurium's metabolite, laudanosine, can be observed.[25] Ketamine should not be used in neurosurgery. In dogs, an 80 per cent increase in CBF and a 16 per cent increase in $CMRO_2$ occur after ketamine injection, and these values remain above control for 30 minutes.[26] In hydrocephalic children, ketamine has been shown to increase CSF pressure two to three times when given either intramuscularly or intravenously.[27]

INHALATION AGENTS

Nitrous oxide is thought to have minimal effect on CBF although animal experiments have demonstrated some increase. The electroencephalogram (EEG) shows progressive loss of alpha rhythm as the concentration is increased above 30 per cent.[28]

All volatile anesthetics are known to be cerebral vasodilators and therefore must be used with caution in the patient with raised ICP.

Enflurane, because it produces epileptiform activity on the EEG, is avoided in neurosurgical patients.[28] Although halothane abolishes autoregulation at 1.0 MAC, the cerebral vasculature remains responsive to changes in $Paco_2$.[29] Prior establishment of hypocapnia minimizes the increase in ICP associated with halothane.[30] After 30 minutes of halothane anesthesia, CBF begins to return toward control values.[31] At 1.0 MAC, isoflurane autoregulation is preserved, but at higher levels, CBF increases. This increase is less than occurs with halothane,[32] and the ICP returns to control levels more rapidly after the establishment of hypocapnia.[33] At higher inspired concentrations, a decrease in $CMRO_2$ is seen which may provide some measure of protection against ischemic insult.[34] In addition, the rapid elimination of isoflurane permits early postoperative neurologic assessment.

Sevoflurane, in animal studies, appears to be similar to isoflurane in its effects on the cerebral circulation. Cerebral metabolism is reduced, and no increase in CBF is seen at concentrations up to 1.0 MAC.[35]

Desflurane also reduces $CMRO_2$ in a similar fashion but is a more potent cerebral vasodilator.[36]

PATIENT POSITION AND AIR EMBOLISM

The airway, circulation, and intracranial pressure are influenced by the patient's position. The sitting position, which is commonly employed for posterior fossa surgery, may produce cardiovascular instability and carries an increased risk of air embolism. Decreases in CBF and spinal cord blood flow occur when the sitting position is used in the presence of elevated ICP.[37]

The reported incidence of air embolism during surgery in the sitting position varies widely. Cucchiara and Bowers, in a study of air embolism in children undergoing suboccipital craniotomy, found the incidence detected by Doppler to be 33 per cent, which is similar to that found in adults.[38] In this study the incidence of hypotension associated with air embolism was 69 per cent in children in contrast to a 36 per cent incidence in adults. Unfortunately, they also reported that attempts to aspirate air from a right atrial catheter were less successful in children. The precordial Doppler has been shown to be more sensitive than pulmonary artery pressure, end-tidal carbon dioxide concentrations, and end-tidal nitrogen in detecting even small volumes of entrained air. However, the noise produced by electrocautery and small changes in the Doppler position or in the patient's systemic blood pressure may alter the sounds and render it less informative.[39]

The high incidence of hypotension associated with air embolism in children requires an immediate response when air embolism is suspected. Nitrous oxide must be discontinued, the operative field flooded with saline, and the head must be lowered. As stated above, attempts to aspirate air from the right atrial catheter are less successful in children.

The prone position is an attractive alternative for posterior fossa and upper cervical spinal cord surgery. Care must be taken to secure the airway and support the anesthetic circuit to prevent accidental extubation. A nasotracheal tube is more easily secured than an oral tracheal tube in this position since the fixation tape is less likely to be loosened by secretions. Depending on the size of the child, either a U-shaped bolster or a Hall-Relton frame can be used to ensure free excursion of the diaphragm without obstruction of the abdominal venous return. If a horseshoe headrest is used, careful padding and positioning of the face are necessary to avoid pressure on the eyes.

When patients are operated upon in the supine position, the bed is usually tilted 15 to 30 degrees head-up, which decreases ICP[40] and increases venous return. Unfortunately, the risk of air embolism is also increased. If the head is to be turned to the side, the lateral decubitus position is preferable to avoid obstruction of the jugular venous system.

GENERAL ANESTHESIA

PREMEDICATION

In the past it has been common to withhold sedative premedication from all neurosurgical patients because it might produce respiratory depression. This approach seems unreasonable except in patients who are obtunded by their raised ICP. Indeed, heavy sedation is often used during their radiologic investigation. Therefore, as with other patients, premedication should be tailored to the patient's needs. Several non-narcotic sedatives are available. The simplest would be midazolam, 0.75 mg/kg orally mixed with an equal volume of sweetening solution, 20 to 30 minutes prior to anesthesia.

ANESTHETIC INDUCTION

For patients who are not obtunded by their raised ICP, either inhalation or intravenous induction is appropriate. If an inhalation technique is chosen, once the patient is deep enough to tolerate intravenous access, anesthetic induction should proceed intravenously with thiopentone and a nondepolarizing muscle relaxant to facilitate intubation. If there is a question of a "full stomach," a rapid-sequence induction with preoxygenation, thiopentone, succinylcholine, and cricoid pressure prior to intubation should be chosen. Although thiopentone reduces ICP, laryngoscopy and intubation may produce significant increases in arterial pressure and ICP. Lidocaine, 1.5 mg/kg intravenously at induction, attenuates the blood pressure response and protects against increases in ICP.[41, 42] Narcotics (e.g., fentanyl 0.002 mg/kg intravenously) are also helpful at this time to attenuate these responses.

ANESTHETIC MAINTENANCE

Surgery for specific lesions may require special consideration from the anesthesiologist and will be discussed separately. As a general principle, anesthesia is maintained with a combination of nitrous oxide and up to 1.0 MAC of a volatile agent augmented with a narcotic and nondepolarizing muscle relaxant.

The development of easily applied monitoring devices in the last decade has greatly added to safety in patient care and the comfort of the anesthesiologist. Minimum monitors now include: esophageal or precordial stethoscope; appropriate-sized blood pressure cuff; electrocardiographic (ECG) oscilloscope; capnograph for continuous assessment of end tidal Pco_2; anesthetic gas analyzer; transcutaneous O_2 saturation and thermistor probe. More extensive surgery will require an arterial cannula for intra-arterial pressure, arterial blood gases and hematocrit, a central venous catheter suitably positioned in the superior vena cava, and a urethral catheter.

Of equal importance and equal difficulty to the maintenance of general anesthesia is the maintenance of blood and fluid homeostasis. Since the demonstration that moderate hyperglycemia augmented ischemic brain damage in animals,[43] lactated Ringer's solution has become the maintenance fluid of choice. The need for blood replacement can only be determined by continuous reference to the information from the available monitors guided by experience. In certain operations, controlled hypotension will be of value. Except in those circumstances in which a short episode of very low systemic blood pressure is required and sodium nitroprusside is appropriate, adequate hypotension can be achieved by the progressive increase in the inspired isoflurane concentration.

SPECIFIC CONSIDERATIONS

SKULL ABNORMALITIES

Craniosynostosis

Craniosynostosis results from premature fusion of single, bilateral, or multiple cranial sutures and may be part of a syndrome involving other abnormalities. Crouzon's syndrome consists of craniosynostosis, maxillary hypoplasia, and shallow orbits with proptosis.

Apert's syndrome has syndactyly as an additional feature.

Surgery is carried out in infancy. Up to 20 per cent of patients will have hydrocephalus, which is seen more commonly in patients with craniofacial syndromes.[44, 45]

Surgical correction varies from simple strip craniectomy for single-suture synostosis to major craniofacial reconstructions required for complex syndromes.

For sagittal craniectomy, the most common procedure, the major anesthetic concerns are positioning (prone) and the potential for rapid blood loss. For craniofacial syndromes, intravenous induction is preferred since nasal obstruction is common. Preservation of CNS homeostasis, blood and fluid replacement, and temperature maintenance are the major intraoperative concerns. Although the supine position is employed, venous air embolism is still a risk.[46] Controlled hypotension should be restricted to primarily facial procedures since the risk of cerebral ischemia may be increased when it is combined with brain retraction.[47] Patients with a difficult airway following facial surgery should be left intubated until the risk of postoperative bleeding and swelling has passed.

Encephalocele

Encephalocele is a herniation of cerebral tissue and meninges through a defect in the skull, which may occur anywhere in the midline from the foramen magnum to the nasal cavity. Anterior encephalocele commonly presents as a mass in the nasopharynx. With large anterior encephaloceles and facial clefts, intubation may be awkward. Posterior encephaloceles, which are more common, present in the neonatal period. The Klippel-Feil deformity and cleft lip and palate are frequently associated with the encephalocele.[48] Defective thermoregulation may be present.[49]

Intubation should be performed with the patient positioned left side down with counterpressure to keep the shoulders back and to prevent the neck from extending. Hydrocephalus, epilepsy, paraplegia, spasticity, and blindness have been reported in survivors.[50]

Arnold-Chiari Malformation

The Arnold-Chiari malformation, the most common anomaly involving the cerebellum, is present in most children with myelomeningocele. It consists of an elongation of the cerebellar vermis and herniation of the caudal vermis and choroid plexus through the foramen magnum, with kinking of the medulla and upper cervical cord.[51] It is often associated with hydrocephalus. In approximately 20 per cent of patients with myelomeningocele, the Arnold-Chiari malformation will become symptomatic and more than half of these before the age of 3 months.[52, 53] The usual signs and symptoms are swallowing difficulty, apneic episodes, stridor, aspiration, arm weakness, and opisthotonos. The gag reflex may be diminished or absent. Due to recurrent aspiration, patients may have pre-existing lung complications. Anesthetic concerns involve hydrocephalus, positioning (prone with neck in flexion), vocal cord paresis, and depressed gag reflex continuing into the postoperative period. Abnormal hypoxic and hypercapnic arousal responses may persist after surgery.[54] It may be necessary to leave an endotracheal tube in place postoperatively, and some patients eventually require tracheotomy and a gastrostomy to decrease the risk of aspiration.

Hydrocephalus

Hydrocephalus is a condition in which there is a disproportionately large volume of CSF relative to the other cranial contents. In noncommunicating hydrocephalus, the CSF is excluded from the subarachnoid space. In communicating hydrocephalus, it flows unimpeded to the spinal subarachnoid space but is excluded from the cerebral subarachnoid sac or cannot be absorbed into the cerebral venous sinuses via the arachnoid villi.

Surgery involves correction of the precipitating cause if possible or a CSF shunting procedure. Ventriculoperitoneal shunt is most commonly performed in noncommunicating hydrocephalus, with pleural or right atrial shunts restricted to those cases in which adhesive peritonitis precludes use of the peritoneal route. Ventriculoatrial shunts are positioned using electrocardiographic control.[55] In communicating hydrocephalus, a lumboperitoneal shunt is often inserted.

The anesthetic considerations relate to the degree of raised ICP. Patients obtunded by their raised ICP will require intravenous lidocaine, narcotic, thiopentone, and a non-depolarizing muscle relaxant with hyperventilation following intubation. Occasionally, the rapid decrease in ICP caused by shunt insertion will result in cardiac dysrhythmias.[56]

Cerebrovascular Abnormalities

Arteriovenous Malformations

Cerebral arteriovenous malformations (AVM) are congenital lesions of the primitive arteriolar-capillary network between the arteries and veins of the brain. Seventy per cent present with intracranial hemorrhage. Some of these patients will be unconscious and require immediate resuscitation prior to transfer to the operating room for evacuation of their expanding space-occupying intracerebral clot. Sympathetic stimulation associated with intubation may result in recurrence or exacerbation of the bleeding from the lesion. Therefore, the usual precautions for elevated ICP and potentially full stomach are required. Other patients will have only signs of subarachnoid bleeding and can be scheduled for surgery after a period of stabilization. They should be sedated preoperatively to facilitate a smooth induction, and the necessary steps to prevent systemic hypertension at the time of intubation should be instituted.

Induced hypotension is of benefit in some cases, particularly if the lesion is deep-seated and difficult to approach. The degree of hypotension required for AVM resections is usually not as low as that required for aneurysm surgery and, in most cases, can be achieved with progressively increased increments of isoflurane.

Arterial Aneurysm

Rupture of an arterial intracranial aneurysm is uncommon in children. Only 1 per cent occur in patients under the age of 15 years.[57] Anesthetic considerations are similar to those for children with AVMs. Hypotensive techniques usually will be required but commonly are more profound and of shorter duration.

Aneurysm of the Vein of Galen

Aneurysm or arteriovenous malformation of the great cerebral vein of Galen is an uncommon vascular lesion. The clinical presentation, anesthetic management, and prognosis are related to the size of the lesion and therefore the age of the patient at presentation. Neonates have the poorest prognosis and present with cranial bruit and severe congestive heart failure. Subendocardial damage due to pressure and volume overload of the neonatal heart, combined with impaired myocardial perfusion, contributes to the high mortality.[58] Although controlled hypotension would be expected to be of benefit in the surgical management of these patients, it is likely to prove dangerous in these neonates. The myocardial perfusion is already at risk because of excessive workload, and the low diastolic pressure will be further decreased by the induced hypotension. Patients who present later in infancy, older children, and teenagers can be managed as are other AVMs.

Moyamoya Disease

Moyamoya disease is a spontaneous progressive occlusion of the internal carotid arteries. Autoregulation appears to be maintained, and the actual reduction in CBF is small because the peripheral resistance vessels are maximally dilated to maintain flow.[59] A decrease in $Paco_2$ or fall in blood pressure may result in ischemia. The surgical treatment consists of one of several operations to revascularize. The anesthetic technique of choice is a primarily narcotic-relaxant technique with a low concentration of a volatile agent to maintain normal blood pressure and normocarbia throughout the procedure.

INTRACRANIAL TUMORS

Tumors of the central nervous system are the second most common malignancy of childhood. The peak incidence is between 5 and 8 years of age, with only 3 per cent occurring before the age of one year.

Anesthesia for these lesions depends upon the site (supratentorial, infratentorial, suprasellar) and the presence of absence of hydrocephalus, which is present in half the cases of brain tumors located near the midline in children. Stereotactic biopsy, which is performed in adults under neuroleptanalgesia, normally requires general anesthesia in children.

Supratentorial Tumors

Children undergoing surgery for supratentorial tumors may or may not have raised ICP. Anesthetic management will follow the general principles, and monitoring will be extensive. A balanced nitrous-narcotic-relaxant technique with low-dose inhalation agent will provide a good surgical field.

Infratentorial Tumors

Surgery for infratentorial neoplasms present additional problems to the anesthesiologist. Some degree of hydrocephalus is usually present, and the tumor may be in close proximity to the vital centers. Although spontaneous ventilation, as an additional monitor of medullary function, was considered desirable in the past, the advent of the operating microscope and modern monitors have eliminated the absolute necessity of this requirement. Today these patients are usually managed following the general principles described above with controlled ventilation. Air embolism, particularly for patients undergoing operation in the sitting position, remains the main complication of these operations.

Suprasellar Tumors

These patients are considered separately because they often have associated endocrine abnormalities. This group of lesions includes craniopharyngioma, optic chiasm glioma, and germ cell tumors and represents 15 per cent of brain tumors in children.[60] It is essential to have a complete endocrinologic assessment preoperatively and steroid pretreatment if necessary.

Transsphenoid resection is rare in small children. Frontal craniotomy is the usual approach. Cardiac arrhythmias, particularly bradycardia, are common during retraction of the frontal lobes and dissection around the optic nerves. The bradycardias can be reversed with atropine if necessary. Postoperative management requires close attention to fluid and electrolyte balance as diabetes insipidus often develops. Continued steroid therapy will be required.

Neurofibromatosis

Neurofibromatosis, or von Recklinghausen's disease, is a disorder of neural crest derivation with proliferation of nerve fibers and Schwann cells. When an intracranial space-occupying lesion forms part of the disorder, the usual precautions should be taken. When it involves the head and neck, careful assessment of the airway for potential intubation difficulty is necessary.

Cervical instability due to tumor infiltration or abnormalities of spinal ligaments leading to atlantoaxial dislocation may be present.[61] Major vessel anomaly and pheochromocytoma must be ruled out preoperatively in patients who present with hypertension. Increased sensitivity to neuromuscular blockers has been reported.[62]

TEMPORAL LOBE EPILEPSY

Temporal lobe epilepsy may present as psychomotor seizures or complex partial seizures. If medical management fails, surgical resection of the area of cortex or a portion of the temporal lobe may be the treatment of choice. In approximately one third of cases considered for surgery, investigation reveals a mass lesion such as a tumor or vascular malformation.[63] When the dominant hemisphere is involved, the laterality of language function and independent memory capability of the contralateral temporal lobe are assessed during the Wada test. The Wada test consists of the intracarotid injection of amobarbital to inactivate the anterior two thirds of one hemisphere followed by the assessment of language and independent memory function in the opposite hemisphere.[64, 65] Since arterial catheterization is required, light sedation with small doses of fentanyl and droperidol, augmented by nitrous oxide and oxygen via nasal tongs or face mask, combined with local anesthesia is usually sufficient. The nitrous oxide is discontinued prior to the injection of the amobarbital, which should be warmed to prevent a shivering response following passage through the hypothalamus. Following the test, the patient can be given a general anesthetic for arteriography.

To minimize the risk of neurologic damage during resection, craniotomy for temporal lobectomy is frequently performed with EEG control and neuroleptanalgesia rather than general anesthesia. Diazepam and barbiturates are not used as premedicants as these will interfere with intraoperative cortical EEG recording. The anesthetic technique is similar to that described for the Wada test, with local anesthetic infiltration into the sites of the pin fixation of the headrest and the operative incision. Nitrous oxide should be discontinued prior to intraoperative cortical recording because of its potential effects on the EEG.[66]

HEAD INJURY

The head-injured child may present with a simple nondisplaced skull fracture and no other injuries or may arrive unconscious with multiple associated injuries. The aim of the anesthetic management is to prevent secondary physiologic brain injury caused by hypoxemia and systemic hypertension or hypotension. Control of the airway is essential to limit secondary head injury in the unconscious patient with depressed respiration. This is often necessary before radiographic examination of the cervical spine. Although awake, blind nasal intubation has been recommended in adults,[67] there are no data that spinal movement under general anesthesia is increased compared with awake tracheal intubation.[68] Neurologic outcomes following intubation under general anesthesia compare favorably with awake tracheal intubations in similar neck-injured patient populations.[69] In the hemodynamically stable patient, pre-oxygenation followed by a rapid-sequence induction including thiopentone, lidocaine, narcotic and muscle relaxant, and laryngoscopy and intubation with the head and neck stabilized in the neutral position by axial traction, would appear to be the safest and most humane technique for children. Anesthesia may then be continued with nitrous oxide, narcotic and muscle relaxant, and hyperventilation to lower the ICP. The hemodynamically unstable patient presents a difficult dilemma for the anesthesiologist. Following fluid resuscitation it may be necessary to reduce the dose of thiopentone in the induction regimen. Subdural hematoma is of special interest. Because of raised ICP, these patients may be normotensive at the time of surgery but suffer a significant fall in blood pressure when the ICP is suddenly lowered by the aspiration of the clot.[70]

CERVICAL SPINE INJURY

Injury to the spinal column in children is relatively uncommon.[71] However, a disproportionate number of these involve the cervical spine. In a reported series of children newborn to 9 years of age, 72 per cent of spinal injuries involved the cervical spine and half of these occurred between the occiput and C2.[72] In addition, several subgroups of pediatric patients are at increased risk of cervical spine injury. Subluxation of C1 on C2 has been reported in Hurler syndrome[73] and atlantoaxial instability in trisomy 21[74] and neurofibromatosis.[75] Cervical instability at the C3-C4 and C4-C5 levels has been reported in athetoid cerebral palsy.[76] The majority of children can be managed with halo-vest or other forms of external immobilization. When early surgery is required, intubation with axial traction under general anesthesia and awake fiberoptic nasal intubation in the older children are acceptable techniques.

MYELOMENINGOCELE

Up to 80 per cent of children with myelomeningocele develop hydrocephalus. Aqueduct stenosis is the cause in 75 per cent.[77] Intubation should be performed with the patient positioned left side down as described for posterior encephaloceles to minimize the risk of trauma to the sac. There is an increased risk of endobronchial intubation in these patients. A study of patients with myelomeningocele demonstrated a 36 per cent incidence of short trachea.[78] Large blood and fluid losses from the operative site and heat loss are the major concerns for the anesthesiologist. Blood and fluid losses are difficult to measure but may be considerable if extensive undermining of the skin or myocutaneous flaps are necessary to close the defect. Changes in vital signs, especially systolic blood pressure, will closely parallel blood volume changes in the neonate. Since the hemoglobin is usually high, colloid solutions such as albumin may be sufficient to maintain the circulating blood volume. Close monitoring is necessary in the postoperative period as associated hydrocephalus and Arnold-Chiari malformation may cause significant hypoventilation or apnea.

NEUROBLASTOMA

Neuroblastoma is one of the most common soft tissue malignant tumors of childhood. It arises from postganglionic adrenergic cells of the sympathetic nervous system. The adrenal glands and the cervical, thoracic, and abdominal sympathetic ganglia are the most frequent primary locations. Neuroblastoma can occur as a "dumbbell," with a primary in the mediastinum or retroperitoneum and extension via the intervertebral foramen into the spinal canal. Excision of the spinal portion usually precedes resection of the primary as manipulation of the extraspinal tumor can produce edema or hemorrhage in the intraspinal component.[79] Increased excretion of catechol metabolites is detectable in most of these patients.[80, 81] Hypertension usually is not a problem and arrhythmias are rare. Coagulation abnormalities are common in children with metastatic neuroblastoma, and disseminated intravascular coagulation has been reported.[82]

The anesthetic considerations depend upon the size and location of the tumor, the stage of the disease, and the extent of the planned surgical excision. Patients with more advanced disease may have received preoperative chemotherapy, with its attendant implications for the anesthesiologist.

REFERENCES

1. Hill A, Volpe JJ: Measurement of intracranial pressure using the Ladd intracranial pressure monitor. J Pediatr 98:974, 1984.
2. Shapiro HM: Intracranial hypertension: therapeutic and anesthetic considerations. Anesthesiology 43:445, 1975.
3. Lofgren J, Zwetnow NN: Cranial and spinal components of the cerebrospinal pressure-volume curve. Acta Neurol Scand 49:575, 1973.
4. Kennedy C, Sokoloff L: An adaptation of the nitrous oxide method to the study of the circulation in children; normal values for cerebral blood flow and cerebral metabolic rate in childhood. J Clin Invest 36:1130, 1957.
5. Lassen NA, Christensen MS: Physiology of cerebral blood flow. Br J Anaesth 48:719, 1976.
6. Lou HC, Lassen NA, Friis-Hansen B: Impaired autoregulation of cerebral blood flow in the distressed newborn infant. J Pediatr 94:118, 1979.
7. Grubb RL Jr, Raichle ME, Eichling JO, et al.: The effects of changes in $PaCO_2$ on cerebral blood volume, blood flow, and vascular mean transit time. Stroke 5:630, 1974.
8. Harbaugh RD, James HE, Marshall LF, et al.: Acute therapeutic modalities for experimental vasogenic cerebral edema. Neurosurgery 5:656, 1979.
9. Cottrell JE, Robustelli AS, Post K, et al.: Furosemide- and mannitol-induced changes in intracranial pressure and serum osmolality and electrolytes. Anesthesiology 47:28, 1977.
10. Samson D, Beyer CW Jr: Furosemide in the intraoperative reduction of intracranial pressure in the patient with subarachnoid hemorrhage. Neurosurgery 10:167, 1982.
11. Pollay M, Fullenwider C, Roberts A, et al.: Effect of mannitol and furosemide on blood-brain osmotic gradient and intracranial pressure. J Neurosurg 59:845, 1983.
12. Eisenberg HM, Barlow CF, Lorenzo AV: Effect of dexamethasone on altered brain vascular permeability. Arch Neurol 23:18, 1970.
13. Shapiro HM, Galindo A, Wyte SR, et al.: Rapid intraoperative reduction of intracranial pressure with thiopentone. Br J Anaesth 45:1057, 1973.
14. Vandesteene A, Trempont V, Engelman E, et al.: Effect of propofol on cerebral blood flow and metabolism in man. Anaesthesia 43(Suppl):42, 1988.
15. Van Hemelrijck J, Fitch W, Mattheussen M, et al.: Effect of propofol on cerebral circulation and autoregulation in the baboon. Anesth Analg 71:49, 1990.
16. Pinaud M, Lelausque J-N, Chettanneau A, et al.: Effects of propofol on cerebral hemodynamics and metabolism in patients with brain trauma. Anesthesiology 73:404, 1990.
17. Cotev S, Shalit MN: Effects of diazepam on cerebral blood flow and oxygen uptake after head injury. Anesthesiology 43:117, 1975.
18. Hoffman WE, Miletich DJ, Albrecht RA: The effects of midazolam on cerebral blood flow and oxygen consumption and its interaction with nitrous oxide. Anesth Analg 65:729, 1986.
19. Jobes DR, Kennell E, Bitner R, et al.: Effects of morphine-nitrous oxide anesthesia on cerebral autoregulation. Anesthesiology 42:30, 1975.
20. Fitch W, Barker J, Jennett WB, et al.: The influence of neuroleptanalgesic drugs on cerebrospinal fluid pressure. Br J Anaesth 41:800, 1969.
21. Junf R, Shah N, Reinsil R, et al.: Cerebrospinal fluid pressure in patients with brain tumors: impact of fentanyl versus alfentanil during nitrous oxide-oxygen anesthesia. Anesth Analg 71:419, 1990.
22. Mayer N, Weinstabl C, Podreka I, Spiss CK: Sufentanil does not increase cerebral blood flow in healthy human volunteers. Anesthesiology 73:241, 1990.
23. Milde LN, Milde JH, Gallagher WJ: Effects of sufentanil on cerebral circulation and metabolism in dogs. Anesth Analg 70:138, 1990.
24. Ducey JP, Deppe SA, Foley KT: A comparison of the effects of suxamethonium, atracurium and vecuronium on intracranial haemodynamics in swine. Anaesth Intens Care 17:448, 1989.
25. Lanier WL, Milde JH, Michenfelder JD: The cerebral effects of pancuronium and atracurium in halothane-anesthetized dogs. Anesthesiology 63:589, 1985.
26. Cawson B, Michenfelder JD, Theye RA: Effects of ketamine on canine cerebral blood flow and metabolism: Modification by prior administration of thiopental. Anesth Analg 50:443, 1971.
27. Crumrine RS, Nulson FE, Weiss MH: Alterations in ventricular fluid pressure during ketamine anesthesia in hydrocephalic children. Anesthesiology 42:758, 1975.
28. Clarke DL, Rosner BS: Neurophysiologic effects of general anesthetics. Anesthesiology 38:564, 1973.
29. Miletich FJ, Ivankovich AD, Albrecht RF, et al.: Absence of autoregulation of cerebral blood flow during halothane and enflurane anesthesia. Anesth Analg 55:100, 1976.
30. Adams RW, Gronert GA, Sundt TM, et al.: Halothane, hypocapnia, and cerebrospinal fluid pressure in neurosurgery. Anesthesiology 37:510, 1972.
31. Albrecht RF, Miletich FJ, Madala LR: Normalization of cerebral blood flow during prolonged halothane anesthesia. Anesthesiology 58:26, 1983.
32. Eger EI II: Isoflurane: A review. Anesthesiology 55:559, 1981.
33. Adams RW, Cucchiara RF, Gronert GA, et al.: Isoflurane and cerebrospinal fluid pressure in neurosurgical patients. Anesthesiology 54:97, 1981.
34. Newberg LA, Michenfelder JD: Cerebral protection by isoflurane during hypoxemia or ischemia. Anesthesiology 59:29, 1983.
35. Scheller MS, Tateishi AC, Drummond JC, Zornow MF: The ef-

fects of sevoflurane on cerebral blood flow, cerebral metabolic rate for oxygen, intracranial pressure, and the electroencephalogram are similar to those of isoflurane in the rabbit. Anesthesiology 68:548, 1988.

36. Lutz LJ, Milde JH, Milde LN: The cerebral functional, metabolic and hemodynamic effects of desflurane in dogs. Anesthesiology 73:125, 1990.

37. Ernst PS, Albin MS, Bunegin L: Intracranial and spinal cord hemodynamics in the sitting position in dogs in the presence and absence of increased intracranial pressure. Anesth Analg 70:147, 1990.

38. Cucchiara RF, Bowers B: Air embolism in children undergoing suboccipital craniotomy. Anesthesiology 57:338, 1982.

39. Matjasko J, Petrozza P, Mackenzie DF: Sensitivity of end-tidal nitrogen in venous air embolism detection in dogs. Anesthesiology 63:418, 1985.

40. Durward QJ, Amacher AL, Del Maestro RF, et al.: Cerebral and cardiovascular responses to changes in head position in patients with intracranial hypertension. J Neurosurg 59:938, 1983.

41. Bedford RF, Winn HR, Tyson G, et al.: Lidocaine prevents increased ICP after endotracheal intubation. In Shulman K, et al. (eds): Intracranial Pressure. 4th ed. New York, Springer Verlag, 1980.

42. Abor-madi MN, Keszler H, Yacoub JM: Cardiovascular reactions to laryngoscopy and tracheal intubation following small and large intravenous doses of lidocaine. Can Anaesth Soc J 24:12, 1977.

43. Pulsinelli WA, Waldman S, Rawlinson D, Plum F: Moderate hyperglycemia augments ischemic brain damage: A neuropathologic study in the rat. Neurology (NY) 32:1239, 1982.

44. Golabi M, Edwards MSB, Ousterhout DK: Craniosynostosis and hydrocephalus. Neurosurgery 21:63, 1987.

45. Collman H, Sorensen N, Kraub J, Muhling J: Hydrocephalus in craniosynostosis. Childs Nerv Syst 4:279, 1988.

46. Harris MM, Strafford MA, Rowe RW, et al.: Venous air embolism and cardiac arrest during craniectomy in a supine infant. Anesthesiology 65:547, 1986.

47. Rosenorn J, Diemer NH: Reduction of regional cerebral blood flow during brain retraction pressure in the rat. J Neurosurg 56:826, 1982.

48. Hendrick EB: Neurosurgery of congenital malformations. In Thompson RA, Green JR (eds): Pediatric Neurology and Neurosurgery. New York, Spectrum Publications, 1987.

49. Cross KW, Hey EN, Kennaird DL, et al.: Lack of temperature control in infants with abnormalities of the central nervous system. Arch Dis Child 46:437, 1971.

50. Karch SB, Urich H: Occipital encephalocele: A morphologic study. J Neurol Sci 15:89, 1972.

51. Ellsmorth CA, Shaw C-M, Sumi SM: Central nervous system developmental abnormalities. In Thompson RA, Green JR (eds): Pediatric Neurology and Neurosurgery. New York, Spectrum, 1978.

52. Park TS, Hoffman HJ, Hendrick EB, et al.: Experience with surgical decompression of the Arnold-Chiari malformation in young infants with myelomeningocele. Neurosurgery 13:147, 1983.

53. Sieben RL, Hamida MB, Shulman K: Multiple cranial nerve deficits associated with the Arnold-Chiari malformation. Neurology 21:673, 1971.

54. Davidson Ward SL, Nickerson BG, van der Hal A, et al.: Absent hypoxic and hypercapnic arousal responses in children with myelomeningocele and apnea. Pediatrics 78:44, 1986.

55. Creighton RE: Paediatric neuroanaesthesia. In Steward DJ (ed): Some Aspects of Paediatric Anaesthesia. Amsterdam, Elsevier/North Holland, 1982.

56. Alfery DD, Shapiro HM, Gagnon RL: Cardiac arrest following rapid drainage of cerebrospinal fluid in a patient with hydrocephalus. Anesthesiology 52:443, 1980.

57. Ostergaard JR, Voldby B: Intracranial arterial aneurysms in children and adolescents. J Neurosurg 58:832, 1983.

58. Jedeikin R, Rowe RD, Freedom RM, et al.: Cerebral arteriovenous malformation in neonates. The role of myocardial ischemia. J Cardiol 4:29, 1983.

59. Taki W, Yonekawa Y, Kobayashi A, et al.: Cerebral hemodynamic change in the child and adult with moyamoya disease. Stroke 21:272, 1990.

60. Sung DI: Suprasellar tumours in children. Cancer 50:1420, 1982.

61. Isu T, Miyasaka K, Abe H, et al.: Atlantoaxial dislocation associated with neurofibromatosis. J Neurosurg 58:451, 1983.

62. Nagao H, Yamashita M, Shinozaki Y, et al.: Hypersensitivity to pancuronium in a patient with von Recklinghausen's disease. Br J Anaesth 55:253, 1983.

63. Drake J, Hoffman HJ, Kobayashi J, et al.: Surgical management of children with temporal lobe epilepsy and mass lesions. Neurosurgery 21:792, 1987.

64. Fisher RS, Uematsu S: Surgical therapy of complex partial epilepsy. Johns Hopkins Med J 151:332, 1982.

65. Blume WT, Grabow JD, Darley FL, et al.: Intracarotid amobarbital test of language and memory before temporal lobectomy for seizure control. Neurology 23:812, 1973.

66. Rasmussen T: Cortical resection in the treatment of focal epilepsy. Adv Neurol 8:197, 1975.

67. Meschino A, Devitt JH, Koch JP, Szalai JP, Schwartz ML: The safety of awake tracheal intubation in cervical spine injury. Can Anaesth Soc J 39:114, 1992.

68. Crosby ET: Tracheal intubation in the cervical spine-injured patient. (Editorial) Can Anaesth Soc J 39:105, 1992.

69. Roen P, Wolfe RE: Therapeutic legends of emergency medicine. J Emerg Med 7:387, 1989.

70. Uchida M, Yamaoka H, Imanishi Y: Hypotension during surgery for subdural hematoma and effusion in infants. Crit Care Med 10:5, 1982.

71. Ruge JR, Sinson GP, McLone DG, Cerullo LJ: Pediatric spinal injury: The very young. J Neurosurg 68:25, 1988.

72. Hadley MN, Zabramski JM, Browner CM, et al.: Pediatric spinal trauma. Review of 122 cases of spinal cord and vertebral column injuries. J Neurosurg 68:18, 1988.

73. Brill CB, Rose JS, Godmilow L, et al.: Spastic quadriparesis due to C1-C2 subluxation in Hurler syndrome. J Pediatr 92:441, 1978.

74. Davidson RG: Atlantoaxial instability in individuals with Down's syndrome: A fresh look at the evidence. Pediatrics 81:857, 1988.

75. Nageb MG, Maxwell RE, Chou SN: Identification and management of high-risk patients with Klippel-Feil syndrome. J Neurosurg 61:523, 1984.

76. Ebara S, Harada T, Yamazaki Y, et al.: Unstable cervical spine in athetoid cerebral palsy. Spine 14:1154, 1989.

77. Stein SC, Schut L: Hydrocephalus in myelomeningocele. Childs Brain 5:413, 1979.

78. Wells TR, Jacobs RA, et al.: Incidence of short trachea in patients with myelomeningocele. Pediatr Neurol 6:109, 1990.

79. King D, Goodman J, Hawk T, et al.: Dumbbell neuroblastomas in children. Arch Surg 110:888, 1975.

80. Wagner HP, Kaser H: The role of surgery, radio- and chemotherapy in the treatment of neuroblastoma and ganglioneuroblastoma. Prog Pediatr Surg 16:1, 1983.

81. Evans AE, D'Angio GJ, Koop CE: Diagnosis and treatment of neuroblastoma. Pediatr Clin North Am 23:161, 1976.

82. Thompson EN, Bosley A: Disseminated intravascular coagulation in association with congenital neuroblastoma. Postgrad Med J 55:814, 1979.

Chapter 50

RADIOSURGERY

PAUL H. CHAPMAN, M.D., and CHRISTOPHER S. OGILVY, M.D.

In 1951, Leksell introduced the term radiosurgery to describe a stereotactic technique for destroying circumscribed intracranial targets with ionizing radiation.[1] Over the ensuing years, technologic innovations have made this concept feasible. Radiosurgery is now an accepted and widely used method for treating a variety of intracranial lesions, especially tumors and vascular malformations, in adults and children. A large dose of highly collimated radiation is delivered in a single fraction to the target volume. Conventional radiotherapy is delivered in many fractions over a period of weeks and typically includes a substantial amount of normal tissue in the radiation beam. To achieve a beneficial effect without harm, one relies on two radiobiologic principles with conventional radiotherapy: (1) abnormal tissue, such as tumor, is relatively more sensitive to radiation than the surrounding brain, and (2) normal tissue is better able to repair itself between radiation doses. The dose per fraction and the period of time (i.e., weeks) over which the total dose is given are important variables in conventional radiotherapy. With radiosurgery, one administers a single dose of radiation that is so large that any difference in sensitivity between target and normal tissue is irrelevant. Moreover, the use of a single fraction precludes any repair processes occurring during treatment. This means that the radiation dose must be confined as precisely as possible to the abnormal tissue. This requires precise aiming, using some form of stereotaxis and a sharply collimated radiation beam. Because it is inevitable that some normal tissue will be in the beam path, multiple radiation portals are used to minimize the dose to any one area outside the target volume.

Radiosurgery is best suited for lesions smaller than 2.5 to 3.0 cm in diameter. It has been observed that the larger the lesion being treated, the smaller the dose of radiation that can be safely given without serious complication. This is true regardless of the type of radiation used, and empiric curves have been derived which describe the relationship between lesion size, radiation dose, and risk of complication (Fig. 50–1).[2, 3] As a result,

for lesions above a certain size, the safe radiation dose is so small that one cannot reasonably expect to provide effective treatment. Although the relationship between risk and efficacy for increasing treatment volumes has been established in a general way, there is still uncertainty as to whether this is influenced by the type of lesion being treated. For example, the complication rate for cavernous angiomas appears to be greater than for arteriovenous malformations (AVMs) of comparable size.[4] The reasons for this are not entirely clear. As one might expect, the location of the lesion is a factor. Treatments in and around the brainstem, for example,

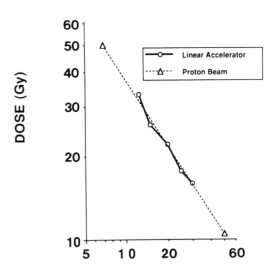

FIGURE 50–1. The relationship between the cross-sectional diameter of treatment volume and radiation dose for a 3 per cent risk of complication. The curves have been empirically derived for both proton and photon irradiation. Note that with increasing treatment volumes, the dose of radiation that can safely be administered is correspondingly smaller. (Reprinted with permission from Flickinger JC, et al.: Estimation of complications for linear accelerator radiosurgery with the integrated logistic formula. Int J Radiat Oncol Biol Phys 19:143, 1990. Pergamon Press Ltd.)

are riskier than those in noneloquent brain areas.[5] Another facet of radiosurgery that remains to be better clarified is the relative sensitivity of various lesions to radiation delivered in a large single fraction at high dose rate. The usual assumptions regarding radiosensitivity, which are based on conventional fractionated treatment, may not be applicable for predicting outcome with radiosurgery.

Children as young as 2 to 3 years are now routinely treated by radiosurgery. There are a number of considerations specific to pediatric patients, such as the need for general anesthesia. A serious concern in very young children is the effect of radiation on the developing brain. This has always been an issue with standard radiotherapy, in which the volume of normal brain irradiated is substantial, and a dose as low as 20 Gy may result in complications.[6] Because radiosurgery utilizes image-based stereotaxic targeting and highly collimated, focused radiation beams, the dose to normal tissue is minimized. This allows one to consider treating children who are too young for conventional radiation. The radiosurgery experience thus far fails to show any relationship between age and complication rate in the pediatric population.[7] However, it may take many more years of experience to identify an age-related complication with long latency or low frequency of occurrence. Radiation-induced neoplasms are also a potential problem, although Steiner has seen no case in 21 years of radiosurgical experience with 2800 patients using the cobalt-60 unit.[8]

RADIATION SOURCES

At the present time, there are at least 135 radiosurgical treatment facilities, either planned or in operation, in North America. Most of these use photon radiation, in the form of either megavoltage x-rays or gamma rays. Three centers utilize charged particles. Although both photons and charged particles are ionizing forms of radiation, there are fundamental differences between them with respect to their physical interaction with tissue.

Photon beams deliver energy to the medium through which they pass in an exponentially decreasing manner. As a result, tissue proximal to a target will receive a higher radiation dose than the target itself. Similarly, tissue beyond the target will also receive some radiation. This is true for both gamma rays and x-rays. Because of the large doses delivered as a single fraction in radiosurgical treatments, it is necessary to distribute the radiation outside the target over as large a volume of normal brain as possible. This is accomplished by using a large number of radiation beams which converge at the target. The linear accelerator employs multiple treatment arcs, the beam diameter being determined by the cross-sectional area of the target volume. In the case of the gamma treatment system, the radiation from 179-201 collimated cobalt-60 sources converge on the stereotaxically defined isocenter. Collimator diameters from 4 to 18 mm are used. Larger volumes require multiple treatment isocenters, and volume shaping is done by selectively blocking individual beam channels.

Charged particles deliver their energy by collision with the atoms of the medium through which they pass. The rate of energy transfer, or linear energy transfer (LET), is relatively constant along the beam path until the particles begin to slow significantly. At that point the LET increases, and this in turn slows the particles even more until they are stopped completely. As a result of this, there is a sharp peak of energy disposition where the charged particle stops. This is known as the Bragg peak (Fig. 50–2).[9] The depth of penetration of a charged particle in tissue, and hence its Bragg peak, will be determined by the initial energy of the particle. If all the particles in the beam have the same known energy, one can precisely deliver a large dose of radiation to the target volume with less radiation of tissue along the beam path. There is also no radiation beyond the Bragg peak and therefore no exit dose. Because the diameter of most lesions treated is greater than the width of the Bragg peak, it is usually necessary to progressively attenuate the energy of the beam with absorbing material to produce a series of peaks that encompass the width of the target volume. The radiation dose to normal tissues can be reduced further by using multiple beam portals (Fig. 50–3). The charged particle beams in use at this time for radiosurgery are protons and helium nuclei.

TUMORS

With the widespread use of radiosurgery in recent years, almost all benign and malignant tumor types

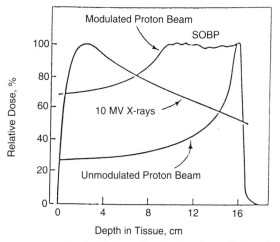

FIGURE 50–2. The depth dose distribution for radiation from a 160-MeV proton beam compared with 10-MeV photons. If the energy of the protons is progressively decreased (modulated) by placing absorbing material in the beam path, the Bragg peak can be spread out (SOBP) to span the entire diameter of a lesion. (From Shipley WU, et al.: Proton radiation as boost therapy for localized prostatic carcinoma. JAMA 241:1912, 1979. Copyright 1979. American Medical Association.)

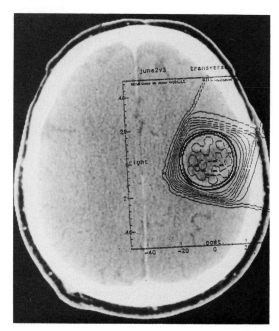

FIGURE 50–3. Dose distribution for treatment of an astrocytoma 3 cm in diameter with 160-MeV protons via three portals. The target volume is circumscribed by the 90 per cent isodose line. Inside this, the radiation dose is uniform to within ±5 per cent. Outside the tumor volume, the dose falls off sharply so that at a distance of 10 to 15 mm from the tumor margin, it is less than 10 per cent of that received by the tumor.

have been treated by this method. In adults, the most commonly treated tumors have been brain metastases,[10, 11] acoustic neuromas,[12] meningiomas,[13] and malignant astrocytomas.[14] There is now sufficient experience with these tumors to begin to analyze the effectiveness of radiosurgery and formulate a systematic approach to treatment. In the case of pediatric brain tumors, the clinical experience is smaller, although an equally wide variety of neoplasms has been treated. As a result, the role of radiosurgery is less certain, vis-à-vis other modes of therapy. The available data must be viewed in this perspective.

Tumor size, location, and histology may all be important considerations in selecting a patient for radiosurgery. With treatment volumes greater than 8 to 14 ml (2.5 to 3.0 cm in diameter), it may be necessary to reduce the radiation dose to the point that a beneficial response is unlikely. If the mass is near eloquent or sensitive structures such as brainstem or optic chiasm, the critical volume may be even less. Craniopharyngioma is a good example of this, in that the intimate relationship of the tumor to optic chiasm, hypothalamus, and medial temporal lobes becomes the limiting factor in its treatability with any type of radiation protocol.[15] In dosimetry planning, one typically requires a margin of several millimeters between the limit of the target volume and some sensitive structure such as the optic chiasm. This also implies that the tumor margin can be clearly distinguished from normal brain. Infiltrative tumors in radiosensitive areas, such as brainstem gliomas, are therefore not good candidates for radiosurgery.

The ability of radiosurgery to treat sharply circumscribed volumes of tissue with relative sparing of surrounding brain makes it of potential value in the treatment of otherwise problematic pediatric neoplasms. For example, even infiltrative tumors may be usefully treated if their location allows one to include an adequate margin in the target volume. In the case of malignant gliomas, survival is a function of tumor dose, and as much as 120 to 160 Gy may be needed to cure a glioblastoma.[16, 17] With fractionated external beam therapy at total doses greater than 60 Gy, brain necrosis is a problem.[18] Early experience suggests that radiosurgery, like brachytherapy, may be a useful adjunct in the treatment of such tumors.[14]

Local recurrence is a feature of pediatric brain tumors.[19] In this situation, radiosurgery may provide effective palliation if the child has already received a full course of conventional radiation. Loeffler treated a variety of recurrent tumors in children 5 to 10 years of age.[20] There were two anaplastic astrocytomas, two ependymomas, one craniopharyngioma, and one pineoblastoma. Of these, three responded completely, two were reduced more than 50 per cent in volume, and one remained stable. There were two deaths from recurrence outside the treatment volume. This small experience is encouraging with respect to salvage therapy when there are otherwise no treatment options. One might also consider radiosurgery for the initial treatment of tumors in very young children, for whom radiotherapy is otherwise contraindicated.

LOW-GRADE ASTROCYTOMAS

Experience in treating benign childhood astrocytomas by radiosurgery is limited and the published information often anecdotal.[21] Extrapolation from adult experience may be helpful but cannot take into account the unique features of typical childhood tumors occurring in the optic pathways, hypothalamus, brainstem, and cerebellum. Pozza et al. have described their radiosurgical experience with the linear accelerator in treating 14 patients with inoperable, low-grade astrocytomas.[22] Nine of these were children 11 to 17 years of age. All tumors were 3 cm or smaller in diameter and radiographically well defined. In the pediatric group, five of the tumors were thalamic, two were pineal, one optic chiasmal, and one parietal. In most cases, the radiation dose was 20 Gy or less, given as one or two fractions. Seventy-nine per cent of the tumors exhibited a ''marked shrinkage'' in volume, with corresponding improvement in clinical condition.

PINEAL TUMORS

A variety of tumors in the pineal region has been treated by radiosurgery, although the patients' ages are not always specified. Casentini treated germinomas in six patients, ages 12 to 29 years.[23] The radiosurgical dose was 10 to 12 Gy supplemented by 24 to 36 Gy of conventionally fractionated therapy. Tumors with diameters up to 25 mm regressed completely with radiosurgery alone, and there were no tumor-related deaths at 14 to 58 months follow-up. Given the radiosensitivity of germinomas, this result is to be expected and does not prove the advantage of radiosurgery over conventional treatment protocols. Based on experience with the Gamma Unit, Moser does not consider germinomas for radiosurgery because treatment volumes greater than 3 cm in diameter are generally required.[24] In treating 20 patients with various pineal area tumors up to 3 cm in diameter, he noted a better outcome for tumors less than 2.1 cm in diameter. In this group, the survivors included two pineocytomas, four benign astrocytomas, and four masses without histologic diagnosis. The only two patients who died had malignant astrocytomas. Of the eight patients with larger tumors, the four who died had either pineocytomas (two), pineoblastoma, or ependymoma. Moser concluded that 2 cm was the effective upper size limit for pineal area tumors treated by radiosurgical techniques. Colombo et al., using a linear accelerator, have reported a good result in a 6-year-old with a pineoblastoma.[21] As with germinomas, the radiosensitivity of pineoblastomas would lead one to expect at least a temporary response, though the role of radiosurgery in the primary therapy of either of these tumors is unclear. Kjellberg has treated two children with pineal masses using the proton beam.[25] One, a 17-year-old, died 5 years after a mass that had not undergone biopsy was treated with 17.5 Gy supplemented by 4.4 Gy of fractionated whole brain radiation. The second, a 7-year-old, died 28 months following treatment of a pineoblastoma with 50 Gy. Steiner points out that a single radiosurgery treatment is more expeditious than fractionated therapy, and if there is no difference in efficacy, the former is preferable on that basis alone.[8] He cautions, however, that malignant pineal tumors should be treated initially by radiosurgery only if their size and geometry allow it, this being the exception rather than the rule.

CRANIOPHARYNGIOMAS

The most extensive published experience concerning the use of radiosurgery to treat craniopharyngiomas is that of Backlund and others utilizing the Gamma Unit.[26, 27] Primary treatment consisted of intracavitary yttrium-90 for cysts and radiosurgery for solid tumor. There were 42 patients with a follow-up of 10 to 23 years. Eight patients had radiosurgery as a component of their treatment, either as the sole modality or in conjunction with yttrium-90. Maximum doses of 20 to 50 Gy were delivered, the periphery of the tumor receiving 10 Gy or less. Of the four patients having radiosurgery alone, three were alive and well and the fourth died of an unrelated cause. Of the four patients in whom yttrium-90 was used as well, all had a satisfactory result. No additional surgery or conventional radiotherapy was required. The authors conclude that this treatment schema is best for tumors that are more than 50 per cent cystic and when there are less than four cysts. Although their experience supports this conclusion, the number of patients whose treatment included radiosurgery is small. The most important aspect of treatment in this series was intracavitary yttrium-90, which was used in 38 of the 42 patients. This method is not widely employed for craniopharyngioma, making it difficult to infer from their experience what the role of radiosurgery might be in the context of other treatment strategies.

CUSHING'S DISEASE

Pituitary adenomas are uncommon in children. They typically present with hormonal hypersecretion and/or pubertal delay. In the pediatric age group, the only type of tumor for which there is substantial radiosurgical experience is that associated with Cushing's disease. Thorén reported treating eight patients, ages 5 to 17 years, with the Gamma Unit.[28] The goal of treatment was to control tumor growth, eliminate hypercortisolism, and maintain normal pituitary function. Radiation doses of 50 to 70 Gy were used. With a follow-up of 2.5 to 6.5 years, complete endocrine remission without relapse was achieved in seven of eight children. Urine cortisols were normal after one month in most. Post-treatment hypopituitarism was a problem. There was deficiency of growth hormone in all eight, thyroid deficiency in two, and hypogonadism in three. The authors conclude that surgical microadenectomy is a better alternative for primary treatment. This experience is similar to that reported for adults by Steiner.[8] Of 90 patients treated for Cushing's disease with the Gamma Unit, there was clinical remission in 76 per cent. Half developed pituitary insufficiency, and some required retreatment for an unsatisfactory response.

As in adults, children with corticotropic pituitary tumors are best treated initially by transsphenoidal adenectomy. This is also true for the other functioning tumors, with the exception of prolactinomas. Seventy per cent of noncorticotropic adenomas in children and adolescents secrete only prolactin.[29] With such tumors, bromocriptine is the first therapeutic consideration. Radiosurgery should generally be reserved for cases in which the primary treatment has failed and the geometry of the tumor will allow it to be radiated with acceptable risk to adjacent structures such as the optic chiasm.

ARTERIOVENOUS MALFORMATIONS (AVM)

MECHANISM OF AVM OBLITERATION USING RADIATION

Despite the type of radiation and delivery system used to treat AVMs, the underlying goal is to induce an inflammatory response in the vessel walls of the malformation, which will result in permanent thickening of pathologic vascular channels with ultimate thrombosis. The proposed pathophysiology of progressive vascular obliteration of AVMs after radiation is described below.

The timing and degree of pathologic changes observed in the walls of vessels vary depending upon total dose of radiation. Qualitative changes can be summarized as follows: The earliest changes occur in small vessels days to weeks after radiation. Endothelial cell swelling occurs with increased nuclear basophilia seen on pathologic specimens. With low doses of radiation, the observed inflammatory changes are reversible, and the vascular walls can return to a normal appearance over time. With large doses of radiation, or with repeated low doses, there is involvement of larger arterioles and associated breakdown of the blood-brain barrier. This stage occurs weeks to months after treatment and is thought to be the pathologic correlate of low-density lesions that appear on CT scans and T1-weighted MRI studies and are associated with increased water content of surrounding brain. Endothelial cell degeneration progresses to necrosis in some areas. There is an increase in interstitial exudate (increased colloids). Diapedesis of leukocytes into the interstitial space occurs. Fissuring of vessel walls and spot hemorrhages also can occur. In response to this injury, there is proliferation of surviving endothelial cells with increased deposition of collagen in the media of vessel walls. Fibrosis of the adventitia also occurs. While intimal proliferation continues as part of the inflammatory and reparative responses, gradual vascular lumen obliteration takes place. Ultimately, there is massive endothelial thickening.

Much of the information regarding vascular changes after radiation has been obtained by histopathologic study of cerebral vasculature from animals exposed to whole-brain x-ray radiation or high-energy protons. The changes seen in animals and human pathologic specimens after x-ray or gamma-ray radiation are virtually identical to changes seen after radiation with high-energy protons.

Despite differences of doses, examination of tissue obtained at autopsy or after surgical removal of an AVM previously treated with x-ray, gamma radiation, or Bragg peak therapy reveals vascular wall morphology similar to changes described in animal studies.

One question that remains unanswered is whether or not focused radiation in children carries with it a higher efficacy. The literature contains several dramatic examples of pediatric patients who have undergone stereotactic radiosurgery that resulted in complete obliteration of large-sized AVMs yet preservation of the normal vasculature through the same area of radiation.[30, 31] Lindquist and Steiner[32] document complete obliteration of lesions in 21 of 22 patients at 2 years after treatment (95.4 per cent). This was in children 13 to 17 years of age. In a group of 31 patients 5 to 12 years of age, only 22 of 28 lesions were completely obliterated (78.5 per cent). Whether or not stereotactic radiosurgery was more effective in the teenage population is difficult to evaluate, and details of lesion size in the two populations of patients are not discussed

in this report. It is hoped that further follow-up will shed light on the issue of whether blood vessels in younger children are more or less susceptible to the effects of focused radiation therapy.

One issue regarding the use of radiosurgery for AVMs in children is the actual risk of the procedure versus the risk of the natural history of the disease. Ondra et al.[33] conducted a 24-year follow-up on patients with cerebral AVMs who had no treatment during follow-up. The annual hemorrhage rate was found to be 4.0 per cent, with an annual morbidity rate of 1.7 per cent and an annual mortality rate of 1.0 per cent. Thus, over a 30-year horizon, the risk of having any hemorrhage is approximately 90 per cent, with the risk of a major or fatal hemorrhage approximately 65 per cent and the risk of a fatal hemorrhage 26 per cent. For children, these longer-range estimates of hemorrhage are important to consider.

The mortality from the first hemorrhage from an AVM is approximately 10 per cent.[34–36] In children, according to one study, a 24 per cent mortality rate was identified for the first hemorrhage from an AVM.[37] These relatively ominous figures argue strongly in favor of treating AVMs when they are discovered in children if the treatment can be offered with a reasonable risk and high efficacy.

RESULTS OF AVM TREATMENT IN CHILDREN USING RADIOSURGERY

A larger number of reports are beginning to appear regarding the results of radiosurgery used to treat AVMs. Usually, several pediatric patients are included in each series of patients reported, and some reports are devoted entirely to results of treatment in children.

Levy et al.[30] reported treatment of 40 patients, ages 6 to 18 years, using heavy charged particle Bragg peak radiosurgery with the helium beam. Three patients had angiographically occult lesions. Of the 37 patients with true AVMs, the volumes treated ranged from 0.265 cm^3 to 60 cm^3, and the doses used ranged from 10 to 45 GyE. Doses were given in 1 to 3 fractions, depending on the size of the lesion. In approximately 70 per cent of patients, angiographic obliteration of lesions occurred by 2 years after the treatment. Neurologic deficits attributed to radiation necrosis occurred in two of 37 patients (5.4 per cent). A third patient with radiation-induced injury was treated for an angiographically occult lesion. Overall, the results are encouraging, even for some of the larger lesions.

Altschuler et al. report the results of treating 18 pediatric patients with the Gamma Knife. Their ages ranged from 34 months to 18 years.[38] The size range of the lesions treated was smaller than for helium beam treated patients and ranged from 7 to 29 mm in diameter (average 17 mm). The doses used ranged from 17.5 to 25 Gy and were based on a predicted risk of radiation necrosis of 3 per cent according to Flickinger's formula.[2] Follow-up angiography was performed at one year in 7 of the 18 patients. Three lesions were completely obliterated, three others were significantly smaller, and one was unchanged. One patient developed an increase in hemiparesis 4 months after treatment (5.5 per cent total). This patient harbored a lesion in the brainstem, and the lesion was totally obliterated on follow-up angiography. Edema was seen surrounding the lesion on MRI studies. Three other patients developed asymptomatic edema of their lesions following treatment based on follow-up MRI studies.

In a separate report on the use of the Gamma Knife to treat AVMs in children, Steiner et al. discuss in detail the results in 54 pediatric patients (aged 5 to 12 years) and 60 adolescents (aged 13 to 17 years).[32]

Of the younger age group, 31 of 54 patients had "optimum treatment," defined as a dose greater than or equal to 25 Gy covering the entire AVM. Angiographic obliteration was observed in 17 of 31 patients (55 per cent) one year after treatment and 22 of 28 (78.5 per cent) 2 years after treatment. In the adolescent group, 23 patients had "optimum treatment," with 56.6 per cent demonstrating angiographic obliteration at one year follow-up and 95.4 per cent obliteration 2 years after treatment.

No hemorrhages were reported in either the pediatric or adolescent group during the follow-up interval. Radiation-induced complications occurred in 1.5 per cent (one patient) of patients between 5 and 12 years of age and in 3.3 per cent (two patients) of the group 13 to 17 years of age. There were no significant cognitive deficits attributed to the radiation and no evidence of endocrine dysfunction. However, as the authors themselves point out, these observations are preliminary. These issues of cognitive deficits and endocrine dysfunction are critical when considering the use of radiation therapy in children. In theory, the incidence of cognitive deficits and endocrine dysfunction would be expected to be lower when focused radiation is used instead of whole-brain radiation, yet the final answer to these issues will require careful, long-term follow-up.

To date, no late radiation-induced tumors have been reported following radiosurgery (of any type). However, the latency for such tumors to develop after standard radiotherapy is on the order of 20 years. Long-term follow-up of radiosurgery-treated patients will determine whether late tumors can be induced by radiosurgery.

Using the linear accelerator adapted with stereotactic targeting, Loeffler et al.[20] reported their initial results treating ten pediatric patients with AVMs. The dose used was 15 to 20 Gy at the 80 to 90 per cent isodose line. The ages of the patients treated ranged from 2 to 20 years. As with other types of radiosurgery, results were encouraging for these smaller lesions. Five of eight lesions underwent complete obliteration at one year. Three patients had asymptomatic edema on CT scan at an interval of 6 to 28 months after treatment. One patient had late onset of headache with lethargy, which required treatment with steroids.

In general, the preliminary results of radiosurgery for AVMs in children appear to parallel what is observed in adults.[39–41] Complication rates can be predicted based on the volume of tissue irradiated and dose of radiation used. The obliteration rates are determined by the total dose used. Therefore, with smaller lesions (less than 2 to 2.5 cm in diameter), reasonable rates of obliteration can be expected (85 to 90 per cent), with a rate of serious, permanent, radiation-induced complications of 1 to 3 per cent.

DECISION-MAKING IN THE MANAGEMENT OF PEDIATRIC AVMs

As in adult patients, several options are available for treatment of AVMs in the pediatric population. Lesions can be embolized via a transvascular route through the femoral artery or embolized at surgery through feeding vessels. Microsurgical techniques alone can be used to extirpate lesions. Radiosurgery offers an effective means of treating appropriately selected patients. In addition, combinations of therapies to include embolization followed by radiosurgery or embolization followed by surgery, and in some cases surgery followed by radiosurgery, are being used to obliterate AVMs.

Regarding radiosurgery, the latent interval of anywhere between 4 months and 3 years is a distinct disadvantage. During this interval, it appears that the incidence of rehemorrhage from lesions is similar to the natural history of the disease and occurs at a rate of approximately 4 per cent per year. In addition, complications from radiosurgery for deep inoperable lesions in children can produce devastating, permanent deficits. Radiosurgery can be used in children to obliterate lesions that are inaccessible surgically or carry a high risk surgically owing to the patient's small blood volume.

The operability or inoperability of a given lesion and the risk associated with the open surgery must be balanced against the risk of radiation necrosis from radiosurgery and the expected risk of future hemorrhage should the lesion not obliterate. One management strategy that can be used in infants is to proceed with a radiosurgical treatment of an appropriately sized AVM in which a reasonable obliteration rate would be predicted. Following treatment, the patient can undergo follow-up with MRI or MRA studies. If the lesion is still patent over 2 to 3 years, open surgery can be considered, at which point the child would be old enough to tolerate the procedure. More recently, advances in endovascular techniques have made it possible to embolize portions of AVMs in an attempt to reduce the overall size and therefore reduce the necessary volume of irradiated tissue during radiosurgery. With this type of treatment plan, permanent agents such as N-butyl-cyanoacrylate (NBCA) glue should be used to minimize the potential recanalization of vessels.

The decision-making process in the management of AVMs in children is often difficult. The safest form of treatment for a given patient should be decided upon by a team composed of neurosurgeons experienced with the management of AVMs as well as a radiation therapist and interventional neuroradiologist experienced in endovascular techniques. The ultimate goal in the overall management of such patients is to minimize the risk while maximizing the potential for obliteration in a given patient.

CAVERNOUS ANGIOMAS

Cavernous angiomas are low-flow vascular lesions that can occur throughout the nervous system. They are defined histologically as vascular channels in direct apposition to each other. The walls of the abnormal vessels have an endothelial lining, and the remainder of the wall is made of collagen. The wall thickness varies significantly between lumens.[42] These lesions are "occult" to angiography due to their slow flow. However, they can hemorrhage and may do so repeatedly.

The typical clinical presentation of supratentorial cavernous angiomas is one of seizures or of a neurologic deficit that progresses in stepwise fashion. Prior to advances in neuro-imaging techniques, patients with cavernous angiomas were often misdiagnosed as having a demyelinating disease due to the stepwise neurologic worsening, with events that can occur months or years apart with improvement in neurologic function between events.

The natural history of cavernous angiomas remains unclear. Two recent retrospective studies demonstrate a hemorrhage rate of 0.25 per cent per patient year in one study and 0.7 per cent per year in another.[43, 44] However, there are clearly patients with these lesions who experience hemorrhage on a frequent basis and require treatment.

When possible, surgical excision is the treatment of choice. These vascular lesions are usually well circumscribed and can be excised with low risk, even when they occur in what appears to be "eloquent" brain tissue. However, some lesions occur deep in the cerebral hemisphere of the brain, and for these, surgery carries a significant morbidity.

For lesions that seem truly inoperable, radiosurgery might be considered. In the report by Levy et al.,[30] three pediatric patients with vascular malformations occult to angiography were treated. Radiation-induced complications occurred in one of these patients. The Gamma Knife has been used to treat these lesions as well. In a report of 24 patients, radiosurgery was used in surgically inaccessible lesions with two or more clinical events consistent with hemorrhage. Of these patients, five experienced radiation-induced complications (21 per cent). Of the five patients with complications, four had lesions in the brainstem.[4]

Although location may explain the relatively high incidence of complications resulting from radiosurgery to treat cavernous angiomas, there may be a basic biologic response of these slow-flow lesions to radiation which makes the surrounding tissue more susceptible to radiation-induced injury. In addition, the end point of therapy for cavernous angiomas using radiosurgery has yet to be accurately defined. Unlike true AVMs, in which angiographic obliteration is used to determine efficacy of treatment, cavernous angiomas have no such solid end point. Cavernous angiomas are known to change in size over time. Increase in size is thought to be a result of small, repeated hemorrhages or possibly recruitment of nearby blood vessels into the malformation. Between hemorrhagic events, cavernous angiomas can decrease in size as a result of clot absorption. Although Kondziolka et al.[4] used reduction of cavernous angioma size on MRI as evidence of effective radiation treatment, this may actually be part of the natural history of these specific lesions.

In general, radiosurgery for cavernous angiomas is discouraged. For certain lesions in the deep white matter or thalamus it might be better to let a pediatric patient live with the natural history of this lesion. As carefully selected lesions are treated, more light should be cast on this critical issue. In addition, with improved neuro-imaging techniques for flow of blood on MRI, stricter criteria for true treatment of cavernous angiomas using radiosurgery may be easier to define.

VENOUS MALFORMATIONS

Venous malformations are thought to be variants of normal venous anatomy. They have a characteristic linear high-density appearance on contrast-enhanced CT and show a linear flow void on MRI studies. Although they can occur in association with cavernous angiomas, the actual morbidity and mortality associated with venous malformations is extremely low. In one retrospective natural history study, there was one hemorrhage in 100 patients.[45] It is generally agreed that radiosurgery should not be used to treat venous malformations.[4] If indeed there is hemorrhage associated with a venous malformation, a high index of suspicion should be held that there is an associated cavernous angioma in the vicinity of the venous malformation.

REFERENCES

1. Leksell L: The stereotactic method and radiosurgery of the brain. Acta Chir Scand 102:316, 1951.
2. Flickinger JC, Schell MC, Larson DA: Estimation of complications for linear accelerator radiosurgery with the integrated logistic formula. Int J Radiat Oncol Biol Phys 19:143, 1990.
3. Marks LB, Spencer DP: The influence of volume on the tolerance of the brain to radiosurgery. J Neurosurg 75:177, 1991.
4. Kondziolka D, Lunsford LD, Coffey RJ, et al.: Stereotactic radiosurgery of angiographically occult vascular malformations: Indications and preliminary experience. Neurosurgery 27:892, 1990.
5. Flickinger JC, Lunsford LD, Kondziolka D, et al.: Radiosurgery and brain tolerance: An analysis of neurodiagnostic imaging changes after Gamma Knife radiosurgery for arteriovenous malformations. Int J Radiat Oncol Biol Phys 23:19, 1992.
6. Edwards MSB, Hudgins RJ, Wilson CB, et al.: Pineal region tumors in children. J Neurosurg 68:689, 1988.
7. Loeffler JS, Siddon RL, Wen PY, et al.: Stereotactic radiosurgery of the brain using a standard linear accelerator: A study of early and late effects. Radiother Oncol 17:311, 1990.
8. Steiner L: Stereotactic radiosurgery with the cobalt 60 gamma unit in the surgical treatment of intracranial tumors and arteriovenous malformations. *In* Schmidek H, Sweet W (eds): Operative

Neurosurgical Techniques: Indications, Methods and Results. New York, Grune & Stratton, vol 2, 1988, pp 515–529.

9. Shipley WU, Tepper JE, Prout GR, et al.: Proton radiation as boost therapy for localized prostatic carcinoma. JAMA 241:1912, 1979.

10. Adler JR, Cox RS, Kaplan I, et al.: Stereotactic radiosurgical treatment of brain metastases. J Neurosurg 76:444, 1992.

11. Loeffler JS, Kooy HM, Wen PY, et al.: The treatment of recurrent brain metastases with stereotactic radiosurgery. J Clin Oncol 8:576, 1990.

12. Flickinger JC, Lunsford LD, Coffey RJ, et al.: Radiosurgery of acoustic neurinomas. Cancer 67:345, 1991.

13. Kondziolka D, Lunsford LD, Coffey RJ, et al.: Stereotactic radiosurgery of meningiomas. J Neurosurg 74:552, 1991.

14. Loeffler JS, Alexander III E, Shea WM, et al.: Radiosurgery as part of the initial management of patients with malignant glioma. J Clin Oncol 10:1379, 1992.

15. Austin-Seymour M, Munzenrider J, Linggood R, et al.: Fractionated proton radiation therapy of cranial and intracranial tumors. Am J Clin Oncol (CCT) 13:327, 1990.

16. Walker MD, Strike TA, Sheline GE: An analysis of dose-effect relationship in the radiotherapy of malignant gliomas. Int J Radiat Oncol Biol Phys 5:1725, 1979.

17. Woo SY, Maor MH: Improving radiotherapy for brain tumors. Oncology 4:41, 1990.

18. Sheline GE, Wara WM, Smith V: Therapeutic irradiation and brain injury. Int J Radiat Oncol Biol Phys 6:1215, 1980.

19. Kun L: Patterns of failure in tumors of the central nervous system. Cancer Treat Symp 2:285, 1983.

20. Loeffler JS, Rossitch E Jr, Siddon R, et al.: Role of stereotactic radiosurgery with a linear accelerator in treatment of intracranial arteriovenous malformations and tumors in children. Pediatrics 85:774, 1990.

21. Colombo F, Benedetti A, Pozza F, et al.: External stereotactic irradiation by linear accelerator. Neurosurgery 16:154, 1985.

22. Pozza F, Colombo F, Chierego G, et al.: Low-grade astrocytomas: treatment with unconventionally fractionated external beam stereotactic radiation therapy. Radiology 171:565, 1989.

23. Casentini L, Colombo F, Pozza F, et al.: Combined radiosurgery and external radiotherapy of intracranial germinomas. Surg Neurol 34:79, 1990.

24. Moser RP, Backlund EO: Stereotactic techniques in the diagnosis and treatment of pineal region tumours. In Neuwelt EA (ed): Diagnosis and Treatment of Pineal Region Tumors. Baltimore, Williams & Wilkins, 1984, pp 236–253.

25. Chapman PH, Linggood RM: The management of pineal area tumors: A recent reappraisal. Cancer 46:1253, 1980.

26. Backlund EO, Axelsson B, Bergstrand C-G, et al.: Treatment of craniopharyngiomas—the stereotactic approach to a ten to twenty years' perspective. I. Surgical, radiological and ophthalmological aspects. Acta Neurochir (Wien) 99:11, 1989.

27. Sääf M, Thorén M, Bergstrand C-G, et al.: Treatment of craniopharyngiomas—the stereotactic approach in a ten to twenty years' perspective. II Psychosocial situation and pituitary function. Acta Neurochir (Wien) 99:97, 1989.

28. Thorén M, Rähn T, Hallengren B, et al.: Treatment of Cushing's disease in childhood and adolescence by stereotactic pituitary irradiation. Acta Paediatr Scand 75:388, 1986.

29. Kane LA, Leinung MC, Scheithauer B, et al.: Noncorticotropic pituitary adenomas in childhood and adolescence. Abstract 269. Proceedings Annual Meeting Endocrine Society, San Antonio, TX, 1992.

30. Levy RP, Fabrikant JI, Frankel KA, et al.: Stereotactic heavy charged particle Bragg peak radiosurgery for the treatment of intracranial arteriovenous malformations in childhood and adolescence. Neurosurgery 24:841, 1989.

31. Fabrikant JI, Frankel DA, Phillips MH, et al.: Stereotactic heavy charged particle Bragg peak radiosurgery for intracranial arteriovenous malformations. In Edwards MS, Hoffman HJ (eds): Cerebral Vascular Disease in Children and Adolescents. Baltimore, Williams & Wilkins, 1988, pp 367–388.

32. Steiner L, Lindquist C: Radiosurgery with focused gamma beam irradiation in children. In Edwards MS, Hoffman HJ (eds): Cerebral Vascular Disease in Children and Adolescents. Baltimore, Williams & Wilkins, 1988, pp 367–388.

33. Ondra SL, Troupp H, George ED, et al.: The natural history of symptomatic arteriovenous malformation of the brain: A 24-year follow-up assessment. J Neurosurg 73:387, 1990.

34. Brown RD, Weibers DO, Forbes G, et al.: The natural history of unruptured intracranial arteriovenous malformations. J Neurosurg 68:352, 1988.

35. Crawford PM, West CR, Chadwick DW, et al.: Arteriovenous malformations of the brain: natural history in unoperated patients. J Neurol Neurosurg Psychiatry 49:1, 1986.

36. Graf CJ, Perret GB, Torner JC: Bleeding from cerebral arteriovenous malformations as part of their natural history. J Neurosurg 58:331, 1983.

37. Humphreys RP, Hendrick EB, Hoffman HJ: Arteriovenous malformations of the brain. Conc Pediatr Neurosurg 8:146, 1988.

38. Altschuler EM, Lunsford LD, Coffey RJ, et al.: Gamma knife radiosurgery for intracranial arteriovenous malformations in childhood and adolescence. Pediatr Neurosci 15:53, 1989.

39. Steinberg GK, Fabrikant JI, Marks MP, et al.: Stereotactic heavy charge particle Bragg peak radiation for intracranial arteriovenous malformations. N Engl J Med 323:96, 1990.

40. Lunsford LD, Kondziolka D, Flickinger JC, et al.: Stereotactic radiosurgery for arteriovenous malformations of the brain. J Neurosurg 75:512, 1991.

41. Betti OO, Munari C, Rosler R: Stereotactic radiosurgery with the linear accelerator: Treatment of arteriovenous malformations. Neurosurgery 24:311, 1989.

42. McCormick WF: The pathology of vascular ("arteriovenous") malformations. J Neurosurg 24:807, 1960.

43. Robinson JR, Awad IA, Little JR: Natural history of the cavernous angioma. J Neurosurg 75:709, 1991.

44. Del Curling O, Kelly DL, Elster AD, et al.: An analysis of the natural history of cavernous angiomas. J Neurosurg 75:702, 1991.

45. Garner TB, Del Curling O, Kelly D, et al.: The natural history of intracranial venous angiomas. J Neurosurg 75:715, 1991.

Chapter 51

TECHNIQUES OF SKULL BASE SURGERY

DEREK A. BRUCE, M.D., IAN R. MUNRO, M.B., and
KENNETH SHAPIRO, M.D.

Many of the lesions that affect the skull base in children occur in the midline or para-midline involving the orbits, nasopharynx, frontal fossa, sphenoid sinus, clivus, petrous apex, and cavernous sinuses. Laterally located lesions are rare. Many of the tumors that occur in this area are at least microscopically benign and often respond poorly to other modes of therapy—radiation or chemotherapy. The techniques of craniofacial surgery introduced by Tessier are now well established,[1] and such surgery frequently involves the craniofacial team working intracranially and in the sinuses—frontal, ethmoidal, and maxillary—simultaneously. This type of surgery has proved that infection can be kept to a minimum, and with careful dural closure, cerebrospinal fluid (CSF) leakage is rare. Derome adapted some of the craniofacial techniques when he described combined transcranial and transsphenoidal surgery for tumors.[2] This chapter considers the surgical techniques and approaches to the midline and para-midline areas of the skull that are of value in treating neoplastic, congenital, traumatic, and infectious lesions of children.

PREOPERATIVE PLANNING

The surgery can be divided conceptually into three stages: exposure, resection, and reconstruction. The last-mentioned is often the most problematic and has to be planned prior to the skin incision since the use of a variety of local and possibly distant tissue transfers may be required to achieve a closure that is infection-resistant, prevents CSF leak, and is cosmetically excellent. The most common tissue transfer is that of flaps of pericranium to reinforce areas of dural opening, replace resected dura, cover bone grafts, and fill in dead

space. Although it is ideal to use vascularized tissue, free pericranium makes an excellent dural substitute and heals well. Part of the preoperative planning is deciding where to base the pericranial flap. There are two main possibilities: (1) to leave the pericranium attached to the temporalis muscle on one or both sides and divide it down the midline or at the junction with the contralateral temporalis muscle, or (2) to divide the pericranium posteriorly and leave it attached to the galea at the supraorbital margins bilaterally (Fig. 51–1). The latter strategy is best when the flaps are required to reinforce the midline dura or skull base or to fill in the sphenoid sinus. A second useful flap, especially in redo operations, where the pericranium may not be available for use as a graft, is the galea-frontalis flap. Drawbacks to the use of this flap are (1) it is very thin in small children and (2) it may leave a cosmetically visible hollow in the scalp of the forehead. Other flaps that may be required are free muscle flaps or pedicle flaps.[3–6]

The ability to make tissue glue has made it possible to resect dura in areas where dural suturing is impossible (e.g., posterior midline frontal fossa or pituitary fossa). Our current formula is shown in Table 51–1. The frozen cryoprecipitate can be made from the designated donor blood, if the blood bank is notified at the time of donation, or from autologous blood donation.

It is extremely common for bone to be required either to replace skull bone involved with tumor or to reconstruct the skull base or the orbits. The use of split cranial bone is standard practice, and this can usually be obtained from the frontal flap itself or from a second craniotomy, usually midline or high parietal (Fig. 51–2). The possible need for extra bone must be considered before the surgery begins so that the patient can be prepped and positioned to permit access to a large enough area of skull to harvest extra bone should that

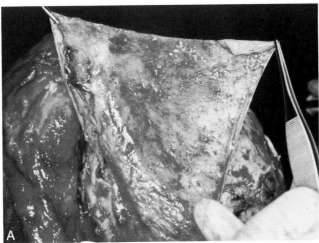
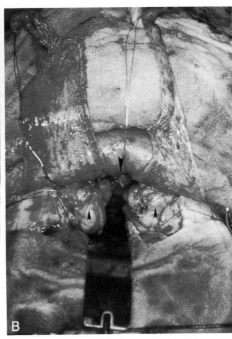

FIGURE 51–1. Pericranial flaps. *A,* Thick pericranial flap based on the temporalis muscle. *B,* Anteriorly based pericranial flap split sagittally to permit "sandwich" coverage of skull base bone graft. Note periorbitum *(small arrowhead)* and nasal cartilage *(large arrowhead).*

prove necessary. The bone is easily split by means of a saw and small sharp osteotomes, and there is rarely a reason for not completely reconstructing the cranium at the time of the initial surgery. If adequate amounts of cranial bone cannot be obtained, rib or iliac crest may be used, as in the past. Both of these donor sites produce significant postoperative pain, and the bone is often absorbed over time. Thus we do not suggest these as donor sites unless no or inadequate amounts of cranial bone can be obtained. Banked bone may be available, or demineralized bone may be used. The fate of this type of bone substitution is not known in the child. If this is the only way to fill a defect, it is best to place the autologous bone in the region of the surgical resection and any bone substitute at the donor site. Acrylic should not be used in proximity to the nasal sinuses because of the increased risk of infection.

Preoperative planning may include examination by members of any combination of the following disciplines: neuro-ophthalmology, neurology, endocrinology, neurosurgery, anthropology, pediatrics, oncology, anesthesiology, craniofacial surgery, dentistry, speech therapy, and social services. Also preoperatively, some or all of the following radiological studies will be necessary: plain skull radiographs, computed tomographic (CT) scan, 3-D reconstruction, cisternography (if a CSF

leak is suspected), facial and dental radiographs, magnetic resonance imaging (MRI) scan and MR angiography, and angiography. When the tumor is highly vascular (e.g., angiofibroma or melanoma), preoperative embolization may be helpful. Surgery should follow within one to two days, before recanalization has occurred.

In children there are concerns that do not exist in the adult. The first of these is the location of the unerupted permanent dentition. The locus of these teeth can be pinpointed on the CT scan prior to surgery, and any maxillary osteotomies have to be superior to this area. Second, the reconstruction of the jaws must be rigid and accurate since any poor alignment will be aggravated by growth. Third, there is an ongoing concern for repeated follow-up of the facial growth in these children to ensure that normal and symmetrical growth is occurring over time. If not, further surgical intervention may be required.

TECHNIQUE

While it seems obvious, the first decision is about the position of the incision. The most frequent is the coronal incision. With any incision, the need to preserve the superficial temporal artery and vein should be paramount in the surgeon's mind, as should the need for access to tissue flaps and additional bone. It is not necessary to shave the hair, and when using a coronal incision, it is neither necessary nor advisable to bring it forward to a peak in the midline. This can increase the risk of hair loss anterior to the incision and has no benefit. We now use a wavy coronal incision, since this minimizes the visibility of the scar when the hair gets wet. The eyes must be protected during the surgery,

TABLE 51–1.   FORMULA FOR FIBRIN GLUE

Syringe 1	Syringe 2
Amicar 0.2 cc of 250 mg/ml Calcium Chloride 10%, 3 cc 1 Vial of topical thrombin, 1000 units	1 unit of frozen cryoprecipitate

The solution from each of the two syringes is delivered to the tissue using three to four times as much of syringe 2 as syringe 1.

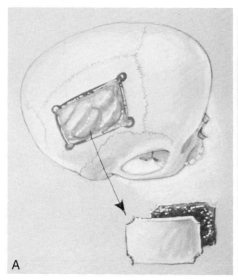

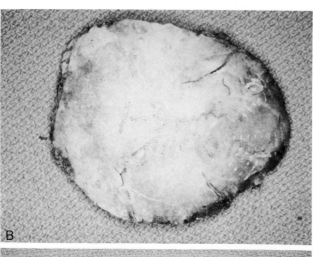

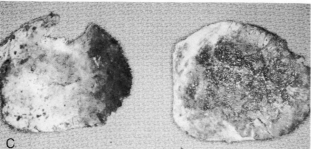

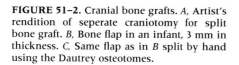

FIGURE 51–2. Cranial bone grafts. *A*, Artist's rendition of seperate craniotomy for split bone graft. *B*, Bone flap in an infant, 3 mm in thickness. *C*, Same flap as in *B* split by hand using the Dautrey osteotomes.

since often the entire face is included in the surgical field. This can be achieved in one of two ways: eye shields may be placed to cover the cornea and sclera or the eyelids may be sutured over ointment. I prefer the latter approach for two main reasons. The first is the concern about adequate corneal oxygenation if the case is a very long one, and the second is that there is less chance that irrigation solutions will collect and produce damage to the cornea. The use of the Colorado microneedle for the skin incision has removed the need for any type of skin clip, thus facilitating the movements of the frontal scalp flap, decreasing the risk of traumatic injury to the eyes by the clips, and avoiding the bleeding that can occur from the scalp at the end of the procedure when the scalp clips are removed.

It is helpful to divide the lesions of the midline skull base into (1) those involving the frontal fossa without invasion of the nasal sinuses, (2) those in the frontal fossa invading the frontal, ethmoid, and sphenoid sinuses, the nasopharynx, and/or the mid and lower clivus, and (3) those in the retropharynx and/or clivus including the upper third (Fig. 51–3). All the lesions in these areas require a midline surgical approach. Lesions that are unilateral (e.g., fibrous dysplasia of the orbit) may require only a unilateral approach.

AREA 1

The common lesions that occur here are frontal ethmoidal and sphenoidal encephaloceles, meningiomas, and mesenchymal chondrosarcomas. The approach is a standard bifrontal craniotomy with a secondary removal, in one piece, of the central portion of the standard bandeau: both medial orbital rims and the residual midline skull down to the foramen cecum. To achieve this it is necessary that the epidural dissection of the orbital roofs and midline frees the dura from the foramen cecum so that the base of the crista galli can be seen. This ensures that the surgeon's line of vision is now straight along the frontal floor, and therefore minimal retraction of the frontal lobes is required. It is this direct access to the frontal floor that is the benefit of this technique. Olfaction can be preserved when the lesion is anterior to the crista galli (e.g., frontal encephalocele), and it is rarely necessary to go intradurally other than at the point at which the encephalocele exits the cranium. This approach allows for the insertion of cranial bone to close the skull defect and to move the nasofrontal angle superiorly and thus improve the cosmetic appearance. It also permits correction of the hypertelorism.[7] In the small infant this usually means infracturing of the lateral walls of the ethmoid sinuses rather than moving the whole orbit as a block.

For more posterior encephaloceles or extradural lesions, it is usually necessary to take down the olfactory bulbs. The dura in this area can usually be sutured directly without a patch and reinforced with tissue glue. The latter is usually done at the end of the procedure. Posterior ethmoidal encephaloceles without involvement of the sphenoid sinus can usually be corrected without removing the midline skull base. The bony defect is dissected out circumferentially, taking great care at the posterior lateral margins where the

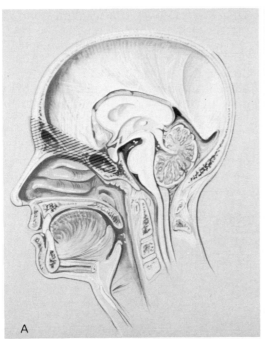

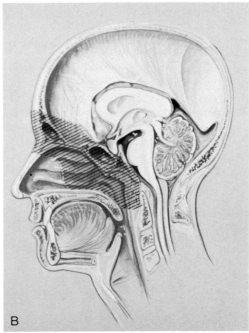

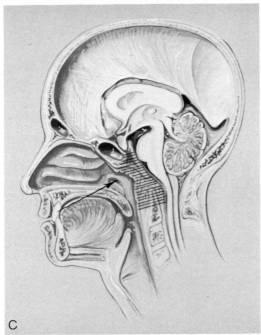

FIGURE 51–3. Division of skull base for consideration of surgical approach. *A,* Frontal base, including the pituitary fossa without pathology in the sinuses. *B,* Frontal base, paranasal sinuses, inferior two thirds of the clivus and nasopharynx. *C,* Retropharynx, clivus including posterior clinoid.

optic nerves are in closest proximity. Depending on the contents of the encephalocele, the dura may be opened at its exit from the cranium, abnormal herniated cerebrum excised, and the dura closed, or if normal brain is herniated (this is unusual), the dura that is herniated may be delivered into the cranium as with sphenoidal lesions (vide infra). Once the bony defect is cleared of tissue, a pericranial graft is placed over the defect to act as a barrier between the intracranial space and the sinuses; a bone graft of cranium is placed to fill the bone defect and wired or screwed into place; and a second layer of pericranium is placed between the bone and the dura. When the encephalocele is through the base of the pituitary fossa (sphenoidal encephalocele), there is usually viable tissue including the pituitary gland and stalk within the extracranial dura (Fig. 51–4). This cannot be safely excised, and the technique for repair is slightly different. The midline skull base anterior to the exit of the encephalocele has to be removed to allow access to the dural sleeve of the encephalocele. This

may be done in one piece using the drill, saw, or osteotomes—taking care in this setting at the anterior lateral margin of the lesions, since this is the location of the optic nerves, which often have no bone between their dural sleeve and the encephalocele. If the anterior floor is to be removed in one piece, it is safer to leave a small shelf of bone at the anterior rim of the cranial defect intact and to remove that last portion with a small rongeur. It is easy to tear the dura at the anterior lateral margin of the encephalocele, at the base of the optic nerves, and this dura should be completely freed from the bone edge prior to removing the bone, since the dura is thin and difficult to suture in this area, and immediately proximal to the area of suture are the optic nerves. If the dura is opened in this area, it is usually possible to obtain a good closure with a piece of Gelfoam and tissue glue. Once the anterior aspect of the bony rim of the encephalocele is removed, the dural neck can be dissected circumferentially and freed from the surrounding bone in preparation for its mobi-

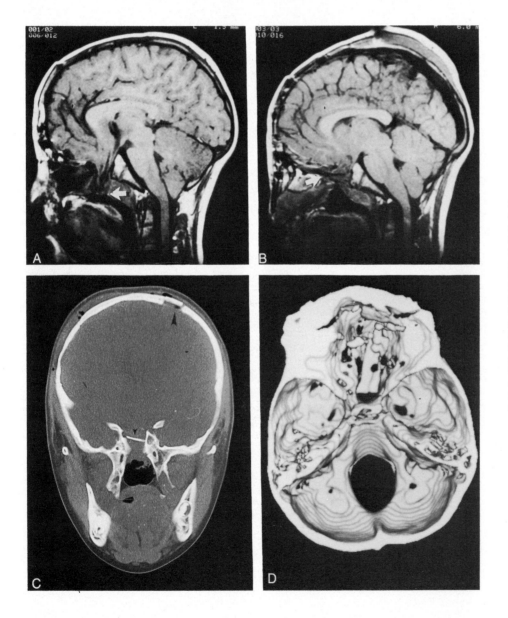

FIGURE 51–4. Sphenoidal encephalocele with nasal obstruction and recurrent meningitis. *A,* Sagittal MRI showing herniated third ventricle, hypothalamus, pituitary gland, and *(arrow)* area of fusion of dura with nasopharyngeal mucosa. *B,* Sagittal MRI scan postoperatively showing reduction of the encephalocele and the bone graft to reconstitute the sellar floor *(arrow). C,* Postoperative coronal CT scan showing bone graft in sellar floor *(small arrowhead)* and area from which split bone was taken *(large arrowhead). D,* Postoperative 3-D CT reconstruction showing bone graft replacing skull base.

lization. Compression of the dural sleeve should be avoided as much as possible to prevent damage to the contents of the dural sac, especially the pituitary stalk and gland. The final area to be freed is where the most inferior portion of the encephalocele is in contact with the mucosa of the pharynx (Fig. 51–4A). In many cases the mucosa is eroded, making this dissection difficult. Gentle superior traction on the dural sac will gradually expose the area of attachment, making it more visible, and permit its freeing usually by blunt dissection. If it is impossible to free the tip of the encephalocele from the mucosa, there are two options: (1) to pass a finger into the oropharynx and elevate the mucosa into the field, thus permitting better visualization of the area of attachment, or (2) to open the dura as inferiorly on the encephalocele as possible, deliver the herniated brain and sac into the cranium and then close the dura. This latter maneuver will increase the risk of damage to the pituitary and stalk, but the encephalocele must be freed so that a bone graft can be placed in contact with the clivus, to close the hole in the base and prevent re-herniation of the encephalocele. Once the inferior dura is freed, the encephalocele is gently delivered by lifting the anterior dura, in a hand-over-hand fashion, from the bony canal until the solid clivus can be seen posterior to the dura. A bone graft can now be placed below the encephalocele to prevent re-herniation (Fig. 51–4B). The bone graft can be shaped to reconstitute the floor of the anterior fossa as well (Fig. 51–4D) and should be secured to the cranial bone as rigidly as possible. Once again the bone graft is sandwiched between two layers of pericranium to seal the intracranial space from the mouth and nose, to reinforce the dura at the base of the encephalocele, and to have the bone graft between two pieces of vascularized tissue. This is the same technique that is used to reconstitute the base after tumor resection in the sphenoid sinus and frontal fossa.

AREA 2

The lesions that involve the frontal fossa of the cranium and the nasal sinuses and medial skull base, including the cavernous sinuses and middle fossae, are predominantly neoplastic, with the rare mucocele or giant aneurysm. The types of tumor found in this area include those arising from dura, bone, cartilage, pituitary tissue, notochord, and mucosa (e.g., meningioma, esthesioneuroblastoma, giant cell tumors of bone, chondrosarcoma, pituitary adenoma, chordoma, angiofibroma, melanoma). Many of these tumors do not destroy the dura and therefore the surgery is all extradural. Some lesions will have destroyed the dura and others will require resection of the dura to obtain a cure. Thus the surgical planning should always include the assumption that dural repair or replacement will be necessary and the source of tissue to ensure a watertight closure preplanned, whether this will be a free muscle flap, temporalis rotation flap, pericranial flap, or another type. Since the main problems with surgical exposure of this area relate to the need for frontal lobe retraction, the small working area, the restricted lateral exposure, and difficulty with control of hemorrhage, the ideal exposure is to permit a direct frontal access to these lesions. The technique described allows for good lateral visualization and adequate access to both the intracranial space, basal skull bone of the frontal and pituitary fossae, clivus and the ethmoid, sphenoid and if necessary maxillary sinuses. The extension of the above exposure, which will now be described, provides access to all these areas with minimal or no facial scars and the ability to reconstitute the patient's preoperative appearance.

Through a wavy, coronal incision a bifrontal craniotomy flap is raised. Once again the preplanning of the development of the pericranial and temporalis flaps is mandatory to obtain a satisfactory and watertight closure with the least risk of infection. Once the frontal bone flap is removed, the subperiosteal dissection of the superior orbits is done along with the extradural dissection of the orbital roofs and freeing of the foramen cecum. The nasal bone is now exposed inferiorly to the junction with the cartilage. The nasal mucosa can be freed either by using a bilateral intranasal incision in the mucosa or by separating the nasal bone from its cartilaginous tip and freeing the mucosa from this area superiorly. The advantage of the latter approach is that it avoids more than one incision and the need to enter the nose. It is difficult when reconstructing the medial canthi to get them in exactly the correct position, and to facilitate this reconstruction, the portions of the nasal bone to which the canthi are attached are freed with the canthi still attached, thus making their return to their original position easier and more accurate. This is easily done with a small drill point, but care must be taken to avoid damaging the lacrimal duct, which is immediately inferior to the bone attachment of the canthus. Once this step is complete and the nasal bone has been separated inferiorly from the nasal cartilage and posteriorly from the mucosa, saw cuts are made through the orbital rims, medial orbital walls, and inferiorly through the skull base at the level of the foramen cecum to allow removal of the midline bone, including the nasal bone, in a single piece (Fig. 51–5). Depending on the location of the tumor and the structures involved, it may be possible to leave the anterior portion of the medial walls of the orbit attached to the midline bone that is removed, thus making the reconstruction easier. To facilitate this, cuts on the floor of the frontal fossa can be made parallel to and immediately lateral to the olfactory bulbs, as would be done for a hypertelorism correction. These are most safely made with the small drill bit or osteotome while the orbital contents are protected by a malleable retractor. Once the central portion is removed (Fig. 51–5), the next step is the removal of the floor of the frontal fossa back to the base of the anterior clinoid processes. If the bone of the anterior portion of the floor of the frontal fossa is involved by the tumor, there is no way to preserve olfaction without the risk of leaving residual tumor. If only the posterior portion of the frontal fossa

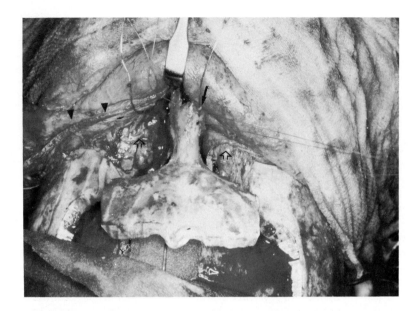

FIGURE 51–5. Removal of midline frontal bone, orbital rims, and nasal bone. The medial canthal bone attachment has been cut free and is marked with wire sutures *(black arrow)*. The periorbitum is visible bilaterally *(white arrows)*, and the reflected anteriorly based pericranial flap is seen *(arrowhead)*.

bone is involved, behind the olfactory fossa, then it is possible to preserve olfaction.[8] To do so, however, requires retraction of a rather bulky portion of central skull base and makes it difficult to seal off the frontal intracranial space from the sinuses at the end of the operation. It is probably not worth the additional risk of infection to preserve smell except in rare cases. The technique for preserving olfaction involves opening the mucosa at the most superior aspect of the nose and dividing it posteriorly, leaving a cuff of mucosa of several millimeters attached below the skull base. The bone through which the olfactory rootlets pass is then freed laterally and posteriorly (this is most easily done using small, sharp, curved Dautrey osteotomes), leaving the dura attached medially, and the whole piece of tissue—which includes a cuff of nasal mucosa, the olfactory nerves, bone, and dura—is retracted superiorly, thus exposing the ethmoid sinuses and the remaining bone that constitutes the posterior portion of the floor of the frontal fossa. This latter bone is now removed with the rongeur, with care to preserve the mucosa of the ethmoid sinuses.

If olfaction is not to be preserved, the dura of the olfactory fossa is opened right against the bone to preserve as much dura as possible. Medially, the dura must be freed off the crista galli, and it is usually necessary to drill down or rongeur away the crista to permit adequate freeing of the olfactory rootlets. The olfactory roots are coagulated and divided until the posterior margin of the fossa is identified. This point is easily recognized by invagination of the dura into the bone and the fact that the dura can now be easily freed from the bone in the midline with no further olfactory roots. Once the dura is free and the roots divided, the dura must now be closed to prevent intradural contamination either by tumor or by infection from the air sinuses. If there is no tumor invasion of the dura in this area, the dura can almost always be closed primarily if it has been correctly dissected off the frontal floor. If

there is inadequate dura to get a watertight closure, a free pericranial patch can be used. This can be reinforced with tissue glue during the final closure.

The remainder of the frontal fossa bone is then removed with a rongeur. The base of the anterior clinoids and the location of the optic nerves as they enter the skull are easily identified if the intraorbital subperiosteal dissection has been carried all the way posteriorly. An instrument can be placed in the orbit to direct the lateral extent of the bone removal. The most likely place for a dural tear is where the dura of the tuberculum sella turns to begin its descent into the pituitary fossa and where the optic nerves enter the dura. Careful freeing of the intracranial dura before the bone is removed will help to avoid a dural tear. If the tumor involves the posterior ethmoid sinuses, the tumor mass will now be visible under the mucosa or, more likely, the mucosa will be deficient and the tumor itself will present in the field (Fig. 51–6). If the tumor has invaded the orbit, the medial orbital wall can now be safely removed since the location of the optic nerve should now be clear (Fig. 51–6E).

If the tumor extends inferiorly to the maxillary sinus or posterolaterally into the pterygoid fossa, better exposure of the middle of the face is required.[9, 10] To accomplish this, either a Weber Ferguson incision or a lateral rhinotomy incision combined with a lower blepharoplasty incision (Fig. 51–7A and B) can be used. This is followed by removal of the front wall of the maxilla, if there is tumor involvement, or by freeing the maxilla above the alveolus and retracting it laterally. In the child, the upper bone cuts must be high enough to avoid the unerupted teeth, and the infraorbital nerve can be spared by mobilizing it and taking the saw cuts posterior and inferior to the nerve. The maxilla can now be hinged laterally to permit direct access to the pterygoid fossa (Fig. 51–7F). It is not necessary to have such a large exposure for all lesions, and in some, the degloving approach through a sublabial

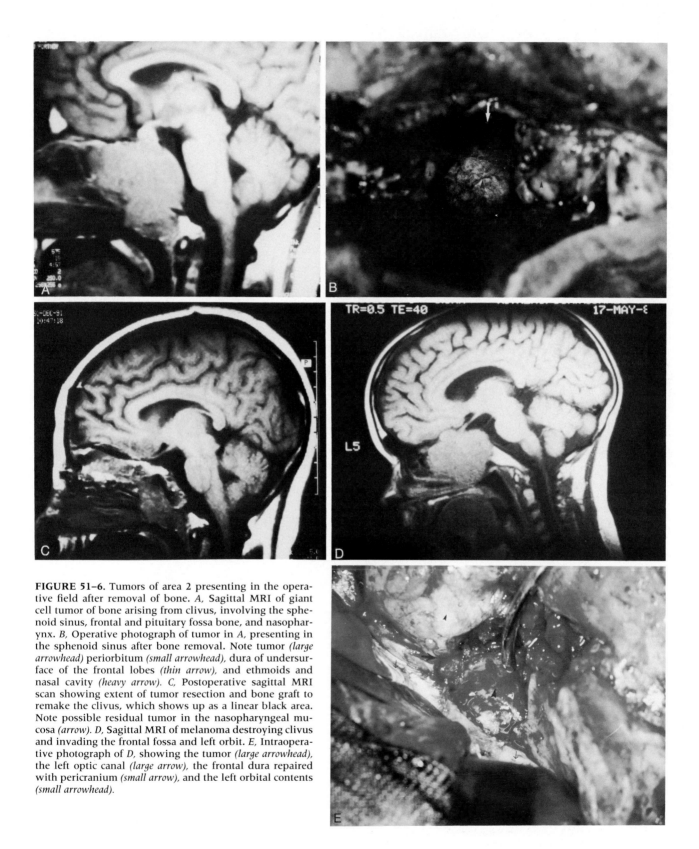

FIGURE 51–6. Tumors of area 2 presenting in the operative field after removal of bone. *A,* Sagittal MRI of giant cell tumor of bone arising from clivus, involving the sphenoid sinus, frontal and pituitary fossa bone, and nasopharynx. *B,* Operative photograph of tumor in *A,* presenting in the sphenoid sinus after bone removal. Note tumor *(large arrowhead)* periorbitum *(small arrowhead),* dura of undersurface of the frontal lobes *(thin arrow),* and ethmoids and nasal cavity *(heavy arrow). C,* Postoperative sagittal MRI scan showing extent of tumor resection and bone graft to remake the clivus, which shows up as a linear black area. Note possible residual tumor in the nasopharyngeal mucosa *(arrow). D,* Sagittal MRI of melanoma destroying clivus and invading the frontal fossa and left orbit. *E,* Intraoperative photograph of *D,* showing the tumor *(large arrowhead),* the left optic canal *(large arrow),* the frontal dura repaired with pericranium *(small arrow),* and the left orbital contents *(small arrowhead).*

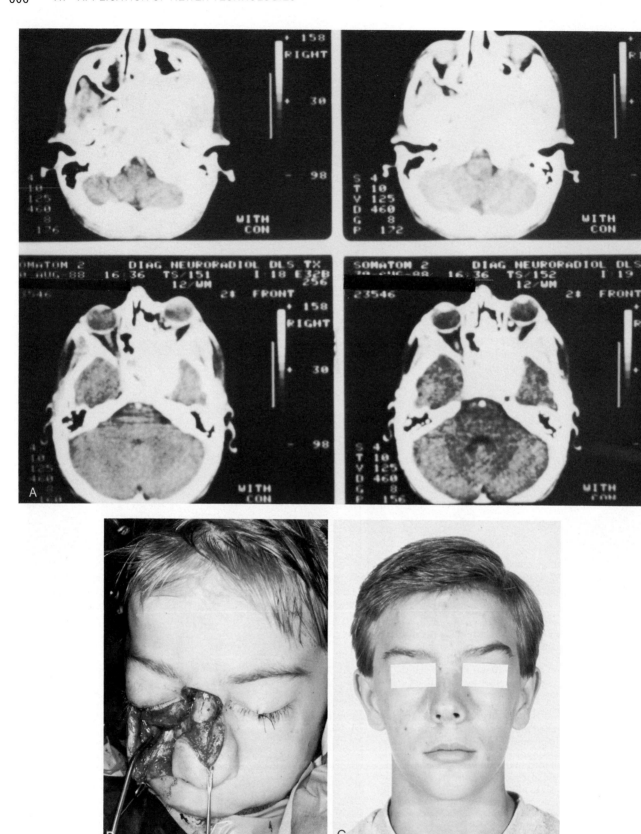

FIGURE 51–7. Extension of the frontonasal approach to include the maxillary sinuses and pterygoid fossa. *A,* Axial CT scan cuts showing large angiofibroma involving the right pterygoid fossa and extending into the cavernous sinus and middle fossa. *B,* Intraoperative photograph showing lateral rhinotomy with inferior blepharoplasty incision in patient whose tumor is shown in *A. C,* Same patient as in *B* 6 months postoperatively showing minimal cosmetic deformity from scar.

Illustration continued on opposite page

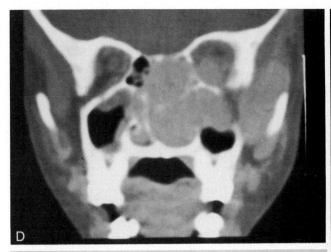

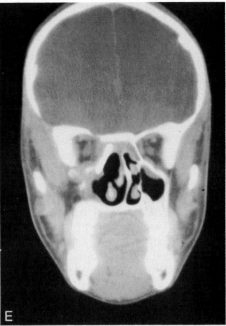

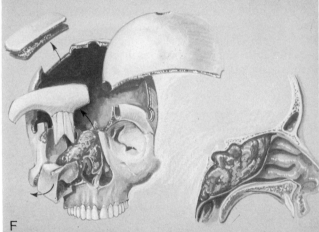

FIGURE 51–7 continued *D,* Coronal CT (patient's right is on right of CT cut) of same patient with angiofibroma showing extension into the right orbit and maxillary sinus. *E,* Postoperative coronal CT scan of same patient (right side of patient is now on the left side of the photograph of the scan) showing resection of tumor and bony reconstruction of the skull base and medial orbital wall. *F,* Artist's depiction of progressive osteotomies that may be required for tumors in area 2.

incision will avoid any scars on the face. The advantage of the use of the facial osteotomies is that the exposure can be tailored to fit the particular lesion, allowing only those areas essential for tumor removal to be disturbed.

Tumor resection can now begin with minimal or no retraction on the frontal lobes, and the vascular supply to the tumor can be divided as the tumor is circumscribed. It is best to preserve the mucosa of the nasopharynx intact as an anterior boundary to the resection. Occasionally there will be tumor invading anteriorly into this mucosa, and a more extensive resection of the mucosa will be required. It is preferable to leave this mucosal barrier until the remainder of the tumor in the sphenoid sinus and clivus has been removed.

If the tumor does not present in the ethmoid sinus, the bony septum of the antrum of the sphenoid sinus has to be removed. The tumor capsule or tumor tissue is now seen, and resection of the tumor begins. The carotid arteries are almost always displaced, and the direction of the displacement of the anterior intracavernous carotid must be known before the tumor is incised since it is possible to open directly into the displaced carotid. If the location of the carotid is in question, a small pencil Doppler can be used over the front of the tumor to identify the vessel. This technique is also useful as the tumor resection is continued more deeply into the sphenoid sinus, since the medial wall of the cavernous sinus may have been destroyed by the tumor, so that the intrapetrous carotid is exposed for most of its course in the lateral extent of the tumor.

In most tumors in children, the dura of the pituitary fossa is intact, and this greatly facilitates the closure. The clivus immediately posterior and superior to the pituitary fossa is impossible to see from this approach, but the rest of the clivus down to the foramen magnum is well visualized and fair lateral vision is possible by moving the microscope. It is extremely difficult and dangerous to enter the cavernous sinus from this approach if the medial wall of the sinus is intact, and this is not recommended since the operator has no access to the carotid artery should severe bleeding occur. Chordomas and angiofibromas rarely invade the cavernous sinus but invaginate themselves between the folds of the dura and can usually be teased out without difficulty.

The clivus can easily be resected down to the foramen magnum (Fig. 51–6*C*) and laterally to the jugular foramina. Once all the obvious tumor has been removed from the posterior pharyngeal area, it is helpful to compress the nasopharyngeal mucosa anteriorly to identify any residual tumor that is within the mucosa. This is most easily done by passing a probe from the ethmoids inferiorly to the pharynx or by passing a finger into the mouth and compressing the nasopharyngeal mucosa posteriorly. If the mucosa is involved by tumor it must be excised. If the dura is intact, there is little concern about leaving an area of mucosal defect since this will heal rapidly from the surrounding intact mucosa. If there is concern about a CSF leak, an effort must be made to close the mucosa with a flap if necessary.

The base should be reconstructed with bone to prevent sagging of the dura between the bone edges, since this can cause headache, and if a dural repair has been performed, the dural sagging may ultimately lead to the development of a meningocele. If the maxilla has been moved, this is replaced and plated back in position (Fig. 51–8A). If the medial orbital walls have been resected, they must be reconstructed to prevent enophthalmos and medial displacement of the orbital contents with resultant diplopia (Fig. 51–8B). Typically there is no

mucosal covering for these bone grafts; they are obtained from either the frontal flap or a second craniotomy.[11] Despite this, we have had no problems with infection of these grafts since the mucosa rapidly covers them. This is also true if grafts have to be used to reconstruct the maxilla, and it is not necessary to utilize the frontalis or pericranial flaps to cover these grafts. The skull base is closed as described previously, and the nasal bone and medial bandeau replaced and rigidly fixed with wire, plates, or screws (Fig. 51–8C). Prior to fixing the frontal nasal bandeau, channels must be cut through the base of the nasal bone to permit the entrance of the pericranial flaps (Fig. 51–8D). The only problem is that this leaves the base of the nose somewhat widened for several months until the base of the flaps involutes. The nasal cartilage must be resutured to the distal nasal bone to prevent collapse of the nasal tip; this is done by making small drill holes at the tip of the nasal bone and securing the cartilage with nonabsorbable sutures. The medial canthi are wired back into position with transnasal wires. At each stage of reconstruction, tissue glue is used to seal that layer and pre-

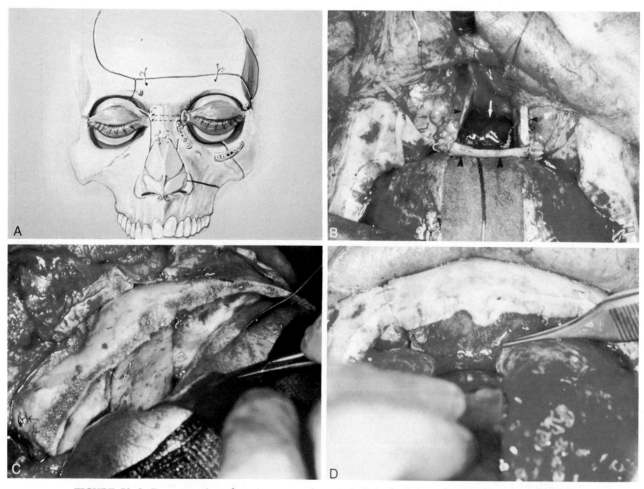

FIGURE 51–8. Reconstruction after tumor resection. *A,* Artist's depiction of reconstituted craniofacial skeleton. *B,* Blood-filled sphenoid after tumor removal *(arrow).* Note split cranial bone to replace orbital walls *(small arrowheads)* and cranial base *(large arrowheads). C,* Replacement of frontal bandeau and skull base before insertion of superior portion of pericranial graft. Rigid fixation with screw *(thin arrow)* and wire *(heavy arrow). D,* Pericranial flap now in place to cover graft.

vent communication between the nose or sinuses and the intracranial space. At the same time, liberal irrigation with hydrogen peroxide, bacitracin solution, and then saline is done to minimize the bacterial count in the tissues.

The frontal bone is then secured into position and the temporalis muscle replaced to prevent any cosmetic defect. If the anterior part of the temporalis muscle has been used as a graft, the posterior portion must be rotated anteriorly to contact the lateral orbital rim and thus prevent a cosmetic defect in the temporal fossa. If the lateral periorbitum has been freed, it will be necessary to reattach the lateral canthal ligament. Any residual defects in the frontal bone can be filled in with the bone dust produced during the opening craniotomy. The frontal burr hole can be obliterated either by a small bone plug or by filling it with bone dust and tissue glue mixture. The galea is closed in two layers with Vicryl or similar absorbable suture and the scalp with a running chromic catgut suture, usually 4-0. Drains are not used, as they tend to encourage suction of sinus or nasal contents into the subgaleal space. Usually no dressing is applied, and Polysporin ointment is placed on the incision. When the surgeon is working in the frontal fossa and sphenoid sinus, a CSF drain is not used either intra- or postoperatively, unless, at the end of the procedure, a known area of dural leak that could not be closed is present.

A modification of this approach has been used to treat fibrous dysplasia of the midline skull base with compression or invasion of the optic foramina (Fig. 51–9). The frontal bone or a portion of it will be involved with fibrous dysplasia and needs to be excised. Thus the craniotomy is planned to remove a flap of normal bone, large enough to produce the required bone grafts for reconstruction. This is usually the continuation of the frontal bone immediately posterior to the involved bone. The displaced dura can now be freed from the fibrous dysplastic bone and resection of the involved bone begun. Subperiorbital dissection of both orbits allows the surgeon to identify the markedly thickened orbital roof and cranial base. As the abnormal bone involving the medial orbital roof is removed, the point of exit of the optic nerve from the apex of the orbit can be easily identified (Fig. 51–9B). The fibrous dysplastic bone can now be removed from around the optic nerve in an anterior to posterior direction. Often the optic canal is up to 2 cm long and the depth of the bone covering the nerve superiorly is also 2 to 3 cm. When the procedure is started intraorbitally, the location of the optic nerve and that of the superior orbital fissure are known, and they can be visualized and irrigated to keep them cool during the resection of the fibrous dysplasia. The abnormal tissue is removed until the dural reflection as the nerve enters the intracranial space is seen. It is easy to make a hole in the dura at this point because the dura is often thin. If that occurs, the leak is best closed with Avitene or Gelfoam and tissue glue. The mass of tissue in the midline, extending into the nose, can be removed on either side of the olfactory apparatus and smell preserved (Fig. 51–9B). As the medial diseased tissue is removed, the optic nerve on the opposite side can be identified as it exits the orbit and can be decompressed (Fig. 51–9B). This approach permits decompression of both optic nerves, resection of the fibrous dysplasia, and reconstruction of the forehead and upper face all in one sitting. Since the dura is not opened, the risk of CSF leakage is minimal. Reconstruction is as described above.

AREA 3

When the lesion involves only the clivus, is on the brain side of the clivus, and does not involve either the soft tissue anterior to the clivus or the sphenoid sinus,

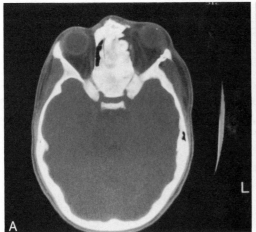
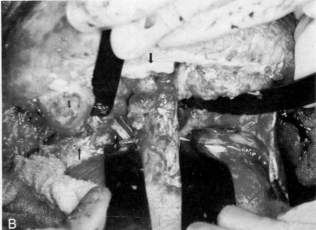

FIGURE 51–9. Fibrous dysplasia involving the midline and both optic canals. Patient had decreasing vision in the left eye. *A,* Axial CT cut showing midline involvement of the ethmoid sinuses, the frontal skull base, and elongation and narrowing of the optic canals, L > R. *B,* Operative photograph of *A* showing left and right optic nerves completely freed of tumor *(large arrowheads),* the left middle fossa dura *(long arrow),* the left orbital contents *(short arrow),* the preserved olfactory rootlets *(small arrowhead),* and the nasion *(thick arrow).*

the easiest approach is transfacial, using a LeFort I osteotomy.[12] In children the foramen magnum is at the level of the hard palate (Fig. 51–10) and the clivus is superior to this, so that the transoral approach makes little sense. In addition, the mouth is small and the tongue relatively large so that prolonged tongue retraction can cause severe swelling and airway obstruction. In addition, the transoral approach usually requires a tracheostomy, further complicating recovery. Since the clivus is cephalic to the hard palate, an approach through the midportion of the face is ideal. In children, a LeFort I osteotomy with division of the palate is a direct route to the clivus, all the way superiorly to the posterior clinoid process. There is no need for a tracheostomy or for significant tongue retraction. It is necessary to prepare a dental splint before the operation to ensure that the proper alignment of the upper and lower teeth is achieved prior to rigid fixation of the maxilla at the end of the procedure.

The incision is a sublabial one with subperiosteal dissection of the soft tissues of the face up to the inferior orbital rims.[13] The important structure to avoid damaging is the infraorbital nerve. The nasal mucosa and septum are separated from the superior surface of the palate and the osteotomy performed high on the maxilla to avoid the unerupted dentition (Fig. 51–11). The palate is then divided, with the incision extending between the upper incisors. The soft palate is then split, and the two halves of the palate can now be retracted laterally to give excellent exposure of the posterior nasopharyngeal mucosa. This is opened in a linear fashion. The microneedle is ideal for this. The mucosa is then dissected off the clivus and the bone resection begun using a small drill bit. If the tumor extends to the upper third of the clivus, the sphenoid sinus, if it is formed, will be entered, and care must be taken to leave the floor of the sella tursica intact as the upper

clivus to the posterior clinoid is removed. Once the clival bone is gone, the tumor is encountered. Often the clivus is involved by tumor, and this usually makes the removal easier.

The amount of destruction of the skull base can be identified from the preoperative studies. If the bone medial to the intrapetrous carotid or foramen lacerum has been destroyed, the surgeon must be careful not to damage the carotid artery during the bone removal. Similarly the bone medial to the jugular foramina may be destroyed, and the jugular bulb can easily be entered with uncontrollable hemorrhage. If the bone of the base is intact, the limits to this approach are at its lateral margins, and for lesions that are predominantly in the lateral two thirds of the petrous bone, this is not a good approach. Superiorly the lateral limits of the exposure are the dural sleeves of the fifth nerves as they enter the petrous bone. With the maxilla split, it is possible to obtain much better lateral exposure than when working through the small mouth of the child and with minimal retraction of the facial tissues.

The dura can be opened for intradural examination. If the lesion does not require resection of the dura, the dura can be closed with small clips in preference to attempts to suture down this deep hole. The closure is reinforced with tissue glue. We try to reconstruct the bony skull base if a large defect is present to help avoid CSF leakage and to prevent dural herniation and pain. The bone and muscle are taken from the temporal region through a small craniotomy to obtain split bone and, after insertion, are held in place with tissue glue. The mucosa is then sutured in two layers if possible, but in children it is usually possible to obtain only a single-layer closure, once again reinforced with tissue glue. The dental splint is then placed over the teeth to get an accurate re-approximation of the maxilla, and the maxilla is rigidly fixed with miniplates and screws.

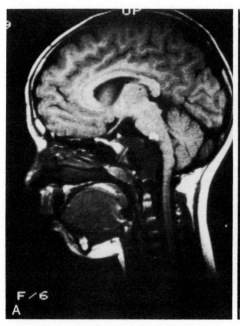 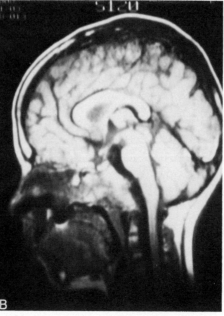

FIGURE 51–10. Tumor of area 3. Six-year-old with chondroid chordoma of clivus, presenting with bilateral sixth nerve palsies. *A,* Preoperative sagittal MRI scan showing the destruction of the clivus, posterior displacement of the pons and medulla with a cystic portion of tumor invaginating into the pons. Note the relationship of the palate to the inferior margin of the clivus. *B,* Four days postoperatively, sagittal MRI with return of the pons and medulla to their correct position and no evidence of residual tumor.

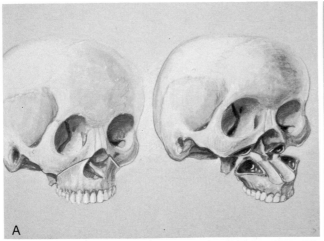

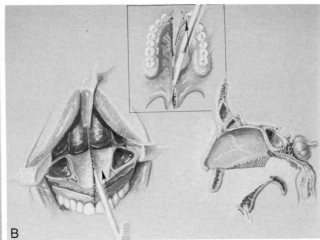

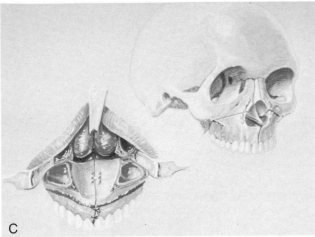

FIGURE 51–11. Artist's depiction of the Le Fort I osteotomy and transclival approach. *A,* Bone cuts in maxilla to avoid unerupted teeth. *B,* Freeing of the mucosa from the hard palate, bisection of the palate, and approach to the intracranial space. *C,* Reconstitution of the maxilla with miniplates.

Wiring of the teeth is not necessary. The mucosal incision is closed with absorbable Vicryl suture. Extubation can be performed at the end of the surgery. Oral hygiene using a water pick and mouth washes is begun. Clear liquids can be taken in 24 hours, and a soft diet is begun in 5 to 7 days. The children are not permitted to eat hard food or food that needs chewing for 6 weeks. Antibiotics are continued intravenously for 3 days. If a CSF drain has been used, this is usually kept in place for 3 or 4 days. The recovery in the absence of tongue swelling and with no tracheostomy is remarkably benign, and the children usually leave the hospital on the fourth to seventh postoperative day. The cosmetic results are excellent (Fig. 51–12), and thus far facial growth has not been a problem.

UNILATERAL LESIONS OF THE CAVERNOUS SINUS, OPTIC FORAMEN, ORBIT, OR PTERYGOID FOSSA

Techniques for unilateral surgery in children are similar to those in adults.[14–16] Typically, a fronto-orbital craniotomy is required. In children it is better to remove the fronto-temporal (pterional) flap as a single flap and then to remove the orbital rim, lateral orbital wall, and, if necessary, the zygoma as a second flap.

This has several benefits. When the lateral orbit and orbital roof are removed with the initial bone flap, a Gigli saw is used to make this cut, and often the periorbitum is lacerated with herniation of the orbital fat. This can interfere with the surgeon's view of the cavernous sinus and optic foramen. Furthermore, when the orbital roof is taken with the initial bone flap, it is hard to preserve a large portion of the posterior and medial portion of the roof. When the orbital rim and lateral wall are taken as a separate flap, since the dura of the frontal lobe can be elevated now that the frontal bone flap is gone, almost all of the orbital roof can be removed still attached to the rim of the orbit. This makes it much easier to reconstruct the orbit to its original size. This is very important since to estimate the correct orbital volume at the time of closure, when the orbital contents are massively swollen, is very difficult and commonly some degree of enophthalmos or exophthalmos results. The frontal sinus is rarely present before the age of 10 years. In older children, if the sinus is opened, it must be obliterated to prevent communication of the air passages with the epidural space postoperatively. To expose the cavernous sinus or lesions that are both intracranial and intraorbital, or for fibrous dysplasia, it is necessary to remove the anterior clinoid process and expose the superior orbital

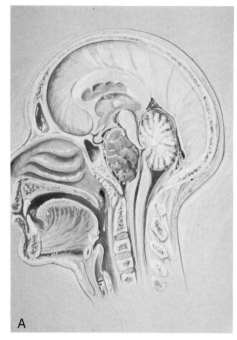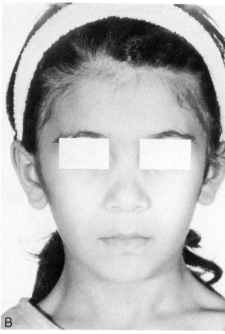

FIGURE 51–12. *A,* Artist's depiction of chordoma shown in Figure 51–10. *B,* Six-year-old patient 2 weeks after Le Fort I osteotomy and transclival resection of chordoma shown in Figure 51–10.

fissure dura and the dura covering the optic nerve. After the orbital portion of the craniotomy, it is easy to drill away the medial aspect of the lesser wing of the sphenoid and to remove the anterior clinoid from its base anteriorly to its tip posteriorly from an extradural approach (Fig. 51–13). This lessens the risk of damage to the third nerve, the optic nerve, and the carotid artery since all these structures remain covered by dura until the bone resection is complete. It also allows for an extradural repair of any entrance into the ethmoid

sinus prior to opening the dura, thus decreasing the risk of CSF leakage and infection.

At the termination of the procedure, the soft tissue repair of the dura or sinuses can be done by rotating a temporalis flap, which in the older child can easily reach to the midline. When the orbital bone is involved, as in meningioma or fibrous dysplasia, the orbit can be reconstructed with split bone grafts. Soft tissue reconstruction requires rotating the temporalis muscle anteriorly to contact the lateral orbit and suturing it in

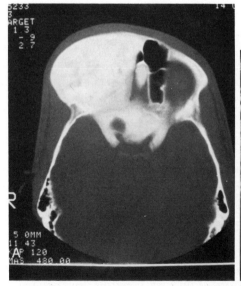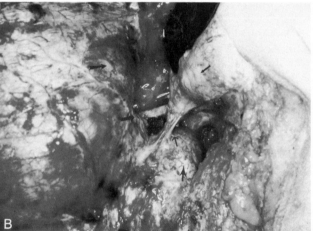

FIGURE 51–13. Unilateral approach to expose the cavernous sinus with resection of the lesser wing of the sphenoid and the anterior clinoid via an epidural approach. The anatomy is especially clear in this case of unilateral fibrous dysplasia. *A,* Axial CT scan showing extensive involvement of the right orbital roof and lesser wing of the sphenoid by fibrous dysplasia. Patient was losing vision in the right eye. *B,* Intraoperative photograph of *A* after removal of all the involved bone. The right optic nerve *(heavy arrow),* the superior orbital fissure *(fine arrow),* orbital contents and dura *(arrow pointing left)* of the frontal *(small arrowhead with long, scalloped tail)* and temporal *(large arrowhead with short tail)* lobes are well seen.

this position to prevent a temporal hollow. The lateral canthus must be reattached to the orbital rim to prevent drooping of the lateral margin of the palpebral fissure. Skin closure is as for the coronal incision.

These techniques allow safe access to the frontobasal areas of the skull and the clivus in children from infancy to teenage. The emphasis is on good exposure with minimal brain retraction, adequate resection of the lesions, and accurate, rigid reconstruction of bone and soft tissues to allow for continued normal growth of the face. The infection rate should be no higher than 5 per cent, and the rate of significant CSF leakage requiring further surgery also should be 5 per cent or less. New cranial nerve deficits are rare unless the lesions are in the cavernous sinus, when risk of damage to the third, fourth, and sixth nerves is similar to that in adults.[16] If transection of any of the nerves occurs it is useful to reconstruct them at the time of the initial surgery.[17]

CONCLUSION

Using the established techniques of craniofacial surgery and modifying them as needed, it is now possible to safely operate on a number of lesions that involve the base of the skull in children. A team approach, as for craniofacial surgery, is imperative if all the precautions that lead to a good result for the child, both immediately and later in life, are to be taken. There are serious concerns in the short run about intraoperative blood loss, infection, CSF leakage, new neurologic deficits, and inadequate tumor removal. Over time the concerns relate to continued facial growth, eruption of dentition, repair of neurologic damage, and finally the risks for tumor recurrence despite such extensive surgery. Only time and careful follow-up will determine whether these surgical procedures are of long-term benefit for the treatment of tumors. In the immediate operative period, experience of the treating team and fastidious attention to all the surgical details comprise the only way to keep the perioperative morbidity to a minimum.

REFERENCES

1. Tessier P: The definitive plastic surgical treatment of severe facial deformities of craniofacial dysostosis, Crouzon's and Apert's disease. Plast Reconstr Surg 48:224, 1971.
2. Derome PJ: The transbasal approach to tumors invading the base of the skull. *In* Schmidek HH, Sweet WH (eds): Operative Neurosurgical Techniques: Indications, Methods and Results, 2nd ed. Vol 1. Orlando, Grune & Stratton, 1988, pp 619–633.
3. Rossen HM, Simeone FA, Bruce DA: Single stage composite resection and reconstruction of malignant anterior skull base tumors. Neurosurgery 18:7, 1986.
4. Rosen HM: The extended trapezius musculocutaneous flap for cranio-orbital, facial reconstruction. Plast Reconstr Surg 75:318, 1985.
5. Sasaki CT, Ariyan S, Spencer D, Buckwalter J: Pectoralis major myocutaneous reconstruction of the anterior skull base. Laryngoscope 95:162, 1985.
6. Jones NF, Sekhar LN, Schramm VL: Free rectus abdominis muscle flap reconstruction of the middle and posterior cranial base. Plast Reconstr Surg 78:471, 1985.
7. Orbital hypertelorism. *In* Jackson IT, Munro IR, Salyer KE, Whitaker LA (eds): Atlas of Craniomaxillofacial Surgery. St. Louis, CV Mosby, 1982, pp 318–413.
8. Fearon J, Bruce DA, Munro IR: The facial split without anosmia: A new technique for anterior cranial base surgery. In press.
9. Sekhar LN, Nanda A, Sen CN, Snyderman CN, Janecka IP: The extended frontal approach to tumors of the anterior, middle and posterior skull base. J Neurosurg 76:198, 1992.
10. Jackson IT, Marsh WR, Bite U, et al.: Craniofacial osteotomies to facilitate skull base tumor resection. Br J Plast Surg 39:153, 160, 1986.
11. Jackson IT, Helden G, Marx R: Skull bone grafts in maxillofacial and craniofacial surgery. J Oral Maxillofac Surg 44:949, 1986.
12. Uttley D, Moore A, Acker DJ: Surgical management of midline skull base tumors: a new approach. J Neurosurg 71:705, 1989.
13. Price JC, Holliday MJ, Johns HE, et al.: The versatile midface degloving approach. Laryngoscope 98:291, 1988.
14. Sekhar LN, Burgess J, Akin O: Anatomical study of the cavernous sinus emphasizing operative approaches and related vascular and neural reconstructions. Neurosurgery 21:806, 1987.
15. Sekhar LN, Sen CN, Jho HD, et al.: Surgical treatment of intracavernous neoplasms: a four year experience. Neurosurgery 24:18, 1989.
16. Sekhar LN, Sen CN: Surgical treatment of tumors involving the cavernous sinus. *In* Wilkens RH, Rengarchy SS (eds): Neurosurgery Update. I: Diagnosis, Operative Technique and Neuro-oncology. New York, McGraw-Hill Inc, 1990, pp 334–345.
17. Sekhar LN, Lanzino G, Sen CN, Pomonis S: Reconstruction of the third through sixth cranial nerves during cavernous sinus surgery. J Neurosurg 76:935, 1992.

ACKNOWLEDGMENT: Special thanks to Mr. Bill Winn for his superb illustrations.

INDEX

Note: Page numbers in italics refer to illustrations; page numbers followed by t refer to tables.

ISBN 0-7216-3767-1

9 780721 637679

90038